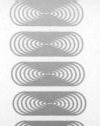

EIGHTH EDITION

Clinical Manifestations and Assessment of Respiratory Disease

Terry Des Jardins, MEd, RRT
Professor Emeritus
Former Director
Department of Respiratory Care
Parkland College
Champaign, Illinois
Faculty/Staff Member
University of Illinois College of Medicine at Urbana–Champaign
Urbana, Illinois

George G. Burton, MD, FACP, FCCP, FAARC
Associate Dean for Medical Affairs
Kettering College
Kettering, Ohio
Clinical Professor of Medicine and Anesthesiology
Wright State University School of Medicine
Dayton, Ohio

Medical Illustrations by

Timothy H. Phelps, MS, FAMI, CMI
Associate Professor
Johns Hopkins University School of Medicine
Baltimore, Maryland

ELSEVIER

ELSEVIER

3251 Riverport Lane
St. Louis, Missouri 63043

Senior Content Strategist: Yvonne Alexopoulos
Content Development Manager: Lisa Newton
Senior Content Development Specialist: Laura Selkirk
Publishing Services Manager: Deepthi Unni
Senior Project Manager: Manchu Mohan
Design Direction: Margaret Reid

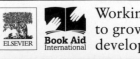
Last digit is the print number: 9 8 7 6 5 4 3 2 1

In Memory of Robert Cohn, MD

Terry Des Jardins, MEd, RRT

George G. Burton, MD

There is a manpower shortage of health care providers who care for the critically ill. This is one of the most pressing issues affecting the future of our aging population and American medicine. ... It has been generally acknowledged ... that the shortages in nursing, respiratory care practitioners, and pharmacists have already reached crisis levels. ... A severe shortage of (pulmonary/critical care physicians) can be expected in the very near future.[1]

> *Respiratory therapists are important for patient outcomes and their roles might even be expanded beyond traditional boundaries. More research is needed to define the ICU multidisciplinary staffing that matches patient needs and optimizes patient outcomes.[2]*

Shortfalls in the pulmonary and critical care physician workforce are estimated to be at least 38% and 22%, respectively, by 2020. Advanced Practice Registered Nurses (APRNs) and Physician Assistants (PAs) are now so entrenched in the medical services they are allowed to act as primary care providers (PCPs), managing everything from diabetes mellitus to heart failure. However, at the time of this writing, the respiratory care profession is in the process of developing a worker with credentials and practice privileges similar to those of the APRN and PA who will be designated as an Advanced Practice Respiratory Therapist (APRT). In the final analysis, respiratory therapists (RTs) are the only ancillary medical professionals with comprehensive training in all aspects of pulmonary medicine, including education and management of patients with chronic lung disease.[3,4]

Three issues will drive the growth of the respiratory care profession into the 21st century: an aging population with complex health care issues, ever more complex and expensive respiratory care technologies, and concern to find the most cost-effective way to face these challenges. It will become increasing clear to respiratory therapy professionals at all levels that pathophysiology drives intelligent therapy—in a very dynamic fashion! What an exciting time for the profession!

[1]Irwin, R. S., Marcus, L., & Lever, A. (2004). The Critical Care Professional Societies address the critical care crisis in the United States. *Chest, 125,* 1512–1513.

[2]Kelly, M. A., Angus, D., Chalfin, D. B., Crandall, E. D., Ingbar, D., Johanson, W., ... Vender, J. S. (2004). The critical care crisis in the United States. *Chest, 125,* 1514–1517.

[3]Fuhrman, T. M., & Aranson, R. (2014). Point: Should Medicare allow respiratory therapists to independently practice and bill for educational activities related to COPD? Yes. *Chest, 145*(2), 210–213.

[4]Barnes, T. A., Kacmarek, R. M., Kageler, W. V., Morris, M. M., & Durbin, C. G, Jr. (2011). Transitioning the respiratory therapy workforce from 2015 and beyond. *Respiratory Care, 56*(5), 681–690.

Consultants

Newborn and Early Childhood Respiratory Disorders

Sue Ciarlariello, MBA, RRT-NPS, RCP, CMTE, FAARC
Director, Respiratory Care and Transport
Dayton Children's Hospital
Dayton, Ohio

Robert Cohn, MD, MBA, FAARC
Associate Vice-President for Medical Affairs
Medical Director, Pulmonary Medicine
Professor, Department of Pediatrics
Wright State University School of Medicine
Dayton Children's Hospital
Dayton, Ohio

Robert J. Fink, MD
Past Medical Director, Pulmonary Medicine
Professor, Department of Pediatrics
Wright State University School of Medicine
Dayton Children's Hospital
Dayton, Ohio

Stacy Hubbard MHA/Ed, RRT-NPS, C-NPT, RCP
Transport and Communication Center Manager
Dayton Children's Hospital
Dayton, Ohio

Neuromuscular Disease

Gabriel Thornton, MD
Pulmonary and Critical Care Medicine Fellow
Northwestern Memorial Hospital, Northwestern Medicine
Chicago, Illinois

Lisa F. Wolfe, MD
Northwestern Medical Group
Pulmonary Critical Care Medicine, Sleep Medicine
Northwestern Memorial Hospital, Northwestern Medicine
Chicago, Illinois

Reviewers

Sara Wing Parker, MPH, RRT-NPS, AE-C
Assistant Clinical Professor
Cardiopulmonary and Diagnostic Sciences
University of Missouri
Columbia, Missouri

Donald J. Raymond, MS, RRT
Program Director, Respiratory Therapy
Chippewa Valley Technical College
Eau Claire, Wisconsin

Richard J. Zahodnic, PhD, RRT-NPS, RPFT, LRT
Program Director
Respiratory Therapy Program
Macomb Community College
Clinton Township, Michigan

Preface

The use of **therapist-driven protocols (TDPs)**—now often called simply **respiratory protocols** is an integral part of respiratory health services. TDPs provide much-needed flexibility to respiratory care practitioners and increase the quality of health care. This is because the respiratory therapy care program can be modified easily and efficiently according to the needs of the patient.

Essential cornerstones to the success of a TDP program are (1) the quality of the respiratory therapist's assessment skills at the bedside and (2) the ability to transfer objective clinical data into a treatment plan that follows agreed-upon guidelines. This textbook is designed to provide the student with the fundamental knowledge and understanding necessary to assess and treat patients with respiratory diseases in order to meet these objectives.

Part I of the textbook, *Assessment of Cardiopulmonary Disease,* contains three sections:

Section I, *Bedside Diagnosis,* consists of three chapters. Chapter 1 describes the knowledge and skills involved in the patient interview. Chapter 2 provides the knowledge and skills needed for the physical examination. Chapter 3 presents a more in-depth discussion of the pathophysiologic basis for commonly observed clinical manifestations of respiratory diseases.

Section II, *Clinical Data Obtained From Laboratory Tests and Special Procedures,* is composed of Chapters 4 through 9. Collectively, these chapters provide the reader with the essential knowledge and understanding base for the assessment of pulmonary function studies, arterial blood gases, oxygenation, the cardiovascular system (including hemodynamic monitoring), radiologic examination of the chest, and other important laboratory tests and procedures.

Section III, *The Therapist-Driven Protocol Program—The Essentials,* consists of Chapters 10, 11, and 12.

Chapter 10, "The Therapist-Driven Protocol Program," provides the reader with the essential knowledge base and step-by-step process needed to assess and implement protocols in the clinical setting. The student is provided with the basic knowledge and helpful tools to (1) gather clinical data systematically, (2) formulate an assessment (i.e., the cause and severity of the patient's condition), (3) select an appropriate and cost-effective treatment plan, and (4) document these essential steps clearly and precisely. At the end of each respiratory disorder chapter, one or more representative case studies demonstrate appropriate TDP assessment, treatment, and charting strategies. Chapter 10 is a cornerstone chapter to the fundamentals necessary for good assessment and critical-thinking skills. The case studies presented at the end of each respiratory disorder chapter often direct the reader back to Chapter 10.

Chapter 11, "Respiratory Insufficiency, Respiratory Failure, and Ventilatory Management Protocols," is a fully up-dated chapter in this eighth edition. This chapter describes how respiratory failure can be classified as (1) hypoxemic (type I) respiratory failure, (2) hypercapnic (type II) respiratory failure, or (3) a combination of both. These categories reflect the pathophysiologic basis of respiratory failure. In addition, this chapter provides the components of mechanical ventilation protocols, including the standard criteria for mechanical ventilation, the clinical indicators for both hypercapnic and hypoxemic respiratory failure, ventilatory support strategies for noninvasive and invasive mechanical ventilation, a mechanical ventilator management protocol, and a mechanical ventilation weaning protocol.

Chapter 12, "Recording Skills and Intraprofessional Communication," provides the basic foundation needed to collect and record respiratory assessments and treatment plans.

Parts II through **XIV** (Chapters 13 through 45) provide the reader with essential information regarding **common respiratory diseases**. Each chapter adheres to the following format: a description of the anatomic alterations of the lungs, etiology of the disease process, an overview of the cardiopulmonary clinical manifestations associated with the disorder, management of the respiratory disorder, one or more case studies, and a brief set of self-assessment questions. A further description of this format follows.

Anatomic Alterations of the Lungs

Each respiratory disease chapter begins with a detailed, color illustration showing the major anatomic alterations of the lungs associated with the disorder. Although a serious effort has been made to illustrate each disorder accurately at the beginning of each chapter, artistic license ("cartooning") has been taken to emphasize certain anatomic points and pathologic processes. The material that follows this section in each respiratory disorder chapter discusses the disease in terms of the following:

1. The common pathophysiologic mechanisms activated throughout the respiratory system as a result of the anatomic alterations
2. The clinical manifestations that develop as a result of the pathophysiologic mechanisms
3. The basic respiratory therapy modalities used to improve the anatomic alterations and pathophysiologic mechanisms caused by the disease

When the anatomic alterations and pathophysiologic mechanisms caused by the disorder are improved, the clinical manifestations also should improve.

Etiology

A discussion of the etiology of the disease follows the presentation of anatomic alterations of the lungs. Various causes, predisposing conditions, and common comorbidities are described.

Overview of the Cardiopulmonary Clinical Manifestations Associated With the Disorder

This section comprises the central theme of the text. The reader is provided with the clinical manifestations commonly associated with the disease under discussion. In essence, the student is given a general "overview" of the signs and symptoms commonly demonstrated by the patient. By having a working knowledge—and therefore a predetermined expectation—of the clinical manifestations associated with a specific respiratory disorder, the respiratory therapist is in a better position to:
1. Gather clinical data relevant to the patient's respiratory status
2. Formulate an objective—and measurable—respiratory assessment
3. Develop an effective and safe treatment plan that is based on a valid assessment

If the appropriate data are not gathered and assessed correctly, the ability to treat the patient effectively is lost. As mentioned earlier, the case studies presented at the end of each respiratory disorder chapter frequently refer the reader back to Chapter 10 for a broader discussion of the signs and symptoms commonly associated with the disease under discussion—the "clinical scenario." When a particular clinical manifestation is unique to the respiratory disorder, however, a discussion of the pathophysiologic mechanisms responsible for the signs and symptoms is presented in the respective chapter.

Because of the dynamic nature of many respiratory disorders, the reader should note the following regarding this section:
• Because the severity of the disease is influenced by a number of factors (e.g., the extent of the disease, age, the general health of the patient), the clinical manifestations may vary considerably from one patient to another. In fact, they may vary in the same patient from one *time* to another. Therefore the practitioner should understand that the patient may demonstrate *all* the clinical manifestations presented or just a *few*.

   For example, many of the clinical manifestations associated with a respiratory disorder may never appear in some patients (e.g., digital clubbing, cor pulmonale, increased hemoglobin level). As a general rule, however, the prototypical patient usually demonstrates most of the manifestations presented during the advanced stages of the disease.
• For a variety of practical reasons, some of the clinical manifestations presented in each chapter may not actually be measured (or measurable) in the clinical setting (e.g., age, mental status, severity of the disorder). They are nevertheless conceptually important and therefore are presented here through extrapolation. For example, the newborn with severe respiratory distress syndrome, who obviously has a restrictive lung disorder as a result of the anatomic alterations associated with the disease, cannot actually perform the maneuvers necessary for a pulmonary function study.
• It should be noted that the clinical manifestations presented in each chapter are based only on the *one respiratory disorder under discussion*. In the clinical setting, however, the patient often has a combination of respiratory problems (e.g., emphysema compromised by pneumonia) and may have manifestations related to each of the pulmonary disorders.

This section does not attempt to present the "absolute" pathophysiologic bases for the development of a particular clinical manifestation. Because of the dynamic nature of many respiratory diseases, the precise cause of some of the manifestations presented by the patient is not always clear. In most cases, however, the primary pathophysiologic mechanisms responsible for the various signs and symptoms are known and understood and are described herein.

Management of the Disease

Each chapter provides a general overview of the current more common therapeutic modalities (treatment protocols) used to offset the anatomic alterations and pathophysiologic mechanisms activated by a particular disorder.

Although several respiratory therapy modalities may be safe and effective in treating a respiratory disorder, the respiratory therapist must have a clear conception of the following:
1. How the therapies work to offset the anatomic alterations of the lungs caused by the disease
2. How the correction of the anatomic alterations of the lungs work to offset the pathophysiologic mechanisms
3. How the correction of the pathophysiologic mechanisms works to offset the clinical manifestations demonstrated by the patient

Without this understanding, the practitioner merely goes through the motions of performing therapeutic tasks without any expected or measurable outcomes.*

Case Study

The case study at the end of each respiratory disease chapter provides the reader with a realistic example of (1) the manner in which the patient may arrive in the hospital with the disorder under discussion; (2) the various clinical manifestations commonly associated with the disease; (3) the way the clinical manifestations can be gathered, organized, and documented; (4) the way an assessment of the patient's respiratory status is formulated from the clinical manifestations; and (5) the way a comprehensive treatment plan is developed from the assessment.

---

*The reader should understand that this book is not a respiratory pharmacology text. Its emphasis is on the appropriate modalities to be used rather than specific pharmacologic agents.

In essence, the case study provides the reader with a good example of the way in which the respiratory therapist would gather clinical data, make an assessment, and treat a patient with the disorder under discussion. In addition, many of the case studies presented in the text describe a respiratory therapist assessing and treating the patient several times—demonstrating the importance of serial assessment and the way therapy is often up-regulated or down-regulated on a moment-to-moment basis in the clinical setting.

Self-Assessment Questions

Each disease chapter concludes with a set of self-assessment questions. Answers appear at the end of the book.

Appendices and Glossary

The appendices and the glossary can be found on the Evolve website for students (http://evolve.elsevier.com/DesJardins/respiratory). The appendices that are on Evolve are as follows:

Appendix I: Symbols and Abbreviations Commonly Used in Respiratory Physiology

Appendix II: Agents Used to Treat Bronchospasm and Airway Inflammation

Appendix III: Antibiotics

Appendix IV: Antifungal Agents

Appendix V: Mucolytic and Expectorant Agents

Appendix VI: Positive Inotropes and Vasopressors

Appendix VII: Diuretic Agents

Appendix VIII: The Ideal Alveolar Gas Equation

Appendix IX: Physiologic Dead Space Calculation

Appendix X: Units of Measure

Appendix XI: Poiseuille's Law

Appendix XII: $PCO_2/HCO_3^-/pH$ Nomogram

Appendix XIII: Calculated Hemodynamic Measurements

Appendix XIV: DuBois Body Surface Area Chart

Appendix XV: Cardiopulmonary Profile

References

A list of references is provided on the Evolve site. The student is also encouraged to review the selected references from uptodate.com, especially the "state-of-the-art" references regarding the respiratory disorders discussed throughout the textbook.

Approach

In writing this textbook, we have tried to present a realistic balance between the often-esoteric language of pathophysiology and the simple, straight-to-the-point approach generally preferred by busy students.

Terry Des Jardins, MEd, RRT
George G. Burton, MD

Acknowledgments

A number of people have provided important contributions to the development of the eighth edition of this textbook. First, for their outstanding input, suggestions, and guidance regarding all the newborn and early childhood respiratory disorders, a very special thank-you goes to Dr. Robert Cohn (deceased), past Director of Pulmonary Medicine; Dr. Robert Fink, past Director of Pulmonary Medicine; and Sue Ciarlariello, recently retired Director of Respiratory Care/Transport/Sleep Center, at Dayton Children's Hospital, Dayton, Ohio. In addition, a special thank-you goes to the many folks at Dayton Children's Hospital who helped secure a number of outstanding items for this new edition—including numerous x-ray films, clinical pictures, clinical charts and forms, and, importantly, the Newborn and Pediatric Protocols, which now appear in Chapters 33 and 34. These protocols will, undoubtedly, enhance the respiratory therapist's ability to understand and better develop effective and safe respiratory treatment plans for the newborn and pediatric patient.

For their work in developing our new Chapter 31, "Neuromuscular Disease," and review of Chapter 32, "Sleep Apnea," we are grateful to Dr. Lisa F. Wolfe, Pulmonary Critical Care Medicine, Sleep Medicine Northwestern Memorial Hospital, Northwestern Medicine Chicago, Illinois, and Dr. Gabriel Thomas, Pulmonary and Critical Care Medicine Fellow, Northwestern Memorial Hospital, Northwestern Medicine, Chicago, Illinois. For his outstanding artistic skills, we are again thankful to Timothy H. Phelps, Associate Professor, Johns Hopkins University School of Medicine, Baltimore, Maryland, for his work on the new color illustrations in Chapters 1, 8, 9, 14, and 15. Tim's artistic skills continue to enhance understanding of the concepts presented in this textbook.

For their very thorough edits, reviews, and helpful suggestions regarding the depth, breadth, and accuracy of the content presented in this textbook, we thank Sara Wing Parker, Associate Clinical Professor, University of Missouri, Columbia, Missouri; Donald J. Raymond, Program Director, Chippewa Valley Technical College, Eau Claire, Wisconsin; and Richard J. Zahodnic, Program Director, Macomb Community College, Clinton Township, Michigan. In addition, a special thank-you again goes to Robert Kacmarek for his review and edits for the common ventilatory management strategies used to treat specific disorders (good starting points) presented in Chapter 11.

For her work on the development of the new Evolve student website test banks, case studies, and PowerPoint presentations, we are very grateful to Sandra T. Hinski, Respiratory Care Program Director, Curriculum Development Facilitator, Gateway Community College, Phoenix, Arizona. For her long hours of preparing the edited manuscripts, we are thankful to Sandy Tuttle, Kettering College, Department of Respiratory Care.

Finally, we are very grateful to the team at Elsevier: Yvonne Alexopoulos, Senior Content Strategist, and Laura Selkirk, Senior Content Development Specialist. Their work and helpful coordination during the long development of this textbook and supplemental student website packages associated with this book is most appreciated.

Terry Des Jardins, MEd, RRT
George G. Burton, MD

Introduction

The Assessment Process—An Overview

Assessment is (1) the process of collecting clinical information about the patient's health status; (2) the evaluation of the data and identification of the specific problems, concerns, and needs of the patient; and (3) the development of a treatment plan that can be managed by the respiratory therapist. The clinical information gathered may consist of subjective and objective data (signs and symptoms) about the patient, the results of diagnostic tests and procedures, the patient's response to therapy, and the patient's general health practices.

The first step in the assessment process is **THINKING**—even before the actual collection of clinical data begins. In other words, the practitioner must first "think" about why the patient has entered the health care facility and about what clinical data will likely need to be collected. Merely obtaining answers to a specific list of questions does not serve the assessment process well. For example, while en route to evaluate a patient who is said to be having an asthma episode, the respiratory therapist might mentally consider the following: What are the likely signs and symptoms that can be observed at the bedside during a moderate or severe asthma attack? What are the usual emotional responses? What are the anatomic alterations associated with an asthma episode that would be responsible for the signs and symptoms observed? Table 1 presents a broader overview of what the practitioner might think about before assessing a patient said to be having an asthma episode.

It should be noted, however, that the respiratory therapist must always be on the alert for the following pitfalls: (1) the patient may have been misdiagnosed as having a certain respiratory problem—such as asthma—when, in fact, the problem is completely different—for example, a spontaneous pneumothorax or pulmonary embolus; (2) there are other abnormal conditions present that further compromise the patient's illness; or (3) there is no history or obvious signs or symptoms to enhance the practitioner's ability to identify the precise cause of the patient's respiratory problem. In short, the respiratory therapist must always be prepared to go through a complete and systematic approach to appropriately assess and treat the patient.

Purpose of Assessment

Relative to the purpose, an assessment may involve asking just two or three specific questions or it may involve an in-depth conversation with the patient. An assessment may involve a comprehensive focus (head-to-toe assessment) or a specific or narrow focus. The purpose of the assessment may include any of the following:

- To obtain a baseline databank about the patient's physical and mental status
- To supplement, verify, or refute any previous data
- To identify actual and potential problems
- To obtain data that will help the practitioner establish an assessment and treatment plan
- To focus on specific problems
- To determine immediate needs and establish priorities
- To determine the cause (etiology) of the problem
- To determine any related or contributing factors, such as comorbidities
- To identify patient strengths as a basis for changing behavior
- To identify the risk for complications
- To recognize complications

Types of Assessment

There are four major types of assessment: initial, focused, emergency, and ongoing.

The *initial assessment* is conducted at the first encounter with the patient. In the hospitalized patient, the initial assessment is typically performed by the admitting nurse and is more comprehensive than subsequent assessments. It starts with the reasons that prompted the patient to seek care and entails a holistic overview of the patient's health care needs. The general objective of the initial assessment is to rule out as well as to identify (rule in) specific problems. The initial assessment most commonly occurs when the patient has sought medical services for a specific problem or desires a general health status examination. The goals of the initial assessment include prevention, maintenance, restoration, or rehabilitation. In general, the thoroughness of the initial assessment is directly related to the length of expected care. In other words, discharge planning should begin at the time of the initial assessment!

The *focused assessment* consists of a detailed examination of the specific problem areas, or patient complaints. The focused assessment looks at clinical data in detail, considers possible causes, looks at possible contributing factors, and examines the patient's personal characteristics that will help—or hinder—the problem. The focused assessment also is used when the patient describes or manifests a new problem. Common patient complaints include pain, shortness of breath, dizziness, and fatigue. The practitioner must be prepared to evaluate the severity of such problems, assess the possible cause, and determine the appropriate plan of action.

TABLE 1 Examples of Topics That Might Be Considered Before Evaluating a Patient Having an Asthma Episode

Questions and/or Considerations	Likely Responses
What are the likely initial observations?	Shortness of breath, use of accessory muscles to breathe, intercostal retractions, pursed-lip breathing; cyanosis, barrel chest
What might be the patient's emotional response to his/her asthma?	Anxiety, concerned, frightened
What anatomic alterations of the lungs are associated with asthma?	Bronchospasm; excessive, thick, white, and tenacious bronchial secretions; air trapping; mucous plugging
What are the known causes of asthma?	*Extrinsic factors:* Pollen, grass, house dust, animal dander *Intrinsic factors:* Infection, cold air, exercise, emotional stress
What are the expected vital signs?	Increased respiratory rate, heart rate, and blood pressure
What are the expected chest assessment findings?	*Breath sounds:* Diminished, wheezing, crackles *Percussion:* Hyperresonant
What are the expected pulmonary function study findings?	*Decreased:* PEFR, FEF_T, FEV_T/FVC *Increased:* RV, FRC
What are the expected acute arterial blood gas findings?	*Early stage:* $\uparrow$ pH, $\downarrow$ $PaCO_2$, $\downarrow$ HCO_3^- (slightly), $\downarrow$ PaO_2, $\downarrow$ SaO_2 and SpO_2 *Late (severe) stage:* $\downarrow$ but normal pH, $\uparrow$ $PaCO_2$, $\uparrow$ HCO_3^- (slightly), $\downarrow$ PaO_2, $\downarrow$ SaO_2 and SpO_2
What are the expected chest radiograph findings?	Translucent lung fields; hyperinflated alveoli; depressed diaphragm
What are the usual respiratory treatments?	Bronchodilator therapy, bronchial hygiene therapy; oxygen therapy
What complications can occur?	Poor response to oxygen and bronchodilator therapy, acute ventilatory failure, severe hypoxia, mechanical ventilation

The *emergency assessment* identifies—or rules out—any life-threatening problems or problems that require immediate interventions. When the patient's medical condition is life threatening or when time is of the essence, the emergency assessment will include only key data needed for dealing with the immediate problem. Additional information can be gathered after the patient's condition has stabilized. The emergency assessment always follows the basic "ABCs" of cardiopulmonary resuscitation (i.e., the securing of the patient's *a*irway, *b*reathing, and *c*irculation).

The *ongoing assessment* consists of the data collection that occurs during each contact with the patient throughout the patient's hospital stay. Depending on the patient's condition, ongoing assessments may take place hourly, daily, weekly, or monthly. In fact, for the critically ill patient, assessments often take place continuously via electronic monitoring equipment. Ongoing assessments also take place while a patient is receiving anesthesia, as well as afterward until the effects of the anesthesia have worn off.

Respiratory therapists routinely make decisions about the frequency, depth, and breadth of the assessment requirements of the patient. To make these decisions effectively, the practitioner must anticipate the potential for a patient's condition to change, the speed at which it could change, and the clinical data that would justify a change. For example, when a patient experiencing an asthma episode inhales the aerosol of a selected bronchodilator, assessment decisions are based on the expected onset of drug action, expected therapeutic effects of the medication, and potential adverse effects that may develop.

Types of Data

Clinical information that is provided by the patient, and that cannot be observed directly, is called *subjective data*. When a patient's subjective data describe characteristics of a particular disorder or dysfunction, they are known as *symptoms*. For example, shortness of breath (dyspnea), pain, dizziness, nausea, and ringing in the ears are symptoms because they cannot be quantitated directly. The patient must communicate to the health care provider the symptoms he/she is experiencing and rate them as to severity. The patient is the only source of information about subjective findings.

Characteristics about the patient that can be observed directly by the practitioner are called *objective data*. When a patient's objective data describe characteristics of a particular disorder or dysfunction, they are known as *signs*. For example, swelling of the legs (pedal edema) is a sign of congestive heart failure. Objective data can be obtained through the practitioner's sense of sight, hearing, touch, and smell. Objective information can be measured (or quantified), and it can be replicated from one practitioner to another—a concept called *interrater reliability*. For example, the respiratory therapist can measure the patient's pulse, respiratory rate, blood pressure, inspiratory effort, and arterial blood gases. Because objective data are factual, they have a high degree of certainty.

Data Collection

To collect data wisely, health care providers must have well-developed skills in observing and listening. In addition, the practitioner must apply his/her mental skills of translation, reason, intuition, and validation to render the clinical data meaningful. Clinically, the collection of data is more useful when the evaluation process is organized into common problem areas, or categories. As the practitioner gathers information in each problem category, a clustering of related data about the patient will be generated. This framework for collecting clinical information enhances the practitioner's ability to establish priorities of care. Furthermore, any time the health care provider interacts with the patient, for any reason, an assessment of the patient's problems, needs, and concerns should be made. To efficiently and correctly gather data, the health care provider must make decisions about what type of assessment is needed, how to obtain the data, the framework and focus of the assessment, and what additional data may be needed before a complete treatment plan can be developed.

Sources of Data

Sources of clinical information include the patient, the patient's significant others, other members of the health care team, the patient's history and physical examination, and results of a variety of clinical tests and procedures. The practitioner must confirm that each data source is appropriate, reliable, and valid for the patient's assessment. *Appropriate* means the source is suitable for the specific purpose, patient, or event. *Reliable* means that the practitioner can trust the data to be accurate and honestly reported. *Valid* means that the clinical data can be verified or confirmed.

The Assessment Process—Role of the Respiratory Therapist

When the lungs are affected by disease or trauma, they are anatomically altered to some degree, depending on the severity of the process. In general, the anatomic alterations caused by an injury or disease process can be classified as resulting in an obstructive lung disorder, a restrictive lung disorder, or a combination of both. Common anatomic alterations associated with obstructive and restrictive lung disorders are illustrated in Fig. 1. Common respiratory diseases and their general classifications are listed in Table 2.

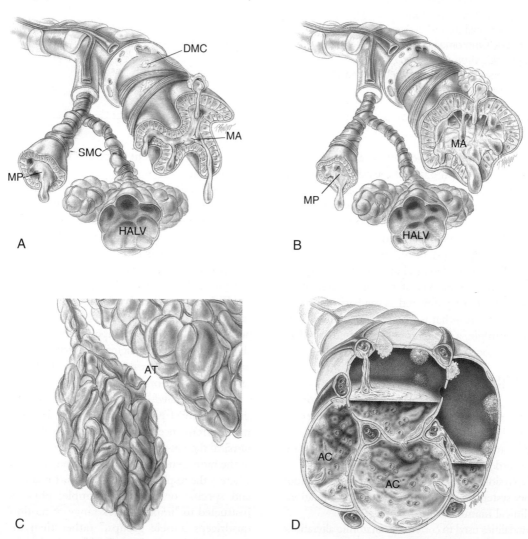

FIGURE 1 (A and B) Common anatomic alterations of the lungs in obstructive lung disorders. (A) Bronchial smooth muscle constriction accompanied by air trapping (as seen in asthma). (B) Tracheobronchial inflammation accompanied by mucus accumulation, partial airway obstruction, and air trapping (as seen in bronchitis). (C and D) Common anatomic alterations of the lungs in restrictive lung disorders. (C) Alveolar collapse or atelectasis (as seen in postoperative patients). (D) Alveolar consolidation (as seen in pneumonia). *AC*, Alveolar consolidation; *AT*, atelectasis; *DMC*, degranulation of mast cell; *HALV*, hyperinflated alveoli; *MA*, mucus accumulation; *MP*, mucus plug; *SMC*, smooth muscle constriction.

Respiratory Disease	Classification		
	Obstructive	Restrictive	Combination
Chronic obstructive pulmonary disease (chronic bronchitis and emphysema)	X		
Asthma	X		
Cystic fibrosis			X
Bronchiectasis			X
Atelectasis		X	
Pneumonia (lung abscess and fungal disease)		X	
Tuberculosis		X	
Pulmonary edema		X	
Flail chest		X	
Pneumothorax		X	
Pleural effusion		X	
Kyphoscoliosis		X	
Cancer of the lungs		X	
Chronic interstitial lung disease			X
Acute respiratory distress syndrome		X	
Meconium aspiration syndrome			X
Transient tachypnea of the newborn			X
Respiratory distress syndrome		X	
Pulmonary air leak syndrome			X
Respiratory syncytial virus			X
Chronic lung disease of infancy (bronchopulmonary dysplasia)			X
Diaphragmatic hernia		X	
Near drowning	X		

TABLE 2 General Classification of Respiratory Diseases

When the normal anatomy of the lungs is altered, certain pathophysiologic mechanisms throughout the cardiopulmonary system are activated. These pathophysiologic mechanisms in turn produce a variety of clinical manifestations specific to the illness. Such clinical manifestations can be readily—and objectively—identified in the clinical setting (e.g., increased heart rate, depressed diaphragm, or an increased functional residual capacity). Because differing chains of events happen as a result of anatomic alterations of the lungs, treatment selection is most appropriately directed at the basic causes of the clinical manifestations—that is, the anatomic alterations of the lungs. For example, a bronchodilator is used to offset the bronchospasm associated with an asthma episode.

The Knowledge Base

A strong knowledge base of the following four factors is essential to good respiratory care assessment and therapy selection skills:

1. Anatomic alterations of the lungs caused by common respiratory disorders
2. Major pathophysiologic mechanisms activated throughout the respiratory system as a result of the anatomic alterations
3. Common clinical manifestations
4. Treatment modalities used to correct the anatomic alterations and pathophysiologic mechanisms caused by the disorder

Specific Components of the Assessment Process

The respiratory therapist with good assessment and treatment selection skills also must be competent in performing the actual assessment process, which has the following components:

1. Quick and systematic collection of the important clinical manifestations demonstrated by the patient
2. Formulation of an accurate assessment of the clinical data—that is, identification of the cause and severity of the data abnormalities
3. Selection of the optimal treatment modalities
4. Quick, clear, and precise documentation of this process

Without this basic knowledge and understanding, the respiratory therapist merely goes through the motions of performing assigned therapeutic tasks with no measurable short- or long-term anticipated outcomes. In such an environment, the practitioner works in an unchallenging, task-oriented rather than goal-oriented manner.

Goal-orientated—patient-oriented—respiratory care became the standard of practice in the early 1990s by analyzing the work performance of other health care disciplines. For example, physical therapists have long been greatly empowered by virtue of the more generic physician's orders under which they work, whereas the respiratory therapists customarily received detailed and specific orders. For example, physical therapists are instructed to "improve back range of motion" or "strengthen quadriceps muscle groups," rather than to "provide warm fomentations to the lower back" or "initiate quadriceps setting exercises with 10-pound ankle weights, four times a day, for 10 minutes." In addition, and, importantly, the physical therapist has long been permitted to start, up-regulate, down-regulate, or discontinue the therapy on the basis of the patient's current needs and capabilities, not on the basis of a 2-hour-, 2-day-, or 2-week-old physician assessment. *Goal achievement,* not task completion, is the way the success of physical therapy is routinely measured.

In the current "sicker in, quicker out" cost-conscious environment, a change has come to respiratory care. Under fixed reimbursement programs, shorter lengths of stay have required hospital administrators and medical staff to examine allocation of health care resources. Recent data suggest that fully one-third of all hospitalized patients receive respiratory care services; therefore such services have come under close scrutiny. Studies using available peer-reviewed clinical practice guidelines have identified tremendous overuse (and, less frequently, underuse) of therapy modalities, and from this misallocation, the now firmly entrenched "therapist-driven protocol" (TDP) approach has emerged as the gold standard of respiratory care practice. Observing that the patient (and more accurately, the pulmonary pathophysiology!) should set the pace, some centers have called these protocols "patient-driven protocols," but the appellation of TDP or just "respiratory therapy protocols" has caught on more strongly. Clinical practice guidelines (CPGs), such as those developed by the American Association of Respiratory Care (AARC) and organizations such as the American Thoracic Society (ATS) and the American College of Chest Physicians (ACCP), are routinely used as the basis for TDPs in respiratory care.

The ACCP defines respiratory care protocols as follows:

> *"Patient care plans which are initiated and implemented by credentialed respiratory care workers. These plans are designed and developed with input from physicians and are approved for use by the medical staff and the governing body of the hospitals in which they are used. They share in common extreme reliance on assessment and evaluation skills. Protocols are by their nature dynamic and flexible, allowing up- or down-regulation of intensity of respiratory services. Protocols allow the respiratory care practitioner authority to evaluate the patient, [to] initiate care, to adjust, discontinue, or restart respiratory care procedures on a shift- by-shift or hour-to-hour basis once the protocol is ordered by the physician. They must contain clear strategies for various therapeutic interventions, while avoiding any misconception that they infringe on the practice of medicine."*

Numerous studies have now shown beyond a shadow of a doubt that when respiratory care protocol guidelines are followed appropriately, the outcomes of respiratory care services improve. This improvement is noted in both clinical and economic ways (e.g., shorter ventilator weaning time in postoperative coronary artery bypass graft [CABG] patients). Under this paradigm, respiratory care that is inappropriately ordered is either withheld or modified (whichever is appropriate), and patients who *need* respiratory care services (but are not receiving them) should now be able to receive care. (Chapters 10 and 11 discuss in detail the structure and implementations of a good TDP program.)

The notion that today's respiratory therapist "might" practice in the TDP setting has passed. Respiratory therapists who find that they are working in an archaic clinical setting—where protocols are not in daily use—should critically reexamine their employment options and career goals! To practice in today's health care environment without the cognitive (thinking) skills used in the protocol-rich environment is no longer acceptable—*and, importantly, can have serious, negative legal consequences*!

Experience, however, indicates that at least *some* respiratory therapists are not entirely comfortable with the new role and responsibility the TDP paradigm has thrust on them. These workers have difficulty separating the contents of *their* "little black bag" of diagnostic and therapeutic modalities from the one traditionally carried and used by the physician. The choice to be a "protocol safe and ready therapist," however, is no longer elective. The profession of respiratory care has changed and moved on. The Clinical Simulation Examination portion of the National Board for Respiratory Care (NBRC) Advanced Practitioner Examination reflects the actual, no longer just "simulated," bedside practice of respiratory care.

Similar to their physical therapist colleagues, today's respiratory therapists are now routinely asked to participate actively in the appropriate allocation of respiratory care services. Modern respiratory therapists must possess the basic knowledge, skills, and personal attributes to collect and assess clinical data and treat their patients effectively. Under the TDP paradigm, specific clinical indicators (clinical manifestations) for a particular respiratory care procedure must first be identified. In other words, a specific treatment plan is only started, up-regulated, down-regulated, or discontinued on the basis of the following:

1. The presence and collection of specific clinical indicators
2. An assessment made from the clinical data (i.e., the cause of the clinical data) that justifies the therapy order or change

In addition, after a particular treatment has been administered to the patient, all treatment outcomes must be measured and documented. Clearly, the success or failure of protocol work depends on accurate and timely patient assessment.

In view of these considerations, today's respiratory therapist *must* have competent bedside pulmonary assessment skills. Fundamental to this process is the ability to systematically gather clinical data, make an assessment, and develop an appropriate, safe, and effective action plan. Typically, once a treatment regimen has been implemented, the patient's progress is monitored on an ongoing assessment basis. In other words, clinical data are, again, collected, evaluated, and acted on based on the patient's response and progress toward a predefined goal.

To be fully competent in the assessment and treatment of respiratory disorders, the respiratory therapist must first have a strong academic foundation in the areas presented in Part I of this textbook. Part I is divided into three sections:

I. Bedside Diagnosis
II. Clinical Data Obtained From Laboratory Tests and Special Procedures
III. The Therapist-Driven Protocol Program—The Essentials

These three sections provide the reader with the essential knowledge base to assess and treat the patient with respiratory disease. The respiratory therapist must master the material in these sections to work efficiently and safely in a good TDP program.

Contents

PART II

Obstructive Lung Disease, 187

PART III

Loss of Alveolar Volume, 273

CHAPTER

1   The Patient Interview

Chapter Objectives

After reading this chapter, you will be able to:

- Describe the major items found on a patient history form.
- Explain the primary tasks performed during the patient interview.
- Describe the internal factors the practitioner brings to the interview.
- Discuss the external factors that provide a good physical setting for the interview.
- Describe the cultural, religious, and spiritual issues in the patient interview.
- Differentiate between open-ended questions and closed or direct questions.
- Describe the nine types of verbal responses.
- Describe the nonproductive verbal messages that should be avoided during the patient interview.
- List the positive and negative nonverbal messages associated with the patient interview.
- Describe how to close the interview.
- Discuss the pitfalls and weaknesses associated with the patient interview.
- Define key terms and complete self-assessment questions at the end of the chapter and on Evolve.

Key Terms

Body language
Clarification
Closed or Direct Questions
Confrontation
Empathy
Explanation
External Factors
Facilitation
Internal Factors
Interpretation
Nonproductive Verbal Messages
Nonverbal Techniques
Open-Ended Questions
Reflection
Silence
Summary

Chapter Outline

Patient History

A complete patient assessment starts and ends with the patient interview. The purpose of the patient history is to gather pertinent historical subjective and objective data, which in turn can be used to develop a more complete picture of the patient's past and present health. In most nonacute clinical settings the patient is asked to fill out a printed history form or checklist. The patient should be allowed ample time to

recall important dates, health-related landmarks, and family history. The patient interview is then used to validate what the patient has written and collect additional data on the patient's health status and lifestyle. Although history forms vary, most contain the following:

- Biographic data (age, gender, occupation)
- The patient's chief complaint or reason for seeking care, including the onset, duration, and characteristics of the signs and symptoms

- Present health or history of present illness
- List of current medications
- Reasons for stopping medications
- Past health, including childhood illnesses, accidents or injuries, serious or chronic illnesses, hospitalizations, operations, obstetric history, immunizations, last examination date, allergies, current medications, and history of smoking or other habits
- The patient's family history
- Review of each body system, including skin, head, eyes, ears, and nose, mouth and throat, respiratory system, cardiovascular system, gastrointestinal system, urinary system, genital system, and endocrine system
- Functional assessment (activities of daily living), including activity and exercise, work performance, sleep and rest, nutrition, interpersonal relationships, and coping and stress management strategies

The Patient Interview

The interview is a meeting between the respiratory care practitioner and the patient. It allows the collection of subjective data about the patient's feelings regarding his/her condition. During a successful interview, the practitioner performs the following tasks:

1. Gathers complete and accurate data about the patient's impressions about his or her health, including a description and chronology of any symptoms
2. Establishes rapport and trust so the patient feels accepted and comfortable in sharing all relevant information
3. Develops and shows interest in, and understanding about, the patient's health state, which in turn enhances the patient's participation in identifying problems

Interview skills are an art form that takes time and experience to develop. The most important components of a successful interview are communication and understanding. Understanding the various signals of communication is the most difficult part. An inability to convey the meaning of messages will lead to miscommunication between the practitioner and the patient.

Communication cannot be assumed just because two people have the ability to speak and listen. Communication is about behaviors—conscious and unconscious, verbal and nonverbal. All of these behaviors convey meaning. The following paragraphs describe important factors that enhance the sending and receiving of information during communication.

Internal Factors

Internal factors encompass what the practitioner brings to the interview—a genuine concern for others, empathy, understanding, and the ability to listen. A genuine liking of other people is essential in developing a strong rapport with the patient. It requires a generally optimistic view of people, a positive view of their strengths, and a nonjudgmental acceptance of their weaknesses. This affection generates an atmosphere of warmth and caring. The patient must feel accepted unconditionally.

Empathy is the art of viewing the world from the patient's point of view while remaining separate from it. Empathy entails recognition and acceptance of the patient's feelings without criticism. It is sometimes described as feeling with the patient rather than feeling like the patient. To have empathy the practitioner needs to listen. Listening is not a passive process. Listening is active and demanding. It requires the practitioner's complete attention. If the examiner is preoccupied with personal needs or concerns, he or she will invariably miss something important. Active listening is a cornerstone to understanding. Nearly everything the patient says or does is relevant.

During the interview the examiner should observe the patient's **body language** and note the patient's facial expressions, eye movement (e.g., avoiding eye contact, looking into space, diverting gaze), pain grimaces, restlessness, and sighing. The examiner should listen to the way things are said. For example, is the tone of the patient's voice normal? Does the patient's voice quiver? Are there pitch breaks in the patient's voice? Does the patient say only a few words and then take a breath? Such behaviors are often in opposition to what the patient is verbalizing, and further investigation may be indicated.

External Factors

External factors, such as a good physical setting, enhance the interviewing process. Regardless of the interview setting (the patient's bedside, a crowded emergency room, an office in the hospital or clinic, or the patient's home), efforts should be made to (1) ensure privacy, (2) prevent interruptions, and (3) secure a comfortable physical environment (e.g., comfortable room temperature, sufficient lighting, absence of noise). The interviewer's use of the *electronic health record* (EHR), also called the *electronic medical record* [EMR]), and its associated hardware can be threatening. In some cases, this may be a potential hazard to good patient communication—especially when combined with the anxiety that is often generated by simply being in the hospital and interacting with the various professional staff members about health issues, test results, and medical procedures; this form of anxiety is often referred to as the "white coat syndrome." In this situation, the patient can be intimidated to the point of "shutting down" and failing to ask questions or learn from the interview. In addition, the interviewer's focus is often shifted from the patient to the EHR and this can cause him/her to overlook important verbal and nonverbal messages. This situation also has the potential to cause patients to think they are not important.

Many respiratory care interviews must be performed in a much more hurried atmosphere than those described in this chapter—that is, relaxed and at the bedside of hospitalized patients. On many occasions, however, time is of the essence. Indeed, in some instances—such as in a "code" situation or emergency room visit—*no* interview may take place at all! Nevertheless, the thoughtful examiner should take away from this section the following conclusion: In any clinical setting, patients should think that their concerns are being heard—and, when things seem rushed, it should be understood that it is only because the urgency of the situation, *at that moment*, demands it! Even in these situations, however, the good interviewer should be able to modify and adapt his/her questions to a given clinical situation and patient ability. For example, if the patient is unable to speak, the respiratory therapist can simply phrase questions so they can be answered (or signed) with a "yes" or "no."

Cultural Sensitivity and Religious and Spirituality Considerations

Culture, religion, and spirituality strongly influence the way in which people think and behave and because of this have a definite and profound effect on their journey through the health care system. For example, in some cultures, the oldest man is the decision-maker for the rest of the family, including the making of health care decisions. In other cultures, elderly patients may be especially upset when an illness or hospitalization interrupts their religious practice. Failure to recognize cultural sensitivities can result in stereotyping, discrimination, racism, and prejudice. Future health care practitioners are now routinely trained in these considerations in "diversity" classes.

Culture can be defined as the values, beliefs, and practices shared by the majority in a group of people. Culture includes language, religious or spiritual practices, foods, social habits, music, and art accepted and expected by a cultural group. Although the terms *religion* and *spirituality* are often used interchangeably, they are different. *Religion* refers to a formalized system of belief and worship (e.g., Catholicism, Protestantism, Hinduism, Buddhism, etc.). *Spirituality* entails the spirit, or soul, and is an element of religion. It is intangible and may include a belief in a higher power, creative force, or divine being or a belief in spirits of departed people and the supernatural.

In the current health care system, all practitioners must work to develop cultural awareness, cultural sensitivity, and cultural competence to deliver effective care. *Cultural awareness* involves the knowledge of the patient's history and ancestry and an understanding of the patient's beliefs, artistic expressions, diets, celebrations, and rituals. *Cultural sensitivity* refers to refraining from using offensive language, respecting accepted and expected ways to communicate, and not speaking disrespectfully of a person's cultural beliefs. *Cultural competence* refers to knowing the health care practitioner's *own* values, attitudes, beliefs, and prejudices while, at the same time, keeping an open mind and trying to view the world through the perspective of culturally diverse groups of people.

All health care practitioners should continue to learn whatever they can about other cultures. When in doubt, the health care practitioner should simply ask the patient's preferences, rather than trying to guess or to stereotype the patient based on previous experiences with other cultures. Although mastery of the subject of diversity will be a lifelong learning process, the following cultural aspects are always a good place to start and should be routinely considered when caring for patients from different cultures:

- What is the patient's preferred method of communication?
- What is the appropriate form of address within the patient's culture?
- Are there potential language barriers (verbal and nonverbal)?
- Is an interpreter needed?
- Is the setting appropriate for the interview? Too private? Too public?
- What roles for women, men, and children are generally accepted within the patient's culture?
- Should a person of the same sex or religious persuasion as the patient be present at the interview?
- Are there religious and/or spiritual beliefs that need to be respected?
- Is direct eye contact considered polite or rude?
- What amount of space between the examiner and the patient is considered appropriate when communicating?
- What are the hidden meanings of nonverbal gestures such as head nodding, smiling, and hand gestures? Are these acceptable or not?
- When, where, and by whom is touch acceptable?
- Who is/are the primary decision-maker(s) within the culture and family?
- What are the appropriate manners and dress attire of a person considered a "professional"?

Health Literacy

Health literacy is defined as the patient's capacity to obtain, process, and understand basic health information and services needed to make appropriate health decisions and follow instructions for treatment. Health literacy includes the patient's ability to read, listen, analyze, and make decisions regarding his/her specific health situations. For example, an individual's degree of health literacy level includes the ability to understand the instructions that accompany prescription drugs, appointment slips, medical education brochures, doctor's directions and consent forms, and the ability to navigate the health care system, including filling out complex forms and locating providers and services.

It is estimated that more than 85% of adults in the United States have basic or below acceptable basic health literacy. In other words, nearly 9 in 10 adults may lack the skills needed to manage their health and prevent disease. Factors that affect health literacy include the patient's literacy skills, communication skills, health knowledge, demographics, culture and linguistic suitability, information dissemination channels, the complexity of the public health infrastructure, the health care provider's communication skills, and the patient's past experiences. In addition, health literacy includes numeracy skills. For example, calculating cholesterol and blood glucose levels, measuring medications, and understanding nutrition labels all require mathematical skills. The understanding of a simple *x-y* plot is beyond most patients and many health professionals. Moreover, choosing among different health plans or comparing prescription drug coverage often involves calculating premiums, copays, and deductibles.

Even for the individual with an advanced health literacy level, the ability to process medical information sometimes can be overwhelming. Medical equipment, techniques, and therapeutic procedures change rapidly. What an individual learned about certain health conditions or biology a few years ago often is outdated and obsolete today. Finally, it should be noted that health information presented during stressful or unfamiliar situations is not likely to be *retained* by the patient. Considerations of short-term or long-term memory problems, especially in older patients, open another set of issues in this category.

Enhancing the Value of the Health History

To enhance the accuracy of written and oral information, the plain language approach is the best strategy. Plain language is a verbal or written communication designed to ensure the intended audience quickly and fully understands the information presented. Plain language avoids verbose, convoluted language, medical terms the patient may not understand, and jargon. It is a language that avoids vagueness, inflated vocabulary, and long-winded written or verbal sentence construction. On the other hand, it is not baby talk, nor is it a simplified version of the English language. It is simply a clear, straightforward form of communication. In fact, in many countries, laws mandate that the public agencies use plain language to increase access to programs and services. The key elements of plain language include:

- Organization of information so that the most important points are presented first
- Extraction and presentation of complex information in small, understandable sections of one at a time
- Use of short sentences and common everyday words
- Use of active voice—for example, Jane changed the flat tire (active) versus the tire was changed by Jane (passive).
- Avoidance of technical terms and jargon
- Use of follow-up questions, such as "Do you understand?" or "Do you have any questions?" when communicating verbally

Finally, language that is plain and easy to understand for one group of people may not be clear and easy to comprehend to another group. Know one's audience and have written material tested and revised when necessary. The primary responsibility for improving health literacy belongs primarily to health professionals, health care facilities, and hospital systems, not the patient!

Techniques of Communication

During the interview, the patient should be addressed by his or her surname and the examiner should introduce himself or herself and state the purpose for being there. The following introduction serves as an example: "Good morning, Mr. Jones. I'm Phil Smith, and I'm your respiratory therapist today. I want to ask you some questions about your breathing so we can plan your respiratory care here in the hospital."

Verbal techniques of communication used by the examiner to facilitate the interview may include the skillful use of open-ended questions or closed or direct questions and responses.

Open-Ended Questions

An **open-ended question** asks the patient to provide narrative information. The examiner identifies the topic to be discussed but only in general terms. This technique is commonly used (1) to begin the interview, (2) to introduce a new section of questions, or (3) to gather further information whenever the patient introduces a new topic. The following are examples of open-ended questions:

"What brings you to the hospital today?"
"Tell me why you have come to the hospital today."

"Can you describe what your breathing has been like today?"
"You said that you have been short of breath. Tell me more about that."

The open-ended question is unbiased; it allows the patient freedom to answer in any way. This type of question encourages the patient to respond at greater length and give a spontaneous account of the condition. As the patient answers, the examiner should stop and listen. Patients often answer in short phrases or sentences and then pause, waiting for some kind of direction from the examiner. What the examiner does next is often the key to the direction of the interview. If the examiner presents new questions on other topics, much of the initial story may be lost. Ideally, the examiner should first respond by saying such things as "Tell me about it" and "Anything else?" The patient will usually add important information to the story when encouraged to expand with more details.

Closed or Direct Questions

A **closed or direct question** asks the patient for specific information. This type of question elicits a short one-word or two-word answer, a yes or no, or a forced choice. The closed question is commonly used after the patient's narrative to fill in any details the patient may have left out. Closed questions are also used to obtain specific facts, such as "Have you ever had this chest pain before?" Closed or direct questions speed up the interview and are often useful in emergency situations when the patient is unable to speak in complete sentences. The use of only open-ended questions is unwieldy and takes an unrealistic amount of time, causing undue stress in the patient. Box 1.1 compares closed and open-ended questions.

Responses: Assisting the Narrative

As the patient answers the open-ended questions, the examiner's role is to encourage free expression but not let the patient digress. The examiner's responses work to clarify the story. There are nine types of verbal responses. In the first five responses the patient leads; in the last four responses the examiner leads.

The first five responses require the examiner's reactions to the facts or feelings the patient has communicated. The examiner's response focuses on the *patient's* frame of reference; the examiner's frame of reference is not relevant. For the last four responses the examiner's reaction is not absolutely required. The frame of reference shifts from the patient's perspective to the examiner's perspective. These responses include the

BOX 1.1 Comparison of Closed and Open-Ended Questions	
Open-Ended Questions	**Closed Questions**
Used for narrative	Used for specific information
Call for long answers	Call for short one- or two-word answers
Elicit feelings, options, ideas	Elicit "cold facts"
Build and enhance rapport	Limit rapport and leave interaction neutral

examiner's thoughts or feelings. The examiner should use these responses only when the situation calls for them. If these responses are used too often, the interview becomes focused more on the examiner than on the patient. The nine responses are described in the following sections.

Facilitation

Facilitation encourages patients to say more, to continue with the story. Examples of facilitating responses include the following: "Mm hmm," "Go on," "Continue," "Uh-huh." This type of response shows patients that the examiner is interested in what they are saying and will listen further. Nonverbal cues, such as maintaining eye contact and shifting forward in the seat, also encourage the patient to continue talking.

Silence

Silent attentiveness is effective after an open-ended question. **Silence** communicates that the patient has time to think and organize what he or she wishes to say without interruption by the examiner.

Reflection

Reflection is used to echo the patient's words. The examiner repeats a part of what the patient has just said to clarify or stimulate further communication. Reflection helps the patient focus on specific areas and continue in his or her own way. The following is a good example:

PATIENT: "I'm here because of my breathing. It's blocked."
EXAMINER: "It's blocked?"
PATIENT: "Yes, every time I try to exhale, something blocks my breath and prevents me from getting all my air out."

Reflection also can be used to express the emotions implicit in the patient's words. The examiner focuses on these emotions and encourages the patient to elaborate:

PATIENT: "I have three little ones at home. I'm so worried they're not getting the care they need."
EXAMINER: "You feel worried and anxious about your children."

The examiner acts as a mirror reflecting the patient's words and feelings. This technique helps the patient elaborate on the problem and, importantly, further helps the examiner ensure that he or she correctly understands what the patient is attempting to communicate.

Empathy

Empathy is defined as the identification of oneself with another and the resulting capacity to feel or experience sensations, emotions, or thoughts similar to those being experienced by another person. It is often characterized as the ability to "put oneself into another's shoes." A physical symptom, condition, or disease frequently has accompanying emotions. Patients often have trouble expressing these feelings. An empathic response recognizes these feelings and allows expression of them:

PATIENT: "This is just great! I used to work out every day, and now I don't have enough breath to walk up the stairs!"

EXAMINER: "It must be hard—you used to exercise every day, and now you can't do a fraction of what you used to do."

The examiner's response does not cut off further communication, which would occur by giving false reassurance (e.g., "Oh, you'll be back on your feet in no time"). Also, it does not deny the patient's feelings nor does it suggest that the patient's feelings are unjustified. An empathic response recognizes the patient's feelings, accepts them, and allows the patient to express them without embarrassment. It strengthens rapport.

Clarification

Clarification is used when the patient's choice of words is ambiguous or confusing:

"Tell me what you mean by bad air."

Clarification is also used to summarize and simplify the patient's words. When simplifying the patient's words, the examiner should ask whether the paraphrase is accurate. The examiner is asking for agreement, and this allows the patient to confirm or deny the examiner's understanding.

Confrontation

In using **confrontation**, the examiner notes a certain action, feeling, or statement made by the patient and focuses the patient's attention on it:

"You said it doesn't hurt when you cough, but when you cough you grimace."

Alternatively, the examiner may focus on the patient's affect:

"You look depressed today."
"You sound angry."

Interpretation

Interpretation links events and data, makes associations, and implies causes. It provides the basis for inference or conclusion:

"It seems that every time you have a serious asthma attack, you have had some kind of stress in your life."

In using this attempt at clarification, the examiner runs the risk for making an incorrect inference. However, if the patient corrects the inference, his/her response often serves to prompt further discussion of the topic.

Explanation

Explanation provides the patient with factual and objective information:

"It is very common for your heart rate to increase a bit after a bronchodilator treatment."

Summary-Making

The **summary** is the final overview of the examiner's understanding of the patient's statements. It condenses the facts and presents an outline of the way the examiner perceives the patient's respiratory status. It is a type of validation in that the patient can agree or disagree with the examiner's summary. Both the examiner and the patient should participate in the summary. The summary signals that the interview is about to end.

Nonproductive Verbal Messages

In addition to the verbal techniques commonly used to enhance the interview, the examiner must refrain from making **nonproductive verbal messages**. These defeating messages restrict the patient's response. They act as barriers to obtaining data and establishing rapport.

Providing Assurance or Reassurance

Providing assurance or reassurance gives the examiner the false sense of having provided comfort. In fact, this type of response probably does more to relieve the examiner's anxiety than that of the patient.

> PATIENT: "I'm so worried about the mass the doctor found on my chest x-ray. I hope it doesn't turn out to be cancer! What happens to your lung?"
> EXAMINER: "Now, don't worry. I'm sure you will be all right. You have a very good doctor."

The examiner's response trivializes the patient's concern and effectively halts further communication about the topic. Instead, the examiner might have responded in a more empathic way:

> "You are really worried about that mass on your x-ray, aren't you? It must be very hard to wait for the lab results."

This response acknowledges the patient's feelings and concerns and, more important, keeps the door open for further communication.

Giving Advice

A key step in professional growth is to know when to give advice and when to refrain from it. Patients will often seek the examiner's professional advice and opinion on a specific topic:

> "What types of things should I avoid to keep my asthma under control?"

This is a straightforward request for information that the examiner has and the patient needs. The examiner should respond directly, and the answer should be based on knowledge and experience. The examiner should refrain from dispensing advice that is based on a hunch or feeling. For example, consider the patient who has just seen the doctor:

> "Dr. Johnson has just told me I may need an operation to remove the mass they found in my lungs. I just don't know. What would you do?"

If the examiner answers, the accountability for the decision shifts from the patient to the examiner. The examiner is not the patient. The patient must work this problem out. In fact, the patient probably does not really want to know what the examiner would do. In this case, the patient is worried about what he or she might have to do. A better response is reflection:

> EXAMINER: "Have an operation?"
> PATIENT: "Yes, and I've never been put to sleep before. What do they do if you don't wake up?"

Now the examiner knows the patient's real concern and can work to help the patient deal with it. For the patient to accept advice, it must be meaningful and appropriate. For example, in planning pulmonary rehabilitation for a male patient with severe emphysema, the respiratory therapist advises him to undertake a moderate walking program. The patient may treat the therapist's advice in one of two ways—either follow it or not. Indeed, the patient may choose to ignore it, thinking that it is not appropriate for him (e.g., he feels he gets plenty of exercise at work anyway).

By way of contrast, if the patient follows the therapist's advice, three outcomes are possible: The patient's condition stays the same, improves, or worsens. If the walking strengthens the patient, the condition improves. However, if the patient was not part of the decision-making process to initiate a walking program, the psychologic reward is limited, promoting further dependency. If the walking program does not improve his condition or compromises it, the advice did not work. Because the advice was not the patient's, he can avoid any responsibility for the failure:

> "See, I did what you advised me to do, and it didn't help. In fact, I feel worse! Why did you tell me to do this anyway?"

Although giving advice might be faster, the examiner should take the time to involve the patient in the problem-solving process. A patient who is an active player in the decision-making process is more likely to learn and modify behavior. The giving of advice is often best spread out over several visits, as rapport develops and diagnostic and therapeutic response data accumulate.

Using Authority

The examiner should avoid responses that promote dependency and inferiority:

> "Now, your doctor and therapist know best."

Although the examiner and the patient cannot have equality in terms of professional skills and experience, both are equally worthy human beings and owe each other respect.

Using Avoidance Language

When talking about potentially frightening topics, people often use euphemisms (e.g., "passed on" rather than "died") to avoid reality or hide their true feelings. Although the use of euphemisms may appear to make a topic less frightening, it does not make the topic or the fear go away. In fact, not talking about a frightening subject suppresses the patient's feelings and often makes the patient more fearful. The use of direct and clear language is the best way to deal with potentially uncomfortable topics.

Distancing

Distancing is the use of impersonal conversation that places space between a frightening topic and the speaker. For example, a patient with a lung mass may say, "A friend of mine has a tumor on her lung. She is afraid that she may need an operation" or "There is a tumor in the left lung." By using "the" rather than "my," the patient can deny any association with the tumor. Occasionally, health care workers also use distancing to soften reality. As a general rule, this technique does not work because it communicates to the patient that the health care practitioner is also afraid of the topic. The use of frank, patient-specific terms usually helps defuse anxiety rather than causing it.

Professional Jargon

What a health care worker calls a myocardial infarction, a patient calls a heart attack. The use of professional jargon can sound exclusionary and paternalistic to the patient. Health care practitioners should always try to adjust their vocabulary to the patient's understanding without sounding condescending. Even if patients use medical terms, the examiner cannot assume that they fully understand the meaning. For example, patients often think the term *hypertension* means that they are very tense and therefore take their medication only when they are feeling stressed, not when they feel relaxed!

Asking Leading or Biased Questions

Asking a patient "You don't smoke anymore, do you?" implies that one answer is better than another. The patient is forced either to answer in a way corresponding to the examiner's values or to feel guilty when admitting the other answer. When responding to this type of question, the patient risks the examiner's disapproval and possible alienation, which are undesirable responses from the patient's point of view. Better to slowly extract the smoke and exercise information slowly (see below), time-consuming as that may be.

Talking Too Much

Some examiners feel that helpfulness is directly related to verbal productivity. If they have spent the session talking, they leave feeling that they have met the patient's needs. In fact, the opposite is true. *The patient needs time to talk.* Some studies have found that "touch" is as important as "talk." As a general rule, the examiner should listen more than talk.

Interrupting and Anticipating

While patients are speaking, the examiner should refrain from interrupting them, even when the examiner believes he/she knows what is about to be said. Interruptions do not facilitate the interview. Rather, they communicate to the patient that the examiner is impatient or bored with the interview. Another trap is thinking about the next question while the patient is answering the last one, or anticipating the answer. Examiners who are overly preoccupied with their role as interviewer are not really listening to the patient. As a general rule, the examiner should allow a second or so of silence between the patient's statement and the next question.

Using "Why" Questions

The examiner should be careful in presenting "why" questions. The use of "why" questions often implies blame; it puts the patient on the defensive:

"Why did you wait so long before calling your doctor?"

"Why didn't you bring your asthma medication with you?"

The only possible answer to a "why" question is "Because …," and this places the patient in an uncomfortable position. To avoid this trap, the examiner might say, "I noticed you didn't call your doctor right away when you were having trouble breathing. I'd like to find out what was happening during this time."

BOX 1.2 Nonverbal Messages of the Interview

Positive	Negative
Professional appearance	Nonprofessional appearance
Sitting next to patient	Sitting behind a desk and/or computer screen
Close proximity to patient	Far away from patient
Turned toward patient	Turned away from patient
Relaxed, open posture	Tense, closed posture
Leaning toward patient	Slouched away from patient
Facilitating gestures	Nonfacilitating gestures
· Nodding of head	· Looking at watch
Positive facial expressions	Negative facial expressions
· Appropriate smiling	· Frowning
· Interest	· Yawning
Good eye contact	Poor eye contact
Moderate tone of voice	Strident, high-pitched voice
Moderate rate of speech	Speech too fast or too slow
Appropriate touch	Overly frequent or inappropriate touch

Nonverbal Techniques of Communication

Nonverbal techniques of communication include physical appearance, posture, gestures, facial expression, eye contact, voice, and touch. Nonverbal messages are important in establishing rapport and conveying feelings. Nonverbal messages may either support or contradict verbal messages—and, thus generate a positive or negative influence on the interview process. Therefore an awareness of the nonverbal messages that may be conveyed by either the patient or the examiner during the interview process is important.

Box 1.2 provides an overview of nonverbal messages that may occur during an interview.

Physical Appearance

The examiner's general personal appearance, grooming, and choice of clothing send a message to the patient. Professional dress codes vary among hospitals and clinical settings. Depending on the setting, a professional uniform can project a message that ranges from comfortable or casual to formal or distant. Regardless of one's personal choice in clothing and general appearance, the aim should be to convey a competent and professional image.

Examiner's Body Posture

An *open position* is one in which a communicator extends the large muscle groups (i.e., arms and legs are not crossed). An open position shows relaxation, physical comfort, and a willingness to share information. A *closed position*, with arms and legs crossed, sends a defensive and anxious message. The examiner should be aware of any posture changes. For example, if the patient suddenly shifts from a relaxed to a tense position, it suggests discomfort with the topic. In addition, the examiner should try to sit comfortably next to the patient during the interview. Sitting too far away or standing over the patient often sends a negative nonverbal message.

Gestures

Gestures send nonverbal messages. For example, pointing a finger may show anger or blame. Nodding of the head or an open hand with the palms turned upward can show acceptance, attention, or agreement. Wringing the hands suggests worry and anxiety. The patient often describes a crushing chest pain by holding a fist in front of the sternum. When a patient has a sharp, localized pain, one finger is commonly used to point to the exact spot.

Facial Expression

An individual's face can convey a wide range of emotions and conditions. For example, facial expressions can reflect alertness, relaxation, anxiety, anger, suspicion, and pain. The examiner should work to convey an attentive, sincere, and interested expression. Patient rapport will deteriorate if the examiner exhibits facial expressions that suggest boredom, distraction, disgust, criticism, and disbelief.

Eye Contact

Lack of eye contact suggests that a person may be insecure, intimidated, shy, withdrawn, confused, bored, apathetic, or depressed. The examiner should work to maintain good eye contact but not stare the patient down with a fixed, penetrating look. Generally, an easy gaze toward the patient's eyes with occasional glances away works well. The examiner, however, should be aware that this approach may not work when interviewing a patient from a culture in which direct eye contact is generally avoided. For example, Asian, Native American, Indochinese, Arab, and some Appalachian people may consider direct eye contact impolite or aggressive, and they may avert their own eyes during the interview.

Voice Style

Nonverbal messages are reflected through the tone of voice, intensity and rate of speech, pitch, and long pauses. These messages often convey more meaning than the spoken word. For example, a patient's voice may show sarcasm, anxiety, sympathy, or hostility. An anxious patient frequently talks in a loud and fast voice. A soft voice may reflect shyness and fear. A patient with hearing impairment generally speaks in a loud voice. Long pauses may have important meanings. For instance, when a patient pauses for a long time before answering an easy and straightforward question, the honesty of the answer may be questionable. Slow speech with long and frequent pauses, combined with a weak and monotonous voice, suggests depression.

Touch

The meaning and social implications of touch are often misinterpreted; they can be influenced by an individual's age, gender, cultural background, past experiences, and the present setting. As a general rule, the examiner should not touch patients during interviews unless he or she knows the patient well and is sure that the gesture will be interpreted correctly. When appropriate, touch (e.g., a touch of the hand or arm) can be effective in conveying empathy.

To summarize, extensive nonverbal messages, communicated by both the examiner and patient, may be conveyed during the interview. Therefore the examiner must be aware of the patient's various nonverbal messages while working to communicate nonverbal messages that are productive and enhancing to the examiner-patient relationship.

Closing the Interview

The interview should end gracefully. If the session has an abrupt or awkward closing, the patient may be left with a negative impression. This final moment may destroy any rapport gained during the interview. To ease into the closing, the examiner might ask the patient one of the following questions:

"Is there anything else that you would like to talk about?"

"Do you have any other questions that you would like to ask me?"

"Are there any other problems that we have not discussed?"

These types of questions give the patient an opportunity for self-expression. The examiner may choose to summarize or repeat what was learned during the interview. This serves as a final statement of the examiner's and the patient's assessment of the situation. Finally, the examiner should thank the patient for the time and cooperation provided during the interview. If appropriate, the examiner should (may) suggest a follow-up visit. If this is not possible, simply telling the patient what is scheduled next—for example, "I see your chest x-ray is scheduled this afternoon" implies a sense of continuity and trust that the examiner is part of the team and knows what is going on!

Pitfalls and Weaknesses Associated With the Patient Interview

The respiratory therapist must be acutely aware of the various pitfalls and weaknesses associated with the patient interview. For example, after completing the interview, the following might be concluded:

A strength of the patient interview is its ownership by the patient—who better than the patient to correctly and completely present his/her side of the story? In turn, this information can be readily transferred and acted on by a skilled examiner, in a cost-effective and timely manner. After all, if anyone knows what is going on, it should be the patient. Right? **WRONG!**

This is because the patient's description of his/her present and past abnormal respiratory conditions—for example, dyspnea, abnormal breathing patterns, cough, sputum production, and pleurisy—can be extremely complex to verbalize, misleading, and often very subjective. Some causes of incorrect information and/or misleading data during the patient interview include the following:

- *The sinister nature of symptoms during the "early stages" of pulmonary disease.* The cardiopulmonary system has an enormous resilience to the early insult of certain pulmonary

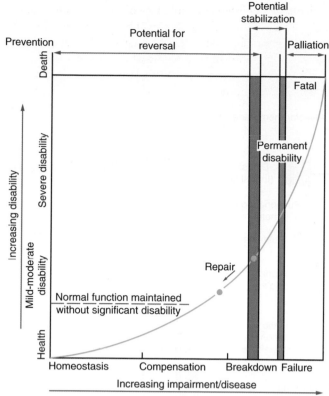

FIGURE 1.1 Graphic Description of Relationship of Symptoms to Extent of Pulmonary Pathology. Early in the process (left side of diagram), when prevention may be possible, the patient may experience few symptoms unless the system is stressed, for example, exercise or sleep. Later in the process (see right side of diagram), small increases in pathologic burden, such as a small pleural effusion in a lung already afflicted with emphysema, may produce extremely severe symptoms, if not death.

diseases. For example, it is not unusual to observe an otherwise healthy young individual who has had long exposures to industrial dust and fumes, has smoked cigarettes for years, or has had a partial or total pneumonectomy readily demonstrate remarkable physical activities such as running, biking, and swimming. This is why, in part, mild injuries to the cardiopulmonary system often go unnoticed during the "early stages" of a particular pulmonary disorder (e.g., chronic obstructive pulmonary disease).

- *The menacing nature of the effect of small pathologic changes during the "late stages" of pulmonary disease.* During the late phases of chronic pulmonary diseases (e.g., chronic obstructive pulmonary disease), even a minor insult, such as mild pneumonia or small pleural effusion, often results in a sudden "system breakdown" and respiratory failure. It should be understood that during the advanced phases of respiratory disorders, the old saying "little things mean a lot," is truly an important and meaningful statement when assessing these patients. Fig. 1.1 illustrates this important nonlinear relationship of symptoms to the extent of pulmonary pathologic condition.

- *The complexity and interdependence of the gas exchange system.* In its simplest form, the purpose of history-taking is to answer these basic questions: "What is going on here?" or, "Why is the patient here?" To answer these types of questions,

the respiratory therapist must work to identify the precise cause and location within the cardiopulmonary system that is responsible for the patient's signs and symptoms. To fully accomplish this, it is critical to understand (1) how each component of the gas exchange system works independently from one another and (2) how each component works to support the other components of the entire system. When any "one" component of the gas exchange system begins to fail, the entire system is affected. Because of the complexity of the gas exchange system, however, the ability to isolate the precise source of the problem can be difficult. A strong knowledge and understanding of the gas exchange system are essential. Fig. 1.2 provides an overview of the major components—that is, the essential knowledge base—of the gas exchange system, which includes:

- Pumps
- Air and blood conducting tubes
- Phyiologic gas exchange membranes

To function properly, each of the components of the cardiopulmonary system must work together in harmony with each other. If any one of the mechanisms fails, the body's ability to efficiently move oxygen and carbon dioxide becomes jeopardized; in short, the failure of only one cardiopulmonary component can create a "Go-no-Go" situation for the entire gas exchange system.

- As illustrated in Fig. 1.3, each component of the gas exchange system is separate and unique in design but strongly interdependent with all the other components to appropriately perform their specific functions. Each cardiopulmonary component must work, or the whole system becomes impaired and, ultimately, causes the entire network to shut down. Throughout the cardiopulmonary system, all the tubes, pumps, and membrane interfaces must all function like gears in a bicycle, simultaneously and continuously. If only one part of the gas exchange system fails, even though the remainder is functioning normally, the total system will be impaired and ultimately fail. Thus one must continually ask this question during the patient assessment: "Is there is any evidence to suggest a malfunction in one or more components of the gas exchange system?

- *The poor memory and/or mental confusion of the patient.* For a variety of reasons, it is not uncommon to elicit incorrect or misleading information during the patient interview. For example, the patient may be confused because of advanced age, poor hearing, hypoxemia, or medications. Or, in some cases, the signs and symptoms associated with the patient pulmonary problem may appear only during physical exertion or exercise. In addition, because of the negative impressions associated with tobacco, many patients who do smoke or have smoked often give ambiguous answers about their smoking history. For example, the following patient-examiner dialog is *not* unusual:

EXAMINER: "Are you a smoker?"
PATIENT: "No."
EXAMINER: "Have you ever smoked?"
PATIENT: "Not for a long time."
EXAMINER: "When did you stop?"
PATIENT: "About 2 weeks ago."
EXAMINER: "Okay. How much did you smoke?"
PATIENT: "Some every day."

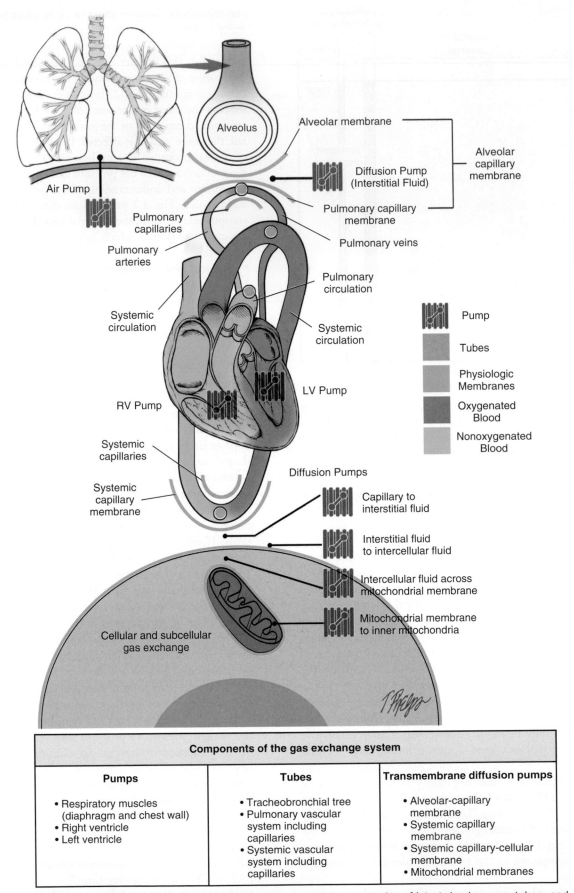

Labels in figure:

Alveolus

Air Pump

Alveolar membrane

Diffusion Pump (Interstitial Fluid)

Alveolar capillary membrane

Pulmonary capillaries

Pulmonary capillary membrane

Pulmonary arteries

Pulmonary veins

Systemic circulation

Pulmonary circulation

Systemic circulation

RV Pump

LV Pump

Systemic capillaries

Systemic capillary membrane

Diffusion Pumps

Capillary to interstitial fluid

Interstitial fluid to intercellular fluid

Intercellular fluid across mitochondrial membrane

Mitochondrial membrane to inner mitochondria

Cellular and subcellular gas exchange

Legend:
Pump
Tubes
Physiologic Membranes
Oxygenated Blood
Nonoxygenated Blood

Components of the gas exchange system

Pumps	Tubes	Transmembrane diffusion pumps
• Respiratory muscles (diaphragm and chest wall) • Right ventricle • Left ventricle	• Tracheobronchial tree • Pulmonary vascular system including capillaries • Systemic vascular system including capillaries	• Alveolar-capillary membrane • Systemic capillary membrane • Systemic capillary-cellular membrane • Mitochondrial membranes

FIGURE 1.2 The cardiorespiratory gas exchange system is seen as a complex of intertwined pumps, tubes, and transmembrane diffusion pumps that serve the demands of the energy "factory" of metabolism at the end-user location, the mitochondria. There, oxygen is consumed and carbon dioxide is produced in the process of energy generation with the formation of adenosine triphosphate (ATP) and water. Disease processes can occur at any one or more of these components of the gas exchange system. *LV,* Left ventricular; *RV,* right ventricular.

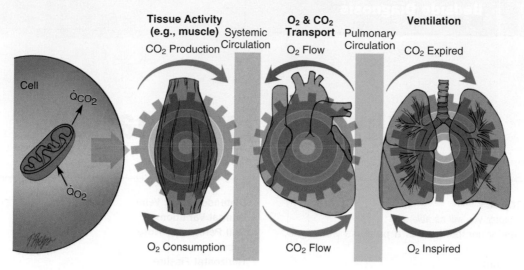

FIGURE 1.3 A Different Model Emphasizing the Interdependence and Interface of Its Major Components of the Gas Exchange System. The major components and functions include the (1) lungs (function: tidal volume [V_T], respiratory frequency [f], oxygen [O_2] intake, and carbon dioxide [CO_2] output), (2) pulmonary circulation (function: recruitment that increased perfusion and ventilation of alveolar capillary units that are quiescent at rest, (3) heart (function: stroke volume [SV] and heart rate [HR]), (4) system circulation (vasodilation and vasoconstriction), and (5) tissue, muscle, and mitochondria activity (O_2 consumption [$\dot{V}O_2$] and CO_2 production [$\dot{V}CO_2$]. Read the figure from right to left to understand the entry of "good" air into the system and left to right to see the process in which CO_2 is removed.

EXAMINER: "How *much* every day?"

PATIENT: "Two packs a day."

Etc. etc. etc.

This whole dialog is much like pulling teeth. Suffice it to say, misleading historical information may be given by the patient on an intentional or nonintentional basis. The former may be in the form of out-and-out lying about historical points; the latter because of inability to recall events from the distant past or because the patient simply does not think such information as "The pneumonia I had twice (!) as a child was important." Encouraging patients to complete an extensive medical history form *before* their first office visit is often a valuable procedure to help streamline the interview process.

A Note of Reassurance

Do not let the foregoing material belittle in any way the value of a carefully obtained history. Thankfully, the history is rarely obtained in a vacuum; it is most often followed by a carefully performed physical examination that will "fill in the blanks" and answer many questions that were prompted by the most careful interviewer.

SELF-ASSESSMENT QUESTIONS

1. During the patient interview, the practitioner states: "You are worried about your child." This type of statement is an example of which of the following techniques:
   a. Reflection
   b. An open-ended question
   c. Confrontation
   d. Facilitation

2. Which of the following is a closed or direct question?
   a. Can you tell me why you appear depressed and angry today?
   b. Have you had this pain before?
   c. How did you first notice the problem?
   d. Why did you wait so long before calling your doctor?

3. Which of the following is considered a negative nonverbal message of the interview?
   a. Nodding of head
   b. Sitting behind a desk
   c. Moderate tone of voice
   d. Sitting next to the patient

4. Which of the following is/are likely to be found on a complete patient history form?
   1. The patient's family history
   2. Activities of daily living
   3. The patient's chief complaint
   4. Review of each body system
      a. 2 and 3 only
      b. 1 and 4 only
      c. 2, 3, and 4 only
      d. 1, 2, 3, and 4

5. Which one of the following is considered a "facilitation" response?
   a. "You feel anxious about your children."
   b. "It must be hard to not be able to do that now."
   c. "Mm hmmm, go on."
   d. "Tell me what you mean by bad air."

CHAPTER

2 The Physical Examination

Chapter Objectives

After reading this chapter, you will be able to:

- Describe the major components of a patient's vital signs, including
  - Body temperature
  - Pulse
  - Respiration
  - Blood pressure
  - Oxygen saturation
- Describe the lung and chest topography, including
  - Thoracic cage landmarks
  - Imaginary lines
  - Lung borders and fissures
- Describe the purpose of inspection
- Describe palpation, including
  - Chest excursion
  - Tactile and vocal fremitus
- Describe percussion, including
  - Abnormal percussion notes
  - Diaphragmatic excursion
- Describe auscultation, including
  - Normal breath sounds
  - Abnormal breath sounds
- Define key terms and complete self-assessment questions at the end of the chapter and on Evolve.

Key Terms

Abnormal Breathing Patterns
Adventitious Lung Sounds
Afebrile
Anterior Axillary Line
Apnea
Auscultation
Biot's Respiration
Blood Pressure (BP)
Body Temperature (T°)
Bradycardia
Bradypnea
Bronchovesicular breath sounds
Cardiac Diastole
Cardiac Output (CO)
Cardiac Systole
Chest Excursion
Constant Fever
Core Temperature
Crackles
Crepitus
Diaphragmatic Excursion
Diastole
Diastolic Blood Pressure
Diminished Breath Sounds
Distended Neck Veins
Diurnal Variations
Dull Percussion Note
Febrile
Horizontal Fissure
Hyperpyrexia
Hyperresonant Note
Hypertension
Hyperthermia
Hyperventilation
Hypotension
Hypothermia
Hypoventilation
Inspection
Intermittent Fever
Kussmaul's Respiration
Lung and Chest Topography
Midaxillary Line
Midclavicular Line
Midscapular Line
Midsternal Line
Mild Hypoxemia
Moderate Hypoxemia
Normal Breath Sounds
Oblique Fissure
Palpation
Pedal (Dorsalis Pedis) Pulse
Percussion
Posterior Axillary Line
Pulse (P)
Pulse Oximetry (SpO$_2$)
Pulse Pressure
Pulsus Alternans
Pulsus Paradoxus
Pyrexia
Relapsing Fever
Remittent Fever
Respiratory Rate
Severe Hypoxemia
Sinus Arrhythmia
Stridor
Subcutaneous Emphysema
Systole
Systolic Blood Pressure
Tachycardia
Tachypnea
Tactile Fremitus
Tripod Position
Tympany
Ultrasonic Doppler
Vasoconstriction

Vital Signs

The four major vital signs—**body temperature (T°)**, **pulse (P)**, respiratory rate (R), and **blood pressure (BP)**—are excellent bedside clinical indicators of the patient's physiologic and psychologic health. In many patient care settings, the oxygen saturation as measured by **pulse oximetry (SpO$_2$)** is considered to be the "fifth vital sign." Table 2.1 shows the normal values that have been established for various age groups.

During the initial measurement of a patient's vital signs, the values are compared with these normal values. After several vital signs have been documented for the patient, they can be used as a baseline for subsequent measurements. Isolated vital sign measurements are not as valuable as a series of measurements. By evaluating a series of values, the practitioner can identify important vital sign trends for the patient. Vital sign trends that deviate from the patient's normal measurements are often more important than an isolated measurement.

Although the skills involved in obtaining the vital signs are easy to learn, interpretation and clinical application require knowledge, problem-solving skills, critical thinking, and experience. Even though vital sign measurements are part of routine bedside care, they provide vital information and should always be considered an important part of the assessment process. The frequency with which vital signs should be assessed depends on the individual needs of each patient.

Body Temperature

Body temperature is routinely measured to assess for signs of inflammation or infection. Even though the body's skin temperature varies widely in response to environmental conditions and physical activity, the temperature inside the body, the **core temperature**, remains relatively constant—about 37°C (98.6°F), with a daily variation of ± 0.5°C (1° to 2°F). Under normal circumstances, the body is able to maintain this constant temperature through various physiologic compensatory mechanisms, such as the autonomic nervous system and special receptors located in the skin, abdomen, and spinal cord.

In response to temperature changes, the receptors sense and send information through the nervous system to the hypothalamus. The hypothalamus, in turn, processes the information and activates the appropriate response. For example, an increase in body temperature causes the blood vessels near the skin surface to dilate, a process called **vasodilation**. Vasodilation, in turn, allows more warmed blood to flow near the skin surface, thereby enhancing heat loss. In contrast, a decrease in body temperature causes **vasoconstriction**, which works to keep warmed blood closer to the center of the body, thus working to maintain the core temperature.

At normal body temperature, the metabolic functions of all body cells are optimal. When the body temperature increases or decreases significantly from the normal range, the metabolic

TABLE 2.1 Average Range of Values for Vital Signs According to Age Group

Age Group	Core Temperature (°F)	Pulse (bpm)	Respirations (breaths/min)	Blood Pressure (mm Hg) Systolic	Diastolic
Newborn	96–99.5	120–170	30–60	45–75	20–50
Infant (1 mo–1 yr)	99.4–99.7	80–160	30–60	75–100	50–70
Toddler (1–3 yr)	99.4–99.7	80–130	25–40	80–110	55–80
Preschooler (3–6 yr)	98.6–99	80–120	20–35	80–110	50–80
Child (6–12 yr)	98.6	65–100	20–30	100–110	60–70
Adolescent (12–18 yr)	97–99	60–90	12–20	110–120	60–65
Adult	97–99	60–100	12–20	110–140	60–90
Older adult (>70 yr)	95–99	60–100	12–20	120–140	70–90

rate and therefore the demands on the cardiopulmonary system also change. For example, during a fever the metabolic rate increases. This action leads to an increase in oxygen consumption and an increase in carbon dioxide production at the cellular level. According to estimates, for every 1°C increase in body temperature, the patient's oxygen consumption increases about 10%. As the metabolic rate increases, the cardiopulmonary system must work harder to meet the additional cellular demands. Hypothermia reduces the metabolic rate and cardiopulmonary demand.

As shown in Fig. 2.1, the normal body temperature is positioned within a relatively narrow range. A patient who has a temperature within the normal range is said to be **afebrile**. A body temperature above the normal range is called **pyrexia** or **hyperthermia**. When the body temperature rises above the normal range, the patient is said to have a *fever* or to be **febrile**. An exceptionally high temperature, such as 41°C (105.8°F), is called **hyperpyrexia**.

The four common types of fevers are **intermittent fever**, **remittent fever**, **relapsing fever**, and **constant fever**. An intermittent fever is said to exist when the patient's body temperature alternates at regular intervals between periods of fever and periods of normal or below-normal temperatures. In other words, the patient's temperature undergoes peaks and valleys, with the valleys representing normal or below-normal temperatures. During a remittent fever, the patient has marked peaks and valleys (more than 2°C [3.6°F]) over a 24-hour period, all of which are above normal—that is, the body temperature does not return to normal between the spikes. A relapsing fever is said to exist when short febrile periods of a few days are interspersed with 1 or 2 days of normal temperature. A continuous fever is present when the patient's body temperature remains above normal with minimal or no fluctuation.

Hypothermia is the term used to describe a core temperature below the normal range. Hypothermia may occur as a result of (1) excessive heat loss, (2) inadequate heat production to counteract heat loss, and (3) impaired hypothalamic thermoregulation. Box 2.1 lists the clinical signs of hypothermia.

Hypothermia may be caused accidentally or may be induced. Accidental hypothermia is commonly seen in the patient who (1) has had an excessive exposure to a cold environment, (2) has been immersed in a cold liquid environment for a prolonged time, or (3) has inadequate clothing, shelter, or heat. It should be noted that geriatric patients generally display a lower temperature than younger adults. In addition, a reduced metabolic rate may compound hypothermia in older patients. Older patients often take sedatives, which further depress the metabolic rate. Box 2.2 lists common therapeutic interventions for patients with hypothermia.

Induced hypothermia refers to the intentional lowering of a patient's body temperature to reduce the oxygen demand of the tissue cells. Induced hypothermia may involve only a portion of the body or the whole body. Induced hypothermia is often indicated before certain surgeries, such as heart or brain surgery, or after return of spontaneous circulation after a cardiac arrest.

BOX 2.1 Clinical Signs of Hypothermia

- Below normal body temperature
- Decreased pulse and respiratory rate
- Severe shivering (initially)
- Patient indicating coldness or presence of chills
- Pale or bluish cool, waxy skin
- Hypotension
- Decreased urinary output
- Lack of muscle coordination
- Disorientation
- Drowsiness or unresponsiveness
- Coma

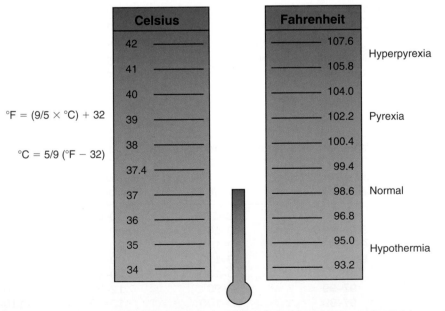

FIGURE 2.1 Range of normal body temperature and alterations in body temperature on the Celsius and Fahrenheit scales. See conversion formulas for Fahrenheit and Celsius scales on the left side of the figure.

Factors Affecting Body Temperature

Table 2.2 lists several factors that affect body temperature. Knowing these factors can help the practitioner better assess the significance of expected or normal variations in a patient's body temperature.

Body Temperature Measurement

The measurement of body temperature establishes an essential baseline for clinical comparison as a disease progresses or as therapies are administered. To ensure the reliability of a temperature reading, the practitioner must (1) select the correct measuring equipment, (2) choose the most appropriate site, and (3) use the correct technique or procedure. The four most commonly used sites are the mouth, rectum, ear (tympanic membrane/auditory canal) and axilla. Any of these sites is satisfactory when the proper technique is used.

BOX 2.2 Common Therapeutic Interventions for Hypothermia

- Remove wet clothing
- Provide dry clothing
- Place patient in a warm environment (slowly increase room temperature)
- Cover patient with warm blankets or electric heating blanket
- Apply warming pads (increase temperature slowly)
- Keep patient's limbs close to body
- Cover patient's head with a cap or towel
- Supply warm oral or intravenous fluids

Additional measurement sites include the esophagus and pulmonary artery. Temperatures measured at these sites, and in the rectum and at the tympanic membrane, are considered core temperatures. The skin, typically that of the forehead or abdomen, also may be used for general temperature purposes. However, practitioners must remember that although skin temperature–sensitive strips or disposable paper thermometers may be satisfactory for general temperature measurements, the patient's precise temperature should always be confirmed—when indicated—with a glass or tympanic thermometer.

Because body temperature is usually measured orally, the practitioner must be aware of certain external factors that can lead to false oral temperature measurements. For example, drinking hot or cold liquids can cause small changes in oral temperature measurements. The most significant temperature changes have been reported after a patient drinks ice water. Drinking ice water may lower the patient's actual temperature by 0.2°F to 1.6°F. Before taking an oral temperature, the practitioner should wait 15 minutes after a patient has ingested ice water. Oral temperature may increase in the patient receiving heated oxygen aerosol therapy and decrease in the patient receiving a cool mist aerosol. Table 2.3 lists the body temperature sites, their advantages and disadvantages, and the equipment used.

Pulse

A pulse is generated through the vascular system with each ventricular contraction of the heart (**systole**). Thus a pulse is a rhythmic arterial blood pressure throb created by the pumping action of the ventricular muscle. Between contractions, the ventricle rests (**diastole**) and the pulsation ceases. The pulse can be assessed at any location where an artery lies close to the skin surface and can be palpated against a firm underlying

---

TABLE 2.2 Factors Affecting Body Temperature

Factor	Effects
Age	Temperature varies with age. For example, the core temperature of the newborn infant is unstable because of immature thermoregulatory mechanisms. It is not uncommon for the elderly person to have a body temperature below 36.4°C (97.6°F). The normal temperature decreases with age.
Environment	Normally, variations in environmental temperature do not affect the core temperature. However, exposure to extreme hot or cold temperatures can alter body temperature. If an individual's core temperature falls to 25°C (77°F), death may occur. Conversely, in conditions of extreme humidity (>80%) and temperatures (>50°C [>122°F]) death may occur.
Time of day	Body temperature normally varies throughout the day, a phenomenon called **diurnal variation**. Typically, an individual's temperature is lowest around 3:00 a.m. and highest between 5:00 p.m. and 7:00 p.m. Approximately 95% of patients have their highest temperature around 6:00 p.m. Body temperature often fluctuates by as much as 2°C (1.8°F) between early morning and late afternoon.
Exercise	Body temperature increases with exercise because exercise increases heat production as the body breaks down carbohydrates and fats to provide energy. During strenuous exercise, the core body temperature can increase to as high as 40°C (104°F).
Stress	Physical or emotional stress may increase body temperature because stress can stimulate the sympathetic nervous system, causing the epinephrine and norepinephrine levels to increase. When this occurs, the metabolic rate increases, causing increased heat production. Stress and anxiety may cause a patient's temperature to increase without an underlying disease.
Hormones	Women normally have greater fluctuations in temperature than do men. The female hormone progesterone, which is secreted during ovulation, causes the temperature to increase 0.3° to 0.6°C (0.5° to 1°F). After menopause, women have the same mean temperature norms as men.

TABLE 2.3 Body Temperature Measurements: Sites, Normal Values, Advantages and Disadvantages, and Equipment Used

Site and Temperature	Advantages and Disadvantages	Equipment
Oral (most common) Average 37°C (98.6°F)	*Advantages:* Convenient, easy access, and patient comfort *Disadvantages:* Affected by ingestion of hot or cold liquids. Contraindicated in patients who cannot follow directions to keep mouth closed, who are mouth breathing, or who might bite down and break the thermometer. Smoking, drinking, and eating can slightly alter the oral temperature, about 1°F lower than rectal temperature.	Glass mercury thermometer, electronic thermometers
Rectal (core) Average 0.7°C (0.4°F) higher than oral	*Advantages:* Very reliable, considered most accurate. *Disadvantages:* Contraindicated in patients with diarrhea, patients who have undergone rectal surgery, or patients who have diseases of the rectum. *General Comment:* Used less often now that tympanic thermometers are available.	Glass mercury thermometer
Ear (tympanic) Also reflects core temperature. Also calibrated to oral or rectal scales	*Advantages:* Convenient, readily accessible, fast, safe, and noninvasive. Does not require contact with any mucous membrane. Infection control is less of a concern. With the advent of the tympanic membrane thermometer, the ear is now a site where a temperature can be easily and safely measured. Reflects the core body temperature because it reflects the tympanic membrane blood supply—the same vascular system that supplies the hypothalamus. Smoking, drinking, and eating do not affect tympanic temperature measurements. Allows rapid temperature measurements in the very young, confused, or unconscious patient. *Disadvantages:* No remarkable disadvantages, assuming site is available.	Tympanic thermometer
Axillary Average 0.6°C (1°F) lower than oral	*Advantages:* Safe and noninvasive. Recommended for infants and children, this is the route of choice in patients whose temperature cannot be measured at other sites. *Disadvantages:* Considered the least accurate and least reliable site because a number of factors can adversely affect the measurement. For example, if the patient has recently been given a bath, the temperature may reflect the temperature of the bathwater. Similarly, body motion and friction applied to dry the patient's skin may influence the temperature.	Glass mercury thermometer

structure, such as muscle or bone. Nine common pulse sites are the temporal, carotid, apical, brachial, radial, femoral, popliteal, **pedal (dorsalis pedis)**, and posterior tibial area (see Fig. 2.2).

In clinical settings the pulse is usually assessed by **palpation**. Initially the practitioner uses the first, second, or third finger and applies light pressure to any one of the pulse sites (e.g., carotid or radial artery) to detect a pulse with a strong pulsation. After locating the pulse, the practitioner may apply a more forceful palpation to count the rate, determine the cardiac rhythm, and evaluate the quality of pulsation. The practitioner then counts the number of pulsations for 15, 30, or 60 seconds and then multiplies appropriately to determine the pulse rate per minute. Shorter measurement time intervals may be used for patients with normal rates or regular cardiac rhythms.

In patients with irregular, abnormally slow, or fast cardiac rhythms, the pulse rates should be counted for 1 minute. To prevent overestimation for any time interval, the practitioner should count the first pulsation as zero and not count pulses at or after the completion of a selected time interval. Counting even one extra pulsation during a 15-second interval leads to an overestimation of the pulse rate by 4. *The characteristics of the pulse are described in terms of rate, rhythm, and strength.*

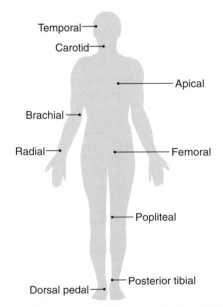

Temporal
Carotid
Apical
Brachial
Radial
Femoral
Popliteal
Posterior tibial
Dorsal pedal

FIGURE 2.2 The nine common pulse measurement sites.

Rate

The normal pulse rate (or heart rate) varies with age. For example, in the newborn the normal pulse rate range is 100 to 180 beats per minute (bpm). In the toddler the normal range is 80 to 130 bpm. The normal range for the child is 65 to 100 bpm, and the normal adult range is 60 to 100 bpm (see Table 2.1).

A heart rate lower than 60 bpm is called **bradycardia**. Bradycardia may be seen in patients with hypothermia and in physically fit athletes. The pulse also may be lower than expected when the patient is at rest or asleep or as a result of head injury, drugs such as beta-blockers (e.g., propranolol), vomiting, or advanced age. A pulse rate greater than 100 bpm in adults is called **tachycardia**. Tachycardia may occur as a result of hypoxemia, anemia, fever, anxiety, emotional stress, fear, hemorrhage, **hypotension**, dehydration, shock, and exercise. Tachycardia is also a common side effect in patients receiving certain medications, such as sympathomimetic agents (e.g., adrenaline or dobutamine).

Rhythm

Normally the ventricular contraction is under the control of the sinus node in the atrium, which generates a normal rate and regular rhythm. Certain conditions and chemical disturbances, such as inadequate blood flow and oxygen supply to the heart or an electrolyte imbalance, can cause the heart to beat irregularly. In children and young adults, it is not uncommon for the heart rate to increase during inspiration and decrease during exhalation. This is called **sinus arrhythmia**.

Strength

The quality of the pulse reflects the strength of left ventricular contraction and the volume of blood flowing to the peripheral tissues. A normal left ventricular contraction combined with an adequate blood volume will generate a strong, throbbing pulse. A weak ventricular contraction combined with an inadequate blood volume will result in a weak, thready pulse. An increased heart rate combined with a large blood volume will generate a full, bounding pulse.

Several conditions may alter the strength of a patient's pulse. For example, heart failure can cause the *strength* of the pulse to vary every other beat while the *rhythm* remains regular. This condition is called **pulsus alternans**. The practitioner may detect a pulse that decreases markedly in strength during inspiration and increases back to normal during exhalation, a condition called **pulsus paradoxus** that is common among patients experiencing a severe asthmatic episode. This phenomenon also can be observed when blood pressure is measured.

Finally, the stimulation of the sympathetic nervous system increases the force of ventricular contraction, increasing the volume of blood ejected from the heart and creating a stronger pulse. Stimulation of the parasympathetic nervous system decreases the force of the ventricular contraction, leading to decreased volume of blood ejected from the heart and a weaker pulse. Clinically, the strength of the pulse may be recorded on a scale of 0 to 4+ (Box 2.3).

For peripheral pulses that are difficult to detect by palpation, an **ultrasonic Doppler** device also may be used. A transmitter

---

BOX 2.3 Scale to Rate Pulse Quality

0: Absent or no pulse detected
1+: Weak, thready, easily obliterated with pressure; difficult to feel
2+: Pulse difficult to palpate; may be obliterated by strong pressure
3+: Normal pulse
4+: Bounding, easily palpated, and difficult to obliterate

---

attached to the Doppler is placed over the artery to be assessed. The transmitter amplifies and transmits the pulse sounds to an earpiece or to a speaker attached to the Doppler device. During normal sinus rhythm, the heart rate also can be obtained through **auscultation** by placing a stethoscope over the apex of the heart.

Respiration

The diaphragm is the primary muscle of respiration. Inspiration is an active process whereby the diaphragm contracts and causes the intrathoracic pressure to decrease. This action, in turn, causes the pressure in the airways to fall below the atmospheric pressure to allow for inflow of air. At the end of inspiration, the diaphragm relaxes and the natural lung elasticity (recoil) causes the pressure in the lung to increase. This action, in turn, causes air to flow out of the lung. Under normal circumstances, expiration is a passive process.

The normal **respiratory rate** varies with age. For example, in the newborn the normal respiratory rate varies between 30 and 60 breaths per minute. In the toddler the normal range is 25 to 40 breaths per minute. The normal range for the preschool child is 20 to 25 breaths per minute, and the normal adult range is 12 to 20 breaths per minute (see Table 2.1).

Ideally the respiratory rate should be counted when the patient is not aware. One good method is to count the respiratory rate immediately after taking the pulse, while leaving the fingers over the patient's artery. As respirations are being counted, the practitioner should observe for variations in the pattern of breathing. For example, an increased breathing rate is called **tachypnea**. Tachypnea is commonly seen in patients with fever, metabolic acidosis, hypoxemia, pain, or anxiety. A respiratory rate below the normal range is called **bradypnea**. Bradypnea may occur with hypothermia, head injuries, and drug overdose. Table 2.4 provides an overview of common normal and **abnormal breathing patterns**.

Blood Pressure

The arterial blood pressure is the force exerted by the circulating volume of blood on the walls of the arteries. The pressure peaks when the ventricles of the heart contract and eject blood into the aorta and pulmonary arteries. The blood pressure measured during ventricular contraction (**cardiac systole**) is the **systolic blood pressure**. During ventricular relaxation (**cardiac diastole**), blood pressure is generated by the elastic recoil of the arteries and arterioles. This pressure is called the **diastolic blood pressure**.

The normal blood pressure in the aorta and large arteries varies with age. For example, in the newborn the normal systolic blood pressure range is 60 to 90 mm Hg. In the toddler the normal range is 80 to 110 mm Hg. The normal range for the child is 100 to 110 mm Hg, and the normal adult range is 110 to 140 mm Hg (see Table 2.1 for normal systolic and diastolic blood pressures according to age). The numeric difference between the systolic and diastolic blood pressure is the **pulse pressure**. For example, a systolic pressure of 120 mm Hg and a diastolic pressure of 80 mm Hg equal a pulse pressure of 40 mm Hg.

Blood pressure is a function of (1) the blood flow generated by ventricular contraction and (2) the resistance to blood flow caused by the vascular system. Thus blood pressure (BP) equals flow ($\dot{V}$) multiplied by resistance (R): BP = $\dot{V} \times R$.

Blood Flow

Blood flow is equal to cardiac output. Cardiac output is equal to the product of (1) the volume of blood ejected from the ventricles during each heartbeat (stroke volume) multiplied by (2) the heart rate. Thus a stroke volume (SV) of 75 mL and a heart rate (HR) of 70 bpm produce a **cardiac output (CO)** of 5250 mL/min, or 5.25 L/min (CO = SV × HR).

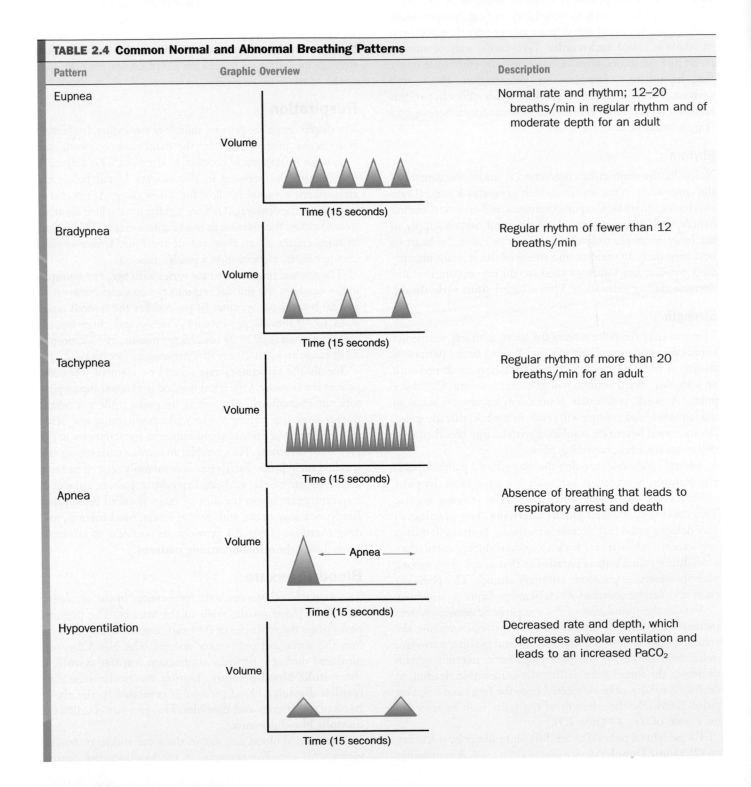

TABLE 2.4 Common Normal and Abnormal Breathing Patterns

Pattern	Graphic Overview	Description
Eupnea		Normal rate and rhythm; 12–20 breaths/min in regular rhythm and of moderate depth for an adult
Bradypnea		Regular rhythm of fewer than 12 breaths/min
Tachypnea		Regular rhythm of more than 20 breaths/min for an adult
Apnea		Absence of breathing that leads to respiratory arrest and death
Hypoventilation		Decreased rate and depth, which decreases alveolar ventilation and leads to an increased $PaCO_2$

TABLE 2.4 Common Normal and Abnormal Breathing Patterns—cont'd

Pattern	Graphic Overview	Description
Hyperventilation	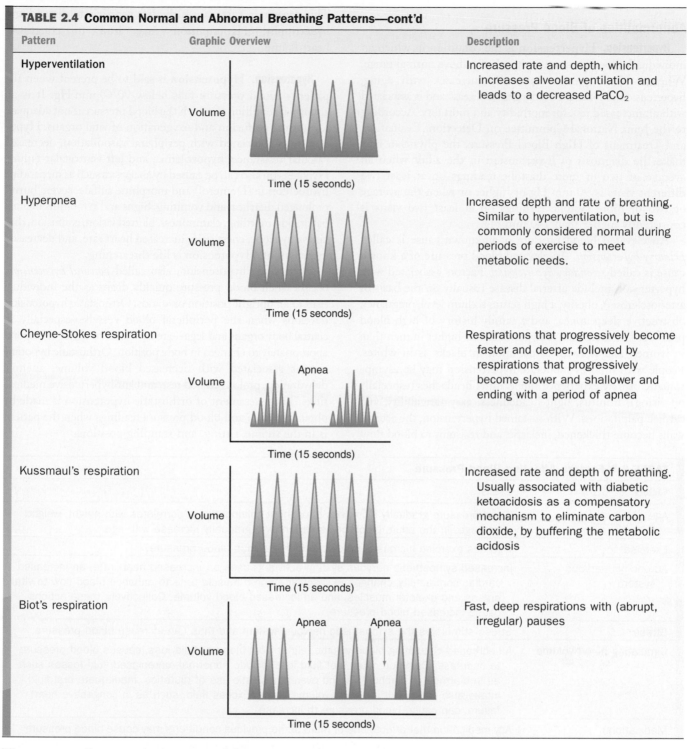	Increased rate and depth, which increases alveolar ventilation and leads to a decreased PaCO$_2$
Hyperpnea		Increased depth and rate of breathing. Similar to hyperventilation, but is commonly considered normal during periods of exercise to meet metabolic needs.
Cheyne-Stokes respiration		Respirations that progressively become faster and deeper, followed by respirations that progressively become slower and shallower and ending with a period of apnea
Kussmaul's respiration		Increased rate and depth of breathing. Usually associated with diabetic ketoacidosis as a compensatory mechanism to eliminate carbon dioxide, by buffering the metabolic acidosis
Biot's respiration		Fast, deep respirations with (abrupt, irregular) pauses

The average cardiac output in the resting adult is approximately 5 L/min.

A number of conditions can alter stroke volume and therefore blood flow. For instance, a decreased stroke volume may develop as a result of poor cardiac pumping (e.g., ventricular failure) or as a result of a decreased blood volume (e.g., during severe hemorrhage). Bradycardia also may reduce cardiac output and blood flow. Conversely, an increased heart rate or blood volume will likely increase cardiac output and blood flow. In addition, an increased heart rate in response to a decreased blood volume (or stroke volume) also may occur as a compensatory mechanism to maintain normal cardiac output and blood flow.

Resistance

The friction between the components of the blood ejected from the ventricles and the walls of the arteries results in a natural resistance to blood flow. Friction between the blood components and the vessel walls is inversely related to the dimensions of the vessel lumen (size). Thus as the vessel lumen narrows (or constricts), vascular resistance increases. As the vessel lumen widens (or relaxes), the resistance decreases. The autonomic nervous system monitors and regulates the vascular tone.

Table 2.5 presents factors that affect the blood pressure.

Abnormalities of Blood Pressure

Hypertension. **Hypertension** is the condition in which an individual's blood pressure is chronically above normal range. Whereas blood pressure normally increases with aging, hypertension is considered a dangerous disease and is associated with an increased risk for morbidity and mortality. According to the Joint National Committee on Detection, Evaluation, and Treatment of High Blood Pressure, the physician may make the diagnosis of hypertension in the adult when an average of two or more diastolic readings on at least two different visits is 90 mm Hg or higher or when the average of two or more systolic readings on at least two visits is consistently higher than 140 mm Hg.

An elevated blood pressure of unknown cause is called *primary hypertension.* An elevated blood pressure of a known cause is called *secondary hypertension.* Factors associated with hypertension include arterial disease (usually on the basis of arteriosclerosis), obesity, a high serum sodium level, pregnancy, obstructive sleep apnea, and a family history of high blood pressure. The incidence of hypertension is higher in men than in women and is twice as common in blacks as in whites. People with mild or moderate hypertension may be asymptomatic or may experience suboccipital headaches (especially on rising), tinnitus, light-headedness, easy fatigability, and cardiac palpitations. With sustained hypertension, the arterial walls become thickened, inelastic, and resistant to blood flow.

This process in turn causes the left ventricle to distend and hypertrophy. Hypertension may lead to congestive heart failure.

Hypotension. **Hypotension** is said to be present when the patient's blood pressure falls below 90/60 mm Hg. It is an abnormal condition in which the blood pressure is not adequate for normal perfusion and oxygenation of vital organs. Hypotension is associated with peripheral vasodilation, decreased vascular resistance, hypovolemia, and left ventricular failure. Hypotension also can be caused by analgesics such as meperidine hydrochloride (Demerol) and morphine sulfate, severe burns, prolonged diarrhea, and vomiting. Signs and symptoms include pallor, skin mottling, clamminess, blurred vision, confusion, dizziness, syncope, chest pain, increased heart rate, and decreased urine output. Hypotension is life threatening.

Orthostatic hypotension, also called *postural hypotension,* occurs when blood pressure quickly drops as the individual rises to an upright position or stands. Orthostatic hypotension develops when the peripheral blood vessels—especially in central body organs and legs—are unable to constrict or respond appropriately to changes in body position. Orthostatic hypotension is associated with decreased blood volume, anemia, dehydration, prolonged bed rest, and antihypertensive medications. The assessment of orthostatic hypotension is made by obtaining pulse and blood pressure readings when the patient is in the supine, sitting, and standing positions.

TABLE 2.5 Factors Affecting Blood Pressure

Factors	Effects
Age	Blood pressure gradually increases throughout childhood and correlates with height, weight, and age. In the adult, blood pressure tends to gradually increase with age.
Exercise	Vigorous exercise increases cardiac output and thus blood pressure.
Autonomic nervous system	Increased sympathetic nervous system activity causes an increased heart rate, an increased cardiac contractility, changes in vascular smooth muscle tone to enhance blood flow to vital organs and skeletal muscles, and an increased blood volume. Collectively, these actions cause increased blood pressure.
Stress	Stress stimulates the sympathetic nervous system and thus can increase blood pressure.
Circulating blood volume	A decreased circulating blood volume, either from blood or fluid loss, causes blood pressure to decrease. Common causes of fluid loss include abnormal, unreplaced fluid losses such as in diarrhea or diaphoresis and overenthusiastic use of diuretics. Inadequate oral fluid intake also can result in a fluid volume deficit. Excess fluid, such as in congestive heart failure, can cause blood pressure to increase.
Medications	Any medication that affects one or more of the previous conditions may cause blood pressure changes. For example, diuretics reduce blood volume; cardiac pharmaceuticals may increase or decrease heart rate and contractility; pain medications may reduce sympathetic nervous system stimulation; and specific antihypertensive agents may also exert their effects.
Normal fluctuations	Under normal circumstances, blood pressure varies from moment to moment in response to a variety of stimuli. For example, an increased environmental temperature causes blood vessels near the skin surface to dilate, causing blood pressure to decrease. In addition, normal respirations alter blood pressure. Blood pressure increases during expiration and decreases during inspiration. Blood pressure fluctuations caused by inspiration and expiration may be significant during a severe asthmatic episode.
Race	Black males over 35 years of age often have elevated blood pressure.
Obesity	Blood pressure is often higher in overweight and obese individuals.
Diurnal (daily diurnal variations)	Blood pressure is usually lowest early in the morning, when the metabolic rate is lowest.

Pulsus Paradoxus

Pulsus paradoxus is defined as a systolic blood pressure that is more than 10 mm Hg lower on inspiration than on expiration. This exaggerated waxing and waning of arterial blood pressure can be detected with a sphygmomanometer or, in severe cases, by palpating the pulse at the wrist or neck. Commonly associated with severe asthmatic episodes, pulsus paradoxus is believed to be caused by the major intrapleural pressure swings that occur during inspiration and expiration. The reason for this phenomenon is described in the following sections.

Decreased Blood Pressure During Inspiration. During inspiration the asthmatic patient frequently relies on use of the *accessory muscles of inspiration*. The accessory muscles help produce an extremely negative intrapleural pressure, which in turn enhances intrapulmonary gas flow. The increased negative intrapleural pressure also causes blood vessels in the lungs to dilate, creating pooled blood. Consequently, the volume of blood returning to the left ventricle decreases, causing a reduction in cardiac output and arterial blood pressure during inspiration.

Increased Blood Pressure During Expiration. During expiration, the patient often activates the *accessory muscles of expiration* in an effort to overcome the increased airway resistance (R_{aw}). The increased power produced by these muscles generates a greater positive intrapleural pressure. Although increased positive intrapleural pressure helps offset R_{aw}, it also works to narrow or squeeze the blood vessels of the lung. This increased pressure on the pulmonary blood vessels enhances left ventricular filling and results in increased cardiac output and arterial blood pressure during expiration.

Oxygen Saturation

Oxygen saturation, often considered the "fifth vital sign," is used to establish an immediate baseline SpO_2 value. It is an excellent monitor by which to assess the patient's response to respiratory care interventions. In the adult, normal SpO_2 values range from 95% to 99%. SpO_2 values of 91% to 94% indicate **mild hypoxemia**. Mild hypoxemia warrants additional evaluation by the respiratory practitioner but does not usually require supplemental oxygen. SpO_2 readings of 86% to 90% indicate **moderate hypoxemia**. These patients often require supplemental oxygen. SpO_2 values of 85% or lower indicate **severe hypoxemia** and warrant immediate medical intervention, including the administration of oxygen, ventilatory support, or both. Table 2.6 presents the relationship of SpO_2 to PaO_2 for the adult and newborn. Table 2.7 provides an overview of the signs and symptoms of inadequate oxygenation. For a more in-depth discussion on oxygenation, see Chapter 6, Assessment of Oxygenation.

Systematic Examination of the Chest and Lungs

The physical examination of the chest and lungs should be performed in a systematic and orderly fashion. The most common sequence is as follows:

TABLE 2.6 SpO_2 and PaO_2 Relationships for the Adult and Newborn

	Adult		Newborn	
Oxygen Status	SpO_2 (%)	PaO_2 (mm Hg)	SpO_2 (%)	PaO_2 (mm Hg)
Normal	95–99	75–100	91–96	60–80
Mild hypoxemia	90–95	60–75	88–90	55–60
Moderate hypoxemia	85–90	50–60	85–89	50–58
Severe hypoxemia	<85	<50	<85	<50

NOTE: The SpO_2 will be lower than predicted when the following are present: low pH, high $PaCO_2$, and high temperature.

TABLE 2.7 Signs and Symptoms of Inadequate Oxygenation

Central Nervous System	
Apprehension	Early
Restlessness or irritability	Early
Confusion or lethargy	Early or late
Combativeness	Late
Coma	Late
Respiratory	
Tachypnea	Early
Dyspnea on exertion (see Chapter 3)	Early
Dyspnea at rest (see Chapter 3)	Late
Use of accessory muscles	Late
Intercostal retractions	Late
Takes a breath between each word or sentence	Late
Cardiovascular	
Tachycardia	Early
Mild hypertension	Early
Arrhythmias	Early or late
Hypotension	Late
Cyanosis	Late
Skin is cool or clammy	Late
Other	
Diaphoresis	Early or late
Decreased urinary output	Early or late
General fatigue	Early or late

- Inspection
- Palpation
- Percussion
- Auscultation

Before the practitioner can adequately inspect, palpate, percuss, and auscultate the chest and lungs, however, he/she must have a good working knowledge of the topographic landmarks of the lung and chest. Various anatomic landmarks and imaginary vertical lines drawn on the chest are used to identify and document the location of specific abnormalities.

Lung and Chest Topography

Thoracic Cage Landmarks

Anteriorly, the first rib is attached to the manubrium just beneath the clavicle. After the first rib is identified, the rest of the ribs can easily be located and numbered. The sixth rib and its cartilage are attached to the sternum just above the xiphoid process (Fig. 2.3).

Posteriorly, the spinous processes of the vertebrae are useful landmarks. For example, when the patient's head is extended forward and down, two prominent spinous processes usually can be seen at the base of the neck. The top one is the spinous process of the seventh cervical vertebra (C-7); the bottom one is the spinous process of the first thoracic vertebra (T-1). When only one spinous process can be seen, it is usually C-7 (see Fig. 2.3).

Imaginary Lines

Various imaginary vertical lines are used to locate abnormalities on chest examination (Fig. 2.4). The vertical **midsternal line,** which is located in the middle of the sternum, equally divides the anterior chest into left and right hemithoraces. The **midclavicular lines,** which start at the middle of either the right or left clavicle, run parallel to the sternum, traditionally down through the male nipple.

On the lateral portion of the chest, three imaginary vertical lines are used. The **anterior axillary line** originates at the anterior axillary fold and runs down along the anterolateral aspect of the chest, the **midaxillary line** divides the lateral chest into two equal halves, and the **posterior axillary line** runs parallel to the midaxillary line along the posterolateral wall of the thorax.

Posteriorly, the **vertebral line** (also called the *midspinal line*) runs along the spinous processes of the vertebrae. The **midscapular line** runs through the middle of either the right or the left scapula parallel to the vertebral line.

Lung Borders and Fissures

Anteriorly, the apex of the lung extends approximately 2 to 4 cm above the medial third of the clavicle. Under normal conditions the lungs extend down to about the level of the sixth rib. Posteriorly, the superior portion of the lung extends to about the level of T-1 and down to about the level of T-10 (Fig. 2.5).

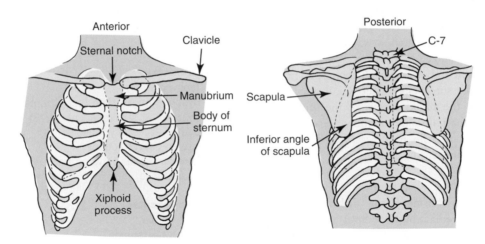

FIGURE 2.3 Anatomic landmarks of the chest.

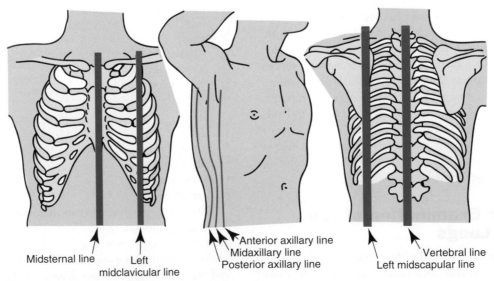

FIGURE 2.4 Imaginary vertical lines on the chest.

The right lung is separated into the upper, middle, and lower lobes by the **horizontal fissure** and the **oblique fissure**. The horizontal fissure runs anteriorly from the fourth rib at the sternal border to the fifth rib at the midaxillary line. The horizontal fissure separates the right anterior upper lobe from the middle lobe. The oblique fissure runs laterally from the sixth or seventh rib and the midclavicular line to the fifth rib at the midaxillary line. From this point, the oblique fissure continues to run around the chest posteriorly and upward to about the level of T-3. Anteriorly, the oblique fissure divides the lower lobe from the lower border of the middle lobe. Posteriorly, the oblique fissure separates the upper lobe from the lower lobe.

The left lung is separated into the upper and lower lobes by the oblique fissure. Anteriorly, the oblique fissure runs laterally from the sixth or seventh rib and the midclavicular line to the fifth rib at the midaxillary line. The fissure continues to run around the chest posteriorly and upward to about the level of T-3.

Inspection

The **inspection** of the patient is an ongoing observational process that begins with the history and continues throughout the patient interview, taking of vital signs, and physical examination. The inspection consists of a series of observations to gather clinical manifestations—signs and symptoms—that are directly or indirectly related to the patient's respiratory status. For example, during the patient interview and physical examination, the respiratory therapist might observe the patient demonstrating an abnormal ventilatory pattern, the use of accessory muscles, pursed-lip breathing, nasal flaring, splinting of the chest, a productive cough, or having clubbed fingers or lip or digital cyanosis.

A more in-depth discussion of the pathophysiologic basis for commonly seen respiratory disease clinical manifestations can be found in Chapter 3, The Pathophysiologic Basis for Common Clinical Manifestations.

Palpation

Palpation is the process of touching the patient's chest to evaluate the symmetry of chest expansion, the position of the trachea, skin temperature, muscle tone, areas of tenderness, lumps, depressions, and tactile fremitus and vocal fremitus. When palpating the chest, the clinician may use the heel or ulnar side of the hand, the palms, or the fingertips. As shown in Fig. 2.6, both the anterior and posterior chest should be palpated from side to side in an orderly fashion, from the apices of the chest down.

To evaluate the position of the trachea, the examiner places an index finger over the sternal notch and gently moves it from side to side. The trachea should be in the midline directly above the sternal notch. A number of abnormal pulmonary conditions can cause the trachea to deviate from its normal position. For example, a tension pneumothorax, pleural effusion,

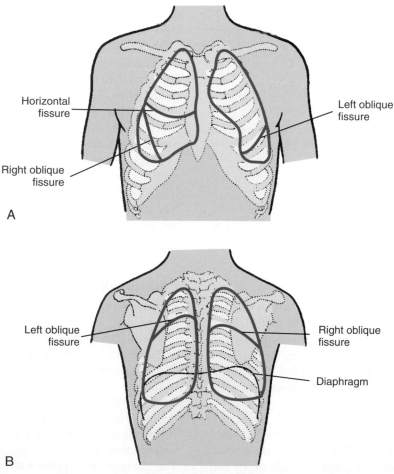

Horizontal fissure

Left oblique fissure

Right oblique fissure

A

Left oblique fissure

Right oblique fissure

Diaphragm

B

FIGURE 2.5 Topographic location of lung fissures projected on the anterior chest (A) and posterior chest (B).

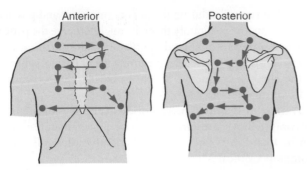

FIGURE 2.6 Path of palpation for vocal or tactile fremitus.

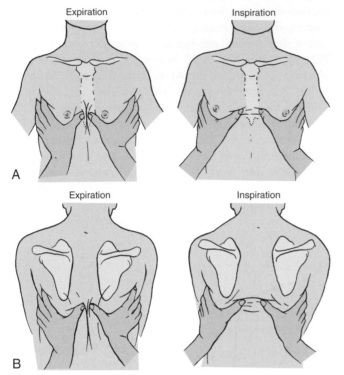

FIGURE 2.7 Assessment of chest excursion. (A) Anterior. (B) Posterior. Note that the thumbs move apart on inspiration as the volume of the thorax increases.

or tumor mass may push the trachea to the unaffected side, whereas atelectasis and pulmonary fibrosis pull the trachea to the affected side.

Chest Excursion

The symmetry of chest expansion is evaluated by lightly placing each hand over the patient's posterolateral chest so that the thumbs meet at the midline at about the T-8 to T-10 level. The patient is instructed to exhale slowly and completely and then inhale deeply. As the patient is inhaling, the examiner evaluates the distance that each thumb moves from the midline. Normally, each thumb tip moves equally about 3 to 5 cm from the midline (Fig. 2.7).

The examiner next faces the patient and lightly places each hand on the patient's anterolateral chest so that the thumbs meet at the midline along the costal margins near the xiphoid process. The patient is again instructed to exhale slowly and completely and then to inhale deeply. As the patient is inhaling,

the examiner observes the distance each thumb moves from the midline. Again, an excursion of 3 to 5 cm from the midline (xiphoid process) is normally seen.

A number of pulmonary disorders can alter the patient's **chest excursion**. For example, bilaterally decreased chest expansion (excursion) may be caused by both obstructive and restrictive lung disorders. An unequal chest expansion may occur when one or more of the following develop in or around one lung only: alveolar consolidation (e.g., pneumonia), lobar atelectasis, pneumothorax, large pleural effusions, or chest trauma (e.g., fractured ribs).

Tactile and Vocal Fremitus

Vibration that can be perceived by palpation over the chest is called **tactile fremitus** (also known as *rhonchial fremitus*). This condition is commonly caused by gas flowing through thick secretions that are partially obstructing the large airways. Tactile fremitus is often noted during inhalation and exhalation and may clear after a strong cough. It is often associated with coarse, low-pitched crackles that are audible without a stethoscope. Vibration that can be perceived by palpation or auscultation over the chest during phonation is called **vocal fremitus.** Sounds produced by the vocal cords are transmitted down the tracheobronchial tree and through the lung parenchyma to the chest wall, where the examiner can feel the vibration. Vocal fremitus can often be elicited by having the patient repeat the phrase "ninety-nine" or "blue moon." These are resonant phrases that produce strong vibrations. Normally, fremitus is most prominent between the scapulae and around the sternum, sites where the large bronchi are closest to the chest wall.

Tactile and vocal fremitus decreases when anything obstructs the transmission of vibration. Such conditions include chronic obstructive pulmonary disease, tumors or thickening of the pleural cavity, pleural effusion, pneumothorax, and a muscular or obese chest wall. Tactile and vocal fremitus increases in patients with alveolar consolidation, atelectasis, pulmonary edema, lung tumors, pulmonary fibrosis, and thin chest walls.

Crepitus (also called **subcutaneous emphysema**) is a coarse, crackling sensation that may be palpable over the skin surface. It occurs when air escapes from the thorax and enters the subcutaneous tissue. It may occur after a tracheostomy and mechanical ventilation, open thoracic injury, or thoracic surgery. In severe cases, crepitus also may be felt over the abdomen, genitalia, extremities, and face.

Percussion

Percussion over the chest wall is performed to determine the size, borders, and consistency of air, liquid, or solid material in the underlying lung. When percussing the chest, the examiner firmly places the distal portion of the middle finger of the nondominant hand between the ribs over the surface of the chest area to be examined. No other portion of the hand should touch the patient's chest. With the end of the middle finger of the dominant hand, the examiner quickly strikes the distal joint of the finger positioned on the chest wall and then quickly withdraws the tapping finger (Fig. 2.8). The examiner should perform the chest percussion in an orderly fashion from top to bottom, comparing the sounds generated

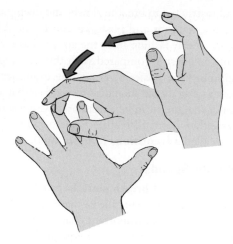

FIGURE 2.8 Chest percussion technique.

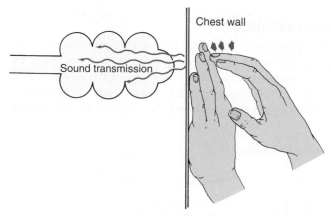

FIGURE 2.10 Chest percussion of a normal lung.

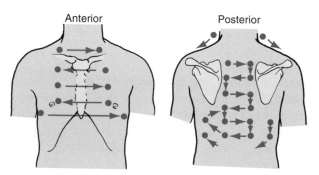

FIGURE 2.9 Path of systematic percussion to include all important areas.

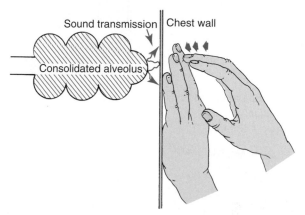

FIGURE 2.11 A short, dull, or flat percussion note is typically produced over areas of alveolar consolidation.

on both sides of the chest, both anteriorly and posteriorly (Fig. 2.9).

In the normal lung the sound created by percussion is transmitted throughout the air-filled lung and is typically described as loud, low in pitch, and long in duration. The sounds elicited by the examiner vibrate freely throughout the large surface area of the lungs and create a sound similar to that elicited by knocking on a watermelon (Fig. 2.10).

Resonance may be muffled somewhat in the individual with a heavily muscular chest wall and in the obese person. When percussing the anterior chest, the examiner should take care not to confuse the normal borders of cardiac dullness with pulmonary pathologic conditions. In addition, the upper border of liver dullness is normally located in the right fifth intercostal space and midclavicular line. Over the left side of the chest, **tympany** (hyperresonance) is produced over the gastric space. When percussing the posterior chest, the examiner should avoid the damping effect of the scapulae.

Abnormal Percussion Notes

A **dull percussion note** is heard when the chest is percussed over areas of pleural thickening, pleural effusion, atelectasis, and consolidation. When these conditions exist, the sounds produced by the examiner do not freely vibrate throughout the lungs. A dull percussion note is described as flat or soft, high in pitch, and short in duration, similar to the sound produced by knocking on a full barrel (Fig. 2.11).

When the chest is percussed over areas of trapped gas, a **hyperresonant note** is heard. These sounds are described as very loud, low in pitch, and long in duration, similar to the sound produced by knocking on an empty barrel (Fig. 2.12). A hyperresonant note is commonly elicited from air trapping in the patient with chronic obstructive pulmonary disease or pneumothorax.

Diaphragmatic Excursion

The relative position and range of motion of the hemidiaphragms also can be determined by percussion. Clinically, this evaluation is called the determination of **diaphragmatic excursion**. To assess the patient's diaphragmatic excursion, the examiner first maps out the lower lung borders by percussing the posterior chest from the apex down and identifying the point at which the percussion note definitely changes from a resonant to flat sound. This procedure is then performed at maximal inspiration and again at maximal expiration. Under normal conditions the diaphragmatic excursion should be equal bilaterally and should measure approximately 4 to 8 cm in the adult.

When severe alveolar hyperinflation is present (e.g., severe emphysema, asthma), the diaphragm is low and flat in position and has minimal excursion. Lobar collapse of one lung may pull the diaphragm up on the affected side and reduce excursion. The diaphragm also may be elevated and immobile in neuromuscular diseases that affect it.

Auscultation

Auscultation of the chest provides information about the heart, blood vessels, and air flowing in and out of the tracheobronchial tree and alveoli. A stethoscope is used to evaluate the frequency, intensity, duration, and quality of the sounds. During auscultation the patient should ideally be in the upright

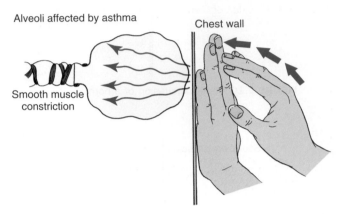

FIGURE 2.12 Percussion becomes more hyperresonant with alveolar hyperinflation.

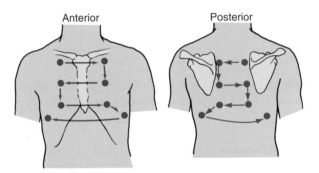

FIGURE 2.13 Path of systematic auscultation to include all important areas. Note the exact similarity of this pathway to that in Fig. 2.6.

position and instructed to breathe slowly and deeply through the mouth. The anterior and posterior chest should be auscultated in an orderly fashion from the apex to base while the right side of the chest is compared with the left (Fig. 2.13). When examining the posterior chest, the examiner should ask the patient to rotate the shoulders forward so that a greater surface area of the lungs can be auscultated. Lung sounds are classified as either normal breath sounds or abnormal lung sounds (also called **adventitious lung sounds**).

Normal Breath Sounds

Three different **normal breath sounds** can be auscultated over the normal chest. They are called *bronchial, bronchovesicular,* and *vesicular breath sounds.* Important characteristics of breath sounds include the pitch (vibration frequency), amplitude or intensity (loudness), and the duration of inspiratory sounds compared with expiration. Fig. 2.14 presents a sound diagram that illustrates the audio characteristics of the normal vesicular breath sound. Table 2.8 provides an overview of the normal breath sounds in regard to their location, pitch, intensity, and sound diagram.

Bronchial Breath Sounds. Bronchial breath sounds are normally auscultated directly over the trachea and are caused by the turbulent flow of gas through the upper airway. Bronchial breath sounds have a harsh, hollow, or tubular quality. They are loud, high in pitch, and about equal in duration in length

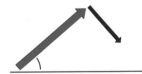

FIGURE 2.14 The normal vesicular breath sound. The blue upward arrow represents *inhalation*. The red downward arrow symbolizes *exhalation*. The length of the arrow signifies *duration*. The thickness of the arrow denotes *intensity* or *loudness*. The angle between the blue inhalation arrow and the horizontal line symbolizes *pitch* (i.e., fast or slow vibration frequency).

TABLE 2.8 Normal Breath Sounds				
Breath Sound	**Location**	**Pitch**	**Intensity**	**Sound Diagram***
Bronchial	Over trachea	High	Loud	
Bronchovesicular	Upper portion of anterior sternum, between scapulae	Moderate	Moderate	
Vesicular	Peripheral lung regions	High	Soft	

*For the sound diagrams above, the blue upward arrow represents *inhalation*. The red downward arrow symbolizes *exhalation*. The length of the arrow signifies *duration*. The thickness of the arrow denotes *intensity* or *loudness*. The angle between the blue inhalation arrow and the horizontal line symbolizes *pitch* (i.e., fast or slow vibration frequency).

of inspiration and expiration. A slight pause occurs between these two components. These sounds are also called *tracheal, tracheobronchial,* and *tubular breath sounds.*

Bronchovesicular Breath Sounds. Bronchovesicular breath sounds are auscultated directly over the mainstem bronchi. They are softer and lower in pitch and intensity than bronchial breath sounds and do not have a pause between the inspiratory and expiratory phase. These sounds are reduced in pitch and intensity as a result of the filtering of sound that occurs as gas moves between the large airways and alveoli. Anteriorly, bronchovesicular breath sounds can be heard directly over the mainstem bronchi between the first and second ribs. Posteriorly, they are heard between the scapulae near the spinal column between the first and sixth ribs, especially on the right side (Fig. 2.15A).

Vesicular Breath Sounds. Vesicular breath sounds are the normal sounds of gas rustling or swishing through the small bronchioles and the alveoli. Under normal conditions, vesicular breath sounds are auscultated over most lung fields, both anteriorly and posteriorly (see Fig. 2.15B). They are primarily heard during inspiration. As the gas molecules enter the alveoli, they are able to spread out over a large surface area and, as a result of this action, create less gas turbulence. Vesicular breath sounds also are heard during the initial third of exhalation as gas leaves the alveoli and bronchioles and moves into the large airways (Fig. 2.16).

Abnormal Lung Sounds. Abnormal lung sounds (ALS) are atypical, or uncharacteristic, lung sounds that are not *normally* heard over a specific area of the thorax. To describe the *pitch* of an ALS, the experts recommend the use of such words as high, moderate, or low—for example, "high-pitched wheezes were auscultated." For *the intensity* or *loudness* of the ALS, words such as faint, soft, mild, moderate, or loud should be used—for example, "loud bronchial breath sounds were auscultated." The part of the respiratory cycle in which the ALS occurs should be recorded—for example, "crackles were heard both during inspiration and expiration." In addition, include mention of when the ALS occurs during

inspiration—for example, "late-inspiratory crackles." Also, document the magnitude of the ALS—for example, "small, scant, or profuse crackles." Always record the precise location over the chest the ALS is auscultated—for example, "expiratory wheezes were noted over the anterior right lower lobe."

Although the experts (American Thoracic Society [ATS] and the American College of Chest Physicians [ACCP] Joint Committee on Pulmonary Nomenclature) have debated for many years the value of some of the terms and adjectives used to describe ALS, they have agreed—for the most part—that several terms or phrases are either ambiguous or very subjective and therefore should not be used for clinical reports, charting, and/or electronic documentation. *Terms, adjectives, and phrases not recommended at present are wet, dry, rales, rhonchi, crepitations, sonorous rales, musical rales, and sibilant rales.*

Currently, the recommended terms, adjectives, and phrases for ALS are the following: fine crackles, medium crackles, or coarse crackles, wheezes, bronchial breath sounds, stridor, pleural friction rub, diminished breath sound, and whispering pectoriloquy. Fig. 2.17 illustrates the general location and cause for these ALS. Table 2.9 provides an overview and description of the common ALS.

Table 2.10 summarizes the common assessment abnormalities found during inspection, palpation, percussion, and auscultation.

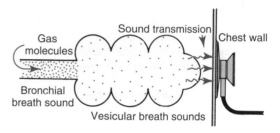

FIGURE 2.16 Auscultation of vesicular breath sounds over a normal lung unit.

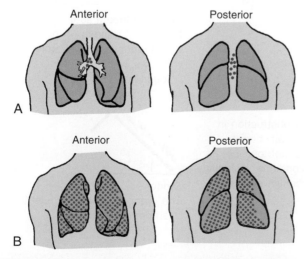

FIGURE 2.15 The location at which bronchovesicular breath sounds (A) and vesicular breath sounds (B) are normally auscultated.

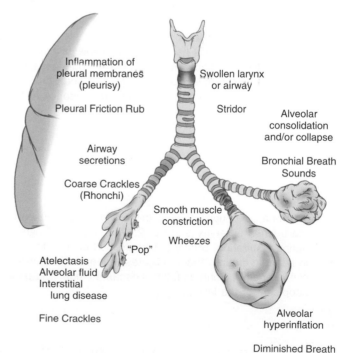

FIGURE 2.17 General location and origin of abnormal lung sounds.

TABLE 2.9 Abnormal Lung Sounds

Abnormal Lung Sound	Sound Diagrams*

Crackles

Crackles (previously called *rales*) can be categorized as fine, medium, and coarse crackles.

Fine crackles are discontinuous, high-pitched, crackling, and popping sounds similar to popping of bubble wrap or the sound created by rolling hair between fingers near one's ear and is heard near the end of inspiration (see Sound Diagram A). Fine crackles are produced by the rapid equalization of gas pressure when collapsed alveoli or terminal bronchioles suddenly snap open (see Fig. 2.17). Fine crackles usually do not clear after a strong cough. Fine crackles are associated with alveolar collapse (atelectasis), interstitial fibrosis, early pulmonary edema, and pneumonia.

Medium crackles are the same as fine crackles but are medium in pitch and have a moist quality as the disease process worsens.

Coarse crackles (previously called *rhonchi*†) are discontinuous, low-pitched, rumbling, bubbling, or gurgling sounds that start early during inspiration and extend into exhalation. These sounds are caused by air moving through excessive airway secretions in the larger airways (see Sound Diagram B). Coarse crackles are commonly associated with severe chronic obstructive pulmonary disease, cystic fibrosis, bronchiectasis, and congestive heart failure (pulmonary edema). Coarse crackles may or may not change in nature after a strong, vigorous cough.

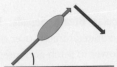

A. **Fine crackles.** The green oval shape represents crackles.

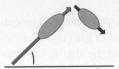

B. **Coarse crackles.** The green oval shape represents crackles.

Wheezing

Wheezing is the characteristic sound produced by airway obstruction. Found in all bronchospasm disorders, it is one of the cardinal findings in asthma (see Fig. 2.17). Wheezes are continuous, high-pitched, musical whistles generally heard on expiration (see Sound Diagram). In severe cases, they may be heard during inspiration. In addition to bronchospasm, other common causes of partial or total airway obstruction include mucosal edema, inflammation, tumors, and foreign bodies.

Partial airway obstruction is often made greater by this mechanism: When the bronchial airway is narrowed, the velocity of air flow through the constricted airway increases, which, in turn, causes the lateral airway wall pressure to decrease. This condition causes the airways to narrow even further and/or collapse. As the airways narrow, they vibrate similar to a reed on a woodwind instrument, thereby producing a wheezing sound (Fig. 2.18).

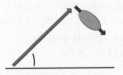

Wheezing
The orange oval shape represents wheezing.

Bronchial Breath Sounds

Bronchial breath sounds have a harsh, hollow, or tubular quality. They are loud, high in pitch, and about equal in duration during inspiration and expiration. The inspiratory phase is louder (see Fig. 2.17 and Sound Diagram). Bronchial breath sounds are associated with alveolar consolidation and atelectasis (Fig. 2.19).

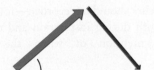

Bronchial breath sound
Note the thickness of the inspiratory and expiratory arrows, which denote loudness.

Stridor

Stridor is a continuous, loud, high-pitched sound caused by an upper obstruction in the trachea or larynx (see Fig. 2.17 and Sound Diagram). It is generally heard during inspiration. Stridor is usually loud enough to hear without a stethoscope, as in infantile croup. Stridor indicates a neoplastic or inflammatory condition, including glottic edema, diphtheria, laryngospasm croup, and papilloma (a benign epithelial neoplasm of the larynx).

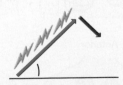

Stridor
The orange shapes represent stridor sounds.

TABLE 2.9 Abnormal Lung Sounds—cont'd

Abnormal Lung Sound	Sound Diagrams*

Pleural Friction Rub

If pleurisy accompanies a respiratory disorder, the inflamed pleural membranes resist movement during breathing and create a peculiar and characteristic sound known as a *pleural friction rub* (see Fig. 2.17 and Sound Diagram). It is a continuous, low-pitched, coarse creaking or grating-type sound reminiscent of that made by a creaking shoe. It is usually heard throughout inspiration and expiration over the area where the patient complains of pain. The intensity of a pleural rub often increases with deep breathing. A pleural friction rub does not clear with cough. A pleural friction rub is associated with pleurisy, tuberculosis, pneumonia, pulmonary fibrosis, pulmonary infarction, or after thoracic surgery.

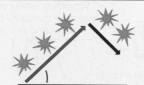

Pleural friction rub
The orange shapes represent pleural friction rub sounds.

Diminished Breath Sounds

Breath sounds are diminished or distant in any respiratory disorder that reduces the sound intensity of air flow as in obesity. In another example, chronic obstructive pulmonary disease leads to air trapping, an increased function residual capacity, and hypoventilation, which, in turn, result in **diminished breath sounds** (Fig. 2.20). Heart sounds also may be diminished in patients with air trapping.

The intensity of breath sounds is also reduced in any condition that causes shallow or slow breathing patterns—for example, drug overdose, major sedation, or neuromuscular diseases such as Guillain-Barré syndrome or myasthenia gravis. Diminished breath sounds are also found in respiratory disorders that cause hypoventilation by compressing the lung, such as flail chest, pleural effusion, and pneumothorax.

Diminished breath sound
Note the decreased angle on the inspiratory and expiratory arrows, which represent decreased intensity or loudness.

Whispering Pectoriloquy

Whispering pectoriloquy is the term used to describe the unusually clear transmission of the whispered voice of a patient as heard through the stethoscope. When the patient whispers "one, two, three," the sounds produced by the vocal cords are transmitted not only toward the mouth and nose but also throughout the lungs. As the whispered sounds travel down the tracheobronchial tree, they remain relatively unchanged, but as the sound disperses throughout the large surface area of the alveoli, it diminishes sharply. Consequently, when the examiner listens with a stethoscope over a normal lung while the patient whispers "one, two, three," the sounds are diminished, distant, muffled, and unintelligible (Fig. 2.21).

When a patient who has atelectasis or consolidated lung areas whispers "one, two, three," the sounds produced are prevented from spreading out over a large alveolar surface area. Even though the consolidated area may act as a sound barrier and diminish the sounds somewhat, the reduction in sound is not as great as it would be if the sounds were allowed to dissipate throughout a normal lung. Consequently, the whispered sounds are much louder and more intelligible over the affected lung areas (Fig. 2.22).

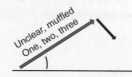

Normal vesicular breath sounds—unclear, muffled words ("one, two, three") auscultated.

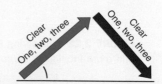

Consolidation and/or atelectasis—clear words ("one, two, three") auscultated.

---

*For the sound diagrams, the blue upward arrow represents *inhalation*. The red downward arrow symbolizes *exhalation*. The length of the arrow signifies *duration*. The thickness of the arrow denotes *intensity* or *loudness*. The angle between the blue inhalation arrow and the horizontal line symbolizes *pitch* (i.e., fast or slow vibration frequency).

†Historically, coarse crackles have also been called *rhonchi*, a term not currently recommended. Coarse crackles often produce palpable vibrations called *tactile fremitus*, also known as *rhonchial fremitus*. Coarse crackles are sometimes referred to as a "death rattle." It is this abnormal lung sound that every practicing respiratory therapist knows all too well—that is, the patient, whose loud, rumbling, gurgling secretions can be heard across the patient's room, which clearly signals the immediate need for tracheal suctioning or chest physical therapy.

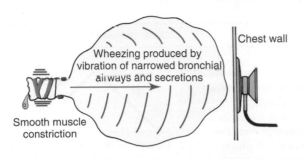

FIGURE 2.18 Wheezing and coarse crackles often develop during an asthmatic episode because of smooth muscle constriction, wall edema, and mucous accumulation.

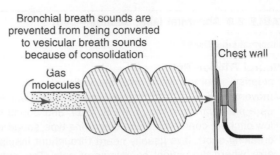

FIGURE 2.19 Auscultation of bronchial breath sounds over a consolidated lung unit.

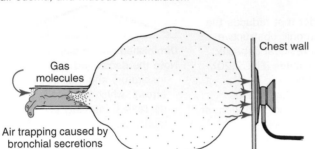

FIGURE 2.20 As air trapping and alveolar hyperinflation develop in obstructive lung diseases, breath sounds progressively diminish.

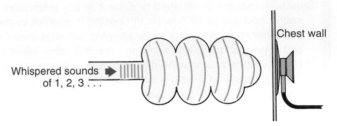

FIGURE 2.21 Whispered voice sounds auscultated over a normal lung are usually faint and unintelligible.

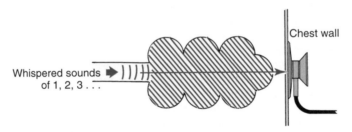

FIGURE 2.22 **Whispering Pectoriloquy.** Whispered voice sounds heard over a consolidated lung are often louder and more intelligible compared with those of a normal lung.

TABLE 2.10 Common Assessment Abnormalities

Finding	Description	Possible Cause and Significance
Inspection		
Pursed-lip breathing	Exhalation through mouth with lips pursed together to slow exhalation.	COPD, asthma. Suggests ↑ breathlessness. Strategy taught to slow expiration, ↓ dyspnea.
Tripod position; inability to lie flat	Leaning forward with arms and elbows supported on overbed table.	COPD, asthma in exacerbation, pulmonary edema. Indicates moderate to severe respiratory distress.
Accessory muscle use; intercostal retractions	Neck and shoulder muscles used to assist breathing. Muscles between ribs pull in during inspiration.	COPD, asthma in exacerbation, secretion retention. Indicates severe respiratory distress, hypoxemia.
Splinting	Voluntary ↓ in tidal volume to ↓ pain on chest expansion.	Thoracic or abdominal incision pain. Chest trauma, pleurisy.
↑ AP diameter	AP chest diameter equal to lateral. Slope of ribs more horizontal (90 degrees) to spine.	COPD, asthma, cystic fibrosis. Lung hyperinflation. Advanced age.
Tachypnea	Rate >20 breaths/min; >25 breaths/min in elderly.	Fever, anxiety, hypoxemia, restrictive lung disease. Magnitude of ↑ above normal rate reflects magnitude of increased work of breathing.

TABLE 2.10 Common Assessment Abnormalities—cont'd

Finding	Description	Possible Cause and Significance
Kussmaul's respiration	Regular, rapid, and deep respirations.	Metabolic acidosis; ↑ in rate aids body in ↑ CO_2 excretion.
Cyanosis	Bluish color of skin best seen in earlobes, under the eyelids, or in nail beds.	↓ Oxygen transfer in lungs, ↓ cardiac output. Nonspecific, unreliable indicator.
Clubbing of fingers	↑ Depth, bulk, sponginess of distal digits of fingers.	Chronic hypoxemia. Cystic fibrosis, lung cancer, bronchiectasis.
Peripheral edema	Pitting edema.	Congestive heart failure, cor pulmonale.
Distended neck veins	Jugular venous distention.	Cor pulmonale, flail chest, pneumothorax.
Cough	Productive or nonproductive.	Bronchial airway and alveolar disease.
Sputum	See Table 3.4.	COPD, asthma, cystic fibrosis, pneumonia.
Abdominal paradox	Inward (rather than normal outward) movement of abdomen during inspiration.	Inefficient and ineffective breathing pattern. Nonspecific indicator of severe respiratory distress.
Palpation		
Tracheal deviation	Leftward or rightward movement of trachea from normal midline position.	Nonspecific indicator of change in position of mediastinal structures. Medical emergency if caused by tension pneumothorax.
Altered tactile fremitus	Increase or decrease in examiner-felt vibrations.	↑ In pneumonia, atelectasis; pulmonary edema; ↓ in pleural effusion, lung hyperinflation; absent in pneumothorax.
Altered chest movement	Unequal or equal but diminished movement of two sides of chest with inspiration.	Unequal movement caused by atelectasis, pneumothorax, pleural effusion, splinting; equal but diminished movement caused by barrel chest, restrictive disease, neuromuscular disease.
Percussion		
Hyperresonance	Loud, lower-pitched sound over areas that normally produce a resonant sound on chest percussion.	Lung hyperinflation (COPD), lung collapse (pneumothorax), air trapping (asthma).
Dullness/flatness	Medium-pitched sound over areas that normally produce a resonant sound on chest percussion.	↑ Density (pneumonia, large atelectasis), ↑ fluid pleural space (pleural effusion).
Auscultation		
Fine crackles	Series of discontinuous short, crackling, and popping sounds, high-pitched sounds heard just before the end of inspiration; result of rapid equalization of gas pressure when collapsed alveoli or terminal bronchioles suddenly snap open; similar sound to that made by rolling hair between fingers just behind ear.	Loss of lung volume (atelectasis), interstitial fibrosis (asbestosis), interstitial edema (early pulmonary edema), alveolar filling (pneumonia), early phase of congestive heart failure.
Coarse crackles	Series of discontinuous short, low-pitched bubbling or gurgling sounds caused by air passing through airway intermittently occluded by mucus, unstable bronchial wall, or fold of mucosa; evident on inspiration and, in more severe cases, expiration; similar sound to blowing through straw under water; increase in bubbling quality with more fluid.	COPD, cystic fibrosis, congestive heart failure, bronchiectasis, pulmonary edema, pneumonia with severe congestion, COPD.
Wheezes	Continuous high-pitched whistling sound caused by rapid vibration of bronchial walls; first evident on expiration but also possibly evident on inspiration as obstruction of airway increases; possibly audible even without a stethoscope.	Bronchospasm (caused by asthma), airway obstruction (caused by mucosal edema, inflammation, foreign body, tumor), COPD.

Continued

TABLE 2.10 Common Assessment Abnormalities—cont'd

Finding	Description	Possible Cause and Significance
Bronchial breath sound	A harsh, hollow, or tubular breath sound. They are loud, high in pitch, and about equal in duration during inspiration and expiration. Inspiration is louder.	Alveolar consolidation and alveolar collapse (atelectasis).
Stridor	Continuous, loud, high-pitched sound caused by a partial obstruction of the larynx or trachea. Generally heard during inspiration.	Croup, epiglottitis, vocal cord edema after extubation, foreign body.
Pleural friction rub	A continuous, low-pitched creaking, or grating sound from roughened, inflamed surfaces of the pleura rubbing together. Generally heard during both inspiration and expiration. There is no change with coughing. The patient is usually uncomfortable, especially on deep inspiration.	Pleurisy, pneumonia, pulmonary fibrosis, pulmonary embolism, and thoracic surgery.
Diminished breath sounds	Diminished or distant breath sounds.	COPD, drug overdose or major sedation, neuromuscular disease (Guillain-Barré or myasthenia gravis), flail chest, pleural effusion, and pneumothorax.
Whispering pectoriloquy	Spoken or whispered syllable more distinct than normal on auscultation.	Alveolar consolidation and alveolar collapse (atelectasis).

AP, Anteroposterior; *COPD*, chronic obstructive pulmonary disease.

SELF-ASSESSMENT QUESTIONS

1. Which of the following pathologic conditions increases vocal fremitus?
   1. Atelectasis
   2. Pleural effusion
   3. Pneumothorax
   4. Pneumonia
       a. 3 only
       b. 4 only
       c. 2 and 3 only
       d. 1 and 4 only

2. A dull or soft percussion note would likely be heard in which of the following pathologic conditions?
   1. Chronic obstructive pulmonary disease
   2. Pneumothorax
   3. Pleural thickening
   4. Atelectasis
       a. 1 only
       b. 2 only
       c. 2 and 3 only
       d. 3 and 4 only

3. Bronchial breath sounds are likely to be heard in which of the following pathologic conditions?
   1. Alveolar consolidation
   2. Chronic obstructive pulmonary disease
   3. Atelectasis
   4. Fluid accumulation in the tracheobronchial tree
       a. 3 only
       b. 4 only
       c. 1 and 3 only
       d. 2 and 4 only

4. Wheezing is:
   1. Produced by bronchospasm
   2. Generally auscultated during inspiration
   3. A cardinal finding of bronchial asthma
   4. Usually heard as high-pitched sounds
       a. 1 only
       b. 1 and 3 only
       c. 2 and 4 only
       d. 1, 3, and 4 only

5. In which of the following pathologic conditions is transmission of the whispered voice of a patient through a stethoscope unusually clear?
   1. Chronic obstructive pulmonary disease
   2. Alveolar consolidation
   3. Atelectasis
   4. Pneumothorax
       a. 1 only
       b. 2 and 3 only
       c. 1 and 4 only
       d. 1, 2, and 3 only

6. Which of the following abnormal breathing patterns is commonly associated with diabetic acidosis?
   a. Orthopnea
   b. Kussmaul's respiration
   c. Biot's respiration
   d. Hypoventilation

CHAPTER 3

The Pathophysiologic Basis for Common Clinical Manifestations

Chapter Objectives

After rteading this chapter, you will be able to:

- Discuss the pathophysiologic basis for abnormal ventilatory patterns, including
  - Effects of lung compliance
  - Airway resistance
  - Peripheral chemoreceptors
  - Central chemoreceptors
  - Pulmonary reflexes
  - Pain, anxiety, and fever
- Describe the function of the accessory muscles of inspiration.
- Describe the function of the accessory muscles of expiration.
- Discuss the effects of pursed-lip breathing.
- Describe the pathophysiologic basis for substernal and intercostal retractions.
- Explain nasal flaring.
- Discuss splinting and decreased chest expansion caused by pleuritic and nonpleuritic chest pain.
- List abnormal chest shape and configurations.
- List abnormal extremity findings.
- Describe normal and abnormal sputum production.
- Define key terms and complete self-assessment questions at the end of the chapter and on Evolve.

Key Terms

Abnormal Ventilatory Patterns
Accessory Muscles of Expiration
Accessory Muscles of Inspiration
Acute-Onset Conditions
Airway Resistance (R_{aw})
Aortic and Carotid Sinus Baroreceptor Reflexes
Borg Dyspnea Scale
Capability-to-Breathe
Cardiac Dyspnea
Cardiopulmonary Exercise Testing
Central Chemoreceptors
Central Cyanosis
Chronic Conditions
Cough
Cyanosis
Demand-to-Breathe
Digital Clubbing
Distended Neck Veins
Dorsal Respiratory Group (DRG)
Dyspnea
Eupnea
Exertional Dyspnea
External Oblique Muscle
Hering-Breuer Reflex
Hemoptysis

Hypothermia
Hysteresis
Inspiratory-to-Expiratory Ratio (I/E Ratio)
intercostal retractions
Internal Oblique Muscle
Irritant Reflex
jungular venous distention
Juxtapulmonary-Capillary Receptors (J Receptors) Reflex
Lung Compliance (C_L)
Modified (British) Medical Research Council (mMRC) Questionnaire
Mucociliary Escalator
Mucous Blanket
Nasal Flaring
Nonpleuritic Chest Pain
Nonproductive Cough
Orthopnea
Paroxysmal Nocturnal Dyspnea
Pectoralis Major Muscle
Peripheral Chemoreceptors
Peripheral Edema
Pitting Edema
Pleural Friction Rub
Pleuritic Chest Pain
Poiseuille's Law
Positional Dyspnea
Productive Cough
Pulmonary Shunting
Pursed-Lip Breathing
Rectus Abdominis Muscles
Renal Dyspnea
Scalene Muscles
Splinting
Sternocleidomastoid Muscles
Substernal
Substernal Retraction
Tidal Volume (V_T)
Transairway Pressure
Transversus Abdominis Muscles
Trapezius Muscles
Tripod Position
Venous Admixture
Ventilation-Perfusion Ratio ($\dot{V}/\dot{Q}$)
Ventral Respiratory Group (VRG)
Work of Breathing (WOB)

Chapter Outline

Normal Ventilatory Pattern
Abnormal Ventilatory Patterns
    Dyspnea
    The Pathophysiologic Basis of Abnormal Ventilatory Patterns

As shown in Box 3.1, there are a variety of clinical manifestations commonly observed in examination of the patient with respiratory disease. For example, the patient often demonstrates an abnormal ventilatory pattern, the use of accessory muscles of inspiration, the use of accessory muscles of expiration, purse-lip breathing, substernal or intercostal retractions, nasal flaring, splinting of the chest, abnormal chest shape, clubbing of the toes and/or fingers, a nonproductive or productive cough, and the appearance of cyanosis. Some of these commonly observed clinical manifestations can be objective—such as observed nasal flaring or the use of accessory muscles of inspiration, whereas other clinical observations can be more subjective—for example, the examiner's documentation of the patient's appearance of cyanosis or of his sputum. To further help in the understanding of these commonly observed clinical manifestations, a more in-depth discussion of their pathophysiologic bases is presented in this chapter.

Normal Ventilatory Pattern

An individual's normal breathing pattern is composed of a **tidal volume (V_T)**, a ventilatory rate, and an **inspiratory-to-expiratory ratio (I/E ratio)**. In normal adults, the V_T is about 500 mL (7 to 9 mL/kg), the ventilatory rate is about 15 (with a range of 12 to 18) breaths per minute, and the I/E ratio is about 1:2. In patients with respiratory disorders, however, an abnormal ventilatory pattern is often present.

Abnormal Ventilatory Patterns

As presented in Chapter 2, The Physical Examination, there are several abnormal breathing patterns frequently seen in the patient with respiratory problems (see Table 2.4). Thus the respiratory therapist must be strongly proficient in the ability to identify and differentiate such ventilatory patterns as bradypnea, tachypnea, apnea, hypoventilation, hyperventilation, Cheyne-Stokes respirations, Kussmaul's respirations, and Biot's respirations. In addition, the respiratory therapist must have a strong understanding of the meaning and use of the word *dyspnea*.

Dyspnea

Dyspnea is a general term often used—although incorrectly—to describe the patient's difficulty in breathing. In fact, the term *dyspnea* is likely the most common symptom the respiratory therapist is asked to evaluate and treat.

Dyspnea is defined as the "breathlessness," or "shortness of breath," or the "labored or difficult breathing" felt and described only by the patient. Although the onset of dyspnea should not be ignored—and it is always a good reason to seek immediate medical attention—dyspnea should not be assumed by the respiratory therapist's impression of the patient's breathing pattern alone.

BOX 3.1 Common Clinical Manifestations Observed During Inspection

- Anxiety
- Abnormal ventilatory pattern findings
- Use of accessory muscles of inspiration
- Use of accessory muscles of expiration
- Pursed-lip breathing
- Substernal or intercostal retractions
- Nasal flaring
- Splinting or decreased chest expansion caused by chest pain
- Abnormal chest shape and configuration
- Abnormal extremity findings:
  - Altered skin color
  - Digital clubbing
  - Pedal edema
- Distended neck veins
- Cough (note characteristics)
- Expectoration of sputum
- Hemoptysis (note volume)

The symptoms of dyspnea ("subjective information") are *sensations* that can be experienced only by the patient who is having breathing difficulties, not by the observation of the hospital care staff. For example, the patient might say: "I just can't seem to get air into my lung!" Or, "Every time I lie down, I get very short of breath." These are clearly sensations.

Signs of dyspnea ("objective information") include audibly labored breathing, hyperventilation, and/or tachypnea, retractions of intercostal spaces, use of accessory muscles, a distressed facial expression, flaring of the nostrils, paradoxical movements of the chest and abdomen, and gasping. These signs of dyspnea are strong indicators of inadequate ventilation and/or an insufficient amount of oxygen in the blood. All of these clinical indicators of inadequate breathing reflecting the patient's reduced capability to breathe should be documented in the patient's chart.

Common types of dyspnea include (1) **positional dyspnea**, which occurs only when the patient is in the reclining position and is also known as **orthopnea**, (2) **cardiac dyspnea**, which is labored breathing caused by heart disease (e.g., congestive heart failure), (3) **exertional dyspnea**, which is provoked by physical exercise or exertion, (4) **paroxysmal nocturnal dyspnea**, which is a form of respiratory distress related to posture (especially reclining while sleeping) and is usually associated with congestive heart failure with pulmonary edema, and (5) **renal dyspnea**, which is difficulty in breathing as a result of kidney disease.

Demand-to-Breathe Versus Capability-to-Breathe

To further our understanding of the sensation of dyspnea, Fig. 3.1 illustrates it as an imbalance of the teeter-totter

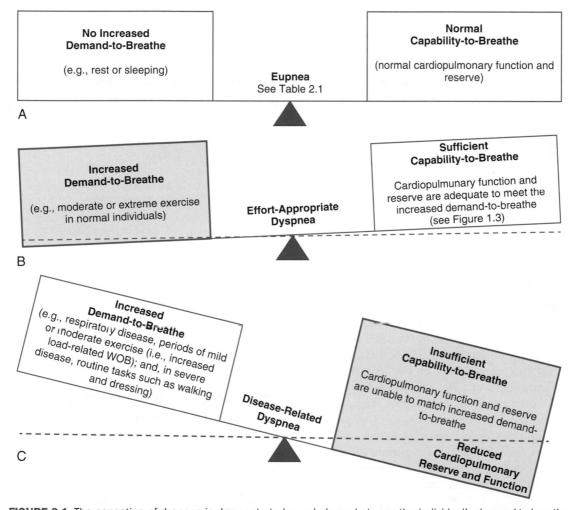

FIGURE 3.1 The sensation of dyspnea is demonstrated as a balance between the individual's demand-to-breathe and capability-to-breathe. In the normal individual, the demand-to-breathe is driven by (1) oxygen consumption ($\dot{V}O_2$), (2) work of breathing required by the task at hand, and (3) the person's physical condition. The capability-to-breathe consists of the individual's integrated function and reserve of the cardiopulmonary system (see Figs. 1.2 and 1.3). At rest and with mild to moderate exercise, the reserve of this system is not rate-limiting for exercise. (A) At rest, there is no increased need-to-breathe and therefore there is no sensation of dyspnea (eupnea). The level teeter-totter beam denotes no dyspnea. (B) During exercise in the normal individual, the $\dot{V}O_2$ increases, but is, up to a point, balanced by normal cardiopulmonary function and reserve, which is adequate to meet the increased metabolic challenge. Although the nonlevel beam denotes dyspnea, this form of dyspnea is normal and can be referred to as *effort-appropriate dyspnea*. (C) Illustrates an increased demand-to-breathe combined with the reduced capability-to-breathe (caused by a decreased cardiopulmonary reserve and function). This condition causes dyspnea and can significantly limit even modest activities of daily living.

relationship between the individual's **demand-to-breathe** and his actual **capability-to-breathe**. For example, during normal periods of eupnea, the individual has no sensation of difficulty breathing and demand-to-breathe matches capability-to-breathe (i.e., the cardiopulmonary system is able to adequately move oxygen into the body and carbon dioxide out of it. In short, the cardiopulmonary function and reserve are in balance with metabolic needs (see Fig. 3.1A). **Eupnea** is defined as the normal breathing rate (between 12 and 20 breaths per minute) and regular rhythm and moderate depth for an adult (see Table 2.1).

During periods of significant exercise, however, the normal individual's capability-to-breathe may be challenged to meet the increased demand-to-breathe as his oxygen consumption increases. When this occurs, the individual may experience dyspnea, depending on metabolic demands and increased *load-related work of breathing* associated with the exercise. This demand-to-breathe sensation is normal and can be considered "effort-appropriate dyspnea" (see Fig. 3.1B).

On the other hand, next consider the severely increased demand-to-breathe and dyspnea that occur in the patient performing mild or moderate exercise with an *abnormal* capability-to-breathe because of a reduced cardiopulmonary function and reserve (e.g., chronic bronchitis, emphysema, or congestive heart failure). In this case, the patient's **work of breathing (WOB)** and required oxygen consumption (in response to the exercise) are both increased. In fact, many patients with severe cardiopulmonary problems frequently remark that they are short of breath when performing even the most routine day-to-day tasks such as walking, climbing stairs, or dressing (see Fig. 3.1C). For further discussion see text and Chapter 4, Pulmonary Function Testing (section on **cardiopulmonary exercise testing**).

Chapter 10, The Therapist-Driven Protocol Program, and Chapter 11, Respiratory Insufficiency, Respiratory Failure, and Ventilatory Management Protocol, will stress the importance of prioritizing patient treatments, and the up- or down-regulating of treatment frequency, dosing, and nature of therapy on the basis of a scheme that in part relies on the severity on the patient's subjective complaints. Not only are severity-based systems used in prioritizing treatments but they are also used in assigning the localization or bedding of patients (e.g., holding areas, intensive care units, step-down units, or rehabilitation units, etc.). Severity-based systems are also an important part of a coding system that determines hospital and physician reimbursement using an alphanumeric coding system (ICD).

The following two methods are commonly used to assess the patient's breathlessness; not surprisingly, they are based on patients' sensation of the severity of their demand-to-breathe—that is, patients' severity assessment of their dyspnea:

- The **Modified (British) Medical Research Council (mMRC) Questionnaire** for Assessing the Severity of Breathlessness in those who can speak (Table 3.1).
- The **Borg Dyspnea Scale** used in patients who cannot communicate because of mouthpieces, endotracheal tubes, tracheotomies, etc. (Table 3.2).

TABLE 3.1 Modified Medical Research Council (mMRC) Dyspnea Scale

mMRC Score	Check the Score Box That Best Applies to You (One Box Only)	
0	I only get breathless with strenuous exercise.	☐
1	I get short of breath when hurrying on level ground or walking up a slight hill.	☐
2	On level ground, I walk slower than people of the same age because of breathlessness or have to stop for breath when walking at my own pace.	☐
3	I stop for breath after walking about 100 m or after a few minutes on level ground.	☐
4	I am too breathless to leave the house or I am breathless when dressing.	☐

Patients choose a score from the right-hand column that reflects their degree (amount) of shortness of breath (dyspnea).

TABLE 3.2 Borg Dyspnea Rating Scale for Use in Patients Unable to Communicate

Scale	Level of Dyspnea
0	No shortness of breath (SOB)
0.5	Slight SOB
1	
2	Mild SOB
3	Moderate SOB
4	
5	Strong or hard breathing
6	
7	Severe breathing or SOB
8	
9	
10	SOB so severe I need to stop and rest

Patients indicate their degree of shortness of breath (dyspnea) by pointing (or having the examiner point) to the appropriate number in the rating scale on the left.

The Pathophysiologic Basis of Abnormal Ventilatory Patterns

Although the precise cause of an **abnormal ventilatory pattern** may not always be known, they are often related to (1) the anatomic alterations of the lungs associated with a specific disorder and (2) the pathophysiologic mechanisms that develop because of the anatomic alterations. Therefore to evaluate and assess the various abnormal ventilatory patterns (rate and volume relationships) seen in the clinical setting, the following pathophysiologic mechanisms that can alter the ventilatory pattern must first be understood:

- Lung compliance
- Airway resistance
- Peripheral chemoreceptors
- Central chemoreceptors
- Pulmonary reflexes
  - Hering-Breuer reflex
  - Deflation reflex

- Irritant reflex
- Juxtapulmonary-capillary receptors (J receptors) reflex
- Reflexes from the aortic and carotid sinus baroreceptors
- Pain, anxiety, and fever

Recall the notion put forward in Chapter 1, The Patient Interview, that respiratory disease processes often start slowly but over time even small pathologic changes can produce remarkable signs and symptoms (see Fig. 1.1). The message is clear: In cardiopulmonary disease, "little things (indeed) do mean a lot." This statement is certainly true for the effects of decreased lung compliance and increased airway resistance on the work of breathing. As discussed in the following section, changes in lung compliance and airway resistance can and do have a profound effect on the patient's ventilatory pattern.

Lung Compliance and Its Effect on the Ventilatory Pattern and Dyspnea

The ease with which the elastic forces of the lungs accept a volume of inspired air is known as **lung compliance (C_L)**. C_L is measured in terms of unit volume change per unit pressure change. Mathematically, it is written as liters per centimeter of water pressure (L/cm H_2O). In other words, compliance determines how much air in liters the lungs will accommodate for each centimeter of water pressure change in distending pressure.

For example, when the normal individual generates a negative intrapleural pressure change of −2 cm H_2O during inspiration, the lungs accept a new volume of about 0.2 L gas. Therefore the C_L of the lungs and thorax is 0.1 L/cm H_2O:

$$C_L = \frac{\Delta V (L)}{\Delta P (cm\ H_2O)}$$
$$= \frac{0.2\ L\ gas}{2\ cm\ H_2O}$$
$$= 0.1\ L/cm\ H_2O.$$

The normal compliance of the lungs is graphically illustrated by the volume-pressure curve seen in (Fig. 3.2). As shown in Fig. 3.3, when C_L increases (e.g., emphysema), the lungs accept a greater volume of gas per unit pressure change. When C_L decreases (e.g., pulmonary fibrosis or atelectasis), the lungs accept a smaller volume of gas per unit pressure change.

Although the precise mechanism is not clear, the fact that certain ventilatory patterns occur when lung compliance is altered is well documented. For example, when C_L decreases, the patient's breathing rate generally increases while the tidal volume simultaneously decreases (Fig. 3.4). This type of breathing pattern is commonly seen in restrictive lung disorders such as pneumonia, pulmonary edema, and acute respiratory distress syndrome. In addition, a rapid breathing rate and reduced tidal volume is also commonly seen during the early stages of an acute asthmatic attack when the alveoli are overinflated—C_L progressively decreases as the alveolar volume increases. Note that the volume/pressure curve flattens at high lung volumes (see Fig. 3.2). C_L is low at both the high and low ends of the normal pressure-volume curve. Note the normal resting tidal volume and where it is placed in the pressure volume curve, very near to the normal functional residual

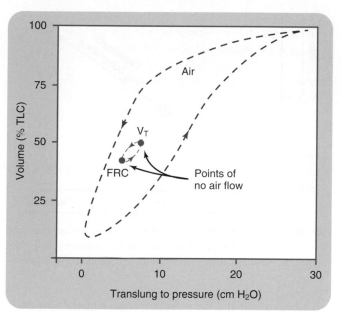

FIGURE 3.2 Inflation-deflation pressure-volume curve (red dotted line). The direction of inspiration and exhalation is shown by the arrows. The difference between the inflation and deflation pressure-volume curve is a result of the variation in surface tension with changes in lung volume. This effect is called **hysteresis**. Also note the normal tidal volume (V_T) pressure-volume curves (blue circle hysteresis) that begin and end at the resting functional residual capacity (FRC). *TLC*, Total lung capacity.

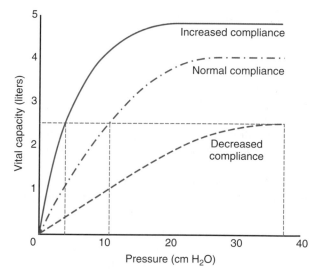

FIGURE 3.3 Effects of increased and decreased compliance on the volume-pressure curve. As the lung compliance decreases, greater pressure change is required to obtain the same volume of 2.5 L (dotted lines).

capacity, illustrated in blue (see Fig. 3.2). It should be noted that, physiologically, we elect to breathe at the most compliant and efficient portion of our lung volume.

Airway Resistance and Its Effect on the Ventilatory Pattern

Airway resistance (R_{aw}) is defined as the pressure difference between the mouth and the alveoli (**transairway pressure**) divided by the flow rate. Therefore the rate at which a certain volume of gas flows through the airways is a function of the

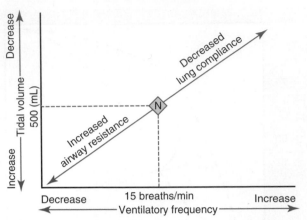

FIGURE 3.4 The effects of increased airway resistance and decreased lung compliance on ventilatory frequency and tidal volume. *N*, Normal resting tidal volume and ventilatory frequency.

pressure gradient and the resistance created by the airways to the flow of gas. Mathematically, R_{aw} is calculated as follows:

$$R_{aw} = \frac{\Delta P (cm\ H_2O)}{\dot{V}(L/s)}.$$

For example, if a patient produces a flow rate of 6 L/s during inspiration by generating a transairway pressure difference of 12 cm H_2O, R_{aw} would be 2 cm H_2O/L/s:

$$R_{aw} = \frac{\Delta P}{\dot{V}}$$
$$= \frac{12\ cm\ H_2O}{6\ L/s}$$
$$= 2\ cm\ H_2O/L/s.$$

Under normal conditions, the R_{aw} in the tracheobronchial tree is about 1.0 to 2.0 cm H_2O/L/s. However, in large airway obstructive pulmonary diseases (e.g., bronchitis, asthma), the R_{aw} may be extremely high. (For a more in-depth discussion on this topic, see Chapter 4, Pulmonary Function Testing.) An increased R_{aw} has a profound effect on the patient's ventilatory patterns. For example, as demonstrated by **Poiseuille's Law** for pressure and flow, even the slightest reduction in airway diameter can have a remarkable effect on the patient's ability to move air in and out of the lungs (Box 3.2).

When airway resistance increases significantly, the patient's ventilatory rate usually decreases while the tidal volume simultaneously increases (see Fig. 3.4). This type of breathing pattern is commonly seen in large airway obstructive lung diseases (e.g., chronic bronchitis, bronchiectasis, asthma, cystic fibrosis, especially during advanced stages of the disease).

The ventilatory pattern adopted by the patient with either a restrictive or an obstructive lung disorder is thought to be based on *minimum work requirements* rather than gas exchange efficiency. In physics, work is defined as the force multiplied by the distance moved (work = force × distance). In respiratory physiology, the change in pulmonary pressure (force) multiplied by the change in lung volume (distance) may be used to quantify the work of breathing (work = pressure × volume).

The patient's customary ventilatory pattern as described previously may not be seen in the clinical setting because of

secondary heart or lung problems. For example, a patient with chronic bronchitis who has "normally" adopted a decreased ventilatory rate and an increased tidal volume because of the increased airway resistance associated with the disorder may demonstrate an *increased* ventilatory rate and a *decreased* tidal volume in response to a secondary pneumonia (a restrictive lung disorder superimposed on a chronic obstructive lung disorder).

Because the patient may adopt a ventilatory pattern based on the expenditure of energy rather than on the efficiency of ventilation, the examiner cannot assume that the ventilatory pattern adopted by the patient in response to a certain respiratory disorder is the most efficient one in terms of physiologic gas exchange.

Peripheral Chemoreceptors and Their Effect on the Ventilatory Pattern

Hypoxemia (defined as $PaO_2 \leq 60$ mm Hg or $SaO_2 \leq 88\%$) and the stimulation of the **peripheral chemoreceptors** (also called *carotid* and *aortic bodies*) is a major cause of dyspnea. The peripheral chemoreceptors are oxygen-sensitive cells that react to a reduction of oxygen in the arterial blood (PaO_2). The peripheral chemoreceptors are located at the bifurcation of the internal and external carotid arteries (Fig. 3.5) and on the aortic arch (Fig. 3.6). Although the peripheral chemoreceptors are stimulated whenever the PaO_2 is less than normal, they are generally most active when the PaO_2 falls below 60 mm Hg ($SaO_2 \leq 88\%$). Suppression of these chemoreceptors, however, is seen when the PaO_2 falls below 30 mm Hg.

When the peripheral chemoreceptors are activated, an afferent (sensory) signal is sent to the respiratory centers of the medulla by way of the glossopharyngeal nerve (cranial nerve IX) from the carotid bodies and by way of the vagus nerve (cranial nerve X) from the aortic bodies. Efferent (motor) signals are then sent to the respiratory muscles, which results in an increased rate of breathing.

It should be noted that in patients who have a chronically high $PaCO_2$ and low PaO_2 (e.g., during the advanced stages of emphysema), the peripheral chemoreceptors are the primary receptor sites for the control of ventilation.

Causes of Hypoxemia

In respiratory disease, a decreased arterial oxygen level (hypoxemia) is the result of a decreased **ventilation-perfusion ratio ($\dot{V}/\dot{Q}$)**, **pulmonary shunting**, and **venous admixture** (see Chapter 11, Pathophysiologic Mechanism of Hypoxemic Respiratory Failure, for a broader discussion of hypoxemia).

Other Factors That Stimulate the Peripheral Chemoreceptors

Although the peripheral chemoreceptors are primarily activated by a decreased arterial oxygen level, they are also stimulated by a decreased pH (increased H^+ concentration). For example, the accumulation of lactic acid (from anaerobic metabolism) or ketoacids (diabetic acidosis) increases the ventilatory rate almost entirely through the peripheral chemoreceptors. The peripheral chemoreceptors are also activated by hypoperfusion, increased temperature, nicotine, and the direct effect of $PaCO_2$. The response of the peripheral chemoreceptors to $PaCO_2$

BOX 3.2 Poiseuille's Law for Flow and Pressure Applied to Bronchial Airways

Poiseuille's law mathematically confirms how small changes in airway diameter can have a profound effect on intrapleural pressure and air flow. For example, consider the mathematics of Poiseuille's law for flow:

$$\dot{V} = \frac{\Delta P r^4 \pi}{8 l \eta}$$

where η = the viscosity of a gas (or fluid), ΔP = the change of pressure from one end of the tube to the other, r = the radius of the tube, l = the length of the tube, $\dot{V}$ = the gas (or fluid) flowing through the tube; and π and 8 = constants, which are excluded from this discussion in the interest of brevity.

The equation shows that flow is directly proportional to P and r^4 and inversely proportional to l and η. Thus flow will decrease in response to either a decreased P or tube radius and flow will increase in response to a decreased tube length and fluid viscosity. In addition, the formula shows that flow will increase in response to an increased P and tube radius or decrease in response to an increased tube length and fluid viscosity. Thus assuming that pressure (P) remains constant, decreasing the radius of a tube by half reduces the gas flow to $\frac{1}{16}$ of its original flow. For example, if the radius of a bronchial tube through which gas flows at a rate of 16 mL/s is reduced from 1 cm to 0.5 cm because of mucosal swelling, the flow rate through the bronchial tube would decrease to 1 mL/s ($\frac{1}{16}$ the original flow rate) as graphically illustrated:

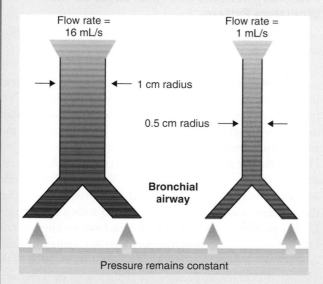

To offset this air flow reduction, Poiseuille's law confirms what pressure changes would be needed to maintain the original air flow. When Poiseuille's law is arranged for pressure, it is written as follows:

$$P = \frac{\dot{V} 8 \eta}{r^4 \pi}$$

Using the previous example of reducing the airway from 1 cm to 0.5 cm, if the original driving pressure (i.e., intrapleural pressure) was 1 cm H_2O to move gas in and out of the lungs, the patient would need to increase the driving pressure to 16 cm H_2O to maintain the same gas flow as illustrated:

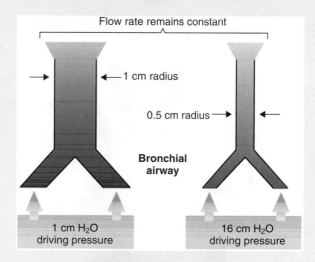

---

stimulation, however, is relatively small compared with the response generated by the **central chemoreceptors**.

Central Chemoreceptors and Their Effect on the Ventilatory Pattern

Although the mechanism is not fully understood, it is now believed that two special respiratory centers in the medulla, the **dorsal respiratory group (DRG)** and the **ventral** **respiratory group (VRG)**, are responsible for coordinating respiration (Fig. 3.7). Both the DRG and VRG are stimulated by an increased concentration of H^+ in the cerebrospinal fluid (CSF). The H^+ concentration of the CSF is monitored by the central chemoreceptors, which are located bilaterally and ventrally in the substance of the medulla. A portion of the central chemoreceptor region is actually in direct contact with the CSF. The central chemoreceptors

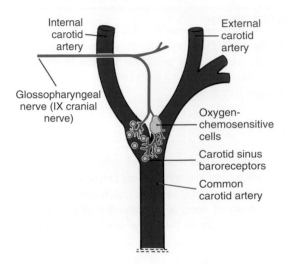

FIGURE 3.5 Oxygen-chemosensitive cells and the carotid sinus baroreceptors are located on the carotid artery.

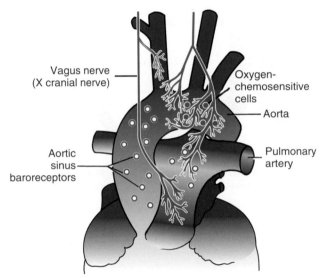

FIGURE 3.6 Oxygen-chemosensitive cells and the aortic sinus baroreceptors are located on the aortic notch and on the proximal pulmonary artery.

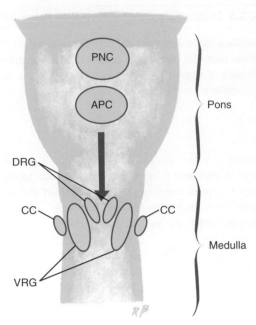

FIGURE 3.7 Schematic illustration of the respiratory components of the lower brain stem (pons and medulla). *APC*, Apneustic center; *CC*, central chemoreceptors; *DRG*, dorsal respiratory group; *PNC*, pneumotaxic center; *VRG*, ventral respiratory group.

transmit signals to the respiratory neurons by the following mechanism:

1. When the CO_2 level increases in the blood (e.g., during periods of hypoventilation), CO_2 molecules readily diffuse across the blood-brain barrier and enter the CSF. The blood-brain barrier is a semipermeable membrane that separates circulating blood from the CSF. The blood-brain barrier is relatively impermeable to ions such as H^+ and HCO_3^- but is very permeable to CO_2.

2. After CO_2 crosses the blood-brain barrier and enters the CSF, it forms carbonic acid:

$$CO_2 + H_2O \Leftrightarrow H_2CO_3^- \Leftrightarrow H^+ + HCO_3^-$$

3. Because the CSF has an inefficient buffering system, the H^+ produced from the previous reaction rapidly increases and causes the pH of the CSF to decrease.

4. The central chemoreceptors react to the liberated H^+ by sending signals to the respiratory components of the medulla, which in turn increases the ventilatory rate.

5. The increased ventilatory rate causes the $PaCO_2$ and, subsequently, the PCO_2 in the CSF to decrease. Therefore the CO_2 level in the blood regulates ventilation by its indirect effect on the pH of the CSF (Fig. 3.8).

Pulmonary Reflexes and Their Effect on the Ventilatory Pattern

Several reflexes may be activated in certain respiratory diseases and influence the patient's ventilatory rate.

Deflation Reflex. When the lungs are compressed or deflated (e.g., atelectasis), an increased rate of breathing is seen. The precise mechanism responsible for this reflex is not known. Some investigators suggest that the increased rate of breathing may simply result from reduced stimulation of the receptors (the **Hering-Breuer reflex**) rather than from stimulation of specific deflation receptors alone. Receptors for the Hering-Breuer reflex are located in the walls of the bronchi and bronchioles. When these receptors are stretched (e.g., during a deep inspiration), a reflex response is triggered to decrease the ventilatory rate. Other investigators, however, feel that the deflation reflex does not result from the absence of receptor stimulation of the Hering-Breuer reflex, because the deflation reflex is not seen when the bronchi and bronchioles are below a temperature of 8°C (46.4°F). The Hering-Breuer reflex does not occur when the bronchi and bronchioles are below this temperature.

Irritant Reflexes. When the lungs are compressed, deflated, or exposed to noxious gases, the irritant receptors are stimulated. The irritant receptors are subepithelial mechanoreceptors located in the trachea, bronchi, and bronchioles. When the receptors are activated, a reflex causes the ventilatory rate to increase. Stimulation of the **irritant reflex** may also produce a cough and bronchoconstriction.

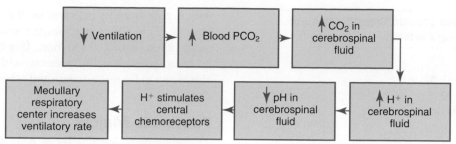

FIGURE 3.8 Sequence of events in alveolar hypoventilation. The central chemoreceptors are stimulated by hydrogen ions (H^+), which increase in concentration as CO_2 moves into the cerebrospinal fluid. In response to this, the central chemoreceptors respond with signals to the respiratory centers in the medulla, increasing the respiratory rate.

Juxtapulmonary-Capillary Receptors. The **juxtapulmonary-capillary receptors**, or **J receptors**, are located in the interstitial tissues between the pulmonary capillaries and the alveoli. Their precise mechanism of action is not known. When the J receptors are stimulated, a reflex triggers rapid, shallow breathing. The J receptors may be activated by the following:

- Pulmonary capillary congestion
- Capillary hypertension
- Edema of the alveolar walls
- Humoral agents (e.g., serotonin)
- Lung deflation
- Emboli in the pulmonary microcirculation

Reflexes From the Aortic and Carotid Sinus Baroreceptors. The normal function of the **aortic and carotid sinus baroreceptors**, also located near the aortic and carotid peripheral chemoreceptors, is to activate reflexes that cause (1) decreased heart rate and ventilatory rate in response to increased systemic blood pressure and (2) increased heart rate and ventilatory rate in response to decreased systemic blood pressure.

Pain, Anxiety, and Fever

An increased respiratory rate may result from chest pain or fear and anxiety associated with the patient's inability to breathe. These symptoms occur in a number of cardiopulmonary pathologic conditions, such as pleurisy, rib fractures, pulmonary hypertension, and angina. An increased respiratory rate also may be caused by fever. Fever is commonly associated with infectious lung disorders such as pneumonia, lung abscess, tuberculosis, and fungal diseases.

Other

Additional illnesses that are not related to the above that increase the demand-to-breathe sensation associated with dyspnea include obesity, physical deconditioning, hypoxia such as seen at high altitude, and metabolic acidosis.

The Onset/Offset Patterns Associated With Various Cardiopulmonary Disorders

Abnormal ventilatory patterns that occur suddenly (minutes to hours maximum) are classified as **acute onset conditions**. Abnormal ventilatory conditions that develop slowly (days to months to years) are classified as **chronic conditions**.

Box 3.3 shows common acute and chronic lung classifications associated with abnormal ventilatory patterns (e.g., dyspnea).

A helpful refinement to the above acute or chronic onset classification tool is to consider the typical *onset/offset* pattern associated with the patient's cardiopulmonary condition. To do this the examiner should first determine how the patient's clinical manifestations developed over time (see Fig. 1.1). Second, the severity of symptoms that appear at that time need to be documented. As discussed earlier, the severity can be rated by the examiner via tools such as the mMRC Dyspnea Evaluation Scale (see Table 3.1) or the Borg Scale discussed earlier in this chapter (see Table 3.2). The final step is to inquire about the *offset pattern* of the condition itself.

Fig. 3.9 provides examples of four basic onset/offset ventilatory patterns of cough, chest pain, or dyspnea. The time scale is dimensionless—that is, in a "minutes" scale for some rapid (acute) onset/offset type illnesses and "years" for the chronic disorders.

Use of the Accessory Muscles of Inspiration

During the advanced stages of chronic obstructive pulmonary disease, the accessory muscles of inspiration are activated when the diaphragm becomes significantly depressed by the increased lung volumes (residual volume [RV], functional residual capacity [FRC], and total lung capacity [TLC]). The **accessory muscles of inspiration** assist or largely replace the diaphragm in creating subatmospheric pressure in the pleural space during inspiration. The major accessory muscles of inspiration are as follows:

- Scalenes
- Sternocleidomastoids
- Pectoralis major muscle groups
- Trapezius muscle groups

Scalenes

The anterior, medial, and posterior **scalene muscles** are separate muscles that function as a unit. They originate on the transverse processes of the second to sixth cervical vertebrae and insert into the first and second ribs (Fig. 3.10). These muscles normally elevate the first and second ribs and flex the neck. When they are used as accessory muscles of inspiration, their primary role is to elevate the first and second ribs.

Sternocleidomastoids

The **sternocleidomastoid muscles** are located on each side of the neck (Fig. 3.11), where they rotate and support the head. They originate from the sternum and clavicle and insert into the mastoid process and occipital bone of the skull.

Normally, the sternocleidomastoid pulls from its sternoclavicular origin, rotates the head to the opposite side, and turns it upward. When the sternocleidomastoid muscle functions as an accessory muscle of inspiration, the head and neck are fixed by other muscles, and the sternocleidomastoid muscle pulls from its insertion on the skull and elevates the sternum. This action increases the anteroposterior diameter of the chest, aiding inspiration. Use of this muscle group is often prominent in patients with end-stage chronic obstructive pulmonary disease and other causes of respiratory distress.

Pectoralis Majors

The **pectoralis major muscles** are powerful, fan-shaped muscles that originate from the clavicle and sternum and insert into the upper part of the humerus. The primary function of the pectoralis muscles is to pull the upper part of the arm to the body in a hugging motion (Fig. 3.12).

When operating as an accessory muscle of inspiration, the pectoralis pulls from the humeral insertion and elevates the chest, resulting in an increased anteroposterior diameter, again aiding inspiratory effort. Patients with advanced chronic obstructive pulmonary disease may secure their arms to something stationary and use the pectoralis major muscles to increase the anteroposterior diameter of the chest (Fig. 3.13). This braced position is called the **tripod position**.

Trapezius

The trapezius is a large, flat, triangular muscle that is situated superficially in the upper part of the back and the back of the neck. The muscle originates from the occipital bone, the ligamentum nuchae, the spinous processes of the seventh cervical vertebra, and all the thoracic vertebrae. It inserts into the spine of the scapula, the acromion process, and the lateral third of the clavicle (Fig. 3.14). The **trapezius muscle** rotates the scapula, raises the shoulders, and abducts and flexes the arm. Its action is typified in shrugging the shoulders (Fig. 3.15). When used as an accessory muscle of inspiration, the trapezius helps elevate the thoracic cage.

Use of the Accessory Muscles of Expiration

Because of the airway narrowing and collapse associated with chronic obstructive pulmonary disorders, the **accessory muscles of expiration** are often recruited when airway resistance becomes significantly elevated. When these muscles actively contract, intrapleural pressure increases and offsets the increased airway resistance. The major accessory muscles of expiration are as follows:
- Rectus abdominis
- External oblique
- Internal oblique
- Transversus abdominis

Rectus Abdominis

A pair of **rectus abdominis muscles** extends the entire length of the abdomen. Each muscle forms a vertical mass about 4 inches wide, separated at the midline by the linea alba. It arises from the iliac crest and pubic symphysis and inserts into the xiphoid process and the fifth, sixth, and seventh ribs. When activated, the muscle assists in compressing the abdominal contents, which in turn push the diaphragm into the thoracic cage (Fig. 3.16).

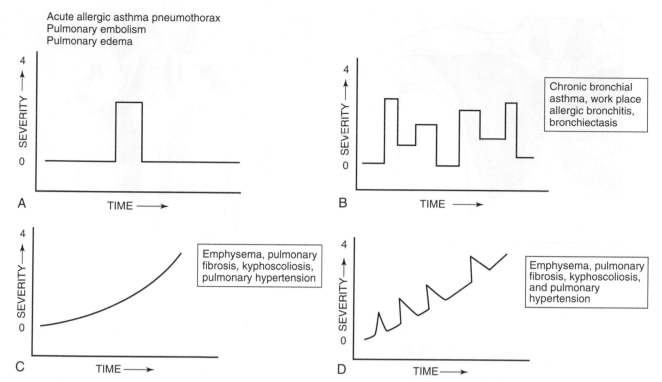

Acute allergic asthma pneumothorax
Pulmonary embolism
Pulmonary edema

A

Chronic bronchial asthma, work place allergic bronchitis, bronchiectasis

B

Emphysema, pulmonary fibrosis, kyphoscoliosis, pulmonary hypertension

C

Emphysema, pulmonary fibrosis, kyphoscoliosis, and pulmonary hypertension

D

FIGURE 3.9 Four basic onset/offset patterns of cardiopulmonary disorders: (A) Sudden crisis onset and offset; (B) sudden repetitive onset and offset; (C) gradual progressive onset without offset (note the similarity to Fig. 1.1); (D) slowly progressive disorder with periodic exacerbations. Severity of symptoms is shown on the upward scale on a 0 to 4+ range (as seen in Table 3.2, the mMRC Dyspnea Evaluation Scale). The horizontal scale is dimensionless—that is, it can range from minutes as in examples A and B to years as in examples C and D.

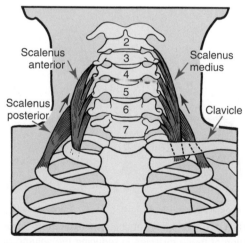

FIGURE 3.10 The scalene muscles (anterior neck). Red arrows indicate upward movement of the ribs.

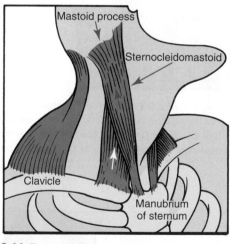

FIGURE 3.11 The sternocleidomastoid muscle. White arrow indicates upward movement of the sternum.

External Obliques

The broad, thin, **external oblique muscle** is on the anterolateral side of the abdomen. The muscle is the longest and most superficial of all the anterolateral muscles of the abdomen. It arises by eight digitations from the lower eight ribs and the abdominal aponeurosis. It inserts in the iliac crest and into the linea alba. The muscle assists in compressing the abdominal contents. This action also pushes the diaphragm into the thoracic cage during exhalation (see Fig. 3.16).

Internal Oblique

The **internal oblique muscle** is in the lateral and ventral part of the abdominal wall directly under the external oblique muscle. It is smaller and thinner than the external oblique. It arises from the inguinal ligament, the iliac crest, and the lower portion of the lumbar aponeurosis. It inserts into the last four ribs and the linea alba. The muscle assists in compressing the abdominal contents and pushing the diaphragm into the thoracic cage (see Fig. 3.16).

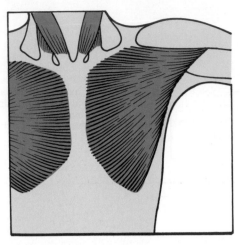

FIGURE 3.12 The pectoralis major muscles (anterior thorax).

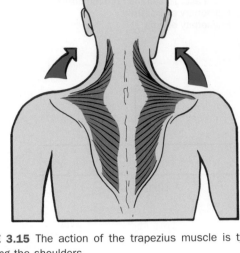

FIGURE 3.15 The action of the trapezius muscle is typified in shrugging the shoulders.

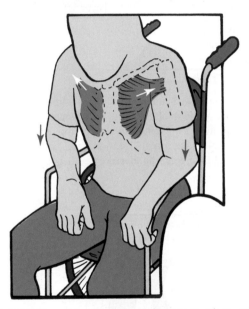

FIGURE 3.13 The way a patient may appear when using the pectoralis major muscles for inspiration. White arrows indicate the elevation of the chest. Downward blue arrows near the patient's elbows indicate how the patient may fix the arms to a stationary object.

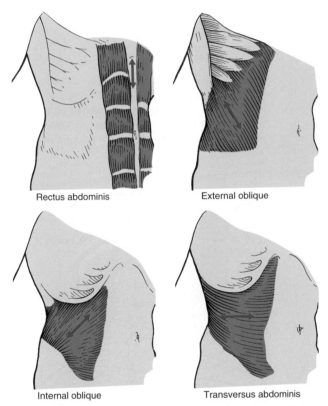

Rectus abdominis

External oblique

Internal oblique

Transversus abdominis

FIGURE 3.16 Accessory muscles of expiration. Arrows indicate the action of these muscles in reducing the volume of the lungs.

Transversus Abdominis

The **transversus abdominis muscle** is found immediately under each internal oblique muscle. It arises from the inguinal ligament, the iliac crest, the thoracolumbar fascia, and the lower six ribs. It inserts into the linea alba. When activated, it constricts the abdominal contents (see Fig. 3.16).

When all four pairs of accessory muscles of exhalation contract, the abdominal pressure increases and drives the diaphragm into the thoracic cage. As the diaphragm moves into the thoracic cage during exhalation, the intrapleural pressure increases and enhances expiratory gas flow (Fig. 3.17).

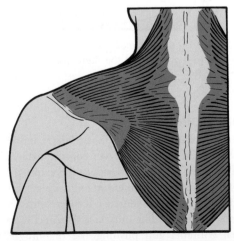

FIGURE 3.14 The trapezius muscles (posterior thorax).

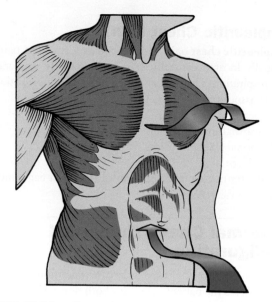

FIGURE 3.17 When the accessory muscles of expiration contract, intrapleural pressure increases, the chest moves outward, and expiratory air flow increases.

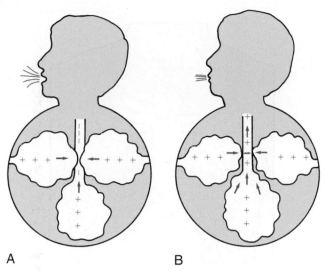

A   B

FIGURE 3.18 (A) Schematic illustration of alveolar compression of weakened bronchiolar airways during normal expiration in patients with chronic obstructive pulmonary disease (e.g., emphysema). (B) Effects of pursed-lip breathing. The weakened bronchiolar airways are kept open by the effects of positive pressure created by pursed lips during expiration.

Pursed-Lip Breathing

Pursed-lip breathing occurs in patients during the advanced stages of obstructive pulmonary disease. It is a relatively simple technique that many patients learn without formal instruction. During pursed-lip breathing the patient exhales through lips that are held in a position similar to that used for whistling, kissing, or blowing through a flute. The positive pressure created by retarding the air flow through pursed lips provides the airways with some stability and an increased ability to resist surrounding intrapleural pressures. This action offsets early airway collapse and air trapping during exhalation. In addition, pursed-lip breathing has been shown to slow the patient's ventilatory rate and generate a ventilatory pattern that is more effective in gas mixing (Fig. 3.18).

Substernal and Intercostal Retractions

Substernal and **intercostal retractions** may be seen in patients with severe restrictive lung disorders such as pneumonia or acute respiratory distress syndrome. In an effort to overcome the low lung compliance, the patient must generate a greater-than-normal negative intrapleural pressure during inspiration. This greater negative intrapleural pressure causes the tissues between the ribs and the substernal area to retract during inspiration (Fig. 3.19). Because the thorax of the newborn is very flexible (as a result of the relatively large amount of cartilage found in the skeletal structure), substernal and intercostal retractions are often seen in newborn respiratory disorders such as respiratory distress syndrome, meconium aspiration syndrome, transient tachypnea of the newborn, bronchopulmonary dysplasia, and congenital diaphragmatic hernia.

Nasal Flaring

Nasal flaring is often seen during inspiration in infants experiencing respiratory distress. It is likely to be a facial reflex that enhances the movement of gas into the tracheobronchial tree. The dilator naris, which originates from the maxilla and inserts into the ala of the nose, is the muscle responsible for this clinical manifestation. When activated, the dilator naris pulls the alae laterally and widens the nasal aperture, providing a larger orifice for gas to enter the lungs during inspiration (see Chapter 33, Newborn Assessment and Management).

Splinting and Decreased Chest Expansion Caused by Pleuritic and Nonpleuritic Chest Pain

Chest pain is one of the most common complaints among patients with cardiopulmonary problems. It can be divided into two categories: pleuritic and nonpleuritic. Unlike cough, dyspnea, and sputum production, it is *not* subtle. Obviously severe resistance to taking a deep breath is a symptom of pleuritic chest pain and is called **splinting**.

Pleuritic Chest Pain (Pleurisy)

Pleuritic chest pain (see Chapter 23, Pneumothorax) is usually described as a sudden, sharp, or stabbing pain. The pain generally intensifies during deep inspiration and coughing and diminishes during breath holding or splinting. The origin of the pain may be the chest wall, muscles, ribs, parietal pleura, diaphragm, mediastinal structures, or intercostal nerves. Because the visceral pleura, which covers the lungs, does not have any sensory nerve supply, pain originating in the parietal region signifies extension of inflammation from the lungs to the contiguous parietal pleura lining the inner surface of the chest wall. This condition is known as *pleurisy* (Fig. 3.20). When a patient with pleurisy inhales, the lung expands, irritating the inflamed parietal pleura and causing pain. On auscultation, a squeaking or grating sound is often heard—known as a **pleural friction rub**. Another good example of a pleural friction rub is the sound made by walking on fresh snow.

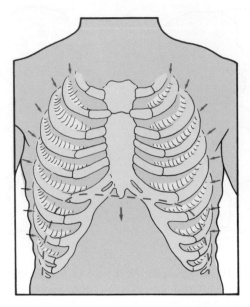

FIGURE 3.19 Intercostal retraction of soft tissues during forceful inspiration.

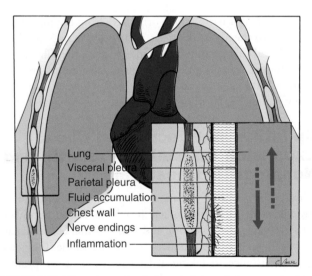

FIGURE 3.20 When the parietal pleura is irritated, the nerve endings in the pleura send pain signals to the brain. Arrows represent inspiration (upward) and expiration (downward).

Because of the nature of the pleuritic pain, the patient usually prefers to lie on the affected side to allow greater expansion of the uninvolved lung and help splint the chest. Pleuritic chest pain is a characteristic feature of the following respiratory diseases:

- Pneumonia
- Pleural effusion
- Pneumothorax
- Pulmonary infarction
- Lung cancer
- Pneumoconiosis
- Fungal diseases
- Tuberculosis

Nonpleuritic Chest Pain

Nonpleuritic chest pain is described as a constant pain that is usually located centrally. It is not generally worsened by deep inspiration. The pain also may radiate. Nonpleuritic chest pain is associated with the following disorders:

- Myocardial ischemia
- Pericardial inflammation
- Pulmonary hypertension
- Esophagitis
- Local trauma or inflammation of the chest cage, muscles, bones, or cartilage

Abnormal Chest Shape and Configuration

During inspection, the respiratory care practitioner systematically observes the patient's chest for both normal and abnormal findings. Is the spine straight? Are any lesions or surgical scars evident? Are the scapulae symmetric? Is there a barrel chest deformity? Common chest deformities are listed in Table 3.3 and illustrated in Fig. 3.21.

Abnormal Extremity Findings

The inspection of the patient's extremities should include the following:

- Altered skin color (e.g., cyanotic, pale, red, purple, etc.)
- Presence or absence of digital clubbing
- Presence or absence of peripheral edema
- Presence or absence of distended neck veins

Altered Skin Color

A general observation of the patient's skin color should be routinely performed. For example, does the patient's skin color appear normal—pink, tan, brown, or black? Is the skin cold or clammy? Does the skin and/or mucous membranes appear ashen or pallid? This appearance could be caused by anemia or acute blood loss. Do the patient's eyes, face, trunk, and arms have a yellow, jaundiced appearance (caused by increased bilirubin in the blood and tissue)? Is there redness of the skin or erythema (often caused by capillary congestion, inflammation, or infection)? Does the patient appear cyanotic?

Cyanosis

Cyanosis is common in severe respiratory disorders. *Cyanosis* is the term used to describe the blue-gray or purplish discoloration of the mucous membranes, fingertips, and toes whenever the blood in these areas contains at least 5 g/dL of reduced hemoglobin. When the normal 14 to 15 g/dL of hemoglobin is fully saturated, the PaO_2 is about 97 to 100 mm Hg and there is about 20 mL/dL of oxygen in the blood. In a typical cyanotic patient with one-third (5 g/dL) of the hemoglobin reduced, the PaO_2 is about 30 mm Hg and there is 13 mL/dL of oxygen in the blood (Fig. 3.22).

The detection and interpretation of cyanosis are problematic in clinical practice, and wide individual variations occur among observers. The recognition of cyanosis depends on the acuity of the observer, the light conditions in the examining room,

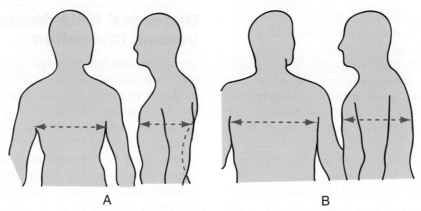

A   B

FIGURE 3.21 (A), Normally, the anteroposterior diameter is about half the lateral diameter (a ratio of 1:2). Because of the air trapping and lung hyperinflation in obstructive pulmonary diseases, the natural tendency of the lungs to recoil is decreased and the normal tendency of the chest to move outward prevails. This condition results in an increased anteroposterior diameter and is referred to as the *barrel chest deformity*. The ratio is nearer to 1:1. (B) The anteroposterior diameter commonly increases with aging. Therefore older individuals may have a slight barrel chest appearance in the absence of any pulmonary disease. Normal infants also usually have an anteroposterior diameter near 1:1.

TABLE 3.3 Common Abnormal Chest Shapes and Configurations

Condition	Description
Kyphosis	A "hunchbacked" appearance caused by posterior curvature of the spine
Scoliosis	A lateral curvature of the spine that results in the chest protruding posteriorly and the anterior ribs flattening out
Kyphoscoliosis	The combination of kyphosis and scoliosis (see Fig. 25.1)
Pectus carinatum	The forward projection of the xiphoid process and lower sternum (also known as "pigeon breast" deformity)
Pectus excavatum	A funnel-shaped depression over the lower sternum (also called "funnel chest")
Barrel chest	In the normal adult, the anteroposterior diameter of the chest is about half its lateral diameter, or 1:2. When the patient has a barrel chest, the ratio is nearer to 1:1 (see Fig. 3.21)

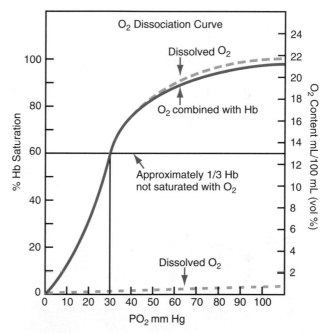

FIGURE 3.22 Cyanosis is likely whenever the blood contains at least 5 g/100 mL of reduced hemoglobin (Hb). In the normal individual who has about 15 g of hemoglobin per 100 mL of blood, a PO_2 of about 30 mm Hg produces 5 g/100 mL of reduced hemoglobin. The hemoglobin, however, is still approximately 60% saturated with oxygen.

and the pigmentation of the patient. Cyanosis of the nail beds is also influenced by temperature, because vasoconstriction induced by cold (i.e., **hypothermia**) may slow circulation to the point at which the blood becomes hypoxic (bluish) in the surface capillaries even though the arterial blood in the major vessels is not lacking in oxygen.

Central cyanosis, as observed on the mucous membranes of the lips and mouth, is almost always a sign of severe hypoxemia and therefore has definite diagnostic value.

In the patient with polycythemia, cyanosis may be present at a PaO_2 well above 30 mm Hg because the amount of reduced hemoglobin is often greater than 5 g/dL in these patients, even when their total oxygen content is within normal limits. *In respiratory disease, cyanosis is the result of (1) a decreased $\dot{V}/\dot{Q}$, (2) pulmonary shunting, (3) venous admixture, and (4) hypoxemia.*

Digital Clubbing

Digital clubbing is sometimes observed in patients with chronic respiratory disorders. Clubbing is characterized by a bulbous swelling of the terminal phalanges of the fingers and toes. The contour of the nail becomes rounded both longitudinally and transversely, which results in an increase in the angle between the surface of the nail and the dorsal surface of the terminal phalanx (Fig. 3.23).

The specific cause of clubbing is unknown. It is a normal hereditary finding in some families without any known history of cardiopulmonary disease. It is believed that the following factors may be causative: (1) circulating vasodilators, such as bradykinin and the prostaglandins, that are released from normal tissues but are not degraded by the lungs because of intrapulmonary shunting, (2) chronic infection, (3) unspecified toxins, (4) capillary stasis from increased venous back pressure, (5) arterial hypoxemia, and (6) local hypoxia. Successful treatment of the underlying disease may result in at least some resolution of the clubbing and return of the digits to normal.

Peripheral Edema

Bilateral, dependent **pitting edema** is commonly seen in patients with congestive heart failure, cor pulmonale, and hepatic cirrhosis. To assess the presence and severity of pitting **peripheral edema**, the health care practitioner places a finger or fingers over the tibia or medial malleolus (2 to 4 inches above the foot), firmly depresses the skin for 5 seconds, and then releases. Normally, this procedure leaves no indentation, although a pit may be seen if the person has been standing all day or is pregnant. If pitting is present, it is graded on the following subjective scale: 1+ (mild, slight depression) to 4+ (severe, deep depression) (Fig. 3.24).

Distended Neck Veins and Jugular Venous Distention

In patients with left-heart failure (congestive heart failure), right-heart failure (cor pulmonale), severe flail chest, pneumothorax, or pleural effusion, flow from the major veins of the chest that return blood to the right side of the heart may be compromised. When this happens, cardiac venous return decreases and central venous pressure increases. This condition is manifested by **distended neck veins** also called **jugular venous distention** (Fig. 3.25). The reduced venous return also may cause the patient's cardiac output and systemic blood pressure to decrease. In severe cases, the veins over the entire upper anterior thorax may be dilated.

Normal and Abnormal Sputum Production

Normal Histology and Mucus Production of the Tracheobronchial Tree

The wall of the tracheobronchial tree is composed of three major layers: an epithelial lining, the lamina propria, and a cartilaginous layer (Fig. 3.26).

The epithelial lining, which is separated from the lamina propria by a basement membrane, is predominantly composed of pseudostratified, ciliated, columnar epithelium interspersed with numerous mucus-secreting glands and serous cells. The ciliated cells extend from the beginning of the trachea to—and sometimes including—the respiratory bronchioles. As the tracheobronchial tree becomes progressively smaller, the columnar structure of the ciliated cells gradually decreases in height. In the terminal bronchioles, the epithelium appears more cuboidal than columnar. These cells flatten even more in the respiratory bronchioles (see Fig. 3.26).

A mucous layer, commonly referred to as the *mucous blanket*, covers the epithelial lining of the tracheobronchial tree (Fig. 3.27). The viscosity of the mucous layer progressively increases from the epithelial lining to the inner luminal surface and has two distinct layers: the sol layer, which is adjacent to the epithelial lining, and the gel layer, which is the more viscous layer adjacent to the inner luminal surface. The mucous blanket

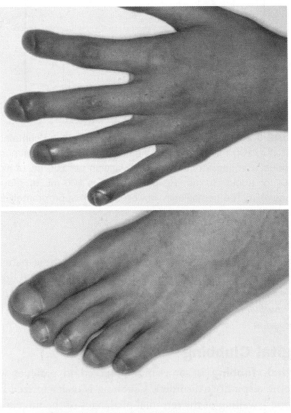

FIGURE 3.23 Digital clubbing and cyanosis.

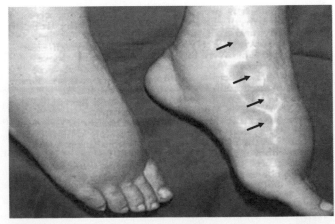

FIGURE 3.24 4+ pitting edema. (From Bloom, A., & Ireland, J. [1992]. *Color atlas of diabetes* [2nd ed.]. London: Mosby-Wolfe.)

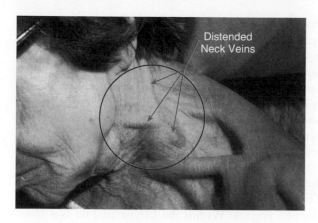

FIGURE 3.25 Distended neck veins (arrows). Prominence of sternocleidomastoid muscle is also seen in the lower portion of this photograph.

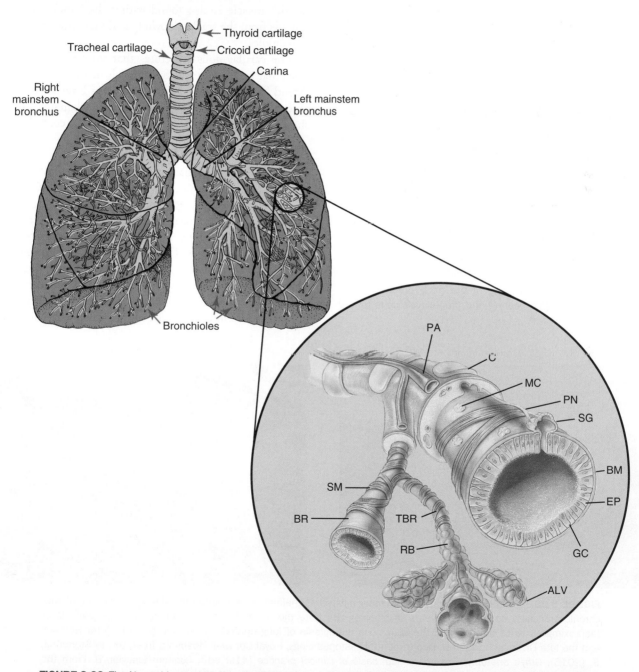

FIGURE 3.26 The Normal Lung. *ALV*, Alveoli; *BM*, Basement Membrane; *BR*, Bronchioles; *C*, Cartilage; *EP*, Epithelium; *GC*, Goblet Cell; *LP*, Lamina Propria; *MC*, Mast Cell; *PA*, Pulmonary Artery; *PN*, Parasympathetic Nerve; *RB*, Respiratory Bronchioles; *SG*, Submucosal Gland; *SM*, Smooth Muscle; *TBR*, Terminal Bronchioles.

is 95% water. The remaining 5% consists of glycoproteins, carbohydrates, lipids, DNA, some cellular debris, and foreign particles.

The mucous blanket is produced by the goblet cells and the submucosal, or bronchial, glands. The goblet cells are located intermittently between the pseudostratified, ciliated columnar cells distal to the terminal bronchioles.

Most of the mucous blanket is produced by the submucosal glands, which extend deeply into the lamina propria and are composed of different cell types: serous cells, mucous cells, collecting duct cells, mast cells, myoepithelial cells, and clear cells, which are probably lymphocytes. The submucosal glands are particularly numerous in the medium-sized bronchi and disappear in the bronchioles. These glands are innervated by parasympathetic (cholinergic) nerve fibers and normally produce about 100 mL of clear, thin bronchial secretions per day.

The mucous blanket is an important cleansing mechanism of the tracheobronchial tree. Inhaled particles stick to the

mucus. The distal ends of the cilia continually strike the innermost portion of the gel layer and propel the mucous layer, along with any foreign particles, toward the larynx. At this point, the cough mechanism moves secretions beyond the larynx and into the oropharynx. This mucociliary mechanism is commonly referred to as the *mucociliary transport* or the **mucociliary escalator**. The cilia move the mucous blanket at an estimated average rate of 2 cm/min. Fig. 3.28A and B shows a microscopic view of normal and abnormal (caused by chronic smoking) pseudostratified columnar ciliated epithelium.

The submucosal layer of the tracheobronchial tree is the lamina propria. Within the lamina propria is a loose, fibrous tissue that contains tiny blood vessels, lymphatic vessels, and branches of the vagus nerve. A circular layer of smooth muscle is also found within the lamina propria. It extends from the trachea down to and including the terminal bronchioles.

The cartilaginous structures that surround the tracheobronchial tree progressively diminish in size as the airways extend into the lungs. The cartilaginous layer is completely absent in bronchioles less than 1 mm in diameter. Fig. 3.29 shows a cross-sectional view of cartilaginous central airway.

Abnormal Sputum Production

Excessive sputum production is commonly seen in respiratory diseases that cause an acute or chronic inflammation of the tracheobronchial tree. Sputum volume, appearance, viscosity, and odor should be part of the objective finding in a good SOAP note (see Chapter 12, Recording Skills and Intraprofessional Communication). Depending on the severity and nature of the respiratory disease, sputum production may take several forms. For example, during the early stages of tracheobronchial inflammation, the sputum is usually clear, thin, and odorless. As the disease intensifies, the sputum becomes yellow-green

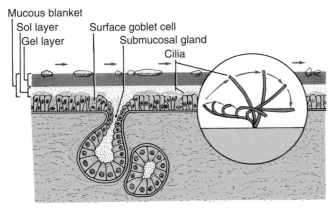

FIGURE 3.27 The epithelial lining of the tracheobronchial tree insert drawing shows cilia beating and propelling mucus toward the mouth.

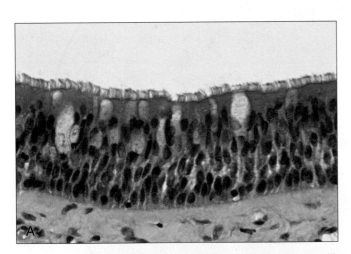
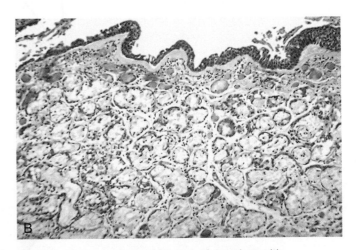

FIGURE 3.28 Normal pseudostratified columnar ciliated epithelium (A) is contrasted with that of a patient with chronic bronchitis secondary to years of smoking (B). Note the marked thickening of the mucous gland layer (approximately twice normal) and the squamous metaplasia of lung epithelium. (A, Courtesy Mr. Peter Helliwell and the late Dr. Joseph Mathew, Department of Histopathology, Royal Cornwall Hospitals Trust, UK. In Standring, S. [2016]. *Gray's anatomy: The anatomical basis of clinical practice* [41st ed.]. London: Elsevier. B, From the Teaching Collection of the Department of Pathology, University of Texas, Southwestern Medical School, Dallas, TX. In Kumar, V. K., Abbas, A. K., & Aster, J. C. [2018]. *Robbins basic pathology* [10th ed.]. Philadelphia, PA: Elsevier.)

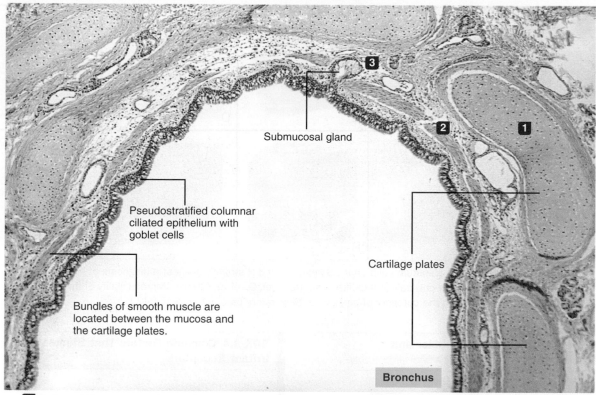

Submucosal gland

Pseudostratified columnar
ciliated epithelium with
goblet cells

Cartilage plates

Bundles of smooth muscle are
located between the mucosa and
the cartilage plates.

Bronchus

1 As bronchi become smaller, irregular cartilage plates are observed. Each cartilage plate, consisting of hyaline cartilage, is surrounded by a bundle of connective tissue fibers blending with the perichondrium.

2 Bundles of smooth muscle fibers are observed between the cartilage plates and the bronchial mucosa. The mucosa is lined by the typical respiratory epithelium.

3 Seromucous glands are observed in the lamina propria with the secretory acini projecting beyond the layer of smooth muscle cell bundles. The excretory ducts open into the bronchial lumen.

FIGURE 3.29 Cross-sectional view of normal cartilaginous central airway. *C,* Cartilage; *E,* epithelial surface; *G,* submucous gland; *L,* lumen; *M,* smooth muscle. Mucus in the lumen does not stain well without special stain preparations. (From Kierszenbaum, A. L., & Tres, L. L. [2016]. *Histology and cell biology: An introduction to pathology* [4th ed.]. Philadelphia, PA: Elsevier.)

and opaque, signifying the early stages of infection. The yellow-green appearance results from an enzyme (myeloperoxidase) released during the cellular breakdown of leukocytes. It also may be caused by retained or stagnant secretions or secretions caused by an acute infection.

Thick and tenacious sputum is commonly seen in patients with chronic bronchitis, chronic obstructive pulmonary disease, bronchiectasis, cystic fibrosis, and asthma. Patients with pulmonary edema expectorate a thin, frothy, pinkish sputum. Technically, this fluid is not true sputum. It results from the movement of plasma and red blood cells across the alveolar-capillary membrane into the alveoli.

Hemoptysis

Hemoptysis is the coughing up of blood or blood-tinged sputum from the tracheobronchial tree. In true hemoptysis the sputum is usually bright red and interspersed with air bubbles.

Clinically, hemoptysis may be confused with hematemesis, which is blood that originates from the upper gastrointestinal tract and usually has a dark, coffee-ground appearance. Repeated expectoration of blood-streaked sputum is seen in chronic bronchitis, bronchiectasis, cystic fibrosis, pulmonary

embolism, lung cancer, necrotizing infections, tuberculosis, and fungal diseases. A small amount of hemoptysis is common after bronchoscopy, particularly when biopsies are performed. *Massive hemoptysis* is defined as coughing up 400 to 600 mL of blood within a 24-hour period. Death from exsanguination resulting from hemoptysis is rare. Table 3.4 provides a general overview and analysis of the types of sputum commonly seen in the clinical setting. Fig. 3.30 is a sputum color chart. Although there is considerable interrater reliability in judging color, its use in recording and charting may be helpful.

Cough

A **cough** is a sudden, audible expulsion of air from the lungs. It is commonly seen in respiratory disease, especially in disorders that cause inflammation of the tracheobronchial tree. In general, a cough is preceded by (1) a deep inspiration, (2) partial closure of the glottis, and (3) forceful contraction of the accessory muscles of expiration to expel air from the lungs. In essence, a cough is a protective mechanism that clears the lungs, bronchi, or trachea of irritants. A cough also prevents the aspiration of foreign material into the lungs. For example, a cough is a common symptom associated with chronic sinusitis

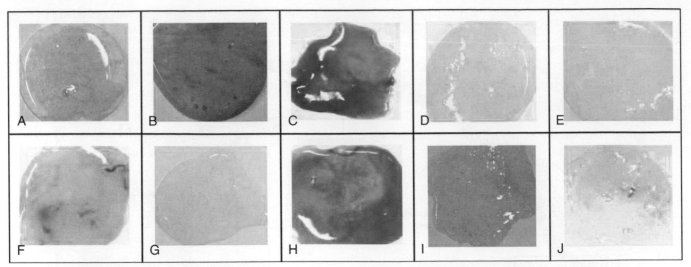

FIGURE 3.30 Illustration of a sputum color chart. Samples C and H strongly suggest a diagnosis of hemoptysis. Samples E and G may well be only saliva. (Modified from Reychler, G., et al. [2016]. Reproducibility of the sputum color evaluation depends on the category of caregivers. *Respiratory Care. 61*, 7, 936-942.)

TABLE 3.4 Analysis of Sputum Color and Characteristics

Color and Characteristics	Indications and Conditions
Brown/dark	Old blood
Bright red (hemoptysis)	Fresh blood (bleeding tumor, tuberculosis)
Clear and translucent	Normal
Copious	Large amount
Frank hemoptysis	Massive amount of blood
Green	Stagnant sputum or gram-negative bacteria
Green and foul smelling	*Pseudomonas* or anaerobic infection
Mucoid (white/gray)	Asthma, chronic bronchitis
Pink, frothy	Pulmonary edema
Tenacious	Secretions that are sticky or adhesive or otherwise tend to hold together
Viscous	Thick, sticky, or glutinous
Yellow or opaque	Presence of white blood cells, bacterial infection

BOX 3.4 Common Factors That Stimulate the Irritant Receptors

- Inflammation
- Infectious agents
- Excessive secretions
- Noxious gases (e.g., cigarette smoke, chemical inhalation)
- Very hot or very cold air
- A mass of any sort obstructing the airway or compressing the lungs
- Mechanical stimulation (e.g., endotracheal suctioning, compression of the airways)

and postnasal drip. The effectiveness of a cough depends largely on the depth of the preceding inspiration and the extent of dynamic compression of the airways.

Although a cough may be voluntary, it is usually a reflex response that arises when an irritant stimulates the irritant receptors (also called *subepithelial mechanoreceptors*). The irritant receptors are located in the pharynx, larynx, trachea, and large bronchi. When stimulated, the irritant receptors send a signal by way of the glossopharyngeal nerve (cranial nerve IX) and vagus nerve (cranial nerve X) to the cough reflex center located in the medulla. The medulla then causes the glottis to close and the accessory muscles of expiration to contract. Box 3.4 lists common factors that stimulate the irritant receptors.

Clinically, a cough is termed *productive* if sputum is produced and *nonproductive* (<25 mL/24 hr) if no sputum is produced.

Nonproductive Cough

Common causes of a **nonproductive cough** include (1) irritation of the airway, (2) inflammation of the airways, (3) mucous accumulation, (4) tumors, and (5) irritation of the pleura.

Productive Cough

For a **productive cough**, the respiratory practitioner should assess the following:

- Is the cough strong or weak? In other words, does the patient have a good or poor ability to mobilize bronchial secretions? A good, strong cough may indicate only deep breathing and cough therapy, whereas an inadequate cough may suggest the need for chest physical therapy or postural drainage.
- A productive cough should be evaluated in terms of its frequency, pitch, and loudness. A brassy cough may indicate a tumor, whereas a barking or hoarse cough indicates croup.
- Finally, the sputum of a productive cough should be monitored and evaluated frequently in terms of amount (teaspoons, tablespoons, cups), consistency (thin, thick, tenacious), odor, and color (see Table 3.4).

SELF-ASSESSMENT QUESTIONS

1. An individual's ventilatory pattern is composed of which of the following?
   1. Inspiratory and expiratory force
   2. Ventilatory rate
   3. Tidal volume
   4. Inspiratory and expiratory ratio
      a. 1 and 3 only
      b. 2 and 3 only
      c. 2, 3, and 4 only
      d. 1, 2, and 3 only

2. What is the average total compliance of the lungs and chest wall combined?
   a. 0.05 L/cm H_2O
   b. 0.1 L/cm H_2O
   c. 0.2 L/cm H_2O
   d. 0.3 L/cm H_2O

3. When lung compliance decreases, which of the following is seen?
   1. Ventilatory rate usually decreases.
   2. Tidal volume usually decreases.
   3. Ventilatory rate usually increases.
   4. Tidal volume usually increases.
      a. 1 only
      b. 2 only
      c. 3 and 4 only
      d. 2 and 3 only

4. What is the normal airway resistance in the tracheobronchial tree?
   a. 0.5 to 1.0 cm $H_2O/L/s$
   b. 1.0 to 2.0 cm $H_2O/L/s$
   c. 2.0 to 3.0 cm $H_2O/L/s$
   d. 3.0 to 4.0 cm $H_2O/L/s$

5. When the systemic blood pressure increases, the aortic and carotid sinus baroreceptors initiate reflexes that cause which of the following?
   1. Increased heart rate
   2. Decreased ventilatory rate
   3. Increased ventilatory rate
   4. Decreased heart rate
      a. 1 only
      b. 2 only
      c. 3 only
      d. 2 and 4 only

6. What is the anteroposterior-transverse chest diameter ratio in the normal adult?
   a. 1:0.5
   b. 1:1
   c. 1:2
   d. 1:3
   e. 1:4

7. Which of the following muscles originate from the clavicle?
   1. Scalene muscles
   2. Sternocleidomastoid muscles
   3. Pectoralis major muscles
   4. Trapezius muscles
      a. 1 only
      b. 2 only
      c. 4 only
      d. 2 and 3 only

8. Which of the following is associated with digital clubbing?
   1. Chronic infection
   2. Local hypoxia
   3. Circulating vasodilators
   4. Arterial hypoxemia
      a. 2 only
      b. 2 and 4 only
      c. 2, 3, and 4 only
      d. 1, 2, 3, and 4

9. Which of the following is associated with pleuritic chest pain?
   1. Lung cancer
   2. Pneumonia
   3. Myocardial ischemia
   4. Tuberculosis
      a. 1 only
      b. 2 only
      c. 1 and 3 only
      d. 1, 2, and 4 only

CHAPTER

4

Pulmonary Function Testing

Chapter Objectives

After reading this chapter, you will be able to:

- Describe the following lung volumes and capacities:
  - List the normal lung volumes and capacities of normal recumbent subjects who are 20 to 30 years of age.
  - Describe the residual volume/total lung capacity ratio (RV/TLC ratio).
  - Identify lung volumes and lung capacity findings characteristic of restrictive lung disorders.
  - List the anatomic alterations of the lungs associated with restrictive lung disorders.
  - Identify forced expiratory volume in 1 second/forced vital capacity ratio lung volumes and capacity findings characteristic of obstructive lung disorders.
  - List the anatomic alterations of the lungs associated with obstructive lung disorders.
- Describe the indirect measurements of the residual volume and lung capacities contained in the total lung capacity (TLC).
- Describe expiratory flow rate and volume measurements and their respective normal values.
- Describe how the FVC, FEV_1, and FEV_1/FVC ratio ($FEV_{1\%}$) are used to differentiate restrictive and obstructive lung disorders.
- Identify forced expiratory flow rate findings characteristic of restrictive lung disorders.
- Identify forced expiratory flow rate findings characteristic of obstructive lung disorders.
- Describe the pulmonary diffusion capacity (DLCO).
- Identify DLCO findings characteristic of restrictive lung disorders.
- Identify DLCO findings characteristic of obstructive lung disorders.
- Describe the following tests used to assess the patient's muscle strength at the bedside:
  - Maximum inspiratory pressure (MIP)
  - Negative inspiratory force
  - Maximum expiratory pressure (MEP)
  - Forced vital capacity (FVC)
  - Maximum volume ventilation
- Describe the role of cardiopulmonary exercise testing (CPET) in the evaluation of pulmonary function.
- Identify other diagnostic tests used to measure airway responsiveness in patients with asthma.
- Define key terms and complete self-assessment questions at the end of the chapter and on Evolve.

Key Terms

Air Trapping
Anaerobic Threshold (AT)
Body Plethysmography
Cardiopulmonary Exercise Testing (CPET)
Closed-Circuit Helium Dilution Test
Exercise or Cold Air Challenge
Expiratory Reserve Volume (ERV)
Flow-Volume Loop
Forced Expiratory Flow 200 to 1200 mL of FVC ($FEF_{200-1200}$)
Forced Expiratory Flow 25% to 75% ($FEF_{25\%-75\%}$)
Forced Expiratory Flow at 50% ($FEF_{50\%}$)
Forced Expiratory Volume in 1 Second (FEV_1)
Forced Expiratory Volume in 1 Second/Forced Vital Capacity Ratio (FEV_1/FVC ratio)
Forced Expiratory Volume in 1 Second Percentage ($FEV_{1\%}$)
Forced Expiratory Volume Timed (FEV_T)
Forced Inspiratory Volume (FIV)
Forced Vital Capacity (FVC)
Functional Residual Capacity (FRC)
Impulse Oscillometry (IOS)
Inhaled Mannitol
Inhaled Methacholine or Histamine
Inspiratory Capacity (IC)
Inspiratory Reserve Volume (IRV)
Lung Capacities
Lung Volumes
Maximum Expiratory Pressure (MEP)
Maximum Inspiratory Pressure (MIP)
Maximum Voluntary Ventilation (MVV)
Obstructive Lung Disorders
Open-Circuit Nitrogen Washout Test
Peak Expiratory Flow Rate (PEFR)
Pulmonary Diffusion Capacity of Carbon Monoxide (DLCO)
Reactance (Xrs)
Residual Volume (RV)
Residual Volume/Total Lung Capacity Ratio (RV/TLC)
Resistance (Rrs)
Respiratory impedance (Zrs)
Restrictive Lung Disorders
Tidal Volume (V_T)
Total Expiratory Time (TET)
Total Lung Capacity (TLC)
Vital Capacity (VC)

Chapter Outline

Normal Lung Volumes and Capacities
    Restrictive Lung Disorders: Lung Volume and Capacity Findings
    Indirect Measurements of the Residual Volume and Lung Capacities Containing the Residual Volume
Forced Expiratory Flow Rate and Volume Measurements
    Forced Vital Capacity
    Forced Expiratory Volume Timed
    Forced Expiratory Volume in 1 Second/Forced Vital Capacity (FEV_1/FVC) Ratio

Pulmonary function studies play a major role in the assessment of pulmonary disease. The results of pulmonary function studies are used to (1) evaluate pulmonary causes of dyspnea, (2) differentiate between obstructive and restrictive pulmonary disorders, (3) assess severity of the pathophysiologic impairment, (4) follow the course of a particular disease, (5) evaluate the effectiveness of therapy, and (6) assess the patient's preoperative status. Pulmonary function studies are commonly subdivided into the following categories: (1) lung volumes and lung capacities, (2) forced expiratory flow rate and volume measurements, (3) pulmonary diffusion capacity measurements, (4) test of respiratory muscle strength, and (5) cardiopulmonary exercise testing.

Pulmonary function tests and studies range from the simple and inexpensive to the complex and expensive. The more complex tests are reserved for use in patients with hard-to-diagnose dyspnea when physical examination, chest imaging studies, and simple pulmonary function studies have not been definitive. A general hierarchy of the increasing expense and complexity of pulmonary function tests is given in Table 4.1.

Normal Lung Volumes and Capacities

As shown in Table 4.2, gas in the lungs is divided into four **lung volumes** and four **lung capacities**. The lung capacities represent different combinations of lung volumes. The amount of air the lungs can accommodate varies with age, weight, height, gender, and, to a much lesser extent, race. Prediction

formulas for normal values exist that take these variables into account. Lung volumes and capacities change as a result of pulmonary disorders. These changes are classified as either restrictive lung disorders or obstructive lung disorders.

Restrictive Lung Disorders: Lung Volume and Capacity Findings

Table 4.3 provides some of the more common restrictive anatomic alterations of the lungs and examples of respiratory disorders that cause them. **Restrictive lung disorders** result in an increased lung rigidity, which in turn decreases lung compliance. When lung compliance decreases, the ventilatory rate increases and the **tidal volume (V_T)** decreases (see Fig. 3.4). Table 4.4 presents an overview of the lung volume and capacity findings characteristic of restrictive lung disorders. Restrictive lung volumes and capacities are associated with pathologic conditions that alter the anatomic structures of the lungs distal to the terminal bronchioles (i.e., the alveoli or the lung parenchyma).

Obstructive Lung Disorders: Lung Volume and Capacity Findings

Table 4.5 provides an overview of the lung volumes and capacity findings characteristic of **obstructive lung disorders**. These lung volume and capacity findings are associated with pathologic conditions that alter the tracheobronchial tree. Table 4.6 provides some of the more common obstructive anatomic alterations of the lungs and examples of respiratory disorders that cause them.

In obstructive lung disorders, the gas that enters the alveoli during inspiration (when the bronchial airways are naturally wider) is prevented from leaving the alveoli during expiration (when the bronchial airways narrow). As a result, the alveoli become overdistended with gas, a condition known as **air trapping**. Fig. 4.1 provides a visual comparison of obstructive and restrictive lung disorders.

Indirect Measurements of the Residual Volume and Lung Capacities Containing the Residual Volume

Because the **residual volume (RV)** cannot be exhaled, the RV and the lung capacities that contain the RV—the **functional residual capacity (FRC)** and **total lung capacity (TLC)**—can be measured indirectly by one of the following methods: the closed-circuit helium dilution test, the open-circuit nitrogen washout test, or body plethysmography. A brief explanation of each of these tests follows.

For the **closed-circuit helium dilution test**, the patient rebreathes both a known volume of gas (V_1) and a known concentration (C_1) of helium (He) for about 7 minutes

TABLE 4.1 General Hierarchy of Expense and Complexity of Pulmonary Function Tests

Cost	Pulmonary Function Test
$	Peak expiratory flow rate determinations
$$	Expiratory only (simple) spirometry*
$$$	Conventional spirometry*
$$$$	Flow-volume loop analysis
$$$$	Complete lung volume studies (open-circuit and closed-circuit)
$$$$	Pulmonary diffusion capacity studies
$$$$	Peak inspiratory and expiratory pressure determinations
$$$$$	Pulmonary mechanics (body plethysmography)
$$$$$	Studies of pulmonary compliance (esophageal balloon)
$$$$$$	Cardiopulmonary exercise tests[†]

*With and without bronchodilator.
[†]With and without arterial blood gas analysis.

TABLE 4.2 Lung Volumes and Capacities of Normal Recumbent Subjects 20 to 30 Years of Age

Measurements	Male (mL)	Female (mL)
Lung Volume Measurements		
Tidal volume (V_T): The volume of gas that normally moves into and out of the lungs in one quiet breath.	500	400–500
Inspiratory reserve volume (IRV): The volume of air that can be forcefully inspired after a normal tidal volume.	3100	1900
Expiratory reserve volume (ERV): The volume of air that can be forcefully exhaled after a normal tidal volume exhalation.	1200	800
Residual volume (RV): The amount of air remaining in the lungs after a forced exhalation.	1200	1000
Lung Capacity Measurements		
Vital capacity (VC): VC = IRV + V_T + ERV. The volume of air that can be exhaled after a maximal inspiration.	4800	3200
Inspiratory capacity (IC): IC = V_T + IRV. The volume of air that can be inhaled after a normal exhalation.	3600	2400
Functional residual capacity (FRC): FRC = ERV + RV. The lung volume at rest after a normal tidal volume exhalation.	2400	1800
Total lung capacity (TLC): TLC = IC + ERV + RV. The maximal amount of air that the lungs can accommodate.	6000	4200
Residual volume/total lung capacity ratio (RV/TLC × 100): The percentage of TLC occupied by the RV.	$\dfrac{1200}{6000}$ = 20% (approx)	$\dfrac{1000}{4200}$ = 25% (approx)

TABLE 4.3 Anatomic Alterations of the Lungs Associated With Restrictive Lung Disorders: Pathology of the Alveoli or Lung Parenchyma

Pathology (Anatomic Alteration of the Alveoli)	Examples of Respiratory Disorders Associated With Specific Pathology
Atelectasis	Pneumothorax, pleural effusion, flail chest, or mucous plugging
Consolidation	Pneumonia, acute respiratory distress syndrome, lung abscess, tuberculosis
Increased alveolar-capillary membrane thickness	Pulmonary edema, pneumoconiosis, tuberculosis, fungal disease

TABLE 4.4 Restrictive Lung Disorders: Lung Volume and Capacity Findings

V_T	IRV	ERV	RV	
N or ↓	↓	↓	↓	
VC	IC	FRC	TLC	RV/TLC
↓	↓	↓	↓	N

ERV, Expiratory reserve volume; *FRC,* functional residual capacity; *IC,* inspiratory capacity; *IRV,* inspiratory reserve volume; *N,* normal; *RV,* residual volume; *TLC,* total lung capacity; *VC,* vital capacity; *V_T,* tidal volume.

TABLE 4.5 Obstructive Lung Disorders: Lung Volume and Capacity Findings

V_T	IRV	ERV	RV	
N or ↑	N or ↓	N or ↓	↑	
VC	IC	FRC	TLC	RV/TLC ratio
↓	N or ↓	↑	N or ↑	N or ↑

ERV, Expiratory reserve volume; *FRC,* functional residual capacity; *IC,* inspiratory capacity; *IRV,* inspiratory reserve volume; *N,* normal; *RV,* residual volume; *TLC,* total lung capacity; *VC,* vital capacity; *V_T,* tidal volume. Note FVC is often reduced (see Fig. 4.5).

TABLE 4.6 Anatomic Alterations of the Lungs Associated With Obstructive Lung Disorders: Pathology of the Tracheobronchial Tree

Pathology (Anatomic Alteration of the Bronchial Airways)	Examples of Respiratory Disorders Associated With Specific Pathology
Excessive mucous production and accumulation	Chronic bronchitis, asthma, respiratory syncytial virus
Bronchospasm	Asthma
Distal airway weakening	Emphysema

(Fig. 4.2). The concentration of He is normally 10%. During the test, the patient is "switched in" to a closed-circuit system at the end of a normal tidal volume breath or at the top of the FRC (see Fig. 4.1). A helium analyzer continuously monitors the helium concentration, and the exhaled carbon dioxide is chemically removed from the system. The gas in the patient's FRC, which at the beginning of the test contained no helium, mixes with the gas in the closed-circuit system. This causes the helium to spread throughout the entire closed-circuit system—the patient's lungs, spirometer, and circuit. When the helium concentration changes by 0.2%, or less, over a 1-second period, the test is completed. The helium concentration at this point is C_2. The final volume of the entire system—the helium circuit and lungs (V_2)—now can be calculated by using the following equation:

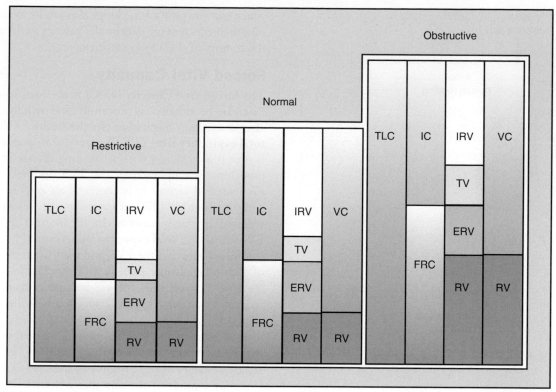

FIGURE 4.1 Visual comparison of lung volumes and capacities in obstructive and restrictive lung disorders. (From Kacmarek, R. M., Stoller, J. K., & Albert, H. J. [2017]. *Egan's fundamentals of respiratory care* [11th ed.]. St. Louis, MO: Elsevier.)

$$V_1 C_1 = V_2 C_2$$

which can be rearranged to solve for V_2 as follows:

$$V_2 = \frac{V_1 C_1}{C_2}.$$

The FRC can be calculated by subtracting the initial spirometer volume (V_1) from the equilibrium volume (V_2) as follows: $FRC = V_2 - V_1$. The RV can be calculated by subtracting the ERV from the FRC: $FRC - ERV$. The TLC can be determined by adding the VC to the RV—$RV + VC$.

For the **open-circuit nitrogen washout test**, the patient inhales and exhales 100% oxygen through a one-way valve for about 7 minutes (Fig. 4.3). At the start of the test, the concentration of nitrogen (N_2) in the alveoli is 79% (C_1). After a few moments into the test, the patient is switched in to the system at the end of a normal tidal volume—or, at the top of the FRC (see Fig. 4.1). At this point, the patient inhales 100% oxygen and exhales nitrogen-rich gas from the FRC. Over the next several minutes, the nitrogen in the patient's FRC progressively washes out. During the washout period, the exhaled gas volume is measured and the average nitrogen concentration is measured with a nitrogen analyzer. The test is terminated when the nitrogen concentration drops to 1.5% or less, at which time a forced expiration is performed and the $F_A N_2$ alveolar 2 is recorded. Based on the initial nitrogen concentration and the final nitrogen concentration, the volume of air in the patient's lungs at the start of the test—that is, the FRC—can be calculated as follows:

$$FRC = \frac{F_E N_2 \text{ final} \times \text{Expired Volume} - N_2 \text{ tissue}}{F_A N_2 \text{ alveolar } 1 - F_A N_2 \text{ alveolar } 2}$$

where:

$F_E N_2$ final = Fraction of N_2 in volume expired.

$F_A N_2$ alveolar 1 = Fraction of N_2 in alveolar gas initially (0.79).

$F_A N_2$ alveolar 2 = Fraction of N_2 in alveolar gas at end of the test (from the final alveolar–end expiratory) sample.

N_2 tissue = Volume of N_2 washed out of blood and tissues. A correction must be made for the N_2 washed out of the blood and tissue. It is estimated that for each minute of oxygen breathing, about 30 to 40 mL of N_2 is removed from the blood and tissue. This value is subtracted from the total volume of N_2 washed out.

Body plethysmography measures the volume of gas in the lungs (thoracic gas volume [VTG]) indirectly by applying a modification of Boyle's law. The patient sits in an airtight chamber called a *plethysmograph* (body box; Fig. 4.4). During the first part of the test, the patient breathes quietly in and out through an open valve (shutter). Once the patient is relaxed, the patient is switched in to the system at the end of a normal tidal volume—that is, at the level at which only the FRC remains in the lungs. At this point, the shutter valve is closed and the patient is instructed to pant against the closed shutter. Pressure and volume changes are monitored during this time. The alveolar pressure changes created by the compression and decompression of the lungs are estimated at the patient's mouth. Because there is no air flow during this period, and because the temperature is kept constant, the pressure and volume changes can be used to calculate the trapped volume—the FRC—by applying Boyle's law. Body plethysmography is generally considered to be the most precise of the three methods for measuring the RV and FRC.

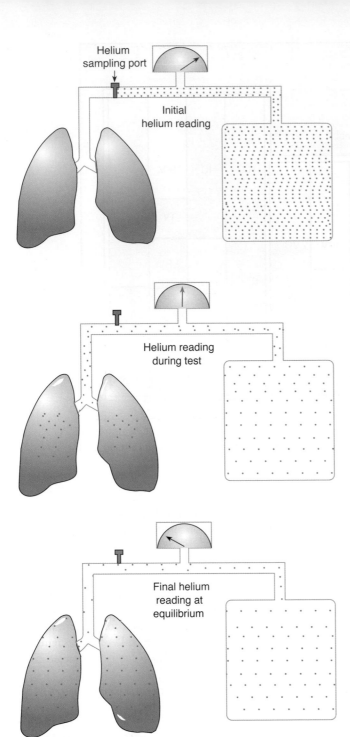

FIGURE 4.2 Helium dilution method for measuring functional residual capacity, residual volume, and total lung capacity. (From Kacmarek, R. M., Stoller, J. K., & Albert, H. J. [2017]. *Egan's fundamentals of respiratory care* [11th ed.]. St. Louis, MO: Elsevier.)

Body plethysmography also can measure *airway resistance* (R_{aw}) and airway conductance ($1/R_{aw}$). Patient claustrophobia in the plethysmograph sometimes limits the application of this valuable test.

Forced Expiratory Flow Rate and Volume Measurements

In addition to the volumes and capacities that can be measured by pulmonary function testing, the flow rate and volume at which gas flows out of the lungs also can be measured. Such measurements provide data on the patency of the airways and the severity of the airway impairment.

Forced Vital Capacity

The **forced vital capacity (FVC)** is the total volume of gas that can be exhaled as forcefully and rapidly as possible after a maximal inspiration. In the healthy individual, the **total expiratory time (TET)** necessary to perform an FVC is 4 to 6 seconds. In obstructive lung disease (e.g., chronic bronchitis or emphysema), the TET increases because of the increased airway resistance and air trapping associated with the disorder. TETs of more than 10 seconds have been reported in these patients. In the normal individual the FVC equals the **vital capacity (VC)**. Clinically, the lungs are considered normal if the FVC and the VC are within 200 mL of each other. In the patient with obstructive lung disease, the FVC is lower than the VC because of increased airway resistance and air trapping associated with maximal effort (Fig. 4.5).

A decreased FVC is also a common clinical manifestation in the patient with a restrictive lung disorder (e.g., pneumonia, acute respiratory distress syndrome, atelectasis). This decrease is mainly a result of the fact that restrictive lung disorders reduce the patient's ability to fully expand the lungs, thus reducing the VC necessary to generate a good FVC exhalation. However, the TET required to perform an FVC exhalation is usually normal or even less than normal because of the high lung elasticity (low lung compliance) associated with restrictive disorders.

A number of pulmonary function values can be calculated from a single FVC maneuver. The most common measurements obtained are as follows:

- Forced expiratory volume timed (FEV_T)
- Forced expiratory volume in 1 second/forced vital capacity ratio (FEV_1/FVC ratio)
- Forced expiratory flow between 200 and 1200 mL of FVC ($FEF_{200-1200}$)
- Forced expiratory flow at 25% to 75% ($FEF_{25\%-75\%}$)
- Peak expiratory flow rate (PEFR)

Forced Expiratory Volume Timed

The maximum volume of gas that can be exhaled over a specific period is the **forced expiratory volume timed (FEV_T)**. This measurement is obtained from an FVC measurement. Commonly used time periods are 0.5, 1.0, 2.0, 3.0, and 6.0 seconds. The most commonly used time period is 1 second (**forced expiratory volume in 1 second [FEV_1]**). In the normal adult, the percentages of the total volume exhaled during these periods are $FEV_{0.5}$, 60%; FEV_1, 83%; FEV_2, 94%; and FEV_3, 97%. In obstructive disease, the FEV_T is decreased because the time necessary to exhale a certain volume forcefully is increased (Fig. 4.6). Although the FEV_T may be normal in restrictive lung disorders (e.g., pneumonia, acute respiratory distress syndrome, atelectasis), it is commonly decreased because of the decreased VC associated with restrictive disorders (similar to the FVC in restrictive disorders). The FEV_T progressively decreases with age (about 23 mL per year after age 18).

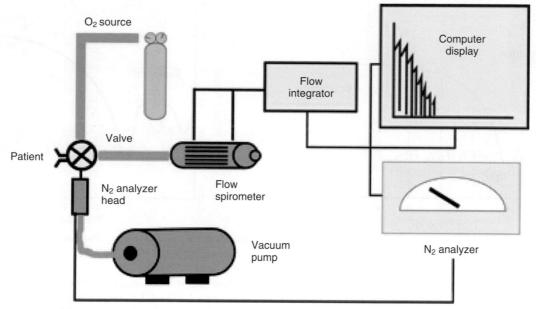

FIGURE 4.3 Open-circuit equipment used for N_2 washout determination of functional residual capacity (FRC). The patient inspires O_2 from a regulated source and exhales past a rapidly responding N_2 analyzer into a pneumotachometer. FRC is calculated from the total volume of N_2 exhaled and the change in alveolar N_2 from the beginning to the end of the test. (From Mottram, C. D. [2018]. *Ruppel's manual of pulmonary function testing* [11th ed.]. St. Louis, MO: Elsevier.)

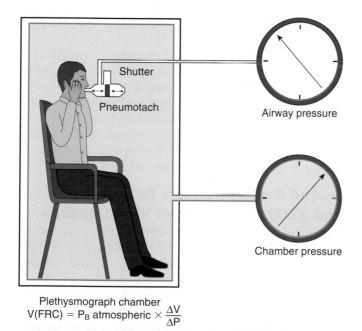

Plethysmograph chamber

$$V(FRC) = P_B \text{ atmospheric} \times \frac{\Delta V}{\Delta P}$$

FIGURE 4.4 Body plethysmography method for measuring lung volumes. V is the change in gas volume in the lungs, as sensed by the chamber pressure manometer. P is the change in pressure produced by the respiratory effort of breathing against the shutter, as sensed by the airway pressure manometer. (From Kacmarek, R. M., Stoller, J. K., & Albert, H. J. [2017]. *Egan's fundamentals of respiratory care* [11th ed.]. St. Louis, MO: Elsevier.)

Forced Expiratory Volume in 1 Second/ Forced Vital Capacity (FEV$_1$/FVC) Ratio

The **FEV$_1$/FVC ratio** compares the amount of air exhaled in 1 second with the total amount exhaled during an FVC maneuver. Because the FEV$_1$/FVC ratio is expressed as a percentage, it is commonly referred to as the **forced expiratory**

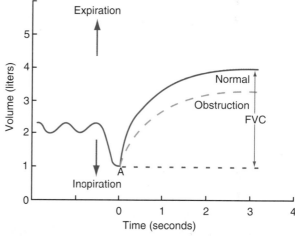

FIGURE 4.5 Forced vital capacity (FVC). A is the point of maximal inspiration and the starting point of an FVC maneuver. Note the reduction in FVC in obstructive pulmonary disease.

volume in 1 second percentage (FEV$_{1\%}$). Simply stated, the FEV$_1$/FVC ratio provides the percentage of the patient's total volume of air forcefully exhaled (FVC) in 1 second. As discussed earlier in the section on FEV$_T$, the normal adult exhales 83% or more of the FVC in 1 second (FEV$_1$). Therefore the FEV$_1$/FVC ratio also should be 83% or greater under normal circumstances. The FEV$_{1\%}$ and the FEV$_1$/FVC ratio progressively decrease with age. According to the Global Initiative for Chronic Obstructive Lung Disease (GOLD), the American Thoracic Society (ATS), and European Respiratory Society (ERS), airway obstruction is considered to be present when the FEV$_1$/FVC ratio is less than 70%.

Clinically, the FVC, FEV$_1$, and FEV$_{1\%}$ are commonly used to assess the severity of a patient's pulmonary disorder and determine whether the patient has an obstructive or a restrictive

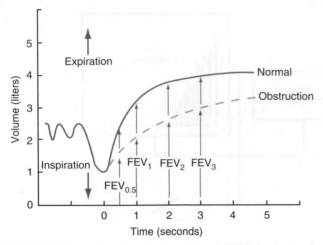

FIGURE 4.6 Forced expiratory volume timed (FEV$_T$). In obstructive pulmonary disease, more time is needed to exhale a specified volume.

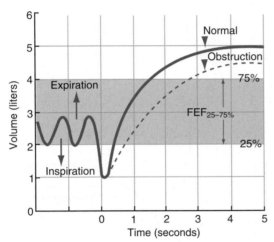

FIGURE 4.7 Forced expiratory flow at 25% to 75% (FEF$_{25\%-75\%}$). This test measures the average rate of flow between 25% and 75% of a forced vital capacity (FVC) maneuver. The flow rate is measured when 25% of the FVC has been exhaled and again when 75% of the FVC has been exhaled. The average rate of flow is derived by dividing the combined flow rates by 2. Note that expiration (in this figure) starts at 1.0 L on the upward axis.

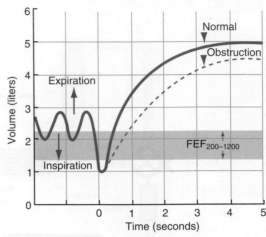

FIGURE 4.8 Forced expiratory flow between 200 and 1200 mL of forced vital capacity (FVC) (FEF$_{200-1200}$). This test measures the average rate of flow between 200 mL and 1200 mL of the FVC. The flow rate is measured when 200 mL has been exhaled and again when 1200 mL has been exhaled. The average rate of flow is derived by dividing the combined flow rates by 2. Note that expiration (in this figure) starts at 1.0 L on the upward axis.

lung disorder. The primary pulmonary function study differences between an obstructive and a restrictive lung disorder are as follows:

- In an obstructive disorder, the FEV$_1$ and FEV$_{1\%}$ are both decreased. The FVC is often normal.
- In a classic restrictive disorder, the FVC and FEV$_1$ are decreased and the FEV$_{1\%}$ is normal or increased.

Forced Expiratory Flow 25% to 75%

The **forced expiratory flow 25%–75% (FEF$_{25\%-75\%}$)** is the average flow rate generated by the patient during the middle 50% of an FVC measurement (Fig. 4.7). This expiratory maneuver is used to evaluate the status of medium to small airways in obstructive lung disorders. The normal FEF$_{25\%-75\%}$ in a healthy man 20 to 30 years of age is about 4.5 L/s (270 L/min). The normal FEF$_{25\%-75\%}$ in a healthy woman 20 to 30

years of age is about 3.5 L/s (210 L/min). The FEF$_{25\%-75\%}$ is somewhat effort-dependent because it depends on the FVC exhaled.

The FEF$_{25\%-75\%}$ progressively decreases in obstructive diseases and with age. The FEF$_{25\%-75\%}$ also may be decreased in moderate or severe restrictive lung disorders. This decrease is believed to be caused primarily by the reduced cross-sectional area of the small airways associated with restrictive lung problems. Clinically, the FEF$_{25\%-75\%}$ is often used to further confirm or rule out the presence of an obstructive pulmonary disease in the patient with a borderline FEV$_{1\%}$ value.

Forced Expiratory Flow Between 200 and 1200 mL of Forced Vital Capacity

The **forced expiratory flow 200–1200 (FEF$_{200-1200}$)** measures the average flow rate between 200 and 1200 mL of an FVC (Fig. 4.8). The first 200 mL of the FVC is usually exhaled more slowly than at the average flow rate because of the normal inertia involved in the respiratory maneuver and the initial slow response time of the pulmonary function equipment. Because the FEF$_{200-1200}$ measures expiratory flows at high lung volumes (i.e., the initial part of the FVC), it provides a good assessment of the large upper airways. The FEF$_{200-1200}$ is relatively effort-dependent.

The normal FEF$_{200-1200}$ for the average healthy man 20 to 30 years of age is about 8 L/s (480 L/min). The normal FEF$_{200-1200}$ in the average healthy woman 20 to 30 years of age is about 5.5 L/s (330 L/min). The FEF$_{200-1200}$ decreases in obstructive lung disorders. The FEF$_{200-1200}$ is a good test to determine the patient's response to bronchodilator therapy. In restrictive lung disorders the FEF$_{200-1200}$ is usually normal because it measures the early expiratory flow rates during the first part of an FVC maneuver (i.e., when the patient's VC is at its highest level). The FEF$_{200-1200}$ progressively decreases with age.

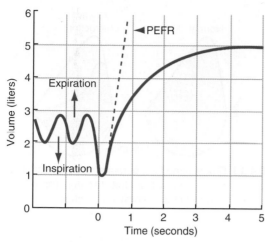

FIGURE 4.9 Peak expiratory flow rate (PEFR). The steepest slope of the ΔV̇/ΔT line is the PEFR (V̇).

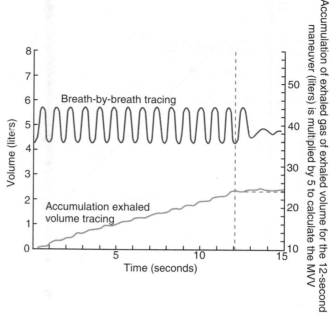

FIGURE 4.10 Volume-time tracing for a maximum voluntary ventilation (MVV) maneuver. Note that the patient actually performs the MVV maneuver for only 12 seconds, not 60 seconds.

Peak Expiratory Flow Rate

The **peak expiratory flow rate (PEFR)** (also known as the *peak flow rate*) is the maximum flow rate generated during an FVC maneuver (Fig. 4.9). The PEFR provides a good assessment of the large upper airways. It is very effort-dependent. The normal PEFR in the average healthy man 20 to 30 years of age is about 10 L/s (600 L/min). The normal PEFR in the average healthy woman 20 to 30 years of age is about 7.5 L/s (450 L/min). The PEFR decreases in obstructive lung diseases. In restrictive lung disorders, the PEFR is usually normal because it measures the early expiratory flow rates during the first part of an FVC maneuver (i.e., when the patient's VC is at its highest level). The PEFR progressively decreases with age.

The PEFR also can be measured easily at the patient's bedside with a hand-held peak flowmeter (e.g., Wright peak flowmeter). The hand-held peak flowmeter is used to monitor the degree of airway obstruction on a moment-to-moment basis and is relatively small, inexpensive, accurate, reproducible, and easy for the patient to use. In addition, the mouthpieces are disposable, thus allowing the safe use of the same peak flowmeter from one patient to another. PEFR measurements should routinely be performed at the patient's bedside to assess the degree of bronchospasm, effect of bronchodilators, and day-to-day progress. The PEFR results generated by the patient before and after bronchodilator therapy can serve as excellent objective data by which to assess the effectiveness of therapy.

Maximum Voluntary Ventilation

The **maximum voluntary ventilation (MVV)** is the largest volume of gas that can be breathed voluntarily in and out of the lungs in 1 minute (Fig. 4.10). The normal MVV in the average healthy man 20 to 30 years of age is about 170 L/min. The normal MVV in the average healthy woman 20 to 30 years of age is about 110 L/min. The MVV progressively decreases in obstructive pulmonary disorders. In restrictive pulmonary disorders, the MVV may be normal or decreased. It is very effort-dependent.

Flow-Volume Loop

The flow-volume loop is a graphic illustration of both a forced vital capacity (FVC) maneuver and a **forced inspiratory volume**

(FIV) maneuver. The FVC and FIV are plotted together as two curves that form what is called a **flow-volume loop**. As shown in Fig. 4.11, the upper half of the flow-volume loop (above the zero-flow axis) represents the maximum expiratory flow generated at various lung volumes during an FVC maneuver plotted against volume. This portion of the curve shows the flow generated between the TLC and RV. An excellent example of this portion of the flow-volume loop is shown in Fig. 4.12, where "chatter" caused by a large pedunculated endobronchial tumor in the trachea was identified using this technology. Poor patient effort also can be identified on the "flow portion" of the flow-volume loop—for example, the upper half of the flow-volume loop (above the zero-flow axis) will show flow decrease, hesitation, or flow stoppage altogether, and there will be variability between successive patient efforts.

The lower half of the flow-volume loop (below the zero-flow axis) illustrates the maximum inspiratory flow generated at various lung volumes during a forced inspiration (called a *forced inspiratory volume [FIV]* plotted against the volume inhaled. This portion of the curve shows the flow generated between the RV and TLC. Depending on the sophistication of the equipment, several important pulmonary function study values can be obtained, including the following:

- FVC
- FEV_T
- $FEF_{25\%-75\%}$
- $FEF_{200-1200}$
- PEFR
- Peak inspiratory flow rate (PIFR)
- **Forced expiratory flow at 50% ($FEF_{50\%}$)**
- Instantaneous flow at any given lung volume during forced inhalation and exhalation

In the normal subject the expiratory flow rate decreases linearly during an FVC maneuver, immediately after the PEFR

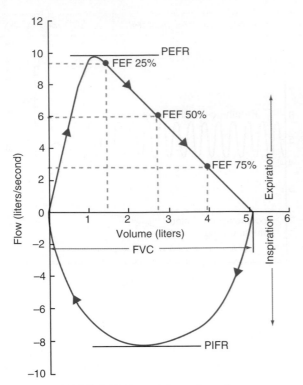

FIGURE 4.11 Normal flow-volume loop.

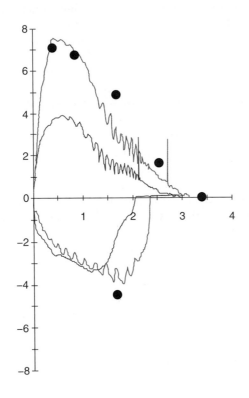

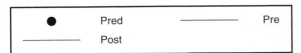

●	Pred	——	Pre
		——	Post

FIGURE 4.12 Flow-volume loop "chatter" seen in a patient with a pedunculated (vibrating) endobronchial tumor.

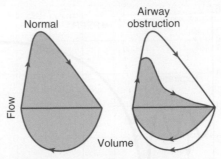

FIGURE 4.13 Flow-volume loop demonstrating the shape change that results from an obstructive lung disorder. The curve on the right represents intrathoracic airway obstruction.

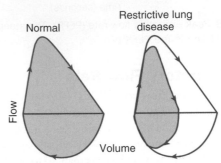

FIGURE 4.14 Flow-volume loop demonstrating the shape change that results from a restrictive lung disorder. Note the symmetric loss of flow and volume.

has been achieved. In the patient with an obstructive lung disease, however, the flow rate decreases in a nonlinear fashion after the PEFR has been reached. This nonlinear flow rate causes a cuplike or scooped-out appearance in the expiratory flow curve when 50% of the FVC has been exhaled. This portion of the flow curve is the $FEF_{50\%}$, or $\dot{V}_{max\,50}$ (Fig. 4.13). Table 4.7 summarizes the forced expiratory flow rate and volume measurements and the normal values found in healthy men and women ages 20 to 30 years.

Table 4.8 provides an overview of the expiratory flow rate measurements characteristic of restrictive lung disorders. In these disorders, flow and volume are, in general, reduced equally. Clinically, this phenomenon is referred to as *symmetric reduction* in flows and volumes. The flow-volume loop is therefore a small version of normal in restrictive pulmonary disease (Fig. 4.14).

Table 4.9 provides an overview of the expiratory flow rate measurements characteristic of obstructive lung disorders. Obstructive lung disorders cause increased airway resistance (R_{aw}) and airway closure during expiration. When R_{aw} becomes high, the patient's ventilatory rate decreases and the tidal volume increases. This ventilatory pattern is thought to be an adaptation to reduce the work of breathing (see Fig. 3.4).

Pulmonary Diffusion Capacity

The **pulmonary diffusion capacity of carbon monoxide (DLCO)** measures the amount of carbon monoxide (CO) that moves across the alveolar-capillary membrane. When the patient has a normal hemoglobin concentration, pulmonary capillary blood volume, and ventilatory status, the only limiting

TABLE 4.7 Normal Forced Expiratory Flow Rate Measurements in Healthy Men and Women 20 to 30 Years of Age

Forced Expiratory Flow Rate Measurement	Men	Women
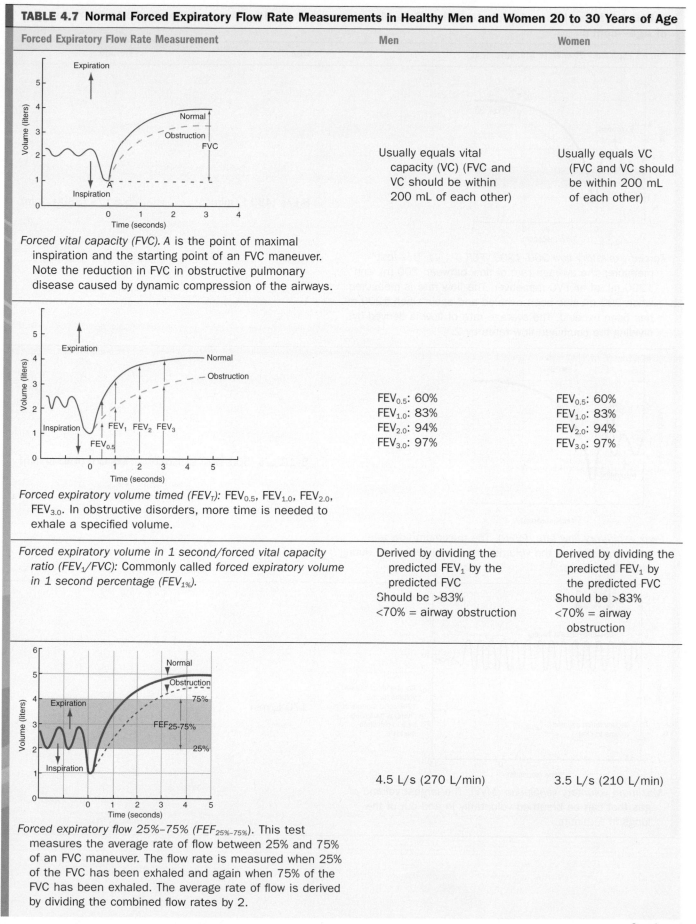_Forced vital capacity (FVC)._ A is the point of maximal inspiration and the starting point of an FVC maneuver. Note the reduction in FVC in obstructive pulmonary disease caused by dynamic compression of the airways.	Usually equals vital capacity (VC) (FVC and VC should be within 200 mL of each other)	Usually equals VC (FVC and VC should be within 200 mL of each other)
Forced expiratory volume timed (FEV$_T$): FEV$_{0.5}$, FEV$_{1.0}$, FEV$_{2.0}$, FEV$_{3.0}$. In obstructive disorders, more time is needed to exhale a specified volume.	FEV$_{0.5}$: 60% FEV$_{1.0}$: 83% FEV$_{2.0}$: 94% FEV$_{3.0}$: 97%	FEV$_{0.5}$: 60% FEV$_{1.0}$: 83% FEV$_{2.0}$: 94% FEV$_{3.0}$: 97%
Forced expiratory volume in 1 second/forced vital capacity ratio (FEV$_1$/FVC): Commonly called _forced expiratory volume in 1 second percentage (FEV$_{1\%}$)._	Derived by dividing the predicted FEV$_1$ by the predicted FVC Should be >83% <70% = airway obstruction	Derived by dividing the predicted FEV$_1$ by the predicted FVC Should be >83% <70% = airway obstruction
Forced expiratory flow 25%–75% (FEF$_{25\%-75\%}$). This test measures the average rate of flow between 25% and 75% of an FVC maneuver. The flow rate is measured when 25% of the FVC has been exhaled and again when 75% of the FVC has been exhaled. The average rate of flow is derived by dividing the combined flow rates by 2.	4.5 L/s (270 L/min)	3.5 L/s (210 L/min)

Continued

Forced Expiratory Flow Rate Measurement	Men	Women
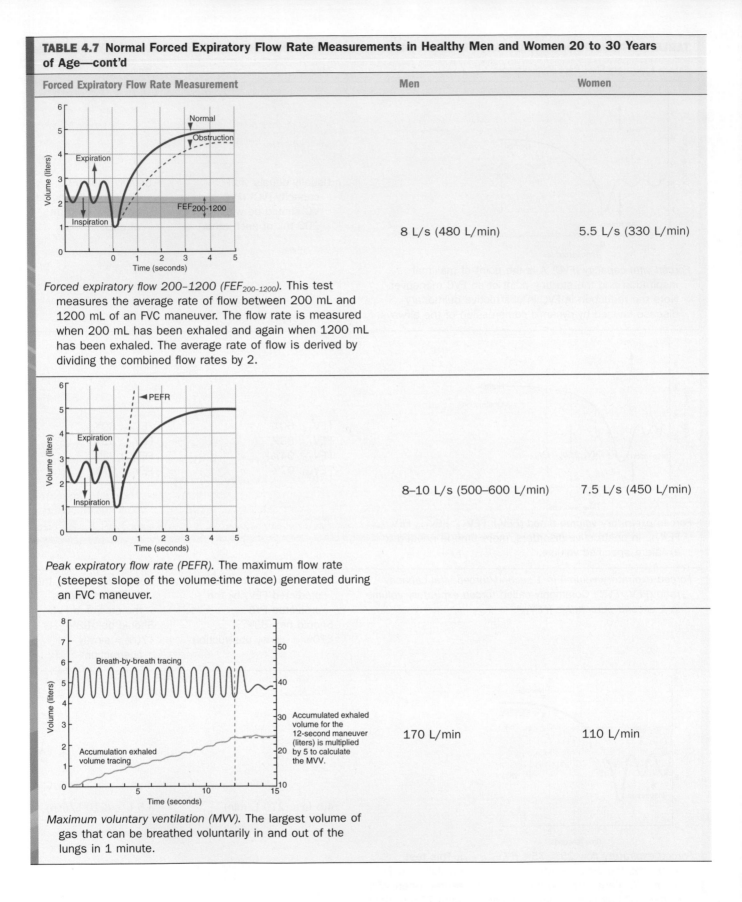 *Forced expiratory flow 200–1200 (FEF$_{200-1200}$).* This test measures the average rate of flow between 200 mL and 1200 mL of an FVC maneuver. The flow rate is measured when 200 mL has been exhaled and again when 1200 mL has been exhaled. The average rate of flow is derived by dividing the combined flow rates by 2.	8 L/s (480 L/min)	5.5 L/s (330 L/min)
Peak expiratory flow rate (PEFR). The maximum flow rate (steepest slope of the volume-time trace) generated during an FVC maneuver.	8–10 L/s (500–600 L/min)	7.5 L/s (450 L/min)
Maximum voluntary ventilation (MVV). The largest volume of gas that can be breathed voluntarily in and out of the lungs in 1 minute.	170 L/min	110 L/min

TABLE 4.8 Restrictive Lung Disease
Forced Expiratory Flow Rate and Volume Findings

FVC	FEV_T	FEV_1/FVC	$FEF_{25\%-75\%}$
↓	N or ↓	N or ↑	N or ↓
$FEF_{50\%}$	$FEF_{200-1200}$	PEFR	MVV
N or ↓	N or ↓	N or ↓	N or ↓

$FEF_{25\%-75\%}$, Forced expiratory flow 25%–75%; $FEF_{50\%}$, forced expiratory flow at 50%; $FEF_{200-1200}$, forced expiratory flow 200–1200 mL of FVC; FEV_1/FVC, forced expiratory volume in 1 second/forced vital capacity ratio; FEV_T, forced expiratory volume timed; FVC, forced vital capacity; MVV, maximum voluntary ventilation; N, normal; PEFR, peak expiratory flow rate.

TABLE 4.9 Obstructive Lung Disease
Forced Expiratory Flow Rate and Volume Findings

FVC	FEV_T	FEV_1/FVC	$FEF_{25\%-75\%}$
↓	↓	↓	↓
$FEF_{50\%}$	$FEF_{200-1200}$	PEFR	MVV
↓	↓	↓	↓

$FEF_{25\%-75\%}$, Forced expiratory flow 25%–75%; $FEF_{50\%}$, forced expiratory flow at 50%; $FEF_{200-1200}$, forced expiratory flow 200–1200 mL of FVC; FEV_1/FVC, forced expiratory volume in 1 second/forced vital capacity ratio; FEV_T, forced expiratory volume timed; FVC, forced vital capacity; MVV, maximum voluntary ventilation; N, normal; PEFR, peak expiratory flow rate.

TABLE 4.10 Pulmonary Diffusion Capacity of Carbon Monoxide

Obstructive lung disorders*	Restrictive lung disorders†
N or ↓	N or ↓

*A decreased DLCO is a hallmark clinical manifestation in emphysema (because of the destruction of the alveolar pulmonary capillaries and decreased surface area for gas diffusion associated with the disease). The DLCO, especially when corrected for alveolar volume (VA), is usually normal in all other obstructive lung disorders.

†This is usually decreased when moderate to severe alveolar atelectasis, alveolar consolidation, or increased alveolar-capillary membrane thickness is present in the restrictive lung disorder.

N, Normal.

factor to the diffusion of carbon monoxide is the alveolar-capillary membrane. Under normal conditions, the average DLCO value for the resting man is 25 mL/min/mm Hg (STPD, A volume of gas, at the standard (S) temperature (T) of 0°C and a barometric pressure (P) of 760 mmHg, and in a dry state (D)). This value is slightly lower in women, presumably because of their smaller normal lung volumes. Table 4.10 provides a general guide to conditions that alter the patient's DLCO.

Assessment of Respiratory Muscle Strength

The most commonly used tests to evaluate the patient's respiratory muscle strength at the bedside are maximum inspiratory pressure (MIP) and maximum expiratory pressure (MEP), forced vital capacity (FVC), and maximum voluntary ventilation (MVV). (See page 61 for discussion of FVC and page 58 for discussion of MVV.)

Maximum inspiratory pressure (MIP), also called *the negative inspiratory force (NIF)*, is the maximum inspiratory pressure the patient is able to generate against a closed airway and is recorded as a negative number in either centimeters of water or millimeters of mercury. The MIP can be measured through an endotracheal tube or by using a mask or mouthpiece and an external pressure gauge. The MIP primarily measures inspiratory muscle strength—that is, the power of the diaphragm and external intercostal muscles.

In the normal healthy adult, the MIP is about −80 to −100 cm H_2O. Ideally, the MIP should be measured at the patient's residual volume. An MIP of −25 cm H_2O or less (more negative) usually indicates adequate muscle strength to maintain spontaneous breathing. An MIP of −20 cm H_2O or greater (less negative) is a strong indicator for the need for ventilatory support (see Protocols 11.1 and 11.2). Reduced MIP values are also commonly seen in patients with neuromuscular disease (e.g., amyotrophic lateral sclerosis [ALS], Guillain-Barré syndrome, or myasthenia gravis), chronic obstructive pulmonary disease (COPD), and chest wall deformities (e.g., kyphoscoliosis).

Maximum expiratory pressure (MEP) is the highest pressure that can be generated during a forceful expiratory effort against an occluded airway and is recorded as a positive number in either centimeters of water or millimeters of mercury. The MEP primarily measures the strength of the abdominal muscles—that is, the rectus abdominis muscles, external abdominis obliquus muscles, internal abdominis obliquus muscles, transversus abdominis muscles, and internal intercostal muscles. Ideally, the MEP is measured at maximal inspiration (near the total lung capacity). The adult normal MEP is greater than 100 cm H_2O in males and greater than 80 cm H_2O in females. Unsatisfactory MEP values are commonly seen in patients with neuromuscular disease (e.g., ALS, Guillain-Barré syndrome, or myasthenia gravis), COPD, and high cervical spine fractures. Finally, it should be noted that a low MEP is associated with a poor or inadequate cough effort. Thus in patients with excessive airway secretions (e.g., chronic bronchitis or cystic fibrosis) a low MEP, accompanied by the inability to effectively mobilize airway secretions, can further complicate the patient's respiratory condition.

Cardiopulmonary Exercise Testing

When one considers the fact that *dyspnea on exertion* is the most common sign of pulmonary disease (see Chapter 3, Dyspnea), it should be noted that the pulmonary function tests, as described in the foregoing text, are all *done at rest*. Tests done during exercise range from simple and inexpensive (e.g., the 6-minute walk used in pulmonary rehabilitation) to the more complex **cardiopulmonary exercise test (CPET)** with or without blood gas analyses. CPET involves treadmill or bicycle ergometer testing while a variety of physiologic parameters are measured and/or calculated (Box 4.1). Contraindications to CPET are listed in Box 4.2.

Although the performance and interpretation of CPET variables are beyond the scope of this volume, evaluation of the physiologic data seen with increasing exercise, at or near the **anaerobic threshold (AT)**, at which minute ventilation as a function of oxygen consumption increases sharply in response to the onset of metabolic acidosis, can assist in the clinical diagnosis of malingering and deconditioning, obesity, hyperventilation/anxiety, coronary artery disease, neuromuscular disease, congestive heart failure/valvular heart disease, interstitial lung disease, obstructive pulmonary disease, pulmonary vascular disease, and for the purpose of disability determinations.

Other Diagnostic Tests for Asthma

Because some patients have clinical manifestations associated with asthma, but otherwise normal lung function between asthma episodes, measurements of airway responsiveness to **inhaled methacholine or histamine**, or an indirect challenge test to **inhaled mannitol**, or to an **exercise or cold air challenge** may be useful in confirming a diagnosis of asthma (see Chapter 14, Asthma). These inhalation challenge tests can be performed only when the patient has an FEV_1 of 80% or greater, to avoid electively inducing significant asthma symptoms in an already compromised patient.

Impulse Oscillometry[1]

Impulse oscillometry (IOS) is a simple, noninvasive, effort-independent test that applies oscillating pressure impulses to the lungs during normal passive breathing. It is used to assess both large and small airway obstructions. A small loudspeaker placed close to the patient's mouthpiece generates the pressure impulses. The pressure impulses are superimposed on the normal tidal volume as the patient inhales and exhales. Pressure-flow transducers measure the impulse changes and, subsequently, separated from the breathing pattern by "signal filtering." The following two types of pressure oscillations are measured during this test:

- **Resistance (Rrs)** pressure oscillations: Oscillations that are in phase with air flow. Resistance represents the energy required to move a pressure wave through the bronchi and bronchioles and to distend the lung parenchyma. Resistance pressure oscillations are determined when the pressure waves are unopposed by airway recoil and are in phase with air flow.
- **Reactance (Xrs)** pressure oscillations: Oscillations that are out of phase with air flow. Reactance represents the energy generated by the elastic recoil of the lungs after distention and inertia.

Respiratory impedance (Zrs) is the sum of all the forces (i.e., $Zrs = Rrs + Xrs$) and is calculated from the ratio of pressure and flow at each frequency during the test.

The pressure oscillations are applied at a fixed (square wave) frequency of 5 Hz, from which all other frequencies of interest are derived. Low-frequency oscillations (5 Hz) penetrate throughout the small airways of the lung periphery, where high-frequency impulses (20 Hz) only reach the proximal airways. When analyzed, these pressure changes separately quantify the degree of obstruction in the central and peripheral airways.

Because the test is easy to administer, it is commonly used with preschool and school-aged children and adults with physical and cognitive limitations (Fig. 4.15). IOS is also used to measure bronchodilator response and bronchoprovocation testing. IOS can also be performed in patients on ventilators and during sleep. Fig. 4.16 shows graphs of IOS and spirometry in patients with normal, obstructive, and restrictive lung disease.

---

[1]In 1956, DuBois et al. described the forced oscillation technique (FOT) as a tool to measure lung function using sinusoidal sound waves of single frequencies generated by a loud speaker and passed into the lungs during tidal breathing. Dubois, A. B., Brody, A. W., Lewis, D. H., et al. (1956). Oscillation mechanics of lungs and chest in man. *Journal of Applied Physiology 8,* 587-594.

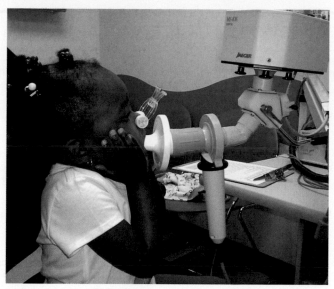

FIGURE 4.15 Impulse oscillometry (IOS) test performed on a 5-year-old child. During the test, the sitting position is preferred. Nose clips should be worn, and the mouthpiece should be positioned so that the neck is slightly extended. Ensure a tight seal between the mouthpiece and lips, and the patient's cheeks should be held firmly by the patient or examiner from behind. The patient is instructed to perform relaxed, normal tidal breathing between 30 and 45 seconds. During this time, about 120 to 150 oscillations are transmitted throughout the lungs while, at the same time, the pressure-flow sensors determine the mean resistance, reactance, and respiratory impedance values between frequencies of 5 and 20 Hz. A minimum of three tests should be performed. If there are breathing segments that contain artifacts (e.g., caused by coughing, gagging, swallowing, air leaks, or tongue obstructions), they should be discarded. (Courtesy Dayton Children's Hospital, Dayton, Ohio.)

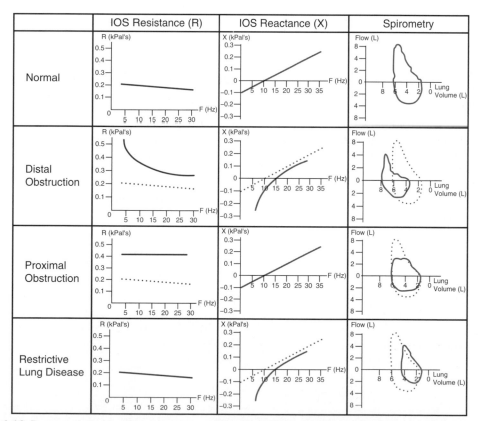

FIGURE 4.16 Representative graphs of impulse oscillometry (IOS) and spirometry in patients with normal, obstructive, and restrictive lung disease. Tracings of lung resistance and reactance in comparison with spirometric flow-volume loop for prototypical patients with normal lung function, distal obstruction, proximal obstruction, and restrictive lung disease. Dotted lines indicate the normal tracing, and solid lines show pathologic tracings.

1. What is the PEFR in the normal healthy woman 20 to 30 years of age?
   a. 250 L/min
   b. 350 L/min
   c. 450 L/min
   d. 550 L/min

2. A restrictive lung disorder is confirmed when the:
   1. FEV_1 is decreased
   2. FVC is increased
   3. FEV_1/FVC ratio is normal or increased
   4. FEV_1 is increased
      a. 1 only
      b. 4 only
      c. 1 and 3 only
      d. 2 and 4 only

3. Which of the following expiratory maneuver findings are characteristic of restrictive lung disease?
   1. Normal FVC
   2. Decreased $FEF_{25\%-75\%}$
   3. Increased PEFR
   4. Decreased FEV_T
      a. 1 and 3 only
      b. 2 and 4 only
      c. 3 and 4 only
      d. 2 and 3 only

4. In an obstructive lung disorder, which of the following occurs?
   1. FRC is decreased
   2. RV is increased
   3. VC is decreased
   4. IRV is increased
      a. 1 and 3 only
      b. 2 and 3 only
      c. 2 and 4 only
      d. 2, 3, and 4 only

5. Under normal conditions, the average DLCO value for the resting man is which of the following?
   a. 10 mL/min/mm Hg
   b. 15 mL/min/mm Hg
   c. 20 mL/min/mm Hg
   d. 25 mL/min/mm Hg

6. What is the vital capacity of the normal recumbent man 20 to 30 years of age?
   a. 2700 mL
   b. 3200 mL
   c. 4000 mL
   d. 4800 mL

7. What is the normal percentage of the total volume exhaled during an FEV_1?
   a. 60%
   b. 83%
   c. 94%
   d. 97%

8. Which of the following can be obtained from a flow-volume loop study?
   1. FVC
   2. PEFR
   3. FEV_T
   4. $FEF_{25\%-75\%}$
      a. 4 only
      b. 1 and 2 only
      c. 1, 3, and 4 only
      d. 1, 2, 3, and 4

9. An obstructive lung disorder is confirmed when the:
   1. FEV_1 is decreased
   2. FVC is increased
   3. FEV_1 is increased
   4. FEV_1/FVC ratio is decreased
      a. 3 only
      b. 4 only
      c. 1 and 3 only
      d. 1 and 4 only

10. Which of the following anatomic alterations of the lungs is or are associated with a restrictive lung disorder?
    1. Bronchospasm
    2. Atelectasis
    3. Distal airway weakening
    4. Consolidation
       a. 1 only
       b. 3 only
       c. 2 and 4 only
       d. 1 and 3 only

CHAPTER

5 Blood Gas Assessment

Chapter Objectives

After reading this chapter, you will be able to:

- Identify the respiratory acid-base disturbances.
- Identify the metabolic acid-base disturbances.
- Identify the combined acid-base disturbances.
- Describe the $PCO_2/pH/HCO_3^-$ relationship.
- Describe the most common acid-base abnormalities seen in the clinical setting.
- Describe the metabolic acid-base abnormalities, including metabolic acidosis, anion gap, and metabolic alkalosis.
- List the causes of metabolic acidosis and metabolic alkalosis.
- Describe the potential common errors in the sampling, analysis, and interpretation of arterial blood gas assessments.
- Define key terms and complete self-assessment questions at the end of the chapter and on Evolve.

Key Terms

Acute Alveolar Hyperventilation
Acute Alveolar Hyperventilation With Partial Renal Compensation
Acute Alveolar Hyperventilation Superimposed on Chronic Ventilatory Failure
Acute Respiratory Acidosis
Acute Respiratory Alkalosis
Acute Ventilatory Failure
Acute Ventilatory Failure With Partial Renal Compensation
Acute Ventilatory Failure Superimposed on Chronic Ventilatory Failure
Anaerobic Metabolism

Anaerobic Threshold
Anion Gap
Chronic Alveolar Hyperventilation With Complete Renal Compensation
Chronic Ventilatory Failure
Chronic Ventilatory Failure With Complete Renal Compensation
Combined Metabolic and Respiratory Acidosis
Combined Metabolic and Respiratory Alkalosis
Compensated Respiratory Acidosis
Compensated Respiratory Alkalosis
Hyperchloremic Metabolic Acidosis
Hypoxemia
Lactic Acidosis
Law of Electroneutrality
Metabolic Acidosis
Metabolic Acidosis With Complete Respiratory Compensation
Metabolic Acidosis With Partial Respiratory Compensation
Metabolic Alkalosis
Metabolic Alkalosis With Complete Respiratory Compensation
Metabolic Alkalosis With Partial Respiratory Compensation

Chapter Outline

Acid-Base Abnormalities
    The $PCO_2/HCO_3^-/pH$ Relationship
    Common Acid-Base Abnormalities Seen in the Clinical Setting
    Metabolic Acid-Base Abnormalities
Errors Associated With Arterial Blood Gas Measurements
Self-Assessment Questions

Acid-Base Abnormalities

As the pathologic processes of a respiratory disorder intensify, the patient's arterial blood gas (ABG) values are usually altered to some degree. Table 5.1 lists the normal ABG values. Box 5.1 provides an overview of the common respiratory and metabolic acid-base disturbances. In the profession of respiratory care, knowledge and understanding of the acid-base disturbances are absolute and unconditional prerequisites to the assessment and treatment of the patient with a respiratory disorder. Because of the fundamental importance of this subject, this chapter provides the following review:

- The $PCO_2/HCO_3^-/pH$ relationship—an essential cornerstone of ABG interpretations

- The most common acid-base abnormalities seen in the clinical setting
- The metabolic acid-base abnormalities
- Errors associated with ABG measurements

The $PCO_2/HCO_3^-/pH$ Relationship

To fully understand the clinical significance of the acid-base disturbances listed in Box 5.1, a fundamental knowledge of the $PCO_2/HCO_3^-/pH$ relationship is essential. The $PCO_2/HCO_3^-/pH$ relationship is graphically illustrated in the $PCO_2/HCO_3^-/pH$ nomogram shown in Fig. 5.1. The $PCO_2/HCO_3^-/pH$ nomogram is an excellent clinical tool to identify acid-base disturbances. See Appendix XII on the Evolve site for a pocket-size $PCO_2/HCO_3^-/pH$ nomogram card that can

TABLE 5.1 Normal Blood Gas Values

Blood Gas Value*	Arterial	Venous
pH	7.35–7.45	7.30–7.40
$PaCO_2$	35–45 mm Hg	42–48 mm Hg
HCO_3^-	22–28 mEq/L	24–30 mEq/L
PaO_2	80–100 mm Hg	35–45 mm Hg

*Technically, only the oxygen (PaO_2) and carbon dioxide ($PaCO_2$) pressure readings are true blood gas values. The pH indicates the balance between the bases and acids in the blood. The bicarbonate (HCO_3^-) reading is an indirect measurement that is calculated from the pH and $PaCO_2$ levels.

BOX 5.1 Acid-Base Disturbance Classifications

Respiratory Acid-Base Disturbances

- Acute alveolar hyperventilation (acute respiratory alkalosis)
- Acute alveolar hyperventilation with partial renal compensation (partially compensated respiratory alkalosis)
- Chronic alveolar hyperventilation with complete renal compensation (compensated respiratory alkalosis)
- Acute ventilatory failure (acute respiratory acidosis)
- Acute ventilatory failure with partial renal compensation (partially compensated respiratory acidosis)
- Chronic ventilatory failure with complete renal compensation (compensated respiratory acidosis)
- Acute alveolar hyperventilation superimposed on chronic ventilatory failure
- Acute ventilatory failure superimposed on chronic ventilatory failure

Metabolic Acid-Base Disturbances

- Metabolic acidosis
- Metabolic acidosis with partial respiratory compensation
- Metabolic acidosis with complete respiratory compensation
- Metabolic alkalosis
- Metabolic alkalosis with partial respiratory compensation
- Metabolic alkalosis with complete respiratory compensation

Combined Acid-Base Disturbances

- Combined metabolic and respiratory acidosis
- Combined metabolic and respiratory alkalosis

Highlighted terms are included in the Key Terms list and glossary.

be cut out, laminated, and used as a handy ABG reference tool in the clinical setting.

How to Read the PCO₂/HCO₃⁻/pH Nomogram

The thick red bar moving from left to right across the PCO_2/HCO_3^-/pH nomogram represents the normal PCO_2 blood buffer line. This red bar is used to identify the pH and HCO_3^- changes that occur immediately in response to an acute increase or decrease in PCO_2. The purple bar is used to identify the pH and HCO_3^- changes that occur in response to acute metabolic acidosis and metabolic alkalosis conditions. The colored areas that surround the red and purple bars are used to identify (1) partial and complete renal compensation, (2) partial and complete respiratory compensation, and (3)

combined metabolic and respiratory acid-base disturbances (see Fig. 5.1).

For example, when the pH, PCO_2, and HCO_3^- values all intersect in the light purple area shown in the upper left-hand corner of the PCO_2/HCO_3^-/pH nomogram, partial renal compensation has occurred in response to a chronically high PCO_2 level. When the HCO_3^- increases enough to move the pH into the light-blue normal bar, complete renal compensation is confirmed. When the pH, PCO_2, and HCO_3^- values all intersect in the green area shown in the lower right-hand corner of the PCO_2/HCO_3^-/pH nomogram, partial renal compensation has occurred in response to a chronically low PCO_2 level. When the HCO_3^- decreases enough to move the pH into the light-blue normal bar, complete renal compensation is confirmed.

When the pH, PCO_2, and HCO_3^- values all intersect in the orange area shown immediately below the red bar on the left side of the PCO_2/HCO_3^-/pH nomogram, combined respiratory and metabolic acidosis is confirmed. When the pH, PCO_2, and HCO_3^- values all intersect in the blue area, shown immediately above the red bar on the right side of the PCO_2/HCO_3^-/pH nomogram, a combined respiratory and metabolic alkalosis is confirmed.

Finally, when the pH, PCO_2, and HCO_3^- values all intersect in the yellow area, shown in the lower left corner of the PCO_2/HCO_3^-/pH nomogram, respiratory compensation has occurred in response to metabolic acidosis. When the pH, PCO_2, and HCO_3^- values all intersect in the pink area, shown in the upper right corner of the PCO_2/HCO_3^-/pH nomogram, respiratory compensation has occurred in response to metabolic alkalosis.

Although it is beyond the scope of this textbook to fully explain how each of the acid-base disturbances listed in Box 5.1 can be identified on the PCO_2/HCO_3^-/pH nomogram, a basic understanding of the following two most commonly encountered PCO_2/HCO_3^-/pH relationships is important: (1) an acute PCO_2 increase and its effects on the pH and HCO_3^- values, and (2) an acute PCO_2 decrease and its effects on the pH and HCO_3^- values.[1]

How Acute PCO₂ Decreases Affect pH and HCO₃⁻ Values

The red normal PCO_2 blood buffer bar shown on the PCO_2/HCO_3^-/pH nomogram is also used to identify the pH and HCO_3^- values that will result immediately in response to a sudden decrease in PCO_2—for example, as a result of alveolar hyperventilation. For example, if the patient's $PaCO_2$ were suddenly to decrease to, say, 25 mm Hg, the pH would immediately increase to about 7.55 and the HCO_3^- level would decrease to about 21 mEq/L. In addition, the PCO_2/HCO_3^-/pH nomogram shows that these ABG values represent acute alveolar hyperventilation (acute respiratory alkalosis). This is shown by the fact that (1) all of the ABG values (i.e., PCO_2, HCO_3^-, and pH) intersect within the red normal PCO_2 blood buffer bar, and (2) the pH and HCO_3^- readings are precisely what are expected for an acute increase in the PCO_2 of 25 mm Hg (Fig. 5.2).

---

[1]For a complete review of the role of the relationship in acid-base balance, see Des Jardins, T. (2019). *Cardiopulmonary anatomy and physiology: essentials of respiratory care* (7th ed.). Clifton Park, NY: Delmar/Cengage Learning.

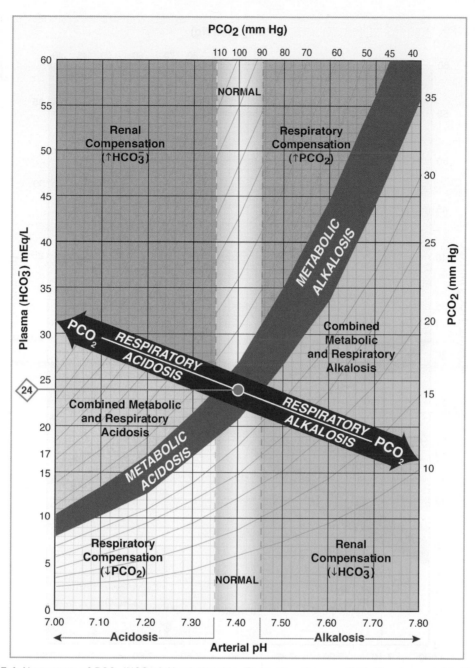

FIGURE 5.1 Nomogram of PCO_2/HCO_3^-/pH relationship. For explanation see text. The green dot in the middle of the red arrow represents the location of values for the normal pH, PCO_2, and HCO_3^- relationship in the arterial blood. (From Terry Des Jardins, with permission.)

How Acute PCO_2 Increases Affect the pH and HCO_3^- Values

As mentioned previously, the red normal PCO_2 blood buffer bar shown on the PCO_2/HCO_3^-/pH nomogram is used to identify the pH and HCO_3^- values that will result immediately in response to a sudden increase in PCO_2, such as a result of net alveolar hypoventilation. For example, if the patient's $PaCO_2$ were to suddenly increase to 60 mm Hg, the pH would immediately fall to about 7.28 and the HCO_3^- level would increase to about 26 mEq/L. Furthermore, the PCO_2/HCO_3^-/pH nomogram shows that these ABG values represent acute ventilatory failure (acute respiratory acidosis). This is shown by the fact that (1) all of the ABG values (i.e., PCO_2, HCO_3^-, and pH) intersect

within the red normal PCO_2 blood buffer bar, and (2) the pH and HCO_3^- readings are precisely what are expected for an acute increase in the PCO_2 of 60 mm Hg (Fig. 5.3).

A Quick Clinical Calculation for the Effect of Acute $PaCO_2$ Changes on pH and HCO_3^-: Rule of Thumb

In addition to using the graphic PCO_2/HCO_3^-/pH nomogram (see Fig. 5.1), the following simple calculations also can be used to estimate the expected pH and HCO_3^- value changes that will occur in response to a sudden increase or decrease in $PaCO_2$.

Acute Increases in $PaCO_2$ (e.g., Acute Hypoventilation). Using the normal ABG values as a baseline (e.g., pH 7.40, $PaCO_2$ 40 mm Hg, and HCO_3^- 24 mEq/L), for every 10 mm Hg

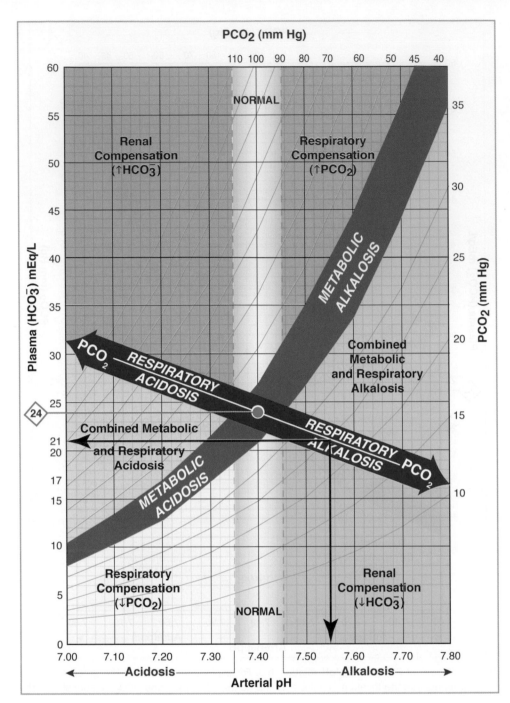

FIGURE 5.2 Acute alveolar hyperventilation is confirmed when the reported PCO_2, pH, and HCO_3^- values all intersect within the red-colored "Respiratory Alkalosis" bar. For example, when the reported PCO_2 is 25 mm Hg at a time when the pH is 7.55 and the HCO_3^- is 21 mEq/L, acute alveolar hyperventilation is confirmed (see black arrows). (From Terry Des Jardins, with permission.)

the $PaCO_2$ increases, the pH will decrease about 0.06 units (from 7.4) and the HCO_3^- will increase about 1 mEq/L (from 24). Or, in another example, for every 20 mm Hg the $PaCO_2$ increases, the pH will decrease about 0.12 units (from 7.40), and the HCO_3^- will increase about 2 mEq/L (from 24). Thus if the patient's $PaCO_2$ suddenly increases to, say, 60 mm Hg, the expected pH change would be about 7.28 and the HCO_3^- would be about 26 mEq/L.

It should be noted, however, that if the patient's PaO_2 is severely low, lactic acid (a metabolic acid) also may be present, resulting in a **combined metabolic and respiratory acidosis**.

In such cases, the patient's pH and HCO_3^- values would both be lower than expected for a particular $PaCO_2$ level.

Acute Decreases in PaCO$_2$ (e.g., Acute Hyperventilation). Using the normal ABG values as a baseline (e.g., pH 7.40, $PaCO_2$ 40 mm Hg, and HCO_3^- 24 mEq/L), for every 5 mm Hg the $PaCO_2$ decreases, the pH will increase about 0.06 units (from 7.40), and the HCO_3^- will decrease about 1 mEq/L. Or, by way of another example, for every 10 mm Hg the $PaCO_2$ decreases, the pH will increase about 0.12 units (from 7.40), and the HCO_3^- will decrease about 2 mEq/L. Thus if the

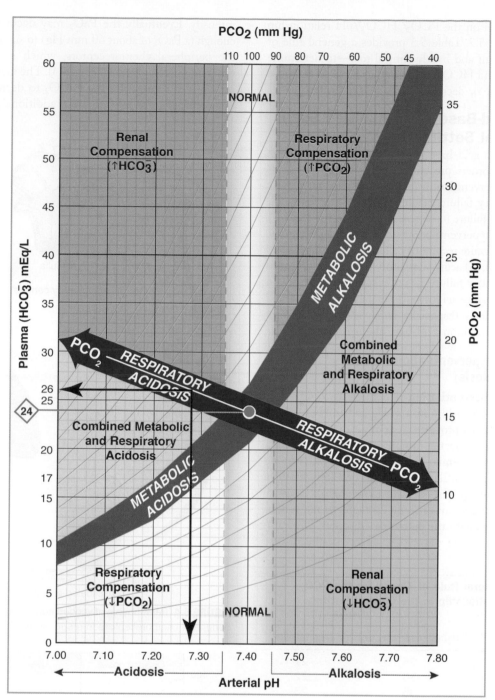

FIGURE 5.3 Acute ventilatory failure is confirmed when the reported PCO_2, pH, and HCO_3^- values all intersect within the red-colored respiratory acidosis bar to the left of the light-blue, vertical bar labeled "normal." For example, when the PCO_2 is 60 mm Hg at a time when the pH is 7.28 and the HCO_3^- is 26 mEq/L, acute ventilatory failure is confirmed (see black arrows). (From Terry Des Jardins, with permission.)

patient's $PaCO_2$ suddenly decreases to, say, 30 mm Hg, the expected pH change would be around 7.52 and the HCO_3^- would be about 22 mEq/L.

Again, it should be noted that if the patient's PaO_2 is also very low, lactic acid may be present. In such cases, the patient's pH and HCO_3^- values would both be lower than expected for a particular $PaCO_2$ level.

Table 5.2 provides a summary of the effects of acute $PaCO_2$ changes on pH and HCO_3^- levels (see previous discussion). Note that the pH and HCO_3^- changes with hypoventilation (increased $PaCO_2$) and hyperventilation (decreased $PaCO_2$)

TABLE 5.2 Summary of Acute $PaCO_2$ Changes on pH and HCO_3^- Levels

If This Happens	Then This Happens	
$PaCO_2$ increases by 10 mm Hg	pH will decrease by 0.06 units	HCO_3^- will Increase by 1 mEq/L
$PaCO_2$ decreases by 5 mm Hg	pH will increase by 0.06 units	HCO_3^- will decrease by 1 mEq/L

are not equal. Based on the $PCO_2/HCO_3^-/pH$ relationship presented in Table 5.2, Table 5.3 provides a general rule of thumb—an excellent and handy clinical tool—to determine the expected pH and HCO_3^- changes that occur in response to an acute increase or decrease in the PCO_2 level.

Common Acid-Base Abnormalities Seen in the Clinical Setting

The most common acid-base abnormalities associated with the respiratory disorders presented in this textbook are (1) acute alveolar hyperventilation (acute respiratory alkalosis), (2) acute ventilatory failure (acute respiratory acidosis), (3) chronic ventilatory failure (compensated respiratory acidosis), (4) acute alveolar hyperventilation superimposed on chronic ventilatory failure (acute respiratory alkalosis on compensated respiratory acidosis), (5) acute ventilatory failure superimposed on chronic ventilatory failure (acute respiratory acidosis on compensated respiratory acidosis), (6) metabolic alkalosis, and (7) metabolic acidosis (especially lactic acidosis). A brief overview of these common acid-base abnormalities follows.

Acute Alveolar Hyperventilation (Acute Respiratory Alkalosis)

Acute alveolar hyperventilation is defined as a pH above 7.45 and a $PaCO_2$ level below 35 mm Hg and an HCO_3^- level down slightly. Table 5.4 provides an example of acute alveolar hyperventilation. The most common cause of acute alveolar hyperventilation is **hypoxemia**. The decreased PaO_2 seen during acute alveolar hyperventilation usually develops from a decreased ventilation-perfusion ratio ($\dot{V}/\dot{Q}$ ratio), capillary shunting (or a relative shunt or shunt-like effect), and venous admixture associated with the pulmonary disorder. The PaO_2 continues to drop as the pathologic effects of the disease

intensify. Eventually the PaO_2 may decline to a point low enough (a PaO_2 of about 60 mm Hg) to significantly stimulate the peripheral chemoreceptors, which in turn causes the ventilatory rate to increase (Fig. 5.4). The increased ventilatory response in turn causes the $PaCO_2$ to decrease and the pH to increase (Fig. 5.5). Box 5.2 lists additional pathophysiologic

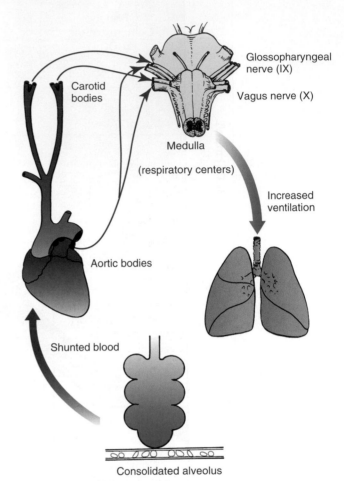

FIGURE 5.4 Relationship of venous admixture to the stimulation of peripheral chemoreceptors in response to alveolar consolidation.

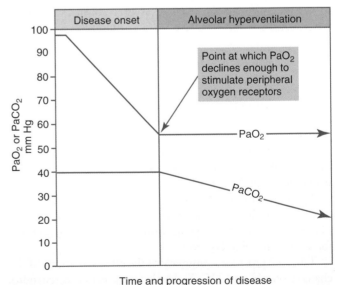

FIGURE 5.5 PaO_2 and $PaCO_2$ trends during acute alveolar hyperventilation.

TABLE 5.3 General Rule of Thumb for the $PCO_2/$ HCO_3^-/pH Relationship in the Clinical Setting

pH (Approximate)	PaCO₂ (Approximate)	mEq/L (Approximate)
7.55	25	21
7.50	30	22
7.45	35	23
7.40 (Normal)	40	24
7.35	50	25
7.30	60	26
7.25	70	27

TABLE 5.4 Acute Alveolar Hyperventilation (Acute Respiratory Alkalosis)

Arterial Blood Gas Changes	Example
pH: Increased	7.52
PaCO₂: Decreased	28 mm Hg
HCO₃⁻: Decreasing but normal	22 mEq/L
PaO₂: Decreased	61 mm Hg (when pulmonary pathologic condition is present)

TABLE 5.5 Acute Ventilatory Failure (Acute Respiratory Acidosis)	
Arterial Blood Gas Changes	Example
pH: Decreased	7.16
$PaCO_2$: Increased	79 mm Hg
HCO_3^-: Decreasing but normal	28 mEq/L
PaO_2: Decreased	57 mm Hg

TABLE 5.6 Chronic Ventilatory Failure (Compensated Respiratory Acidosis)	
Arterial Blood Gas Changes	Example
pH: Normal	7.36
$PaCO_2$: Increased	79 mm Hg
HCO_3^-: Increased (significantly)	43 mEq/L
PaO_2: Decreased	61 mm Hg

BOX 5.2 Pathophysiologic Mechanisms That Lead to a Reduction in $PaCO_2$

- Decreased lung compliance
- Stimulation of the central chemoreceptors
- Activation of the deflation reflex
- Activation of the irritant reflex
- Stimulation of the J receptors
- Pain and anxiety

BOX 5.3 Respiratory Diseases Associated With Chronic Ventilatory Failure During Advanced Stages

Chronic Obstructive Pulmonary Disorders (Most Common)
- Chronic bronchitis
- Emphysema
- Bronchiectasis
- Cystic fibrosis

Restrictive Respiratory Disorders
- Tuberculosis
- Fungal diseases
- Kyphoscoliosis
- Chronic interstitial lung diseases
- Bronchopulmonary dysplasia

mechanisms in respiratory disorders that can contribute to an increased ventilatory rate and a reduction in $PaCO_2$.

Acute Ventilatory Failure (Acute Respiratory Acidosis)

Acute ventilatory failure is defined as a pH below 7.35, a $PaCO_2$ level above 45 mm Hg, and an HCO_3^- level slightly increased. Table 5.5 provides an example of acute ventilatory failure. Acute ventilatory failure is a condition in which the lungs are unable to meet the metabolic demands of the body in terms of CO_2 homeostasis and typically tissue oxygenation. In other words, the patient is unable to provide the muscular, mechanical work necessary to move gas into and out of the lungs to meet the normal CO_2 production of the body. This condition leads to an increased $PACO_2$ and subsequently an increased $PaCO_2$. The increased $PACO_2$ causes a decrease in the PAO_2, which in turn leads to a decreased PaO_2 in the arterial blood.

Acute ventilatory failure is not associated with a typical ventilatory pattern. For example, the patient may demonstrate apnea, severe hyperpnea, or tachypnea. The bottom line is that acute ventilatory failure can develop in response to any ventilatory pattern that does not provide adequate *alveolar* ventilation. When an increased $PaCO_2$ is accompanied by acidemia (decreased pH), acute ventilatory failure, or respiratory acidosis, is said to exist. Clinically, this is a medical emergency that may require mechanical ventilation.

Chronic Ventilatory Failure (Compensated Respiratory Acidosis)

Chronic ventilatory failure (compensated respiratory acidosis) is defined as a greater than normal $PaCO_2$ level with a normal pH status and, typically, a decreased PaO_2 on room air. Table 5.6 provides an example of chronic ventilatory failure. Although chronic ventilatory failure is most commonly seen in patients with severe chronic obstructive pulmonary disease, it is also seen in several chronic restrictive lung disorders (e.g., severe tuberculosis, kyphoscoliosis). Box 5.3 lists common

respiratory diseases associated with chronic ventilatory failure during the advanced stages of the disorder.

The basic pathophysiologic mechanisms that produce ABGs associated with chronic ventilatory failure are as a respiratory disorder gradually worsens, the work of breathing progressively increases to a point at which more oxygen is consumed than is gained. Although the exact mechanism is unclear, the patient slowly develops a breathing pattern that uses the least amount of oxygen for the energy expended. In essence, the patient selects a breathing pattern based on *work efficiency* rather than *ventilatory efficiency*. (See the discussion of airway resistance and its effect on the ventilatory pattern in Chapter 3, The Pathophysiologic Basis for Common Clinical Manifestations.) As a result, the patient's alveolar ventilation slowly decreases, which in turn causes the PaO_2 to decrease and the $PaCO_2$ to increase further (Fig. 5.6). As the $PaCO_2$ increases, the pH falls.

When an individual hypoventilates for a long period, the kidneys work to correct the decreased pH by retaining HCO_3^-. Renal compensation in the presence of chronic hypoventilation can be shown when the calculated HCO_3^- and pH readings are higher than expected for a particular PCO_2 level. For example, in terms of the absolute $PCO_2/HCO_3^-/pH$ relationship, when the PCO_2 level is about 70 mm Hg, the HCO_3^- level should be about 27 mEq/L and the pH should be about 7.22 according to the normal blood buffer line (see Fig. 5.3).

If the HCO_3^- and pH levels are greater than these values (i.e., the pH and HCO_3^- readings cross a PCO_2 isobar[2] above

---

[2]The isobars on the $PCO_2/HCO_3^-/pH$ nomogram illustrate the pH changes that develop in the blood as a result of metabolic changes (i.e., HCO_3^- changes) or a combination of metabolic and respiratory (CO_2) changes.

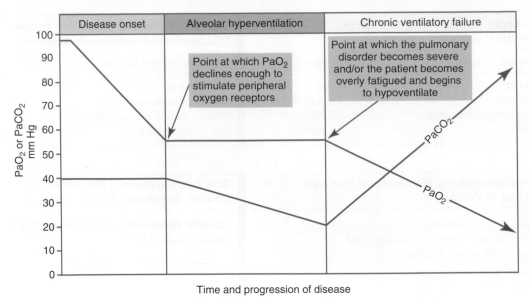

Point at which PaO$_2$ declines enough to stimulate peripheral oxygen receptors

Point at which the pulmonary disorder becomes severe and/or the patient becomes overly fatigued and begins to hypoventilate

PaO$_2$ or PaCO$_2$ mm Hg

PaCO$_2$

PaO$_2$

Time and progression of disease

FIGURE 5.6 PaO$_2$ and PaCO$_2$ trends during acute or chronic ventilatory failure.

the normal blood buffer line in the upper left-hand corner of the nomogram), renal retention of HCO_3^- (partial renal compensation) has occurred (see Fig. 5.3, purple area, upper left quadrant). When the HCO_3^- level increases enough to return the acidic pH to normal, complete renal compensation is said to have occurred (chronic ventilatory failure) (see Fig. 5.3, normal area).

Thus the following should be understood. The lungs play an important role in maintaining the PaCO$_2$, HCO_3^-, and pH levels on a moment-to-moment basis. The kidneys play an important role in maintaining the HCO_3^- and pH levels during long periods of hyperventilation or hypoventilation.

Acute Ventilatory Changes Superimposed on Chronic Ventilatory Failure

Because acute ventilatory changes (i.e., hyperventilation or hypoventilation) are frequently seen in patients who have chronic ventilatory failure (compensated respiratory acidosis), the respiratory therapist must be familiar with and be on the alert for **acute alveolar hyperventilation superimposed on chronic ventilatory failure** and **acute ventilatory failure (hypoventilation) superimposed on chronic ventilatory failure**.

Like any other person (healthy or unhealthy), the patient with chronic ventilatory failure also can experience acute periods of hyperventilation. For example, the patient with chronic ventilatory failure can acquire an acute shunt-producing disease (e.g., pneumonia) and hypoxemia. Some of these patients have the mechanical reserve to increase their alveolar ventilation significantly in an attempt to maintain their baseline PaO$_2$. However, in regard to the patient's baseline PaCO$_2$ level, the increased alveolar ventilation is often excessive.

When excessive alveolar ventilation occurs, the patient's PaCO$_2$ rapidly decreases. This action causes the patient's PaCO$_2$ to decrease from its normally "high baseline" level. As the PaCO$_2$ decreases, the arterial pH increases. As this condition intensifies, the patient's baseline ABG values can

TABLE 5.7 Acute Alveolar Hyperventilation Superimposed on Chronic Ventilatory Failure (Acute Hyperventilation on Compensated Respiratory Acidosis)

Arterial Blood Gas Changes	Example
pH: Increased	7.52
PaCO$_2$: Increased	51 mm Hg
HCO$_3^-$: Increased	40 mEq/L
PaO$_2$: Decreased	46 mm Hg

quickly change from chronic ventilatory failure to acute alveolar hyperventilation superimposed on chronic ventilatory failure. Table 5.7 provides an example of acute alveolar hyperventilation superimposed on chronic ventilatory failure.

A clinician who does not know the history of the patient with acute alveolar hyperventilation superimposed on chronic ventilatory failure might initially interpret the ABG values as signifying partially compensated metabolic alkalosis with severe hypoxemia (see Box 5.1). However, the clinical situation that offsets this interpretation is the presence of marked hypoxemia. A low oxygen level is not normally seen in patients with pure metabolic alkalosis. Thus whenever the ABG values appear to reflect partially compensated metabolic alkalosis but the condition is accompanied by significant hypoxemia, the respiratory therapist should be alert to the possibility of *acute alveolar hyperventilation superimposed on chronic ventilatory failure.*

Often patients with chronic ventilatory failure do not have the mechanical reserve to meet the hypoxemic challenge of a respiratory disorder. When these patients attempt to maintain their baseline PaO$_2$ by increasing their alveolar ventilation, they often consume more oxygen than is gained or become fatigued or experience a combination of both. When this happens, the patient begins to breathe less. This action causes the PaCO$_2$ to increase and eventually to rise above the patient's normally high PaCO$_2$ baseline level. This action causes the patient's arterial pH level to fall or become acidic. In short, the patient's baseline ABG values shift from chronic ventilatory failure to **acute ventilatory failure superimposed on chronic ventilatory failure**. Table 5.8 provides an example of acute ventilatory failure superimposed on chronic ventilatory failure. Table 5.9 provides an overview summary of acute ventilatory failure superimposed on chronic ventilatory failure and acute alveolar hyperventilation superimposed on chronic ventilatory failure, in relationship to typical baseline ABG values of a patient with chronic ventilatory failure.

Metabolic Acid-Base Abnormalities

Metabolic acid-base disturbances are subdivided into the following two categories: metabolic acidosis and metabolic alkalosis (see Box 5.1). An overview of the metabolic acid-base disturbances are presented in the following section.

Metabolic Alkalosis

The presence of other bases not related to either a decreased $PaCO_2$ level or renal compensation also can be identified by using the $PCO_2/HCO_3^-/pH$ nomogram illustrated in Fig. 5.1. The presence of **metabolic alkalosis** is verified when the calculated HCO_3^- and pH readings are both higher than expected for a particular $PaCO_2$ level in terms of the absolute $PCO_2/HCO_3^-/pH$ relationship. For example, according to the normal blood buffer line, an HCO_3^- reading of 35 mEq/L and a pH level of 7.54 would both be higher than expected in a patient who has a $PaCO_2$ level of 40 mm Hg (see Fig. 5.1). This extremely common condition is known as metabolic alkalosis. Table 5.10 provides an example of metabolic alkalosis. Box 5.4 provides common causes of metabolic alkalosis.

Metabolic Acidosis

The presence of other acids not related to an increased $PaCO_2$ level also can be identified by using the isobars of the $PCO_2/$

HCO_3^-/pH nomogram shown in Fig. 5.1. The presence of other acids is verified when the calculated HCO_3^- reading and pH level are both lower than expected for a particular $PaCO_2$ level in terms of the absolute $PCO_2/HCO_3^-/pH$ relationship. For example, according to the normal blood buffer line, an HCO_3^- reading of 15 mEq/L and a pH of 7.20 would both be less than expected in the patient with a PCO_2 of 40 mm Hg. This condition is referred to as **metabolic acidosis**. Table 5.11 provides an example of metabolic acidosis. Note that if the PaO_2 is normal, which generally rules out lactic acidosis, the precise cause of the metabolic acidosis is not readily known. Box 5.4 provides common causes of metabolic acidosis.

Lactic Acidosis (Metabolic Acidosis). Because acute tissue hypoxia and acute hypoxemia are commonly associated with any of the respiratory disorders presented in this textbook, acute metabolic acidosis, or **lactic acidosis**, (caused by lactic acid) often further compromises the patient's ABG status. This is because oxygenation is inadequate to meet tissue metabolism, so alternative biochemical reactions that do not use oxygen are activated. This is called **anaerobic metabolism** (non–oxygen-using). It is commonly seen in cardiopulmonary exercise testing (CPET) as occurring at the **anaerobic threshold**, where the $\dot{V}CO_2$ increases more rapidly than normal as a function of work done (as measured in the CPET continuously by the $\dot{V}O_2$). Lactic acid is the end-product of this

---

BOX 5.4 Common Causes of Metabolic Acid-Base Abnormalities

Metabolic Acidosis
- Lactic acidosis (most common)
- Ketoacidosis (most commonly associated with diabetes mellitus)
- Salicylate intoxication (aspirin overdose)
- Renal failure
- Chronic diarrhea

Metabolic Alkalosis
- Hypokalemia
- Hypochloremia
- Gastric suctioning
- Vomiting
- Excessive administration of corticosteroids
- Excessive administration of sodium bicarbonate
- Diuretic therapy
- Hypovolemia

TABLE 5.8 Acute Ventilatory Failure Superimposed on Chronic Ventilatory Failure (Acute Hypoventilation on Compensated Respiratory Acidosis)

Arterial Blood Gas Changes	Example
pH: Decreased	7.28
$PaCO_2$: Increased	99 mm Hg
HCO_3^-: Increased	45 mEq/L
PaO_2: Decreased	34 mm Hg

TABLE 5.9 Overview Examples of Acute Changes in Chronic Ventilatory Failure

Acute Ventilatory Failure on Chronic Ventilatory Failure	Chronic Ventilatory Failure (Baseline Values)	Acute Alveolar Hyperventilation on Chronic Ventilatory Failure
7.28 ⟵	pH 7.36	⟶ 7.52
99 ⟵	$PaCO_2$ 79	⟶ 51
45 ⟵	HCO_2^- 43	⟶ 40
34 ⟵	PaO_2 61	⟶ 46

TABLE 5.10 Metabolic Alkalosis

Arterial Blood Gas Changes	Example
pH: Increased	7.56
$PaCO_2$: Normal	44 mm Hg
HCO_3^-: Increased	36 mEq/L
PaO_2: Normal	94 mm Hg

TABLE 5.11 Metabolic Acidosis

Arterial Blood Gas Changes	Example
pH: Decreased	7.26
$PaCO_2$: Normal	37 mm Hg
HCO_3^-: Decreased	16 mEq/L
PaO_2: Normal (or decreased if lactic acidosis is present)	94 mm Hg (or 37 mm Hg if lactic acidosis is present)

TABLE 5.12 Lactic Acidosis (Metabolic Acidosis)

Arterial Blood Gas Changes	Example
pH: Decreased	7.21
$PaCO_2$: Normal or decreased	35 mm Hg
HCO_3^-: Decreased	14 mEq/L
PaO_2: Decreased	34 mm Hg

process. When acidic ions move into the blood, the pH decreases. Thus whenever moderate to *severe* acute hypoxemia is present, the possible presence of lactic acid should be suspected. For example, when acute alveolar hyperventilation is caused by a sudden drop in PaO_2, the patient's pH may be lower than expected for a particular decrease in $PaCO_2$ level. Table 5.12 provides an example of lactic acidosis.

Anion Gap. The **anion gap** is used to assess if the patient's metabolic acidosis is caused by the accumulation of fixed acids (lactic acids, ketoacids, or salicylate intoxication) or an excessive loss of HCO_3^-.

The **law of electroneutrality** states that the total number of plasma positively charged ions (cations) must equal the total number of plasma negatively charged ions (anions) in the body fluids. To calculate the anion gap, the most commonly measured cations are sodium (Na^+) ions. The most commonly measured anions are the chloride (Cl^-) ions and bicarbonate (HCO_3^-) ions. The normal plasma concentrations of these cations and anions are the following:

Na^+: 140 mEq/L
Cl^-: 105 mEq/L
HCO_3^-: 24 mEq/L

The anion gap is the calculated difference between the Na^+ ions and the sum of the HCO_3^- and Cl^- ions:

$$\text{Anion gap} = Na^+ - (Cl^- + HCO_3^-)$$
$$= 140 - (105 + 24)$$
$$= 140 - 129$$
$$= 11\,\text{mEq/L}$$

The normal range for the anion gap is 9 to 14 mEq/L. When the anion gap is greater than 14 mEq/L, metabolic acidosis is present—that is, an elevated anion gap caused by the accumulation of fixed acids in the blood. Fixed acids produce H^+ ions that chemically react with and are buffered

by the plasma HCO_3^-. This action causes the HCO_3^- level to fall and the anion gap to increase.

Clinically, when the patient demonstrates both metabolic acidosis and an increased anion gap, the source of the fixed acids must be identified for the patient to be appropriately treated. For example, metabolic acidosis caused by lactic acids requires oxygen therapy to reverse the accumulation of the lactic acids. Metabolic acidosis caused by ketone acids requires insulin therapy to help facilitate the movement of glucose into the cells and normalize metabolism.

It is interesting to note that metabolic acidosis caused by an excessive loss of HCO_3^- (e.g., from renal disease or severe diarrhea) does not cause an increase in the anion gap. This is because as the HCO_3^- level decreases, the Cl^- level usually increases to maintain electroneutrality. In short, for every HCO_3^- ion lost, a Cl^- anion takes its place (i.e., the law of electroneutrality). This action maintains a normal anion gap. Metabolic acidosis caused by decreased HCO_3^- with an increased Cl^- is commonly called **hyperchloremic metabolic acidosis**.

Thus when metabolic acidosis is accompanied by an increased anion gap, the most likely cause of the acidosis is the accumulation of fixed acids. When metabolic acidosis is seen with a normal anion gap, the most likely cause of the acidosis is an excessive loss of HCO_3^- (e.g., caused by renal failure or severe diarrhea).

Errors Associated With Arterial Blood Gas Measurements

Because an ABG error can occur before, during, or after the analysis of the sample, the respiratory therapist must always be on alert for ABG results that do not fit the patient's current clinical condition. Accurate and efficient ABG samplings, along with the correct analysis and interpretation of ABG values, are no simple matters, as anyone who has performed these procedures can testify. Fast and precisely accurate ABG results are often life-critical!

In general, the types of ABG errors can be classified as (1) preanalytic errors, (2) analytic errors, (3) postanalytic errors, and (4) interpretation errors. *Preanalytic errors* include errors that occur either before or after the sample analysis—for example, improper sample or data handling. *Analytic errors* include errors that occur during the actual analysis of the ABG sample—for example, blood gas machine malfunctions and poor individual technique. *Postanalytic errors* include the recording of the ABG results after analysis—for example, incorrect patient name or FIO_2 setting. *Interpretation errors* are the incorrect classification of any ABG results (see Box 5.1). Table 5.13 provides an overview of common errors of ABG measurements.

The "take home message" from this brief section is to be aware of the common sources of ABG errors and be ready to repeat the test if the ABG data do not correlate with the clinical situation. Unexpected or questionable ABG results should always be thoroughly investigated. Failure to do so is unacceptable! Noninvasive "reality checks" on ABG results include observation of the patient's sensorium and vital signs, presence or absence of cyanosis, and the timely readings from pulse oximeters and transcutaneous PO_2 and PCO_2 electrodes.

TABLE 5.13 Common Errors of Arterial Blood Gas Measurements

Errors	pH	PaCO$_2$	PaO$_2$
Preanalytic Errors Include			
Air in syringe or icing plastic syringes	↑	↓	↑
Venous blood sample or contamination	↓	↑	↓
(In fact, sometimes venous blood *will* pulsate; e.g., in pulmonary hypertension or CHF.)			
Anticoagulant type or concentration	↑↓	↓	↑
Metabolic effects (e.g., delay in running the blood sample)	↓	↑	↓
Misidentification of patient			
Inappropriately transported sample			
Analytic Errors Include			
Poor quality assurance (QA) and quality control (QC) programs*			
Malfunctioning PO$_2$ and PCO$_2$ electrodes			
Out-of-date reagents (cleaning, rinse, and calibration solutions)			
Postanalytic Errors Include			
Incorrect patient name/location/demographics on report			
Typographic and transcription errors (e.g., 74 instead of 47 mm Hg)			
Incorrect FIO$_2$ or ventilator setting on patient chart			
Failure to wait at least 20 minutes after an FIO$_2$ or ventilator setting change before sampling			
Incorrect sampling time recorded			
Failure to notify appropriate personnel of critical results (e.g., impending ventilatory failure and/or acute ventilatory failure)			
Slow turnaround time for results to get back to the patient's bedside to be interpreted by the medical staff			
Interpretation Errors Include			
The incorrect interpretation of *any* of the acid-base disturbances discussed in this chapter (see Box 5.1)			
Interpretation errors can result in serious harm and/or death to the patient (e.g., failure to correctly identify impending ventilatory failure, or acute ventilatory failure, or to identify a mixed acid-base disorders)			

*NOTE: Two quick internal checks of blood gas accuracy entail (1) calculating the Henderson-Hasselbalch equation to determine if the measured arterial blood gas (ABG) values correlate and (2) calculating the alveolar-arterial oxygen gradient for the same purpose. The Henderson-Hasselbalch equation ensures that the pH, PCO$_2$, and HCO$_3^-$ determinations are at least internally consistent. The alveolar-arterial oxygen gradient ensures that the FIO$_2$, PaO$_2$, and PaCO$_2$ calculations are at least reasonable. For a complete review of these two equations, see Des Jardins, T. (2019). *Cardiopulmonary anatomy and physiology: essentials of respiratory care* (7th ed.). Clifton Park, NY: Delmar/Cengage Learning.

SELF-ASSESSMENT QUESTIONS

1. During acute alveolar hyperventilation, which of the following occurs?
1. HCO$_3^-$ decreases.
2. PaCO$_2$ increases.
3. HCO$_3^-$ increases.
4. PaCO$_2$ decreases.
   a. 2 only
   b. 3 only
   c. 1 and 4 only
   d. 2, 3, and 4 only

2. When lactic acidosis is present, which of the following will occur?
1. pH will likely be lower than expected for a particular PaCO$_2$.
2. HCO$_3^-$ will likely be higher than expected for a particular PaCO$_2$.
3. pH will likely be higher than expected for a particular PaCO$_2$.
4. HCO$_3^-$ will likely be lower than expected for a particular PaCO$_2$.
   a. 2 only
   b. 3 only
   c. 2 and 3 only
   d. 1 and 4 only

3. What is the clinical interpretation of the following ABG values (in addition to hypoxemia)?

pH: 7.17
PaCO$_2$: 77 mm Hg
HCO$_3^-$: 27 mEq/L
PaO$_2$: 54 mm Hg

a. Acute alveolar hyperventilation superimposed on chronic ventilatory failure
b. Acute ventilatory failure
c. Acute alveolar hyperventilation
d. Acute ventilatory failure superimposed on chronic ventilatory failure

4. A 74-year-old man with a long history of emphysema and chronic bronchitis enters the emergency department in respiratory distress. His respiratory rate is 34 breaths per minute and labored. His heart rate is 115 beats per minute, and his blood pressure is 170/120. What is the clinical interpretation of the following ABG values (in addition to hypoxemia)?

pH: 7.51
PaCO$_2$: 68 mm Hg
HCO$_3^-$: 52 mEq/L
PaO$_2$: 49 mm Hg

a. Acute alveolar hyperventilation superimposed on chronic ventilatory failure
b. Acute ventilatory failure
c. Acute alveolar hyperventilation
d. Acute ventilatory failure superimposed on chronic ventilatory failure

5. Which of the following is classified as metabolic acidosis?
a. pH 7.23; PaCO$_2$ 63; HCO$_3^-$ 26; PaO$_2$ 52
b. pH 7.16; PaCO$_2$ 38; HCO$_3^-$ 13; PaO$_2$ 86
c. pH 7.56; PaCO$_2$ 27; HCO$_3^-$ 23; PaO$_2$ 101
d. pH 7.64; PaCO$_2$ 49; HCO$_3^-$ 51; PaO$_2$ 91

6. Which of the following cause metabolic acidosis?
1. Hypokalemia
2. Renal failure
3. Excessive administration of sodium bicarbonate
4. Hypochloremia
a. 1 only
b. 2 only
c. 1 and 4 only
d. 2 and 3 only

7. Using the general rule of thumb for the PCO$_2$/HCO$_3^-$/pH relationship, if the PaCO$_2$ suddenly increased to 90 mm Hg in a patient who normally has a pH of 7.40, a PaCO$_2$ of 40 mm Hg, and an HCO$_3^-$ of 24 mEq/L, the pH will decrease to approximately what level?
a. 7.15
b. 7.10
c. 7.05
d. 7.00

8. Which of the following is classified as metabolic alkalosis?
a. pH 7.23; PaCO$_2$ 63; HCO$_3^-$ 26; PaO$_2$ 52
b. pH 7.16; PaCO$_2$ 38; HCO$_3^-$ 13; PaO$_2$ 86
c. pH 7.56; PaCO$_2$ 27; HCO$_3^-$ 23; PaO$_2$ 101
d. pH 7.64; PaCO$_2$ 44; HCO$_3^-$ 46; PaO$_2$ 91

9. Lactic acidosis develops from which of the following?
1. Inadequate tissue oxygenation
2. Renal failure
3. An inadequate insulin level
4. Anaerobic metabolism
5. An inadequate glucose level
a. 1 only
b. 2 only
c. 1 and 4 only
d. 3 and 5 only

10. Metabolic alkalosis can develop from which of the following?
1. Hyperchloremia
2. Hypokalemia
3. Hypochloremia
4. Hyperkalemia
a. 4 only
b. 1 and 3 only
c. 1 and 4 only
d. 2 and 3 only

11. During acute alveolar hypoventilation, the blood:
1. HCO$_3^-$ increases
2. pH decreases
3. PCO$_2$ increases
4. HCO$_3^-$ decreases
a. 2 only
b. 4 only
c. 2 and 3 only
d. 1, 2, and 3 only

12. During acute alveolar hyperventilation, the blood:
1. PCO$_2$ increases
2. HCO$_3^-$ increases
3. HCO$_3^-$ decreases
4. pH increases
a. 2 only
b. 4 only
c. 1 and 3 only
d. 3 and 4 only

13. In chronic hypoventilation, kidney compensation has likely occurred when the:
1. HCO$_3^-$ is higher than expected for a particular PaCO$_2$
2. pH is lower than expected for a particular PaCO$_2$
3. HCO$_3^-$ is lower than expected for a particular PaCO$_2$
4. pH is higher than expected for a particular PaCO$_2$
a. 1 only
b. 2 only
c. 1 and 4 only
d. 3 and 4 only

14. Which of the following represents acute alveolar hyperventilation?
a. pH 7.56; PaCO$_2$ 51; HCO$_3^-$ 44
b. pH 7.45; PaCO$_2$ 37; HCO$_3^-$ 25
c. pH 7.53; PaCO$_2$ 46; HCO$_3^-$ 29
d. pH 7.58; PaCO$_2$ 26; HCO$_3^-$ 21

15. Which of the following represents compensated metabolic alkalosis?
a. pH 7.55; PaCO$_2$ 21; HCO$_3^-$ 19
b. pH 7.52; PaCO$_2$ 45; HCO$_3^-$ 29
c. pH 7.45; PaCO$_2$ 26; HCO$_3^-$ 18
d. pH 7.45; PaCO$_2$ 61; HCO$_3^-$ 41

CHAPTER

6 Assessment of Oxygenation

Chapter Objectives

After reading this chapter, you will be able to:

- Describe the two ways in which oxygen is carried in the blood.
- Calculate the oxygen tension–based indices equations.
- Calculate the oxygen saturation–based and content-based indices equations.
- Describe the clinical significance of pulmonary shunting.
- List factors that increase and decrease the oxygen content and oxygen-transport calculations.
- Discuss mechanisms by which specific respiratory diseases alter oxygen transport studies.
- Differentiate between hypoxemia and hypoxia.
- Classify the severity of mild, moderate, and severe hypoxemia.
- Describe the four types of hypoxia.
- List common causes for each type of hypoxia.
- Describe the pathophysiologic conditions associated with chronic hypoxia.
- Define key terms and complete self-assessment questions at the end of the chapter and on Evolve.

Key Terms

Alveolar-Arterial Oxygen Tension Difference (P[A-a]O$_2$)
Anemic Hypoxia
Arterial-Venous Oxygen Content Difference (C[a-$\overline{v}$]O$_2$)
Circulatory Hypoxia
Cor Pulmonale
Erythropoietin
Histotoxic Hypoxia
Hypoxemia
Hypoxia
Hypoxic Hypoxia
Hypoxic Vasoconstriction of the Lungs
Ideal Alveolar Gas Equation to Determine PAO$_2$
Intracellular Oxygen Tension (icO$_2$)
Lactic Acid

Mild Hypoxemia
Mixed Venous Blood C$\overline{v}$O$_2$
Mixed Venous Oxygen Saturation (S$\overline{v}$O$_2$)
Moderate Hypoxemia
Nanostraws
Oxygen Consumption ($\dot{V}$O$_2$)
Oxygen Content of Arterial Blood (Cao$_2$)
Oxygen Content of Mixed Venous Blood (C$\overline{v}$O$_2$)
Oxygen Content of Pulmonary Capillary Blood (Cco$_2$)
Oxygen Extraction Ratio (O$_2$ER)
Oxyhemoglobin Dissociation Curve
Oxyhemoglobin Equilibrium Curve
PaO$_2$/FIO$_2$ Ratio
PaO$_2$/PAO$_2$ Ratio
Polycythemia
Pulmonary Capillary Blood (CcO$_2$)
Pulmonary Shunt Fraction ($\dot{Q}_S/\dot{Q}_T$)
Severe Hypoxemia
Thermodilution
Total Oxygen Delivery (DO$_2$)

Chapter Outline

Oxygen Transport Review
    Oxygen Dissolved in the Blood Plasma
    Oxygen Bound to Hemoglobin
Total Oxygen Content of Blood
    Case Example
Oxyhemoglobin Dissociation Curve
Oxygenation Indices
    Oxygen Tension–Based Indices
    Oxygen Saturation–Based and Content-Based Indices
Hypoxemia Versus Hypoxia
    Pathophysiologic Conditions Associated With Chronic Hypoxia
    True Hypoxia—Can It Be Measured?
Self-Assessment Questions

Oxygen transport between the lungs and the metabolizing cells is a function of the blood itself and the cardiovascular system (blood vessels and heart). Oxygen is carried in the blood in two ways: as dissolved oxygen in the blood plasma and oxygen bound to the hemoglobin (Hb). Most oxygen is carried to the tissue cells bound to hemoglobin. The following pages provide the essential knowledge cornerstones needed to effectively and safely assess the patient's oxygenation status.

Oxygen Transport Review

Oxygen Dissolved in the Blood Plasma

A small amount of oxygen that diffuses from the alveoli to the pulmonary capillary blood remains in the dissolved form. The term *dissolved* means that the gas molecule (in this case oxygen) maintains its exact molecular structure and freely moves throughout the plasma of the blood in its normal gaseous state. Clinically, it is the dissolved oxygen that is measured to assess the patient's partial pressure of oxygen (PO_2).

At normal body temperature, about 0.003 mL of oxygen will dissolve in each 100 mL of blood for every 1 mm Hg of PO_2. Therefore in the normal individual with an arterial PaO_2 of 100 mm Hg, only about 0.3 mL of oxygen exists in the dissolved form in every 100 mL of plasma (0.003×100 mm Hg $= 0.3$ mL). Clinically, this is written as 0.3 mL/dL.[1] Relative to the total oxygen transport, only a small amount of oxygen is carried to the tissue cells in the form of dissolved oxygen.

Oxygen Bound to Hemoglobin

In the healthy individual, over 98% of the oxygen that diffuses into the pulmonary capillary blood chemically combines with hemoglobin. Clinically, the weight measurement of hemoglobin, in reference to 100 mL of blood, is known as the *grams per deciliter* (g/dL).[2] The normal hemoglobin value for men is 14 to 16 g/dL. The normal hemoglobin value for women is 12 to 15 g/dL. The normal hemoglobin value for infants is 14 to 20 g/dL.

Each gram of hemoglobin is capable of carrying about 1.34 mL of oxygen. Therefore if the hemoglobin level is 12 g/dL and the hemoglobin is fully saturated with oxygen (i.e., carrying all the oxygen that is physically possible), about 16.08 O_2 mL/dL will be bound to the hemoglobin:

$$O_2 \text{ bound to Hb} = 1.34 \text{ mL } O_2 \times 12 \text{ g/dL Hb}$$
$$(12 \text{ g per 100 mL of blood})$$
$$= 16.08 \text{ mL/dL } O_2$$
$$(16.08 \text{ mL of } O_2 \text{ per 100 mL of blood}).$$

However, because of normal physiologic shunts (e.g., Thebesian venous drainage and bronchial venous drainage), the actual normal hemoglobin saturation is only about 97% (see chapter 11, Pathophysiologic mechanisms of Hyoxemic Respiratory Failure). Therefore the final amount of arterial oxygen shown in the previous calculation must be adjusted by 97% as follows:

$$O_2 \text{ bound to Hb} = 16.08 \text{ mL/dL } O_2 \times 0.97 = 15.60 \text{ mL/dL } O_2.$$

Total Oxygen Content of Blood

To calculate the total amount of oxygen in each 100 mL of blood, the dissolved oxygen and the oxygen bound to the hemoglobin must be added together. The following case example summarizes the mathematics required to determine the total oxygen content of the patient's blood.

Case Example

A 44-year-old woman with a long history of asthma arrives in the emergency department in severe respiratory distress. Her vital signs are respiratory rate 36 breaths per minute, heart rate 130 bpm, and blood pressure 160/95 mm Hg. Her hemoglobin concentration is 10 g/dL, and her PaO_2 is

55 mm Hg (SaO_2 85%). On the basis of these data, the patient's total oxygen content is determined as follows:

1. Dissolved O_2

$$55 \, (PaO_2) \times 0.003 \, (\text{dissolved } O_2) = 0.165 \text{ mL/dL } O_2$$

2. Oxygen bound to hemoglobin

$$10 \text{ g/dL} \times 1.34 \times 0.85 \, (SaO_2) = 11.39 \text{ mL/dL } O_2$$

3. Total oxygen content

$$11.39 + 0.165 = 11.55 \text{ mL/dL } O_2$$

The total oxygen content can be calculated in the patient's arterial blood (CaO_2), venous blood ($C\overline{v}O_2$), and pulmonary capillary blood, also known as the **oxygen content of capillary blood (CcO_2)**. The mathematics for these calculations is as follows:

1. **CaO_2: Oxygen content of arterial blood**

$$CaO_2 = (Hb \times 1.34 \times SaO_2) + (PaO_2 \times 0.003)$$

2. **$C\overline{v}O_2$: Oxygen content of venous blood**

$$C\overline{v}O_2 = (Hb \times 1.34 \times S\overline{v}O_2) + (P\overline{v}O_2 \times 0.003)$$

3. **CcO_2: Oxygen content of pulmonary capillary blood**

$$CcO_2 = (Hb \times 1.34^3) + PAO_2{}^4 \times 0.003$$

As will be shown later in this chapter, various mathematical manipulations of the CaO_2, $C\overline{v}O_2$, and CcO_2 values are used in several different oxygen transport studies that provide important clinical information regarding the patient's ventilatory and cardiac status.

Oxyhemoglobin Dissociation Curve

As shown in Fig. 6.1, the **oxyhemoglobin dissociation curve** (HbO_2 curve), also called the **oxyhemoglobin equilibrium curve**, is an S-shaped curve on a nomogram that illustrates the *percentage of hemoglobin that is saturated with oxygen* (left side of the graph) related to oxygen at a specific oxygen partial pressure (PO_2) (bottom portion of the graph). On the right side of the graph, the precise oxygen content that is carried by the hemoglobin, for a particular oxygen partial pressure at a normal pH, is provided.

The steep portion of the oxyhemoglobin dissociation curve falls between 10 and 60 mm Hg, and the upper flat portion falls between 70 and 100 mm Hg. The steep part of the curve demonstrates that oxygen quickly combines with hemoglobin as the PO_2 increases or, the converse, quickly breaks away (or dissociates) from the hemoglobin as the PO_2 decreases.[5] It is also interesting to note that very little additional oxygen combines with hemoglobin between a PO_2 of 60 and 100 mm Hg. In fact, a PO_2 increase from 60 to 100 mm Hg increases the total saturation of hemoglobin by only 7% (from 90% to 97% saturated) (see Fig. 6.1).

---

[3]It is assumed that the hemoglobin saturation with oxygen in the pulmonary capillary blood is 100%.
[4]See Appendix VIII on the Evolve site.
[5]For a more in depth discussion of the oxyhemoglobin dissociation curve, see Des Jardins. Cardiopulmonary Anatomy and Physiology–Essentials of Respiratory Care, 7th edition, Cengage Learning, Clifton Park, NY.

---

[1]Previously the quantity of oxygen in 100 mL of blood was written as volumes percent (vol%) of oxygen. Thus in this case, 0.3 vol%.
[2]Also abbreviated as grams percent of hemoglobin (g% Hb).

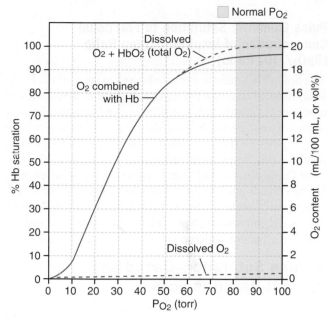

FIGURE 6.1 Oxyhemoglobin dissociation curve at a normal pH.

Oxygenation Indices

A number of oxygen transport measurements are available to assess the oxygenation status of the critically ill patient. Results from these studies can provide important information to adjust therapeutic interventions. The oxygen transport studies can be divided into the oxygen tension–based indices and the oxygen saturation–based and content-based indices.[6]

Oxygen Tension–Based Indices

Arterial Oxygen Tension (PaO$_2$)

The PaO$_2$ has withstood the test of time as a good indicator of the patient's oxygenation status. In general, an appropriate PaO$_2$ on an inspired low oxygen concentration almost always indicates good tissue oxygenation. The PaO$_2$, however, can be misleading in a number of clinical situations. For example, the PaO$_2$ may give a "falsely normal" impression of true tissue oxygenation when the patient has (1) a low hemoglobin concentration, (2) a decreased cardiac output or reduced blood flow to specific organs (e.g., the heart), (3) peripheral shunting, or (4) been exposed to carbon monoxide. In all of these cases, the PaO$_2$ may be at an appropriate level (normal PaO$_2$) but the actual oxygen content available for tissue metabolism—the oxygen bound to the hemoglobin—is inadequate.

Alveolar-Arterial Oxygen Tension Difference (P[A-a]O$_2$)

The **alveolar-arterial oxygen tension difference (P[A-a]O$_2$)** is the oxygen tension difference between the alveoli and arterial blood. The P(A-a)O$_2$ is also known as the *alveolar-arterial oxygen tension gradient*. The information required for the P(A-a)O$_2$ is obtained from (1) the patient's calculated alveolar

oxygen tension (PAO$_2$), which is derived from the **ideal alveolar gas equation to determine PAO$_2$** and (2) the patient's PaO$_2$, which is obtained from an arterial blood gas analysis.

The ideal alveolar gas equation is written as follows:

$$PAO_2 = FIO_2 \, (P_B - PH_2O) - PaCO_2 \div RQ.$$

where P$_B$ is the barometric pressure, PAO$_2$ is the partial pressure of oxygen within the alveoli, PH$_2$O is the partial pressure of water vapor in the alveoli (which is 47 mm Hg), FIO$_2$ is the fractional concentration of inspired oxygen, PaCO$_2$ is the partial pressure of arterial carbon dioxide, and RQ is the respiratory quotient. The RQ is the ratio of carbon dioxide production ($\dot{V}CO_2$) divided by **oxygen consumption ($\dot{V}O_2$)**. Under normal circumstances, about 250 mL of oxygen per minute is consumed by the tissue cells and about 200 mL per minute of carbon dioxide is excreted into the lung. Thus the RQ is normally about 0.8 but can range from 0.7 to 1.0. Clinically, a value of 0.8 is generally used for the RQ.

For example, if the patient is receiving an FIO$_2$ of 0.30 on a day when the barometric pressure is 750 mm Hg, and if the patient's PaCO$_2$ is 70 mm Hg and PaO$_2$ is 60 mm Hg, the P(A-a)O$_2$ can be calculated as follows:

$$
\begin{aligned}
PAO_2 &= FIO_2 \, (P_B - PH_2O) - PaCO_2 \div RQ \\
&= 0.30 \, (750 - 47) - 70 \div 0.8 \\
&= (0.30)(703) - 87.5 \\
&= 123.4^7 \text{ mm Hg.}
\end{aligned}
$$

Using the PaO$_2$ obtained from the arterial blood gas, the P(A-a)O$_2$ can now easily be calculated as follows:

$$
\begin{array}{r}
123.4 \text{ mm Hg (PAO}_2) \\
-60.0 \text{ mm Hg (PaO}_2) \\
\hline
= 63.4 \text{ mm Hg [P(A-a)O}_2]
\end{array}
$$

The normal P(A-a)O$_2$ on room air at sea level ranges from 7 to 15 mm Hg and should not exceed 30 mm Hg. Although the P(A-a)O$_2$ is very useful in patients breathing a low FIO$_2$, it loses some of its sensitivity in patients breathing a high FIO$_2$. The P(A-a)O$_2$ increases at high oxygen concentrations. Because of this, the P(A-a)O$_2$ has less value in the critically ill patient who is breathing a high oxygen concentration. The normal value for the P(A-a)O$_2$ on 100% oxygen is between 25 and 65 mm Hg. *The critical value is greater than 350 mm Hg.*

The P(A-a)O$_2$ increases in response to (1) oxygen diffusion disorders (e.g., chronic interstitial lung diseases), (2) ventilation-perfusion ratio mismatching, (3) right-to-left intracardiac shunting (e.g., a patent ventricular septum), and (4) age. *The P(A-a)O$_2$ is normal when alveolar hypoventilation is the cause of the patient's hypoxemia.*

Arterial-Alveolar Pressure Ratio (PaO$_2$/PAO$_2$ Ratio)

The **PaO$_2$/PAO$_2$ ratio** (also called *the a-A ratio or PaO$_2$/PAO$_2$ index*) reflects the amount of alveolar oxygen that moves into the arterial blood, not the calculated difference between alveolar and arterial pressure. The normal range for the young adult

---

[6]See Appendix XV on the Evolve site for a representative example of a cardiopulmonary profile sheet used to monitor the oxygen transport status of the critically ill patient.

[7]Blood gases and blood-derived values are customarily rounded up or down to the nearest whole number in clinical practice.

is 0.75 to 0.95. *The critical value is less than 0.75.* With pulmonary shunting, diffusion defects, and ventilation-perfusion mismatching, the PaO_2/PAO_2 ratio decreases in proportion to the amount of lung abnormality. Clinically, the PaO_2/PAO_2 ratio is most reliable when (1) the ratio is less than 0.55, (2) the FIO_2 is greater than 0.30, and (3) the PaO_2 is less than 100 mm Hg. Because of its reliability, the PaO_2/PAO_2 ratio is useful in following the patient's oxygenation status as the FIO_2 changes. In clinical practice, the FIO_2 often varies a great deal, and use of the ratio corrects for this problem and allows comparison of one blood gas with another.

Assuming that the cardiovascular system is otherwise stable, the PaO_2/PAO_2 ratio is an excellent clinical indicator of pulmonary shunting. It also changes minimally with FIO_2 changes and is not affected by $PaCO_2$ changes. It also may be used to predict the FIO_2 needed to obtain a desired PaO_2 level.

Thus using the data obtained for the case example presented previously in which the $PaO_2 = 60$ mm Hg and $PAO_2 = 123.4$ mm Hg, the patient's PaO_2/PAO_2 ratio would be calculated as follows:

$$PaO_2/PAO_2 \text{ ratio} = 60/123.4$$
$$= 0.49.$$

Arterial Oxygen Tension to Fractional Concentration of Inspired Oxygen Ratio (PaO_2/FIO_2 Ratio)

The **PaO_2/FIO_2 ratio** (also called *oxygenation ratio*) is useful in determining the extent of lung diffusion defects—for example, in acute respiratory distress syndrome (ARDS) (see Chapter 28, Acute Respiratory Distress Syndrome) or ventilator-induced lung injury (VILI) associated with mechanical ventilation (see Chapter 11, Respiratory Insufficiency, Respiratory Failure, and Ventilatory Management Protocols). On room air, the normal PaO_2/FIO_2 ratio range is between 350 and 450.[8] A PaO_2/FIO_2 ratio less than 200 indicates poor lung function. The PaO_2/FIO_2 ratio also decreases with ventilation-perfusion mismatching, pulmonary shunting, and diffusion defects.

The PaO_2/FIO_2 ratio is a relatively easy calculation to use when the PaO_2 is less than 100 mm Hg. For example, a PaO_2 of 75 mm Hg divided by an FIO_2 of 1.0 is 75 (75/1.0 = 75). However, a major limiting factor associated with use of the PaO_2/FIO_2 ratio is that changes in $PaCO_2$ can cause false readings. For example, if the $PaCO_2$ increases from 40 to 70 mm Hg during a period of hypoventilation, the PaO_2 decreases by about the same amount that the $PaCO_2$ increases (e.g., from 85 to 55 mm Hg). Thus if the patient was breathing an FIO_2 of 0.4, the PaO_2/FIO_2 ratio is 55/0.40 = 138. This low value of 138 suggests that the diffusion of oxygen is more impaired than the actual lung oxygenation status, which in this case is: 85/0.40 = 212. Thus caution should be used when using the PaO_2/FIO_2 ratio in patients who are hypoventilating and retaining CO_2.

Pulse Oximetric Saturation to Fractional Concentration of Inspired Oxygen Ratio (SpO_2/FIO_2 Ratio)

The SpO_2/FIO_2 ratio is commonly used in place of the PaO_2/FIO_2 ratio to facilitate the early recognition, diagnosis, and treatment of patients with lung diffusion problems such as acute respiratory distress syndrome (ARDS) and ventilator-induced lung injuries (VILI) (see VILI in Chapter 11, Respiratory Insufficiency, Respiratory Failure, and Ventilatory Management Protocols, and ARDS in Chapter 28, Acute Respiratory Distress Syndrome). Studies have shown there is a very high correlation between the SpO_2/FIO_2 ratio and the PaO_2/FIO_2 ratio—and, importantly, SpO_2/FIO_2 can be obtained without having the patient undergo an arterial blood gas stick.

Oxygen Saturation–Based and Content-Based Indices

The oxygen saturation–based and content-based indices can serve as excellent indicators of the individual's cardiac and ventilatory status. These oxygenation indices are derived from the patient's total **oxygen content in the arterial blood (CaO_2)**, **mixed venous blood ($C\bar{v}O_2$)**, and **pulmonary capillary blood (CcO_2)**. As explained earlier in this chapter, the CaO_2, $C\bar{v}O_2$, and CcO_2 are calculated using the following formulas:

$$CaO_2 = (Hb \times 1.34 \times SaO_2) + (PaO_2 \times 0.003)$$
$$C\bar{v}O_2 = (Hb \times 1.34 \times S\bar{v}O_2) + (P\bar{v}O_2 \times 0.003)$$
$$CcO_2 = (Hb \times 1.34) + (PAO_2 \times 0.003).$$

Clinically, the most common oxygen saturation–based and content-based indices are (1) total oxygen delivery (DO_2), (2) arterial-venous oxygen content difference ($C[a\text{-}\bar{v}]O_2$), (3) oxygen consumption ($\dot{V}O_2$), (4) oxygen extraction ratio (O_2ER), (5) **mixed venous oxygen saturation ($S\bar{v}O_2$)**, and (6) **pulmonary shunt fraction ($\dot{Q}_S/\dot{Q}_T$)**.[9]

Total Oxygen Delivery (DO_2)[10]

Total oxygen delivery (DO_2) is the amount of oxygen delivered to the peripheral tissue cells. The DO_2 is calculated as follows:

---

[9]The availability of the oxygen saturation–based and content-based indices that require the venous oxygen content—the $C(a\text{-}\bar{v})O_2$, $\dot{V}O_2$, O_2ER, $S\bar{v}O_2$, and $\dot{Q}_S/\dot{Q}_T$—may not be readily available because of the high risk to benefit ratio associated with the insertion of the pulmonary artery catheter needed to obtain venous blood. (See section on pulmonary artery catheter, page 97.)

[10]**Important Clinical Note:** It is important to understand that the formula used to calculate total oxygen delivery is one in which factors are *multiplied 3 times (!)* rather than added—in short, small decreases or increases in these factors have a marked influence on the final product. For example, consider the following: An elderly two-pack-per-day smoking gentlemen presents with dyspnea. His PaO_2 is 65 mm Hg on room air. He is mildly anemic (Hb = 9.0 g/dL) and has an SpO_2 of 90%. His carboxyhemoglobin level is (3.0%), which in turn makes the true SaO_2 87% (90% − 3% = 87%). He is on a beta-blocker for his hypertension, which reduces his cardiac output to 3.0 L/min. In addition, he has mild metabolic alkalosis (pH 7.48) from chronic diuretic therapy, which causes a leftward shift in his oxyhemoglobin dissociation curve. Inserting these figures into the total oxygen delivery calculation results in a markedly reduced oxygen delivery (oxygen transport) of about 321 mL of oxygen per minute. Couple this situation with fever and pain, which increase oxygen consumption, and we see real trouble ahead!

---

[8]The precise normal room air breathing PaO_2/FIO_2 ratio range is 380 to 476 (80 mm Hg/0.21 = 380; 100 mm Hg/0.21 = 476).

$$DO_2 = \dot{Q}_T \times (CaO_2 \times 10).$$

where $\dot{Q}_T$ is total cardiac output (L/min),[10] CaO_2 is oxygen content of arterial blood (milliliters of oxygen per 100 mL of blood), and the factor 10 is used to convert the CaO_2 to milliliters of oxygen *per liter* of blood.

For example, if the patient has a cardiac output of 3 L/min and a CaO_2 of 10.5 mL/dL, the DO_2 is 315 mL of oxygen per minute:

$$\begin{aligned} DO_2 &= \dot{Q}_T \times (CaO_2 \times 10) \\ &= 3\,L/min \times (10.5 \times 10) \\ &= 315\,mL\,O_2/min \end{aligned}$$

Normally, the DO_2 is about 1000 mL of oxygen per minute. Box 6.1 provides factors that increase and decrease the DO_2. Clinically, the **thermodilution** method is used to measure the patient's cardiac output. A bolus of solution of known volume and temperature is injected into the right atrium, and the resultant change in blood temperature is detected by a thermistor previously placed in the pulmonary artery with a special catheter (see Chapter 7, Assessment of the Cardiovascular System, for more discussion on hemodynamics).

Arterial-Venous Oxygen Content Difference (C[a-$\overline{v}$]O$_2$)[11]

The **arterial-venous oxygen content difference (C[a-$\overline{v}$]O$_2$)** is the difference between the CaO_2 and the $C\overline{v}O_2$ ($CaO_2 - C\overline{v}O_2$). Therefore if the patient's CaO_2 is 15 mL/dL, the $C\overline{v}O_2$ is 8 mL/dL, and the $C(a-\overline{v})O_2$ is 7 mL/dL:

$$\begin{aligned} C(a-\overline{v})O_2 &= CaO_2 - C\overline{v}O_2 \\ &= 15 - 8 \\ &= 7\,mL/dL\,O_2 \end{aligned}$$

Normally, the $C(a-\overline{v})O_2$ is about 5 mL/dL O$_2$. The $C(a-\overline{v})O_2$ is useful in assessing the patient's cardiopulmonary status because oxygen changes in the mixed venous blood ($C\overline{v}O_2$) often occur earlier than oxygen changes in arterial blood gas. Box 6.2 provides factors that increase and decrease the $C(a-\overline{v})O_2$.

Oxygen Consumption ($\dot{V}O_2$)[12]

Oxygen consumption ($\dot{V}O_2$), also known as *oxygen uptake*, is the amount of oxygen consumed by the peripheral tissue cells during a 1-minute period. The $\dot{V}O_2$ is calculated as follows:

$$\dot{V}O_2 = \dot{Q}_T[C(a-\overline{v})O_2 \times 10]$$

where $\dot{Q}_T$ is the total cardiac output (L/min), $C(a-\overline{v})O_2$ is the arterial-venous oxygen content difference, and the factor 10 is used to convert the $C(a-\overline{v})O_2$ to mL O$_2$/L.

Therefore if a patient has a cardiac output of 4 L/min and a $C(a-\overline{v})O_2$ of 6 mL/dL, the total amount of oxygen consumed by the tissue cells in 1 minute would be 240 mL:

$$\begin{aligned} \dot{V}O_2 &= \dot{Q}_T[C(a-\overline{v})O_2 \times 10] \\ &= 4\,L/min \times 6\,mL/dL \times 10 \\ &= 240\,mL\,O_2/min \end{aligned}$$

Normally, the $\dot{V}O_2$ is about 250 mL of oxygen per minute. It is often reported as a function of body weight (i.e., mL/kg or mL/lb). Box 6.3 provides factors that increase and decrease the $C(a-\overline{v})O_2$.

Oxygen Extraction Ratio (O$_2$ER)[13]

The **oxygen extraction ratio (O$_2$ER)**, also known as the *oxygen coefficient ratio* or *oxygen utilization ratio*, is the amount of oxygen consumed by the tissue cells divided by the total amount

---

[11]$C(a-\overline{v})O_2$ may not be readily available because of the high risk to benefit ratio associated with the insertion of the pulmonary artery catheter needed to obtain venous blood. (See section on pulmonary artery catheter, page 97.)

[12]The determination of $\dot{V}O_2$ may not be readily available because of the high risk to benefit ratio associated with the insertion of the pulmonary artery catheter needed to obtain venous blood. (See section on pulmonary artery catheter, page 97.)

[13]The determination of O$_2$ER may not be readily available because of the high risk to benefit ratio associated with the insertion of the pulmonary artery catheter needed to obtain venous blood. (See section on pulmonary artery catheter, page 97.)

BOX 6.3 Factors That Increase and Decrease the $\dot{V}O_2$

Factors That Increase the $\dot{V}O_2$
- Seizures
- Exercise
- Hyperthermia
- Increased body size

Factors That Decrease the $\dot{V}O_2$
- Skeletal muscle relaxation (e.g., induced by drugs)
- Peripheral shunting (e.g., sepsis)
- Certain poisons (e.g., cyanide)
- Hypothermia
- Decreased body size

BOX 6.4 Factors That Increase and Decrease the O_2ER

Factors That Increase the O_2ER
- Respiratory disease (e.g., asthmatic episode, pneumonia, emphysema)*
- Decreased cardiac output
- Periods of increased oxygen consumption
- Exercise
- Seizures
- Shivering
- Hyperthermia
- Anemia
- Decreased arterial oxygenation

Factors That Decrease the O_2ER
- Improvement of respiratory disease (e.g., reverse alveolar atelectasis or asthmatic episode)*
- Increased cardiac output
- Skeletal muscle relaxation (e.g., induced by drugs)
- Peripheral shunting (e.g., sepsis, trauma)
- Certain poisons (e.g., cyanide)
- Hypothermia
- Increased hemoglobin
- Increased arterial oxygenation

*See Table 6.3, page 89.

of oxygen delivered. The O_2ER is calculated by dividing the $C(a\text{-}\overline{v})O_2$ by the CaO_2. Therefore if a patient has a CaO_2 of 15 mL/dL and a $C\overline{v}O_2$ of 10 mL/dL, the O_2ER would be 33%:

$$O_2ER = \frac{CaO_2 - C\overline{v}O_2}{CaO_2}$$
$$= \frac{15\text{ mL/dL} - 10\text{ mL/dL}}{15\text{ mL/dL}}$$
$$= \frac{5\text{ mL/dL}}{15\text{ mL/dL}}$$
$$= 0.33$$

Normally, the O_2ER is about 25%. Box 6.4 provides factors that increase and decrease the O_2ER.

Mixed Venous Oxygen Saturation ($S\overline{v}O_2$)[14]

When a patient has a normal arterial oxygen saturation (SaO_2) and hemoglobin concentration, the mixed venous oxygen saturation ($S\overline{v}O_2$) is often used as an early indicator of changes in the patient's $C(a\text{-}\overline{v})O_2$, $\dot{V}O_2$, and O_2ER, which are measures of net tissue oxygenation. The $S\overline{v}O_2$ can signal changes in the patient's $C(a\text{-}\overline{v})O_2$, $\dot{V}O_2$, and O_2ER earlier than arterial blood gases because the PaO_2 and SaO_2 levels are often normal during early tissue oxygenation changes. Normally, the $S\overline{v}O_2$ is about 75%. The $S\overline{v}O_2$ can be measured directly by obtaining a venous blood sample from a pulmonary arterial catheter or derived as follows:

$$S\overline{v}O_2 = \frac{DO_2 - \dot{V}O_2}{DO_2}$$

where the DO_2 is the total oxygen delivery and the $\dot{V}O_2$ is the oxygen consumption. Thus if the patient has a normal DO_2 of 1000 mL O_2/min, and a normal $\dot{V}O_2$ of 250 mL O_2/min, the $S\overline{v}O_2$ is 0.75:

$$S\overline{v}O_2 = \frac{DO_2 - \dot{V}O_2}{DO_2}$$
$$= \frac{1000 - 250}{1000}$$
$$= \frac{750}{1000}$$
$$= 0.75.$$

Box 6.5 lists factors that increase and decrease the $S\overline{v}O_2$. Table 6.1 summarizes the way various clinical factors alter the patient's DO_2, $\dot{V}O_2$, $C(a\text{-}\overline{v})O_2$, O_2ER, and $S\overline{v}O_2$.

A simple but helpful way to visualize the $S\overline{v}O_2$ is to consider this oxygen index as reflecting the oxygen that is "left over" in the mixed venous blood after it has been used by the tissues in satisfying the metabolic needs of the body. This can be used as a good, quick estimate of the *overall success* of the gas exchange mechanism described in Chapter 3, The Pathophysiologic Basis for Common Clinical Manifestations.

Pulmonary Shunt Fraction ($\dot{Q}_S/\dot{Q}_T$)[15]

Because pulmonary shunting and venous admixture are frequent complications in respiratory disorders, knowledge of the degree of shunting is desirable in developing patient care plans. The amount of intrapulmonary shunting can be calculated by using the classic shunt equation:

$$\frac{\dot{Q}_S}{\dot{Q}_T} = \frac{CcO_2 - CaO_2}{CcO_2 - C\overline{v}O_2}$$

where $\dot{Q}_S$ is the cardiac output that is shunted, $\dot{Q}_T$ is the total cardiac output, CcO_2 is the oxygen content of pulmonary

---

[14]The determination of $S\overline{v}O_2$ may not be readily available because of the high risk to benefit ratio associated with the insertion of the pulmonary artery catheter needed to obtain venous blood. (See section on pulmonary artery catheter, page 97.)

[15]The measurement of $\dot{Q}_S/\dot{Q}_T$ may not be readily available because of the high risk to benefit ratio associated with the insertion of the pulmonary artery catheter needed to obtain venous blood. (See pulmonary artery catheter, page 97.)

BOX 6.5 Factors That Increase and Decrease the S$\bar{v}O_2$

Factors That Increase the S$\bar{v}O_2$
- Improvement of respiratory disease (e.g., reverse alveolar atelectasis or asthmatic episode)*
- Increased cardiac output
- Increased concentration of oxygen (FIO$_2$)
- Skeletal muscle relaxation (e.g., induced by drugs)
- Peripheral shunting (e.g., sepsis)
- Certain poisons (e.g., cyanide)
- Hypothermia

Factors That Decrease the S$\bar{v}O_2$
- Respiratory disease (e.g., asthmatic episode, pneumonia, emphysema)*
- Decreased cardiac output
- Decreased concentration of oxygen (FIO$_2$)
- Periods of increased oxygen consumption
- Exercise
- Seizures
- Shivering
- Hyperthermia

*See Table 6.3, page 89.

TABLE 6.1 Clinical Factors That Affect Oxygen Transport Calculations*

Oxygen Transport Study	Equation	Factors That Increase Value	Factors That Decrease Value
Total oxygen delivery (DO$_2$)	$DO_2 = \dot{Q}_T \times (CaO_2 \times 10)$	Increased blood oxygenation Increased hemoglobin Increased cardiac output	Decreased blood oxygenation Decreased hemoglobin Decreased cardiac output
Arterial-venous oxygen content difference (C[a-$\bar{v}$]O$_2$)	$C(a-\bar{v})O_2$	Decreased cardiac output Increased O$_2$ consumption Exercise Seizures Shivering Hyperthermia	Increased cardiac output Skeletal muscle relaxation Induced by drugs Peripheral shunting Sepsis Trauma Certain poisons Cyanide Hypothermia
Oxygen consumption (V̇O$_2$)	$\dot{V}O_2 = \dot{Q}_T[C(a-\bar{v})O_2 \times 10]$	Exercise Seizures Shivering Hyperthermia	Skeletal muscle relaxation induced by drugs Peripheral shunting Sepsis Trauma Certain poisons Cyanide Hypothermia
Oxygen extraction ratio (O$_2$ER)	$O_2ER = \dfrac{CaO_2 - C\bar{v}O_2}{CaO_2}$	Increased cardiac output Skeletal muscle relaxation induced by drugs Peripheral shunting Sepsis Trauma Certain poisons Cyanide Hypothermia Increased hemoglobin Increased arterial oxygenation	Decreased cardiac output Increased O$_2$ consumption Exercise Seizures Shivering Hyperthermia Anemia Decreased arterial oxygenation
Mixed venous oxygen saturation (S$\bar{v}O_2$)	$S\bar{v}O_2 = \dfrac{DO_2 - \dot{V}O_2}{DO_2}$	Decreased cardiac output Increased O$_2$ consumption Exercise Seizures Shivering Hyperthermia	Increased cardiac output Skeletal muscle relaxation induced by drugs Peripheral shunting Sepsis Trauma Certain poisons (cyanide) Hypothermia
Pulmonary shunt fraction ($\dot{Q}_S/\dot{Q}_T$)	$\dfrac{\dot{Q}_S}{\dot{Q}_T} = \dfrac{CcO_2 - CaO_2}{CcO_2 - C\bar{v}O_2}$	See Table 6.3	N/A

*The availability of the oxygen saturation–based and content-based indices that require the venous oxygen content—the C(a-$\bar{v}$)O$_2$, V̇O$_2$, O$_2$ER, S$\bar{v}$O$_2$, and $\dot{Q}_S/\dot{Q}_T$—may not be readily available because of the risk to benefit ratio associated with the insertion of the pulmonary arterial catheter needed to obtain mixed venous blood.

capillary blood, CaO_2 is the oxygen content of arterial blood, and $C\bar{v}O_2$ is the oxygen content of mixed venous blood.

To obtain the data necessary to calculate the patient's intrapulmonary shunt, the following information must be gathered:
- Barometric pressure
- PaO_2
- SaO_2 (arterial oxygen saturation)
- $PaCO_2$
- $P\bar{v}O_2$
- $S\bar{v}O_2$ (mixed venous oxygen saturation)
- Hemoglobin concentration
- PAO_2 (partial pressure of alveolar oxygen)[16]
- FIO_2 (fractional concentration of inspired oxygen)

A clinical example of the shunt calculation follows:

Shunt Study Calculation in an Automobile Accident Victim

A 22-year-old man is on a volume-cycled mechanical ventilator on a day when the barometric pressure is 755 mm Hg. The patient is receiving an FIO_2 of 0.60. The following clinical data are obtained:
- Hb: 15 g/dL
- PaO_2: 65 mm Hg (SaO_2: 90%)
- $PaCO_2$: 56 mm Hg
- $P\bar{v}O_2$: 35 mm Hg ($S\bar{v}O_2$: 65%)

With this information the patient's PAO_2, CcO_2, CaO_2, and $C\bar{v}O_2$ now can be calculated. (The clinician should remember that PH_2O represents alveolar water vapor pressure and is always 47 mm Hg.)

1.
$$PAO_2 = (PB - P_{H_2O})\, FIO_2 - PaCO_2\,(1.25)$$
$$= (755 - 47)\,0.60 - 56\,(1.25)$$
$$= (708)\,0.60 - 70$$
$$= 424.8 - 70$$
$$= 354.8$$

2.
$$CcO_2 = (Hb \times 1.34) + (PAO_2 \times 0.003)$$
$$= (15 \times 1.34) + (354.8 \times 0.003)$$
$$= 20.1 + 1.064$$
$$= 21.164\ (mL/dL\ O_2)$$

3.
$$CcO_2 = (Hb \times 1.34) + (PAO_2 \times 0.003)$$
$$= (15 \times 1.34) + (354.8 \times 0.003)$$
$$= 20.1 + 1.064$$
$$= 21.164\ (mL/dL\ O_2)$$

4.
$$C\bar{v}O_2 = (Hb \times 1.34 \times S\bar{v}O_2) + (P\bar{v}O_2 \times 0.003)$$
$$= (15 \times 1.34 \times 0.65) + (35 \times 0.003)$$
$$= 13.065 + 0.105$$
$$= 13.17\ (mL/dL\ O_2)$$

TABLE 6.2 Clinical Significance of Pulmonary Shunting

Degree of Pulmonary Shunting (%)	Clinical Significance
Below 10%	Normal lung status
10%–20%	Indicates a pulmonary abnormality but is not significant in terms of cardiopulmonary support
20%–30%	May be life threatening, possibly requiring cardiopulmonary support
Greater than 30%	Serious life-threatening condition, almost always requiring cardiopulmonary support

With this information the patient's intrapulmonary shunt fraction now can be calculated:

$$\frac{\dot{Q}_S}{\dot{Q}_T} = \frac{CcO_2 - CaO_2}{CcO_2 - C\bar{v}O_2}$$
$$= \frac{21.164 - 18.285}{21.164 - 13.17}$$
$$= \frac{2.879}{7.994}$$
$$= 0.36$$

Therefore 36% of the patient's pulmonary blood flow is perfusing lung alveoli that are not being ventilated.

Table 6.2 shows the clinical significance of pulmonary shunting. Table 6.3 summarizes how specific respiratory diseases alter the oxygen saturation–based and content-based indices.[17]

Hypoxemia Versus Hypoxia

Hypoxemia refers to an abnormally low arterial oxygen tension (PaO_2) and is frequently associated with **hypoxia**, which is an inadequate level of tissue oxygenation (see the following discussion). Although the presence of hypoxemia strongly suggests tissue hypoxia, it does not necessarily mean the absolute existence of tissue hypoxia. For example, the reduced level of oxygen in the arterial blood may be offset by an increased cardiac output or an increased hemoglobin level. However, in sick patients, these compensatory mechanisms often are not available. A good example would be an anemic patient on beta-adrenergic blockers such as propranolol or an elderly patient with reduced cardiac function.

Hypoxemia is commonly classified as **mild hypoxemia, moderate hypoxemia,** or **severe hypoxemia** (Table 6.4). Clinically, the presence of mild hypoxemia generally stimulates

---

[16]See Appendix VIII on the Evolve site.

[17]Note in Table 6.3 that virtually every respiratory disorder presented in this textbook causes the $\dot{Q}_S/\dot{Q}_T$ to increase and the DO_2 to decrease.

TABLE 6.3 Oxygenation Index Changes Commonly Seen in Specific Respiratory Diseases

Respiratory Diseases	Oxygenation Indices					
Pulmonary disorder	SⱽO2 (75%)	DO2* (1000 mL O2/min)	V̇O2 (250 mL O2/min)	C(a-v̄)O2 5 mL/dL	O2ER (25%)	Q̇s/Q̇t (<10%)
Obstructive airway disease	↓	↓	~†	~	↑	↑
Chronic bronchitis						
Emphysema						
Asthma						
Cystic fibrosis						
Bronchiectasis						
Loss of volume	↓	↓	~	~	↑	↑
Atelectasis						
Infectious pulmonary diseases	↓	↓	~	~	↑	↑
Pneumonia						
Tuberculosis						
Pulmonary vascular diseases	↓	↓	~	↑†	↑	↑
Pulmonary edema						
Pulmonary embolism						
Chest and pleural trauma	↓	↓	~	↑†	↑	↑
Flail chest						
Pneumothorax						
Disorders of the pleura and chest wall	↓	↓	~	~	↑	↑
Pleural disease (e.g., hemothorax)						
Kyphoscoliosis						
Lung cancer	↓	↓	~	~	↑	↑
Diffuse alveolar disease	↓	↓	~	~	↑	↑
Interstitial lung disease						
Acute respiratory distress syndrome						
Neurorespiratory disorders	↓	↓	~	~	↑	↑
Sleep apnea						
Amyotrophic lateral sclerosis (ALS)						
Newborn and childhood diseases	↓	↓	~	~	↑	↑
Meconium aspiration syndrome						
Transient tachypnea of the newborn						
Respiratory distress syndrome						
Pulmonary air leak syndrome						
Respiratory syncytial virus infection						
Bronchopulmonary dysplasia						
Congenital diaphragmatic hernia						
Croup syndrome						

*The DO2 may be normal in patients with an increased cardiac output, an increased hemoglobin level (polycythemia), or a combination of both. For example, a normal DO2 is often seen in patients with chronic obstructive pulmonary disease and polycythemia. When the DO2 is normal, the patient's O2ER is usually normal.

†~ Unchanged.

‡The increased C(a-v̄)O2 is associated with a decreased cardiac output.

the oxygen peripheral chemoreceptors to increase the patient's breathing rate and heart rate (see Fig. 3.5).

Hypoxia refers to low or inadequate oxygen for aerobic cellular metabolism. Hypoxia is characterized by tachycardia, hypertension, peripheral vasoconstriction, dizziness, and mental confusion. Table 6.5 provides an overview of the four main types of hypoxia. When hypoxia exists, alternative anaerobic mechanisms are activated in the tissues that produce dangerous metabolites, such as **lactic acid**, as waste products. Lactic acid is a nonvolatile acid and causes the pH to decrease.

Pathophysiologic Conditions Associated With Chronic Hypoxia

Cor Pulmonale

Cor pulmonale is the term used to denote pulmonary arterial hypertension, right ventricular hypertrophy, increased right ventricular work, and ultimately right ventricular failure. The three major mechanisms involved in producing cor pulmonale in chronic pulmonary disease are (1) the increased viscosity of the blood associated with polycythemia, (2) the increased pulmonary vascular resistance caused by hypoxic vasoconstriction, and (3) the obliteration of the pulmonary capillary bed, particularly in emphysema. Items 1 and 2 are discussed in greater depth in the following paragraphs.

Polycythemia

When pulmonary disorders produce chronic hypoxia, the renal cells release higher than normal amounts of the hormone **erythropoietin**, which in turn stimulates the bone marrow to increase red blood cell production. Red blood cell production is known as *erythropoiesis*. An increased level of red blood cells is called **polycythemia**. The polycythemia that results from hypoxia is an adaptive mechanism that increases the oxygen-carrying capacity of the blood.

Unfortunately, the advantage of the increased oxygen-carrying capacity in polycythemia is at least partially offset by the increased viscosity of the blood when the hematocrit reaches 50% to 60%. Because of the increased viscosity of the

blood, a greater driving pressure is needed to maintain a given flow.

Hypoxic Vasoconstriction of the Lungs

Hypoxic vasoconstriction of the pulmonary vascular system (**hypoxic vasoconstriction of the lungs**) commonly develops in response to the decreased PAO_2 that occurs in chronic respiratory disorders. The decreased PAO_2 causes the smooth muscles of the pulmonary arterioles to constrict. The exact mechanism of this phenomenon is unclear. However, the PAO_2 (and not the PaO_2) is known to chiefly control this response.

The early effect of hypoxic vasoconstriction is to direct blood away from the hypoxic regions of the lungs and thereby offset the shunt effect. However, when the number of hypoxic regions becomes significant, such as during the advanced stages of emphysema or chronic bronchitis, a generalized pulmonary vasoconstriction develops, causing the pulmonary vascular resistance to increase substantially. Increased pulmonary vascular resistance leads to pulmonary hypertension, increased work of the right side of the heart, right ventricular hypertrophy, and cor pulmonale.

The cor pulmonale associated with chronic respiratory disorders may develop from the combined effects of polycythemia and pulmonary arterial vasoconstriction. Both of these conditions occur as a result of chronic hypoxia. Clinically, cor pulmonale leads to the accumulation of venous blood in the large veins. This condition causes (1) the neck veins to become distended (see Fig. 3.25), (2) the extremities to show signs of peripheral edema and pitting edema (see Fig. 3.24), and (3) the liver to become enlarged and tender.

TABLE 6.4 Hypoxemia Severity Classifications*	
Classification	PaO$_2$ (mm Hg) (Rule of Thumb)
Normal	80–100
Mild hypoxemia	60–80
Moderate hypoxemia	40–60
Severe hypoxemia	<40

*The hypoxemia classifications provided in this table are generally accepted in clinical practice. Minor variations of these values are found in the literature. As a general rule of thumb, however, the hypoxemia classifications and PaO$_2$ range(s) presented in this table are useful guidelines.

TABLE 6.5 Types of Hypoxia		
Hypoxia	Descriptions	Common Causes
Hypoxic hypoxia (also called *hypoxemic hypoxia*)	Inadequate oxygen at the tissue cell caused by low arterial oxygen tension (PaO$_2$)	Low PAO$_2$ caused by: Hypoventilation High altitude Diffusion impairment Interstitial fibrosis Interstitial lung disease Interstitial pulmonary edema Pneumoconiosis Ventilation-perfusion mismatch Pulmonary shunting
Anemic hypoxia	PaO$_2$ is normal, but the oxygen-carrying capacity and thus the oxygen content of the blood is inadequate	Decreased hemoglobin concentration Anemia Hemorrhage Abnormal hemoglobin Carboxyhemoglobin Methemoglobin
Circulatory hypoxia (also called *stagnant* or *hypoperfusion hypoxia*)	Blood flow to the tissue cells is inadequate; therefore adequate oxygen is not available to meet tissue needs	Hypotension Slow flow or stagnant (pooling) of peripheral blood Arterial-venous shunts
Histotoxic hypoxia	Impaired ability of the tissue cells to metabolize oxygen	Cyanide poisoning

True Hypoxia—Can It Be Measured?

Our understanding of oxygen transport and cellular utilization of oxygen may be on the threshold of greatly increased depth and scientific sophistication. In the past decade, a number of cell-permeable phosphorescence-based probes for imaging of **intracellular oxygen tension (icO2)** have been developed. These probes are 1/600th of the diameter of a human hair. Once placed they can aid in the analysis of true tissue hypoxia and gradients across the cellular, nuclear, and mitochondrial membranes and can evaluate oxygenation responses to pharmacologic and oxygen therapy manipulations with high cellular component resolution. That is, you will be able to analyze tissue oxygen at the mitochondrial level. The technology of the probes themselves, called **nanostraws**, is remarkable and too complex to describe in detail here. The operational performance of this technology is still being evaluated in individual cell and tissue models, but it is clear that the next edition of this volume may well describe oxygen-related physiology at the "end-user level," *where it counts*—that is, in the powerhouse of the cell, the mitochondria themselves!

SELF-ASSESSMENT QUESTIONS

1. A 46-year-old woman with severe asthma arrives in the emergency department with the following clinical data:
   Hb: 11 g/dL
   PaO_2: 46 mm Hg
   SaO_2: 70%
   Based on these clinical data, what is the patient's CaO_2?
   a. 6.75 mL/dL O_2
   b. 10.50 mL/dL O_2
   c. 12.30 mL/dL O_2
   d. 15.25 mL/dL O_2

2. If the patient has a cardiac output of 6 L/min and a CaO_2 of 12 mL/dL, what is the DO_2?
   a. 210 mL O_2/min
   b. 345 mL O_2/min
   c. 540 mL O_2/min
   d. 720 mL O_2/min

3. If the patient's CaO_2 is 11 mL/dL and the $C\overline{v}O_2$ is 7 mL/dL, what is the $C(a-\overline{v})O_2$?
   a. 4 mL/dL O_2
   b. 7 mL/dL O_2
   c. 11 mL/dL O_2
   d. 15 mL/dL O_2

4. Clinically, the patient's $C(a-\overline{v})O_2$ increases in response to which of the following?
   1. Hypothermia
   2. Decreased cardiac output
   3. Seizures
   4. Cyanide poisoning
   a. 2 only
   b. 4 only
   c. 2 and 3 only
   d. 1 and 4 only

5. If a patient has a cardiac output of 6 L/min and a $C(a-\overline{v})O_2$ of 4 mL/dL, what is the $\dot{V}O_2$?
   a. 160 mL O_2/min
   b. 180 mL O_2/min
   c. 200 mL O_2/min
   d. 240 mL O_2/min

6. Clinically, the $\dot{V}O_2$ decreases in response to which of the following?
   1. Exercise
   2. Hyperthermia
   3. Body size
   4. Peripheral shunting
   a. 2 only
   b. 4 only
   c. 1 and 3 only
   d. 2, 3, and 4 only

7. If the patient's CaO_2 is 12 mL/dL and the CvO_2 is 7 mL/dL, what is the O_2ER?
   a. 0.27
   b. 0.33
   c. 0.42
   d. 0.53

8. Clinically, the $S\overline{v}O_2$ decreases in response to which of the following?
   a. Increased cardiac output
   b. Seizures
   c. Peripheral shunting
   d. Hypothermia

9. In the patient with severe emphysema, which of the following oxygenation indices are commonly seen?
   1. Decreased $S\overline{v}O_2$
   2. Increased $\dot{V}O_2$
   3. Decreased $C(a-\overline{v})O_2$
   4. Increased O_2ER
   a. 1 only
   b. 3 only
   c. 1 and 4 only
   d. 2 and 3 only

10. In the patient with pulmonary edema, which of the following oxygenation indices are commonly seen?
    1. Increased O_2ER
    2. Decreased $S\overline{v}O_2$
    3. Increased $\dot{V}O_2$
    4. Decreased $\dot{V}O_2$
    a. 2 only
    b. 4 only
    c. 1 and 2 only
    d. 1, 2, and 3 only

Case Study: Gunshot Victim (Questions 11 to 15)

A 37-year-old woman is on a volume-cycled mechanical ventilator on a day when the barometric pressure is 745 mm Hg. The patient is receiving an FIO_2 of 0.50. The following clinical data are obtained:

Hb: 11 g/dL
PaO_2: 60 mm Hg (SaO_2 90%)
$P\overline{v}O_2$: 35 mm Hg ($S\overline{v}O_2$ 65%)
$PaCO_2$: 38 mm Hg
Cardiac output: 6 L/min

11. Based on this information, calculate the patient's total oxygen delivery.
    a. 510 mL O_2/min
    b. 740 mL O_2/min
    c. 806 mL O_2/min
    d. 930 mL O_2/min

12. Based on this information, calculate the patient's arterial-venous oxygen content difference.
    a. 2.45 mL/dL O_2
    b. 3.76 mL/dL O_2
    c. 4.20 mL/dL O_2
    d. 5.40 mL/dL O_2

13. Based on this information, calculate the patient's intrapulmonary shunt fraction.
    a. 22%
    b. 26%
    c. 33%
    d. 37%

14. Based on this information, calculate the patient's oxygen consumption.
    a. 170 mL O_2/min
    b. 200 mL O_2/min
    c. 230 mL O_2/min
    d. 280 mL O_2/min

15. Based on this information, calculate the patient's oxygen extraction ratio.
    a. 16%
    b. 24%
    c. 26%
    d. 28%

CHAPTER

7 Assessment of the Cardiovascular System

Chapter Objectives

After reading this chapter, you will be able to:

- Describe the electrocardiogram pattern of a normal cardiac cycle.
- Evaluate and identify arrhythmias.
- Describe the noninvasive hemodynamic monitoring assessments.
- Evaluate the basic pathophysiologic mechanisms associated with an increased heart rate (pulse), cardiac output, and blood pressure and a decreased perfusion state.
- Describe invasive hemodynamic monitoring assessment methods.
- Describe how the hypoxemia, acidemia, or pulmonary vascular obstruction associated with respiratory disease alters the hemodynamic status.
- Define key terms and complete self-assessment questions at the end of the chapter and on Evolve.

Key Terms

Arterial Catheter (Systemic)
Asystole (Cardiac Standstill)
Atrial Fibrillation
Atrial Flutter
Atrial "Kick"
Bigeminy
Capillary Refill Test
Cardiac Arrest
Central Venous Catheter
Central Venous Pressure (CVP) Catheter
Coronary Angiography
Electrocardiograph (ECG) Patterns
Hemodynamics
Invasive Hemodynamic Monitoring Assessments
Noninvasive Hemodynamic Monitoring Assessments
P Wave
Premature Ventricular Contraction (PVC)

Pulmonary Artery Catheter (Swan-Ganz Catheter)
Pulmonary Capillary Wedge Pressure (PWCP)
Pulseless Electrical Activity (PEA)
QRS Complex
Sinus Arrhythmia
Sinus Bradycardia
Sinus Tachycardia
Thermodilution Catheter
T wave
Trigeminy
Ventricular Fibrillation
Ventricular Tachycardia

Chapter Outline

The Electrocardiogram
Common Heart Arrhythmias
  Sinus Bradycardia
  Sinus Tachycardia
  Sinus Arrhythmia
  Atrial Flutter
  Atrial Fibrillation
  Premature Ventricular Contractions
  Ventricular Tachycardia
  Ventricular Fibrillation
  Asystole (Cardiac Standstill)
Noninvasive Hemodynamic Monitoring Assessments
  Heart Rate (Pulse), Cardiac Output, and Blood Pressure
  Perfusion State
Invasive Cardiovascular Monitoring Assessments
  Pulmonary Artery Catheter
  Systemic Arterial Catheter
  Central Venous Pressure Catheter
Cardiovascular (Hemodynamic) Monitoring in Respiratory Diseases
Self-Assessment Questions

Because the transport of oxygen to the tissue cells and the delivery of carbon dioxide to the lungs are functions of the cardiovascular system, a basic knowledge and understanding of (1) normal electrocardiogram (ECG) patterns, (2) common heart arrhythmias, (3) **noninvasive hemodynamic monitoring assessments**, (4) **invasive hemodynamic monitoring**

assessments, and (5) determinants of cardiac output are essential components of patient assessment.[1]

The Electrocardiogram

Because the respiratory care practitioner frequently works with critically ill patients who are on cardiac monitors, a basic understanding of normal and common abnormal **electrocardiograph (ECG) patterns** is important. An ECG monitors, both visually and on recording paper, the electrical activity of the heart.

---

[1]See Appendix XV on the Evolve site for an example of a cardiopulmonary profile sheet used to monitor the hemodynamic status of the critically ill patient.

Fig. 7.1 illustrates the ECG pattern of a normal cardiac cycle. The **P wave** reflects depolarization of the atria. The **QRS complex** represents the depolarization of the ventricles, and the **T wave** represents ventricular repolarization.

In normal adults the heart rate is between 60 and 100 beats per minute (bpm). In normal infants the heart rate is 130 to 150 bpm. A number of methods can be used to calculate the heart rate. For example, when the rhythm is regular, the heart rate can be determined at a glance by counting the number of large boxes (on the electrocardiograph [ECG] strip) between two QRS complexes and then dividing this number into 300. Therefore if an ECG strip consistently shows four large boxes between each pair of QRS complexes, the heart rate is 75 bpm ($300 \div 4 = 75$). When the rhythm is irregular, the heart rate can be determined by counting the QRS complexes on a 6-second strip and multiplying by 10. The following heart arrhythmias are commonly seen and should be recognized by the respiratory care practitioner.

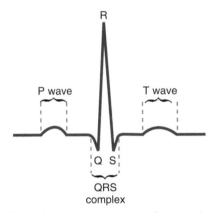

FIGURE 7.1 Electrocardiographic pattern of a normal cardiac cycle.

Common Heart Arrhythmias[2]

Sinus Bradycardia

In **sinus bradycardia** the heart rate is less than 60 bpm. *Bradycardia* means "slow heart." Sinus bradycardia has a normal P-QRS-T pattern, and the rhythm is regular (Fig. 7.2). Healthy athletes often demonstrate this finding because of increased cardiac stroke volume and other poorly understood mechanisms. Common pathologic causes of sinus bradycardia include a weakened or damaged sinoatrial (SA) node, severe or chronic hypoxemia, increased intracranial pressure, obstructive sleep apnea, and certain drugs (most notably the beta-blockers). Sinus bradycardia may lead to decreased cardiac output and blood pressure. In severe cases, sinus bradycardia may lead to a decreased vascular perfusion state and tissue hypoxia. The patient may demonstrate a weak pulse, poor capillary refill, cold and clammy skin, and a depressed sensorium.

Sinus Tachycardia

In **sinus tachycardia** the heart rate is greater than 100 bpm. *Tachycardia* means "fast heart." Sinus tachycardia has a normal P-QRS-T pattern, and the rhythm is regular (Fig. 7.3). Sinus tachycardia is the normal physiologic response to stress and exercise. Common abnormal causes of sinus tachycardia include hypoxemia, severe anemia, hyperthermia, massive hemorrhage, pain, fear, anxiety, hyperthyroidism, and sympathomimetic or parasympatholytic drug administration.

[2]For a complete review of common heart arrhythmias, see Des Jardins, T. (2019). *Cardiopulmonary anatomy and physiology: essentials of respiratory care* (7th ed.). Clifton Park, NY: Delmar/Cengage Learning.

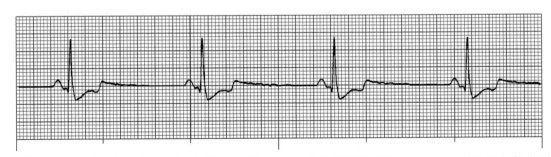

FIGURE 7.2 Sinus bradycardia at about 40 bpm. (From Aehlert, B. [2018]. *ECGs made easy* [6th ed.]. St. Louis, MO: Elsevier.)

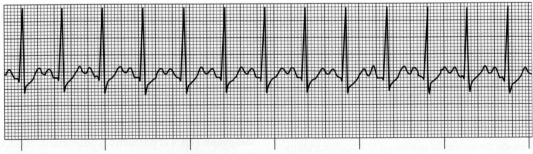

FIGURE 7.3 Sinus tachycardia at about 125 bpm. (From Aehlert, B. [2018]. *ECGs made easy* [6th ed.]. St. Louis, MO: Elsevier.)

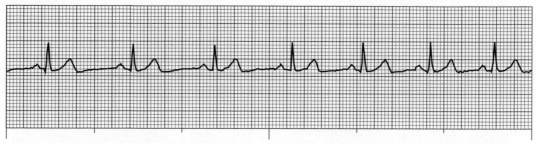

FIGURE 7.4 Sinus arrhythmia at 63 to 81 bpm. (From Aehlert, B. [2018]. *ECGs made easy* [6th ed.]. St. Louis, MO: Elsevier.)

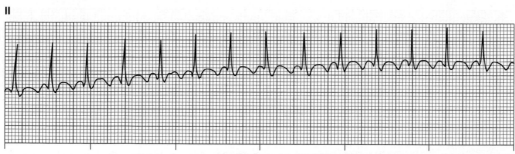

FIGURE 7.5 Atrial flutter. (From Aehlert, B. [2018]. *ECGs made easy* [6th ed.]. St. Louis, MO: Elsevier.)

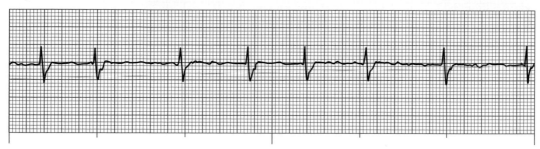

FIGURE 7.6 Atrial fibrillation with a ventricular response of 63 to 100 bpm. (From Aehlert, B. [2018]. *ECGs made easy* [6th ed.]. St. Louis, MO: Elsevier.)

Sinus Arrhythmia

In **sinus arrhythmia** the heart rate varies by more than 10% from beat to beat. The P-QRS-T pattern is normal (Fig. 7.4), but the interval between groups of complexes (i.e., the R-R interval) varies. Sinus arrhythmia is a normal rhythm in children and young adults. The patient's pulse will often increase during inspiration and decrease during expiration. No treatment is required unless significant alteration occurs in the patient's arterial blood pressure.

Atrial Flutter

In **atrial flutter** the normal P wave is absent and replaced by two or more regular sawtooth waves. The QRS complex is normal, and the ventricular rate may be regular or irregular, depending on the relationship of the atrial to the ventricular beats. Fig. 7.5 shows an atrial flutter with a regular rhythm with a 2:1 conduction ratio (i.e., two atrial beats for every one ventricular beat). The atrial rate is usually constant, between 250 and 350 bpm, whereas the ventricular rate is in the normal range or elevated. Causes of atrial flutter include hypoxemia, a damaged SA node, and congestive heart failure.

Atrial Fibrillation

In **atrial fibrillation**, the atrial contractions are disorganized and ineffective, and the normal P wave is absent (Fig. 7.6). The atrial rate ranges from 350 to 700 bpm. The QRS complex is normal, and the ventricular rate ranges from 100 to 200 bpm. Causes of atrial fibrillation include hypoxemia and a damaged SA node. Atrial fibrillation may reduce the cardiac output by 20% because of a loss of atrial filling (the so-called **atrial kick**). Atrial fibrillation is frequently seen in sleep apnea (see Chapter 32, Sleep Apnea).

Premature Ventricular Contractions

A **premature ventricular contraction (PVC)** is not preceded by a P wave. The QRS complex is wide, bizarre, and unlike the normal QRS complex (Fig. 7.7). The regular heart rate is altered by the PVC. The heart rhythm may be very irregular when there are many PVCs. PVCs can occur at any rate. PVCs often occur in pairs. A PVC also may be seen after every normal heartbeat—an arrhythmia called *bigeminal PVCs* or **bigeminy**. A PVC also may be seen after every two normal heartbeats—an arrhythmia called *trigeminal PVCs* or **trigeminy**.

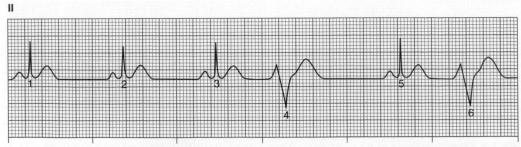

FIGURE 7.7 Sinus rhythm with premature ventricular complexes (PVCs). The fourth and sixth beats are very different in appearance from the normal conducted sinus beats. Beats 4 and 6 are PVCs. They are not preceded by P waves. (From Grauer, K. [1998]. *A practical guide to ECG interpretation* [2nd ed.]. St. Louis, MO: Mosby.)

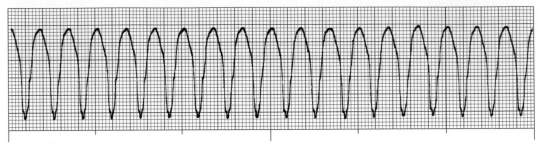

FIGURE 7.8 Ventricular tachycardia. (From Aehlert, B. [2004]. *ECG study cards.* St. Louis, MO: Elsevier.)

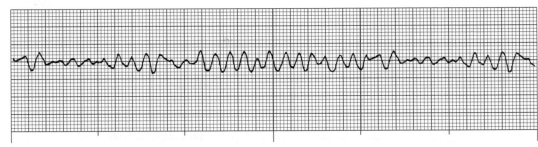

FIGURE 7.9 Ventricular fibrillation. (From Aehlert, B. [2018]. *ECGs made easy* [6th ed.]. St. Louis, MO: Elsevier.)

Common causes of PVCs include intrinsic myocardial disease, hypoxemia, acidemia, hypokalemia, and congestive heart failure. PVCs also may be a sign of theophylline or alpha-stimulant or beta-agonist toxicity.

Ventricular Tachycardia

In **ventricular tachycardia** the P wave is generally indiscernible, and the QRS complex is wide and bizarre in appearance (Fig. 7.8). The T wave may not be separated from the QRS complex. The ventricular rate ranges from 150 to 250 bpm, and the rate is regular or slightly irregular. The patient's blood pressure is usually decreased during ventricular tachycardia. In fact, ventricular tachycardia may result in a lack of a palpable pulse and a blood pressure of zero. Clinically, the respiratory therapist should note that the treatment and management for ventricular tachycardia—with and without a pulse—is different, but both are medical emergencies.

Ventricular Fibrillation

Ventricular fibrillation is characterized by chaotic electrical activity and cardiac activity. The ventricles literally quiver out of control with no perfusion beat-producing rhythm (Fig. 7.9). During ventricular fibrillation, there is no cardiac output or blood pressure, and the patient will die in minutes without

treatment. Ventricular fibrillation is treated with cardiopulmonary resuscitation (CPR) and electric shock (defibrillation). These actions often allow the normal heart rhythm to resume.

Asystole (Cardiac Standstill)

Asystole (cardiac standstill) is the complete absence of electrical and mechanical activity. As a result, the cardiac output stops and the blood pressure falls to zero. The ECG tracing appears as a flat line and indicates severe damage to the heart's electrical conduction system (Fig. 7.10). Occasionally, periods of disorganized electrical and mechanical activity may be generated during long periods of asystole; this is referred to as an *agonal rhythm* or a *dying heart*. Defibrillation is not effective for this rhythm—CPR and Advanced Cardiovascular Life Support (ACLS) medications are required.

Noninvasive Hemodynamic Monitoring Assessments

Hemodynamics describes forces that influence the circulation of blood. The general hemodynamic status of the patient can be monitored noninvasively at the bedside by assessing the heart rate (via an ECG monitor, auscultation, or pulse),

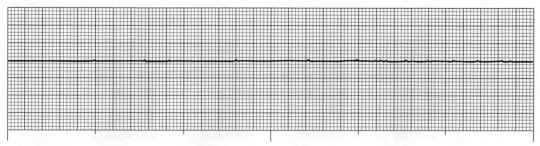

FIGURE 7.10 Asystole. (From Aehlert, B. [2018]. *ECGs made easy* [6th ed.]. St. Louis, MO: Elsevier.)

blood pressure, and perfusion state. During the acute stages of respiratory disease, the patient frequently demonstrates the hemodynamic changes described in the following paragraphs.

The most common causes of **cardiac arrest** are ventricular fibrillation, asystole, and **pulseless electrical activity (PEA)**– also called electrical mechanical dissociation. Advanced Cardiac Life Support (ACLS) and Pediatric Advanced Life Support (PALS) guidelines for cardiac arrest appear in Chapter 33 and Chapter 34. The role of the Respiratory Therapist in these conditions should focus on airway management. Recent literature suggests that the survival and neurological sequelae of cardiac standstill are basically equal whether intubation or bag-mask ventilation is used. The provision of an adequate airway, ventilation, oxygenation, chest compressions and defibrillation are more important than administration of medications and take precedence over initiating an intravenous line or injecting pharmacologic agents. Doses of medication may be administered via an endotracheal tube, but are 2.0-2.5 times the intravenous dose.

Heart Rate (Pulse), Cardiac Output, and Blood Pressure

Abnormal heart rate, pulse, and blood pressure findings frequently develop during the acute stages of pulmonary disease. Tachycardia can result from the indirect response of the heart to hypoxic stimulation of the peripheral chemoreceptors, primarily the carotid bodies. When the carotid bodies are stimulated, reflex signals are sent to the respiratory muscles, which in turn activate the *pulmonary reflex;* this triggers tachycardia and an increased cardiac output and blood pressure. The increased cardiac output is a compensatory mechanism that at least partially counteracts the hypoxemia produced by the pulmonary shunting in respiratory disorders.

Other causes of increased heart rate, cardiac output, and blood pressure include severe anemia, high fever, anxiety, and hyperthyroidism. When the heart rate increases beyond 150 to 175 bpm, cardiac output and blood pressure begin to decline (Starling's relationship). Bradycardia (reduced heart rate), reduced cardiac output, and hypotension may be seen in acute myocardial infarction. Most severe cardiac arrhythmias result in measurable hypotension.

Perfusion State

The perfusion of the body state can be evaluated by examining the patient's skin color, capillary refill, and sensorium. Under normal conditions the patient's nail beds and oral mucosa are pink. If these areas appear cyanotic or mottled, poor perfusion and tissue hypoxia are likely to be present. When the nail beds are compressed to expel blood, they should refill and turn pink within 2 seconds when the pressure is released (**capillary refill test**). If the nail beds remain white, perfusion is inadequate. Under normal conditions the patient's skin should be dry and warm. When the skin is diaphoretic (wet), cool, or clammy, local perfusion is inadequate. Finally, when the patient is disoriented as to person, place, and time, a decreased perfusion state and cerebral hypoxia may be present.

Invasive Cardiovascular Monitoring Assessments

Invasive monitoring is used in the assessment and treatment of critically ill patients. Invasive cardiovascular monitoring includes the measurement of (1) intracardiac pressures and flows via a **pulmonary artery catheter**, (2) arterial pressure via an **arterial catheter (systemic)**, (3) central venous pressure via a **central venous catheter** and (4) coronary artery pathology (e.g., the use of the procedure **coronary angiography** in severe arteriosclerotic heart disease and angina pectoris). Monitoring of these parameters provides rapid and precise measurements (assessment data) of the patient's cardiovascular function, which in turn are used to down-regulate or up-regulate the patient's treatment plan in a timely manner.

Pulmonary Artery Catheter

Right-heart catheterization assists in the diagnosis and management of heart valve problems, congestive heart failure, and pulmonary hypertension. The **pulmonary artery catheter (Swan-Ganz catheter)** is a balloon-tipped, flow-directed catheter that is inserted at the patient's bedside; the respiratory therapist monitors the pressure waveform as the catheter, with the balloon inflated, is guided by blood flow through the right atrium and right ventricle into the pulmonary artery (Fig. 7.11).

The pulmonary artery catheter is used to directly measure the (1) right atrial pressure (via the proximal port), (2) pulmonary artery pressure (via the distal port), (3) left atrial pressure (indirectly via the **pulmonary capillary wedge pressure [PCWP]**), (4) cardiac output via the **thermodilution** technique,[3] and (5) oxygenation levels in the central venous blood to be used for oxygen transport studies ($C[a\text{-}\bar{v}]O_2$, $\dot{V}O_2$, O_2ER, $S\bar{v}O_2$, and $\dot{Q}_s/\dot{Q}_T$) (see Chapter 6, Assessment of Oxygenation).

The insertion of a pulmonary catheter is not without risks and can be life-threatening. For example, it can lead to

---

[3]Thermodilution is a method of cardiac output determination. A bolus of a solution of known volume and temperature is injected into the right atrium, and the resultant change in blood temperature is detected by a thermistor previously placed in the pulmonary artery with a catheter.

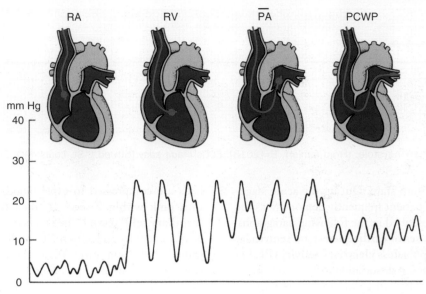

RA   RV $\overline{PA}$ PCWP

FIGURE 7.11 Insertion of the pulmonary catheter (shown in blue in the illustration). The preferred insertion site is the right internal jugular (IJ) vein. Other possible sites are the basilic, brachial, femoral, subclavian, or internal insertion sites. As the catheter advances, pressure readings and waveforms are monitored to determine the catheter's position as it moves through the right atrium (RA), right ventricle (RV), mean pulmonary artery ($\overline{PA}$), and finally into a pulmonary capillary wedge pressure (PCWP) position. Immediately after a PCWP reading, the balloon is deflated to allow blood to flow past the tip of the catheter. When the balloon is deflated, the catheter continuously monitors the pulmonary artery pressure.

arrhythmias, rupture of the pulmonary artery, thrombosis, infection, pneumothorax, and bleeding. Because of the high risk to benefit ratio associated with the insertion of the pulmonary artery catheter, its use is reserved for only the most critically ill patients.

Systemic Arterial Catheter

The systemic arterial catheter (referred to as an *a-line*) is the most commonly used mode of invasive hemodynamic monitoring. It is generally inserted in the radial artery for patient comfort and convenient access. The indwelling arterial catheter allows (1) continuous and precise measurements of systolic, diastolic, and mean blood pressure; (2) accurate information regarding fluctuations in blood pressure; and (3) guidance in the decision to up-regulate or down-regulate therapy—for example, in hypotension or hypertension. The arterial catheter is also useful in patients who require frequent or repeated arterial blood gas samples (e.g., the patient being mechanically ventilated). The blood samples are readily available, and the patient is not subjected to the pain of repeated arterial punctures.

Central Venous Pressure Catheter

The **central venous pressure (CVP) catheter** readily measures the CVP and the right ventricular filling pressure. It serves as an excellent monitor of right ventricular function. An increased CVP reading is commonly seen in patients who (1) have left ventricular heart failure (e.g., pulmonary edema), (2) are receiving excessively high positive-pressure mechanical breaths, (3) have cor pulmonale, or (4) have a severe flail chest, pneumothorax, or pleural effusion.

Table 7.1 summarizes the hemodynamic parameters that can be measured directly. Table 7.2 lists the hemodynamic

TABLE 7.1 Hemodynamic Values Measured Directly

Hemodynamic Value	Abbreviation	Normal Range
Central venous pressure	CVP	0–8 mm Hg
Right atrial pressure	RAP	0–8 mm Hg
Mean pulmonary artery pressure	$\overline{PA}$	10–20 mm Hg
Pulmonary capillary wedge pressure (also called *pulmonary artery wedge, pulmonary artery occlusion*)	PCWP PAW PAO	4–12 mm Hg
Cardiac output	CO	4–6 L/min

TABLE 7.2 Hemodynamic Values Calculated From Direct Hemodynamic Measurements

Hemodynamic Value	Abbreviation	Normal Range
Stroke volume	SV	40–80 mL
Stroke volume index	SVI	40 ± mL/beat/m^2
Cardiac index	CI	3.0 ± 0.5 L/min/m^2
Right ventricular stroke work index	RVSWI	7–12 g/m^2
Left ventricular stroke work index	LVSWI	40–60 g/m^2
Pulmonary vascular resistance	PVR	50–150 dynes × s × cm^{-5}
Systemic vascular resistance	SVR	800–1500 dynes × s × cm^{-5}

TABLE 7.3 Hemodynamic Changes Commonly Seen in Respiratory Diseases

Disorder	Cardiovascular Indices											
	CVP	RAP	$\overline{PA}$	PCWP	CO	SV	SVI	CI	RVSWI	LVSWI	PVR	SVR
Chronic obstructive pulmonary disease (COPD) Chronic bronchitis Emphysema Cystic fibrosis Bronchiectasis	↑	↑	↑↑	~	~	~	~	~	↑	~	↑	~
Pulmonary edema (cardiogenic)	~	↑	↑	↑↑	↓	↓	↓	↓	↑	↓	↑	↓
Pulmonary embolism	↑	↑	↑↑	↓	↓	↓	↓	↓	↑	↓	↑	~
Acute respiratory distress syndrome (ARDS)—severe	~↑	~↑	~↑	~	~	~	~	~	~↑	~	~↑	~
Lung collapse Flail chest Pneumothorax Pleural disease (e.g., hemothorax)	↑	↑	↑	↓	↓	↓	↓	↓	↑	↓	↑	↓
Kyphoscoliosis	↑	↑	↑	~	~	~	~	~	↑	~	↑	~
Pneumoconiosis	↑	↑	↑↑	~	~	~	~	~	↑	~	↑	~
Chronic interstitial lung diseases	↑	↑	↑↑	~	~	~	~	~	↑	~	↑	~
Cancer of the lung (tumor mass)	↑	↑	↑	↓	↓	↓	↓	↓	↑	~	↑	~
Hypovolemia	↓↓	↓	↓	↓	↓	↓	↓	↓	↓	↓	~	↑
Hypervolemia (burns)	↑↑	↑	↑	↑	↑	↑	↑	↑	↑	↑	~	~
Right-heart failure (cor pulmonale)	↑↑	↑↑	↓	↓	~	~	~	~	~	~	~	~

~, Unchanged; *CI*, cardiac index; *CO*, cardiac output; *CVP*, central venous pressure; *LVSWI*, left ventricular stroke work index; $\overline{PA}$, mean pulmonary artery pressure; *PCWP*, pulmonary capillary wedge pressure; *PVR*, pulmonary vascular resistance; *RAP*, right atrial pressure; *RVSWI*, right ventricular stroke work index; *SV*, stroke volume; *SVI*, stroke volume index; *SVR*, systemic vascular resistance.

parameters that can be calculated from results obtained from these direct measurements.

Cardiovascular (Hemodynamic) Monitoring in Respiratory Diseases

Because respiratory disorders can have a profound effect on the cardiopulmonary system, the data generated by the previously described invasive cardiovascular monitors can be used in the assessment and treatment of these patients. For example, respiratory diseases associated with severe or chronic hypoxemia, acidemia, or pulmonary vascular obstruction can increase the pulmonary vascular resistance (PVR) significantly. An increased

PVR, in turn, can lead to a variety of secondary hemodynamic changes such as increased CVP, right atrial pressure (RAP), mean pulmonary artery pressure (PA), right ventricular stroke work index (RVSWI), and decreased cardiac output (CO), stroke volume (SV), stroke volume index (SVI), cardiac index (CI), and left ventricular stroke work index (LVSWI). Table 7.3 lists common hemodynamic changes seen in pulmonary diseases discussed in this volume.

Other noninvasive methods used to assess cardiac pathophysiology include cardiac ultrasound and echocardiography, which are discussed in Chapter 8, Radiologic Examination of the Chest.

SELF-ASSESSMENT QUESTIONS

1. In which of the following arrhythmias is there no cardiac output or blood pressure?
   a. Ventricular flutter
   b. Arial fibrillation
   c. Premature ventricular contractions
   d. Ventricular fibrillation

2. The general hemodynamic status of the patient can be monitored noninvasively at the patient's bedside by assessing which of the following?
   1. Perfusion state
   2. Heart rate
   3. Pulse rate
   4. Blood pressure
      a. 4 only
      b. 2 and 3 only
      c. 2, 3, and 4 only
      d. 1, 2, 3, and 4

3. Cardiac output and blood pressure begin to decline when the heart rate increases beyond which of the following?
   a. 125 to 150 bpm
   b. 150 to 175 bpm
   c. 175 to 200 bpm
   d. 200 to 250 bpm

4. An increased central venous pressure reading is commonly seen in the patient who:
   1. Has a severe pneumothorax
   2. Is receiving high positive-pressure breaths
   3. Has cor pulmonale
   4. Is in left-sided heart failure
      a. 3 only
      b. 4 only
      c. 2, 3, and 4 only
      d. 1, 2, 3, and 4

5. What is the normal range of the mean pulmonary artery pressure?
   a. 0 to 5 mm Hg
   b. 5 to 10 mm Hg
   c. 10 to 20 mm Hg
   d. 20 to 30 mm Hg

6. What is the normal range for the pulmonary capillary wedge pressure?
   a. 0 to 4 mm Hg
   b. 4 to 12 mm Hg
   c. 12 to 20 mm Hg
   d. 20 to 25 mm Hg

7. The hemodynamic indices in patients with chronic obstructive pulmonary disease commonly show which of the following?
   1. Increased central venous pressure
   2. Decreased right atrial pressure
   3. Increased mean pulmonary artery pressure
   4. Decreased pulmonary capillary wedge pressure
   5. Increased cardiac output
      a. 3 only
      b. 1 and 3 only
      c. 2 and 4 only
      d. 3, 4, and 5 only

8. The hemodynamic indices in patients with pulmonary edema commonly show which of the following?
   1. Decreased central venous pressure
   2. Increased right atrial pressure
   3. Decreased mean pulmonary artery pressure
   4. Increased pulmonary capillary wedge pressure
   5. Decreased cardiac output
      a. 1 and 3 only
      b. 2, 3, and 5 only
      c. 2, 4, and 5 only
      d. 1, 2, 4, and 5

9. Atrial flutter is defined as a constant atrial rate of:
   a. 100 to 150 bpm
   b. 150 to 250 bpm
   c. 250 to 350 bpm
   d. 350 to 450 bpm

10. In sinus arrhythmia, the heart rate varies by more than:
    a. 5%
    b. 10%
    c. 15%
    d. 20%

CHAPTER 8

Radiologic Examination of the Chest

Chapter Objectives

After reading this chapter, you will be able to:

- Describe the fundamentals of radiography.
- Differentiate among the standard positions and techniques of chest radiography.
- Define the radiologic terms commonly used during inspection of the chest radiograph.
- Describe the three steps to evaluate technical quality of the radiograph.
- Describe a logical, systematic sequence of radiograph examination.
- Describe the push-pull notion of malposition of thoracic structures.
- Describe the application and diagnostic value of the following radiologic procedures:
  - Computed tomography (CT)
  - Positron emission tomography (PET)
  - Positron emission tomography and computed tomography scan (PET/CT scan)
  - Magnetic resonance imaging (MRI)
  - Pulmonary angiography
  - Ventilation-perfusion scan
  - Fluoroscopy
  - Bronchography
  - Ultrasound Imaging
  - Echocardiography
- Describe the principles and techniques of radiation safety.
- Describe the respiratory therapist's role in chest radiology.
- Define key terms and complete self-assessment questions at the end of the chapter and on Evolve.

Key Terms

Air Cyst
Anteroposterior Radiograph
Bleb
Bronchogram
Bronchography
Bullae
Cardiothoracic Ratio
Cavity
Color Doppler
Computed Tomography (CT)
Computed Tomography Pulmonary Angiogram (CTPA)
Consolidation
Doppler Echocardiogram
Echocardiogram
Fetal Echocardiogram
Fluoroscopy
High-Resolution CT (HRCT) Scans
Hilar Displacement
Homogeneous Density

Honeycombing
Hot Spots in Chest PET Scan
Infiltrates
Interstitial Density
Lateral Decubitus Radiograph
Lateral Radiograph
Lesion
Lung Tissue Markings
Lung Window CT Scan
Magnetic Resonance Imaging (MRI)
Mediastinal Window CT Scan
Opacity
Pleural Density
Pleural Nodule
Positron Emission Tomography (PET)
Positron Emission Tomography and Computed Tomography Scan (PET/CT Scan)
Posteroanterior Radiograph
Power Doppler
Pulmonary Angiography
Pulmonary Mass
"Push-Pull" Abnormal Positioning of Chest Structures
Radiodensity
Radiolucency
Rib Series (Radiograph)
Spectral Doppler
Spiral Computed Tomography Pulmonary Angiogram Scan
Stress Echocardiogram
Subcutaneous Emphysema
Tracheal Shift
Transesophageal Echocardiogram (TEE)
Translucency
Transthoracic Echocardiogram (TTE)
Ultrasound Imagining
Ventilation-Perfusion Lung Scan

Chapter Outline

Fundamentals of Radiography
Standard Positions and Techniques of Chest Radiography
    Posteroanterior Radiograph
    Anteroposterior Radiograph
    Lateral Radiograph
    Lateral Decubitus Radiograph
Inspecting the Chest Radiograph
    Technical Quality of the Radiograph
    Sequence of Examination
    Computed Tomography
    Positron Emission Tomography
    Positron Emission Tomography and Computed Tomography
      Scan

Radiography is the making of a photographic image of the internal structures of the body by passing x-rays through the body to an x-ray film, or radiograph. In patients with respiratory disease, radiography plays an important role in the diagnosis of lung disorders, the assessment of the extent and location of the disease, and the evaluation of the subsequent progress of the disease.

Fundamentals of Radiography

X-rays are created when fast-moving electrons with sufficient energy collide with matter in any form. Clinically, x-rays are produced by an electronic device called an *x-ray tube*.

The x-ray tube is a vacuum-sealed glass tube that contains a cathode and a rotating anode. A tungsten plate approximately a half-inch square is fixed to the end of the rotating anode at the center of the tube. This tungsten plate is called the *target*. Tungsten is an effective target metal because of its high melting point, which can withstand the extreme heat to which it is subjected, and because of its high atomic number, which makes it more effective in the production of x-rays.

When the cathode is heated, electrons "boil off." When a high voltage (70 to 150 kV) is applied to the x-ray tube, the electrons are driven to the rotating anode, where they strike the tungsten target with tremendous energy. The sudden deceleration of the electrons at the tungsten plate converts energy to x-rays. Although most of the electron energy is converted to heat, a small amount (less than 1%) is transformed to x-rays and allowed to escape from the tube through a set of lead shutters called a *collimator*. From the collimator the x-rays travel through the patient to the x-ray film.

The ability of the x-rays to penetrate matter depends on the density of the matter. For chest radiographs the x-rays must also pass through bone, air, soft tissue, and fat. Dense objects such as bone absorb more x-rays (preventing penetration) than objects that are not as dense, such as blood and the air-filled lungs.

After passing through the patient, the x-rays strike the x-ray film. X-rays that pass through low-density objects strike the film at full force and produce a black image on the film. X-rays that are absorbed by high-density objects (such as bone) either do not reach the film at all or strike the film with less force. Relative to the density of the object, these objects appear as light gray to white on the film.

Standard Positions and Techniques of Chest Radiography

Clinically, the standard radiograph of the chest includes two views: a **posteroanterior radiograph** and a lateral projection

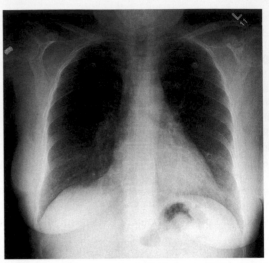

FIGURE 8.1 Standard posteroanterior chest radiograph with the patient's lungs in full inspiration.

(either a left or right **lateral radiograph**) with the patient in the standing position. When the patient is seriously ill or immobilized, an upright radiograph may not be possible. In such cases, a supine **anteroposterior radiograph** is obtained at the patient's bedside. A lateral radiograph is rarely obtainable under such circumstances.

Posteroanterior Radiograph

The standard PA chest radiograph is obtained by having the patient stand (or sit) in the upright position. The anterior aspect of the patient's chest is pressed against a film cassette holder, with the shoulders rotated forward to move the scapulae away (aside) from the lung fields. The distance between the x-ray tube and the film is 6 feet. The x-ray beam travels from the x-ray tube, through the patient from back to front, and to the x-ray film.

The x-ray examination is usually performed with the patient's lungs in full inspiration to show the lung fields and related structures to their greatest possible extent. At full inspiration, the diaphragm is lowered to approximately the level of the ninth to eleventh ribs posteriorly (Fig. 8.1). For certain clinical conditions, radiographs are sometimes taken at the end of both inspiration and expiration. For example, in patients with obstructive lung disease an expiratory radiograph also may be made to evaluate diaphragmatic excursion and the symmetry or asymmetry of such excursion (Fig. 8.2).

Anteroposterior Radiograph

A supine AP radiograph may be taken in patients who are debilitated, immobilized, or too young to tolerate the PA procedure. The AP radiograph is usually taken with a portable x-ray unit at the patient's bedside. The film is placed behind the patient's back, with the x-ray unit positioned in front of the patient, approximately 48 inches from the film.

Compared with the PA radiograph, the AP radiograph has disadvantages. For example, the heart and superior portion of the mediastinum are significantly magnified in the AP radiograph. This is because the heart is positioned in front of the thorax as the x-ray beams pass through the chest in the anterior-to-posterior direction, causing the image of the heart to be enlarged (Fig. 8.3).

The AP radiograph frequently has less resolution and more distortion. Because the patient is often unable to sustain a maximal inspiration, the lower lung lobes frequently appear hazy, erroneously suggesting pulmonary congestion or pleural effusion. Finally, because the AP radiograph is commonly taken in the intensive care unit, extraneous shadows, such as those produced by ventilator tubing and indwelling lines, are

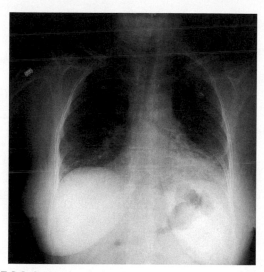

FIGURE 8.2 A posteroanterior chest radiograph of the same patient shown in Fig. 8.1 during expiration.

often present (Fig. 8.4). The position in which the chest x-ray is taken will be at the discretion of the radiology technician, unless specifically ordered to do otherwise.

Lateral Radiograph

The lateral radiograph is obtained to complement the PA radiograph. It is taken with the side of the patient's chest compressed against the cassette. The patient's arms are raised, with the forearms resting on the head.

To view the right lung and heart, the patient's right side is placed against the cassette. To view the left lung and heart, the patient's left side is placed against the cassette. Therefore a right lateral radiograph would be selected to view a density or **lesion** that is known to be in the right lung. If neither lung is of particular interest, a left lateral radiograph is usually selected to reduce the magnification of the heart. The lateral radiograph provides a view of the structures behind the heart and left diaphragmatic dome. It is combined with the PA radiograph to give a three-dimensional view of the cardiac and pulmonary structures or of any abnormal densities (Fig. 8.5).

Lateral Decubitus Radiograph

The **lateral decubitus radiograph** is obtained by having the patient lie on the left or right side rather than standing or sitting in the upright position. The naming of the decubitus radiograph is determined by the side on which the patient lies; thus a right lateral decubitus radiograph means the patient's right side is down.

The lateral decubitus radiograph is useful in the diagnosis of a suspected or known fluid accumulation in the pleural space (e.g., a pleural effusion; see Chapter 24, Pleural Effusion and Empyema) that is not easily seen in the PA radiograph. A pleural effusion, which is usually more thinly spread out over the diaphragm in the upright position, collects in the gravity-dependent areas while the patient is in the lateral decubitus position, allowing the fluid to be more readily seen (Fig. 8.6).

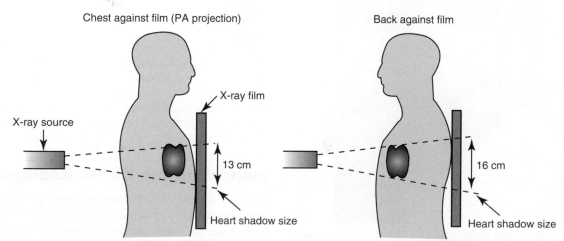

FIGURE 8.3 Compared with the posteroanterior (PA) chest radiograph, the heart is significantly magnified in the anteroposterior (AP) chest radiograph. In the PA radiograph, the ratio of the width of the heart to the thorax is normally less than 1:2. The reason the heart appears larger in the AP radiograph is that it is positioned in front of the thorax as the x-ray beams pass through the chest in the anterior-to-posterior direction. This allows more space for the heart shadow to "fan out" before it reaches the x-ray film.

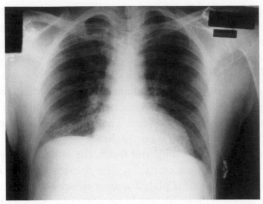

FIGURE 8.4 Anteroposterior (AP) chest radiograph. The diaphragms are elevated, the lower lung lobes appear hazy, the ratio of the width of the heart to the thorax is greater than 2:1 (i.e., the width of the heart is greater than 50% of the width of the thorax), and an extraneous object is apparent outside the patient's left lateral chest (probably an electrocardiograph lead). X-ray examinations using portable devices are frequently performed on patients too ill to be transported to the radiology department. These films, in the best of circumstances, are of poorer quality than erect films taken with standard x-ray apparatus. The films are usually AP projections taken with the x-ray unit in front of and the film plate behind the patient. Overexposure, underexposure, malpositioning, marginal cutoffs, and motion artifacts are often present. In this setting, major events such as partial pneumothoraces, pleural effusions, and infiltrates in dependent parts of the lung may go unrecognized. Therefore careful clinical correlation with the patient's pathophysiology and symptomatology is imperative.

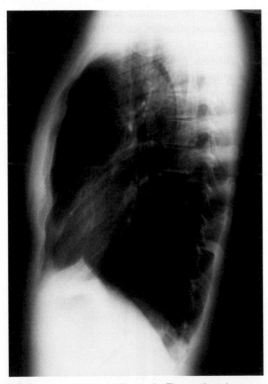

FIGURE 8.5 Lateral chest radiograph. The patient has an overexpanded lung and chest wall (barrel chest deformity) consistent with his known emphysema.

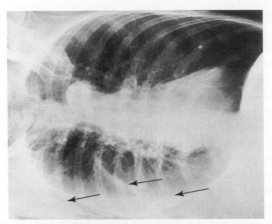

FIGURE 8.6 Right lateral decubitus view. Subpulmonic pleural effusion. Subdiaphragmatic fluid has run up the lateral chest wall, producing a band of soft tissue density. The medial curvilinear shadow (arrows) indicates fluid in the lips of the major fissure.

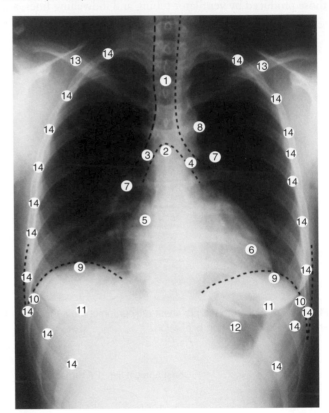

FIGURE 8.7 Normal posteroanterior chest radiograph. *1,* Trachea (note vertebral column in middle of trachea in this correctly centered and exposed film); *2,* carina; *3,* right mainstem bronchus; *4,* left mainstem bronchus; *5,* right atrium; *6,* left ventricle; *7,* hilar vasculature; *8,* aortic knob; *9,* diaphragm; *10,* costophrenic angles; *11,* breast shadows; *12,* gastric air bubble; *13,* clavicle; *14,* rib.

Inspecting the Chest Radiograph

Before the respiratory therapist can effectively identify abnormalities on a chest radiograph, he or she must be able to recognize the normal anatomic structures. Fig. 8.7 represents a normal PA chest radiograph with identification of important anatomic landmarks. Fig. 8.8 labels the anatomic structures seen on a lateral chest radiograph.

Table 8.1 lists some of the more important radiologic terms used to describe abnormal chest x-ray findings.

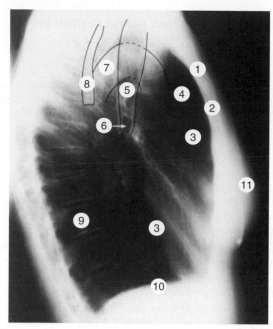

FIGURE 8.8 Normal lateral chest radiograph. *1,* Manubrium; *2,* sternum; *3,* cardiac shadow; *4,* retrosternal air space in the lung; *5,* trachea; *6,* bronchus, on end; *7,* aortic arch (ascending and descending); *8,* scapulae; *9,* vertebral column; *10,* diaphragm; *11,* breast shadow.

Technical Quality of the Radiograph

The *first step* in examining a chest radiograph is to evaluate its technical quality. Was the patient in the correct position when the radiograph was taken? To verify the proper position, check the relationship of the medial ends of the clavicles to the vertebral column. For the PA radiograph the vertebral column should be precisely in the center between the medial ends of the clavicles and the distance between the right and left costophrenic angles and the spine should be equal. Even a small degree of patient rotation relative to the film can create a false image, erroneously suggesting tracheal deviation, cardiac displacement, or cardiac enlargement.

Second, the exposure quality of the radiograph should be evaluated. Normal exposure is verified by determining whether the spinal processes of the vertebrae are visible to the fifth or sixth thoracic level (T-5 to T-6). X-ray equipment is now available that allows the vertebrae to be seen down to the level of the cardiac shadow. The degree of exposure can be evaluated further by comparing the relative densities of the heart and lungs. For example, because the heart has a greater density than the air-filled lungs, the heart appears whiter than the lung fields. The heart and lungs become more radiolucent (darker) with greater exposure of the radiograph. A radiograph

TABLE 8.1 Common Radiologic Terms

Term	Definition
Air cyst	A thin-walled radiolucent area surrounded by normal lung tissue.
Bleb	A superficial air cyst protruding into the pleura; also called *bullae.*
Bronchogram	An outline of air-containing bronchi beyond the normal point of visibility. An air bronchogram develops as a result of an infiltration or consolidation that surrounds the bronchi, producing a contrasting air column on the radiograph—that is, the bronchi appear as dark tubes surrounded by a white area produced by the infiltration or consolidation.
Bullae	A large, thin-walled radiolucent area surrounded by normal lung tissue.
Cavity	A radiolucent (dark) area surrounded by dense tissue (white). A cavity is the hallmark of a lung abscess. A fluid level may be seen inside a cavity.
Consolidation	The act of becoming solid; commonly used to describe the solidification of the lung caused by a pathologic engorgement of the alveoli, as occurs in acute pneumonia.
Homogeneous density	Refers to a uniformly dense lesion (white area); commonly used to describe solid tumors, fluid-containing cavities, or fluid in the pleural space.
Honeycombing	A coarse reticular (netlike) density commonly seen in pneumoconiosis.
Infiltrate	Any poorly defined radiodensity (white area); commonly used to describe an inflammatory lesion.
Interstitial density	A density caused by interstitial thickening.
Lesion	Any pathologic or traumatic alteration of tissue or loss of function of a part.
Opacity	State of being opaque (white); an opaque area or spot; impervious to light rays or, by extension, x-rays; opposite of translucent or radiolucent.
Pleural density	A radiodensity caused by fluid, tumor, inflammation, or scarring.
Pulmonary mass	A lesion in the lung that is 6 cm or more in diameter; commonly used to describe a pulmonary tumor.
Pulmonary nodule	A lesion in the lung that is less than 6 cm in diameter and composed of dense tissue; also called a *solitary pulmonary nodule* or *"coin"* lesion because of its rounded, coinlike appearance.
Radiodensity	Dense areas that appear white on the radiograph; the opposite of radiolucency.
Radiolucency	The state of being radiolucent; the property of being partly or wholly permeable to x-rays; commonly used to describe darker areas on a radiograph such as an emphysematous lung or a pneumothorax.
Translucent (translucency)	Permitting the passage of light (or in this case, x-rays); commonly used to describe darker areas of the radiograph.

TABLE 8.2 Examples of Factors That "Push or Pull" Anatomic Structures Out of Their Normal Position in the Chest Radiograph

Structure	Examples of Abnormal Position	Lesion

Mediastinum and hilar region
  Trachea
  Carina
  Heart
  Major vessels
	Leftward shift	Pulled left by left upper lobe tuberculosis, atelectasis, or fibrosis
		Pushed left by right upper lobe emphysematous bullae, fluid, gas, or tumor

Left diaphragm	Upward shift	Pulled up by left lower lobe atelectasis or fibrosis Pushed up by distended gastric air bubble
Horizontal fissure	Downward shift	Pulled down by right middle lobe or right lower lobe atelectasis Pushed down by right upper lobe neoplasm
Left lung	Rightward shift	Pulled right by right lung collapse, atelectasis, or fibrosis Pushed right by left-sided tension pneumothorax or hemothorax

that has been overexposed is said to be "heavily penetrated" or "burned out." Conversely, the heart and lungs on an underexposed radiograph may appear denser and whiter. The lungs may erroneously appear to have infiltrates, and there may be little or no visibility of the thoracic vertebrae.

Third, the level of inspiration at the moment the radiograph was taken should be evaluated. At full inspiration, the diaphragmatic domes should be at the level of the ninth to eleventh ribs posteriorly. On radiographs taken during expiration, the lungs appear denser, the diaphragm is elevated, and the heart appears wider and enlarged (see Fig. 8.2).

Sequence of Examination

Although the precise sequence in examining a chest radiograph is not important, the inspection should be done in a systematic manner to avoid errors of omission. A common preference is an "inside-out" approach to inspecting the chest radiograph, which entails beginning with the mediastinum and proceeding outward to the peripheral extrathoracic soft tissue. Some practitioners prefer the reverse. The following sequence reflects an "inside-out" method.

Mediastinum

The mediastinum should be inspected for width, contour, and shifts from the midline. The respiratory therapist should inspect the anatomy of the mediastinum, including the trachea, carina, cardiac borders, aortic arch, and superior vena cava (see Fig. 8.7).

Trachea

On the PA projection, the trachea should appear as a translucent column overlying the vertebral column. The diameter of the right and left bronchi progressively tapers for a short distance beyond the carina, which then disappears (see Fig. 8.7). A number of clinical conditions can cause the trachea to shift from its normal position. For example, fluid or gas accumulation in the pleural space causes **tracheal shift** away from the affected area. Atelectasis or fibrosis usually causes the trachea to shift toward the affected area. The trachea also may be displaced by tumors of the upper lung regions.

Anatomic structures in the chest (e.g., the trachea) move out of their normal position because they are either **"pushed or pulled"** in a given direction. In other words, they may be moved up or down or from side to side by lesions "pushing or pulling" in that direction. Table 8.2 lists examples of factors that push or pull the trachea and other anatomic structures out of their normal position in the chest radiograph.

Heart

On the PA projection, the ratio of the width of the heart to the thorax (the **cardiothoracic ratio**) is normally less than 1:2. In other words, the width of the heart should be less than 50% of the width of the thorax. A small portion of the heart should be visible on the right side of the vertebral column. Two bulges should be seen on the right border of the heart. The upper bulge is the superior vena cava; the lower bulge is the right atrium. Three bulges are normally seen on the left side of the heart. The superior bulge is the aorta, the middle bulge is the main pulmonary artery, and the inferior bulge is the left ventricle (see Fig. 8.7). See Table 8.2 for examples of factors that push or pull the heart out of its normal position in the chest radiograph.

Hilum

The right and left hilar regions should be evaluated for change in size or position (**hilar displacement**). Normally, the left hilum is about 2 cm higher than the right (see Fig. 8.7). An increased density of the hilar region may indicate engorgement of hilar vessels caused by pulmonary hypertension. Vertical displacement of the hilum suggests volume loss from one or more upper lobes of the lung on the affected side. In infectious lung disorders such as histoplasmosis or tuberculosis, the lymph nodes around the hilar region are often enlarged, calcified, or both. Malignant pulmonary lesions, including hilar malignant lymphadenopathy, also may be seen. See Table 8.2 for additional factors that push or pull structures in the hilar region out of their normal position in the chest radiograph.

Lung Parenchyma (Tissue)

The lung parenchyma should be systematically examined from top to bottom, one lung compared with the other. Normally, **lung tissue markings** can be seen throughout the film (see Fig. 8.7). The absence of tissue markings may suggest a pneumothorax, recent pneumonectomy, or chronic obstructive lung disease (e.g., emphysema) or may be the result of an overexposed radiograph. An excessive amount of tissue markings may indicate fibrosis, interstitial or alveolar edema, lung compression, or an underexposed radiograph. The periphery of the lung fields should be inspected for abnormalities that obscure the interface of the lung with the pleural space, mediastinum, or diaphragm. Abnormal lung tissue markings are call **infiltrates**. See Table 8.2 for additional examples of factors that push or pull the lung tissue out of its normal position in the chest radiograph.

Pleura

The peripheral borders of the lungs should be examined for pleural thickening, presence of fluid (pleural effusion) or air (pneumothorax) in the pleural space, or mass lesions (see Fig. 8.7). The costophrenic angles should be inspected. Blunting of the costophrenic angle suggests the presence of fluid. A lateral decubitus radiograph may be required to confirm the presence of fluid (see Fig. 8.6).

Diaphragms

Both the right and left hemidiaphragms should have an upwardly convex, dome-shaped contour. The right and left costophrenic angles should be clear. Normally, the right diaphragm is about 2 cm higher than the left because of the liver below it (see Fig. 8.7). Chronic obstructive pulmonary diseases (e.g., emphysema) and diseases that cause gas or fluid to accumulate in the pleural space (e.g., pneumothorax or pleural effusion) flatten and depress the normal curvature of the diaphragm. Abnormal elevation of one diaphragm may result from excessive gas in the stomach, collapse of the middle or lower lobe on the affected side, pulmonary infection at the lung bases, phrenic nerve damage, or spinal curvature. See Table 8.2 for additional examples of factors that push or pull the diaphragm out of its normal position in the chest radiograph.

Gastric Air Bubble

The area below the diaphragm should be inspected. A stomach air bubble is commonly seen under the left hemidiaphragm (see Fig. 8.7). Free air may appear under either diaphragm after abdominal surgery or in patients with peritoneal abscess.

Bony Thorax

The ribs, vertebrae, clavicles, sternum, and scapulae should be inspected. The intercostal spaces should be symmetric and equal over each lung field (see Fig. 8.7). Intercostal spaces that are too close together suggest a loss of muscle tone, commonly seen in patients with paralysis involving one side of the chest. In chronic obstructive pulmonary disease, the intercostal spaces are generally far apart because of alveolar hyperinflation. Finally, the ribs should be inspected for deformities or fractures. If a rib fracture is suspected but not seen on the standard chest radiograph, a special **rib series** (radiographs that focus on the ribs) may be necessary.

Extrathoracic Soft Tissues

The soft tissue external to the bony thorax should be closely inspected. If the patient is a female (or an obese male), the outer boundaries of the breast shadows may be seen (see Fig.

8.7). If the patient has undergone a mastectomy, there will be a relative hyperlucency on the side of the mastectomy. Large breasts can create a significant amount of haziness over the lower lung fields, giving the false appearance of pneumonia or pulmonary congestion. Although nipple shadows are easily identified when they are bilaterally symmetric, one may become less visible when the patient is slightly rotated. The other nipple then appears abnormally opaque and may be mistaken for a **pulmonary nodule**. Fatty tissue in the chest wall in obese patients also may be seen. After a tracheostomy or pneumothorax, subcutaneous air bubbles (called **subcutaneous emphysema**) often form in the soft tissue, especially if the patient is on a positive-pressure ventilator.

Computed Tomography

The same basic principles used in film radiography apply to **computed tomography (CT)** scanning—that is the absorption of x-rays by tissues that contain anatomic structures and organs of different atomic number. A CT scan provides a series of cross-sectional (transverse) pictures (called *tomograms*) of the structures within the body at numerous levels. The procedure is painless and noninvasive and requires no special preparation. The patient simply lies on the examination table, and this moves the patient through the opening of the CT scanner. The major components of a CT scanner are (1) an x-ray tube, which rotates in a continuous 360-degree motion around the patient to image the body in cross-sectional slices; (2) an array of x-ray detectors opposite the x-ray tube, which record the x-rays that pass through the body; and (3) a computer, which converts the different x-ray absorption levels to cross-sectional images based on the density of the structures being scanned (Fig. 8.9). This cross-sectional slice is called an *axial view* or *computerized axial tomogram*.

Up to 250 images, about 1 mm apart, can be generated on a chest CT scan. These "cuts" are often called **high-resolution CT (HRCT) scans** (also called *spiral, volume,* or *helical scans*). In essence, each CT scan provides an image of what a "slice" through the body looks like at specific points—similar to cutting a piece of fruit in half and viewing the

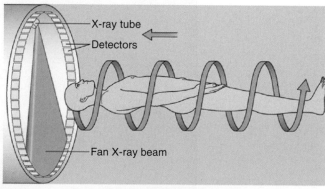

FIGURE 8.9 The principle of spiral computed tomography. The patient moves into the scanner with the x-ray tube continuously rotating and the detectors acquiring information. The rapidity of data acquisition allows a complete examination of the thorax to be performed in a single breath hold. (From Spiro, S. G., Silvestri, F. A., & Agusti, A. [2012]. *Clinical respiratory medicine* [4th ed.]. St. Louis, MO: Elsevier.)

cross-section of the structures inside the fruit. Dense structures, such as bone, appear white on the tomogram, whereas structures with a relatively low density, such as the lungs, appear dark or black. Therefore a dense tumor in the lungs would appear as a white object surrounded by dark lung parenchyma.

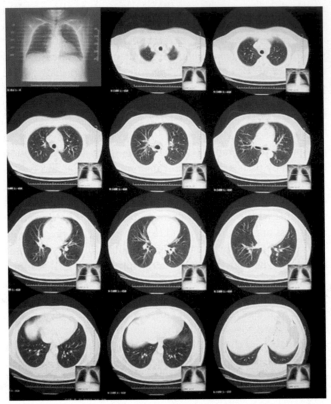

FIGURE 8.10 Overview of normal lung window computed tomography scan. The apex appears in the two views in the upper right corner of this figure; the diaphragm at the base of the lungs appears in the lower right view.

The resolution of a CT scan can be adjusted to primarily view (1) lung tissue—commonly called a **lung window CT scan**—or (2) bone and mediastinal structures—commonly called a **mediastinal window CT scan**. In a mediastinal window CT scan, the lung tissue is overexposed and appears mostly black; the bones and mediastinal organs appear mostly white. Fig. 8.10 provides an overview of a normal lung window CT scan. Fig. 8.11 shows a close-up of one "slice" of a normal lung window CT scan. Fig. 8.12 provides a close-up view of one slice of a normal mediastinal window CT scan.

Finally, for poorly defined lesions evident on the standard radiograph, the CT scan is a useful supplement in determining the precise location, size, and shape of the lesion. The CT scan is especially helpful in confirming the presence of a mediastinal mass, small pulmonary nodules, small lesions of the bronchi, pulmonary cavities, a small pneumothorax, pleural effusion, and small tumors (as small as 0.3 to 0.5 cm). The CT scan can be done with contrast material in the vessels to delineate vascular structures.

Positron Emission Tomography

Positron emission tomography (PET) shows the metabolic activity of the tissues and organs scanned and the anatomic structures themselves. Used in conjunction with a chest x-ray and CT scan for comparison, the PET scan is an excellent diagnostic tool for early detection of malignant lesions. The unique aspect of the PET scan is its ability to evaluate highly metabolic cells that may be cancerous. In other words, the PET scan is able to detect cancerous cells in the tissues of the body before changes develop in the anatomic shape of the organ itself.

Before undergoing the scan, the patient is injected intravenously with a solution of glucose that has been tagged with a radioactive chemical isotope (generally fluorine-18 fluorodeoxyglucose or F18-FDG compound). Cancer cells metabolize glucose at extremely high rates. The PET scan measures the

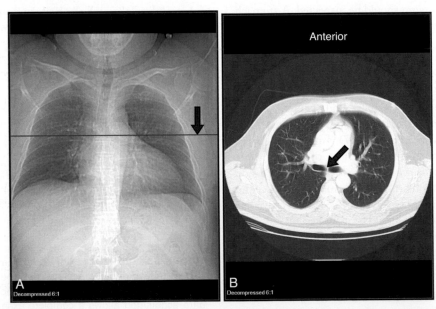

FIGURE 8.11 Close-up of a normal lung window computed tomography (CT) scan. (A) The red arrow indicates the portion of the chest undergoing CT scanning. (B) The actual cross-sectional slice or axial view of the chest. Note the carina and both mainstem bronchi (arrow).

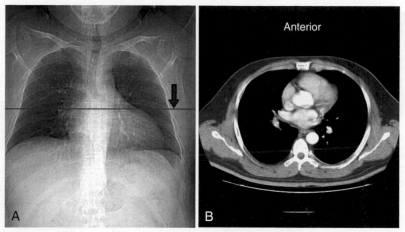

FIGURE 8.12 Close-up of normal computed tomography (CT) mediastinal window. (A) The red arrow indicates the portion of the chest the CT scan is taken. (B) The actual cross-sectional slice or axial view of the chest. Note that the lungs are overexposed and appear mostly black. The bone and mediastinal organs appear mostly white.

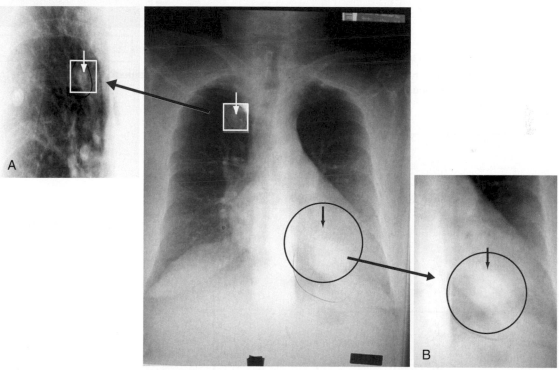

FIGURE 8.13 Chest radiograph identifying two suspicious findings: in the right upper lobe (white arrows) (A) and in the left lower lobe (B), just behind the heart (red arrows).

way cells burn glucose. If present, the cancer cells rapidly consume the tagged glucose. As the glucose molecules break down, end-products that emit positrons are produced. The positrons collide with electrons that give off gamma rays. The gamma rays are converted to dark spots on the PET scan image. These dark spots are commonly referred to as **hot spots.** The presence of a hot spot on a PET scan is likely to confirm a rapidly growing tumor.

Clinically, a PET scan is an excellent tool to rule out suspicious findings (i.e., a possible malignant lesion) that are identified on either the chest radiograph or CT scan. For example, Fig. 8.13 shows a chest radiograph that identifies two suspicious findings: one small nodule in the right upper lung lobe and a larger density in the left lower lung lobe, just

behind the heart. Fig. 8.14 shows two CT scans that also identify the two suspicious findings and their precise location. Figs. 8.15, 8.16, and 8.17 show PET scan images that all confirm a hot spot (likely to be cancer) in the lower left lobe. However, the PET scan image shown in Fig. 8.18 confirms that the nodule in the right upper lobe is benign (i.e., no hot spot noted).

Although the PET scan is relatively painless (i.e., tantamount to the discomfort associated with an intravenous needle insertion), it is lengthy. It may take up to 90 minutes to complete the scan. After the injection, the patient quietly rests in a reclining chair for 30 to 60 minutes before the scan is performed. This allows time for the body to absorb the compound. This step may be difficult or impossible for patients

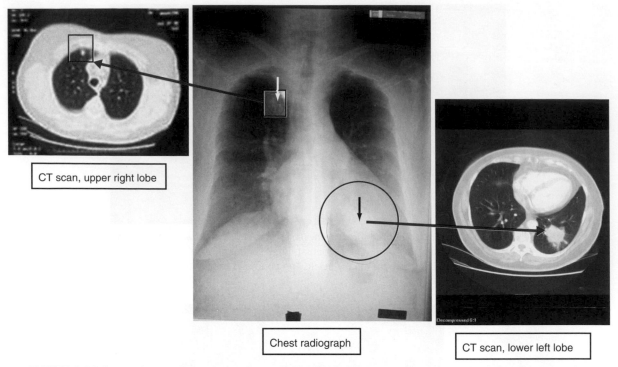

CT scan, upper right lobe

Chest radiograph

CT scan, lower left lobe

FIGURE 8.14 Same chest radiograph as shown in Fig. 8.13. Note that the computed tomography scan also identifies the suspicious nodules and their precise location.

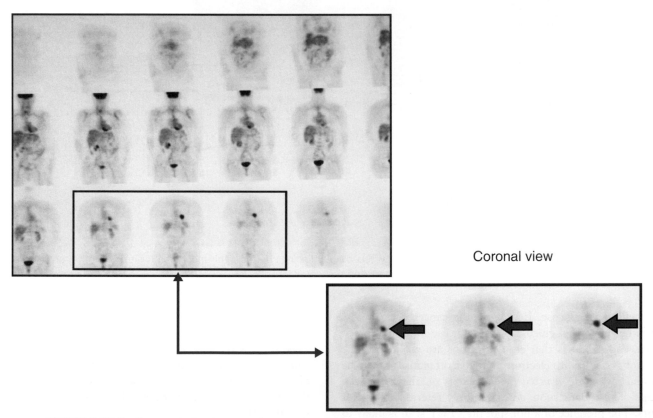

Coronal view

FIGURE 8.15 Positron emission tomography scan: coronal views. The last three views show a hot spot in left lower lobe.

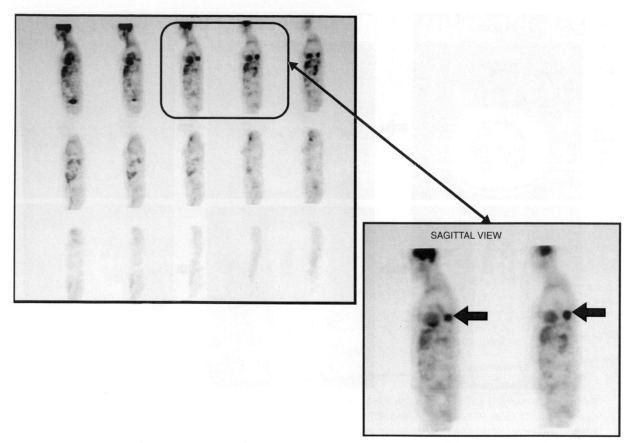

FIGURE 8.16 Positron emission tomography scan: sagittal view. The encircled images show a hot spot in the lower left lobe.

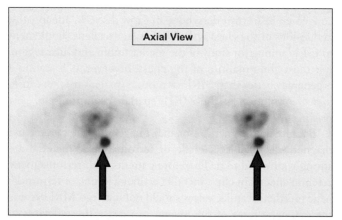

FIGURE 8.17 Positron emission tomography scan: axial view. A hot spot is further confirmed in left lower lobe.

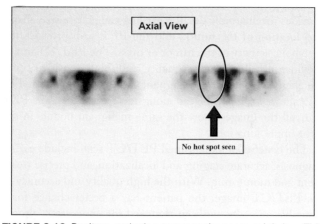

FIGURE 8.18 Positron emission tomography scan: axial view. This image confirms that the small nodule identified in the upper right lobe in the chest radiograph and computed tomography scan is benign (i.e., no hot spot is evident).

who are unable to remain motionless for long periods. PET scans are very expensive to perform, compared with CT or **magnetic resonance imaging (MRI)** studies.

Positron Emission Tomography and Computed Tomography Scan

As described in the preceding sections, PET and CT are both standard imaging tools used by the radiologist to pinpoint the location of cancer or infection within the body before developing a treatment strategy. Individually, however, each scan has its own benefits and limitations. For example, the PET scan detects the metabolic activity of growing cancer cells in the body, and the CT scan provides a detailed picture

of the pulmonary anatomy that shows the precise location, size, and shape of a tumor or mass. By contrast, because the PET scan and CT scan are done at different times and locations, variations in the patient's body position often make the interpretation of the two images difficult.

Technology has now been developed that allows both the PET scan and the CT scan to be merged and performed at the same time. The image produced is called a **positron emission tomography and computed tomography scan (PET/CT scan)** (also known as a *PET/CT fusion*). The PET/CT scan provides an image far superior to that afforded by either

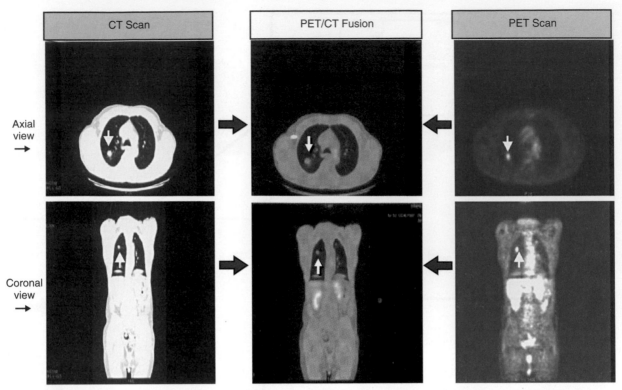

| CT Scan | PET/CT Fusion | PET Scan |

Axial view →

Coronal view →

FIGURE 8.19 Merged positron emission tomography (PET) and computed tomography (CT) scan (PET/CT scan) (center). The CT scan, PET/CT fusion, and PET scan are all showing the same malignant nodule in the right upper lobe (white arrow). *NOTE:* The PET/CT fusion is normally presented in color (e.g., red, blue, yellow).

technology independently. When combined, the CT scan provides the anatomic detail regarding the precise size, shape, and location of the tumor, and the PET scan provides the metabolic activity of the tumor or mass. The PET/CT image provides excellent image quality and high sensitivity and specificity in detecting malignant lesions in the chest. Fig. 8.19 shows a PET/CT scan alongside a CT scan and a PET scan; all the images show the same malignant nodule in the right upper lung lobe.

The benefits of a combined PET/CT scan include earlier diagnosis, accurate staging and localization, and precise treatment and monitoring. With the high quality and accuracy of the PET/CT image, the patient has a better chance for a favorable outcome, without the need for unnecessary procedures. In addition, the PET/CT scan provides early detection of the recurrence or metastasis of cancer, revealing tumors that might otherwise be obscured by scars from previous surgery or radiation therapy. Thus the combined PET/CT scan provides the radiologist with a more complete overview of what is occurring in the patient's body, both anatomically and metabolically at the same time.

Magnetic Resonance Imaging

MRI uses magnetic resonance as its source of energy to take cross-sectional (transverse, sagittal, or coronal) images of the body. It uses no ionizing radiation. The patient is placed in the cylindric imager, and the body part in question is exposed to a magnetic field and radiowave transmission. The MRI produces a high-contrast image that can detect subtle lesions (Fig. 8.20).

MRI is superior to CT scanning in identifying complex congenital heart disorders, bone marrow diseases, adenopathy, and lesions of the chest wall. MRI is an excellent supplement to CT scanning for study of the mediastinum and hilar region. For most abnormalities of the chest, however, CT scanning is generally better than MRI for motion (patient motion causes loss of resolution in the MRI), spatial resolution, and cost reasons.

Because the magnetic resonance imager generates an intense magnetic field, objects made of ferromagnetic material are strongly attracted to it. Therefore patients with ferromagnetic cerebral aneurysm clips, metallic artificial joints, or ferromagnetic prosthetic cardiac valves should not undergo MRI because the magnetic force of the imager can cause these devices to heat, shift, and harm the patient. The magnetic force of the imager also can interfere with the normal function of cardiac pacemakers and most ventilators.

Pulmonary Angiography

Pulmonary angiography is useful in identifying pulmonary emboli or arteriovenous malformations. It involves the injection of a radiopaque contrast medium through a catheter that has been passed through the right side of the heart and into the pulmonary artery. The injection of the contrast material into the pulmonary circulation is followed by rapid serial pulmonary angiograms. The pulmonary vessels are filled with radiopaque contrast material and therefore appear white. Fig. 8.21 shows an abnormal angiogram in which the major blood vessels appear *absent* distal to pulmonary emboli in the left lung. Today, the spiral (helical) volumetric **computed tomography**

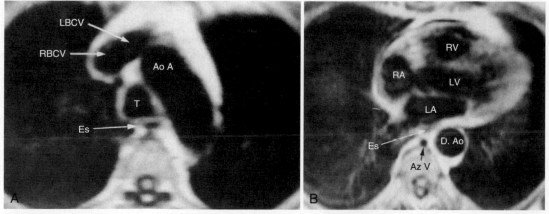

FIGURE 8.20 Anatomy of mediastinum on magnetic resonance imaging scan. (A) *Ao A,* Aortic arch; *Es,* esophagus; *LBCV,* left brachiocephalic vein; *RBCV,* right brachiocephalic vein; *T,* trachea. (B) *Az V,* Azygos vein; *D. Ao,* descending aorta; *Es,* esophagus; *LA,* left atrium; *LV,* left ventricle; *RA,* right atrium; *RV,* right ventricle. (From Armstrong, P., Wilson, A. G., & Dee, P. [1990]. *Imaging of diseases of the chest.* St. Louis, MO: Mosby.)

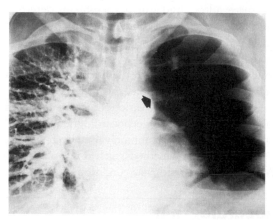

FIGURE 8.21 Abnormal pulmonary angiogram. Radiopaque material injected into the blood is prevented from flowing into the left lung past the pulmonary embolism (arrow). No vascular structures are seen distal to obstruction.

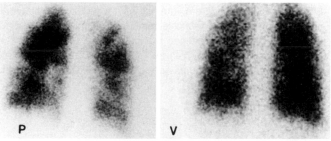

FIGURE 8.22 Fat embolism in a patient with dyspnea and hypoxemia after a recent orthopedic procedure. Perfusion (P) and ventilation (V) radionuclide scans show multiple peripheral subsegmental perfusion defects suggestive of fat embolism. (From Hansell, D. M., Lynch, D., McAdams, H. P., et al. [2010]. *Imaging of diseases of the chest* [5th ed.]. Philadelphia, PA: Elsevier.)

pulmonary angiogram (CTPA) (also called a *CT pulmonary angiogram*) with intravenous contrast has largely replaced pulmonary angiography and is fast becoming the first-line test for diagnosing suspected pulmonary embolism. The CTPA is now a preferred choice of imaging in the diagnosis of a pulmonary embolism, because the only invasive requirement for the scan is an insertion of an intravenous line (see Chapter 21).

Ventilation-Perfusion Lung Scan

A **ventilation-perfusion lung scan** can be used in determining the presence of a pulmonary embolism. The perfusion scan is obtained by injecting small particles of albumin, called *macroaggregates,* tagged with a radioactive material such as iodine-131 or technetium-99m. After injection the radioactive particles are carried in the blood to the right side of the heart, from which they are distributed throughout the lungs by the blood flow in the pulmonary arteries. The radioactive particles that travel through unobstructed arteries become trapped in the pulmonary capillaries because they are 20 to 50 μm in diameter, and the diameter of the average pulmonary capillary is approximately 8 to 10 μm.

The lungs are then scanned with a gamma camera that produces a picture of the radioactive distribution throughout the pulmonary circulation. The dark areas show good blood flow, and the white or light areas represent decreased or complete absence of blood flow. The macroaggregates eventually break down, pass through the pulmonary circulation, and are excreted by the liver. The injection of these radioactive particles has no significant effect on the patient's hemodynamics because the patent pulmonary capillaries far outnumber those "embolized" by the radioactive particles. In addition to pulmonary emboli, a perfusion scan defect (white or light areas) may be caused by a lung abscess, lung compression, loss of the pulmonary vascular system (e.g., emphysema), atelectasis, or alveolar **consolidation**.

The perfusion scan is supplemented with a ventilation scan. During the ventilation scan the patient breathes a radioactive gas such as xenon-133 from a closed-circuit spirometer. A gamma camera is used to create a picture of the gas distribution throughout the lungs. A normal ventilation scan shows a uniform distribution of the gas, with the dark areas reflecting the presence of the radioactive gas and therefore good ventilation. White or light areas represent decreased or complete absence of ventilation. Fig. 8.22 presents an abnormal perfusion scan and a normal ventilation scan of a patient with a severe pulmonary embolism. An abnormal ventilation scan also may be caused by airway obstruction (e.g., mucous plug or

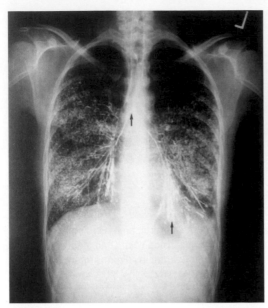

FIGURE 8.23 Bronchogram obtained using contrast medium in a patient with a history of bronchiectasis. Arrows indicate the carina and the dilated and thickened bronchi leading to the posterior basilar segment of the left lower lobe. (From Rau, J. L., Jr., & Pearce, D. J. [1984]. *Understanding chest radiographs.* Denver, CO: Multi-Media Publishing.)

bronchospasm), loss of alveolar elasticity (e.g., emphysema), alveolar consolidation, or pulmonary edema.

This test is slowly being replaced by more sensitive and rapid tests, such as the **spiral computed tomography pulmonary angiogram scan**.

Fluoroscopy

Fluoroscopy is a technique by which x-ray motion pictures of the chest are taken. Fluoroscopy subjects the patient to a larger dose of x-rays than does standard radiography. Therefore it is used only in selected cases, as in the assessment of abnormal diaphragmatic movement (e.g., unilateral phrenic nerve paralysis) or for localization of lesions to be biopsied during fiberoptic bronchoscopy.

Bronchography

Bronchography entails the instillation of a radiopaque material into the lumen of the tracheobronchial tree. A chest radiograph is then taken, providing a film called a **bronchogram**. The contrast material provides a clear outline of the trachea, carina, right and left mainstem bronchi, and segmental bronchi. Bronchography is occasionally used to diagnose bronchogenic carcinoma and determine the presence or extent of bronchiectasis (Fig. 8.23). CT of the chest has largely replaced this technique. Radiation safety techniques need to be used by the respiratory therapist assisting in the performance of this technique.

Ultrasound

Ultrasound imaging (also called *ultrasound scanning* or *sonography*) is a quick, noninvasive diagnostic examination that produces images of organs and structures inside the body.

The ultrasound transducer, which is placed on the skin over the area to be examined, sends ultrasound waves into the body. The sound waves bounce off the organs, tissue, or fluid like an echo and return to the transducer. The transducer processes the reflected waves, and a computer transforms the waves into an image of the structures being examined. Because the ultrasound uses high-frequency sound waves, as opposed to ionizing radiation, it is a safe tool for examination.

As shown in Fig. 8.24, an ultrasound is most associated with the test used to examine a baby in pregnant women. However, it is also very commonly used to examine a large multiplicity of other organs and conditions throughout the body. For example, chest ultrasound is used to examine the trachea, lungs, mediastinum, heart and its large vessels, esophagus, thymus, and lymph nodes. In addition, the chest ultrasound is often used to assess the presence of fluid in the pleural space or other areas of the chest, especially when the amount of fluid is small. When there is a large amount of fluid in the pleural space, ultrasound can be helpful in determining if the fluid is an *exudate* (e.g., fluid caused by inflammatory or cancerous conditions) or a *transudate* (e.g., caused by fluid that has leaked from blood or lymph vessels). The chest ultrasound is also used to help guide a needle during a thoracentesis or to obtain a lung biopsy sample, assess the movement of the diaphragm, and diagnose a variety of heart conditions (see the following section on the echocardiogram).

The echocardiogram is commonly used in conjunction with other types of diagnostic methods, such as CT scanning, x-rays, and MRI to assess a particular condition.

Echocardiogram

An **echocardiogram** (also called *cardiac echo* or simply *echo*) is a type of ultrasound that produces images of the heart (Fig. 8.25). Today, echocardiography is a very common, noninvasive diagnostic tool for real-time imaging of cardiac structures and function. For example, the echocardiogram is used to assess the extent of an enlarged heart, the size and shape the ventricular cavities, the thickness and integrity of the interaterial and intraventricular septa, the origin of an abnormal heart sound, the functional status of the heart's valves, the cause of unexplained chest pain or pressure, and the source of an irregular heartbeat. It may be performed at the patient's bedside and thus has been increasingly used in the intensive care setting.

An echocardiogram is also used to calculate the heart's pumping capacity, including the stroke volume, cardiac output, ejection fraction, and diastolic function. In pregnant women known to be at high risk, a pediatric cardiologist who is specially trained in fetal cardiac evaluation commonly performs a **fetal echocardiogram** to detect congenital heart defects. The test is typically performed by placing the transducer over the mother's abdomen to visualize the fetal heart. Box 8.1 provides an overview of some of the specific problems that can be identified with the echocardiogram.

The different types of echocardiograms are as follows:
- **Transthoracic echocardiogram (TTE):** Provides a noninvasive, highly accurate, and quick examination of the heart. The transducer is placed on the patient's chest while

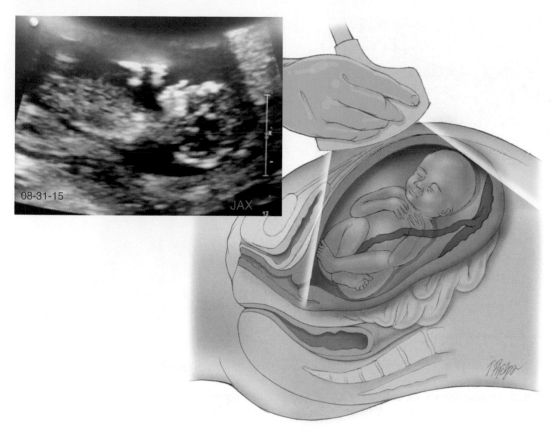

FIGURE 8.24 Fetal Ultrasound.

ultrasound waves create images of the heart. It is the standard method to view the heart. The transthoracic echocardiogram is the most common echocardiogram method.

- **Transesophageal echocardiogram (TEE):** Commonly used when the quality of the transthoracic echocardiogram images is poor. A flexible tube containing a transducer is passed down the esophagus and positioned close to the heart. The TEE provides a cleaner and sharper image of the heart because the various structures between the outside of the chest and heart (i.e., sternum, ribs, and lung) are not between the transducer and the heart. Conscious sedation and localized numbing medication are usually applied during this procedure.
- **Stress echocardiogram:** Is performed before and after the patient's heart is stressed by either exercise or the injection of an agent that stimulates the heart to beat harder and faster.
- **Doppler echocardiogram:** A special ultrasound method used to examine both the direction and velocity of blood flow through the heart chambers, heart valves, and great vessels. There are three types of Doppler ultrasounds:
  - **Color Doppler** uses a computer to convert Doppler measurements into an array of colors to show the speed and direction of blood flow through a blood vessel. Fig. 8.26 provides a color Doppler recording of a severe mitral regurgitation.
  - **Power Doppler** is a newer technique that is used to obtain images that are difficult to obtain with the

standard color Doppler. This method provides greater detail of blood flow, especially in vessels that are located inside an organ or have little or minimal blood flow. The power Doppler, however, does not determine the direction of blood flow. The determination of blood flow is done with color Doppler and spectral Doppler (see later).
  - **Spectral Doppler** displays blood flow measurements graphically, in terms of the distance traveled per unit of time, rather than as a color picture. It also can convert blood flow information into a distinctive sound that can be heard with every heartbeat.
- **Three-dimensional echocardiography** (also called *four-dimensional echocardiography* when the image is moving)—is now possible. This method uses an array of ultrasound probes to create detailed images to assess cardiac pathology, valvular defects, and cardiomyopathies. Real-time three-dimensional echocardiography is used to guide the physician to the location to obtain a right ventricular endomyocardial biopsy or to reach the precise position for the placement of catheter-delivered valvular devices.

Although echocardiography does not offer continuous monitoring and assessment of the cardiac function, the portability of the equipment readily provides quality studies at the patient's bedside. However, it may be difficult to obtain a satisfactory image of the patient who has excessive chest bandages, is obese, is unable to turn or maintain a certain position, or has air trapping in the lungs (e.g., emphysema).

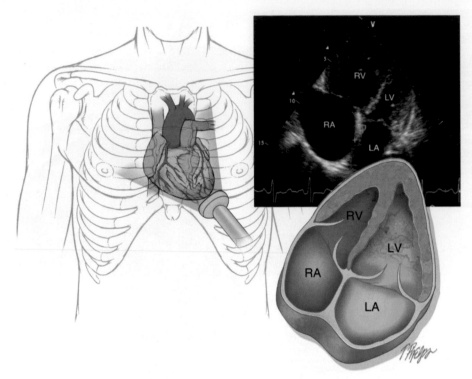

FIGURE 8.25 Echocardiogram. *LA,* Left atrium; *LV,* left ventricle; *RA,* right atrium; *RV,* right ventricle. (Echocardiogram from Kacmarek, R. M., Stoller, J. K., & Heuer A. J. [2017]. *Egan's fundamentals of respiratory care* [11th ed.]. St. Louis, MO: Elsevier.)

BOX 8.1 Specific Conditions That Can Be Identified With the Echocardiogram

- Pericardial effusion
- Cardiac tamponade
- Idiopathic congestive cardiomyopathy
- Hypertrophic cardiomyopathy
- Mitral valve regurgitation
- Mitral valve prolapse
- Aortic regurgitation
- Aortic stenosis
- Vegetation on the valves

- Intracardiac masses
- Ischemic heart muscle
- Left ventricular aneurysm
- Ventricular thrombi
- Proximal coronary disease
- Congenital heart disease
- Interventricular thickness
- Pericarditis
- Aortic dissection

Radiation Safety

All health care workers near the area where an x-ray is being generated must observe the proper safety precautions. The potential harmful effects caused by radiation are directly related to the amount of the exposure, the duration of the exposure, and the area of the body exposed. Simply stated, the less time one is exposed to radiation, the lower is the radiation dose; the further one is away from the radiation source, the lower is the radiation dose; and the more shielding between the health care worker and the radiation source, the better.

Radiation shields include both fixed protective barriers (e.g., lead screens) and personal protective equipment (e.g., lead gowns). Even though it is the responsibility of the radiographer to manage the radiation dose and ensure the safety for both the patient and the surrounding staff, it is also the responsibility of every health care practitioner in the immediate vicinity to take all the appropriate safety precautions necessary. For example, many respiratory therapy departments require their respiratory therapists to wear radiation badges. Other protection strategies include:

- If pregnant, leave the area
- Have only the personnel needed for the x-ray procedures present in the room
- When in the room during the x-ray procedures, stand behind portable or fixed lead panels, or wear the following:
  - Lead aprons
  - Lead safety glasses
  - Thyroid shields
  - Leaded gloves

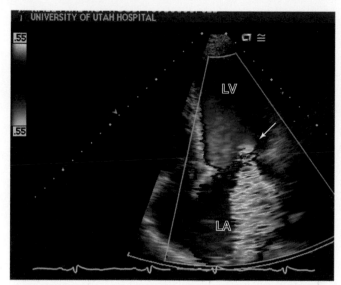

FIGURE 8.26 Color Doppler recording demonstrating severe mitral regurgitation. The regurgitant jet seen in the left atrium (LA) is represented in blue because blood flow is directed away from the transducer. The yellow components are the mosaic pattern traditionally assigned to turbulent or high-velocity flow. The arrow points to the hemisphere of blood accelerating proximal to the regurgitant orifice (proximal isovelocity surface area [PISA]). The size of the PISA can be used to help grade the severity of regurgitation. *LA,* Left atrium; *LV,* left ventricle. (Courtesy Sheldon E. Litwin, MD, Division of Cardiology, University of Utah. In Benjamin, I. J., Griggs, R. C., Wing, E. J., et al. [2016]. *Andreoli and Carpenter's Cecil essentials of medicine* [9th ed.]. Philadelphia, PA: Elsevier.)

Radiation Safety Techniques

The role of the respiratory therapist is important. The intent of this chapter is not to suggest that the respiratory therapist function as a "junior radiologist." Instead, the following areas *are* worthy of consideration. The therapist must:

- Understand the *language* of radiologic interpretation as discussed in this chapter, including the indications for and complications of the radiologic procedures described.
- Recognize good versus poor *radiologic technique* in the performance of chest x-rays. Do these studies need to be repeated? If so, and recognized in advance, they can be requested by the therapist and avoid a premature physician visit.
- Understand the *exact location of cardiopulmonary structures* identified in the chest x-ray.
- Understand ways in which the respiratory therapist can assist in *preparing the patient* for radiologic procedures, such as patient positioning, preprocedure suctioning, etc.
- Understand the principles and practice of *radiation safety;* particularly in procedures with high exposure risk, including bronchoscopy, lung biopsy, and administration of radioactive substances such as in PET scanning.

SELF-ASSESSMENT QUESTIONS

1. Clinically, the standard radiograph of the chest includes which of the following?
   1. Anteroposterior radiograph
   2. Lateral decubitus radiograph
   3. Lateral radiograph
   4. Posteroanterior radiograph
      a. 1 only
      b. 4 only
      c. 3 and 4 only
      d. 1 and 2 only

2. Compared with the posteroanterior radiograph, the anteroposterior radiograph:
   1. Magnifies the heart
   2. Is usually more distorted
   3. Frequently appears more hazy
   4. Often has extraneous shadows
      a. 2 only
      b. 3 and 4 only
      c. 1, 3, and 4 only
      d. 1, 2, 3, and 4

3. To view the right lung and the heart in the lateral radiograph, the:
   a. Left side of the patient's chest is placed against the cassette
   b. Anterior portion of the patient's chest is placed against the cassette
   c. Right side of the patient's chest is placed against the cassette
   d. Posterior portion of the patient's chest is placed against the cassette

4. A right lateral decubitus radiograph means that the:
   a. Right side of the chest is down
   b. Posterior side of the chest is up
   c. Left side of the chest is down
   d. Anterior side of the chest is up

5. A leftward shift of the mediastinum is commonly seen on the chest radiograph in response to which of the following?
   1. Left upper lobe atelectasis
   2. Right upper lobe gas
   3. Left upper lobe fibrosis
   4. Right upper lobe tumor
      a. 1 and 3 only
      b. 3 and 4 only
      c. 2, 3, and 4 only
      d. 1, 2, 3, and 4

6. **The normal exposure of the radiograph is verified by determining whether the spinal processes of the vertebrae are visible to which level?**
   a. C-1 to C-3
   b. C-3 to C-5
   c. T-2 to T-4
   d. T-5 to T-6

7. **The lung in a radiograph that is described as being "heavily penetrated" is which of the following?**
   1. Darker in appearance
   2. More translucent
   3. Whiter in appearance
   4. More opaque in appearance
      a. 3 only
      b. 4 only
      c. 3 and 4 only
      d. 1 and 2 only

8. **When the radiograph is taken at full inspiration, the diaphragmatic domes should be at the level of the:**
   a. First to fourth ribs posteriorly
   b. Fourth to sixth ribs posteriorly
   c. Sixth to ninth ribs posteriorly
   d. Ninth to eleventh ribs posteriorly

9. **Which of the following involves x-ray motion pictures of the chest?**
   a. Bronchography
   b. Fluoroscopy
   c. Magnetic resonance imaging
   d. Computed tomography

10. **Magnetic resonance imaging is superior to computed tomography scanning for identifying which of the following?**
    1. Lesions of the chest
    2. Bone marrow diseases
    3. Congenital heart disorders
    4. Adenopathy
       a. 3 and 4 only
       b. 2 and 3 only
       c. 2, 3, and 4 only
       d. 1, 2, 3, and 4

CHAPTER

9 Other Important Tests and Procedures

Chapter Objectives

After reading this chapter, you will be able to:

- Describe the diagnostic value of the sputum examination.
- Describe the diagnostic tests and procedures presented in this chapter.
- Describe the components of hematology testing.
- Describe the role of platelets.
- Identify the blood chemistry tests commonly monitored in respiratory care.
- Identify the electrolytes commonly monitored in respiratory care.
- Recognize abnormal results of the following tests: arterial blood gases, complete blood count, platelet count, and electrolytes.
- Define key terms and complete self-assessment questions at the end of the chapter and on Evolve.

Key Terms

Acid-Fast Smear and Culture
AIDS
Alveolar Proteinosis
Anemia (Types of)
Anergy
B Cells
Band Forms
Basophils
Bronchoalveolar Lavage
Bronchoscopy
Complete Blood Count (CBC)
Culture and Sensitivity Studies
Cytology
Diagnostic Bronchoscopy
Electrolytes
Endobronchial Ultrasound (EBUS)
Endoscopic Examinations
Eosinophils
Exudate
Glucose
Gram Staining
Granular Leukocytes
Hematocrit (Hct)
Hemoglobin (Hb)

Leukocytosis
Lung Biopsy
Lymphocytes
Macrophages
Mediastinoscopy
Monocytes
Navigational Bronchoscopy
Neutrophils
Nongranular Leukocytes
Open Lung Biopsy
Phagocytosis
Platelets
Pleurodesis
Red Blood Cell Indices
Sclerosants
Skin Tests
Sputum Examination
T Cells
Therapeutic Bronchoscopy
Thoracentesis
Thrombocytopenia
TomoTherapy
Transbronchial Lung Biopsy
Transudate
Video-Assisted Thoracoscopy Surgery (VATS)

Chapter Outline

Sputum Examination
Skin Tests
Endoscopic Examinations
    Bronchoscopy
    Mediastinoscopy
    Lung Biopsy
Video-Assisted Thoracoscopy Surgery
    Navigational Bronchoscopy
Thoracentesis
Pleurodesis
Hematology, Blood Chemistry, and Electrolyte Findings
    Hematology
    Blood Chemistry
    Electrolytes
Self-Assessment Questions

As already discussed throughout the first seven chapters of this textbook, the correct assessment associated with patients with pulmonary disease depends on a variety of important diagnostic studies and bedside skills. In addition to the clinical data obtained at the patient bedside (i.e., the patient interview and the physical examinations) and from standard laboratory tests and special procedures (i.e., pulmonary function studies, arterial blood gases, hemodynamic monitoring, and the radiologic examination of the chest), a number of other important tests are often required to diagnose and treat the patient appropriately. Additional important diagnostic studies include the sputum examination, skin tests, endoscopic examinations, lung biopsy, thoracentesis, and hematology, blood chemistry, and electrolyte tests.

Sputum Examination

A sample for **sputum examination** can be obtained by expectoration, tracheal suction, or bronchoscopy (discussed later). In addition to the analysis of the amount, quality, and color of the sputum (previously discussed in Chapter 3, The Pathophysiologic Basis for Common Clinical Manifestations), the sputum sample may be examined for (1) culture and sensitivity, (2) Gram stain, (3) acid-fast smear and culture, and (4) cytology.

For a **culture and sensitivity study**, a single sputum sample is collected in a sterile container. This test is performed to diagnose bacterial infection, select an antibiotic, and evaluate the effectiveness of antibiotic therapy. The turnaround time for this test is 48 to 72 hours. **Gram staining** of sputum is performed to classify bacteria into *gram-negative* organisms and *gram-positive* organisms. The results of the Gram stain tests guide therapy until the culture and sensitivity results are obtained. Box 9.1 presents common organisms associated with respiratory disorders. All but the viral organisms can be seen on a Gram stain.

The **acid-fast smear and culture** is performed to determine the presence of acid-fast bacilli (e.g., *Mycobacterium tuberculosis*). A series of three early morning sputum samples is tested. The respiratory therapist should take care in obtaining a clean sample that is not contaminated. **Cytology** examination entails the collection of a single sputum sample in a special container with fixative solution. The sample is evaluated under a microscope for the presence of abnormal cells that may indicate a malignant condition.

The amount, color, and components of the sputum are often important in the assessment and diagnosis of many respiratory disorders, including tuberculosis, pneumonia, cancer of the lungs, and pneumoconiosis. Table 9.1 provides an overview of sputum characteristics that correlate with clinical disease states.

Skin Tests

Skin tests are commonly performed to evaluate allergic reactions or exposure to tuberculous bacilli or fungi. Skin tests entail the intradermal injection of an antigen. A positive test result indicates that the patient has been exposed to the antigen. However, it does not mean that active disease is actually present. A negative test result indicates that the patient has had no exposure to the antigen. A negative test result also may be seen in patients with a depression of cell-mediated immunity (**anergy**), such as that which develops in human immunodeficiency virus (HIV) infections.

Endoscopic Examinations

The various **endoscopic examinations** are discussed in this section.

Bronchoscopy

Bronchoscopy is a well-established diagnostic and therapeutic tool used by a number of medical specialists, including those in intensive care units, special procedure rooms, and outpatient settings. With minimal risk to the patient—and without interrupting the patient's ventilation—the flexible fiberoptic bronchoscope allows direct visualization of the upper airways (nose, oral cavity, and pharynx), larynx, vocal cords, subglottic area, trachea, bronchi, lobar bronchi, and segmental bronchi down to the third or fourth generation. Under fluoroscopic

---

BOX 9.1 Common Organisms Associated With Respiratory Disorders

Gram-Negative Organisms
- *Klebsiella*
- *Pseudomonas aeruginosa*
- *Haemophilus influenzae*
- *Legionella pneumophila*

Gram-Positive Organisms
- Streptococcus (80% of all bacterial pneumonias)
- Staphylococcus

Viral Organisms
- *Mycoplasma pneumoniae*
- Respiratory syncytial virus

TABLE 9.1 Sputum Correlations*

Sputum Characteristics	Correlations
Yellow sputum	Acute infection
Green sputum	Associated with old, retained secretions. Green and foul-smelling secretions are frequently found in patients with anaerobic or *Pseudomonas* infection, such as in bronchiectasis, cystic fibrosis, and lung abscess
Thick, stringy, and white or mucoid sputum	Bronchial asthma
Brown sputum	Presence of old blood
Red sputum	Fresh blood

*See also Chapter 2, The Physical Examination.

control, more peripheral areas can be examined or treated (Fig. 9.1). Bronchoscopy may be diagnostic or therapeutic.

A **diagnostic bronchoscopy** is usually performed when an infectious disease is suspected and not otherwise diagnosed or to obtain a lung biopsy sample when the abnormal lung tissue is located on or near the bronchi. Diagnostic bronchoscopy is indicated for a number of clinical conditions, including further inspection and assessment of (1) abnormal radiographic findings (e.g., question of bronchogenic carcinoma or the extent of a bronchial tumor or mass lesion), (2) persistent atelectasis, (3) excessive bronchial secretions, (4) acute smoke inhalation injuries, (5) intubation damage, (6) bronchiectasis, (7) foreign bodies, (8) hemoptysis, (9) lung abscess, (10) major thoracic trauma, (11) stridor or localized wheezing, and (12) unexplained cough.

A videotape or colored picture of the bronchoscopic procedure also may be obtained to record any abnormalities. When abnormalities are found, additional diagnostic procedures include brushings, biopsies, needle aspirations, and washings. For example, a common diagnostic bronchoscopic technique, termed **bronchoalveolar lavage (BAL)**, involves injecting a small amount (30 mL) of sterile saline through the bronchoscope and then withdrawing the fluid for examination of cells. BAL is commonly used to diagnose *Pneumocystis jiroveci* pneumonia.

Therapeutic bronchoscopy includes (1) suctioning of excessive secretions or mucous plugs, especially when lung atelectasis is present or forming as in **alveolar proteinosis**, (2) the removal of foreign bodies or malignant lesions obstructing the airway, (3) selective lavage (with normal saline or mucolytic agents), and (4) management of life-threatening hemoptysis. Although the virtues of therapeutic bronchoscopy are well established, routine respiratory therapy modalities at the patient's bedside (e.g., chest physical therapy, intermittent percussive ventilation, postural drainage, deep breathing and coughing techniques, and positive expiratory pressure therapy) are considered the first line of defense in the treatment of atelectasis from retained secretions. Clinically, therapeutic bronchoscopy is commonly used in the management of bronchiectasis, alveolar proteinosis (with lavage), lung abscess, smoke inhalation and thermal injuries, and lung cancer (see Airway Clearance Therapy Protocol 10.2, page 136).

Endobronchial Ultrasound

An **endobronchial ultrasound (EBUS)** examination may be performed during a bronchoscopy to help establish the stage of lung cancer and, importantly, establish if—and how—the cancer may have spread. An EBUS can provide an accurate staging of a lung cancer and can help reduce the amount of tissue that needs to be removed during surgery. Traditionally, accurate staging has often required invasive tests such as mediastinoscopy, thoracoscopy, or thoracotomy. An EBUS may provide sufficient information to stage a cancer without these invasive procedures. It also spares the patient from undergoing unnecessary surgery when it is determined that the cancer also can be better treated in another way, such as with chemotherapy or radiation.

During an EBUS procedure, an ultrasound probe is used to send sound waves through the walls of the airways into the surrounding areas, lungs, and mediastinum. When abnormal areas are detected, a small sample of tissue is taken with a thin needle guided by the ultrasound (**transbronchial lung biopsy**). The sample is then sent to a laboratory to determine the presence of malignancy or other abnormalities.

There are four primary reasons for which an EBUS is recommended:

- To detect the presence of tumors or pathologically enlarged lymph nodes
- To diagnose tumors within the lung or mediastinum
- To diagnose lymph node abnormalities in the mediastinum or hila

In addition to diagnosing and staging lung cancer, an EBUS examination also may be used to identify specific infections or help diagnose other lung conditions such as sarcoidosis.

Mediastinoscopy

Mediastinoscopy includes the insertion of a scope (mediastinoscopy scope) through a small incision in the suprasternal notch. The scope is then advanced into the mediastinum (Fig. 9.2). The test is used to inspect and perform biopsy of lymph nodes in the anterior mediastinal area. This procedure is performed to diagnose carcinoma, granulomatous infections, and sarcoidosis. Mediastinoscopy is done in the operating room while the patient is under general anesthesia.

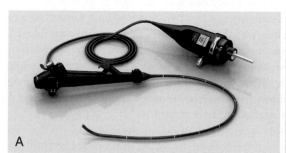
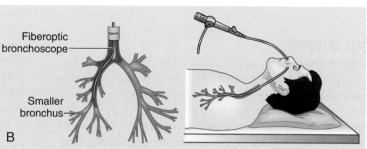

FIGURE 9.1 Fiberoptic bronchoscope. (A) The transbronchoscopic balloon-tipped catheter and the flexible fiberoptic bronchoscope. (B) The catheter is introduced into a small airway and the balloon inflated with 1.5 to 2 mL of air to occlude the airway. Bronchoalveolar lavage is performed by injecting and withdrawing 30-mL aliquots of sterile saline solution, gently aspirating after each instillation. Specimens are sent to the laboratory for analysis. (A, Courtesy Olympus America Inc., Melville, New York. B, From Lewis, S. M., Dirksen, S. R., Heitkemper, M. M., et al. [2014]. *Medical-surgical nursing* [9th ed.]. St. Louis, MO: Elsevier.)

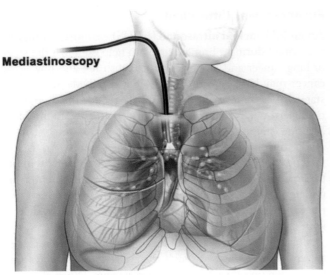

Mediastinoscopy

FIGURE 9.2 Mediastinoscopy. (Courtesy Wenda Speers.)

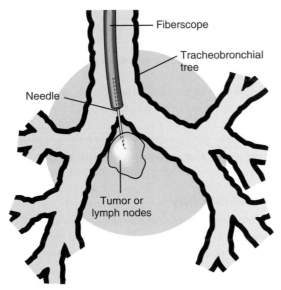

— Fiberscope

— Tracheobronchial tree

Needle —

Tumor or lymph nodes

FIGURE 9.3 Transbronchial needle biopsy. The diagram shows a transbronchial biopsy needle penetrating the bronchial wall and entering a mass of subcarinal lymph nodes or tumor. (Redrawn from DuBois, R. M., & Clarke, S. W. [1987]. *Fiberoptic bronchoscopy in diagnosis and management.* Orlando, FL: Grune and Stratton.)

Lung Biopsy

A **lung biopsy** sample can be obtained by means of a transbronchial needle biopsy or an open-lung biopsy. A **transbronchial lung biopsy** entails passing a forceps or needle through a bronchoscope to obtain a specimen (Fig. 9.3). An **open-lung biopsy** involves surgery to remove a sample of lung tissue. An incision is made over the area of the lung from which the tissue sample is to be collected. In some cases, a large incision may be necessary to reach the suspected problem area. After the procedure, a chest tube is inserted for drainage and suction for 7 to 14 days. An open-lung biopsy is usually performed when either a bronchoscopic biopsy or needle biopsy

under ultrasound or CT guidance has been unsuccessful or cannot be performed or when a larger piece of tissue is necessary to establish a diagnosis.

An open biopsy requires general anesthesia and is more invasive and thus more likely to cause complications, which include pneumothorax, bleeding, bronchospasm, cardiac arrhythmias, and infection. A needle lung biopsy is contraindicated in patients with lung bullae, cysts, blood coagulation disorders of any type, severe hypoxia, pulmonary hypertension, or cor pulmonale.

A lung biopsy is usually performed to diagnose abnormalities identified on a chest radiograph or computed tomography (CT) scan that are not readily accessible by other diagnostic procedures, such as bronchoscopy. A lung biopsy is especially useful in investigating peripheral lung abnormalities, such as recurrent infiltrates and pleural or subpleural lesions. Additional conditions under which a lung biopsy may be performed include metastatic cancer to the lung and pneumonia with abscess formation.

The tissues from a lung biopsy are sent to a pathology laboratory for examination of malignant cells. Other samples may be sent to a microbiology laboratory to determine the presence of infection and to characterize it. Lung biopsy results are usually available in 2 to 4 days. In some cases, however, it may take several weeks to confirm (by culture) certain infections, such as tuberculosis.

Video-Assisted Thoracoscopy Surgery

In **video-assisted thoracoscopy surgery (VATS)**, a small incision is made in the chest wall, and a device called a *thoracoscope* is inserted (Fig. 9.4). This device is equipped with a fiberscope that can examine the pleural cavity. The results are displayed on a video monitor (as in bronchoscopy). When pleural lesions are identified, biopsy can be performed under video guidance. This procedure is helpful in the diagnosis of tuberculosis, mesothelioma, and metastatic cancer.

Navigational Bronchoscopy

Although the standard bronchoscope is typically used to examine lung lesions, many bronchoscopes are unable to find or reach tissue located in the periphery of the lung, where smaller bronchi are not wide enough to permit passage of a normal endoscope. Over two-thirds of lung tumors are located in the lung periphery. **Navigational bronchoscopy** (also called *electromagnetic navigation bronchoscopy*) is a diagnostic and treatment procedure that combines electromagnetic navigation with real-time virtual three-dimensional (3D) CT imaging that allows the physician to reach these distal tumors, take a biopsy, and administer treatment.

Before navigational bronchoscopy is administered, a routine CT scan is performed to locate any masses or infiltrate in the lung. The CT scan is then loaded into a computer and is used to create a virtual, 3D "road map" of the lung. The lesions are marked on a virtual map, and an action plan is then made to "navigate" through the lung to reach the lesions.

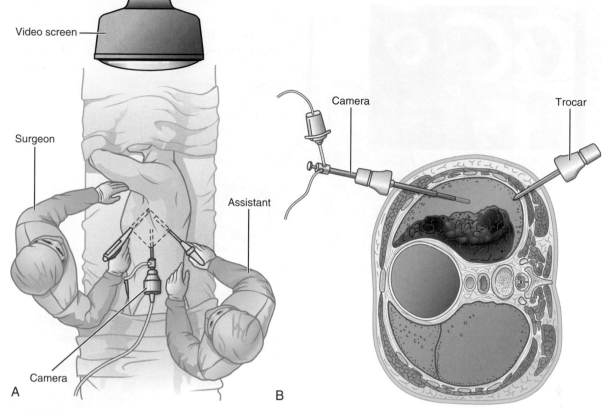

FIGURE 9.4 Different views of video-assisted thoracic surgery (VATS). (A) Patient is positioned in a 30-degree semi-supine position. (B) Transverse plane view. (From Good, V. S., & Kirkwood, P. L. [2018]. *Advanced critical care nursing* [2nd ed.]. St. Louis, 2018, Elsevier.)

As shown in Fig. 9.5, during the procedure, the patient lies on a low-frequency electromagnetic bed. A bronchoscope, which contains an extended working channel and locatable guide, is inserted into the patient's nasal airway, trachea, and into the bronchus. The electromagnetic bed allows the physician to view the locatable guide in real time and to carefully navigate the scope deep into the lung. The physician is able to control the movement and direction of the locatable guide as it moves into the distal airways. When the lesion is reached, the physician can easily perform a biopsy of the lesion for testing, stage lymph nodes, insert markers to guide radiotherapy, or guide brachytherapy catheters.

Navigational bronchoscopy also can be used in conjunction with external beam radiation therapy, such as **TomoTherapy**,[1] which is used to treat peripheral tumors with a precise dose of radiation while reducing radiation exposure to surrounding healthy tissue. The advantages of the navigational bronchoscopy procedure include the following:

- Minimally invasive compared with percutaneous lung biopsy procedures.
- Reaches tumors located in the periphery of the lungs
- Requires less time for recovery
- Can be done on an outpatient basis

Thoracentesis

Thoracentesis (also called *thoracocentesis*) is a procedure in which excess fluid accumulation (pleural effusion) between the chest cavity and lungs (pleural space) is aspirated through a needle inserted through the chest wall (Fig. 9.6). A chest radiograph, CT scan, or ultrasound scan may be used to confirm the precise location of the fluid. Once the fluid has been located, thoracentesis can be performed for diagnostic or therapeutic purposes.

Diagnostic thoracentesis may be performed to identify the cause of a pleural effusion. The analysis of the pleural fluid is extremely useful in the diagnosis and staging of a suspected or known malignancy. A pleural biopsy also may be performed during a thoracentesis to collect a tissue sample from the inner lining of the chest wall. Therapeutic thoracentesis may be performed to relieve shortness of breath or pain caused by a large pleural effusion, to remove air trapped between the lung and chest wall, or to administer medication directly into the lung cavity to treat the cause of the fluid accumulation

---

[1]TomoTherapy is a type of therapy in which radiation is aimed at a tumor from many different directions. The patient lies on a table and is moved through a donut-shaped device. The radiation source in the machine rotates around the patient in a spiral pattern. Before radiation, a 3D image of the tumor is taken. This helps the physician find the highest dose of radiation that can be used to kill tumor cells while causing less damage to nearby tissue. Tomotherapy is a type of intensity-modulated radiation therapy (IMRT), also called *helical tomotherapy*.

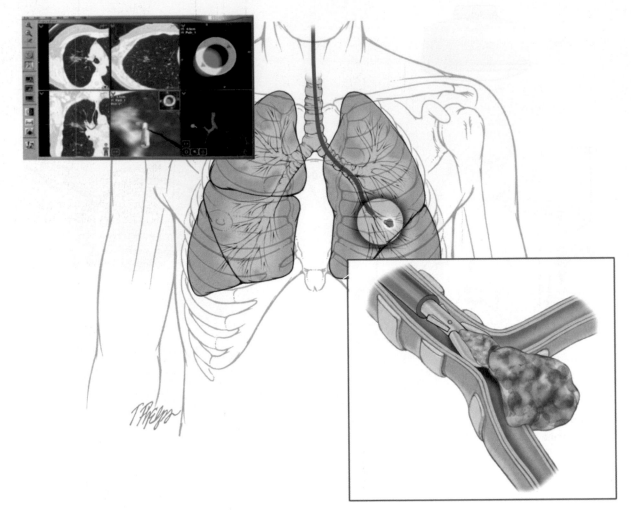

FIGURE 9.5 CT-guided navigational bronchoscopy.

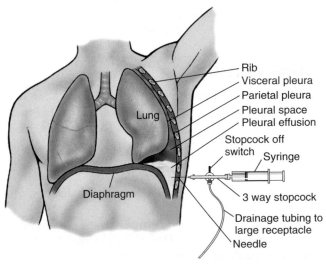

Rib
Visceral pleura
Parietal pleura
Pleural space
Pleural effusion
Stopcock off switch
Syringe
3 way stopcock
Drainage tubing to large receptacle
Needle
Lung
Diaphragm

FIGURE 9.6 Thoracentesis. A catheter is positioned in the pleural space to remove accumulated fluid. Pleural fluid is seen as the yellow shadow at the base of the left lung. (From Monahan, F. D., Neighbors, M., Sands, J. K., et al. [2007]. *Phipps' medical-surgical nursing health and illness perspectives* [8th ed.]. St. Louis, MO: Elsevier.)

or to treat the malignancy. The fluid in the lung cavity is classified as either a **transudate** or an **exudate** (see Chapter 24, Pleural Effusion and Empyema).

The thoracentesis procedure is generally performed while the patient is in an upright position, leaning forward slightly, typically over a bedside table. Using a local anesthetic, the physician inserts a large-bore thoracentesis needle (16 to 19 gauge), or needle-catheter, between the ribs over the fluid accumulation. The needle or catheter is connected to a small tube with a three-way stopcock, which in turn is attached to either a large syringe or a vacuum and collection bottle. Depending on the purpose of the thoracentesis, up to 1500 mL may be withdrawn. Once the fluid has been collected, the needle or catheter is removed and a bandage is placed over the puncture site. The patient is usually instructed to lie on the puncture site side for about an hour to allow the puncture site to seal.

A thoracentesis is usually a safe procedure. However, a chest radiograph is generally obtained shortly after the procedure to ensure that no complications have developed. Complications may include pneumothorax, postaspiration pulmonary edema (which sometimes occurs when large amounts of fluid are aspirated too rapidly), infection, bleeding, and organ damage.

Pleurodesis

Pleurodesis is performed to prevent the recurrence of a pneumothorax or pleural effusion. Pleurodesis is achieved by injecting any number of agents (called *sclerosing agents* or **sclerosants**) into the pleural space through a chest tube. There is no one sclerosant that is more effective or safer than the others. Common sclerosant chemicals include a slurry of talc, bleomycin, nitrogen mustard, doxycycline, povidone-iodine, or quinacrine. The instilled sclerosing agents cause irritation and inflammation (pleuritis) between the parietal and the visceral layers of the pleura. This action causes the pleurae to stick together and thereby prevents subsequent gas or fluid accumulation.

A chemical pleurodesis is considered to be the standard of care for patients with malignant pleural effusions. Because chemical pleurodesis is a painful procedure, the patient is premedicated with a sedative and analgesics. A local anesthetic also may be instilled into the pleural space or added to the sclerosant. Although complications of pleurodesis are uncommon, risks include the following:

- Superinfection
- Bleeding
- Acute respiratory distress syndrome
- Pneumothorax and respiratory failure
  Complications may be specific for each sclerosant:
- Talc and doxycycline can cause fever and pain.
- Quinacrine can cause low blood pressure, fever, and hallucinations.
- Bleomycin can cause fever, pain, and nausea.
  Pleurodesis may fail because of the following complications:
- Trapped lung, in which the lung is enclosed in scar or tumor tissue ("plural peel")
- Formation of isolated pockets (loculation) within the pleural space
- Loss of lung flexibility (elasticity)
- Production of large amounts of pleural fluid
- Extensive spread (metastasis) of pleural cancer
- Improper positioning, blockage, or kinking of the chest tube

Hematology, Blood Chemistry, and Electrolyte Findings

Abnormal hematology, blood chemistry, or electrolyte values assist the respiratory care practitioner and physician in the assessment of cardiopulmonary disorders. Knowledge of these laboratory tests provides a greater understanding of the clinical manifestations of a particular cardiopulmonary disorder.

Hematology

The most frequent laboratory **hematology** test is the **complete blood count (CBC)**. The CBC includes the red blood cell (RBC) count, **hemoglobin (Hb)**, **hematocrit (Hct)**, the total WBC count, and at least an estimate of the platelet count. Various **types of anemia** (e.g., iron deficiency, pernicious anemia, and sickle cell anemia) are all diagnosed by visual examination of the peripheral blood smear (Table 9.2).

Red Blood Cell Count

The RBCs (erythrocytes) constitute the major portion of the blood cells. The healthy man has about 5 million RBCs in each cubic millimeter (mm^3) of blood. The healthy woman has about 4 million RBCs in each cubic millimeter of blood. Clinically, the hemoglobin, the total number of RBCs and the **red blood cell indices** are useful in assessing the patient's overall oxygen-carrying capacity (see Chapter 6). The RBC indices are helpful in the identification of specific RBC deficiencies.

White Blood Cell Count

The major functions of the white blood cells (WBCs) (leukocytes) are to (1) fight against infection, (2) defend the body by phagocytosis against foreign substances, and (3) produce (or at least transport and distribute) antibodies in the immune response. The WBCs are far less numerous than the RBCs, averaging 5000 to 10,000 cells per cubic millimeter of blood. There are two types of WBCs: granular leukocytes and nongranular leukocytes. Because the general function of the leukocytes is to combat inflammation and infection, the clinical diagnosis of an injury or infection often entails a differential WBC count, which is the determination of the number of each type of cell in 100 WBCs. Box 9.2 shows a normal differential count. Table 9.3 provides an overview of cell types and common causes for their increase (**leukocytosis**).

Granular Leukocytes. The **granular leukocytes** (also called *granulocytes*) are so classified because of the granules present in their cytoplasm. The granulocytes are further divided into the following three types according to the staining properties of the granules: **neutrophils**, **eosinophils**, and **basophils**. Because these cells have distinctive multilobar nuclei, they are often referred to as *polymorphonuclear leukocytes.*

Neutrophils. The neutrophils make up about 60% to 70% of the total number of WBCs. They have granules that are neutral and therefore do not stain with an acid or a basic dye. The neutrophils are the first WBCs to arrive at the site of infection or inflammation, usually appearing within 90 minutes of the injury. They represent the primary cellular defense against bacterial organisms through the process of **phagocytosis** (ingestion of foreign material). The neutrophils are one of

---

BOX 9.2 Normal Differential White Blood Cell Count

Granular Leukocytes
- Neutrophils 60% to 70%
- Eosinophils 2% to 4%
- Basophils 0.5% to 1%

Nongranular Leukocytes
- Lymphocytes 20% to 25%
- Monocytes 3% to 8%

TABLE 9.2 Red Blood Cell Indices

Index	Description
Hematocrit (Hct)	The Hct is the volume of red blood cells (RBCs) in 100 mL of blood and is expressed as a percentage of the total volume in whole blood. In the healthy man, the Hct is about 45%; in the healthy woman, the Hct is about 42%. In the healthy newborn, the Hct ranges from 45% to 60%. The Hct is also called the *packed cell volume* (PCV).
Hemoglobin (Hb)	Most of the oxygen that diffuses into the pulmonary capillary blood rapidly moves into the RBCs and chemically attaches to the Hb. Each RBC contains about 280 million Hb molecules. The Hb value is reported in grams per 100 mL of blood (also referred to as grams percent of hemoglobin [g% Hb]). The normal Hb value for men is 14 to 16 g%. The normal Hb value for women is 12 to 15 g%. Hb constitutes about 33% of the RBC weight.
Mean cell volume (MCV)	The MCV is the actual size (volume) of the RBCs and is used to classify anemias. It is an index that expresses the volume of a single red cell and is measured in cubic microns. The normal MCV is 87 to 103 μm^3 for both men and women.
Mean corpuscular hemoglobin concentration (MCHC)	The MCHC is a measure of the concentration or proportion of Hb in an average (mean) RBC. The MCHC is derived by dividing the g% Hb by the Hct. For example, if a patient has 15 g% Hb and an Hct of 45%, the MCHC is 33%. The normal MCHC for men and women ranges from 32% to 36%. The MCHC is most useful in assessing the degree of anemia because the two most accurate hematologic measurements (Hb and Hct—not RBC) are used for the test.
Mean cell hemoglobin (MCH)	The MCH is a measure of weight of Hb in a single RBC. This value is derived by dividing the total Hb (g% Hb) by the RBC count. The MCH is useful in diagnosing severely anemic patients but not as good as the MCHC because the RBC count is not always accurate. The normal range for the MCH is 27 to 32 pg/RBC.
Types of Anemias	
Normochromic (normal Hb) and normocytic (normal cell size) anemia	Normochromic anemia is most commonly caused by excessive blood loss. The amount of Hb and the number of RBCs are decreased, but the individual size and content remain normal. Clinically, the laboratory report reveals the following: Hct: Below normal Hb: Below normal MCV: Normal MCHC: Normal MCH: Normal
Hypochromic (decreased Hb) microcytic (small cell size) anemia	In hypochromic anemia, the size of the RBCs and the Hb content are decreased. This form of anemia is commonly seen in patients with chronic blood loss, iron deficiency, chronic infections, and malignancies. Clinically, the laboratory report reveals the following: Hct: Below normal Hb: Below normal MCV: Below normal MCHC: Below normal MCH: Below normal
Macrocytic (large cell size) anemia	Macrocytic anemia is commonly caused by folic acid and vitamin B_{12} deficiencies. Patients with macrocytic anemia produce fewer RBCs, but the RBCs that are present are larger than normal. Clinically, the laboratory report reveals the following: Hct: Below normal Hb: Below normal MCV: Above normal (because of the larger RBC size) MCHC: Above normal (because of the larger RBC size)

several types of cells called *phagocytes* that ingest and destroy bacterial organisms and particulate matter. The neutrophils also release an enzyme called *lysozyme*, which destroys certain bacteria. An increased neutrophil count is associated with (1) bacterial infection, (2) physical and emotional stress, (3) tumors, (4) inflammatory or traumatic disorders, (5) some leukemias, (6) myocardial infarction, and (7) burns.

Early (immature) forms of neutrophils are nonsegmented and are called **"band" forms**. They almost always signify

TABLE 9.3 Common Causes of White Blood Cell Increase

Cell Type	Causes of Increase
Neutrophil	Bacterial infection, inflammation
Eosinophil	Allergic reaction, parasitic infection
Basophil	Myeloproliferative disorders
Monocyte	Chronic infections, malignancies
Lymphocyte	Viral infections

infection if elevated above 10% of the differential. More mature forms of neutrophils have segmented nuclei. They may increase even in the absence of infection (e.g., with stress [exercise] or the use of corticosteroid medication).

Eosinophils. The cytoplasmic granules of eosinophils stain red with the acid dye eosin. These leukocytes make up 2% to 4% of the total number of WBCs. Although the precise function of the eosinophils is unknown, they are thought to play an important role in the breakdown of protein material. It is known, however, that the eosinophils are activated by allergies (such as an allergic asthmatic episode) and parasitic infections. Their role in the pathogenesis of asthma (see Chapter 14, Asthma) appears to be increasingly important, e.g., eosinophilic asthma. Eosinophils are thought to detoxify the agents or chemical mediators associated with allergic reactions. An increased eosinophil count also may be associated with lung cancer, chronic skin infections (e.g., psoriasis, scabies), polycythemia, and tumors.

Basophils. The **basophils** make up only about 0.5% to 1.0% of the total WBC count. The granules of the basophils stain blue with a basic dye. The precise function of the basophils is not clearly understood. Increased basophils are primarily associated with certain myeloproliferative disorders. It is thought that the basophils are involved in allergic and stress responses. They are also considered to be phagocytic and contain heparin, histamines, and serotonin.

Nongranular Leukocytes. There are two groups of **nongranular leukocytes**: the **monocytes** and **lymphocytes**. The term *mononuclear leukocytes* is also used to describe these cells because they do not contain granules but have spheric nuclei.

Monocytes. The monocytes are the second order of cells to arrive at the inflammation site, usually appearing about 5 hours or more after the injury. After 48 hours, however, the monocytes are usually the predominant cell type in the inflamed area. The monocytes are the largest of the WBCs and make up about 3% to 8% of the total leukocyte count. The monocytes are short-lived, phagocytic WBCs, with a half-life of about 1 day. They circulate in the bloodstream, from which they move into tissues—at which point they may mature into long-living macrophages (also called *histiocytes*).

Macrophages are large wandering cells that engulf larger and greater quantities of foreign material than the neutrophils. When the foreign material cannot be digested by the macrophages, the macrophages may proliferate to form a capsule that surrounds and encloses the foreign material (e.g., fungal spores). Although the monocytes and macrophages do not respond as quickly to an inflammatory process as the neutrophils, they are considered one of the first lines of cellular inflammatory defense. Therefore an elevated number of monocytes suggests infection and inflammation. The monocytes play an important role in chronic inflammation and are also involved in the immune response and malignancies.

Lymphocytes. Increased lymphocytes are typically seen in viral infections (e.g., infectious mononucleosis). The lymphocytes are also involved in the production of antibodies, which are special proteins that inactivate antigens. For a better understanding of the importance of the lymphocytes and the clinical significance of their destruction or depletion (e.g., in acquired immunodeficiency syndrome [**AIDS**]), a brief review of the role and function of the lymphocytes in the immune system is in order.

The lymphocytes can be divided into two categories: **B cells** and **T cells**. These cells can be identified with an electron microscope according to certain distinguishing surface marks, called *rosettes*. T cells have a smooth surface; B cells have projections. B cells make up 10% to 30% of the total lymphocytes; T cells account for 70% to 90% of the total lymphocytes.

The B cells, which are formed in the bone marrow, further divide into either plasma cells or memory cells. The plasma cells secrete antibodies in response to foreign antigens. The memory cells retain the ability to recognize specific antigens long after the initial exposure and therefore contribute to long-term immunity against future exposures to invading pathogens.

The T cells, which are formed in the thymus, are further divided into four functional categories: (1) cytotoxic T cells (also called *killer lymphocytes* or *natural killer cells*), which attack and kill foreign or infected cells; (2) helper T cells, which recognize foreign antigens and help activate cytotoxic T cells and plasma cells (B cells); (3) inducer T cells, which stimulate the production of the different T-cell subsets; and (4) suppressor T cells, which work to suppress the responses of the other cells and help provide feedback information to the system.

The T cells also may be classified according to their surface antigens (i.e., the T cells may display either T4 or T8 surface antigen). The T4 surface antigen subset, which makes up 60% to 70% of the circulating T cells, consists mainly of the helper and inducer cells. The T8 surface antigen subset consists mainly of the cytotoxic and suppressor cells.

Sequence of the Lymphocytic Response to Infection. Initially, the macrophages attack and engulf the foreign antigens. This activity in turn stimulates the production of T cells and, ultimately, the antibody-producing B cells (plasma cells). The T4 cells play a pivotal role in the overall modulation of this immune response by (1) secreting a substance called *lymphokine*, which is a potent stimulus to T-cell growth and differentiation; (2) recognizing foreign antigens; (3) causing clonal proliferation of T cells; (4) mediating cytotoxic and suppressor functions; and (5) enabling B cells to secrete specific antibodies.

Because T cells (especially the T4 lymphocytes) have such a central role in this complex immune response, it should not be difficult to imagine the devastating effect that would ultimately follow from the systematic depletion of T lymphocytes. For example, virtually all the infectious complications of HIV/AIDS may be explained with reference to the effect that HIV has on the T cells. A decreased number of T cells increases the patient's susceptibility to a wide range of opportunistic infections and neoplasms. In the healthy subject, the T4/T8 ratio is about 2.0. In the patient with HIV/AIDS, the T4/T8 ratio is usually 0.5 or less.

Platelet Count. **Platelets** (also called *thrombocytes*) are the smallest of the formed elements in the blood. They are round or oval, flattened, and disk-shaped in appearance. Platelets are produced in the bone marrow and possibly in the lungs. Platelet activity is essential for blood clotting. The normal platelet count is 150,000 to 350,000/mm³.

A deficiency of platelets leads to prolonged bleeding time and impaired clot retention. A low platelet count (**thrombocytopenia**) is associated with (1) massive blood transfusion, (2) pneumonia, (3) cancer chemotherapy, (4) infection, (5) allergic conditions, and (6) toxic effects of certain drugs (e.g., heparin, isoniazid, penicillins, prednisone, streptomycin). A high platelet count (thrombocythemia) is associated with (1) cancer, (2) trauma, (3) asphyxiation, (4) rheumatoid arthritis, (5) iron deficiency, (6) acute infections, (7) heart disease, (8) tuberculosis, and (9) polycythemia vera.

A platelet count of less than 20,000/mm³ is associated with spontaneous bleeding, prolonged bleeding time, and poor clot retraction. The precise platelet count necessary for hemostasis is not firmly established. Generally, platelet counts greater than 50,000/mm³ are not associated with spontaneous bleeding. Therefore various diagnostic or therapeutic procedures, such as bronchoscopy or the insertion of an arterial catheter, are usually considered safe when the platelet count is greater than 50,000/mm³.

Blood Chemistry

A basic knowledge of blood chemistry, normal values, and common health problems that alter these values is an important cornerstone of patient assessment. Table 9.4 lists the blood chemistry tests monitored in respiratory care.

Electrolytes

For the cells of the body to function properly, a normal concentration of **electrolytes** must be maintained, especially for normal cardiac function. Therefore the monitoring of electrolytes is extremely important in the patient whose body fluids are being endogenously or exogenously manipulated (e.g., intravenous therapy, renal disease, diarrhea). Table 9.5 lists electrolytes monitored in respiratory care. Normal values for blood sodium, potassium, chloride, and bicarbonate should be memorized by the respiratory care practitioner.

TABLE 9.4 Blood Chemistry Tests Monitored in Respiratory and Cardiac Care

Chemical	Normal Value	Common Abnormal Findings
Glucose	70–110 mg/dL	Hyperglycemia (excess glucose level) Diabetes mellitus Acute infection Myocardial infarction Thiazide and loop diuretics Hypoglycemia (low glucose level) Pancreatic tumors or liver disease Pituitary or adrenocortical hyperfunction
Lactic dehydrogenase (LDH)	80–120 Wacker units	Increases are associated with the following: Myocardial infarction Chronic hepatitis Pneumonia Pulmonary infarction
Serum glutamic oxaloacetic transaminase (SGOT)	8–33 U/mL	Increases are associated with the following: Myocardial infarction Congestive heart failure Pulmonary infarction
Aspartate aminotransferase (AST)	7–40 units/L (0.12–0.67 µKat/L)	Increases are associated with the following: Acute aminotransferase hepatitis Liver disease Myocardial infarction Pulmonary infection
Alanine aminotransferase (ALT) (previously called serum glutamic pyruvic transaminase [SGPT])	5–36 units/L (0.08–0.6 µKat/L)	Increases are associated with the following: Liver damage Inflammation Shock
Bilirubin	*Adult:* 0.1–1.2 mg/dL *Newborn:* 1–12 mg/dL	Increases are associated with the following; Massive hemolysis Hepatitis
Blood urea nitrogen (BUN)	8–18 mg/dL	Increases are associated with acute or chronic renal failure
Serum creatinine	0.6–1.2 mg/dL	Increases are associated with renal failure

TABLE 9.5 Electrolytes Commonly Monitored in Respiratory Care

Electrolyte	Normal Value	Common Abnormal Findings	Clinical Manifestations
Sodium (Na^+)	136–142 mEq/L	Hypernatremia (excess Na^+) Dehydration Hyponatremia (low Na^+) Sweating Burns Loss of gastrointestinal secretions Use of some diuretics Excessive water intake	Desiccated mucous membranes Flushed skin Great thirst Dry tongue Abdominal cramps Muscle twitching Poor perfusion Vasomotor collapse Confusion Seizures
Potassium (K^+)	3.8–5.0 mEq/L	Hyperkalemia (excess K^+) Renal failure Muscle tissue damage Hypokalemia (low K^+) Diuretic therapy Endocrine disorder Diarrhea Reduced intake or loss of K^+ Chronic stress	Irritability Nausea Diarrhea Weakness Ventricular fibrillation Metabolic alkalosis Muscular weakness Malaise Cardiac arrhythmias Hypotension
Chloride (Cl^-)	95–103 mEq/L	Hyperchloremia (excess Cl^-) Renal tubular acidosis Hypochloremia (low Cl^-) Alkalosis—associated frequently with hypokalemia; that is, hypokalemic, hypochloremic metabolic alkalosis	Deep, rapid breathing Weakness Disorientation Metabolic alkalosis Muscle hypertonicity Tetany Depressed ventilation (respiratory compensation)
Calcium (Ca^{++})	4.5–5.4 mEq/L	Hypercalcemia (excess Ca^{++}) Malignant tumors Bone fractures Diuretic therapy Excessive use of antacids or milk consumption Vitamin D intoxication Hyperparathyroidism Hypocalcemia (low Ca^{++}) Respiratory alkalosis Pregnancy Vitamin D deficiency Diuretic therapy Hypoparathyroidism	Lethargy, weakness Hyporeflexia Constipation, anorexia, renal stones Mental deterioration Paresthesia, cramping of muscles, stridor, seizures, mental disturbance, Chvostek's sign, Trousseau's sign

SELF-ASSESSMENT QUESTIONS

1. In the healthy woman, what is the hematocrit (Hct)?
   a. 31%
   b. 38%
   c. 42%
   d. 45%

2. Which of the following represent the primary defense against bacterial organisms through phagocytosis?
   a. Eosinophils
   b. Neutrophils
   c. Monocytes
   d. Basophils

3. What is the normal hemoglobin value for men?
   a. 10 to 12 g%
   b. 12 to 14 g%
   c. 14 to 16 g%
   d. 16 to 18 g%

4. What percent of the normal white blood cell count are neutrophils?
   a. 20% to 25%
   b. 40% to 50%
   c. 60% to 70%
   d. 75% to 85%

5. In the healthy man, what is the red blood cell count?
   a. 5,000,000/mm^3
   b. 6,000,000/mm^3
   c. 7,000,000/mm^3
   d. 8,000,000/mm^3

6. What is the normal white blood cell count?
   a. 1000 to 5000/mm^3
   b. 5000 to 10,000/mm^3
   c. 10,000 to 15,000/mm^3
   d. 15,000 to 20,000/mm^3

7. Which of the following are activated by allergies (such as an allergic asthmatic episode)?
   a. Eosinophils
   b. Neutrophils
   c. Monocytes
   d. Basophils

8. Various clinical procedures such as bronchoscopy or the insertion of an arterial catheter are generally safe when the platelet count is *no lower* than which of the following?
   a. 100,000/mm^3
   b. 75,000/mm^3
   c. 50,000/mm^3
   d. 20,000/mm^3

9. Which of the following are associated with hyperglycemia?
   1. Diabetes mellitus
   2. Myocardial infarction
   3. Thiazide and loop diuretics
   4. Acute infection
      a. 2 and 4 only
      b. 2, 3, and 4 only
      c. 1, 2, and 3 only
      d. 1, 2, 3, and 4

10. Which of the following are clinical manifestations associated with hyponatremia?
    1. Seizures
    2. Confusion
    3. Muscle twitching
    4. Abdominal cramps
       a. 2 and 4 only
       b. 2, 3, and 4 only
       c. 1, 2, and 3 only
       d. 1, 2, 3, and 4

CHAPTER 10

The Therapist-Driven Protocol Program

Chapter Objectives

After reading this chapter, you will be able to:

- Describe the therapist-driven protocol (TDP) program and the role of the respiratory care practitioner now and in the future.
- Discuss the knowledge base required for a successful TDP program.
- Explain the assessment process skills required for a successful TDP program.
- Describe the essential cornerstones (Protocols) for a successful TDP program.
- List the anatomic alterations of the lungs commonly seen in clinical practice.
- Describe the clinical scenarios—chain of events—activated by the common anatomic alterations of the lungs.
- Identify the most common anatomic alterations associated with the respiratory disorders presented in this textbook.
- Understand in depth the differences between obstructive and restrictive pathophysiology.
- Identify the bases for resistance to development of protocol programs, and outline steps to overcome them.
- Define key terms and complete self-assessment questions at the end of the chapter and on Evolve.

Key Terms

Aerosolized Medication Therapy Protocol
Airway Clearance Therapy Protocol
Anatomic Alterations of the Lung
Assess, Treat, and Teach Protocols
Atelectasis
Bronchospasm
Clinical Manifestation
Clinical Scenarios
Diagnostic Coding
Discharge Planning
Disease-Specific Protocols
Distal Airway and Alveolar Weakening
Evidence-Based Clinical Practice Guidelines
Excessive Bronchial Secretions
Increased Alveolar-Capillary Membrane Thickness
Length of Stay (LOS)
Lung Expansion Therapy Protocol
Oxygen Therapy Protocol
Pathophysiologic Mechanisms
Patient-Driven Protocols
Patient Education
Patient Focused Protocols
Patient Protection and Affordable Care Act
Protocol Competency Testing
Readmission Prevention Teams
Severity Assessment
TDP Safe and Ready Respiratory Therapist
Therapist-Driven Protocol (TDPs)

Chapter Outline

The "Knowledge Base" Required for a Successful Therapist-Driven Protocol Program
The "Assessment Process Skills" Required for a Successful Therapist-Driven Protocol Program
    Severity Assessment
The Essential Cornerstones of a Successful Therapist-Driven Protocol Program
    Summary of a Good Therapist-Driven Protocol Program
Common Anatomic Alterations of the Lungs
    Clinical Scenarios Activated by Common Anatomic Alterations of the Lungs
Self-Assessment Questions

There is an emerging consensus that the United States health care system is broken and new and innovative solutions to the problem must be sought. The US Department of Health and Human Services (DHHS), **Patient Protection and Affordable Care Act**, often called the *Affordable Care Act (ACA),* was made law in 2010 and came into effect in 2014.

One of the earliest effects of the ACA was to institute a system whereby hospitals would be penalized for what were designated as conditions subject to wasteful excess and excessive use of resources—particularly in the general area of **length of stay (LOS)**. Of the seven "index conditions" monitored, five involve significant use of respiratory care services: acute pneumonia, chronic obstructive pulmonary disease exacerbations, postoperative infections, ventilator-associated pneumonia, congestive heart failure/pulmonary edema, and myocardial infarction. Put simply, it was implied that LOS was a good easy surrogate measure for quality of care; if a patient's hospital stay was significantly longer than a "benchmark" (chosen by the DHHS), how could the quality of care and use of precious resources be anything *but* substandard?

Over the past several years, the following troubling concerns have been noted:

- Many hospitals have not been proactive in securing their institutions from possible penalties for exceeding the LOS benchmark—for example, a 5.4-day LOS instead of 5.0 days—and the financial penalties were significant; some hospitals have already found this out with penalties in the neighborhood of hundreds of thousands of dollars!

- Many hospital leaders do not know how close their institutions were to the penalty threshold, nor did they appear to be aware of the generally poor results of attempts to remediate the problem published in the current literature—remedies such as, **patient education**, transition clinics, focused **discharge planning**, and **readmission prevention teams**. All have pros and cons, but none has been extremely successful.

What *has* worked has been precision in discharge **diagnostic coding** (ICD-10) and cost-effective use of therapeutic modalities. Among the latter are respiratory care services. This latter area is where the **therapist-driven protocol (TDP)** approach is attractive and where acceptance of its overall effectiveness will be more widely recognized sooner or later.

Clearly, TDPs (also called: **patient-driven protocols,** or **patient focused protocols**) have proved to be an important and integral part of respiratory care health services, resulting in superior cost-effective clinical outcomes. According to the American Association for Respiratory Care (AARC), Guidelines for Respiratory Care Departments Protocol Program Directors,[1] the purposes of respiratory TDPs are to:

- Deliver individualized diagnostic and therapeutic respiratory care to patients
- Assist the physician with evaluating patients' respiratory care needs and optimize the allocation of respiratory care services
- Determine the indications for respiratory therapy and the appropriate modalities for providing high-quality, cost-effective care that improves patient outcomes and decreases length of stay
- Empower respiratory therapists to allocate care using sign- and symptom-based algorithms for respiratory treatment

To support the AARC's purpose statement on TDPs, the American College of Chest Physicians (ACCP) initially defined **respiratory therapy protocols** as follows, with subsequent approval by the National Association of Medical Directors of Respiratory Care (NAMDRC):

TDPs are patient care plans which are initiated and implemented by credentialed respiratory care workers. These plans are designed and developed with input from physicians, and are approved for use by the medical staff and the governing body of the hospitals in which they are used. They share in common extreme reliance on assessment and evaluation skills.

Protocols are by their nature dynamic and flexible, allowing up- or down-regulation of intensity of respiratory services. Protocols allow the respiratory therapist authority to evaluate the patient, initiate care, and to adjust, discontinue, or restart respiratory care procedures on a shift-by-shift or hour-to-hour basis once the protocol is ordered by the physician. They must contain clear strategies for various therapeutic interventions, while avoiding any misconception that they infringe on the practice of medicine. All programs must comply with Federal and State regulations and standards including those published by their State Licensing Boards.

TDPs provide the respiratory therapist with a wide-ranging flexibility to both assess and treat the patient—but *only* within preapproved and clearly defined boundaries outlined by the physician, the medical staff, and the hospital. In addition, respiratory TDPs give the therapist specific authority to (1) gather clinical information related to the patient's respiratory status, (2) make an assessment of the clinical data collected, and (3) start, increase, decrease, or discontinue certain respiratory therapies on a moment-to-moment, hour-to-hour, shift-by-shift, or day-to-day basis. The innate beauty of respiratory TDPs is that (1) the physician should always be in the "information loop" regarding patient care and (2) therapy can be quickly modified in response to the specific and immediate needs of the patient. Numerous clinical research studies have verified these facts: respiratory TDPs (1) significantly improve selected respiratory therapy outcomes and (2) provided appreciably lower therapy costs.

Unfortunately, the implementation of TDPs throughout the United States continues to be slow. In 2008 the AARC Protocol Implementation Committee conducted a survey to evaluate the barriers to implementation. Over 450 respiratory managers responded to the survey. Despite the overwhelming evidence that protocols clearly improve outcomes and reduce cost, the survey showed that less than 50% of respiratory care nationwide was provided by protocols. About 75% of the respondents had at least one protocol in operation. The majority of the respondent hospitals did not have a *comprehensive* (All-Service, All-Modality) program in place. According to the study, the department medical directors, managers, nurses, and administrators were not perceived as barriers.

Of significant interest was the fact that the biggest barrier to the implementation of protocols was perceived to be the medical staff itself. The primary reason for the medical staff's resistance was their perception that "staff therapists did not have the skills (i.e., assessment skills) to function under protocols." The AARC Protocol Implementation Committee stated that "[this] perception must change...."[2] To address this concern, many respiratory care departments have established mandatory **protocol competency testing** on a periodic basis to ensure their employees are **"TDP safe and ready respiratory therapists"**—that is, up-to-date on the medical staff and specific hospital-approved TDPs used in their place of work. It goes beyond what the respiratory therapy student learns at school, and beyond what is being tested on the National Board for Respiratory Care (NBRC) examinations. It gets right at the issue of the individual therapist's assessment and treatment (i.e., protocol) skills in this hospital at this point in time.

As of the date of this writing there has been some, but far from complete, improvement in this diagnosis/delivery paradox. Overlap of many of the functions potentially seen as within the scope of practice of the respiratory therapist is now being assumed by the physical therapist and certified nurse practitioner. The Advanced Practice Respiratory Therapist (APRT) is a long way from being fully implemented. Only a handful of therapist training programs in this county are training at

---

[1]Available online at http://www.aarc.org.

[2]The AARC Protocol Implementation Committee has developed a PowerPoint presentation of the complete survey, which is intended to assist in understanding the barriers and developing successful strategies to implement protocol utilization (http://www.aarc.org; search for AARC Protocol Implementation Committee).

the level of competency required in the knowledge and skills base described in the following material. Furthermore, the NBRC has not yet developed, let alone implemented, a certifying examination at the APRT level. In fact, licensure at the level of TDP competency is currently available in only a handful of states.

TDPs must be recognized as different from **disease-specific protocols** (sometimes called disease management protocols), which involve the diagnosis and treatment of *individual diseases* rather than the use of modalities or medications—for example, an Initial Asthma Management Protocol such as might be used in an emergency department (see Chapter 14, Asthma). Respiratory therapists may be asked to be familiar with certain disease-specific protocols, depending on their work site, but at this juncture should be *required* to be competent in the use of *all* the general modality-specific TDPs (i.e., Oxygen Therapy Protocol, Airway Clearance Therapy Protocol, Lung Expansion Therapy Protocol, Aerosolized Medication Therapy Protocol, and Mechanical Ventilation Protocol).

The essential components of a good TDP program do not come easy. This is because a strong TDP program promises that the respiratory therapist who is identified as "TDP safe and ready" will be qualified to (1) systematically collect the appropriate clinical data, (2) formulate a uniform and accurate assessment, and (3) select a uniform and optimal treatment plan within the limits set by the protocol (Fig. 10.1).

The converse, however, is also true: When the respiratory therapist is *not* TDP safe and ready, the systematic collection of clinical data is not done at all or is incomplete. As a result, nonuniform or inaccurate assessments are made, resulting in nonuniform or inaccurate treatment selections (Fig. 10.2). This inappropriate and ineffective type of respiratory therapy leads to the misallocation of care, the administration of unneeded care, and—most important—the nonprovision of needed patient care. The bottom line is poor-quality patient care and unnecessary costs. To be sure, the development and implementation of a strong TDP program require a good deal of fundamental knowledge, training, and practice, but the benefits are worth the price. The essential components of a good TDP program are discussed in the following paragraphs.

The "Knowledge Base" Required for a Successful Therapist-Driven Protocol Program

As shown in Fig. 10.3 the essential knowledge base for a successful TDP program includes (1) the anatomic alterations of the lungs caused by common respiratory disorders, (2) the major pathophysiologic mechanisms activated throughout the respiratory and cardiac systems as a result of the anatomic alterations, (3) the common clinical manifestations that develop as a result of the activated pathophysiologic mechanisms, and (4) the treatment modalities used to correct them. *In other words, the clinical manifestations demonstrated by the patient do not arbitrarily appear but are the result of specific anatomic lung alterations and pathophysiologic events.*

Hence, it is essential that the respiratory therapist knows and understands that certain anatomic alterations of the lung will lead to specific and often predictable clinical manifestations. Each respiratory disease presented in this textbook describes these four essential knowledge components necessary for TDPs to successfully work in the modern health care setting. In the clinical setting, this knowledge base enhances the assessment process essential to a good TDP program.

The "Assessment Process Skills" Required for a Successful Therapist-Driven Protocol Program

Using the knowledge base described previously, the respiratory therapist must be competent in performing the actual assessment process. This means that the practitioner can (1) quickly

RCP STAFF	HOSPITAL SHIFTS 365 DAYS/YR	THERAPIST-DRIVEN PROTOCOL PROGRAM		
		Clinical Data	Assessment	Tx Selection
TDP SAFE AND READY	Days Evenings Nights	Systematic Collection of Clinical Data	Uniform and Accurate Assessment	Uniform and Optimal Tx Selections

FIGURE 10.1 The promise of a good therapist-driven protocol program.

RCP STAFF	HOSPITAL SHIFTS 365 DAYS/YR	NO THERAPIST-DRIVEN PROTOCOL PROGRAM		
		Clinical Data	Assessment	Tx Selection
			Nonuniform and Inaccurate	Nonuniform and Nonoptimal
NOT TDP SAFE AND READY	Days Evenings Nights	Incomplete or NO Collection of Clinical Data	Assessment Assessment Assessment	Tx Selection Tx Selection Tx Selection

FIGURE 10.2 No assessment program in place.

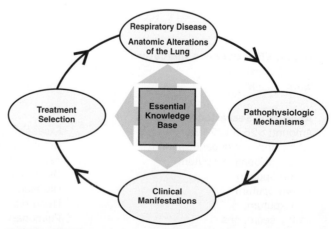

FIGURE 10.3 Foundations for a strong therapist-driven protocol program. Overview of the essential knowledge base for outcome assessment of respiratory disease.

and systematically gather the clinical information demonstrated by the patient, (2) formulate an accurate assessment of the clinical data (i.e., identify the cause and severity of the problem), (3) select an optimal treatment modality, and (4) document the use and evaluation of this process quickly, clearly, and precisely. In the clinical setting, the practice and mastery of the assessment process are absolutely central and essential to the success of a good TDP program (Fig. 10.4). Simply stated, immediately after the respiratory therapist identifies the clinical manifestations (clinical indicators) present, an assessment of the data must be performed and a treatment plan must be formulated. For the most part, the initial assessment is primarily directed at the anatomic alterations of the lungs that are causing the clinical indicators (e.g., **bronchospasm**) and the severity of the clinical indicators.

For example, an appropriate assessment for the clinical cause and indicator of wheezing might be bronchospasm—the anatomic alteration of the lungs. If the therapist assesses the cause of the wheezing correctly as bronchospasm, the correct treatment selection would be a bronchodilator treatment from the **Aerosolized Medication Therapy Protocol**, Protocol 10.4, page 144. If, however, the cause of the wheezing is correctly assessed to be excessive airway secretions, the appropriate treatment plan would entail a specific treatment modality found in the **Airway Clearance Therapy Protocol**, such as deep breathing and coughing or chest physical therapy, Protocol 10.2, page 140.

Table 10.1 illustrates common clinical manifestations (i.e., clinical indicators), initial assessments, and treatment selections routinely made by the TDP-practicing respiratory therapist.

Severity Assessment

The frequency at which a respiratory therapy modality is to be administered is just as important to quality cost-efficient

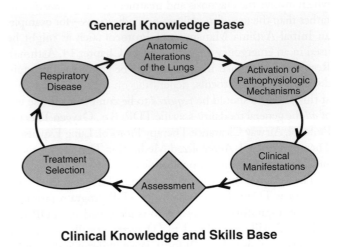

FIGURE 10.4 Overview of TDP program. The way knowledge, outcome assessment, and a therapist-driven protocol program interface between each other.

TABLE 10.1 Clinical Manifestations, Assessments, and Treatment Selections Commonly Made by the Respiratory Therapist

Clinical Data (Indicators)	Assessments	Treatment Selections
Vital Signs		
↑ Breathing rate, blood pressure, pulse	Respiratory distress and dyspnea	Treat underlying cause
Abnormal Airway Indicators		
Wheezing	Bronchospasm	Bronchodilator treatment
Inspiratory stridor	Laryngeal edema	Racemic epinephrine
Coarse crackles	Secretions in large airways	Airway clearance therapy
Fine and medium crackles	Secretions in distal airways	Treat underlying cause, such as congestive heart failure
		Hyperinflation therapy
Cough Effectiveness Indicators		
Strong cough	Good ability to mobilize secretions	None
Weak cough	Poor ability to mobilize secretions	Airway clearance therapy
Abnormal Secretion Indicators		
Amount: >25 mL/24 h	Excessive bronchial secretions	Airway clearance therapy
White and translucent sputum	Normal sputum	None
Yellow or opaque sputum	Acute airway infection	Treat underlying cause
Green sputum	Old, retained secretions and infections	Airway clearance therapy
Brown sputum	Old blood	Airway clearance therapy
Red sputum	Fresh blood	Notify physician
Frothy secretions	Pulmonary edema	Treat underlying cause, such as congestive heart failure
		Hyperinflation therapy

TABLE 10.1 Clinical Manifestations, Assessments, and Treatment Selections Commonly Made by the Respiratory Therapist—cont'd

Clinical Data (Indicators)	Assessments	Treatment Selections
Abnormal Lung Parenchyma Indicators		
Bronchial breath sounds	Atelectasis	Hyperinflation therapy, oxygen treatment
Dull percussion note	Infiltrates or effusion	Treat underlying cause
Opacity on chest radiograph	Fibrosis	No specific treatment
Restrictive pulmonary function test values	Consolidation	No specific, effective respiratory care treatment
Depressed diaphragm on radiograph	Air trapping and hyperinflation	Treat underlying cause
Abnormal Pleural Space Indicators		
Hyperresonant percussion note	Pneumothorax	Evacuate air* and hyperinflation treatment
Dull percussion note	Pleural effusion	Evacuate fluid* and hyperinflation treatment
Abnormalities of Chest Shape and Motion		
Paradoxical movement of the chest wall	Flail chest	Mechanical ventilation†
Barrel chest	Air trapping (hyperinflation)	Treat underlying cause, such as asthma
Posterior and lateral curvature of spine	Kyphoscoliosis	Airway clearance therapy
Arterial Blood Gases—Ventilatory		
pH ↑, $PaCO_2$ ↓, HCO_3^- ↓	Acute alveolar hyperventilation	Treat underlying cause
pH N, $PaCO_2$ ↓, HCO_3^- ↓↓†	Chronic alveolar hyperventilation	Generally none
pH ↓, $PaCO_2$ ↑, HCO_3^- ↑	Acute ventilatory failure	Mechanical ventilation*
pH N, $PaCO_2$ ↑, HCO_3^- ↑↑	Chronic ventilatory failure	Low-flow oxygen, bronchial hygiene
Sudden Ventilatory Changes on Chronic Ventilatory Failure (CVF)		
pH ↑, $PaCO_2$ ↑, HCO_3^- ↑↑, PaO_2 ↓	Acute alveolar hyperventilation on CVF	Treat underlying cause
pH ↓, $PaCO_2$ ↑↑, HCO_3^- ↑ PaO_2 ↓	Acute ventilatory failure on CVF	Mechanical ventilation*
Metabolic		
pH ↑, $PaCO_2$ N or ↑, HCO_3^- ↑, PaO_2 N	Metabolic alkalosis	Give potassium†— Hypokalemia
		Give chloride†—Hypochloremia
pH ↓, $PaCO_2$ N or ↓, HCO_3^- ↓, PaO_2 ↓	Metabolic acidosis	Give oxygen—Lactic acidosis
pH ↓, $PaCO_2$ N or ↓, HCO_3^- ↓, PaO_2 N	Metabolic acidosis	Give insulin*—Ketoacidosis
pH ↓, $PaCO_2$ N or ↓, HCO_3^- ↓, PaO_2 N	Metabolic acidosis	Renal therapy
Indication for Mechanical Ventilation		
pH ↑, $PaCO_2$ ↓, HCO_3^- ↓, PaO_2 ↓	Impending ventilatory failure	Mechanical ventilation
pH ↓, $PaCO_2$ ↑, HCO_3^- ↑, PaO_2 ↓	Ventilatory failure	Mechanical ventilation
pH ↓, $PaCO_2$ ↑, HCO_3^- ↑, PaO_2 ↓	Apnea	Mechanical ventilation
Oxygenation Status		
PaO_2 <80 mm Hg	Mild hypoxemia	Oxygen therapy and treat underlying cause
PaO_2 <60 mm Hg	Moderate hypoxemia	
PaO_2 <40 mm Hg	Severe hypoxemia	
Oxygen Transport Status		
↓ PaO_2, anemia, ↓ cardiac output	Inadequate oxygen transport	Oxygen therapy and treat underlying cause

*These procedures should be performed only as ordered by the physician. It should be noted that some of the treatment options are not included in respiratory protocols and may not necessarily be administered by respiratory therapists.
†Significant.

care as the current selection of the respiratory therapy modality itself. Often the frequency of treatment must be up-regulated or down-regulated on a shift-by-shift, hour-to-hour, minute-to-minute, or even (in life-threatening situations) second-to-second basis. Such frequency changes must be made in response to a **severity assessment**.

In a good TDP program, the well-seasoned respiratory therapist routinely and systematically documents many severity assessments throughout each working day. For the new practitioner, however, a predesigned *Severity Assessment Rating Form* may be used to enhance this important part of the assessment process. One excellent, semiquantitative method of accomplishing this is illustrated in Table 10.2. The clinical application of severity assessment using this scale is provided in the following case example:

Severity Assessment Case Example

A 67-year-old man arrived in the emergency department in respiratory distress. The patient was well known to the therapist-driven protocol (TDP) team; he had been diagnosed with chronic bronchitis several years before this admission (3 points). The patient had no recent surgery history, and he was ambulatory, alert, and cooperative at the time of admission (0 points). He complained of dyspnea and was using his accessory muscles of inspiration (3 points). Auscultation revealed bilateral coarse crackles over both lung fields (3 points). His cough was weak and productive of thick gray sputum (3 points). A chest radiograph revealed pneumonia (consolidation) in the left lower lobe (3 points). On room air his arterial blood gas values were pH 7.52, $PaCO_2$ 54, HCO_3^- 41, and PaO_2 52, suggesting an ABG-based diagnosis of acute alveolar hyperventilation superimposed on chronic ventilatory failure (3 points).

Using the Severity Assessment Form shown in Table 10.2, the following treatment selection and administration frequency would be appropriate:

Total score: 17 (moderate)
Treatment selection: Chest physical therapy
Frequency of administration: Four times a day; and as needed

The Essential Cornerstones of a Successful Therapist-Driven Protocol Program

Although there are many "assess and treat" respiratory care protocols (now more appropriately called **Assess, Treat, and Teach Protocols**) used throughout the health care industry today, the following respiratory protocols provide the essential foundation of a successful TDP program[3]:

- **Oxygen Therapy Protocol** (Protocol 10.1, page 138)
- **Airway Clearance Therapy Protocol** (Protocol 10.2, page 140)
- **Lung Expansion Therapy Protocol** (Protocol 10.3, page 142)

- **Aerosolized Medication Therapy Protocol** (Protocol 10.4, page 144)

The vast majority of the daily work performed by the respiratory therapist involves assessments and treatments associated with the cornerstone protocols mentioned previously.[4] Done well, they are the essential foundations of a good TDP program. For example, a patient experiencing a severe asthmatic episode would probably demonstrate a variety of objective and subjective clinical indicators to justify the assessments that call for the administration of oxygen therapy (e.g., to treat hypoxemia), an aerosolized bronchodilator (e.g., to treat bronchospasm), air clearance therapy (e.g., to mobilize the thick white secretions associated with asthma), and mechanical ventilation (e.g., to treat acute ventilatory failure).

As shown in the algorithms in Protocols 10.1 through 10.4,[5] a step-by-step, branching logic process directs the practitioner to (1) gather clinical data (clinical indicators), (2) make assessment decisions based on the clinical data, and (3) either start, up-regulate, down-regulate, or discontinue a treatment modality. In fact, the primary reasons a good TDP program works is because a specific treatment modality cannot be started, stopped, or modified unless there are specific and measurable clinical indicators identified to justify the assessment and treatment decision.[6]

The treatment selections outlined in each of the previously mentioned protocols are based on current AARC Clinical Practice Guidelines (CPGs), which provide the most recent scientific evidence that justifies the administration of a specific treatment modality. Using the evidence-based methods mandated by the scientific community, **evidence-based clinical practice guidelines** provide the indications, contraindications, hazards and complications, assessment of need, assessment of outcome, and appropriate monitoring techniques used for specific therapy modalities. *In other words, the CPGs are the gold standards used by the respiratory therapy profession to start, adjust, or discontinue a specific treatment modality.* In Box 10.1 (see page 147), excerpts from the AARC's CPG on oxygen therapy for adults in the acute care facility provide a representative example of a CPG and, more importantly, describe current thinking on the scientific basis for the Oxygen Therapy (see Protocol 10.1, page 138).

On occasion, several different treatment selections may be listed under each of the protocols. In essence, the various treatment selections serve as a "therapy selection menu." When the patient demonstrates the clinical indications associated

---

[3]The "teach" edition reflects the recognition that has been given to patient education as an important part of the hospital stay.

[4]Sample protocols for mechanical ventilation are provided in Chapter 11, Respiratory Insufficiency, Respiratory Failure and Ventilatory Management Protocols, page 169.

[5]Protocols for mechanical ventilation are provided in Chapter 11, Respiratory Insufficiency, Respiratory Failure and Ventilatory Management Protocols.

[6]The authors would like to thank the Respiratory Care Department at the Kettering Health Network, in Dayton, Ohio, for providing the use of their Oxygen Therapy Protocol, Airway Clearance Therapy Protocol, Lung Expansion Protocol, and Aerosolized Medication Therapy Protocol. The Kettering Health Network (KHN) protocols shown here serve only as examples. The modalities and medications reflect only those that KHN is currently using in their patient care. This is particularly true in the case of ventilators discussed in Chapter 11, Respiratory Insufficiency, Respiratory Failure, and Ventilatory Management Protocols, where clearly not *every* ventilator or ventilator modality is being used by the KHN.

TABLE 10.2 Respiratory Care Protocol Severity Assessment

Item	0 Points	1 Point	2 Points	3 Points	4 Points
Respiratory history	Negative for smoking or history not available	Smoking history <1 pack a day	Smoking history >1 pack a day	Pulmonary disease	Severe or exacerbation
Surgery history	No surgery	General surgery	Lower abdominal	Thoracic or upper abdominal	Thoracic with lung disease
Level of consciousness	Alert, oriented, cooperative	Disoriented, follows commands	Obtunded, uncooperative	Obtunded	Comatose
Level of activity	Ambulatory	Ambulatory with assistance	Nonambulatory	Paraplegic	Quadriplegic
Respiratory pattern	Normal rate 8–20/min	Respiratory rate 20–25/min	Patient complains of dyspnea	Dyspnea, use of accessory muscles, prolonged expiration	Severe dyspnea, use of accessory muscles, respiratory rate >25, and/or swallow
Breath sounds	Clear	Bilateral crackles	Bilateral fine, medium, or coarse crackles	Bilateral wheezing; fine, medium, or coarse crackles	Absent and/or diminished bilaterally and/or severe wheezing; fine, medium, or coarse crackles
Cough	Strong, spontaneous, nonproductive	Excessive bronchial secretions and strong cough	Excessive bronchial secretions but weak cough	Thick bronchial secretions and weak cough	Thick bronchial secretions but no cough
Chest radiograph	Clear	One lobe: Infiltrates, atelectasis, consolidation, or pleural effusion	Same lung, two lobes: Infiltrates, atelectasis, consolidation, or pleural effusion	One lobe in both lungs: Infiltrates, atelectasis, consolidation, or pleural effusion	Both lungs, more than one lobe: Infiltrates, atelectasis, consolidation, or pleural effusion
Arterial blood gases and/or oxygen saturation measured by pulse oximeter (SpO_2)	Normal	Normal pH and $PaCO_2$ but PaO_2 60–80 and/or SpO_2 91%–96%	Normal pH and $PaCO_2$ but PaO_2 40–60 and/or SpO_2 85%–90%	Acute respiratory alkalosis, PaO_2 <40 and/or SpO_2 80%–84%	Acute respiratory failure, PaO_2 <80 and/or SpO_2 <80%

Severity Index		
Total Score	**Severity Assessment**	**Treatment Frequency**
1–5	Unremarkable	As needed
6–15	Mild	Two or three times a day
16–25	Moderate	Four times a day or as needed
>26	Severe	Two to four times a day and as needed; alert attending physician

with any of these protocols, the respiratory therapist is expected to select and administer the most efficient and most cost-effective treatment listed in that protocol. As already discussed, the treatment selection decision and the frequency with which the therapy is to be administered are based on (1) the identification of the appropriate clinical indicators, (2) the severity of the abnormality suggested by the clinical information, (3) the

patient's ability to perform or tolerate the therapy, (4) the patient's response to the therapy, and (5) the local cost-effective conditions where appropriate.

In another example, the implementation of the Lung Expansion Therapy Protocol, Protocol 10.3 (see pages 142), would probably be indicated after thoracic surgery to prevent, or correct **atelectasis**. While a patient is on a mechanical

OXYGEN THERAPY PROTOCOL[1]

Box 1	Box 2	Box 3
Indications • Room air PaO_2 <60 mm Hg • Room air SaO_2 <90% • Acute hypoxia is suspected • After severe trauma • Intraoperative and postoperative state • Acute myocardial infarction (only if SaO_2 <90%) • Hypoxia suggested in sleep study or CPET • Low cardiac output state • Hemoglobin <8.0 g/dL	**Device Selection Guidelines (determined from narrative portion of protocol)** If heated humidified high-flow nasal cannula (HHHFNC) system is used, adequate flow must be provided to minimize patient WOB. Use pulse oximetry whenever FIO_2 in use is ≥0.44. High-flow systems include variable concentration nonrebreathing mask (can achieve FIO_2 ≥0.90). Nasal cannula is titrated in increments of 1.0 to 2.0 liters per minute.	**Assess Outcomes— Goals Achieved?** • At discharge, ensure patient's SpO_2 is ≥91% or back to preadmission baseline level at discharge. • Beware of signs of oxygen toxicity.

[1]The AARC has developed protocols pertinent to the topic of Oxygen Therapy. These include: Oxygen Protocol, Oxygen Protocol Addendum for Pulmonary Thromboendarterectomy (PET), Oxygen Delivery Device Protocol, Oxygen to Treat Pneumothorax Protocol, and Oximetry Protocol.

PROTOCOL 10.1 *Continued on page 139*

ventilator, positive end-expiratory pressure (PEEP) is a time-honored way of treating this condition. If the patient was still breathing but was unconscious or unable to follow directions, a continuous positive airway pressure (CPAP) mask would be a more appropriate treatment selection (under the same protocol) than, say, incentive spirometry, even though both are designed to treat or prevent atelectasis. In this example, although treatment with CPAP mask therapy would be more expensive, it would be more appropriate than the less expensive incentive spirometry, which would require that the patient be alert.

Remember, the treatment portion of a protocol is based on the therapy that will *best* work to correct or offset the anatomic alterations and pathophysiologic mechanisms caused by the respiratory disorder in a timely and cost-efficient manner. Finally, even when a patient is transferred to the intensive care unit, intubated, and placed on a mechanical ventilator, the respiratory therapist *usually* must still administer one or more of the first four respiratory therapy treatment protocols listed in this section. For example, the patient would probably need CPAP, PEEP, or other lung expansion or airway clearance therapies to offset any alveolar atelectasis caused by airway mucous plugs via the Lung Expansion Therapy Protocol. The patient might require a bronchodilator agent to offset bronchospasm via the Aerosolized Medication Therapy Protocol.

Summary of a Good Therapist-Driven Protocol Program

As illustrated in Fig. 10.5, the essential components of a good TDP program are as follows. Every respiratory care plan must be directly linked to (1) a physician's order, (2) specific clinical indicators (obtained from the patient's chart, physical examination, and laboratory and x-ray results—all identified and documented), (3) a bedside respiratory assessment and severity assessment must be performed (diagnosis), (4) a treatment selection that is both therapeutic and cost-effective, and finally, (5) the evaluation of the patient's response to the treatment must be routinely performed.

This step-by-step process mandates that the respiratory therapist (1) has a strong knowledge base of the major respiratory disorders, and (2) is competent in the actual assessment process. Fig. 10.6 provides an assessment form with common examples for each category (i.e., clinical indicators, respiratory assessments, and treatment plans). The data documented in Fig. 10.6 can be easily transferred to the subjective-objective evaluation, assessment, and treatment (SOAP) format. The SOAP format used in the assessment of respiratory diseases is discussed in more detail in Chapter 12, Recording Skills and Intraprofessional Communication.[7]

---

[7]The memorization of the protocols, algorithms, or specific medications presented in this chapter is not recommended. This is because protocols frequently change as updated CPGs become available, and local institutional practice mandates vary. However, it is important to commit to memory the *kinds* of protocols available in your institution (e.g., Oxygen Therapy Protocol) and the *types* of therapy used in them (e.g., ultra-high-flow oxygen therapy, hyperbaric oxygen therapy, etc.). The protocols in this textbook reflect the availability of modalities from the Respiratory Care Department at Kettering Health Network, and Dayton Children's Hospital, in Dayton, Ohio, which have recently been modified to reflect the most recent AARC CPGs.

OXYGEN THERAPY PROTOCOL,[1] *cont'd*

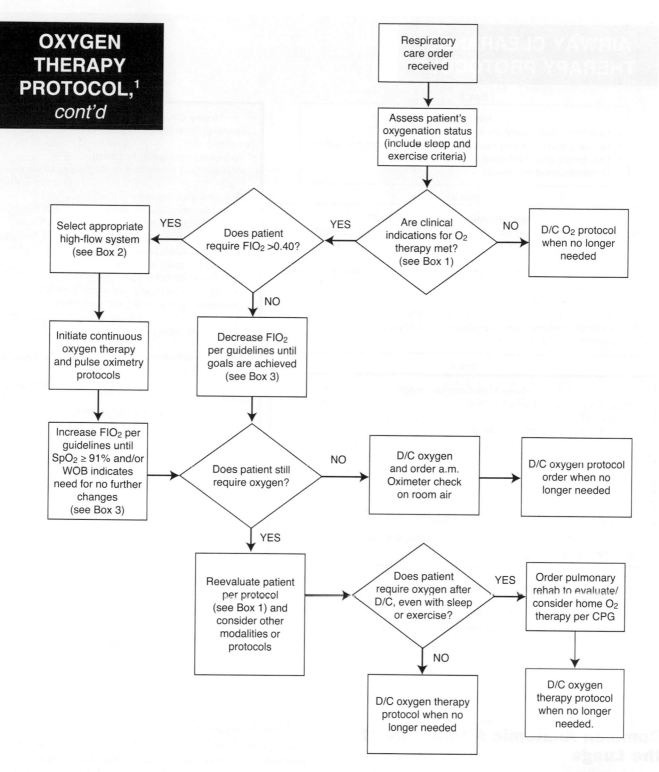

Respiratory care order received

↓

Assess patient's oxygenation status (include sleep and exercise criteria)

↓

Are clinical indications for O₂ therapy met? (see Box 1) — NO → D/C O₂ protocol when no longer needed

YES ↓

Does patient require FIO₂ >0.40? — YES → Select appropriate high-flow system (see Box 2)

↓ (YES)

Initiate continuous oxygen therapy and pulse oximetry protocols

↓

Increase FIO₂ per guidelines until SpO₂ ≥ 91% and/or WOB indicates need for no further changes (see Box 3)

Does patient require FIO₂ >0.40? — NO → Decrease FIO₂ per guidelines until goals are achieved (see Box 3)

↓

Does patient still require oxygen? — NO → D/C oxygen and order a.m. Oximeter check on room air → D/C oxygen protocol order when no longer needed

YES ↓

Reevaluate patient per protocol (see Box 1) and consider other modalities or protocols

→ **Does patient require oxygen after D/C, even with sleep or exercise?** — YES → Order pulmonary rehab to evaluate/consider home O₂ therapy per CPG → D/C oxygen therapy protocol when no longer needed.

NO ↓

D/C oxygen therapy protocol when no longer needed

PROTOCOL 10.1

AIRWAY CLEARANCE THERAPY PROTOCOL[2]

Box 1

Indications
- To restore mucociliary blanket (bland aerosol)
- To hydrate and remove retained secretions (bland aerosol/IPV)
- To improve cough effectiveness/expectoration
- To prevent/treat atelectasis

Box 3

Assess Outcomes—Goals Achieved?
- Achieve optimal hydration with reduction in sputum volume ≤5 mL/day
- Breath sounds change from diminished to adventitious with coarse crackles cleared by cough
- Decreased respiratory rate and patient's subjective impression of improved sputum clearance
- Resolution/improvement in CXR
- Improvement in vital signs, e.g., temperature, and measures of gas exchange
- If on ventilator, reduced airway resistance and improved compliance
- Improvement in bedside in PFTs

Box 4

Care Plan Considerations
- Discontinue therapy if improvement is observed and sustained over a 24-hour period.
- Patients with chronic pulmonary disease, including cystic fibrosis, bronchiectasis, chronic neuromuscular disorders and selected COPD patients with excessive secretions/secretion control, who continue to have problems should continue on therapy at home at a frequency no less than effective in the hospital.
- Lung Expansion Therapy Protocol should be considered for patients considered at high risk for development of pulmonary complications. (See indications in Protocol 10.3.)
- Many of the Protocols listed in Box 2 are available for home use in simplified and patient acceptable form.

Box 2

Airway Clearance Therapy Selections
Objective: To enhance mobilization of bronchial secretions
- To increase bronchial hydration
  Increase fluid intake to 6 to 10 glasses of water a day
  Bland aerosol therapy
  Ultrasonic nebulization (USN) (Note: USN has become obsolete because they are no longer manufactured and seldom, if ever, used today.)
  Cough and deep breathing (C & DB)
- Techniques used to enhance:
  Incentive spirometry (IS)
  Oscillatory positive expiratory pressure (OPEP)
  Intermittent percussive ventilation (IPV)
  Positive expiratory pressure (PEP) Therapy Flutter Valve (Acapella)
- Vibrating mesh therapy
- Chest physical therapy (CPT)
- Postural drainage (PD)
- Percussion, vibration, and postural drainage and percussion (PD & P)
- Suctioning (*NOTE:* In some hospitals, suctioning cannot be performed without TDPs or direct physician order.)
- Mucolytic therapy (see Protocol 10.4)
- Assist physician in bronchoscopy

[2]The AARC has developed protocols that are pertinent to the topic of Airway Clearance Therapy. These include Secretion Clearance Protocol, Secretion Clearance Device Selection Protocol, Cough Assist Protocol, and Airway Management Protocol for Artificial Airways. Other KHN Protocols cross-referenced here include Suctioning Protocol (not shown) and Aerosolized Medication Protocol (see Protocol 10.4).

PROTOCOL 10.2 *Continued on page 141*

Common Anatomic Alterations of the Lungs

Although the respiratory therapist may at some time treat one or two cases of every respiratory disorder presented in this textbook, most of the therapist's professional career will be caring for patients with only a few of them. For example, the *diagnosis–related group* (DRG) system, which uses the most current edition of the *International Statistical Classification of Diseases and Related Health Problems* (ICD-10) identification listings, shows the following short list of respiratory disorders: *chronic bronchitis, emphysema, asthma, pneumonia, atelectasis, acute respiratory distress syndrome (ARDS), interstitial fibrosis, pulmonary edema/congestive heart failure, and acute and chronic respiratory failure with and without ventilatory support.*

From this relatively short list of respiratory disorders identified through the DRG system, an even shorter list of the most common anatomic alterations of the lungs treated by the respiratory therapist can be derived. This list includes (1) atelectasis (e.g., which can occur from mucous plugging, upper abdominal surgery, pleural effusion, or pneumothorax), (2) alveolar consolidation (e.g., pneumonia), (3) increased alveolar-capillary membrane thickness (e.g., ARDS, pneumoconiosis, or pulmonary edema), (4) bronchospasm (e.g., asthma or bronchitis), (5) excessive bronchial secretions (e.g., chronic bronchitis, asthma, pulmonary edema, and bronchiectasis), and (6) **distal airway and alveolar weakening** (e.g., emphysema). Each of these anatomic alterations of the lung leads to a chain of events that can be summarized in the following clinical scenarios based on their most prominent pathophysiology.

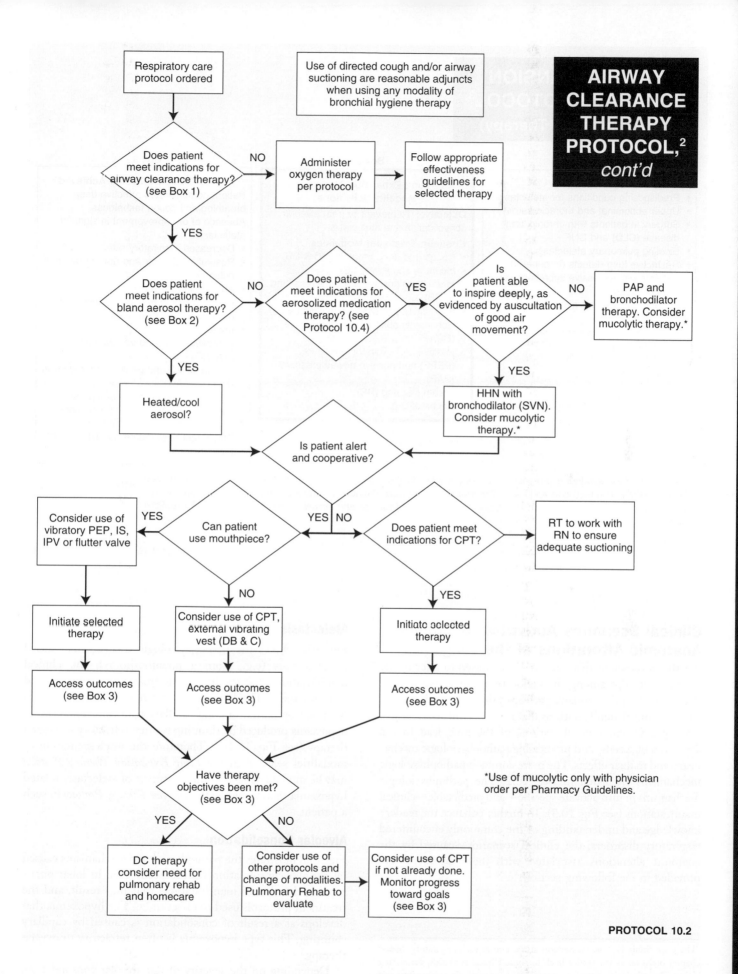

AIRWAY CLEARANCE THERAPY PROTOCOL,[2] cont'd

Respiratory care protocol ordered

Use of directed cough and/or airway suctioning are reasonable adjuncts when using any modality of bronchial hygiene therapy

Does patient meet indications for airway clearance therapy? (see Box 1) — NO → Administer oxygen therapy per protocol → Follow appropriate effectiveness guidelines for selected therapy

YES

Does patient meet indications for bland aerosol therapy? (see Box 2) — NO → Does patient meet indications for aerosolized medication therapy? (see Protocol 10.4) — YES → Is patient able to inspire deeply, as evidenced by auscultation of good air movement? — NO → PAP and bronchodilator therapy. Consider mucolytic therapy.*

YES

Heated/cool aerosol?

YES → HHN with bronchodilator (SVN). Consider mucolytic therapy.*

Is patient alert and cooperative?

Consider use of vibratory PEP, IS, IPV or flutter valve ← YES — Can patient use mouthpiece? — YES | NO → Does patient meet indications for CPT? → RT to work with RN to ensure adequate suctioning

NO

Initiate selected therapy

Consider use of CPT, external vibrating vest (DB & C)

YES

Initiate selected therapy

Access outcomes (see Box 3)

Access outcomes (see Box 3)

Access outcomes (see Box 3)

Have therapy objectives been met? (see Box 3)

YES

NO

DC therapy consider need for pulmonary rehab and homecare

Consider use of other protocols and change of modalities. Pulmonary Rehab to evaluate

Consider use of CPT if not already done. Monitor progress toward goals (see Box 3)

*Use of mucolytic only with physician order per Pharmacy Guidelines.

PROTOCOL 10.2

LUNG EXPANSION THERAPY PROTOCOL[3]
(Hyperinflation Therapy)

Box 1	Box 2	Box 3
Indications	**Lung Expansion Therapy Modality Selections**	**Assess Outcomes/Goals Achieved?**

Box 1

Indications

- Predisposing conditions for atelectasis
- Upper abdominal and thoracic surgery
- Surgery in patients with chronic lung disease (CLD) and CHF
- Existing pulmonary atelectasis
- Restrictive lung defects (in general)
- Patients with excessive secretions (see Protocol 10.2)
- Patients with chronic neuromuscular conditions

Box 2

Lung Expansion Therapy Modality Selections

Objective: To prevent or treat alveolar consolidation and atelectasis

Common Treatment Modalities

- Cough and deep breathing (C & DB)
- Incentive spirometry (IS)
- Intermittent positive pressure breathing (IPPB)
- Intermittent percussive ventilation (IPV)
- Continuous positive airway pressure (CPAP)
- Positive and expiratory pressure (PEEP) and positive airway pressure (PAP)
- Breath stacking (BS)
- Sip breathing

Box 3

Assess Outcomes/Goals Achieved?

Patient demonstrates affective deep breathing and cough techniques.
Absence of or improvement in signs of atelectasis:

- Decreased respiratory rate
- Resolution of fever and normalization of pulse rate
- Absent coarse crackles
- Improvement in previously absent or diminished breath sounds
- Improved CXR
- Improved PaO_2 and decreased $P(A-a)O_2$
- Increased VC and peak expiratory flows (PF)
- Return of FRC or VC to preoperative values in absence of lung resection

Improved inspiratory muscle function:

- Attainment of preadmission NIF and IC
- Increased FVC

[3]The AARC has developed protocols that are pertinent to the topic of Lung Expansion Therapy. These include Secretion Clearance Protocols Atelectasis Prophylaxis, Prophylactic Protocol Addendum for Post-Operative Laparotomy, Chest Trauma, and Rib Fracture, IPPB Protocol, Cough Assist Protocol, and Airway Management Protocol for Artificial Airways.

PROTOCOL 10.3 *Continued on page 143*

Clinical Scenarios Activated by Common Anatomic Alterations of the Lungs

For the purposes of this text, we have chosen to refer to the interrelationships among the major **anatomic alterations of the lung**, the predominant **pathophysiologic mechanisms**, and the **clinical manifestations** that result as **clinical scenarios**. The specific anatomic alterations of the lung lead to the activation of specific and predictable pathophysiologic mechanisms and to their effects. The more common pathophysiologic mechanisms are listed in Box 10.2. The pathophysiologic mechanisms in turn activate specific—and predictable—clinical manifestations (see Fig. 10.3). To further enhance the reader's knowledge and understanding of the commonly encountered respiratory disorders, the clinical scenarios—caused by the anatomic alterations associated with these disorders—are provided in the following section.[8]

---

[8]The Case Study Discussion Section at the end of each respiratory disease chapter often refers the reader back to these clinical scenarios, correlating various clinical manifestations to specific pathophysiologic mechanisms and alterations of the lungs.

Atelectasis

Fig. 10.7 shows the pathophysiologic mechanisms caused by atelectasis (e.g., from a pneumothorax), the clinical manifestations that result, and the treatment protocols used to offset them. The hypoxemia that results from atelectasis is caused by partial or total capillary shunting. The type of hypoxemia produced by shunting is often refractory to oxygen therapy (see Fig. 11.1C). Therefore the implementation of modalities selected in the *Lung Expansion Therapy Protocol* may be more beneficial in the treatment of atelectasis-related hypoxemia than would be the *Oxygen Therapy Protocol* in such a patient.

Alveolar Consolidation

Fig. 10.8 illustrates the pathophysiologic mechanisms caused by alveolar consolidation (as classically seen in lobar pneumonia), the clinical manifestations that may result, and the treatment protocols used to offset them. The hypoxemia that develops as a result of consolidation is caused by capillary shunting. This type hypoxemia is often refractory to oxygen therapy.

Depending on the severity of the alveolar consolidation, the *Lung Expansion Therapy Protocol* or the *Oxygen Therapy*

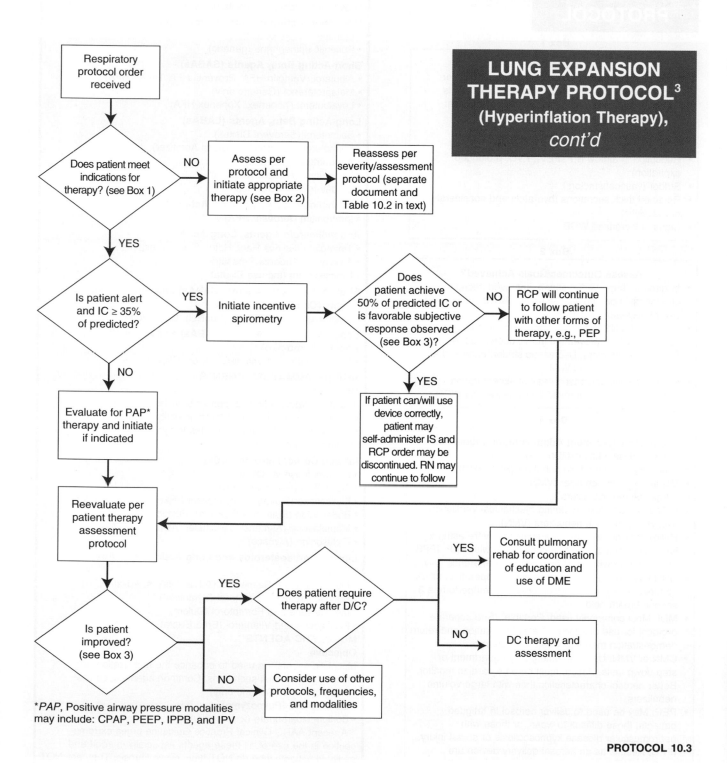

LUNG EXPANSION THERAPY PROTOCOL[3]
(Hyperinflation Therapy),
cont'd

Respiratory protocol order received

Does patient meet indications for therapy? (see Box 1) — NO → Assess per protocol and initiate appropriate therapy (see Box 2) → Reassess per severity/assessment protocol (separate document and Table 10.2 in text)

YES

Is patient alert and IC ≥ 35% of predicted? — YES → Initiate incentive spirometry → Does patient achieve 50% of predicted IC or is favorable subjective response observed (see Box 3)? — NO → RCP will continue to follow patient with other forms of therapy, e.g., PEP

NO

Evaluate for PAP* therapy and initiate if indicated

YES

If patient can/will use device correctly, patient may self-administer IS and RCP order may be discontinued. RN may continue to follow

Reevaluate per patient therapy assessment protocol

Is patient improved? (see Box 3) — YES → Does patient require therapy after D/C? — YES → Consult pulmonary rehab for coordination of education and use of DME

NO → DC therapy and assessment

NO → Consider use of other protocols, frequencies, and modalities

*PAP, Positive airway pressure modalities may include: CPAP, PEEP, IPPB, and IPV

PROTOCOL 10.3

AEROSOLIZED MEDICATION THERAPY PROTOCOL

Box 1

Indications

The primary indication for aerosolized bronchodilator therapy is reversible reactive airway disease. This is detected through the following signs and symptoms:

- C/O dyspnea
- Wheezing
- Pulmonary hyperinflation
- Reduction in airflow (PF, FEV_1, FVC, prolonged expiration)
- Stridor (vasoconstrictors)
- Retained thick secretions (hydration and consideration of mucolytic)
- Signs of increased WOB

Box 2

Assess Outcomes/Goals Achieved?

- In general: Improved dyspnea, improved secretion clearance, improved vital signs and ABGs, decreased use of accessory muscles
- For bronchodilators: ≥15% improvement in baseline FEV_1 or FVC, improvement in PF, decreased WOB
- For vasoconstrictors: Decreased stridor, improved air movement, decreased WOB
- For mucolytics: Increased ease of expectoration, decreased ronchi, improved CXR, decreased WOB

Box 4

Common Treatment Administration Modalities

- Metered dose inhaler (MDI) with spacer
- Small-volume hand-held nebulizer (SVN/HHN)
- Vibrating mesh nebulizer (VMN)
- Large-volume nebulizers
- In-line aerosol delivery during mechanical ventilation with vibrating mesh nebulizers (VMN)
- Heliox may be used as an adjunct in severe asthma.
- Nebulizers may be used in conjunction with PEP, IPPB, and IPV. Use with IPPB by physician preference only.
- HHN used in patients who are alert, cooperative, follow commands, are able to deep breathe, and perform a 3 second breath hold
- MDI: Most commonly used. Portable. (See separate protocol for use of spacer.) Patient education and return demonstration mandatory before discharge.
- CMN or VMN: Useful in emergency department or step-down units. Patient must be on a cardiac monitor. Better aerosol characteristics than with large volume nebulizers.
- PEP: May be used to deliver aerosol in fatigued patients, those difficult to wean, or those with neuromuscular disease kyphoscoliosis or spinal injury.
- IPPB: Results as an aerosol delivery device are controversial.
- IPV: Can be used in conjunction with airway clearance therapy.

MDI, SVN, LVN, or VMN are considered devices of choice for COPD and stable asthma patients.

Box 3

AEROSOLIZED MEDICATION THERAPY SELECTIONS*

BRONCHODILATOR AGENTS

Objective

Bronchodilator agents are used to offset bronchial smooth muscle constriction. Common agents used are:

Ultra-Short-Acting Bronchodilator Agents
- Epinephrine (Adrenalin)
- Racemic epinephrine (generic)

Short-Acting Beta₂ Agents (SABAs)
- Albuterol (Ventolin HFA, Proventil HFA, ProAir HFA)
- Metaproterenol (Generic only)
- Levalbuterol (Xopenex, Xopenex HFA)

Long-Acting Beta₂ Agents (LABAs)
- Salmeterol (Serevent Diskus)
- Formoterol (Perforomist, Foradil Aerolizer)
- Arformoterol (Brovana)
- Indacaterol (Arcapta Neohaler)
- Olodaterol (Striverdi Respimat)

Anticholinergic Agents Short Acting
- Ipratropium (Atrovent HFA)

Anticholinergic Agents, Long Acting
- Tiotropium (Spiriva HandiHaler, Spiriva Respimat)
- Aclidinium (Tudorza Pressair)
- Umeclidinium (Incruse Ellipta)

Short-Acting Beta₂ Agents (SABAs) and Anticholinergic Agents (Combined)
- Ipratropium and Albuterol (DuoNeb, Combivent)

Long-Acting Beta₂ Agents (LABAs) and Anticholinergic Agents (Combined)
- Umeclidinium and Vilanterol (Anoro Ellipta)

ANTIINFLAMMATORY AGENTS

Objective

Antiinflammatory agents suppress bronchial inflammation and edema. They also are used for their ability to enhance the responsiveness of B₂ receptor sites to sympathomimetic agents. Common agents used are:

Inhaled Corticosteroids (ICSs)
- Beclomethasone (QVAR)
- Flunisolide (Aerospan HFA)
- Fluticasone (Flovent HFA, Flovent Diskus, Arnuity Ellipta)
- Budesonide (Pulmicort Flexhaler, Pulmicort Respules)
- Mometasone (Asmanex Twisthaler, Asmanex HFA)
- Ciclesonide (Alvesco)

Inhaled Corticosteroids and Long-Acting Beta₂ Agents (Combined)
- Fluticasone and Salmeterol (Advair Diskus, Advair HFA)
- Budesonide and Formoterol (Symbicort)
- Mometasone and Formoterol (Dulera)
- Fluticasone and Vilanterol (Breo Ellipta)

MUCOLYTIC AGENTS**

Objective

Mucolytic agents are used to enhance the mobilization and thinning of bronchial secretions. Common agents used are:
- Acetylcysteine (Generic only)
- Dornase alfa (Pulmozyme)
- Sodium bicarbonate (2% solution)

**A recent AARC Clinical Practice Guideline urges extreme caution in the use of all these agents especially in adult and pediatric patients who do NOT have cystic fibrosis. They are NOT recommended to improve clearance in patients with neuromuscular disease or in the treatment of atelectasis.

*For the complete listing, doses, and administration of agents approved by the FDA, visit the Drugs@FDA website (www.accessdata.fda.gov/scripts/cder/drugsatfda/).

PROTOCOL 10.4 *Continued on page 145*

Therapeutic Dosage Selection*

The therapeutic dosage is the amount of agent required to provide improvement (see Box 2). Guidelines are as follows:

- Patient responds to first treatment: Continue q4h + q2h PRN with 5 mg albuterol in 2.5 mL NS. May substitute 0.5 mg ipratropium for patients with COPD or previous history of successful ipratropium use.
- Patient responds to second treatment: Continue q4h + q2h PRN with 10 mg albuterol in 2.5 mL NS. May substitute 0.5 mg ipratropium for patients with COPD or previous history of successful ipratropium use.
- Patient responds to third treatment: Continue q4h + q2h PRN with 15 mg albuterol in 2.5 mL NS. May substitute 0.5 mg ipratropium for patients with COPD or previous history of successful ipratropium use.
- PRN treatments are appropriate when moderate to severe symptoms reoccur within the 2-hour period. The physician and/or RN should be notified if the patient continues to require PRN dosing.
- Nonresponse may indicate that the patient is bronchodilator-resistant. Alternative diagnoses such as pulmonary fibrosis, cystic fibrosis, bronchiectasis, and end-stage COPD.

*Modified from UC San Diego Respiratory Care Department and AARC Clinical Practice Guidelines.

Hazards/Complications of Therapy

- Hypoventilation or hyperventilation: During therapy
- Cardiac arrhythmias or tachycardia
- Worsening hypoxemia
- Acute hypertension
- Muscular tremors
- Pneumothorax from hyperinflation
- Transmission of infection because of poor device cleaning
- Inappropriate patient technique including abuse
- Complications of specific pharmacologic agents
- Repeated exposure to aerosols has been reported to produce asthmatic symptoms in caregivers.

PROTOCOL 10.4 *Continued on page 146*

Protocol may be beneficial. In general, however, there is no effective, *specific* respiratory care treatment modality for alveolar consolidation. With pneumonia, the great temptation for the respiratory therapist is to do too much, such as instituting lung expansion therapy, bronchodilator therapy, and airway clearance therapy. Such treatment protocols generally are not indicated, especially during the early consolidation stages of the disease process. Appropriate antibiotics (prescribed by the physician), bed rest, fluids, and supplementary oxygen are all that are usually needed. When pneumonia is in its resolution stage, however, the patient may experience excessive secretions and atelectasis, accompanied by bronchoconstriction. At this time, other treatment modalities may be indicated.

Increased Alveolar-Capillary Membrane Thickness

Fig. 10.9 illustrates the major pathophysiologic mechanisms caused by **increased alveolar-capillary membrane thickness** (as seen in postoperative ARDS, pulmonary edema, asbestosis, and chronic interstitial lung disease), the clinical manifestations that develop, and the treatment protocols used to offset them. The hypoxemia that develops as a result of an increased alveolar-capillary membrane thickness is caused by an alveolar-capillary diffusion block. This type of hypoxemia often responds

favorably to the *Oxygen Therapy Protocol* and the *Lung Expansion Protocol*.

Bronchospasm

Fig. 10.10 shows the major pathophysiologic mechanisms activated by **bronchospasm** (as seen in asthma), the clinical manifestations that result, and the appropriate treatment protocols used to offset them. The *Aerosolized Medication Therapy Protocol* (bronchodilator therapy) is the primary treatment modality used to offset the anatomic alterations of bronchospasm (the original cause of the pathophysiologic chain of events). The *Oxygen Therapy Protocol* and *Mechanical Ventilation Protocol*[9] are secondary treatment modalities used to offset the mild, moderate, or severe clinical manifestations associated with bronchospasm.

Excessive Bronchial Secretions

Fig. 10.11 illustrates the major pathophysiologic mechanisms caused by **excessive bronchial secretions** (e.g., as seen in chronic bronchitis, cystic fibrosis, and asthma), the clinical manifestations that result, and the appropriate treatment protocols used to correct them. The *Airway Clearance Therapy Protocol* is the

[9]The mechanical ventilation protocols are presented in Chapter 11, Respiratory Insufficiency, Respiratory Failure, and Ventilatory Management Protocols.

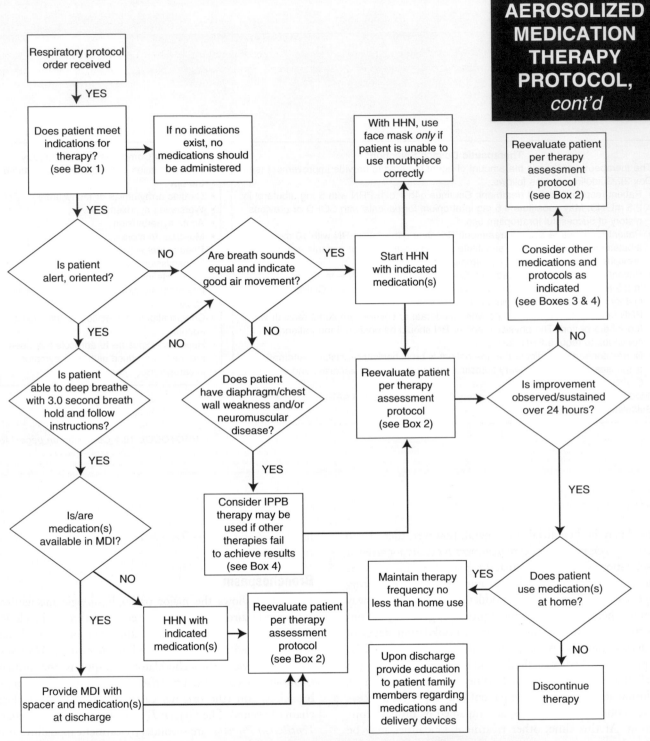

The AARC has developed protocols that are pertinent to the topic of Aerosolized Medication Therapy: IPPB Protocol, Secretion Clearance Protocol, Metered Dose Inhaler (MDI) Protocol, Small Volume Nebulizer (SVN) Protocol, Therapeutic Effective Dosage Protocol, DNA-ase Protocol, Inhaled Antibiotics Protocol, MDI Protocol for Ventilated Patients, and several protocols for infants and pediatric patients (see Part XIII).

Also see Strickland, S. L., et al. (2015). AARC clinical practice guideline: Effectiveness of pharmacologic airway clearance therapies in hospitalized patients. *Respiratory Care 60*, 7, 1071-1077.

NOTE: Standard algorithmic protocol format is such that boxes = start, mandated action and/or end points and diamonds = a yes or no decision is required.

PROTOCOL 10.4

BOX 10.1 American Association for Respiratory Care Clinical Practice Guideline for Oxygen Therapy in the Acute Care Facility (Excerpts)*

Indications

- Documented hypoxemia. Defined as a decreased PaO_2 in the blood below normal range.
- PaO_2 <60 mm Hg or SaO_2 <90% in persons breathing room air.
- Acute care situations in which hypoxemia is suspected.
- Severe trauma.
- Acute myocardial infarction.
- Short-term therapy or surgical intervention (e.g., postanesthesia recovery, hip surgery).

Contraindications

- No specific contraindications to oxygen therapy exist when indications are present.

Precautions and/or Possible Complications

- PaO_2 >60 mm Hg may depress ventilation in some patients with elevated $PaCO_2$.
- FIO_2 >0.50, may cause absorption atelectasis, oxygen toxicity, and/or ciliary or leukocyte depression.
- Supplemental oxygen should be administered with caution to patients with paraquat poisoning or to those receiving bleomycin.
- During laser bronchoscopy, minimal FIO_2 should be used to avoid intratracheal ignition.
- Fire hazard is increased in the presence of increased oxygen concentration.
- Bacterial contamination associated with nebulizers or humidifiers is a possible hazard.

Assessment of Need

- Need is determined by measurement of inadequate oxygen tension and/or saturation, by invasive or noninvasive methods, and/or by the presence of clinical indicators.

Assessment of Outcome

- Outcome is determined by clinical and physiologic assessment to establish adequacy of patient response to therapy.

Monitoring
Patient

- Clinical assessment, including cardiac, pulmonary, and neurologic status.
- Assessment of physiologic parameters (PaO_2, SaO_2, SpO_2) in conjunction with the initiation of therapy or:
  - Within 12 hours of initiation with FIO_2 <0.40
  - Within 8 hours with FIO_2 ≥0.40 (including postanesthesia recovery)
  - Within 72 hours in acute myocardial infarction
  - Within 2 hours for any patient with principal diagnosis of chronic obstructive pulmonary disease

Equipment

- All oxygen delivery systems should be checked at least once per day.
- More frequent checks are needed in systems:
  - Susceptible to variation in oxygen concentration (e.g., hood, high-flow blending systems)
  - Applied to patients with artificial airways
  - Delivering a heated gas mixture
  - Applied to patients who are clinically unstable or who require FIO_2 >0.50
- Care should be taken to avoid interruption of oxygen therapy in situations including ambulation or transport for procedure.

From Kalstrom, T. J.; American Association for Respiratory Care (AARC). (2002). AARC clinical practice guideline: Oxygen therapy for adults in the acute care facility—2002 revision and update. *Respiratory Care 47*, 6, 717-720. See this article for the complete guidelines.

*See http://www.aarc.org/ (Clinical Practice Guidelines) for the most recent and complete list of clinical practice guidelines.

BOX 10.2 Pathophysiologic Mechanisms Commonly Activated in Respiratory Disorders

- Decreased ventilation-perfusion ($\dot{V}/\dot{Q}$) ratio
- Alveolar diffusion block
- Decreased lung compliance
- Stimulation of oxygen receptors
- Deflation reflex
- Irritant reflex
- Pulmonary reflex
- Increased airway resistance
- Air trapping and alveolar hyperinflation

primary treatment modality used to offset the anatomic alterations associated with excessive bronchial secretions.

Distal Airway and Alveolar Weakening

Fig. 10.12 illustrates the major pathophysiologic mechanisms caused by distal airway and alveolar weakening (e.g., pulmonary emphysema), the clinical manifestations that result, and the appropriate treatment protocols used to offset them. Pulmonary rehabilitation and oxygen therapy may be all the practitioner can provide to treat the symptoms associated with distal airway and alveolar weakening.

Text continued on p. 152

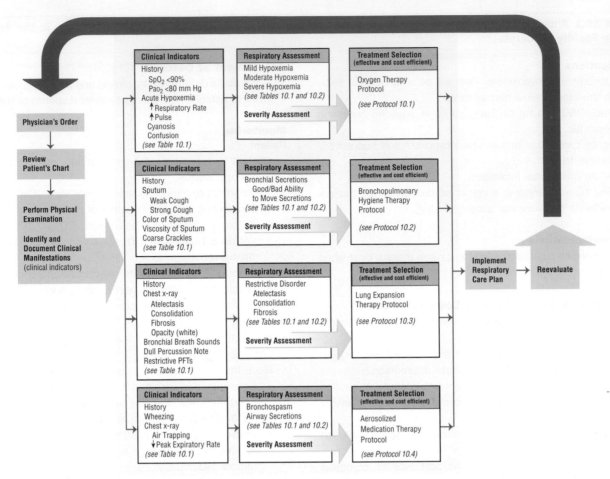

FIGURE 10.5 Overview of the essential components of a good therapist-driven protocol program.

| Patient Identification Box | Date:_____ | Admitting Diagnosis:_____ |
| | Time:_____ | Attending Physician:_____ |

Clinical Indicators
(see Table 10.1)

Oxygen Therapy	Bronchopulmonary Hygiene Therapy	Lung Expansion Therapy	Aerosolized Medication
Examples:	Examples:	Examples:	Examples:
☐ History	☐ History	☐ History	☐ History
☐ SpO₂ <90%	☐ Sputum	☐ Chest x-ray	☐ Wheezing
☐ Pao₂ <80 mm Hg	☐ Weak cough	☐ Atelectasis	☐ Chest x-ray
☐ Acute hypoxemia	☐ Color of sputum	☐ Consolidation	☐ Air trapping
☐ ≠ Respiratory rate	☐ Viscosity of sputum	☐ Fibrosis	☐ Obstructive PFT values
☐ ≠ Pulse	☐ Coarse crackles	☐ Opacity (white)	
☐ Cyanosis		☐ Bronchial breath sounds	
☐ Confusion		☐ Restrictive PFT values	
☐ Other			

Respiratory Assessments
(see Tables 10.1 and 10.2)

Oxygen Therapy	Bronchopulmonary Hygiene Therapy	Lung Expansion Therapy	Aerosolized Medication
Examples:	Examples:	Examples:	Examples:
☐ Mild hypoxemia	☐ Excessive sputum production	☐ Atelectasis	☐ Bronchospasm
☐ Moderate hypoxemia	☐ Thick secretions	☐ Consolidation	☐ Thick secretions
☐ Severe hypoxemia	☐ Weak cough	☐ Weak diaphragm	☐ Bronchial edema
Severity Score:_____	Severity Score:_____	Severity Score:_____	Severity Score:_____

Treatment Plans

Oxygen Therapy (see Protocol 10.1)	Bronchopulmonary Hygiene Therapy (see Protocol 10.2)	Lung Expansion Therapy (see Protocol 10.3)	Aerosolized Medication (see Protocol 10.4)
Examples:	Examples:	Examples:	Examples:
☐ Nasal cannula	☐ Deep breath and cough	☐ Incentive spirometry	☐ SABA
☐ Oxygen mask	☐ Chest physical therapy	☐ CPAP	☐ LABA
☐ 28% Venturi mask	☐ Postural drainage	☐ PEEP	☐ Corticosteroids
Frequency:_____	Frequency:_____	Frequency:_____	Frequency:_____

| Reevaluation Date:_____ | Therapist Signature:_____ |

FIGURE 10.6 Therapist-driven protocol program assessment form.

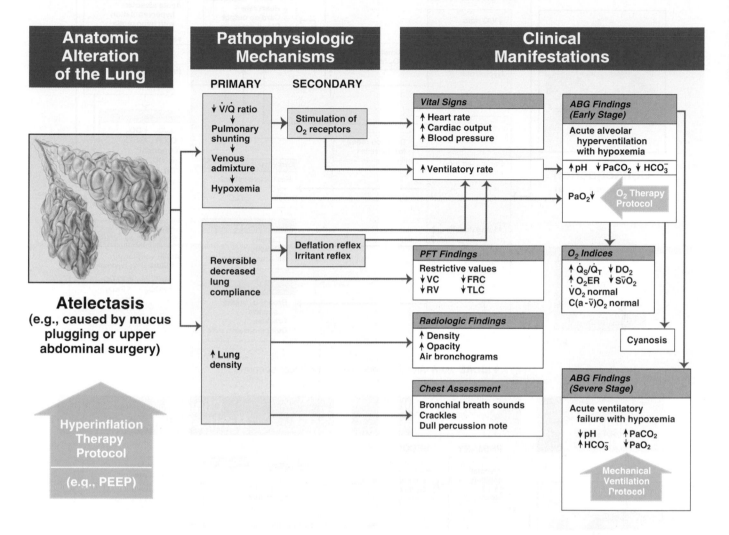

FIGURE 10.7 Atelectasis clinical scenario.

Key to Abbreviations in Figures 10.7 through 10.12

ABG	= Arterial blood gas	MVV	= Maximum voluntary ventilation
ARDS	= Acute respiratory distress syndrome	O_2ER	= Oxygen extraction ratio
CPAP	= Continuous positive airway pressure	PD	= Postural drainage
CPT	= Chest physical therapy	PEEP	= Positive end-expiratory pressure
DO_2	= Total oxygen delivery	PEFR	= Peak expiratory flow rate
ERV	= Expiratory reserve volume	PFT	= Pulmonary function test
FEF	= Forced expiratory flow, midexpiratory phase	$\dot{Q}_S/\dot{Q}_T$	= Shunt fraction
FEV_1	= Forced expiratory volume in 1 second	RV	= Residual volume
FEV_T	= Forced expiratory volume timed	$S\bar{v}O_2$	= Mixed venous oxygen saturation
FRC	= Functional residual capacity	TLC	= Total lung capacity
FVC	= Forced vital capacity	VC	= Vital capacity
IC	= Inspiratory capacity	$\dot{V}/\dot{Q}$	= Ventilation-perfusion ratio

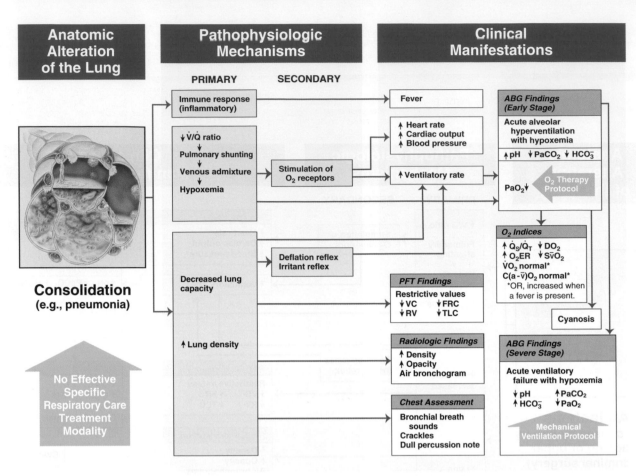

FIGURE 10.8 Alveolar consolidation clinical scenario.

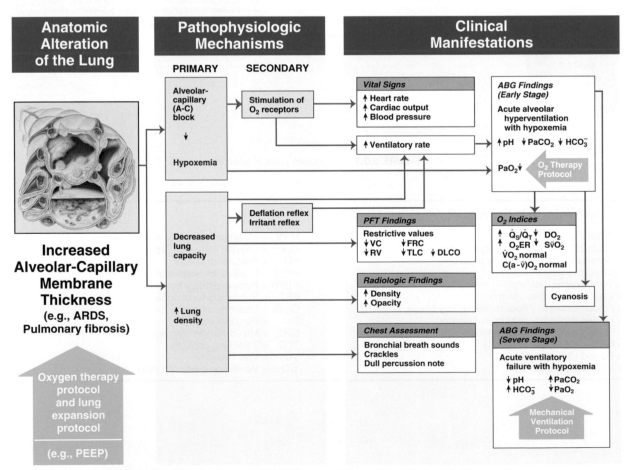

FIGURE 10.9 Increased alveolar-capillary membrane thickness clinical scenario.

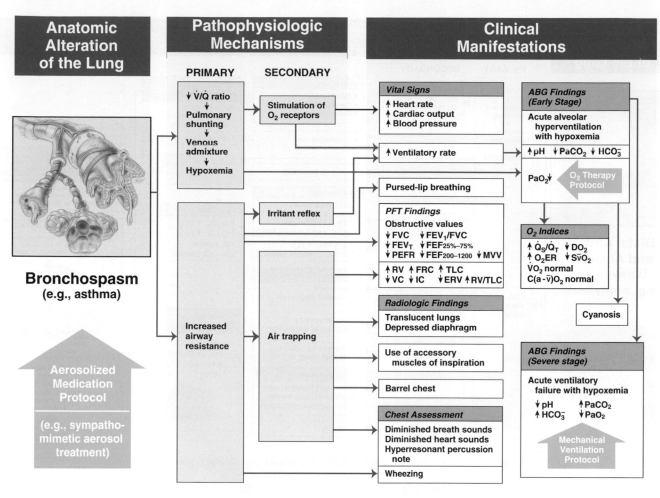

FIGURE 10.10 Bronchospasm clinical scenario.

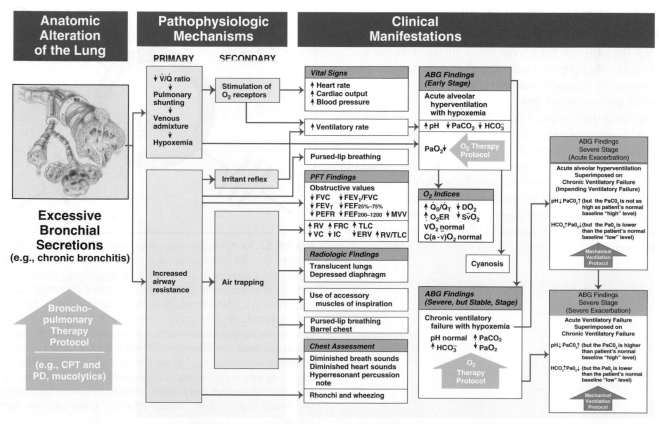

FIGURE 10.11 Excessive bronchial secretions clinical scenario.

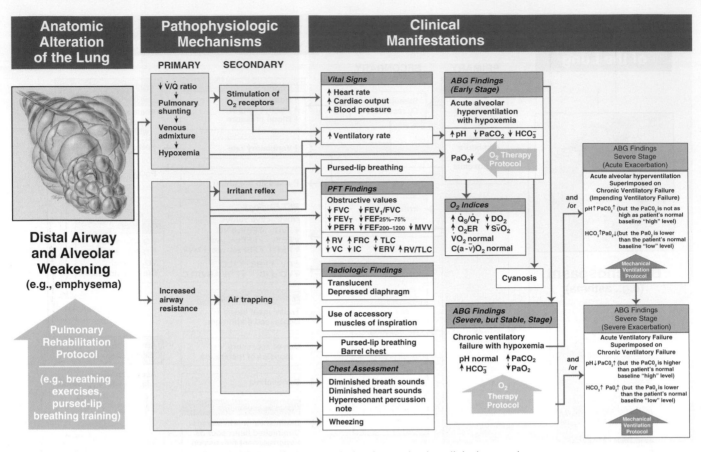

FIGURE 10.12 Distal airway and alveolar weakening clinical scenario.

Overview of Common Anatomic Alterations Associated With Respiratory Disorders

When the safe and ready respiratory therapist knows and understands the chain of events (clinical scenarios) that develop in response to common anatomic alterations of the lungs, an accurate assessment and appropriate treatment protocol design can be easily determined. Table 10.3 provides an overview of the most common anatomic alterations associated with the respiratory disorders presented in this textbook.

Fig. 10.13 provides a three-component overview model of a prototype airway to further enhance the reader's visualization of anatomic alterations of the lungs commonly associated with obstructive respiratory disorders (e.g., asthma, bronchitis, or emphysema) and the treatment plans commonly used to offset them.

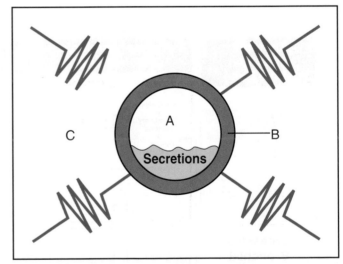

FIGURE 10.13 A three-component model of a prototype airway. Therapy may be directed at any or all components. (A) Airway lumen. (B) Airway wall. (C) Supporting structures. Therapy for A includes deep breathing and coughing, smoking cessation, suctioning, mucolytics, bland aerosols, systemic and parenteral hydration, and therapeutic bronchoscopy. Therapy for B includes bronchodilators, aerosolized antiinflammatory agents, aerosolized antibiotics, and aerosolized decongestants. Therapy for C includes pursed-lip breathing exercises (e.g., when the elastic recoil of the lungs is absent in emphysema—as represented by the broken spring in the upper left corner) and removal of external factors compressing the airway (e.g., bullae, pleural effusion, pneumothorax, tumor masses).

TABLE 10.3 Common Anatomic Alterations of the Lungs Associated With Respiratory Disorders

Respiratory Disorder	Atelectasis	Alveolar Consolidation	Increased Alveolar-Capillary Membrane Thickness	Bronchospasm	Excessive Bronchial Secretions	Distal Airway Weakening
Chronic bronchitis				X*	X	
Emphysema				X	X*	X
Asthma				X	X	
Cystic fibrosis	X*			X*	X	
Bronchiectasis	X	X		X	X	
Atelectasis	X					
Pneumonia		X			X*	
Tuberculosis		X	X			
Pulmonary edema	X		X		X	
Pulmonary embolism	X			X		
Flail chest	X	X				
Pneumothorax	X					
Pleural diseases	X					
Kyphoscoliosis	X				X*	
Cancer of the lung	X	X			X	
Interstitial lung diseases			X	X*		
Acute respiratory distress syndrome	X*	X	X			
Guillain-Barré syndrome	X*	X*			X*	
Myasthenia gravis	X*	X*			X*	
Meconium aspiration syndrome	X	X			X	
Transient tachypnea of newborn			X		X	
Respiratory distress syndrome	X	X			X	
Pulmonary air leak syndromes	X					
Respiratory syncytial virus	X	X			X	
Bronchopulmonary dysplasia	X		X		X	
Congenital diaphragmatic hernia	X					
Near drowning	X	X	X	X	X	
Smoke inhalation and thermal injuries	X	X	X	X	X	

*Common secondary anatomic alterations of the lungs associated with this disorder.

SELF-ASSESSMENT QUESTIONS

1. Which of the following pathophysiologic mechanisms is/are associated with the "atelectasis" clinical scenario?
   1. Air trapping
   2. Decreased ventilation-perfusion ratio
   3. Deflation reflex
   4. Irritant reflex
      a. 1 and 4 only
      b. 2 and 3 only
      c. 1 and 4 only
      d. 2, 3, and 4 only

2. Which of the following clinical manifestations is/are associated with the "excessive bronchial secretions" clinical scenario?
   1. Translucent radiographs
   2. Increased forced vital capacity
   3. Pursed-lip breathing
   4. Air bronchograms
      a. 1 and 4 only
      b. 1 and 3 only
      c. 2, 3, and 4 only
      d. 1, 2, 3, and 4

3. Which of the following clinical manifestations is/are associated with the "atelectasis" clinical scenario?
   1. Increased opacity in chest x-ray
   2. Decreased forced vital capacity
   3. Bronchial breath sounds
   4. Diminished heart sounds
      a. 1 and 4 only
      b. 2 and 3 only
      c. 1, 2, and 3 only
      d. 2, 3, and 4 only

4. Which of the following pathophysiologic mechanisms is/are associated with the "bronchospasm" clinical scenario?
   1. Air trapping
   2. Decreased ventilation-perfusion ratio
   3. Increased airway resistance
   4. Irritant reflex
      a. 1 and 4 only
      b. 2 and 3 only
      c. 2, 3, and 4 only
      d. 1, 2, 3, and 4

5. Which of the following clinical manifestations is/are associated with the "distal airway and alveolar weakening" clinical scenario?
   1. Diminished breath sounds
   2. Decreased residual volume
   3. Pursed-lip breathing
   4. Dull percussion note
      a. 1 and 4 only
      b. 1 and 3 only
      c. 2, 3, and 4 only
      d. 1, 2, 3, and 4

6. According to the American Association for Respiratory Care (AARC), the purpose(s) of respiratory TDPs is/are to:
   1. Deliver individualized diagnostic and therapeutic respiratory care to patients
   2. Assist the physician with evaluating patients' respiratory care needs and optimize the allocation of respiratory care services
   3. Determine the indications for respiratory therapy and the appropriate modalities for providing high-quality, cost-effective care that improves patient outcomes and decreases length of stay
   4. Empower respiratory therapists to allocate care using sign- and symptom-based algorithms for respiratory treatment
      a. 1 only
      b. 3 only
      c. 1, 2, and 3 only
      d. 1, 2, 3, and 4

7. A patient experiencing a severe asthmatic episode would probably demonstrate a variety of objective clinical indicators to justify the assessments that call for the administration of which of the following protocols:
   1. Oxygen Therapy Protocol
   2. Airway Clearance Therapy Protocol
   3. Aerosolized Medication Therapy Protocol
   4. Lung Expansion Therapy Protocol
      a. 1 and 3 only
      b. 3 and 4 only
      c. 1, 2, and 4 only
      d. 1, 2, and 3 only

8. On the previous page, the Aerosolized Medication Protocol appears with one or more steps left out. Which steps have been omitted?
   1. Discharge training/documentation has been left out
   2. Effect of treatment with MDI/spacer has not been evaluated
   3. Failure to be able to breath hold has not been related to muscle weakness, following the finding of a reduced inspiratory capacity
   4. Use of additional protocols has not been considered in view of the patient's failure to improve on aerosol therapy via small-volume nebulizer treatment or intermittent positive-pressure breathing
      a. 1 and 3 only
      b. 2 and 4 only
      c. 2, 3, and 4 only
      d. 1, 2, 3, and 4

9. A patient with recent thoracic surgery, who has developed both left and right lower lung lobe atelectasis, would *most* likely benefit from which of the following protocols?
   a. Oxygen Therapy Protocol
   b. Airway Clearance Therapy Protocol
   c. Aerosolized Medication Therapy Protocol
   d. Lung Expansion Therapy Protocol

10. An obese 37-year-old man enters the emergency department in respiratory distress. He stated that he had been bedridden for the past 8 days with the flu. He thought he was getting better but had been short of breath for the past 2 days. His vital signs are blood pressure 175/125, respiratory rate 25 breaths/min, and heart rate 110 bpm. He has bilateral bronchial breath sounds over the lower lobes and dull percussion notes over the bases. His arterial blood gases show that he has acute alveolar hyperventilation with moderate hypoxemia. His chest x-ray image revealed bilateral atelectasis throughout his right and left lower lobes. Which of the following protocols would initially be the *most* beneficial?
   a. Oxygen Therapy Protocol
   b. Airway Clearance Therapy Protocol
   c. Aerosolized Medication Therapy Protocol
   d. Lung Expansion Therapy Protocol

CHAPTER

11 Respiratory Insufficiency, Respiratory Failure, and Ventilatory Management Protocols

Chapter Objectives

After reading this chapter, you will be able to:

- Define respiratory failure.
- Identify the six major anatomic alterations of the lungs and subsequent clinical scenarios that can lead to respiratory failure.
- Differentiate between the two major classifications of respiratory failure.
- Describe hypoxemic respiratory failure (type I) (oxygenation failure).
- List respiratory disorders associated with hypoxemic respiratory failure.
- Discuss the pathophysiologic mechanisms of hypoxemic respiratory failure.
- Describe the benefit of the alveolar-arterial oxygen radiant $[P(A-aO)_2]$ in the treatment of respiratory failure.
- Describe hypercapnic respiratory failure (type II) (ventilatory failure).
- Describe the pathophysiologic mechanisms of hypercapnic respiratory failure.
- List respiratory disorders associated with hypercapnic respiratory failure.
- Differentiate the types of ventilatory failure.
- Describe the major components of a mechanical ventilation protocol.
- Identify good "starting points" for selection of ventilator modes and settings.
- Describe the benefits of ventilator graphics in modern ventilator management.
- Describe the etiology, pathogenesis, and presentation of ventilator-induced/ventilator-associated lung injury (VILI/VALI)
- Discuss the concept and application of lung-protective strategies in mechanical ventilation.
- Define key terms and complete self-assessment questions at the end of the chapter and on Evolve.

Key Terms

Absolute Shunt
Acute Alveolar Hyperventilation Superimposed on Chronic
  Ventilatory Failure
Acute Ventilatory Failure
Acute Ventilatory Failure Superimposed on Chronic
  Ventilatory Failure

Adaptive Support Ventilation (ASV)
Alveolar-Arterial Oxygen Tension Difference $[P(A-a)O_2]$
Alveolar Flooding
Alveolar Hypoventilation
Anatomic Shunt
Apnea
ARDSNet Protocol
Arterial Oxygen Tension (PaO_2)
Arterial Oxygen Tension to Fractional Inspired Oxygen Ratio
  (PaO_2/FIO_2)
Arterial to Alveolar Oxygen Tension Ratio (PaO_2/PAO_2 ratio)
Barotrauma
Bohr Equation
Capillary Shunt
Chronic Ventilatory Failure
Continuous Positive Airway Pressure (CPAP) Ventilation
Dead Space/Tidal Volume Ratio (V_D/V_T) Ratio
Diffusion Defect
Hypercapnic Respiratory Failure (Type II)
Hypoxemic (Type I) Respiratory Failure
Impending Ventilatory Failure
Intermittent Mandatory Ventilation (IMV)
Invasive Mechanical Ventilation
Maximum Inspiratory Pressure (MIP)
Mechanical Dead Space
Neurally Adjusted Ventilatory Assist (NAVA)
Noninvasive Ventilation (NIV)
Patient-Ventilator Interaction
Permissive Hypercapnia
Pressure Time Index (PTI)
Prone Positioning
Prophylactic Ventilatory Support
Protective Lung Strategies
Pulmonary Shunting
Rapid Shallow Breathing Index (RSBI)
Relative Shunt
Respiratory Failure
Richmond Agitation Sedation Scale
Shunt-Like Effect
Spontaneous Breathing Trial (SBT)
Static Lung Compliance (C_L)
Type III Respiratory Failure
Venous Admixture
Ventilator-Associated Lung Injury (VALI)

Ventilator-Induced Lung Injury (VILI)
Ventilation-Perfusion Mismatch
Ventilatory Failure
Volutrauma

Chapter Outline

Respiratory failure (also called *ventilatory failure*) is a general term used to describe the inability of the respiratory system to establish and maintain adequate oxygen uptake and carbon dioxide removal from the body. The arterial blood gas (ABG) criteria for respiratory failure in the normal individual are an arterial partial pressure of oxygen (PaO_2) less than 60 mm Hg, an arterial partial pressure of carbon dioxide ($PaCO_2$) greater than 50 mm Hg, or a mixture of both. These ABG values constitute the *definition* for respiratory failure. Additional objective findings include cardiac arrhythmias, both hypertension and preterminally hypotension, coma, and death. Subjective findings (symptoms) of respiratory failure include dyspnea, anxiety, restlessness, and rapid and shallow breathing. Respiratory failure is a life-threatening clinical condition that the respiratory therapist must be 100% proficient in consistently recognizing, assessing, and managing.

Virtually every respiratory disorder presented in this textbook can result in respiratory failure. Each respiratory disorder can cause one or more of the *anatomic alterations of the lung*, which in turn activate specific and very predictable *pathophysiologic mechanisms* and *clinical manifestations* that can progressively worsen if not identified and treated. The interrelationship between the anatomic alterations of the lungs, the pathophysiologic mechanisms, and the clinical manifestations are collectively referred to as *clinical scenarios* (see Chapter 10, The Therapist-Driven Protocol Program).

As discussed in detail in Chapter 10, there are six basic anatomic alterations of the lungs, which in turn cause six different clinical scenarios that can result in respiratory failure. These scenarios are (1) *atelectasis* (see Fig. 10.7), (2) *alveolar consolidation* (see Fig. 10.8), (3) *increased alveolar-capillary membrane thickness* (see Fig. 10.9), (4) *bronchospasm* (see Fig. 10.10), (5) *excessive bronchial secretions* (see Fig. 10.11), and (6) *distal airway and alveolar weakening* (see Fig. 10.12).

Classifications of Respiratory Failure

On the basis of the ABG values, respiratory failure is commonly classified as (1) hypoxemic respiratory failure (also called *type I respiratory failure*), (2) hypercapnic respiratory failure (also called *type II respiratory failure*), or (3) a combination of both. The term *hypoxemic respiratory failure* is used when the primary problem is inadequate oxygenation exchange between the alveoli and the pulmonary capillary system, which results in a decreased PaO_2. The term *hypercapnic respiratory failure* is used when the primary problem is alveolar hypoventilation, which results in an increased $PaCO_2$ and, without supplemental oxygen, a decreased PaO_2.

In the clinical setting, hypercapnic respiratory failure is commonly called **ventilatory failure**. Based on the $PaCO_2$ and pH values, ventilatory failure is further classified as being either **acute ventilatory failure** (high $PaCO_2$ and low pH) or **chronic ventilatory failure** (high $PaCO_2$ and normal pH). Because acute ventilatory changes (i.e., hyperventilation or hypoventilation) are often seen in patients with chronic ventilatory failure, the patient also may present with either (1) **acute alveolar hyperventilation superimposed on chronic ventilatory failure** or (2) **acute ventilatory failure superimposed on chronic ventilatory failure**.

The different types of respiratory failures are described in the following section.

Hypoxemic Respiratory Failure—Type I (Oxygenation Failure)

Hypoxemic respiratory failure (type I) is used to describe a patient whose primary problem is inadequate oxygenation. Patients with hypoxemic respiratory failure typically demonstrate hypoxemia—a low PaO_2—and a normal or low $PaCO_2$ value.[1] The low $PaCO_2$ is usually attributable to the alveolar hyperventilation associated with hypoxemia (see Figs. 3.5 and 3.6). Box 11.1 provides a listing of common respiratory disorders that can cause hypoxemic respiratory failure. The major pathophysiologic causes of hypoxemic respiratory failure

---

[1]Key clinical indicators of hypoxemic respiratory failure include a decreased **arterial oxygen tension (PaO_2)**, an increased alveolar-arterial oxygen tension gradient [$P(A-a)O_2$], a decreased **arterial-to-alveolar oxygen tension ratio (PaO_2/PAO_2 ratio)**, a decreased **arterial oxygen tension to fractional inspired oxygen ratio (PaO_2/FIO_2 ratio** (see Table 11.8), and/or an increased pulmonary shunt ($\dot{Q}_s/\dot{Q}_T$). See Table 11.11 for clinical indicators of hypoxemic respiratory failure, page 164.)

The results of alveolar hypoventilation are hypoxia, hypercapnia, respiratory acidosis, and, in severe cases, pulmonary hypertension with cor pulmonale. It should be emphasized, however, that even though alveolar hypoventilation causes hypoxemia, the alveoli are still able to efficiently transfer oxygen into the pulmonary capillary blood—assuming the inspired oxygen can be delivered to the alveoli. Thus treatment of alveolar hypoventilation primarily consists of ventilatory support.

Pulmonary Shunting. **Pulmonary shunting** is defined as that portion of the cardiac output that moves from the right side to the left side of the heart without being exposed to alveolar oxygen (PAO_2). Pulmonary shunting is divided into the following two categories: (1) absolute shunt and (2) relative shunt. As discussed in more detail in the following section, all forms of pulmonary shunting lead to venous admixture and a decreased PaO_2 level.

Absolute Shunt. **Absolute shunts** (also called *true shunts*) are classified as either an anatomic shunt or a capillary shunt. Both types, anatomic and capillary shunts, are classified under the general heading of absolute shunts.

Anatomic shunts occur when blood flows from the right side of the heart to the left side without coming in contact with an alveolus for gas exchange (Fig. 11.1B). In the healthy lung, there is a normal anatomic shunt of about 3% of the cardiac output. This normal shunting is caused by nonoxygenated blood completely bypassing the alveoli and entering (1) the pulmonary vascular system by means of the *bronchial venous drainage* and (2) the left atrium by way of the *thebesian veins.* These natural anatomic shunts explain the small normal difference between the partial pressure of oxygen in the alveoli (PAO_2) and the arterial blood (PaO_2)—that is, the normal $P(A-a)O_2$ difference of 7 to 15 mm Hg.

Common abnormal causes of anatomic shunt include the following:
- Congenital heart disease
- Intrapulmonary fistula
- Vascular lung tumors

Capillary shunts are caused by (1) alveolar collapse or atelectasis, (2) alveolar fluid accumulation, or (3) alveolar consolidation or pneumonia (see Fig. 11.1C).

The sum of both the anatomic shunt and capillary shunt makes up the absolute (also called the *true shunt*). The patient with absolute shunting responds poorly to oxygen therapy because of the two pathologic mechanisms:

are (1) *alveolar hypoventilation,* (2) *pulmonary shunting,* and (3) *ventilation-perfusion ($\dot{V}/\dot{Q}$) mismatch.* Although less common, a decrease in inspired oxygen pressure (PIO_2) (e.g., exposure at high altitudes) also can cause hypoxemic respiratory failure.

The primary pathophysiologic mechanisms of hypoxemic respiratory failure are discussed in more detail in the following sections.

Pathophysiologic Mechanisms of Hypoxemic Respiratory Failure

Alveolar hypoventilation develops when the minute volume of alveolar ventilation ($\dot{V}_A$) is not adequate for the body's metabolic needs. It is characterized by an increased $PaCO_2$ level and, without supplemental oxygen, a decreased PaO_2. Common causes of alveolar hypoventilation include central nervous system depressants, head trauma, chronic obstructive pulmonary disease (COPD), obesity, sleep apnea, and neuromuscular disorders (e.g., amyotrophic lateral sclerosis [ALS], myasthenia gravis, or Guillain-Barré syndrome). The current epidemic of opioid and sedative substance abuse has increased the number of cases of alveolar hypoventilation to a frightening extent. Box 11.2 lists the substances currently monitored by authorities with urinary or blood screening.

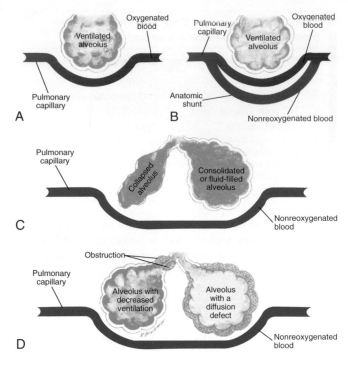

FIGURE 11.1 Pulmonary shunting. (A) Normal alveolar-capillary unit. (B) Anatomic shunt. (C) Types of capillary shunt. (D) Types of relative or shunt-like effect.

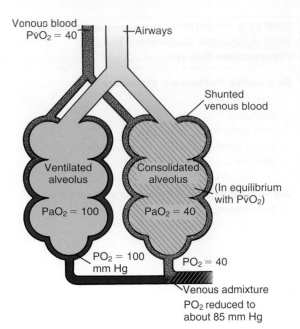

FIGURE 11.2 Venous admixture occurs when reoxygenated blood mixes with nonreoxygenated blood distal to the alveoli. Technically, the PO_2 in the pulmonary capillary system will not equilibrate completely because of the normal $P(A-a)O_2$. The PO_2 in the pulmonary capillary system is normally a few millimeters of mercury less than the PO_2 in the alveoli.

1. In an *anatomic shunt* the alveolar oxygen does not come in direct contact with the shunted blood—that is, the nonoxygenated blood *completely bypasses* the ventilated alveoli and mixes downstream with the oxygenated blood.

2. When a *capillary shunt* is present, the nonoxygenated blood passes alveoli that are not ventilated and, as a result, moves downstream as venous blood and mixes with the oxygenated blood (see section on Venous Admixture).

The patient with absolute shunting is refractory to oxygen therapy. In other words, the reduced arterial oxygen level caused by this type of pulmonary shunting cannot be easily treated by increasing the concentration of oxygen for these two major reasons: (1) because of the pathology associated with an absolute shunt, the alveoli are unable to accommodate any form of ventilation, and (2) the blood that bypasses the normal, functional alveoli is unable to carry more oxygen once it has become fully saturated, except for a very small amount of oxygen that dissolves in the plasma ($PO_2 \times 0.003 =$ Dissolved O_2).

Relative Shunt. When pulmonary capillary perfusion is in excess of alveolar ventilation, a **relative shunt** (also referred to as a **shunt-like effect**) is said to be present (see Fig. 11.1D). A relative shunt can be caused by an airway obstruction, an alveolar-capillary **diffusion defect**, or a combination of both.

Airway obstruction leads to poor ventilation of the distal airways. As a result, the pulmonary capillary blood flow is greater than the alveolar ventilation—in short, a decreased V̇/Q̇ ratio exists. This condition results in a relative shunt, or shunt-like effect, which in turn causes the PaO_2 to fall (see Fig. 11.1D). Common respiratory disorders that cause airway obstruction include emphysema, chronic bronchitis, asthma, and cystic fibrosis.

Alveolar-capillary diffusion defects occur when an abnormality in the structure of the alveolar-capillary membranes slows the movement of oxygen between the alveoli and the pulmonary capillary blood. Under these conditions, the pulmonary capillary blood passing by the alveolus does not have enough time to equilibrate with the alveolar oxygen tension. This condition results in a relative shunt, or shunt-like effect, which in turn causes the PaO_2 to fall (see Fig. 11.1D).

Common causes of diffusion defects include interstitial pulmonary edema and interstitial lung disorders (e.g., asbestosis, scleroderma, or idiopathic pulmonary fibrosis). Relative shunting also may occur after the administration of drugs that cause an increase in cardiac output or dilation of the pulmonary vessels. *Unlike an absolute shunt, which is refractory to oxygen therapy, conditions that cause a shunt-like effect are more easily corrected (at least partially) by oxygen therapy and alveolar expansion techniques such as continuous positive airway pressure (CPAP) or positive end-expiratory pressure (PEEP).*

Table 11.1 illustrates the type of pulmonary shunting associated with common respiratory disorders.

Venous Admixture. **Venous admixture** is defined as the mixing of shunted, nonoxygenated blood with reoxygenated blood distal to the alveoli—that is, downstream in the pulmonary venous system in route to the left side of the heart (Fig. 11.2). When venous admixture occurs, the shunted—nonoxygenated—blood gains oxygen molecules while at the same time the reoxygenated blood loses oxygen molecules. This process continues until (1) the PO_2 throughout all the plasma of the newly mixed blood is in equilibrium and (2) all the hemoglobin molecules carry the same number of oxygen molecules.

TABLE 11.1 Type of Pulmonary Shunting Associated With Common Respiratory Diseases

Respiratory Diseases	Capillary Shunt	Relative or Shunt-Like Effect
Chronic bronchitis		X
Emphysema		X
Asthma		X
Croup/epiglottitis		X
Sleep apnea		X
Bronchiectasis*	X	X
Cystic fibrosis*	X	X
Interstitial lung disease*	X	X
Cancer of the lungs	X	X
Guillain-Barré syndrome	X	X
Myasthenia gravis	X	X
Pneumonia	X	
Tuberculosis	X	
Pulmonary edema	X	
Flail chest	X	
Pneumothorax	X	
Kyphoscoliosis	X	
Interstitial lung disease	X	
Acute respiratory distress syndrome	X	
Pleural diseases	X	
Respiratory distress syndrome	X	
Near drowning	X	
Smoke inhalation	X	
Atelectasis	X	

*Relative or shunt-like effect is most common.

The final result of venous admixture is (1) a "downstream" blood mixture that has a higher PO_2 and CaO_2 than the original shunted, nonoxygenated blood and (2) a lower PO_2 and CaO_2 than the original reoxygenated blood—in other words, a blood mixture with PaO_2 and CaO_2 values somewhere between those of original values of the reoxygenated and nonoxygenated blood. The overall final outcome of venous admixture is a reduced PaO_2 and CaO_2 level returning to the left side of the heart via the systemic venous system. Clinically, it is this oxygen mixture that is evaluated downstream (e.g., from the radial artery) to assess the patient's ABGs.

To calculate the amount of a patient's pulmonary shunting, see the discussion of pulmonary shunt fraction in Chapter 6, Assessment of Oxygenation, page 86.

Ventilation-Perfusion ($\dot{V}/\dot{Q}$) Ratio Mismatch

Under normal conditions, the overall alveolar ventilation is about 4 L/min and pulmonary capillary blood flow is about 5 L/min, making the average overall ratio of alveolar ventilation to blood flow about 4:5 or 0.8. This relationship is expressed as the *ventilation-perfusion ($\dot{V}/\dot{Q}$) ratio* (Fig. 11.3).

In some disorders, such as pulmonary embolism (see Chapter 21, Pulmonary Vascular Disease: Pulmonary Embolism and Pulmonary Hypertension), the lungs receive less blood flow in relation to ventilation. When this condition develops, the $\dot{V}/\dot{Q}$ ratio increases. A larger portion of the alveolar ventilation therefore will not be physiologically effective and the patient

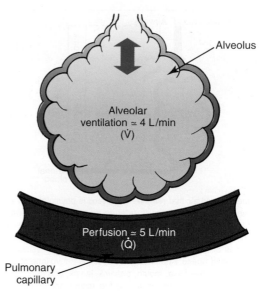

FIGURE 11.3 The normal overall pulmonary ventilation-perfusion ratio ($\dot{V}/\dot{Q}$) is approximately 0.8.

will be said to demonstrate "wasted" or dead-space ventilation (Fig. 11.4).

In other lung disorders (e.g., asthma, emphysema, pulmonary edema, or pneumonia), the lungs receive relatively less ventilation in relation to blood flow. When this condition develops, the $\dot{V}/\dot{Q}$ ratio decreases. A decreased ratio leads to a relative shunt, or shunt-like effect, which in turn leads to venous admixture and a decreased PaO_2 (see Fig. 11.1D).

Ratio of Dead Space to Tidal Volume

In the clinical setting, the patient's alveolar dead space is often expressed as the **dead space/tidal volume (V_D/V_T) ratio**. The V_D/V_T ratio provides a good reference of the patient's wasted ventilation (i.e., both the anatomic and alveolar dead space) per each breath. The calculation of the V_D/V_T ratio requires both a sample of the patient's arterial CO_2 ($PaCO_2$) and the mixed expired CO_2 ($P_{\bar{E}}CO_2$). The $PaCO_2$ is obtained from a routine ABG sample, and the $P_{\bar{E}}CO_2$ is collected in a sampling bag or balloon or estimated via capnography. The calculation of the V_D/V_T ratio uses a modified form of the **Bohr equation**, which assumes that there is no CO_2 in the inspired gas. The V_D/V_T ratio is written as follows:

$$\frac{V_D}{V_T} = \frac{PaCO_2 - P_{\bar{E}}CO_2}{PaCO_2}$$

where $PaCO_2$ is the arterial CO_2 tension, and $P_{\bar{E}}CO_2$ is the expired CO_2 tension. Thus if a patient has a $PaCO_2$ of 40 mm Hg and a $P_{\bar{E}}CO_2$ of 30 mm Hg, the V_D/V_T ratio would be calculated as follows:

$$\frac{V_D}{V_T} = \frac{PaCO_2 - P_{\bar{E}}CO_2}{PaCO_2}$$
$$= \frac{40 - 30}{40}$$
$$= \frac{10}{40}$$
$$= 0.25 \text{ or } 25\%$$

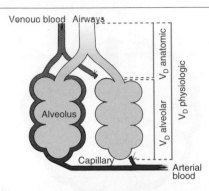

Only the inspired air that reaches the alveoli is physiologically effective. This portion of the inspired gas is referred to as *alveolar ventilation*. The volume of inspired air that does not reach the alveoli is not physiologically effective. This portion of gas is referred to as *dead-space ventilation*. There are three types of dead spaces: anatomic, alveolar, and physiologic.

Anatomic Dead Space. Anatomic dead space is the volume of gas in the conducting airways: the nose, mouth, pharynx, larynx, and lower portions of the airways down to but not including the respiratory bronchioles. The volume of the anatomic dead space is approximately equal to 1 mL/lb (2.2 mL/kg) of normal body weight.

Alveolar Dead Space. When an alveolus is ventilated but not perfused with blood, the volume of air in the alveolus is dead space—that is, the air within the alveolus is not physiologically effective in terms of gas exchange. The amount of alveolar dead space is unpredictable.

Physiologic Dead Space. The physiologic dead space is the sum of the anatomic and alveolar dead space. Because neither of these two forms of dead space is physiologically effective in terms of gas exchange, the two forms are combined and are referred to as the physiologic dead space (PDS) (see Append IX: Physiologic Dead Space Calculation on the Evolve site.)

FIGURE 11.4 Dead-space ventilation ($\dot{V}_2$).

The V_D/V_T ratio in the normal adult breathing spontaneously ranges between 20% and 40%. For patients receiving mechanical ventilation, the normal V_D/V_T ratio ranges between 40% and 60%, because of the **mechanical dead space** added by the endotracheal tube, etc. The V_D/V_T ratio increases with diseases that cause significant dead space, such as pulmonary embolism.

Decreased Partial Pressure of Inspired Oxygen (Decreased PIO₂)

Hypoxemia also can develop from decreases in inspired concentrations of oxygen. For example, hypoxemia can develop at high altitudes. This is because the partial pressure of inspired oxygen progressively decreases in response to the falling barometric pressure that occurs at high altitudes. The higher the altitude above sea level, the lower is the barometric pressure. The lower the barometric pressure, the lower is the partial pressure of inspired oxygen. For example, at an altitude of 18,000 to 19,000 feet, the barometric pressure is about half the sea-level value of 760 mm Hg (380 mm Hg).

The barometric pressure on the summit of Mount Everest (altitude 29,028 feet) is about 250 mm Hg (the atmospheric PO_2 is about 43 mm Hg). To compensate for this, it is not

uncommon for a mountain climber to use an oxygen mask. At an altitude of about 65,000 feet, the barometric pressure falls below the pressure of water vapor, and tissue fluids begin to "boil" or "vaporize." Airlines correct for the decreased barometric pressure by pressurizing their cabins.[2] However, the individual with chronic hypoxemia may still require supplemental oxygen during the flight. The effects of chronic hypoxia and hyperoxia are being increasingly more appreciated, and steps to remedy the problems range from high-flow oxygen therapy, pressurized hospital rooms, hyperbaric oxygen therapy, and—recently reported—even the use of oxygen generators in some carriages in a train[3] running from China to Lhasa, Tibet. This train frequently passes through altitudes near 5000 meters, and supplemental oxygen is bled into the carriage to relieve the symptoms of altitude sickness of passengers.

Identifying the Pathophysiologic Mechanisms of Acute Hypoxemic Respiratory Failure

To more effectively treat the patient, the **alveolar-arterial oxygen tension difference [P(A-a)O₂]** is used clinically to identify the primary *cause* of the hypoxemic respiratory failure— *alveolar hypoventilation, pulmonary shunting,* or $\dot{V}/\dot{Q}$ *mismatch.* The clinical determination of the P(A-a)O₂ is made by subtracting the PaO₂ (obtained from an ABG value) from the PAO₂, which is obtained from the *ideal alveolar gas equation:*

$$PAO_2 = FIO_2 (P_B - PH_2O) - PaCO_2/RQ$$

where P_B is the barometric pressure, PAO₂ is the partial pressure of oxygen within the alveoli, PH₂O is the partial pressure of water vapor in the alveoli (which is 47 mm Hg), FIO₂ is the fractional concentration of inspired oxygen, PaCO₂ is the partial pressure of arterial carbon dioxide, and RQ is the respiratory quotient. The RQ is the ratio of carbon dioxide production ($\dot{V}CO_2$) divided by *oxygen consumption* ($\dot{V}O_2$).

Under normal circumstances, about 250 mL of oxygen per minute is consumed by the tissue cells and about 200 mL of carbon dioxide is excreted into the lung. Thus the RQ is normally about 0.8, but can range from 0.7 to 1.0. Clinically, 0.8 is generally used for the RQ. For example, consider the following case example:

Case Example

If a patient is receiving an FIO₂ of 0.30 on a day when the barometric pressure is 750 mm Hg, and if the patient's PaCO₂ is 70 mm Hg and PaO₂ is 60 mm Hg, the P(A-a)O₂ can be calculated as follows:

$$PAO_2 = FIO_2 (P_B - PH_2O) - PaCO_2/RQ$$
$$= 0.30 (750 - 47) - 70/0.8$$
$$= (703) 0.30 - 87.5$$
$$= 123.4 \text{ mm Hg.}$$

---

[2]Most commercial jet aircraft fly at cruising altitudes between 30,000 and 40,000 feet. The barometric pressure (P_B) at sea level is about 760 mm Hg (14.7 psi). At 30,000 feet above sea level, the P_B is about 226 mm Hg (4.4 psi); at 40,000 feet, the P_B is about 104 mm Hg (2.7 psi). To prevent people from losing consciousness from the lack of oxygen at these high cruising altitudes, the plane's cabin is pressurized to an altitude between 6000 and 8000 feet, which provides a barometric pressure between 609 mm Hg (11.8 psi) and 563 mm Hg (10.9 psi), respectively.

[3]In the Chinese train, the ambient oxygen is increased by only 3 percentage points (from 21% to 24%), but this is enough to result in symptomatic improvement for its passengers. It is not practical to pressurize whole buildings in a process called *oxygen conditioning*, but pressurization of entire hospital rooms is now being done at selected sites.

TABLE 11.2 Causes of Hypoxemic Respiratory Failure

Cause of Hypoxemic Respiratory Failure	Pathophysiologic Mechanism	P(A-a)O$_2$ Findings	General Response to Oxygen Therapy	Examples
Alveolar hypoventilation	Decreased minute ventilation: Increased PaCO$_2$, decreased PaO$_2$	Normal	Fair/good, with ventilatory support or increased alveolar ventilation	Drug overdose Oversedation Obesity Head trauma Myasthenia gravis Guillain-Barré syndrome
Pulmonary shunting	Venous admixture (venous blood mixing with arterial blood)	Increased	Poor	Atelectasis Pneumonia Alveolar fibrosis ARDS Pulmonary edema
Ventilation-perfusion mismatch	Venous admixture (nonoxygenated blood mixing with arterial blood)	Increased	Good	Emphysema Chronic bronchitis Asthma Pulmonary embolus
Decrease in inspired oxygen (decreased FIO$_2$ or PIO$_2$)	Decreased oxygen concentration or decreased inspired oxygen pressure (e.g., decreased barometric pressure)	Normal	Good	High altitude Low oxygen content of gas mixture Enclosed breathing spaces (suffocation)

ARDS, Acute respiratory distress syndrome.

Using the PaO$_2$ obtained from the ABG, the P(A-a)O$_2$ now can be easily calculated as follows:

$$123.4 \text{ mm Hg (PAO}_2)$$
$$\underline{- 60.0 \text{ mm Hg (PaO}_2)}$$
$$63.4 \text{ mm Hg [P(A-a)O}_2]$$

The normal P(A-a)O$_2$ on room air at sea level ranges from 7 to 15 mm Hg and should not exceed 30 mm Hg. Although the P(A-a)O$_2$ may be useful in patients breathing a low FIO$_2$, it loses some of its sensitivity in patients breathing a high FIO$_2$. The P(A-a)O$_2$ increases at high oxygen concentrations. Because of this, the P(A-a)O$_2$ has less value in the critically ill patient who is breathing a high oxygen concentration. *The normal P(A-a)O$_2$ for an FIO$_2$ of 1.0 is between 25 and 65 mm Hg. The critical value of the P(A-a)O$_2$ on the 100% oxygen is greater than 350 mm Hg.*

When conditions such as obesity or drug overdose lead to alveolar hypoventilation and subsequent hypoxemic respiratory failure, the (P[A-a]O$_2$) is normal, thus indicating that the lungs are normal but alveolar *ventilation* is not. In these cases, the treatment management is directed at a ventilatory support strategy. These patients readily respond to ventilator therapy and *not* to oxygen therapy alone.

When $\dot{V}/\dot{Q}$ mismatch, pulmonary shunting, or diffusion blockade is the primary cause of the hypoxemic respiratory failure, the (P[A-a]O$_2$) is elevated. In these cases, the administration of oxygen is used to identify the specific pathologic basis of the hypoxemic respiratory failure—that is, a $\dot{V}/\dot{Q}$ mismatch or pulmonary shunting. The patient with a $\dot{V}/\dot{Q}$ mismatch shows significant improvement with oxygen therapy, indicating that the patient's $\dot{V}/\dot{Q}$ status may not have been permanently altered. For example, the use of bronchodilators may improve the patient's bronchoconstriction

and thus improve his alveolar hypoventilation and his altered $\dot{V}/\dot{Q}$ status. By contrast, the patient with an absolute shunt shows little to no improvement with oxygen therapy, even at an FIO$_2$ of 1.0. In these cases, the treatment needs to focus on the cause of the intrapulmonary shunting. For example, therapeutic efforts are directed at opening collapsed alveoli (in cases of atelectasis or **alveolar flooding**), reducing pulmonary edema, or mobilizing excessive secretions that lead to atelectasis. The (PA-Pa) is a helpful tool in the early diagnosis of the patient's disease process (and in following its progress), especially when the FIO$_2$ varies during the course of therapy.

Summary of Causes of Hypoxemic Respiratory Failure. Table 11.2 summarizes the major causes of hypoxemic respiratory failure, the pathophysiologic mechanisms involved, the typical P(A-a) O$_2$ findings, the expected patient response to oxygen therapy, and types of patients who demonstrate the mechanism.

Hypercapnic Respiratory Failure—Type II (Ventilatory Failure)

Hypercapnic respiratory failure (type II) is the phrase used when the primary problem is alveolar hypoventilation. Patients with hypercapnic respiratory failure demonstrate an increased PaCO$_2$ and, without supplemental oxygen, a decreased PaO$_2$.[4] The major pathophysiologic mechanisms that result in hypercapnic respiratory failure are (1) alveolar hypoventilation,

---

[4] In addition to the patient's ABG status discussed here, key clinical indicators of hypercapnic respiratory failure are also reflected in the patient's tidal volume (V$_T$), respiratory rate (breaths per minute), maximum inspiratory pressure (MIP), vital capacity (VC), and work of breathing (e.g., minute ventilation and dead-space/tidal volume ratio [V$_D$/V$_T$ ratio]). For further discussion of these important points, see Table 11.9, Criteria for Instituting Mechanical Ventilation, page 169.

BOX 11.3 Respiratory Disorders Associated With Hypercapnic Respiratory Failure* (Ventilatory Failure)

Pulmonary Disorders
- Emphysema
- Chronic bronchitis
- Asthma
- Cystic fibrosis

Respiratory Center Depression
- Drug overdose
- Cerebral trauma or infarction
- Bulbar poliomyelitis
- Encephalitis

Neuromuscular Disorders
- Myasthenia gravis
- Guillain-Barré syndrome
- Spinal cord trauma
- Muscular dystrophy

Pleural and Chest Wall Disorders
- Flail chest
- Pneumothorax
- Pleural effusion
- Kyphoscoliosis
- Obesity

Sleep Apnea

*It should be noted that any of the pulmonary disorders associated with hypoxemic respiratory failure can—when severe enough—lead to hypercapnic respiratory failure.

TABLE 11.3 Acute Ventilatory Failure (Acute Respiratory Acidosis)

Arterial Blood Gas Changes	Example
pH: Decreased	7.17
$PaCO_2$: Increased	79 mm Hg
HCO_3^-: Increased (but normal)	28 mEq/L
PaO_2: Decreased	49 mm Hg*

*Moderate to severe hypoxemia.

TABLE 11.4 Chronic Ventilatory Failure (Compensated Respiratory Acidosis)

Baseline Arterial Blood Gas Values*	
ABG Changes	Example
pH: Normal	7.37
$PaCO_2$: Increased	77 mm Hg
HCO_3^-: Increased (significantly)	43 mEq/L
PaO_2: Decreased	61 mm Hg

ABG, Arterial blood gas.
*NOTE: Chronic ventilatory failure ABG baseline values are much different than the ABG baseline values of the normal individual (e.g., pH: 7.35–7.45; $PaCO_2$: 35–45; HCO_3^-: 22–26; PaO_2: 80–100).

(2) increased dead-space disease, and (3) severe $\dot{V}/\dot{Q}$ ratio mismatch. Box 11.3 provides common respiratory disorders associated with hypercapnic respiratory failure.

Types of Ventilatory Failure

In the clinical setting, *hypercapnic respiratory failure* is commonly referred to as *ventilatory failure*. Based on the arterial blood $PaCO_2$ and pH values, ventilatory failure can be further classified as either (1) acute ventilatory failure (high $PaCO_2$ and low pH) or (2) chronic ventilatory failure (high $PaCO_2$ and normal pH).

In addition, chronic ventilatory failure is often complicated by conditions that cause the patient to either *hyperventilate* or *hypoventilate*—that is, on top of (in addition to) their chronic ventilatory failure. In these cases, the patient is said to have either (1) acute alveolar hyperventilation superimposed on chronic ventilatory failure or (2) acute ventilatory failure (hypoventilation) superimposed on chronic ventilatory failure. The different classifications of ventilatory failure are discussed in more detail in the following paragraphs.

Acute ventilatory failure (also called *acute respiratory acidosis*) is a condition in which the lungs are unable to meet the metabolic demands of the body in terms of CO_2 removal. As a result, the $PaCO_2$ rises and, without supplemental oxygen, the PaO_2 falls. When an increased $PaCO_2$ level is accompanied by acidemia

(decreased pH), *acute ventilatory failure,* or *acute respiratory acidosis,* is said to exist. Table 11.3 shows an ABG example of acute ventilatory failure. Clinically, this is a life-threatening medical emergency that requires ventilatory support.

Chronic ventilatory failure (also called *compensated respiratory acidosis*) is defined as a greater-than-normal $PaCO_2$ level with a normal pH status. The renal system has compensated for the low pH by retaining bicarbonate (HCO_3^-) and adding it to the patient's blood. Although chronic ventilatory failure is most commonly seen in patients with severe COPD (e.g., chronic bronchitis, emphysema, or cystic fibrosis), it is also seen in several chronic restrictive lung disorders (e.g., obesity, severe tuberculosis, fungal disease, kyphoscoliosis, or interstitial lung disease). Table 11.4 shows an ABG example of chronic ventilatory failure with hypoxemia. Clinically, this is a life-threatening medical emergency that requires ventilatory support.

Acute Alveolar Hyperventilation Superimposed on Chronic Ventilatory Failure

Like any other patient (healthy or unhealthy), the patient with chronic ventilatory failure also can acquire a new—that is, additional—acute shunt-producing disease (e.g., pneumonia or pulmonary edema). This is not unusual in the real world of clinical medicine. For example, when such patients have the mechanical reserve to increase their alveolar ventilation significantly in an attempt to maintain their baseline PaO_2, their $PaCO_2$ often decreases from their normally high baseline level. This action causes their pH to increase. As this condition intensifies, the patient's baseline ABG values can quickly change from chronic ventilatory failure to that of acute alveolar hyperventilation superimposed on chronic ventilatory failure (Table 11.5).

TABLE 11.5 Acute Alveolar Hyperventilation Superimposed on Chronic Ventilatory Failure*

Arterial Blood Gas Changes	Example
pH: Increased	7.51
$PaCO_2$: Increased (but lower than patient's typical elevated baseline level)	52 mm Hg
HCO_3: Increased (significantly) (but lower than patient's typical elevated baseline level)	40 mEq/L
PaO_2: Decreased (but lower than patient's typical low baseline level)	49 mm Hg

*This condition is often seen in patients with acute bronchitis, pneumonia, or pulmonary edema that exacerbates their chronic obstructive pulmonary disease.

TABLE 11.6 Acute Ventilatory Failure Superimposed on Chronic Ventilatory Failure

Arterial Blood Gas Changes	Example
pH: Decreased	7.28
$PaCO_2$: Increased (but higher than patient's typical elevated baseline level)	97 mm Hg
HCO_3^-: Increased (significantly) (but higher than patient's typical elevated baseline level)	44 mEq/L
PaO_2: Decreased (but lower than patient's typical low baseline level)	39 mm Hg

Acute Ventilatory Failure (Hypoventilation) Superimposed on Chronic Ventilatory Failure

When the patient with chronic ventilatory failure *does not* have the additional mechanical reserve to meet the hypoxemic challenge of a new respiratory disorder, the patient begins to breathe less efficiently—that is, the patient hypoventilates.[5] This action causes the $PaCO_2$ to increase above the patient's already high $PaCO_2$ baseline level.

As the $PaCO_2$ suddenly increases, the patient's arterial pH level falls, or becomes acidic. As this condition intensifies, the patient's baseline ABG values change from chronic ventilatory failure to acute ventilatory failure superimposed on chronic ventilatory failure—acute on chronic ventilatory failure (Table 11.6).

Table 11.7 provides a summary overview of the ABG findings for (1) chronic ventilatory failure, (2) acute hyperventilation superimposed on chronic ventilatory failure, and (3) acute ventilatory failure superimposed on chronic ventilatory failure.

Mechanical Ventilation

Before a decision can be made to commit the patient to any form of mechanical ventilation, the respiratory therapist must

[5]Often the patient initially demonstrates acute alveolar hyperventilation superimposed on chronic ventilatory failure before becoming fatigued, when acute ventilatory failure superimposed on chronic ventilatory failure develops. Clinically, this condition is called **impending ventilatory failure**.

TABLE 11.7 Examples of Acute Changes Superimposed on Chronic Ventilatory Failure

Acute Ventilatory Failure on Chronic Ventilatory Failure		Chronic Ventilatory Failure (Baseline Values)		Acute Alveolar Hyperventilation on Chronic Ventilatory Failure
7.28	←	pH 7.37	→	7.51
97	←	$PaCO_2$ 77	→	52
44	←	HCO_3^- 43	→	40
39	←	PaO_2 61	→	49

first answer these questions: Are key clinical indicators of respiratory failure present? Does the patient meet the standard criteria for mechanical ventilation? Does the patient primarily have hypoxemic respiratory failure, hypercapnic respiratory failure, or a combination of both? Which ventilatory support strategy would best serve the patient's short-term or long-term ventilatory needs? Should noninvasive ventilation or invasive ventilation be used? How can the lung be best protected from the harmful effects of mechanical ventilation? Finally, what will be the most effective strategies to "liberate" him from mechanical ventilation?

To satisfactorily answer these questions, it is essential that the respiratory therapist must again use good clinical judgment skills, which are based on the ability to (1) collect all the clinical data relevant to the patient's respiratory status, (2) formulate an objective and measurable respiratory assessment, (3) select and implement a safe and effective ventilatory management plan, and (4) clearly and correctly document the subjective and objective data, assessment, and ventilatory support plan that he has selected in pursuit of these goals.

Standard Criteria for Instituting Mechanical Ventilation

The four standard criteria for mechanical ventilation are (1) apnea, (2) acute ventilatory failure, (3) impending ventilatory failure, and (4) severe refractory hypoxemia. To help determine if the mechanical ventilation should be invasive or noninvasive, the respiratory therapist should also establish if the patient is able to protect his/her own airway during mechanical ventilation with the modality under consideration. **Apnea** is defined as the complete absence of spontaneous ventilation, which is an absolute indication for invasive mechanical ventilation. Apnea causes the PaO_2 to rapidly decrease and the $PaCO_2$ to increase. Death will ensue in minutes unless an airway is established and ventilation is provided.

Acute ventilatory failure is defined as a sudden increase in $PaCO_2$ to greater than 50 mm Hg with an accompanying low pH value (<7.30). *Impending ventilatory failure* occurs when the patient demonstrates a significant increase in the work of breathing with borderline acceptable ABG values. Severe refractory hypoxemia (PaO_2 <40 mm Hg, SaO_2 <75%) reflects a critically low oxygenation status that does not respond well to oxygen therapy. Severe refractory hypoxemia is often seen in cases of severe pneumonia, interstitial lung diseases, and acute respiratory distress syndrome (ARDS). The PaO_2/FIO_2 ratio may be used to judge the degree of severity and

TABLE 11.8 Refractory Hypoxemia

Classifications That May Suggest the Need for Treatment Modalities in Addition to Oxygen

Classification	PaO_2/FIO_2 Ratio
Normal	350–450 (room air)
Mild (acute) lung injury (acute respiratory distress syndrome)	200–300
Moderate lung injury	100–200
Severe lung injury	<100

TABLE 11.9 Criteria for Instituting Mechanical Ventilation and the Primary Type of Respiratory Failure Associated With These Conditions

Criteria for Instituting Mechanical Ventilation	Primary Type of Respiratory Failure
1. Apnea	Hypercapnic
2. Acute ventilatory failure	Respiratory failure
3. Impending ventilatory failure	
4. Severe refractory hypoxemia	Hypoxemic Respiratory failure

TABLE 11.10 Key Clinical Indicators of Hypercapnic Respiratory Failure (Ventilatory Failure)

Clinical Indicator*	Normal Value	Critical Value
Alveolar Ventilation		
$PaCO_2$ (acute change)	35–45 mm Hg	>50 mm Hg and rising
pH	7.35–7.45	<7.20
Lung Expansion		
Tidal volume (V_T)	5–8 mL/kg	<3–5 mL/kg
Respiratory rate (breaths/min)	12–20/min	>30/min, or <10/min
Muscle Strength		
Maximum inspiratory pressure (MIP, cm H_2O)	−80 to 100 cm H_2O	<−20 cm H_2O
Vital capacity (VC)	65–75 mL/kg	<10–15 mL/kg
Work of Breathing		
Minute ventilation ($\dot{V}E$)	5–6 L/min	>10 L/min
V_D/V_T (%)	25%–40%	>60%

*See a detailed discussion of these clinical indications for hypercapnic respiratory failure in Chapter 4, Pulmonary Function Assessment, and Chapter 5, Arterial Blood Gas Assessment.

TABLE 11.11 Key Clinical Indicators of Hypoxemic Respiratory Failure (Oxygenation Failure)

Clinical Indicator*	Normal Value	Critical Value
Oxygenation Status		
PaO_2 (mm Hg)	80–100	<60 on FIO_2 >0.50
$P(A-a)O_2$ on 100%	25–65	>350
PaO_2/PAO_2 ratio	0.75–0.95	<0.75
PaO_2/FIO_2 ratio	350–450	<200
$\dot{Q}_S/\dot{Q}_T$ (%)	<5	>20

*See a detailed discussion of these oxygen clinical indications in Chapter 6, Oxygenation Assessment.

need for other treatments of this disorder (Table 11.8). Table 11.9 presents the basic criteria for instituting mechanical ventilation and the primary type of respiratory failure associated with these conditions.

Prophylactic Ventilatory Support

In addition to the four standard primary criteria for mechanical ventilation, the decision to place the patient on ventilatory support may be based on prophylactic reasons. For example, **prophylactic ventilatory support** is sometimes provided to patients in postanesthesia and surgery recovery, particularly in patients with preexisting cardiopulmonary disease, who (especially while still sedated) are at high risk for postoperative complications such as atelectasis, aspiration pneumonia, or ARDS. In addition, prophylactic ventilatory support is often provided to nonsurgical patients who are high risk for pulmonary complications, such as hypercapnic respiratory failure or hypoxemic respiratory failure in COPD, pulmonary, fibrosis, and left articular failure. As discussed in the following section, noninvasive ventilation also belongs in this category of ventilatory support.

Key Clinical Indicators for Ventilatory Support in Hypercapnic and Hypoxemic Respiratory Failure

There are a variety of key clinical indicators (laboratory and bedside) that can be used to help establish the need for ventilatory support. In addition, these clinical indicators can be used to determine the primary type of respiratory failure and the ventilatory strategy that may be used to most safely and effectively ventilate the patient. Table 11.10 lists key clinical indicators for ventilatory support associated with hypercapnic respiratory failure. Table 11.11 provides key clinical indicators

associated with ventilatory support for hypoxemic respiratory failure.

Ventilatory Support Strategy

The selection of a ventilatory support strategy is based on the type of respiratory failure the patient demonstrates. For example, *hypoxemic respiratory failure* is treated with various oxygen therapy modalities to manage the patient's oxygenation status. Table 11.12 provides common oxygen treatment modalities for specific causes of hypoxemia.

By contrast, *hypercapnic respiratory failure* is treated with ventilatory support techniques to manage the patient's $PaCO_2$ levels and acid-base status. Both oxygen and ventilatory support modalities are used when the patient demonstrates both hypoxemic and hypercapnic respiratory failure (sometimes referred to as **Type III respiratory failure**). Depending on the clinical situation, either noninvasive ventilation or invasive

TABLE 11.12 Common Oxygen Treatment Modalities for Specific Causes of Hypoxemia

Cause of Hypoxemia	Treatment
Alveolar hypoventilation—examples: COPD Drug overdose	Ventilatory support—increased alveolar ventilation
Decreased ventilation/perfusion ratio—examples: COPD Asthma Pulmonary edema	Ventilatory support: Oxygen CPAP PEEP
Pulmonary shunting—examples: Pneumonia Atelectasis ARDS	Oxygen via: CPAP PEEP
Decreased barometric pressure High attitude	Oxygen Move to lower altitude

ARDS, Acute respiratory distress syndrome; *COPD*, chronic obstructive pulmonary disease; *CPAP*, continuous positive airway pressure; *PEEP*, positive end-expiratory pressure.

BOX 11.4 Benefits of Noninvasive Ventilation

- Avoids endotracheal intubation
- Reduces problems associated with intubation—for example, airway trauma, increased risk for aspiration, and nosocomial pneumonia
- Maximizes patient comfort
- Decreases mortality
- Increases alveolar ventilation
- Improves alveolar oxygen (PAO_2) and carbon dioxide ($PACO_2$) status
- Opens and/or prevents alveolar collapse
- Reduces the work of breathing
- Decreases oxygen consumption
- Decreases muscle fatigue

ventilation can be used as a ventilatory support strategy in all these types of respiratory failure.

Noninvasive Ventilation

Noninvasive ventilation (NIV) is defined as any mode of ventilatory support that does not require an invasive artificial airway (i.e., endotracheal tube or tracheostomy tube). As shown in Box 11.4, NIV has many benefits and is often the first choice for ventilatory support. NIV systems include **continuous positive airway pressure (CPAP) ventilation** delivered through a nasal or oral mask alone (which is a means to maintain or restore functional residual capacity) or in combination with any mode of pressure-limited or volume-limited ventilation. Both hypoxemic and hypercapnic types of respiratory failure can be managed effectively by NIV.

The primary indication for NIV is *hypercapnic respiratory failure* secondary to COPD exacerbation. NIV is also beneficial for a variety of other respiratory disorders when patient are able to protect their airway, including (1) asthma, (2) mild to moderate atelectasis, (3) community-acquired pneumonia, (4) cardiogenic pulmonary edema, (5) ARDS, (6) obesity-hypoventilation syndrome, and (7) neuromuscular diseases such as myasthenia gravis or Guillain-Barré syndrome.

Although NIV is a very safe and effective means of ventilatory support, it may be *poorly tolerated, contraindicated, or even harmful* in patients with (1) respiratory arrest, (2) cardiac arrest, (3) nonrespiratory organ failure (e.g., severe encephalopathy, severe gastrointestinal bleeding, or hemodynamic instability) (4) upper airway obstruction, (5) excessive or viscous airway secretions, (6) a poor ability to clear secretions, (7) an improperly fitting mask, (8) facial or head trauma or surgery, (9) profound refractory hypoxemia, (10) cardiovascular instability (e.g., hypotension, dysrhythmias, or acute myocardial infarction), (11) an inability to cooperate (e.g., impaired mental status, somnolence), (12) extreme obesity, or (13) the anticipation of a slowly resolving respiratory condition. In these cases, invasive ventilation is required.

Invasive Mechanical Ventilation

Invasive mechanical ventilation is defined as mechanical ventilation via an endotracheal or tracheostomy tube. Both hypoxemic and hypercapnic types of respiratory failure can be managed effectively by invasive mechanical ventilation. Mechanical ventilation protocols are discussed in the following sections.

Mechanical Ventilation Protocols

It is interesting to note that many medical centers have started their therapist-driven protocol (TDP) programs with a Mechanical Ventilation Protocol rather than with one of the relatively simple protocols described in Chapter 10, The Therapist-Driven Protocol Program (e.g., Oxygen Therapy Protocol, Airway Clearance Protocol, Lung Expansion Protocol, or Aerosolized Medical Protocol). The decision to proceed in this manner often appears to be based on humanistic, pathophysiologic, and economic grounds. Indeed, who could defend practices that are unnecessary (if not harmful), uncomfortable, and costly to patients requiring ventilator support?

Unquestionably, the high-technology, high-risk, high-visibility portion of respiratory therapy work is embedded in ventilator management. Much of the success of the TDP movement has occurred because of the dramatic ways in which standardized, data-driven algorithms have improved patient outcomes. Most dramatic reported outcomes include shortened ventilator weaning times, reduction of nosocomial infections, and reduced complications associated with mechanical ventilation (e.g., barotrauma).

Although most Mechanical Ventilation Protocols require the respiratory therapist to select a ventilator mode on the basis of specific patient needs, it is not the intent of this textbook to fully review or discuss the various types, modes, and weaning strategies. Table 11.13, however, does provide an overview of common ventilatory management strategies and good starting points used to treat specific pulmonary disorders.

TABLE 11.13 Common Ventilatory Management Strategies Used to Treat Specific Disorders (Good Starting Points)

Disorder	Disease Characteristics	Ventilator Mode	Tidal Volume and Respiratory Rate	Flow Rate	I/E Ratio	FIO₂	General Goals and/or Concerns
Normal lung mechanics	Normal compliance and airway resistance	Volume ventilation in the AC or SIMV mode	4–8 mL/kg of ideal body weight	60–80 L/min	1:2	Low to moderate	Care to ensure plateau pressure of ≤30 cm H_2O.
But patient has apnea (e.g., drug overdose or abdominal surgery)		or pressure ventilation—either PRVC or PC	10–12 breaths/min or slower rates (6–10 breaths/min) when SIMV mode is used				Small tidal volumes (<7 mL/kg) should be avoided, because atelectasis can develop.
Chronic obstructive pulmonary disease (e.g., chronic bronchitis or emphysema)	High lung compliance and high airway resistance	Volume ventilation in the AC or SIMV mode	Good starting point: 4–8 mL/kg and a rate of 10–12 breaths/min	60–100 L/min	1:4	Low to moderate	Air trapping and auto-PEEP can occur when expiratory time is too short. The preferred method of managing auto-PEEP is to increase expiratory time.
		or pressure ventilation—either PRVC or PC	Good starting point: (8–10 mL/kg) and slightly slower rate (8–10 breaths/min) with increased flow rates to allow adequate expiratory time				In severe cases the development of auto-PEEP may be inevitable. With controlled ventilation, a small amount of PEEP to offset auto-PEEP may be cautiously applied.
		Noninvasive positive pressure ventilation (NPPV) by nasal or full face mask is a good alternative during acute exacerbation.					Inspiratory flow up to 100 L/min may be helpful in decreasing inspiratory time and increasing expiratory time.
							Tidal volume or rate may be decreased to reduce inspiratory and increase expiratory time.
							Care to avoid overventilation in COPD patients with chronically high $PaCO_2$ levels

TABLE 11.13 Common Ventilatory Management Strategies Used to Treat Specific Disorders (Good Starting Points)—cont'd

Disorder	Disease Characteristics	Ventilator Mode	Tidal Volume and Respiratory Rate	Flow Rate	I/E Ratio	FIO$_2$	General Goals and/or Concerns
Acute asthmatic episode	High airway resistance (bronchospasm and excessive thick airway secretions)	The SIMV mode is recommended to avoid patient triggering at an increased rate—leading to a decrease in expiratory time and further air trapping.	Good starting point: 8–4 to 8 mL/kg and rate of 10–12 breaths/min When air trapping is extensive, a lower tidal volume (5–6 mL/kg) and slower rate may be required.	60 L/min	1:2 or 1:3	Start at 100% and titrate downward as pulse oximetry findings and arterial blood gas values permit.	In severe cases the development of auto-PEEP may be inevitable. With controlled ventilation, a small amount of PEEP to offset auto-PEEP may be cautiously applied.
Acute respiratory distress syndrome	Diffuse, uneven alveolar injury	Volume ventilation in the AC or SIMV mode or pressure ventilation—either PRVC or PC	Typically started at low tidal volumes and higher respiratory rate. Initial tidal volume set at 8 mL/kg and adjusted downward to 6 mL/kg. May be as low as 4 mL/kg. Respiratory rates as high as 35 breaths/min may be required.	60–80 L/min	1:1 or 1:2. Do what is necessary to meet a rapid respiratory rate.	FIO$_2$ less than 0.6 if possible.	The goal is to limit transpulmonary pressure and the resultant barotrauma caused by overdistending portions of the lungs. Maintaining a plateau pressure of 30 cm H$_2$O or less is preferred. PEEP is usually required with a low tidal volume to prevent atelectasis. The PaCO$_2$ may be allowed to increase (**permissive hypercapnia**). The hypercapnia is not a therapeutic goal, it is a final tradeoff and may be accepted as a lung protective strategy when lower airway pressures are necessary.
Postoperative ventilatory support (e.g., coronary artery bypass surgery, heart valve and replacement)	Often normal compliance and airway resistance	SIMV with pressure support or AC volume ventilation are acceptable modes or pressure ventilation—either PRVC or PC	Good starting point: 4–8 mL/kg and a rate of 10–12 breaths/min	60 L/min	1:2	Low to moderate	PEEP or CPAP of 3–5 cm H$_2$O may be applied to offset the development of atelectasis.
Neuromuscular disorders (e.g., myasthenia gravis or Guillain-Barré syndrome)	Normal compliance and airway resistance	Volume ventilation in the AC or SIMV mode or pressure ventilation—either PRVC or PC	Good starting point: 4–8 mL/kg and a rate of 10–12 breaths/min	60 L/min	1:2	Low to moderate	PEEP of 3–5 cm H$_2$O may be applied to offset the development of atelectasis.

AC, Assist-control; *breaths/min,* breaths per minute; *CPAP,* continuous positive airway pressure; *PC,* pressure control; *PEEP,* positive end-expiratory pressure; *PRVC,* pressure-regulated volume control; *SIMV,* synchronized intermittent mandatory ventilation.

Protocol 11.1 provides a good example of a Ventilator Initiation and Management Protocol. Protocol 11.2 illustrates an example of a Ventilator Weaning Protocol.[6]

Mechanical Ventilation Discontinuation (Weaning)

Because of the many hazards and complications associated with mechanical ventilation, the patient should be weaned from the ventilator as soon as possible. Once the reason for ventilatory support has been resolved, the vast majority of patients on ventilators can be removed from the ventilator quickly and easily. However, about 15% to 20% of ventilated patients need a more systematic approach to discontinuing the ventilatory support. About 5% require days to weeks to be weaned from mechanical ventilation. Less than 1% are ultimately proven to be *ventilator-dependent* or "unweanable" patients.

Conditions that prolong ventilatory-dependence include abnormal respiratory, cardiovascular, neurologic, or psychologic factors. Thus before ventilator weaning can be initiated, the respiratory therapist must first determine if any of these factors are present—that is, conditions that could lead to an unsuccessful attempt. The bottom line is this: For the best possibility of a successful ventilator weaning outcome, the respiratory therapist must fully assess and confirm that the patient has an acceptable balance between ventilatory demands and ventilatory muscle capabilities.

Fig. 11.5 again illustrates how the need for ventilatory support depends on the critical balance between the patient's ventilatory muscle demands (i.e., workloads) and the patient's ventilatory muscle capabilities. For an additional description and visual reinforcement of the important relationship between patient's ventilatory muscle demands and the patient's ventilatory muscle capabilities, see the patient's increased "need-to-breathe" and the patient's actual "capability-to-breathe" (see Fig. 3.1).

Clinical Indicators for the Readiness of Ventilator Discontinuance

Once the original reason for placing the patient on the ventilator has been resolved, there are a number of bedside studies that can be used to help determine the patient's readiness to be weaned from the ventilator (Table 11.14). It should be strongly stressed, however, that none of the currently used indices is

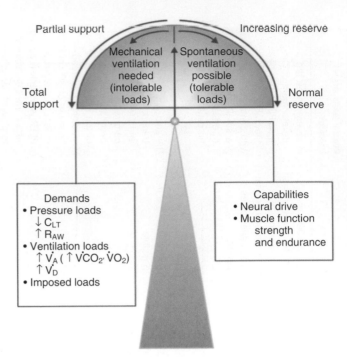

C_{LT} = total lung compliance

FIGURE 11.5 Ventilatory failure and the need for ventilator support. (Modified from MacIntyre, N. R. [1995]. Respiratory factors in weaning from mechanical ventilatory support. *Respiratory Care 40*, 244-259.)

100% reliable in confirming the patient's readiness for a successful ventilator weaning attempt. Good clinical judgement and common sense also must be added to the mix. That said, common tools used to assess the patient's readiness for ventilator weaning include the arterial oxygen tension to fractional concentration of oxygen ratio (PaO_2/FIO_2 ratio), the alveolar-to-arterial partial pressure of oxygen difference [$P(A-a)O_2$], the **maximum inspiratory pressure (MIP)**, the airway occlusion pressure at 0.1 second ($P_{0.1}$), the $P_{0.1}$/MIP ratio, the vital capacity (VC), spontaneous minute ventilation (VEsp), maximum voluntary ventilation (MVV), the **pressure time index (PTI)**,[7] and the **rapid shallow breathing index (RSBI)**.[8] The *cuff-leak test* is another semiquantitative measure of readiness to discontinue ventilator support. If the patient can breathe around a deflated endotracheal tub cuff, he or she probably will be able to breathe even easier once it is removed.

---

[6]The authors would like to thank the Respiratory Care Department at the Kettering Health Network (KHN), in Dayton, Ohio, for providing their Ventilator Initiation, Management, and Weaning Protocols. In addition, the authors ask the reader to note a difference in the Protocols presented in this chapter compared with earlier editions of this volume. Simple branching logic algorithms, as seen in the Protocols in Chapter 10, The Therapist-Driven Protocol Program, are no longer used. They are replaced by a series of steps, which follow one on the other, recycling back and forth between steps if needed. Some steps in these protocols are missing because there is *no* precise descriptive significant ventilator management activities in these sections that are not disease-specific. Kettering Health Network (KHN) maintains disease-specific critical care and ventilator care management competencies required for therapists treating patients with end-stage COPD, severe pneumonia, aspiration pneumonia, congestive heart failure/cardiogenic pulmonary edema, ARDS and VILI/VALI (see VILI/VALI discussion on page 174).

[7]The pressure time index (PTI) is a measure of strength and endurance combined into one value. It combines the strength measurement of esophageal pressure and the maximum inspiratory pressure with the endurance value of respiratory time fraction. The normal range is 0.5 to 1.2. Criteria for successful ventilator weaning are less than 0.15 to 0.18.

[8]The rapid shallow breathing index (RSBI) is the ratio of the spontaneous respiratory frequency (f) to tidal volume (V_T) and is calculated as follows (the RSBI is also abbreviated as f/V_T):

$$RSBI = f \ (breaths/min)/V_T \ (L)$$

The normal range is 60 to 90 breaths/min per liter. The successful discontinuance from mechanical ventilation is more likely to occur when the RSBI is less than 105 breaths/min per liter within the first minute of a spontaneous breathing trial.

VENTILATOR INITIATION AND MANAGEMENT PROTOCOL

Purpose:
The respiratory therapist will use the following protocol to determine the most appropriate ventilator mode types and settings to maintain and manage oxygenation, ventilation, ventilator-patient synchrony, safety, and comfort for patients who meet acceptable indications for mechanical ventilation.

Sequential Approach:

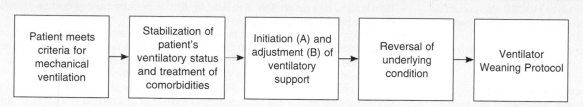

Patient meets criteria for mechanical ventilation → Stabilization of patient's ventilatory status and treatment of comorbidities → Initiation (A) and adjustment (B) of ventilatory support → Reversal of underlying condition → Ventilator Weaning Protocol

---

STEP 1: Patient meets criteria for mechanical ventilation

1. Acute respiratory failure (hypoxic/hypercapnic)
2. Apnea or impending respiratory failure
3. Acute exacerbation of COPD or other pulmonary disease
4. Neuromuscular disease with alveolar hypoventilation
5. Cardiac or respiratory arrest
6. Postoperative patients requiring ongoing sedation

Key Point(s):

1. STEP 1
1. Patient meets criteria for mechanical ventilation as above.
2. Obtain physician orders for initiation of mechanical ventilation

STEP 1
1. Criteria as previously
2. Ensure physician orders are entered and correct for initiation of mechanical ventilation and that they reflect attending physician's preferences for management, techniques if any

---

2. STEP 2
Not addressed in this Protocol

STEP 2
NA

---

3. STEP 3A
Initiation of ventilator support
Selection of ventilator breath delivery

TYPE/TARGET:
Should be based on patient needs and pathophysiology. In addition to ventilation and oxygenation needs, patient comfort and ventilator synchrony should also be optimized.

STEP 3A
- Volume control ventilation (VCV): Tidal volume (V_T) and flow are set parameters and remain constant. Because VCV uses a constant flow, it has the potential to produce an uneven distribution of gas. The constant flow pattern may cause patient-ventilator asynchrony because the patient cannot control flow rate to meet needs. Monitored peak pressure.
- Pressure control ventilation (PCV): Inspiratory pressure and I-time are set parameters and remain constant. PCV uses a rapidly decelerating flow pattern, which may provide a more even gas distribution and may promote better patient-ventilator synchrony. Monitor V_T closely, because of its variability.
- Dual control ventilators (VC+, AF, and PRVC): Volume and I-time are set parameters. Volume is delivered at lowest pressure possible and is pressure regulated. Flow rapidly decelerates and may provide a more even gas distribution and patient-ventilator synchrony.
- Spontaneous breath types (PAV+, CPAP, MMV) are generally not considered in ventilator initiation, but typically used in the liberation or weaning phase.

PROTOCOL 11.1 *Continued on page 170*

Selection of Ventilator MODES:
Selection of MODES also should be based on patient's needs when initiating mechanical ventilation. Patient comfort and synchrony should be considered, to optimize compliance with therapy.

Selection of SETTINGS of ventilator parameters in various modes.

- See Menu I for selection of MODES.
- Tidal volume (V_T) set on IBW. 6 to 8 mL/kg IBW is preferred and should be adjusted to keep the plateau pressure <30 cm H_2O.
- Respiratory rate (RR) initially set between 12 and 20 breaths per minute and adjusted to keep minute ventilation (MV) <10 lpm. When setting in bi-level, ≤18 bpm is preferred. In APRV, no higher than 12 bpm is preferred, so as to encourage spontaneous respirations and to avoid unwanted gas trapping and excessive intrathoracic pressures.
- Positive end-expiratory pressure (PEEP): Note frequency of this ancillary setting in various Modes (see Menu I). Initial settings around 5 cm H_2O and titrated in 2 cm H_2O. *An optimal PEEP study is highly recommended.* Ideally used in cases of pneumonia, atelectasis, ARDS, and other situations in which patients are at risk for loss of FRC. In such cases, PEEP is generally set 2 to 4 cm H_2O above the lower inflection point on the pressure volume curve.
- In patients with refractory hypoxemia, the **ARDSnet*** oxygen-sparing algorithm is to be followed.

ARDSNET* PEEP/FIO$_2$ Titration Scale

Lower PEEP/Higher FIO$_2$

FIO$_2$	0.3	0.4	0.4	0.5	0.5	0.6	0.7	0.7	0.8	0.9	0.9	0.9	0.9	1.0
PEEP	5	5	8	8	10	10	10	12	14	14	14	16	18	18–24

Higher PEEP/Lower FIO$_2$

FIO$_2$	0.3	0.3	0.3	0.3	0.3	0.4	0.4	0.5	0.5	0.5	0.8	0.8	0.9	1.0
PEEP	5	8	10	12	14	14	16	16	18	20	22	22	22	24

- Other important ventilator settings: See MENU II when manipulating the follow settings: PF, PS, IT, Pressure Rise Time/Ramp, and Trigger Sensitivity.

STEP 3B Adjustment of ventilatory support:
1. Obtain plateau pressure to determine resistance and compliance measurements.
2. Obtain ABG 30 minutes after placing patient on ventilator.

STEP 3B
1. Plateau pressure: To monitor resistance and compliance changes, baseline P_{plat} measurements need to be obtained and documented after ventilator initiation and no less than once a shift thereafter. Ideally, P_{plat} is kept at ≤30 cm H_2O.
2. After accessing the ABG results, if indicated, determine target PaCO$_2$ and calculate target MV. *NOTE: Caution must be used in selecting ventilator settings in patients with chronic hypercapnia.*
- Consider use of permissive hypercapnia.
- Recalculate P(A-a)O$_2$ to see if $\dot{V}/\dot{Q}$ ratio has changed significantly since placing the patient on the ventilator.
- Ensure that the new PaO$_2$ is not excessive (>80 mm Hg) or lower than desired (<55 mm Hg).

*see ARDSnet in Chapter 28

PROTOCOL 11.1 *Continued on page 171*

STEP 4
Not addressed in this Protocol.

STEP 4
Some disease-specific treatment protocols are available in various hospital departments. Use of ventilator graphics and appropriate humidification techniques (see specific departmental protocols) is mandated.

STEPS 5 and 6
Not addressed in this Protocol

STEPS 5 and 6
See Protocol 11.2.

MENU I (Protocol 11.1)

MODE	Parameter(s) Selected	Patient Initiated (Yes or No)	Additional Needs	Benefits and Hazards
AC or CMV	Rate and V_T or IP	No	PEEP to maintain/ restore FRC	Prolonged AC can lead to muscle atrophy
SIMV	Rate and V_T or IP	Yes: TC or PS supported	PEEP	Spontaneous breathing is allowed, may lead to ventilator asynchrony
Bi-level	Incorporates two levels of PEEP (P_H and P_L) T_H and T_L, RR, I-time, I/E	Yes	Can support spontaneous breaths with PS or TC	Permits alveolar recruitment
Airway pressure release ventilation (APRV)	Same as bi-level automatically incorporates two levels of PEEP (P_H and P_L)	Yes	Can be supported by PS or TC	Gas trapping and high intrathoracic pressures if RR >12
Proportional assist ventilation + (PAV+)	Automatically calculates WOB; provides a set portion of WOB for ventilatory needs	Yes	Requires use of ventilator graphics	—
Mandatory minute ventilation (MMV)	Set target $\dot{V}E$, RR and VT set to match target $\dot{V}E$	Yes	PEEP	—
Volume support (VS)	Target V_T pressures will be adjusted to meet target	Yes	PEEP	—
Pressure support (PS) or (CPAP)	Operating pressure	Yes	PEEP	—

MENU II (Protocol 11.1)

Initial Ventilator Settings in Various Modes

- *Peak flow (PF):* When VCV is used, the PF should be set to achieve an appropriate I/E ratio for the patient's condition and to achieve patient-ventilator synchrony. Caution must be used in setting PF because flow that is too slow can produce a sensation of air hunger in the patient, and a PF that is too excessive can produce airway turbulence and create discomfort/asynchrony. *NOTE:* It is strongly advised to always choose breath types that allow *patient control* of PF rates to promote optimal patient-ventilator synchrony.
- *Pressure support (PS):* If PS is used when supporting spontaneous breaths, PS should be set for the patient to achieve tidal volumes of 5 to 6 mL/kg IBW. If used with bi-level, caution must be taken when setting PS to achieve these spontaneous volumes at PEEP high because volumes may be excessive at PEEP low and result in increased intrathoracic pressures and pulmonary overdistention. Recent research suggests using TC in bi-level is a better option than PS.
- *Inspiratory time (IT):* Used in pressure-regulated breath types and generally titrated to optimize gas exchange longer. IT is preferred in refractory hypoxemia; shorter IT is preferred in patients with unwanted intrinsic PEEP or with COPD. ITs resulting in inverse I/E ratios require attending physician affirmation. Peek and plateau pressure monitoring is important.
- *Pressure rise time (REMP):* Rise time refers to the time required to reach pressure target, peak inspiratory flow, or transition from PEEP high to PEEP low. Rise time titration with ramping may help with patient-ventilator asynchrony.
- *Trigger sensitivity:* Sensitivity may be set for pressure or flow, appropriate so as to maximize patient's synchrony and inspiratory efforts.

PROTOCOL 11.1

VENTILATOR WEANING PROTOCOL

Purpose

This protocol will be used to facilitate timely liberation from mechanical ventilation using the **spontaneous breathing trial (SBT)** and the prolonged spontaneous breathing trial (SPBT). *NOTE: The RCP is to ensure the nurse has initiated an SBT before weaning between 0500 and 0900 each morning.*

Key Point(s):

STEP 1: *Assess* the following criteria. Patient must meet *all* criteria to advance to Step 2, unless protocol override from the physician.
- Determine pass/fail

1. Weaning trial criteria
   - Resolution of acute phase of disease and comorbidities (if possible)
   - PO_2/FIO_2 >150 mm Hg with FIO_2 <0.8
   - BP and hemodynamic status stable off vasopressors if possible
   - HR >50 and <130 bpm, temperature (core) <38°C
   - pH >7.25 in last 24 hours
   - Cough/gag reflex present
   - Able to initiate spontaneous respiration
   - RASS (see Table 11.14) at −1 or −2 unless otherwise approved by physician
   - Hemoglobin >7.0 g/dL

   If patient passes Step 1, proceed to Step 2

STEP 2: Spontaneous breathing trial
- Obtain the patient parameters in the CPAP/PS mode after 5 minutes to determine readiness for PSBT trial.
- Determine pass/fail

2. Patient is placed on CPAP ≤8 with pressure support 5 cm H_2O for duration of 5 minutes.

   Parameter Goals:
   - MV <10 lpm
   - V_T target >5 mL/kg IBW
   - RR <30 breaths/min
   - RSBI <100 (Rate ÷ V_T in liters)
   - SpO_2 greater ≥92%
   - Signs of distress must be absent

   If patient passes Step 2, proceed to Step 3

   NOTE: All failures will be reassessed in 3 hours. Second failure will be reassessed in 24 hours.

PROTOCOL 11.2 *Continued on page 172*

Additional criteria used to evaluate the patient's readiness to be weaned from the ventilator include the patient's (1) cardiovascular stability (e.g., heart rate, blood pressure, cardiac output, and cardiac rhythms), (2) psychologic condition (e.g., fear, anxiety, and stress), and (3) central nervous system functions (e.g., stable ventilatory drive, adequate secretion clearance [i.e., coughing, deep breathing, or gag reflex and swallowing]), and (4) level of alertness and agitation before weaning. Table 11.15 shows the *Richmond Agitation-Sedation Scale (RASS)*, which is a commonly used scale for measuring the agitation or sedation level of the patient, is incorporated in Protocol 11.2.[9]

Once it has been determined that a ventilation weaning attempt should be started, most experts[10] agree that one (or a sequence of more than one) of the following three basic methods for discontinuing ventilatory support should be implemented:

- Spontaneous breathing trials (SBT) with or without CPAP
- Synchronized **intermittent mandatory ventilation** (SIMV)
- Pressure support ventilation (PSV)

Other techniques that may enhance the patient's discontinuance from mechanical ventilation include *volume-support ventilation (VSV)*, **adaptive support ventilation (ASV)**, and continuous positive airway pressure (CPAP). Protocol 11.2 provides an example of a Ventilator Weaning Protocol.

Ventilator Graphics

Once the selection of a ventilatory support strategy has been determined, the matching of the various ventilator parameters to the patient's specific ventilatory needs often can be a challenge. The reality is this: Mechanical ventilators—for all their strengths and virtues—only do what they are programmed to do. Thus the respiratory therapist must continually monitor and assess **patient-ventilator interaction** and, importantly, routinely determine if the ventilator settings are allowing a good, or poor, patient-ventilator interaction. A therapeutically

---

[9]Other scales used to measure the patient's alertness include the Ramsay scale, the Agitation-Sedation Scale, and the COMFORT scale for pediatric patients.

[10]American College of Chest Physicians (ACCP), American Association for Respiratory Care (AARC), and the Society of Critical Care Medicine (SCCM) Evidence-Based Weaning Guidelines Taskforce.

STEP 3A:

1. Prolonged spontaneous breathing trial (PSBT). Spontaneous mode to be in one of the following: Tube compensation (TC), PS 5 to 6, PAV+, or T-piece adapter with oxygen.

Discontinuation Criteria Include:

a. Hemodynamic stability
b. Change in mental status
c. Onset or worsening of discomfort
d. Diaphoresis
e. Signs of increased shortness of breath (SOB)
f. Acceptable RSBI
g. Negative inspiratory pressure (NIP)
h. ABG, if indicated/ordered
• Determine pass/fail:

All criteria must be within acceptable parameters before extubation. If goals are not met, consider other respiratory protocols and implement as indicated.

2. Extubate the patient.

3. Follow results of postextubation ABG, if drawn.

STEP 3A. PSBT guidelines:

1. Place patient in spontaneous mode, or T-piece or PAV+ for a minimum of 30 minutes.

Parameter goals:

• Minute volume <10 lpm
• V_T ≥5 mL/kg IBW
• RR <30
• RSBI <100
• SpO_2 ≥91%
• HR <120

   a. As defined in Step 1
   e. No use of accessory muscles, thoracoabdominal paradox
   f. RSBI <100. *NOTE:* RSBI research was conducted using T-piece adapters and results obtained with no ventilator support. If RSBI is in the higher range on pressure-supported breaths, it may be beneficial to measure on TC to ensure the most accurate assessment of patient status.
   g. NIP ≥ –20 cm H_2O
   h. pH >7.32, $PaCO_2$ increased <10 mm Hg above pretrial baseline; SpO_2 ≥91%

2. If patient passes, check for an extubation order. Before extubation, an airway leak test is strongly recommended to check for airway patency. To perform, deflate cuff on airway and observe for audible air leak and large loss of V_T. If minimal or no leak exists, document and notify attending physician of findings.
   • If patient fails, support with mode of ventilation that will offload muscles.

3. Other protocols may be indicated to either enhance the weaning process or treat the patient effectively after extubation. Please refer to KHN Respiratory Protocols on the Cardiopulmonary intranet site.

4. Extubation is only to be completed with a physician order. Perform cuff leak test before extubating

5. Patient must be assessed using Respiratory Protocol Assessment within 1 hour of extubation to determine postextubation respiratory needs (refer to RP-6 on Cardiopulmonary intranet for details of assessment).

Richmond Agitation-Sedation Scale (RASS)* (see Table 11.14)

Score Term Description
• +4 Combative. Overtly combative, violent, immediate danger to staff
• +3 Very agitated. Pulls or removes tube(s) or catheter(s); aggressive
• +2 Agitated. Frequent nonpurposeful movement, fights ventilator
• +1 Restless. Anxious but movements not aggressively vigorous
• 0 Alert and calm
• –1 Drowsy, not fully alert, but has sustained awakening (eye-opening/eye contact) for *voice* (>10 seconds)
• –2 Light sedation, briefly awakens with eye contact to voice (<10 seconds)
• –3 Moderate sedation, movement or eye opening to voice (but no eye contact)
• –4 Deep sedation, no response to voice, but movement or eye opening to physical stimulation (e.g., sternal rub or shaking of upper body)
• –5 Unarousable, no response to *voice* or *physical stimulation*

PROTOCOL 11.2

Does expiratory flow curve return to baseline?

A. Presence of Auto-PEEP Because of a Variable Airway Obstruction: Measure and evaluate auto-PEEP. Does the patient need to be suctioned? Is the inspiratory flow adequate for the rate and tidal volume? Is there bronchospasm present? Is there underlying lung disease present?

Does shape of inspiratory curve match that selected on the ventilator?

B. Inadequate Inspiratory Flow Rate: Increase flow rate or consider changing flow pattern. Consider changing mandatory breath type to pressure control.

Is expiratory flow curve not "square"?

C. Fixed Airway Obstruction: Is the endotracheal tube size appropriate? Is the patient's HME occluded? Change expiratory filter or evaluate need for a larger endotracheal/tracheostomy tube.

Is the "trigger" (flow or pressure) matched with an immediate rise in flow? Does the pressure drop (flow change) match the sensitivity?

D. Ventilator Sensitivity Inadequate: Increase driving pressure if possible. Evaluate function of inspiratory gas source. Evaluate ventilator for proper function of sensitivity setting. Consider changing ventilator modes.

Does baseline PEEP match the ventilator setting? Does the tidal volume waveform return to baseline?

Correct problem, evaluate prior step for correction of irregular waveform.

Does the peak of the tidal volume graphic match the ventilator setting?

E. Potential Leak in Ventilator Circuit: Check integrity of cuff on artificial airway. Check integrity of ventilator circuit. Investigate and correct.

Does PV loop look "ideal"?

F. Evaluate PV Loop:
- Has the loop become more "horizontal" (loss of compliance) since previous evaluations? Evaluate for optimal PEEP setting.
- Does the waveform have a "duckbill" shape on the right representing hyperinflation? Consider decreasing tidal volume.
- Is there an increase in airway resistance represented by a "wide" PV loop? Consider bronchodilator therapy.

Ventilator is properly set.

---

effective and comfortable patient-ventilator interaction is always the goal.

Fortunately, the visual graphics that are now available on mechanical ventilators provide the respiratory therapist with a wealth of important and helpful information. For example, the pressure-volume and flow-volume loops are especially beneficial in assessing the patient's work of breathing (WOB), alveolar overdistention, lung compliance, airway/system resistance, delayed or premature ventilator cycling, or inadequate inspiratory efforts to trigger a ventilator breath. Ventilator graphics are useful in the detection of excessive secretions in the airway and the patient's response to bronchodilator therapy (problems of airway resistance) and problems related to worsening lung compliance. Fig. 11.6 illustrates the ventilator graphic display of normal airway expiratory resistance, high expiratory resistance (and prolonged expiration), and shortened expiratory time, which worsens auto-PEEP.

Ventilator Hazards

Barotrauma and Volutrauma

Although mechanical ventilators provide important and lifesaving support to the patient, they can be very dangerous. Care must be taken to set all the ventilator parameters to achieve the best and, importantly, the "safest" patient-ventilator interaction possible. This is because certain ventilator settings can quickly lead to specific lung injuries referred to as **ventilator-induced lung injury (VILI)** or **ventilator-associated lung injury (VALI)**. The term *VILI* is used when it can be proved the mechanical ventilation caused the acute lung injury. In contrast, the term *VALI* is used when the causative relationship cannot be verified. In most clinical situations, the term VALI is the best term because it is virtually impossible to prove the cause of a lung injury outside the research laboratory.

The histologic changes associated with VALI are proportional to the duration and magnitude of the volume and

TABLE 11.14 Clinical Indicators Used to Predict Readiness for Ventilator Discontinuance

Clinical Indicator	Criterion for Ventilator Discontinuance
Ventilation	
pH	≤7.35
$PaCO_2$	<50 mm Hg
Oxygenation	
PaO_2 (mm Hg)	≥60%
SaO_2	>90%
SvO_2	≥60%
$P(A-a)O_2$ on 100% oxygen	<350
PaO_2/PAO_2 ratio	<0.75
PaO_2/FIO_2 ratio	<200
$\dot{Q}_s/\dot{Q}_T$ (% shunt)	<15%–20%
FIO_2	≤0.40–0.50
PEEP	≤5–8 cm H_2O
Ventilation Mechanics	
Respiratory rate (f)	12–30 (breaths/min)
Tidal volume (V_T)	>5 mL/kg
Vital capacity (VC)	>10–15 mL/kg
Static lung compliance (CL)	>25 mL/cm H_2O
Minute ventilation (V_E)	<10 L/min
Deadspace to tidal volume ratio (V_D/V_T)	<0.55–0.60
Airway resistance (R_{aw})	<15 cm H_2O/L/s
Rapid shallow breathing index (RSBI)	<105
Respiratory Muscle Strength	
Airway occlusion pressure ($P_{0.1}$)	<6
Maximum inspiratory pressure (MIP)	<−20 to −30 cm H_2O
$P_{0.1}$/MIP	<0.30
Pressure time index (PTI)	<0.15–0.18
Maximum voluntary ventilation (MVV)	>20 L/min (>2 × V_E)
Cardiovascular Stability	
Heart rate	<60 or >120
Blood pressure	<90/60 or >180/110
Cardiac index	<2.1
Cardiac rhythm	Tachycardia, bradycardia, multiple premature ventricular contractions, heart block
Hemoglobin	Anemia, <10 g%
Level of Alertness or Agitation	
Richmond Agitation-Sedation Scale (RASS)	Zero is ideal (see Protocol 11.2)
Psychologic Factors	
Fear, anxiety, and stress	Low is ideal

TABLE 11.15 The Richmond Agitation-Sedation Scale

Score	Term	Description
+4	Combative	Overtly combative or violent; immediate danger to staff
+3	Very agitated	Pulls on or removes tube(s) or catheter(s) or has aggressive behavior toward staff
+2	Agitated	Frequent nonpurposeful movement or patient-ventilator dyssynchrony
+1	Restless	Anxious or apprehensive but movements not aggressive or vigorous
0	Alert and calm	Spontaneously pays attention to caregiver
−1	Drowsy	Not fully alert, but has sustained (>10 seconds) awakening, with eye contact, to voice
−2	Light sedation	Briefly (<10 seconds) awakens with eye contact to voice
−3	Moderate sedation	Any movement (but no eye contact) to voice
−4	Deep sedation	No response to voice, but any movement to physical stimulation
−5	Unarousable	No response to voice or physical stimulation

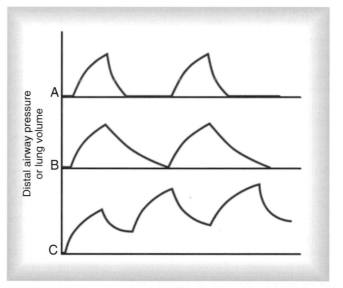

FIGURE 11.6. Causes of auto-PEEP. (A) When airway resistance is normal and expiratory time is long enough, distal airway pressure and lung volume return to normal after a positive pressure breath. (B) High expiratory resistance prolongs exhalation to the point at which air-trapping begins and causes auto-PEEP. (C) Shortening the expiratory time aggravates the problem and worsens auto-PEEP. (Modified from Benson, M. S., Pierson, D. J. [1988]. Auto-PEEP during mechanical ventilation of adults. *Respiratory Care 33,* 557.)

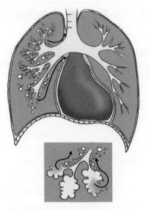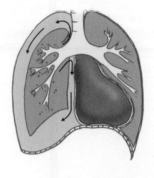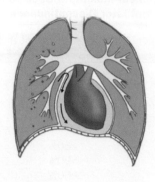

A Interstitial emphysema   B Pneumothorax   C Pneumopericardium

FIGURE 11.7. Barotrauma. (Modified from Korones, S. B. [1986]. *High-risk newborn infants* [4th ed.]. St. Louis, Mosby.)

pressures used in mechanical ventilation. The most common forms of VALI are *barotrauma* and *volutrauma*. **Barotrauma** is defined as the overexpansion of the alveolar structure (referred to as *alveolar strain*), alveolar rupture, and air leakage caused by high ventilator volumes and pressures. Other possible causes of baroatrauma include high ventilator rates (frequencies), high inspiratory flow rates, and inverse I/E ratios. Clinical examples of barotrauma include interstitial emphysema, emphysema, pneumothorax, pneumopericardium (Fig. 11.7).

Note that this listing of VALI "causes" does *not* include oxygen toxicity, which is often confused with VILI/VALI, and ARDS, a diagnosis most accurately based on its cellular morphology.

Similar to barotrauma, **volutrauma** is caused by high ventilator pressures and volumes, but in the case of volutrauma, alveolar rupture does not occur. Volutrauma is described as the result of microscopic release of alveolar-capillary membrane inflammatory mediators (e.g., cytokines, complement, prostanoids, and leukotrines) caused by high lung volumes and pressures. The released mediators in turn lead to increased alveolar-capillary permeability, pulmonary edema, and impaired transmembrane oxygen delivery. Ventilator patients who demonstrate poor ventilator-patient synchrony, declining lung compliance, increased pulmonary shunting, falling PaO_2/PAO_2 ratios, and an increased WOB may all be suffering from VALI.

Studies have suggested that ventilator plateau pressures (P_{plat}) is the most reliable single measurement to assess the risk for barotrauma in ventilated patients. Monitoring of peak airway pressures is also helpful, especially in patients in whom pulmonary compliance is a problem.

Lung Protective Strategies

The generally accepted **lung protective strategies** to avoid and treat VALI are low tidal volumes, low peak and plateau pressures, and permissive hypercapnia. A good example of this ventilation strategy can be reviewed under the General Management section in Chapter 28, Acute Respiratory Distress Syndrome. The use of NIV before, during, and after intubation makes good physiologic sense and in selected cases is definitely

---

BOX 11.5 Protective Lung Strategies—Preventive and Therapeutic*

Ventilator Strategies
- Ventilator settings
  - Low tidal volumes
  - Low inspiratory flow rate
  - Avoid spontaneous breathing as much as possible
  - Early use of assisted breathing techniques
- Noninvasive ventilation (NIV)
- **Neurally Adjusted Ventilatory Assist (NAVA)**
- Use of "best PEEP" based on detrimental PEEP titration
- Rigorous use of ventilator graphics
- Consider use of chest computed tomography and ultrasound

Other Techniques and Strategies
- High-frequency ventilation
- **Prone positioning** (controversial).
  - Use if PaO_2/FIO_2 <150 or best PEEP >10 cm H_2O
- Permissive hypercapnia
- Careful control of fluid therapy/monitor central venous pressure
- Careful early use of sedation and paralysis
- Use of low-dose corticosteroids early and late

Data from Gutierrez TM, Pelosi P, Rocco PRM: Ventilator-induced lung injury, *Eur Respir Mon* 55: 1–18, 2012.
*Best modes/modalities still not agreed upon.

---

helpful. Box 11.5 provides an overview of common lung protective strategies.

Ventilator Malfunctions

Finally, an important hazard of mechanical ventilation is ventilator malfunction—problems with the ventilator itself. Although this is rare, ventilator malfunction is a possibility and always should be under the respiratory therapist's surveillance. Suspect ventilators should be switched out immediately.

Charting the Progress of Ventilated Patients

The sicker the patient, the more carefully done must be the charting of the patient's progress or lack of it. Box 11.6 lists some areas in which the Protocol Therapist may wish to add terms like "Doing Well" or "Not Doing Well" to the Assessment portion of his Progress Note. Items that appear in such an assessment will obviously call for up-regulation, down-regulation, or change of the patient's respiratory care program, and use of such terms is thus strongly encouraged.

BOX 11.6 Status Reporting in Ventilated Patients
Items Worth Reporting in the Assessment Portion of Progress Notes

"Doing Well"	"Not Doing Well"
Decreased WOB	Increased WOB
Decreased dyspnea	Increased dyspnea
Improved mental status	Mental status worse or not improved
Not anxious or restless	Increased anxiety and restlessness
Improved acid-base status	Worse acid-base status (name the abnormality)
Improved $P(A-a)O_2$	Worsening or unimproved $P(A-a)O_2$
CXR improved	CXR worse or unchanged
Weaning parameters improved	Weaning parameters unimproved or worse

CXR, Chest x-ray; *WOB*, work of breathing.

SELF-ASSESSMENT QUESTIONS

1. Which of the following pulmonary condition(s) respond poorly to oxygen therapy?
   1. Chronic obstructive pulmonary disease
   2. Atelectasis
   3. Asthma
   4. Consolidation
      a. 1 only
      b. 3 only
      c. 2 and 4 only
      d. 1 and 3 only

2. A 68-year-old man presents in the emergency department with paralysis of the lower extremities that has progressively worsened over the past several hours. Arterial blood gases on room air are as follows: pH 7.12, $PaCO_2$ 86, HCO_3^- 27, PaO_2 39, and SaO_2 70%. Which of the following is indicated?
   a. Oxygen with nonrebreathing mask
   b. Oxygen with continuous positive airway pressure
   c. Bronchodilator therapy
   d. Ventilatory support with oxygen

3. A relative shunt is caused by:
   1. Alveolar-capillary defect
   2. Atelectasis
   3. Airway obstruction
   4. Consolidation
      a. 2 only
      b. 1 and 3 only
      c. 2, 3, and 4 only
      d. 1, 2, 3, and 4

4. A 76-year-old woman in the intensive care unit is in respiratory distress. She appears cyanotic and short of breath. Her vital signs are as follows: blood pressure 186/115, heart rate 125, and a respiratory rate of 35 and shallow. Her PaO_2 is 81 on an FIO_2 of 0.40. Her PaO_2/PAO_2 ratio is 0.90, and her $\dot{Q}_S/\dot{Q}_T$ is 4%. Her $PaCO_2$ is 67, and her maximum inspiratory pressure (MIP) is −12 cm H_2O. Based on this information, which of the following is the primary problem?
   a. Hypercapnic respiratory failure
   b. Hypoxemic respiratory failure
   c. Both hypoxemic and respiratory failure
   d. Severe refractory hypoxemia

5. Which of the following indicate(s) the need for ventilatory support?
   1. VC: 65 mL/kg
   2. $\dot{Q}_S/\dot{Q}_T$: <5
   3. MIP: ≥ −20 (less negative)
   4. $P(A-a)O_2$: >350
      a. 1 and 3 only
      b. 2 and 4 only
      c. 3 and 4 only
      d. 1, 2, and 3 only

6. One cause of hypoxemic respiratory failure is alveolar hypoventilation. Which of the following best describes the pathophysiologic mechanism of alveolar hypoventilation?
   a. Venous blood mixing with arterial blood
   b. Decreased oxygen concentration
   c. Decreased minute ventilation
   d. Nonoxygenated blood mixing with arterial blood

7. An 81-year-old man with a long history of chronic obstructive pulmonary disease presents in the emergency department in respiratory distress. He is pursed-lip breathing and using his accessory muscles of inspiration. His heart rate is 125, and his blood pressure is 176/105. His arterial blood gases on a 2-L nasal cannula are as follows: pH 7.54, $PaCO_2$ 56, HCO_3^- 46, and PaO_2 41. Based on this information, which of the following best identifies the arterial blood gas status?
   a. Acute ventilatory failure
   b. Acute alveolar hyperventilation
   c. Acute alveolar hyperventilation superimposed on chronic ventilatory failure
   d. Acute ventilatory failure superimposed on chronic ventilatory failure

8. The $P(A-a)O_2$ finding is increased in which of the following conditions?
   1. Alveolar atelectasis
   2. Drug overdose
   3. Consolidation
   4. Obesity
      a. 1 and 3 only
      b. 2 and 4 only
      c. 1 and 2 only
      d. 2 and 3 only

9. A 67-year-old man with chronic obstructive pulmonary disease presented in the emergency department with acute alveolar hyperventilation superimposed on chronic ventilatory failure. He was taken to the intensive care unit and placed on a noninvasive ventilation (NIV) system with supplemental oxygen at an FIO_2 of 0.40. Arterial blood gas values are as follows: pH 7.22, $PaCO_2$ 84, HCO_3^- 33, PaO_2 43, SaO_2 71%. At this time, which of the following would be the most appropriate treatment?
   a. Change the patient to invasive ventilation
   b. Increase the FIO_2
   c. Recommend a sedative
   d. Change the NIV mask

10. A 57-year-old woman presents in the coronary care unit in respiratory distress. She is alert and appropriately answering the doctor's questions. Her vital signs are as follows: heart rate 145, blood pressure 170/110, and respiratory rate 32. She appears cyanotic, and her breath sounds reveal bilateral crackles. Arterial blood gases on a nonrebreathing oxygen mask are pH 7.51, $PaCO_2$ 27, HCO_3^- 21, and PaO_2 46. Based on this information, which of the following would you recommend to initially treat the patient?
   a. Invasive ventilation
   b. Continuous positive airway pressure mask
   c. Noninvasive ventilation
   d. Nonrebreathing oxygen mask

CHAPTER 12

Recording Skills and Intraprofessional Communication

Chapter Objectives

After reading this chapter, you will be able to:

- Describe the clinical importance of good charting skills.
- Differentiate among the following types of patient records:
  - Traditional charting
  - Problem-oriented medical records (POMRs), and include SOAPIER progress notes
  - Computer documentation
- Discuss the importance of the Health Insurance Portability and Accountability Act.
- Define key terms and complete self-assessment questions at the end of the chapter and on Evolve.

Key Terms

Block Chart
Computer Base Health Records
Cost-Effective Respiratory Care
Electronic Health Records
Electronic Medical Records
Electronic Patient Medical Charts
Department of Health and Human Services (DHHS)
Health Insurance Portability and Accountability Act (HIPAA)
Legal Document
Patient-Focused Respiratory Care Protocols
Problem-Oriented Medical Record (POMR)
SOAP
SOAPIER
Source-Oriented Record
Telemedicine
Therapist-Driven Protocols (TDPs)
Traditional Record

Chapter Outline

Types of Patient Records
   Traditional Chart
   Problem-Oriented Medical Record
   Computer Documentation
Telemedicine
Health Insurance Portability and Accountability Act
Self-Assessment Questions

Because all health care workers share information through written or electronic communication, the respiratory therapist must understand the way to document and use the patient's medical records effectively and efficiently. The process of adding documentary information to the patient's chart is called *charting, recording,* or *documenting.* Good charting should allow the provision of basic clinical information necessary for ongoing critical thinking and further implementation of assessment skills—that is, good charting should be an effective way to summarize pertinent clinical data, analyze and assess it (i.e., determine the cause of the clinical data), record the formulation of an appropriate treatment plan, and document adjustments made in the treatment plan (and to the effectiveness of these changes) after they have been implemented.

Good charting enhances communication and continuity of care among all members of the health care team. There is a definite and direct relationship between the quality of charting (communication) and the quality of patient care. Good charting also provides a permanent record of past and current assessment data, treatment plans, therapy given, and the patient's response to various therapeutic modalities. This information may be used by various governmental agencies and accreditation teams to evaluate the quality of the institution's patient care and determine that care was given appropriately. Accurate and legible records are the only means by which hospitals can prove that they are providing appropriate **cost-effective respiratory care** and meeting established standards.

Most health care reimbursement plans (e.g., Medicare and Medicaid) are based on diagnosis-related groups (DRGs). Under these plans, remuneration is based on disease diagnoses. Most private insurance companies use uniformly similar illness categories when setting hospital payment rates. Before providing reimbursement, insurance companies carefully review the patient's medical record when assessing whether appropriate and efficient care was given.

Finally, the patient's chart is a legal document that can be called into court. Even though the physician or institution owns the original record, the patient, lawyers, and courts can gain access to it on demand. As an instrument of continuous patient care and as a **legal document**, the patient's chart therefore should contain all pertinent respiratory care assessments, planning, interventions, and evaluations.

Types of Patient Records

Three basic methods are used to record assessment data: the traditional chart, the **problem-oriented medical record (POMR)**, and computer documentation.

Traditional Chart

The **traditional record** (also called **block chart** or **source-oriented record**) is divided into distinct areas or blocks, with emphasis placed on specific information. The traditional record is commonly seen in the patient's chart as full-colored sheets of block information. Typical blocks of information include the admission sheet, physician's order sheet, progress notes, history and physical examination, medication sheet, nurses' admission information, nursing care plans, nursing notes, graphs and flowsheets, laboratory and x-ray reports, and discharge summary. The order, content, and number of blocks vary among institutions. The traditional chart makes locating special areas of interest (e.g., x-ray records, pulmonary function test results) easier, but it also makes it more difficult to review a particular event sequence readily and efficiently or to follow the overall progress of the patient, without going back and forth among the specialty blocks.

Problem-Oriented Medical Record

The organization of the **problem-oriented medical record (POMR)** is based on an objective, scientific, problem-solving method. The POMR is one of the most important medical records used by the health care practitioner to (1) systematically gather clinical data, (2) formulate an assessment (i.e., the cause of the clinical data), and (3) systematically develop an appropriate treatment plan. A number of good POMR methods are available for recording assessment data. Regardless of the method selected, it is essential that one method be adopted and used consistently.

A good POMR method should take a systematic approach in documenting the following:

- The subjective and objective information collected
- An assessment based on the subjective and objective data
- The treatment plan (with measurable target outcomes described)
- An evaluation of the patient's response to the treatment plan
- A section to record any adjustments made to the original treatment plan

One of the most common POMR methods is the **SOAPIER** progress note, often abbreviated in the clinical setting to a **SOAP** progress note.[1] *SOAPIER* is an acronym for seven specific aspects of charting that systematically review one health problem.

S *Subjective* information refers to information about the patient's feelings, concerns, or sensations presented by the patient, for example:

"I coughed hard all night long."

"My chest feels very tight."

"I feel very short of breath."

Only the patient can provide subjective information. Some cases may not involve subjective information. For instance, a comatose, intubated patient on a mechanical ventilator is unable to provide subjective data.

O *Objective* information is the data the respiratory therapist can measure, factually describe, or obtain from other professional reports or test results. Objective data include the following:

- Heart rate
- Respiratory rate
- Blood pressure
- Temperature
- Breath sounds
- Cough effort and efficiency
- Sputum production (volume, consistency, color, and odor)
- Arterial blood gas (ABG) and pulse oximetry data
- Pulmonary function study results
- X-ray reports
- Hemodynamic data
- Chemistry results

A *Assessment* refers to the practitioner's professional conclusion about the cause of the subjective and objective data presented by the patient. In the patient with a respiratory disorder, the cause is usually related to a specific anatomic alteration of the lung. The assessment, moreover, provides the specific reason why the respiratory therapist is working with the patient. For example, the presence of wheezes are objective data (the clinical indicator) to verify the assessment (the cause) of bronchial smooth muscle constriction; an ABG with a pH of 7.18, a $PaCO_2$ of 80 mm Hg, an HCO_3^- of 29 mm/L, and a PaO_2 of 54 mm Hg are the objective data to verify the assessment of acute ventilatory failure with moderate hypoxemia. The presence of coarse crackles is a clinical indicator to verify the assessment of secretions in the large airways.

P *Plan* is/are the therapeutic interventions chosen to remedy the cause identified in the assessment. For example, an assessment of bronchial smooth muscle constriction justifies the administration of a bronchodilator; the assessment of acute ventilatory failure justifies mechanical ventilation.

I *Implementation* is the actual administration of the specific therapy plan. It documents exactly what was done, when, and by whom. These data are often recorded in the "Progress Notes" of the Traditional Chart.

E *Evaluation* is the collection and reporting of measurable data regarding the effectiveness of the therapy plan and the patient's response to it. For example, an ABG assessment may reveal that the patient's PaO_2 did not increase to a safe level in response to oxygen therapy. The terms *better* or *worse* are often used in this section of the chart.

R *Revision* refers to any changes that may be made to the original therapy plan in response to the evaluation. For example, if the PaO_2 does not increase appropriately after the implementation of oxygen therapy, the respiratory therapist might further increase the patient's FIO_2 until the desired PaO_2 is reached.

For the new practitioner, a predesigned SOAP form is especially useful in the (1) rapid collection and systematic organization of important clinical data, (2) formulation of an assessment (i.e., the cause of the clinical data), and (3) development of a treatment plan. For example, consider the case example and SOAP progress note shown in Fig. 12.1.

---

[1]The authors fully expect that the student will become proficient in the development and automatic use of good "SOAP notes" as a result of reading—and studying—this textbook.

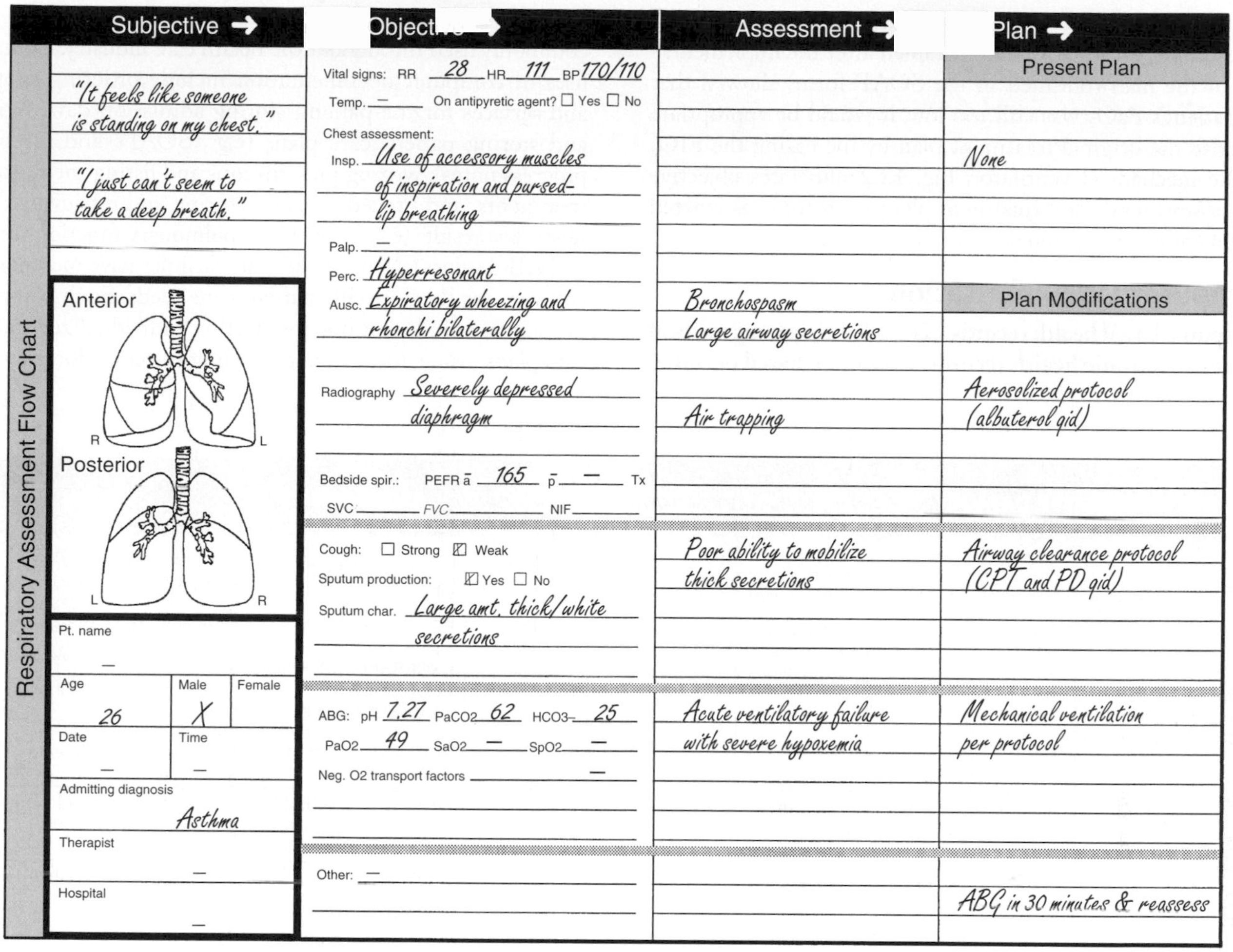

Respiratory Assessment Flow Chart

Subjective → | **Objective →** | **Assessment →** | **Plan →**

Subjective:

"It feels like someone is standing on my chest."

"I just can't seem to take a deep breath."

Anterior

R L

Posterior

L R

Pt. name —
Age 26 | Male X | Female
Date — | Time —
Admitting diagnosis: Asthma
Therapist —
Hospital —

Objective:

Vital signs: RR _28_ HR _111_ BP _170/110_
Temp. — On antipyretic agent? ☐ Yes ☐ No

Chest assessment:
Insp. Use of accessory muscles of inspiration and pursed-lip breathing
Palp. —
Perc. Hyperresonant
Ausc. Expiratory wheezing and rhonchi bilaterally

Radiography Severely depressed diaphragm

Bedside spir.: PEFR ā _165_ p̄ _—_ Tx
SVC ___ FVC ___ NIF ___

Cough: ☐ Strong ☑ Weak
Sputum production: ☑ Yes ☐ No
Sputum char. Large amt. thick/white secretions

ABG: pH _7.27_ PaCO2 _62_ HCO3- _25_
PaO2 _49_ SaO2 _—_ SpO2 _—_
Neg. O2 transport factors ___

Other: —

Assessment:

Bronchospasm
Large airway secretions

Air trapping

Poor ability to mobilize thick secretions

Acute ventilatory failure with severe hypoxemia

Plan:

Present Plan

None

Plan Modifications

Aerosolized protocol (albuterol qid)

Airway clearance protocol (CPT and PD qid)

Mechanical ventilation per protocol

ABG in 30 minutes & reassess

FIGURE 12.1 Completed predesigned SOAP form (see SOAP Case Example).

Although the SOAP form or format may not be automatically transferable into the computer-based record (see later), it is an instrument of tremendous help in organizing otherwise often disorganized and incomplete "progress notes" in the traditional hospital record.

Although the SOAP form may initially appear long and time-consuming, the experienced respiratory therapist and assessor can typically condense and abbreviate SOAP information in a few minutes (primarily at the patient's bedside) in just a few short statements. Typically, a written SOAP form uses only 1 to 3 inches of space in the patient's chart. For example, the information presented in Fig. 12.1 may actually be documented in the patient's chart in the following abbreviated form.[2]

SOAP Case Example*

A 26-year-old man arrived in the emergency department having a severe asthmatic episode. On observation, his arms were fixed to the bed rails, he was using his accessory muscles of inspiration, and he was using pursed-lip breathing. The patient stated that "it feels like somcone is standing on my chest.

I just can't seem to take a deep breath." His heart rate was 111 beats per minute, and his blood pressure was 170/110. His respiratory rate was 28 and shallow. Hyperresonant notes were produced on percussion. Auscultation revealed expiratory wheezing and coarse crackles bilaterally. His chest x-ray film revealed a severely depressed diaphragm and alveolar hyperinflation. His peak expiratory flow was 165 L/min. Even though his cough effort was weak, he produced a large amount of thick white secretions. His arterial blood gases showed pH of 7.27, PaCO2 of 62, HCO$_3^-$ of 25, and PaO2 of 49 (on room air).

*Subjective and objective data presented in bold.

S—"It feels like someone is standing on my chest. I can't take a deep breath."

O—Use of acc. mus. of insp.; HR 111, BP 170/110, RR 28 & shallow, pursed-lip; hyperresonance; exp. whz; diaph. & alv. hyperinfl.; PEFR 165; wk. cough; lg. amt. thick/white sec.; pH 7.27, PaCO$_2$ 62; HCO$_3^-$ 27; PaO$_2$ 49.

A—Bronchospasm; hyperinflation; poor ability to mob. tk. sec.; acute vent. fail. with severe hypox.

P—Aerosolized Medication Protocol (albuterol qid); Airway Clearance Protocol (CPT & PD qid), Mechanical Ventilation Protocol, ABG 30 min.

After the treatment has been administered, another abbreviated SOAP note should be made to determine whether the

[2]*Thinking* in the SOAP format is every bit as important as writing a progress note in it. We hope that instructors who read this chapter will share our enthusiasm when teaching students to present and discuss cases, report at shift change times, justify treatment plan changes, etc.

treatment plan needs to be up-regulated or down-regulated. For example, if the ABG data obtained after the implementation of the plan (outlined in the SOAP form) showed that the patient's PaO_2 was still too low, it would be appropriate to revise the original treatment plan by increasing the FIO_2 on the mechanical ventilator. Fig. 12.2 illustrates objective data, assessments, and treatment plans commonly associated with respiratory disorders.

Computer Documentation

Computer-based health records (also called **electronic medical records, electronic health records, computer-based personal records**, and **electronic patient medical charts**) are now commonly used throughout the health care industry. Common uses of computer documentation include ordering supplies and services for the patient; storing admission data; writing and storing patient care plans (e.g., SOAPs and physician progress notes); writing prescriptions and listing medications, treatments, and procedures; and storing and retrieving diagnostic test results (e.g., x-ray films, pulmonary function studies, and ABG values). Many health care facilities have incorporated software for their specific patient care needs. Such computer programs include options for starting individualized patient care plans, using automated card filing systems, documenting

A — RESPIRATORY CARE POCKET PROTOCOL CARD

OBJECTIVE DATA — Clinical manifestations (clinical indicators) that commonly develop in response to respiratory disease						ASSESSMENT	PLAN
Chest Assessment				Chest Radiograph	Bedside Spirometry	COMMON CAUSES/ SEVERITY OF CLINICAL INDICATORS	TREATMENT SELECTION (PHYSICIAN ORDERED*)
Inspection	Palpation	Percussion	Auscultation				
• Barrel chest • Use of accessory muscles • Pursed-lip breathing • Cyanosis	May show ↓ chest excursion	May be hyper-resonant	• Wheezes • Prolonged exhalation	May be normal or show over-expansion	↓ PEFR ↓ FEV₁ SVC > FVC	BRONCHOSPASM e.g., Asthma EXCESSIVE BRONCHIAL SECRETIONS e.g., Bronchitis or Cystic Fibrosis BRONCHIAL TUMOR	Bronchodilator therapy Bronchial hygiene therapy General management/ comfort
• Dyspneic • Cyanosis	Usually normal	Usually normal	Inspiratory stridor	Laryngeal narrowing	Not indicated	LARYNGEAL EDEMA e.g., Croup or Post-extubation Edema	Cool, bland aerosol therapy Racemic epinephrine
Sputum production	May be normal	May be normal	Crackles	May be normal	↓ PEFR ↓ FEV₁	LARGE AIRWAY SECRETIONS e.g., Bronchitis or Cystic Fibrosis	Bronchial hygiene therapy
• Use of accessory muscles of inspiration • Pursed-lip breathing • Barrel chest • Cyanosis	↓ Tactile and vocal fremitus	Hyper-resonant	• ↓Breath sounds • ↓Heart sounds • Prolonged exhalation	• ↓ Diaphragm • Translucency • Over-expanded	↓ PEFR ↓ FVC ↓ FEV₁/FVC	AIR TRAPPING (Hyperinflation) e.g., • COPD • Asthma • Bronchitis • Emphysema	Treat underlying cause, if possible, e.g., • Bronchospasm • Airway secretions
• May appear dyspneic • Cyanosis	↑ Tactile and vocal fremitus	Dull	• Bronchial breath sounds • Crackles • Whispered pectoriloquy	• Opacity	↓ VC	CONSOLIDATION e.g., Pneumonia ATELECTASIS e.g., Post-op or mucus plugs INFILTRATION e.g., Pneumoconiosis	• Antibiotic agents* • Lung expansion Tx • Bronchial hygiene therapy when atelectasis is caused by mucus accumulation/ mucus plugs
• Rapid shallow breath • Cyanosis • Frothy pink secretions	Usually normal	Dull	• Crackles • May be: wheezes	• Enlarged heart • Infiltrates "Butterfly"	↓ VC	PULMONARY EDEMA • Left heart failure	• Lung expansion Tx • Positive inotropic agents* • Diuretics*
• Cyanosis • Rapid shallow breath • Unilateral expansion	• Usually normal • Tracheal shift	Hyper-resonant	Absent or ↓ breath sounds	• Pneumothorax • Translucency • Mediastinum shift • ↓Diaphragm	Not indicated	AIR PRESSURE IN INTRAPLEURAL SPACE GREATER THAN ATMOSPHERE • Tension pneumothorax	Chest tube to evacuate air* Lung expansion Tx
• Cyanosis • Rapid shallow breath • Unilateral expansion	• Usually normal • May be tracheal shift	Dull	↓Breath sounds	• Opacity • Obscured diaphragm	↓ VC	FLUID IN INTRAPLEURAL SPACE • Pleural effusion • Empyema	• Treat underlying cause • Thoracentesis* • Lung expansion Tx
Paradoxical chest movement	Tender	Not indicated	Varies	• Rib fractures • Opacity (e.g., ARDS and/or atelectasis)	Not possible	DOUBLE FRACTURES OF THREE OR MORE ADJACENT RIBS • Flail chest	• Stabilization of chest mechanical ventilation* • Lung expansion Tx

FIGURE 12.2 Respiratory care protocol guide. (Used with permission from Terry Des Jardins.)

B Respiratory Care Pocket Protocol Card

Objective Data (Clinical manifestations or clinical indicators)	ASSESSMENT COMMON CAUSES/SEVERITY OF CLINICAL INDICATORS	Plan TREATMENT SELECTION (PHYSICIAN ORDERED*)
Cough effort: ○ Strong ○ Weak Sputum production: ○ No ○ Yes Sputum characteristics: • Amount > 25 mL/24 hrs. _____ • White and translucent sputum _____ • Yellow/opaque sputum _____ • Green sputum _____ • Brown sputum _____ • Red sputum _____ • Frothy secrecion _____	Patient's ability to mobilize secretions: ○ Good ○ Poor • Excessive bronchial secretions _____ • Normal sputum _____ • Acute airway infection _____ • Old, retained secretions and infections _____ • Old blood _____ • Fresh blood _____ • Pulmonary edema _____	Bronchial hygiene therapy • Bronchial hygiene therapy • None • Treat underlying cause • Bronchial hygiene therapy • Bronchial hygiene therapy • Notify physician • Treat underlying cause, e.g., CHF
Arterial blood gas status - Ventilatory • $pH\uparrow$, $PaCO_2\downarrow$, $HCO_3\downarrow$ _____ • pH normal, $PaCO_2\downarrow$, $HCO_3\downarrow\downarrow$* _____ • $pH\downarrow$, $PaCO_2\uparrow$, $HCO_3\uparrow$ _____ • pH normal, $PaCO_2\uparrow$, $HCO_3\uparrow\uparrow$ _____	• Acute alveolar hyperventilation _____ • Chronic alveolar hyperventilation _____ • Acute ventilatory failure _____ • Chronic ventilatory failure _____	• Treat underlying cause, if possible, e.g., pneumonia, pain. • Generally none (occurs normally at high altitude) • Mechanical ventilation* • Low flow oxygen, bronchial hygiene, nocturnal ventilation
Sudden ventilatory changes or chronic ventilatory failure: • $pH\uparrow$, $PaCO_2\uparrow$, $HCO_3\uparrow\uparrow$, $PaO_2\downarrow$ _____ • $pH\uparrow$, $PaCO_2\uparrow\uparrow$, $HCO_3\uparrow$, $PaO_2\downarrow$ _____	• Acute alveolar hyperventilation on chronic ventilatory failure _____ • Acute ventilatory failure on chronic ventilatory failure _____	• Treat the underlying cause, if possible, e.g., pneumonia • Mechanical ventilation*
Indicators for mechanical ventilation: • $pH\uparrow$, $PaCO_2\downarrow$, $HCO_3\downarrow$, $PaO_2\downarrow$ but pt is fatigued _____ • $pH\downarrow$, $PaCO_2\uparrow$, $HCO_3\uparrow$, $PaO_2\downarrow$ hypoventilation _____ • $pH\downarrow$, $PaCO_2\uparrow$, $HCO_3\uparrow$, $PaO_2\downarrow$ apnea _____	• Impending ventilatory failure • Ventilatory failure • Apnea	• Mechanical ventilation*
Metabolic: • $pH\uparrow$, $PaCO_2$ normal or $\uparrow$, $HCO_3\uparrow$, PaO_2 normal _____ • $pH\downarrow$, $PaCO_2$ normal or $\downarrow$, $HCO_3\downarrow$, $PaO_2\downarrow$ _____ • $pH\downarrow$, $PaCO_2$ normal or $\downarrow$, $HCO_3\downarrow$, PaO_2 normal _____ • $pH\downarrow$, $PaCO_2$ normal or $\downarrow$, $HCO_3\downarrow$, PaO_2 normal _____	• Metabolic alkalosis: • Hypokalemia _____ • Hypochloremia _____ • Metabolic acidosis: • Lactic acidosis _____ • Ketoacidosis _____ • Renal failure _____	• Potassium administration* • Chlorine administration* • Oxygen administration, cardiovascular support* • Insulin administration* • Renal failure management*
Ventilatory and metabolic: • $pH\downarrow$, $PaCO_2\uparrow$, $HCO_3\downarrow$ _____ • $pH\uparrow$, $PaCO_2\downarrow$, $HCO_3\uparrow$ _____	• Combined metabolic and respiratory acidosis • Combined metabolic and respiratory alkalosis	• Mechanical ventilation* • Treat the underlying cause of metabolic acidosis (see above) • Treat the underlying cause for acute alveolar hyperventilation • Treat the underlying cause for metabolic alkalosis (see above)
Oxygenation status: • $PaO_2 < 80$mm Hg _____ • $PaO_2 < 60$mm Hg _____ • $PaO_2 < 40$mm Hg _____	• Mild hypoxemia • Moderate hypoxemia • Severe hypoxemia	• Oxygen therapy • Treat the underlying cause of hypoxemia
Negative oxygen transport indicators: ○ $\downarrow PaO_2$ ○ Anemia ○ Blood loss ○ $\downarrow$Cardiac output ○ CO poisoning ○ Abnormal Hb	Oxygen transport status: ○ Adequate ○ Inadequate	• Treat the underlying cause, if possible, e.g., ○ Oxygen therapy ○ Blood replacement* ○ Positive inotropic agents*

* Significant

FIGURE 12.2, cont'd

acuity levels, and providing a mechanism to electronically record ongoing assessment data. There are literally hundreds of electronic medical chart solutions available today, targeted at every size and type of medical setting.

With all the patient information in a central location, computer documentation provides easy access to patient data. It greatly reduces the chance for errors, and updated patient information can be easily entered in real time. Computer-based records do away with the need to make phone calls to other departments to gather patient information or order patient supplies or services. In addition, electronic documentation eliminates the need to read through the entire chart to evaluate the patient's progress or to review specific data such as medication listings, treatments, diagnostic test results, and procedures. The patient's clinical information is permanently recorded, and other health care departments can review it and communicate with one another.

Basic computer knowledge and skills are usually taught through the institution's in-service education department. Each nursing station usually has multiple data entry stations, laptops, and tablets available for charting. Printers are also readily accessible throughout institutions and clinics. The entire patient record or just a part of it may be retrieved and printed. Today, many health care practitioners use hand-held bedside computer documentation systems. Bedside computer devices, referred to as *point-of-care (POC) systems*, commonly include specific clinical prompts for data entry, which result in records that are more accurate and complete.

Good charting skills are essential to critical thinking and patient assessment—they provide the basic means to collect clinical data, analyze it, assess it, and formulate a treatment plan. Furthermore, good charting skills document the effectiveness of patient care and adjustments of the treatment plan in response to its effectiveness. Without good charting systems and skills, the practitioner merely administers health care without a predetermined (and recorded) goal.

Historically, respiratory therapists have focused on treating patients with specific disease entities and implementing physicians' orders. Little planning was done by respiratory therapists to individualize their treatments for a specific patient. Today, a systematic, patient-specific problem-solving approach to respiratory care, based on broad theoretic knowledge, combined with technical expertise and communication skills, is essential and is the focus of this textbook. Indeed, in some quarters, the old term "**therapist-driven protocols**" (**TDPs**) (see page 132) has been replaced with "**patient-focused respiratory care protocols**" emphasizing this way of thinking.

Telemedicine

Telemedicine (also referred to as "*telehealth*" or "*e-health*") uses modern audiovisual technology that allows health care professionals an excellent way to evaluate, diagnose, and treat patients in remote locations. For example, telemedicine allows the health care practitioner the ability to (1) conduct real-time interactive videoconferencing with patients, other caregivers, and consultants; (2) send and receive patient medical files, radiologic images, and health informatics data; (3) perform remote monitoring (e.g., vital signs or sleep apnea episodes); (4) attend medical education seminars; (5) consult with other experts when needed; and (6) attend patient case conferences (grand rounds) without having to travel from one location to another or to take away valuable time from their patients.

Telemedicine provides the health care practitioner, the patient, and the patient's medical staff an effective and efficient way for everyone to communicate without having to leave their respective locations. Physician's management of patient's care (e.g., needed medications, tests, and therapy) is all conducted in a timely manner. In addition, telemedicine eliminates the possible transmission of infectious diseases between the patient and health care worker. This is especially an issue where methicillin-resistant *Staphylococcus aureus* (MRSA) is a concern. Today, telemedicine is being used daily, across dozens of countries, in hundreds of ways, including telenursing, telepharmacy, telecardiology, telepsychiatry, teleradiology, telepathology, teledermatology, teleaudiology, and teledentistry.

Health Insurance Portability and Accountability Act

In 2003 the **Department of Health and Human Services (DHHS)** proposed national rules that outlined the ways in which a patient's medical files should be used or shared with others. These rules were adopted as federal standards after the passage of the **Health Insurance Portability and Accountability Act (HIPAA)**. Presently, HIPAA requires that all health care practitioners who have access to patient medical records prove that they have a plan to protect the privacy of the records. In essence, the HIPAA regulations protect the patient's privacy with specific rules outlining when, how, and what type of health care information can be shared. HIPAA gives the patient the right to know about and to control how his or her personal medical records will be used. The following provides a general overview of the HIPAA regulations:

- Both the health care provider and a representative of the insurance company must explain to patients how they plan to disclose any medical records.
- Patients may request copies of all their medical information and make appropriate changes to it. Patients also may ask for a history of any unusual disclosures.
- The patient must give formal consent should anyone want to share any health information.
- The patient's health information is to be used only for health purposes. Without the patient's consent, medical records cannot be used by either (1) a bank to determine whether to give the patient a loan or (2) a potential employer to determine whether to hire the patient.
- When the patient's health information is disclosed, only the minimum necessary amount of information should be released.
- Records dealing with a patient's mental health get an extra level of protection.
- The patient has the right to complain to the DHHS about violations of HIPAA rules.

One disadvantage of the HIPAA regulations, according to many health care practitioners, is that the health care provider must allocate large sums of money to comply with the HIPAA rules—dollars that might be better spent elsewhere. Critics also argue that this cost will probably be passed on to the consumer. In addition, many health care providers think that the quality of patient care will be compromised as a result of HIPAA, making it more difficult for various health care practitioners to obtain vital information regarding patient care.

For example, consider the potential HIPAA-related problems for a health care team in a Miami, Florida, hospital that is trying to obtain the pharmaceutical history—in a timely fashion—of an elderly, unconscious, non-intoxicated car accident victim whose medical records are in a Detroit, Michigan, hospital. Proponents of the HIPAA regulations argue that the urgent sharing of this patient's health record would be a trade-off made to ensure the *privacy* of his health care information and to treat him in a most effective manner. Regardless of the pros or cons of HIPAA regulations, the respiratory therapist—like all other health care providers—must comply with the current HIPAA regulations. The reader is advised to stay current on the "privacy" aspects of the HIPAA regulations because the entire HIPAA system is under close legislative scrutiny and debate at the present time.

SELF-ASSESSMENT QUESTIONS

1. What is the process of adding written information to the patient's chart called?
   1. Recording
   2. Critical thinking
   3. Documenting
   4. Charting
      a. 2 only
      b. 3 and 4 only
      c. 1 and 3 only
      d. 1, 3, and 4 only

2. The admission sheet, physician's order sheet, and history sheet are all what type of patient records?
   1. Source-oriented record
   2. Problem-oriented medical record
   3. Block chart
   4. Traditional chart
      a. 2 only
      b. 4 only
      c. 3 and 4 only
      d. 1, 3, and 4 only

3. Which of the following is based on a sequential, objective, scientific, problem-solving method?
   1. Source-oriented record
   2. Problem-oriented medical record
   3. Block chart
   4. Traditional chart
      a. 1 only
      b. 2 only
      c. 4 only
      d. 3 and 4 only

4. According to the respiratory care protocol guide (see Fig. 12.2), bronchial breath sounds and dull percussion notes are associated with which of the following clinical assessments?
   1. Air trapping
   2. Bronchospasm
   3. Atelectasis
   4. Consolidation
      a. 2 only
      b. 3 only
      c. 1 and 2 only
      d. 3 and 4 only

5. Good charting should be an effective way to do the following:
   a. _____
   b. _____
   c. _____
   d. _____

6. A good problem-oriented medical record (POMR) should include a systematic approach that documents the following:
   a. _____
   b. _____
   c. _____
   d. _____
   e. _____

7. Define the following components of a SOAP progress note and list one or more examples.
   S _____
   Example(s):_____

   O _____
   Example(s):_____

   A _____
   Example(s):_____

   P _____
   Example(s):_____

8. According to the Respiratory Care Protocol guide (see Fig. 12.2), what are the three major indicators (assessments) for mechanical ventilation?

a. _____
_____
_____

b. _____
_____
_____

c. _____
_____
_____

9. A patient arterial blood gas values reveal pH of 7.56, $PaCO_2$ of 24, HCO_3^- of 20, and PaO_2 of 52. Based on the blood gas values, identify the indication(s) for initiation of mechanical ventilation.

Answer:_____
_____
_____
_____

10. Case: A 36-year-old woman is in the emergency department in respiratory distress. Her heart rate is 136 beats/min, and her blood pressure is 165/120 mm Hg. Her respiratory rate is 32 breaths/min, and her breathing is labored. The patient states that "It feels like a rope is around my neck." Expiratory wheezing and rhonchi are auscultated bilaterally. Her arterial blood gas values reveal a pH of 7.56, a $PaCO_2$ of 28, HCO_3^- of 21, and a PaO_2 of 47 (on room air). Her cough effort is strong, and she is producing a moderate amount of thin white secretions. Her peak expiratory flow rate is 185 L/min, and her chest x-ray film demonstrates a moderately depressed diaphragm and alveolar hyperinflation.

With this clinical information, provide SOAP documentation for the patient (use Fig. 12.2 for assistance).

S _____
_____
_____

O _____
_____
_____

A _____
_____
_____

P _____
_____
_____

PART II

Obstructive Lung Disease

Obstructive lung diseases are characterized by a variety of pathologic conditions, such as bronchial inflammation, excessive airway secretions, mucous plugging, bronchospasm, and distal airway weakening, that cause a reduction of air flow into and out of the lungs. Gas flow reduction is especially decreased during exhalation. The most common obstructive lung disorders are *chronic bronchitis, emphysema,* and *asthma.*

As shown in the Venn diagram,[1] although chronic bronchitis (subset 3), emphysema (subset 4), and asthma (subset 9) may appear alone, they often appear in combination. For example, when chronic bronchitis and emphysema appear together as one disease complex (subset 5), the patient is said to have *chronic obstructive pulmonary disease (COPD).*

Asthma is represented by subset 9, which by definition is associated with reversible air flow obstruction and

therefore is not considered to be COPD. In some cases, however, it is virtually impossible to differentiate patients with partially reversible air flow obstruction from the patient with chronic bronchitis or emphysema who has partially reversible air flow obstruction and hyperreactivity. Thus asthma patients with unremitting asthma are classified as having COPD (subsets 6, 7, and 8).

Chronic bronchitis and *emphysema* with air flow obstruction are commonly seen together (subset 5 and called COPD), and some patients also may have asthma associated with these two disorders (subset 8). Patients with asthma exposed to chronic irritation, such as from cigarette smoke, may develop a chronic productive cough, a feature associated with chronic bronchitis (subset 6). Such patients are said to have asthmatic bronchitis, or the asthmatic form of COPD. Patients with *chronic bronchitis* and/or *emphysema*, without air flow obstruction are not classified as having COPD (subsets 1, 2, and 11). The patient demonstrating overlapping signs and symptoms of both asthma and emphysema (subset 7) is discussed on page 228.

Finally, other obstructive lung disorders include *cystic fibrosis* and *bronchiectasis* (less common) and are not generally included in this definition (subset 10).

---

[1]A Venn diagram, or set diagram, is a diagram that shows all possible logical relations among a finite collection of sets (aggregation of things). The Venn diagrams were first conceived around 1880 by John Venn. They are used to teach elementary set theory and illustrate simple set relationships in probability, logic, statistics, linguistics, and computer science.

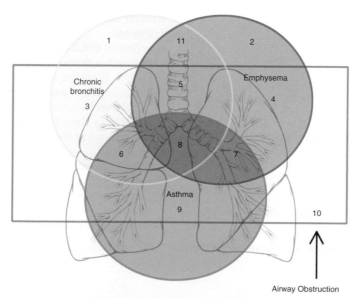

Airway Obstruction

The Venn diagram shown above illustrates all the possible subsets of patients with chronic bronchitis, emphysema, or asthma (see description of subsets above).

CHAPTER 13

Chronic Obstructive Pulmonary Disease, Chronic Bronchitis, and Emphysema

Chapter Objectives

After reading this chapter, you will be able to:

- Describe the American Thoracic Society (ATS) guidelines for chronic obstructive pulmonary disease (COPD), chronic bronchitis, and emphysema.
- Describe the Global Initiative for Chronic Obstructive Lung Disease (GOLD) definition of COPD.
- Explain the anatomic alterations of the lungs associated with chronic bronchitis and emphysema.
- Describe the etiology and epidemiology of COPD.
- Discuss the risk factors associated with COPD.
- Describe the GOLD guidelines for the diagnosis and assessment of COPD.
- Identify the key distinctive differences between chronic bronchitis and emphysema—the "pink puffer" and the "blue bloater."
- Describe the cardiopulmonary clinical manifestations associated with chronic bronchitis and emphysema (COPD).
- Describe the GOLD global strategy for the diagnosis, management, and prevention of COPD.
- Describe the clinical strategies, rationales, and cost implications of the SOAPs presented in the case studies.
- Define key terms and complete self-assessment questions at the end of the chapter and on Evolve.

Key Terms

All-Cause Readmission Prevention Program (ACRPP)
Alpha₁-Antitrypsin Deficiency
American Thoracic Society (ATS)
Asthma and COPD Overlap Syndrome (ACOS)
Biomass in Cooking and Heating
"Blue Bloater"
Bullectomy
Centriacinar Emphysema
Centrilobular Emphysema
Chronic Bronchitis
Chronic Obstructive Pulmonary Disease (COPD)
COPD Assessment Test (CAT)
Endobronchial One-Way Valves or Lung Coils
End-of-Life Care (Palliative) Care
Emphysema
Global Initiative for Chronic Obstructive Lung Disease (GOLD)
Hoover sign

Lung Transplantation
Lung Volume Reduction Surgery (LVRS)
MM Alpha₁-Antitrypsin Phenotype
Modified British Medical Research Council (mMRC) Breathlessness Scale
MZ Alpha₁-Antitrypsin Phenotype
Panacinar Emphysema
Panlobular Emphysema
"Pink Puffer"
Pulmonary Rehabilitation
Spirometry Test
ZZ Alpha₁-Antitrypsin Phenotype

Chapter Outline

Anatomic Alterations of the Lungs Associated With Chronic Bronchitis
Anatomic Alterations of the Lungs Associated With Emphysema
Etiology and Epidemiology
Risk Factors
Diagnosis and Assessment of Chronic Obstructive Pulmonary Disease
  Spirometry
  Severity Assessment of Chronic Obstructive Pulmonary Disease
Key Distinguishing Features Between Emphysema and Chronic Bronchitis
Overview of the Cardiopulmonary Clinical Manifestations Associated With Chronic Bronchitis and Emphysema
General Management of Chronic Obstructive Pulmonary Disease
Overview of GOLD's Management of Stable Chronic Obstructive Pulmonary Disease
  Reduce Exposure to Risk Factors
  Management of Acute Chronic Obstructive Pulmonary Disease Exacerbations
  Respiratory Care Treatment Protocols
  Implications of the GOLD Guidelines for Respiratory Care
Case Studies
  Chronic Bronchitis
  Emphysema
  Example of Classic Chronic Obstructive Pulmonary Disease
Self-Assessment Questions

188

The **American Thoracic Society (ATS)** guidelines for **chronic obstructive pulmonary disease (COPD)**, **chronic bronchitis**, and **emphysema** provide the following definitions:

> *Chronic obstructive pulmonary disease is a preventable and treatable disease state characterized by airflow limitation that is not fully reversible. The airflow limitation is usually progressive, is associated with an abnormal inflammatory response of the lungs to noxious particles or gases, and is primarily caused by cigarette smoking. Although COPD affects the lungs, it also produces significant systemic consequences.*
>
> *Chronic bronchitis is defined clinically as chronic productive cough for 3 months in each of 2 successive years in a patient in whom other causes of productive chronic cough have been excluded.*
>
> *Emphysema is defined pathologically as the presence of permanent enlargement of the air spaces distal to the terminal bronchioles, accompanied by destruction of bronchiole walls and without obvious fibrosis.*

In patients with COPD, both chronic bronchitis and emphysema are present. However, the relative contribution of each to the disease process is often difficult to discern. Note that the ATS definition for chronic bronchitis is based on the major clinical manifestation associated with the disease (i.e., productive cough). Also note that the ATS definition for emphysema is based on the pathologic findings or the anatomic alterations of the lung associated with the disorder.

The **Global Initiative for Chronic Obstructive Lung Disease (GOLD)** now provides the following working definition[1]:

> *Chronic obstructive pulmonary disease (COPD) is a common, preventable and treatable disease that is characterized by persistent respiratory symptoms and airflow limitation that is caused by airway and/or alveolar abnormalities usually caused by significant exposure to noxious particles or gases.*

Note that the GOLD definition does not use the terms *chronic bronchitis* and *emphysema*. GOLD explains that *emphysema*, or destruction of the gas-exchanging surfaces of the lung (alveoli), is a pathologic (i.e., anatomic alteration of the lung) term that is often—but incorrectly—used clinically and describes only one of the several structural abnormalities present in the patient with COPD. Chronic bronchitis, or the presence of cough and sputum production (i.e., clinical manifestations) for at least 3 months in each of 2 consecutive years, remains a clinically and epidemiologically useful term but is present in only a minority of subjects when this definition is used.

The bottom line is this: even though chronic bronchitis and emphysema can each develop alone, they often occur together as one disease entity. When this happens, the disease entity is called *chronic obstructive pulmonary disease (COPD)*. In other words, *COPD* is a term referring to two lung diseases—chronic bronchitis and emphysema—occurring simultaneously. Patients with COPD demonstrate a variety of clinical manifestations associated with both disorders,

although the relative contribution of each respiratory disorder is often difficult to ascertain. For this reason, chronic bronchitis, emphysema, or a combination of both disorders (COPD) are treated as one disease entity in the clinical setting.[2]

Anatomic Alterations of the Lungs Associated With Chronic Bronchitis

The conducting airways (particularly the bronchi) are the primary structures that undergo change in chronic bronchitis. As a result of chronic inflammation, the bronchial walls are narrowed by vasodilation, congestion, and mucosal edema. This condition is often accompanied by bronchial smooth muscle constriction. In addition, continued bronchial irritation causes the submucosal bronchial glands to enlarge and the number of goblet cells to increase, resulting in excessive mucous production. The number and function of cilia lining the tracheobronchial tree are diminished, and the peripheral bronchi are often partially or totally occluded by inflammation and mucous plugs, which in turn leads to hyperinflated alveoli (Fig. 13.1). Fig. 13.2 shows two microscopic views of chronic bronchitis.

To summarize, the following major pathologic or structural changes are associated with chronic bronchitis:

- Chronic inflammation and thickening of the walls of the peripheral airways.
- Excessive mucous production and accumulation.
- Partial or total mucous plugging of the airways.
- Smooth muscle constriction of bronchial airways (bronchospasm)—a variable finding.
- Air trapping and hyperinflation of alveoli may occur in late stages.

Anatomic Alterations of the Lungs Associated With Emphysema

Emphysema is characterized by a weakening and permanent enlargement of the air spaces distal to the terminal bronchioles and by destruction of the alveolar walls. As these structures enlarge and the alveoli coalesce, many of the adjacent pulmonary capillaries also are affected, resulting in a decreased surface area for gas exchange across the alveolar-capillary membrane. Furthermore, the distal airways, weakened in the process, tend to collapse during expiration in response to increased intrapleural pressure. This traps gas in the alveoli. There are two major types of emphysema: panacinar (panlobular) emphysema and centriacinar (centrilobular) emphysema.

In **panacinar emphysema**, or **panlobular emphysema**, there are an abnormal weakening and enlargement of all alveoli distal to the terminal bronchioles, including the respiratory bronchioles, alveolar ducts, alveolar sacs, and alveoli; the entire acinus is affected by dilatation and destruction. The alveolar-capillary surface area is significantly decreased (Fig. 13.3). Panlobular emphysema is commonly found in the lower parts

---

[1]Modified from GOLD, Global Strategy for the Diagnosis, Management, and Prevention of Chronic Obstructive Pulmonary Disease, Revised 2018. (http://www.goldcopd.org). GOLD is recognized as a worldwide leading authority for the diagnosis, management, and prevention of COPD.

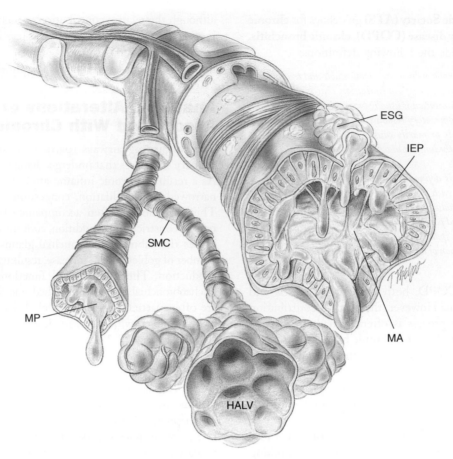

FIGURE 13.1 Chronic bronchitis, one of the most common airway diseases. *SMC,* Smooth muscle constriction; *ESG,* enlarged submucosal gland; *HALV,* hyperinflation of alveoli (distal to airway obstruction); *IEP,* inflammation of epithelium; *MA,* mucous accumulation; *MP,* mucous plug.

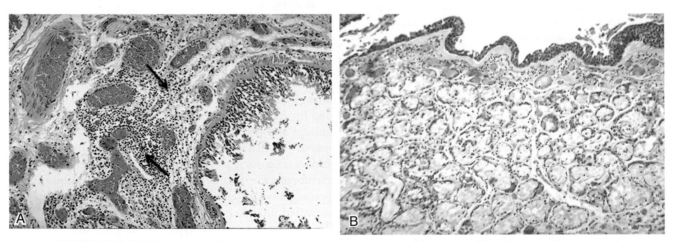

FIGURE 13.2 (A) Chronic bronchitis, microscopic. This bronchus (lower right corner) has increased numbers of chronic inflammatory cells (arrows) in the submucosal bronchial region. (B) Chronic bronchitis. The lumen of the bronchus is above. Note the marked thickening of the mucous gland layer (approximately twice normal) and squamous metaplasia of lung epithelium. (A, From Klatt, E. C. [2015]. *Robbins and Cotran Atlas of Pathology* [3rd ed.]. Philadelphia, PA: Elsevier. B, From the Teaching Collection of the Department of Pathology, University of Texas, Southwestern Medical School, Dallas, Texas. In Kumar, V., Abbas, A. K., Aster, J. C. [2018]. *Robbins Basic Pathology* [10th ed.]. Philadelphia, PA: Elsevier.)

of the lungs and is sometimes associated with a deficiency of the protease inhibitor alpha₁-antitrypsin. Panlobular emphysema is one of the more severe types of emphysema and therefore the most likely to produce significant clinical manifestations.

In **centriacinar emphysema,** or **centrilobular emphysema,** the pathologic issues involve the respiratory bronchioles in the proximal (central) portion of the acinus. The respiratory bronchiolar walls enlarge, become confluent, and are then destroyed. A rim of parenchyma remains relatively unaffected

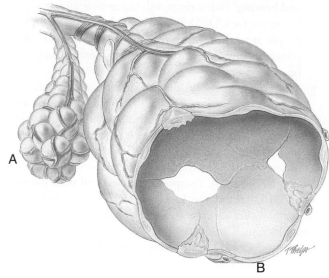

FIGURE 13.3 Panlobular emphysema. (A) Normal alveoli for comparison purposes. (B) Panlobular emphysema. Abnormal weakening and enlargement of all air spaces distal to the terminal bronchioles.

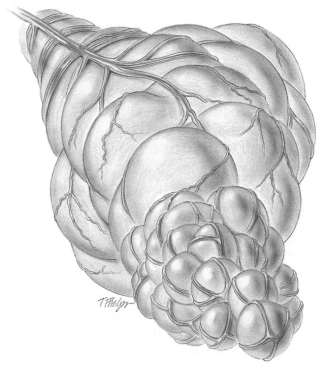

FIGURE 13.4 Centrilobular emphysema. Abnormal weakening and enlargement of the respiratory bronchioles and alveoli in the proximal portion of the acinus.

(Fig. 13.4). Centriacinar emphysema is the most common form of emphysema and is strongly associated with cigarette smoking and with chronic bronchitis. Fig. 13.5 shows a microscopic view of pulmonary emphysema.

To summarize, the following are the major pathologic or structural changes associated with emphysema:

- Permanent enlargement and destruction of the air spaces distal to the terminal bronchioles
- Destruction of the alveolar-capillary membrane

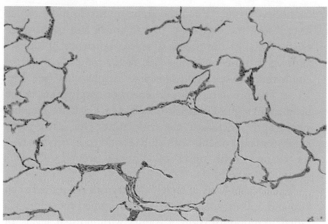

FIGURE 13.5 Pulmonary emphysema, microscopic. There is loss of alveolar ducts and alveoli with emphysema, and the remaining air spaces become dilated. There is less surface area for gas exchange. Emphysema leads to loss of lung parenchyma, loss of elastic recoil, increased lung compliance, and increased pulmonary residual volume with increased total lung capacity, mainly from an increased residual volume. (From Klatt, E. C. [2015]. *Robbins and Cotran atlas of pathology* [3rd ed.]. Philadelphia, PA: Elsevier.)

- Weakening of the distal airways, primarily the respiratory bronchioles
- Air trapping and hyperinflation

Etiology and Epidemiology

Although the precise incidence of COPD is not known, it is estimated that 10 to 15 million people in the United States have chronic bronchitis, emphysema, or a combination of both. Most authorities agree that COPD is underdiagnosed. It is felt that if one takes into account the numbers of people who have not been "officially" diagnosed with COPD, the incidence would be more than 20 million people in the United States. It is generally accepted that more people have chronic bronchitis than emphysema. For example, the National Center for Health Statistics estimates that in the United States about 9.5 million people have chronic bronchitis and 4.1 million people have emphysema. COPD-related deaths claim that 138,000 Americans each year. It is the third leading cause of death in the United States. Recent data show that COPD prevalence and mortality are now about equal in men and women, which likely reflects the changing patterns of smoking.

Risk Factors

According to GOLD, although the current understanding of the risk factors associated with COPD is incomplete, the following factors influence the development and progression of COPD:

- *Genetic factors:* **Alpha₁-antitrypsin deficiency** (also known as alpha₁-proteinase inhibitor deficiency, A₁AD, AATD, ATT deficiency, AP₁ deficiency, and alpha₁ inherited emphysema) is a genetic disorder affecting the lung, liver, and, rarely, the skin. Alpha₁-antitrypsin is made in the liver, and one of its functions is to protect the lungs from neutrophil elastase, an enzyme that can break down connective tissue. When the alpha$_1$-antitrypsin deficiency level is low, the elastase is free to attack and destroy the elastic tissue of the lungs. A severe deficiency of alpha$_1$-antitrypsin poses a strong risk factor for early onset of emphysema—especially panacinar emphysema (see Fig. 13.3). The premature development of emphysema is the hallmark of alpha$_1$-antitrypsin deficiency. Cigarette smoking significantly increases the risk factor for early-onset emphysema in patients with alpha$_1$-antitrypsin deficiency—for example, the onset of dyspnea around 30 years of age.

The normal level of alpha$_1$-antitrypsin ranges between 150 and 350 mg/dL (1.5 to 3.5 g/L) when measured via radial immunodiffusion. Patients with normal levels of alpha$_1$-antitrypsin are referred to genetically as having an **MM alpha$_1$-antitrypsin phenotype** or simply an M phenotype (homozygote). The phenotype associated with severely low serum concentrations is the **ZZ alpha$_1$-antitrypsin phenotype**, or simply Z. The heterozygous offspring of parents with the M and Z phenotypes have an **MZ alpha$_1$-antitrypsin phenotype**. The **MZ alpha$_1$-antitrypsin phenotype** results in an intermediate deficiency of alpha$_1$-antitrypsin. The precise effect of the intermediate level of alpha$_1$-antitrypsin is unclear. It is strongly recommended, however, that individuals with this phenotype do not smoke or work in areas having significant environmental air pollution. Although alpha$_1$-antitrypsin deficiency is considered to be rare, it is estimated that 80,000 to 100,000 individuals in the United States have severe deficiency of alpha$_1$-antitrypsin.

- *Age and gender:* As a person ages, the risk for COPD increases. Although the precise connection between age and COPD is unclear, it is suggested it may be related to the sum of cumulative exposures throughout life. In the past, COPD was greater among men than women. However, more recent data indicate that the prevalence of COPD between men and women is about equal, likely reflecting the changing patterns of tobacco smoking.
- *Lung growth and development:* Any condition that affects lung growth during gestation and childhood (e.g., low birth weight, respiratory infections) has the potential for increasing an individual's risk for developing COPD (see Chapter 33, The Newborn Disorders).
- *Exposure to particles*
  - *Tobacco smoke:* Cigarette smoking is the most commonly encountered risk factor for COPD worldwide. Other types of tobacco (e.g., pipe, cigar, water pipe) and marijuana are also risk factors for COPD. Passive exposure to cigarette smoke also may cause COPD. Smoking during pregnancy may affect lung growth and development of the fetus.
  - *Occupational exposure:* Organic and inorganic dusts and chemical agents and fumes (e.g., asbestos, coal dust, moldy hay, bird droppings, or paints) may cause COPD.
  - *Indoor air pollution:* Wood, animal dander and dung, crop residues, and coal, commonly burned in open fires or poorly functioning stoves, may lead to very high levels of indoor pollution. Research data continue to grow that indoor pollution from **biomass in cooking and heating**[3] in poorly ventilated areas is an important risk factor for COPD. It is estimated that about 3 billion people around the world use biomass and coal as their primary source of energy for cooking, heating, and basic household needs.
  - *Outdoor air pollution:* Although high levels of air pollution (e.g., silicates, sulfur dioxide, the nitrogen oxides, and ozone) are known to be harmful to individuals with existing heart and lung disease, the role of outdoor pollution in causing COPD is unclear.
- *Socioeconomic status:* Poverty is clearly a risk factor for COPD, although the precise components associated with poverty and COPD are unclear. Likely factors include exposure to indoor and outdoor air pollutants, crowding, poor nutrition, and infection. The data strongly suggest that the risk for developing COPD is inversely related to an individual's socioeconomic status.
- *Asthma/bronchial hyperreactivity:* Asthma may be a risk factor for the development of COPD.
- *Chronic bronchitis:* May be a risk factor for the development of COPD. In other words, chronic bronchitis may lead to emphysema. When both chronic bronchitis and emphysema are present, the patient is said to have COPD.
- *Respiratory infections:* A history of severe childhood respiratory infections is associated with decreased lung function and increased respiratory complications in adulthood. Susceptibility to respiratory infections may lead to COPD. Tuberculosis has been shown to be a risk factor for COPD.

Diagnosis and Assessment of Chronic Obstructive Pulmonary Disease

According to GOLD, the diagnosis of COPD should be considered in any patient who is over 40 years of age and who has dyspnea, chronic cough or sputum production, and a history of exposure to risk factors for the disease—especially cigarette smoking—and a family history of COPD. The key indicators for considering a COPD diagnosis are shown in Fig. 13.6. Although these indicators are not diagnostic by themselves, the presence of any combination of these clinical markers significantly increases the possibility of a diagnosis of COPD. A **spirometry test** is required to confirm the diagnosis of COPD, showing the presence of a postbronchodilator FEV$_1$/FVC of less than 0.70 (see following section).

Spirometry

The three main spirometric tests used to measure the severity of airflow limitation in the patient with suspected COPD are the *forced vital capacity (FVC), forced expiratory volume in 1 second (FEV$_1$), and forced expiratory volume in 1 second/forced vital capacity ratio (FEV$_1$/FVC ratio)*. Clinically, the FEV$_1$/FVC ratio is also commonly called the *forced expiratory volume 1 second percentage (FEV$_1$%)*. Fig. 13.7 illustrates a normal FEV$_1$ and an FEV$_1$ that is typically seen in the spirogram of

---

[3]Biomass energy sources include the burning of garbage, crop residue, landfill, alcohol fuels, and wood.

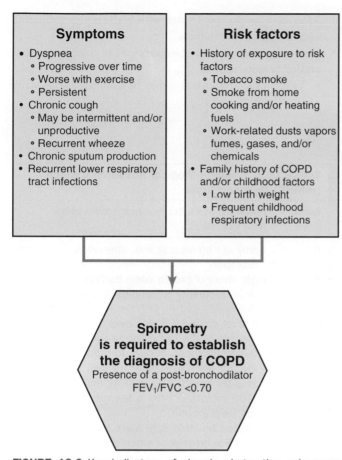

Symptoms	Risk factors

• Dyspnea
  ∘ Progressive over time
  ∘ Worse with exercise
  ∘ Persistent
• Chronic cough
  ∘ May be intermittent and/or unproductive
  ∘ Recurrent wheeze
• Chronic sputum production
• Recurrent lower respiratory tract infections
	• History of exposure to risk factors
	  ∘ Tobacco smoke
	  ∘ Smoke from home cooking and/or heating fuels
	  ∘ Work-related dusts vapors fumes, gases, and/or chemicals
	• Family history of COPD and/or childhood factors
	  ∘ Low birth weight
	  ∘ Frequent childhood respiratory infections

Spirometry is required to establish the diagnosis of COPD
Presence of a post-bronchodilator
$FEV_1/FVC < 0.70$

FIGURE 13.6 Key indicators of chronic obstructive pulmonary disease (COPD) in patients over age 40. The diagnosis of COPD entails documentation of symptoms (clinical indicators), risk factors, and the final confirmation of spirometry with the presence of a postbronchodilator $FEV_1/FVC < 0.70$. *Note:* The above indicators are not diagnostic by themselves. However, the presence of multiple key indicators increases the likelihood of a diagnosis of COPD. A pulmonary function study is required to establish a diagnosis of COPD. (Data from GOLD, Global Strategy for the Diagnosis, Management, and Prevention of Chronic Obstructive Pulmonary Disease. Revised 2017. Retrieved from http://www.goldcopd.org.)

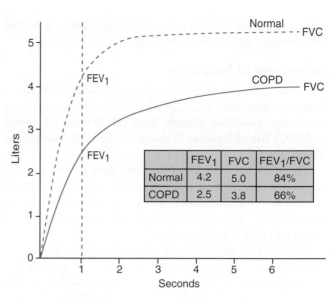

	FEV_1	FVC	FEV_1/FVC
Normal	4.2	5.0	84%
COPD	2.5	3.8	66%

Postbronchodilator FEV_1 is recommended for the diagnosis and assessment of severity of COPD

FIGURE 13.7 Normal spirogram and spirogram typical of patients with mild to moderate chronic obstructive pulmonary disease.

TABLE 13.1 Severity of Airflow Limitation in Chronic Obstructive Pulmonary Disease Based on Postbronchodilator FEV_1

(Only in Patients With FEV_1/FVC Ratio <0.70)		
GOLD 1	Mild	$FEV_1 \geq 80\%$ predicted
GOLD 2	Moderate	FEV_1 50%–79% predicted
GOLD 3	Severe	FEV_1 30%–49% predicted
GOLD 4	Very Severe	$FEV_1 \leq 29\%$ or less than predicted

Modified from GOLD, Global Strategy for the Diagnosis, Management, and Prevention of Chronic Obstructive Pulmonary Disease, Revised 2018. http://www.goldcopd.org.

patients with mild to moderate COPD. The presence of a postbronchodilator FEV_1/FVC ratio of less than 0.70 is required to establish the diagnosis of COPD in the patient who also has the key symptoms and risk factors associated with COPD (see Fig. 13.6).

Severity Assessment of Chronic Obstructive Pulmonary Disease

According to GOLD, before an effective treatment plan for COPD can be outlined, a thorough COPD assessment must first be performed. The primary goals of COPD assessment are to (1) establish the degree of airflow limitation, (2) determine the effect of the COPD on the patient's health status, and (3) ascertain the risk for future events (e.g., exacerbations or hospital admissions).

To achieve this goal, GOLD recommends the assessment of the following features of the disease independently:
• Airflow limitation
• Symptoms
• Exacerbation risk
• Comorbidities

Assessment of Airflow Limitation

As shown in Table 13.1, GOLD has established a classification chart of airflow limitation severity in COPD. This classification chart defines the severity of the disease according to airflow limitation. The primary pulmonary functions test (PFT) measurements used to evaluate the patient's airflow limitation are the *forced expiratory volume in one second (FEV₁)* and the *forced expiratory volume in one second (FEV₁) to forced vital capacity ratio (FEV₁/FVC ratio)*. Spirometry should be performed after the administration of a short-acting inhaled bronchodilator to minimize variability.

It should be noted that assessing the degree of reversibility of airflow limitation before and after bronchodilator or corticosteroids is no longer recommended. The degree of reversibility has not been shown to help in the diagnosis of COPD, differentiate the COPD diagnosis from asthma, or predict the patient's possible response to long-term treatment. Because there is only a weak correlation among the patient's FEV₁, symptoms, and impairment of the patient's health status, a formal symptomatic assessment is required.

Assessment of Symptoms

There are several validated questionnaires available to assess symptoms in patients with COPD. GOLD recommends using either the **Modified British Medical Research Council (mMRC) Breathlessness Scale** or the **COPD Assessment Test (CAT)**.

The mMRC questionnaire relates well to other health conditions and predicts future mortality risks. An mMRC score of less than 1 is classified as a low-risk patient; a score greater than 2 is considered a high-risk patient. Table 13.2 shows an mMRC questionnaire.

The CAT is an eight-item one-dimensional assessment of health status in COPD. This questionnaire is applicable worldwide, and validated translations are available in a wide range of languages. A score less than 10 is classified as a low-risk patient; a score greater than 10 is identified as a high-risk patient. Fig. 13.8 shows an example of the CAT assessment.

Assessment of Exacerbation Risk

According to GOLD, a COPD exacerbation is defined as "acute worsening of respiratory symptoms that result in additional therapy." An exacerbation event is classified as either mild, moderate, or severe as follows:

- *Mild exacerbation:* Treated with short-acting bronchodilators (SABDs) only
- *Moderate exacerbation:* Treated with SABDs plus antibiotics and/or oral corticosteroids
- *Severe exacerbation:* Patient requires visit to emergency room and/or hospitalization
  - Severe exacerbations also may be associated with acute ventilatory failure.

TABLE 13.2 Modified Medical Research Council (mMRC) Dyspnea Scale

mMRC Score	Check the Score Box That Best Applies to You (One Box Only)	
0	I only get breathless with strenuous exercise.	☐
1	I get short of breath when hurrying on level ground or walking up a slight hill.	☐
2	On level ground, I walk slower than people of the same age because of breathlessness or have to stop for breath when walking at my own pace.	☐
3	I stop for breath after walking about 100 meters or after a few minutes on level ground.	☐
4	I am too breathless to leave the house or I am breathless when dressing.	☐

For each item below, place a mark (X) in the box that best describes you currently. Be sure to only select one response for each question.

Example: I am very happy ⓪ⓧ②③④⑤ I am very sad — SCORE

I never cough	⓪①②③④⑤	I cough all the time
I have no phlegm (mucus) in my chest at all	⓪①②③④⑤	My chest is completely full of phlegm (mucus)
My chest does not feel tight at all	⓪①②③④⑤	My chest feels very tight
When I walk up a hill or one flight of stairs I am not breathless	⓪①②③④⑤	When I walk up a hill or one flight of stairs I am very breathless
I am not limited doing any activities at home	⓪①②③④⑤	I am very limited doing activities at home
I am confident leaving my home despite my lung condition	⓪①②③④⑤	I am not at all confident leaving my home because of my lung condition
I sleep soundly	⓪①②③④⑤	I don't sleep soundly because of my lung condition
I have lots of energy	⓪①②③④⑤	I have no energy at all

TOTAL SCORE

FIGURE 13.8 COPD Assessment tests. (Courtesy GlaxoSmithKline. In Jones PW, et al: Development and first validation of the COPD assessment test, *European Respiratory Journal* 34(3): 648-654, 2009.)

The best predictor for the risk for exacerbations is the patient's history of exacerbations, including hospitalizations. A history of two or more exacerbations per year is considered a high risk for more exacerbations. In addition, the risk for exacerbation is significantly higher in patients identified as GOLD 3 (severe) and GOLD 4 (very severe) (see Table 13.1).

Assessment of Comorbidities

Patients with COPD often have additional diseases that further worsen their condition. Common comorbidities associated with COPD include cardiovascular disease, skeletal muscle dysfunction, metabolic syndrome, osteoporosis, depression, anxiety, and lung cancer. Having COPD itself can also have significant extrapulmonary (systemic) effects, including weight loss and nutritional abnormalities. Comorbidities in patients with COPD should be evaluated and treated appropriately. The diagnosis, assessment of severity, and management of specific comorbidities in patients with COPD are the same as in any other patient.

To summarize, to assess the severity of the patient's COPD—and, importantly, to subsequently develop a pharmacologic treatment algorithm that is specifically designed to meet the patient's needs (discussed later in this chapter)—GOLD recommends that the patient undergo the following:

1. Spirometry to determine the severity of airflow limitation
2. An assessment of either the patient's dyspnea (using mMRC), or symptoms (using CAT)
3. A full history of the patient's exacerbations, including hospitalizations
4. Consideration of the effect of any associated comorbidities

By establishing the patient's spirometric values, current symptoms, exacerbation history, and comorbidities, the ability to diagnosis, prognosticate, and develop an effective and helpful therapeutic treatment plan for the patient is quickly and systematically secured. GOLD has developed an outstanding combined COPD Assessment Tool that can be used to quickly gather, organize, and manage all of the COPD patient's relative clinical information.

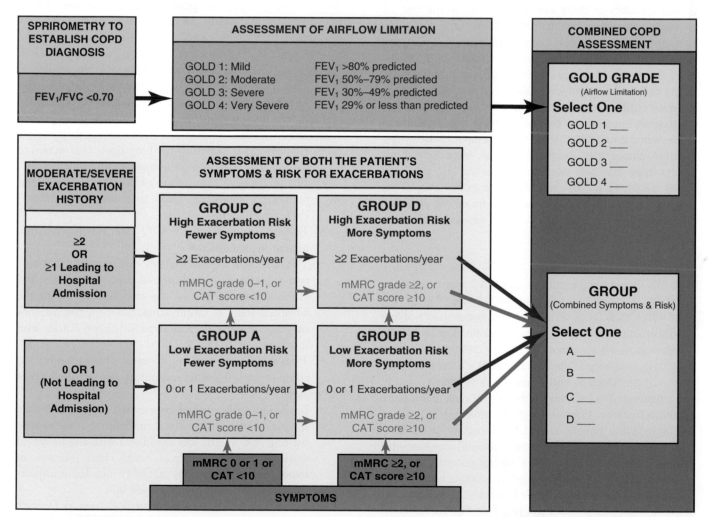

FIGURE 13.9 Combined COPD Assessment Tool. (Data from GOLD, Global Strategy for the Diagnosis, Management, and Prevention of Chronic Obstructive Pulmonary Disease. Revised 2018. Retrieved from http://www.goldcopd .org.)

Combined COPD Assessment Tool. A representative example of GOLD's Combined COPD Assessment Tool is shown in Fig. 13.9.

- The *GOLD* numbers (1, 2, 3, or 4) represent the severity of the patient's airflow limitation.
- The *Groups A, B, C,* and *D* are derived from the patient's present "dyspnea," or "symptoms," and past history of "exacerbations" values.

The patient's GOLD score (i.e., 1, 2, 3 or 4), in conjunction with the patient's symptoms and exacerbation history values, provides the practicing clinician a consistent and simple tool to quickly assess the severity of the patient's COPD and, as discussed later in this chapter, provides the basis to develop an effective pharmacologic treatment plan. Box 13.1 provides two case examples that demonstrate the application of the Combined Assessment Tool.

BOX 13.1 Combined Chronic Obstructive Pulmonary Disease Assessment Case Examples

Case 1

A 73-year-old male COPD patient has a "symptom CAT" score of 16, an FEV$_1$ of 55% (GOLD Grade 2) of predicted, and a history of three exacerbations within the last 12 months. Based on this information, the symptom CAT score shows that the patient is more symptomatic (CAT ≥10) and therefore should be placed in either Group B or Group D.

Between groups B and D, the GOLD Grade of 2 (moderate airflow limitation) indicates Low Exacerbation Risk—which suggests the patient should be placed in Group B. However, because the patient had three exacerbations in the last 12 months, the correct placement is Group D—which shows High Exacerbation Risk, More Symptoms, and more than two exacerbations in the last year (see Fig. 13.9). As will be discussed later in this chapter, an effective and helpful pharmacologic treatment algorithm now can be established based on this assessment information (see Fig. 13.18).

Case 2

A 67-year-old female patient with COPD has a "dyspnea mMRC" score of 1, a "symptom CAT" score of 8, an FEV$_1$ of 44% (GOLD Grade 3) of predicted, and a history of four exacerbations within the last 12 months. Based on this information, the symptom CAT score shows that the patient is "less symptomatic" (mMRC 1 and CAT <10) and therefore should be placed in either Group C or Group A.

Between Groups C and A, the GOLD Grade of 3 (severe airflow limitation) indicates "High Exacerbation Risk"—which suggests the patient should be placed in Group C. In addition, the fact that the patient has had four exacerbations in the last 12 months further confirms that the correct placement for this patient is Group C, which shows High Exacerbation Risk, Fewer Symptoms, and more than two Exacerbations in the last year (see Fig. 13.9). As will be discussed later in this chapter, an effective and helpful pharmacologic treatment algorithm now can be established based on this assessment information (see Fig. 13.18).

Additional Screening Methods Used to Diagnosis Chronic Obstructive Pulmonary Disease. Table 13.3 provides additional diagnostic procedures that may be considered in the diagnosis and assessment of COPD.

Key Distinguishing Features Between Emphysema and Chronic Bronchitis

Even though chronic bronchitis and emphysema often occur as one disease complex referred to as COPD, they can develop alone. A complete presentation of all the specific signs and symptoms associated with emphysema and chronic bronchitis are provided in the Overview of the Cardiopulmonary Clinical Manifestations section on page 199.

An abbreviated and handy overview of the key distinguishing features between emphysema and chronic bronchitis is provided as follows.

Clinically, the patient with emphysema is sometimes classified as a **"pink puffer,"** or a patient with type A COPD; and the patient with chronic bronchitis is sometimes classified as a **"blue bloater,"** or a patient with type B COPD. These general, older terms are primarily based on the clinical manifestations commonly associated with each respiratory disorder.

- *Pink puffer (Type A Chronic Obstructive Pulmonary Disease):* The term *pink puffer* is derived from the reddish complexion and the "puffing" (pursed-lip breathing) commonly seen in the patient with emphysema. The major pathophysiologic mechanisms responsible for the red complexion and puffing are the following:
  - Emphysema is caused by the progressive destruction of the distal airways and pulmonary capillaries.
  - The progressive elimination of the distal airways and pulmonary capillaries leads to ventilation-perfusion ($\dot{V}/\dot{Q}$) mismatches.
  - To compensate for these $\dot{V}/\dot{Q}$ ratio mismatches, the patient hyperventilates.
  - The increased respiratory rate, in turn, works to maintain a relatively normal arterial oxygenation level and causes a ruddy or flushed skin complexion. During the advanced stage of emphysema, however, the patient's oxygenation status decreases and the carbon dioxide level increases.
  - Thus the patient with emphysema, who has both a red complexion and a rapid respiratory rate, is called a *pink puffer*.
  - In addition to the marked dyspnea and ruddy complexion, the pink puffer tends to be thin (because of the muscle wasting and weight loss associated with the increased work of breathing), has a barrel chest (because of hyperinflated lungs), uses accessory muscles of inspiration, and exhales through pursed lips.
- *Blue bloater (Type B Chronic Obstructive Pulmonary Disease):* The term *blue bloater* is derived from the cyanosis—the bluish color of the lips and skin—commonly seen in the patient with chronic bronchitis. The bluish complexion is caused by the following:

TABLE 13.3 Additional Tests to Consider in Assessment and Diagnosis of Chronic Obstructive Pulmonary Disease

Imaging	A chest x-ray is not helpful to establish a diagnosis of COPD However, it may be valuable in ruling out other diagnoses or establishing the presence of significant comorbidities, such as pneumonia, pulmonary fibrosis, bronchiectasis, pleural disease, kyphoscoliosis, and cardiac diseases. Radiologic changes associated with COPD include lung hyperinflation, hyperlucency of the lungs, and rapid tapering of the vascular markings. Computed tomography scanning may be helpful in the detection of bronchiectasis lung cancer in the patient with COPD
Lung volumes and diffusing capacity	A complete measurement of lung volumes, capacities, and airflow limitations can provide additional information concerning the severity of the disease. Measurement of the diffusing capacity (DLCO) provides further information on the functional effect of emphysema in COPD. The DLCO also may explain the breathlessness in some patients that appears out of proportion to the degree of airflow limitation.
Oximetry and arterial blood gas measurement	Oximetry is commonly used to assess the patient's arterial oxygen saturation and the need for supplemental oxygen therapy. Oximetry is recommended to assess all patients with clinical signs that suggest respiratory failure or right-heart failure When the peripheral arterial oxygen saturation (SpO_2) is <92%, an arterial or capillary blood gases should be assessed. For example, an ABG of a patient with "stable" COPD could be pH 7.36, $PaCO_2$ 79, HCO_3^- 43, and PaO_2 61; or An ABG example that shows the patient with COPD is in "impending ventilatory failure" (or acute alveolar hyperventilation on top of chronic ventilatory failure) could be pH 7.52, $PaCO_2$ 52, HCO_3^- 40, and PaO_2 46 (mild or moderate acute exacerbation); or An ABG example that shows the patient with COPD is in "acute ventilatory failure" (on top of chronic ventilatory failure) could be pH 7.28, $PaCO_2$ 99, HCO_3^- 45, and PaO_2 34 (severe acute exacerbation) (see Chapter 5 for further discussion).
Exercise testing and assessment of physical activity	Objectively measured exercise activities, such as self-paced shuttle walk test, or the unpaced 6-minute walk test, are powerful indicators of the patient's health status. Walking tests are useful in assessing the disability and risk for mortality, and are used to measure the effectiveness of pulmonary rehabilitation. Laboratory testing using cycle or treadmill ergometry are useful in identifying coexisting or alternative conditions (e.g., cardiac disease).
Alpha$_1$-antitrypsin deficiency (AATD) screen	When a younger patient (<45 years old) presents with a history and clinical indicators associated with COPD, an AATD screen should be considered. A serum concentration below 15% to 20% of normal value is highly suggestive of emphysema caused by AATD.

- Unlike emphysema, the pulmonary capillaries in the patient with chronic bronchitis are not damaged. The patient with chronic bronchitis responds to the increased airway obstruction by decreasing ventilation and increasing cardiac output—that is, a decreased $\dot{V}/\dot{Q}$ ratio.
- The chronic hypoventilation and increased cardiac output (decreased $\dot{V}/\dot{Q}$ ratio) leads to a decreased arterial oxygen level, an increased arterial carbon dioxide level, and a compensated (normal) pH—or chronic ventilatory failure arterial blood gas (ABG) values (also called *compensated respiratory acidosis*). The respiratory drive is depressed in patients with chronic ventilatory failure.
- The persistent low $\dot{V}/\dot{Q}$ ratio and depressed respiratory drive both contribute to a chronically reduced arterial oxygenation level and polycythemia that in turn causes cyanosis. In addition, the blue bloater tends to be stocky and overweight, has a chronic productive cough, and frequently has swollen ankles and legs and distended neck veins as a result of pulmonary hypertension and right-sided heart failure (cor pulmonale).

Table 13.4 provides an overview of the more common distinguishing features between emphysema and chronic bronchitis.

The clinical features of emphysema and chronic bronchitis are not always clear-cut because many patients have a combined disease process, COPD. This is especially the case during the late stages of emphysema and chronic bronchitis.[4]

---

[4]It should be noted that the current definition for these respiratory disorders (i.e., chronic bronchitis and emphysema), even if occurring as a singular disease, is often called COPD if there is airflow limitation.

TABLE 13.4 Key Features Distinguishing Emphysema From Chronic Bronchitis*

Clinical Manifestation	Emphysema (Type A COPD: Pink Puffer)	Chronic Bronchitis (Type B COPD: Blue Bloater)
Inspection		
Body build	Thin	Stocky, overweight
Barrel chest	Common, classic sign	Normal
Respiratory pattern	Hyperventilation and marked dyspnea; often occurs at rest Late stage: Diminished respiratory drive and hypoventilation	Diminished respiratory drive Hypoventilation common, with resultant hypoxia and hypercapnia
Pursed-lip breathing	Common	Uncommon
Cough	Uncommon	Common; classic sign
Sputum	Uncommon	Common; classic sign Copious amounts, purulent
Cyanosis	Uncommon (reddish skin)	Common
Peripheral edema	Uncommon	Common Right-sided heart failure
Neck vein distention	Uncommon	Common Right-sided heart failure
Use of accessory muscles	Common	Uncommon
Auscultation	Decreased breath sounds, decreased heart sounds, prolonged expiration	Wheezes, crackles, depending on severity of disease
Percussion	Hyperresonance	Normal
Laboratory Tests		
Chest radiograph	Hyperinflation, narrow mediastinum, normal or small vertical heart, low flat diaphragm, presence of blebs or bullae	Congested lung fields, densities, increased bronchial vascular markings, enlarged horizontal heart
Polycythemia	Uncommon	Common
Infections	Occasionally	Common
Pulmonary Function Study		
DLCO and DL/VA	Decreased	Often normal
Other		
Pulmonary hypertension	Uncommon	Common
Cor pulmonale	Uncommon	Common Right-sided heart failure

*The clinical features of emphysema and chronic bronchitis are not always clear-cut because many patients have a combined disease process (COPD; this is especially the case during the late stages of emphysema and chronic bronchitis).

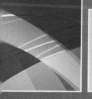

OVERVIEW of the Cardiopulmonary Clinical Manifestations Associated with Chronic Bronchitis and Emphysema (Chronic Obstructive Pulmonary Disease)[1]

The following clinical manifestations result from the pathophysiologic mechanisms caused (or activated) by excessive bronchial secretions (see Fig. 10.11) and bronchospasm (see Fig. 10.10)—the major anatomic alterations of the lungs associated with chronic bronchitis (see Figs. 13.1 and 13.2), and the clinical manifestations activated by distal airway and alveolar weakening (see Fig. 10.12)—the major anatomic alterations of the lungs associated with emphysema (see Figs. 13.3, 13.4, and 13.5).

CLINICAL DATA OBTAINED AT THE PATIENT'S BEDSIDE

Vital Signs	Chronic Bronchitis and Emphysema
Heart rate and respiratory rate	Stable patients: Normal vital signs
	Exacerbations: Usually acute increase in heart rate and respiratory rate (tachypnea)
	Classic signs of hypoxemia

Chest Assessment Findings Inspection	Emphysema	Chronic Bronchitis
General body build	Thin, underweight	Stocky, overweight
Altered sensorium—anxiety, irritability	Common during severe stage	Common during moderate and severe stage
	Classic sign of hypoxemia	Classic sign of hypoxemia
Barrel chest	Classic sign	Occasionally
Digital clubbing	Late stage	Common
Cyanosis	Uncommon—often reddish skin	Common
Peripheral edema and venous distention	End-stage emphysema	Common
		Because polycythemia and cor pulmonale are common in chronic bronchitis, the following are often seen:
		• Distended neck veins
		• Pitting edema
		• Enlarged and tender liver
Use of accessory muscles	Common, especially during exacerbations	Uncommon
		End stage in some chronic bronchitis
Hoover sign: The inward movement of the lower lateral chest wall during each inspiration—indicates severe hyperinflation	Common—severe stage	Uncommon
Pursed-lip breathing	Common	Uncommon
Cough	Uncommon during mild and moderate stage	Classic sign
	Some coughing during severe stage with infection	More severe in the mornings
Sputum	Uncommon	Common
	Little, mucus	Classic sign; copious amounts, purulent (see sputum examination)
Palpation of the chest	Decreased tactile fremitus	Normal
	Decreased chest expansion	
	Point of maximal impulse (PMI) often shifts to the epigastric area	
Percussion of the chest	Hyperresonance	Normal
	Decreased diaphragmatic excursion	
Auscultation of the chest	Diminished breath sounds	Crackles
	Prolonged expirations	Wheezes
	Diminished heart sounds	

[1]Chronic bronchitis and emphysema frequently occur together as a disease complex referred to as chronic obstructive pulmonary disease (COPD). Patients with COPD typically demonstrate clinical manifestations of both chronic bronchitis and emphysema.

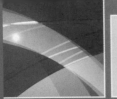

OVERVIEW of the Cardiopulmonary Clinical Manifestations Associated With Chronic Bronchitis and Emphysema (Chronic Obstructive Pulmonary Disease)—cont'd

CLINICAL DATA OBTAINED FROM LABORATORY AND SPECIAL PROCEDURES

Pulmonary Function Test Findings
Moderate to Severe Chronic Bronchitis and Emphysema
(Obstructive Lung Pathophysiology)

Pulmonary function tests are the cornerstone to the diagnostic evaluation of patients with suspected COPD. The most important values measured are the forced expiratory volume in 1 second (FEV_1), the forced vital capacity (FVC), and the FEV_1/FVC ratio.

FORCED EXPIRATORY VOLUME AND FLOW RATE FINDINGS

FVC	FEV_T	FEV_1/FVC ratio	$FEF_{25\%-75\%}$
↓	↓	↓	↓

$FEF_{50\%}$	$FEF_{200-1200}$	PEFR	MVV
↓	↓	↓	↓

LUNG VOLUME AND CAPACITY FINDINGS

V_T	IRV	ERV	RV^2
N or ↑	N or ↓	N or ↓	Normal or ↑

VC	IC	FRC^2	TLC^2	RV/TLC ratio^2
↓	N or ↓	↑	N or ↑	N or ↑

Diffusion Capacity (DLCO)[3]

Emphysema	Chronic Bronchitis
Decreased	Normal

A decreased DLCO is a classic diagnostic sign of emphysema

Arterial Blood Gases
Chronic Bronchitis and Emphysema

MILD TO MODERATE STAGES (GOLD 1 AND 2)
Acute Alveolar Hyperventilation With Hypoxemia[4]
(Acute Respiratory Alkalosis)

pH	$PaCO_2$	HCO_3^-	PaO_2	SaO_2 or SpO_2
↑	↓	↓ (but normal)	↓	↓

SEVERE STAGES (GOLD 3 AND 4)
Chronic Ventilatory Failure With Hypoxemia[5]
(Compensated Respiratory Acidosis)

pH	$PaCO_2$	HCO_3^-	PaO_2	SaO_2 or SpO_2
N	↑	↑ (significantly)	↓	↓

ACUTE VENTILATORY CHANGES SUPERIMPOSED ON CHRONIC VENTILATORY FAILURE[6]

Because acute ventilatory changes are frequently seen in patients with chronic ventilatory failure, the respiratory therapist must be familiar with—and alert for—the following two dangerous ABG findings:

- Acute alveolar hyperventilation superimposed on chronic ventilatory failure that should further alert the respiratory therapist to document the following important arterial blood gas assessment: possible *impending acute ventilatory failure.*
- Acute ventilatory failure (acute hypoventilation) superimposed on chronic ventilatory failure.

Oxygenation Indices[7] for Chronic Bronchitis and Emphysema
Moderate to Severe Stages

$\dot{Q}_S/\dot{Q}_T$	$DO_2{}^8$	$\dot{V}O_2$	$C(a-\bar{v})O_2$	O_2ER	$S\bar{v}O_2$
↑	↓	N	N	↑	↓

---

[2]Air trapping, and a subsequent increase in the RV and FRC, is uncommon in patients with only chronic bronchitis.

[3]The most accurate way to express DLCO as the DLCO corrected for alveolar volume (D_L/V_A). This measure is always reduced in severe emphysema and reflects the loss of alveolar-capillary membrane.

[4]See Fig. 5.2 and Table 5.4 and related discussions for the acute pH, $PaCO_2$, and HCO_3^- changes associated with acute alveolar hyperventilation.

[5]See Table 5.6 and related discussion for the pH, $PaCO_2$, and HCO_3^- changes associated with chronic ventilatory failure.

[6]See Table 5.7, Table 5.8, and Table 5.9 and related discussion for the pH, $PaCO_2$, and HCO_3^- changes associated with acute ventilatory changes superimposed on chronic ventilatory failure.

[7]DO_2, Total oxygen delivery; $C(a-\bar{v})O_2$, arterial-venous oxygen difference; O_2ER, oxygen extraction ratio; $\dot{Q}_S/\dot{Q}_T$, pulmonary shunt fraction; $S\bar{v}O_2$, mixed venous oxygen saturation; $\dot{V}O_2$, oxygen consumption.

[8]The DO_2 may be normal in patients who have compensated to the decreased oxygenation status with (1) an increased cardiac output, (2) an increased hemoglobin level, or (3) a combination of both. When the DO_2 is normal, the O_2ER is usually normal.

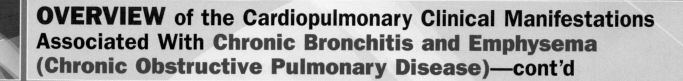

OVERVIEW of the Cardiopulmonary Clinical Manifestations Associated With Chronic Bronchitis and Emphysema (Chronic Obstructive Pulmonary Disease)—cont'd

Hemodynamic Indices[9] for Chronic Bronchitis and Emphysema
Moderate to Severe Stages

CVP	RAP	$\overline{PA}$	PCWP	CO	SV
↑	↑	↑	N	N	N

SVI	cardiac index	RVSWI	LVSWI	PVR	SVR
N	N	↑	N	↑	N

Laboratory Tests and Procedures

Test

	Emphysema	Chronic Bronchitis
Hematocrit and hemoglobin	Normal—mild to moderate stage Elevated—late stage	Polycythemia common during early and late stages
Electrolytes (abnormal)	Late stage: Hypochloremia (Cl⁻) when chronic ventilatory failure is present Hypernatremia (Na⁺)	Early and late stages: Hypochloremia (Cl⁻) (when chronic ventilatory failure is present) Hypernatremia (Na⁺)
Sputum examination (culture)	Normal	*Streptococcus pneumoniae* *Haemophilus influenzae* *Moraxella catarrhalis*

Radiology Findings

Test	Findings
	Chronic Bronchitis

Chest radiograph	Lungs may be clear if only large bronchi are affected.
	Occasionally:
	    Translucent (dark) lung fields
	    Depressed or flattened diaphragms
	Common:
	    Right ventricle (cor pulmonale) and/or left ventricle enlargement
	No radiographic abnormalities may be present in chronic bronchitis if only the large bronchi are affected. This often explains why the diagnosis is delayed. Although the situation is uncommon, if the more peripheral bronchi are involved, air trapping may occur. This is revealed on x-ray film as areas of translucency or areas that are darker in appearance. In addition, because of the increased functional residual capacity, the diaphragms may be depressed or flattened and are seen as such on the radiograph (Fig. 13.10).
	Because bronchial wall thickening is common in chronic bronchitis, increased, diffuse, fibrotic-appearing lung markings are often seen. This is commonly referred to as a *dirty chest x-ray*.
	Finally, because right and left ventricular enlargement and failure are commonly associated with chronic bronchitis, in the late stage an enlarged heart may be seen on the chest radiograph.

Bronchogram Computed tomography (CT) scan	Although bronchograms are rarely done today, small spikelike protrusions ("train tracks" appearance of airways) from the larger bronchi often could be seen on the bronchograms of patients with chronic bronchitis. It is believed that the spikes result from pooling of the radiopaque medium in the enlarged ducts of the mucous glands (Fig. 13.11). Since the advent of the CT examination, bronchograms are seldom done today on patients with chronic bronchitis. A "thin-section" CT examination is even more helpful.

Continued

[9]CO, Cardiac output; CVP, central venous pressure; LVSWI, left ventricular stroke work index; $\overline{PA}$, mean pulmonary artery pressure; PCWP, pulmonary capillary wedge pressure; PVR, pulmonary vascular resistance; RAP, right atrial pressure; RVSWI, right ventricular stroke work index; SV, stroke volume; SVI, stroke volume index; SVR, systemic vascular resistance.

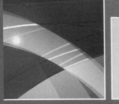

OVERVIEW of the Cardiopulmonary Clinical Manifestations Associated With Chronic Bronchitis and Emphysema (Chronic Obstructive Pulmonary Disease)—cont'd

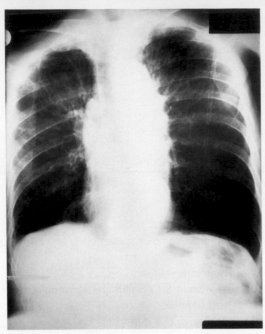

FIGURE 13.10 Chest x-ray film from a patient with chronic bronchitis. Note the translucent (dark) lung fields at the bases, depressed diaphragms, and long and narrow heart.

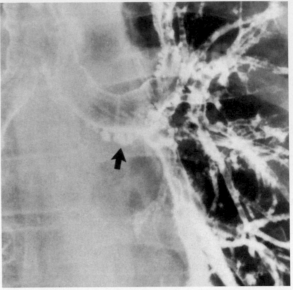

FIGURE 13.11 Chronic bronchitis. Bronchogram with localized view of left hilum. Rounded collections of contrast lie adjacent to bronchial walls and are particularly well demonstrated below the left mainstem bronchus (arrow) in this film. They are caused by contrast in dilated mucous gland ducts. (From Hansel, D. M., Armstrong, P., Lynch, D. A., et al. [2005]. *Imaging of the diseases of the chest* [4th ed.]. St. Louis, MO: Elsevier.)

Test	Findings
	Emphysema
Chest radiograph	Common:
	Translucent (dark) lung fields
	Depressed or flattened diaphragms
	Long and narrow heart (pulled downward by diaphragms)
	Increased retrosternal air space (lateral radiograph)
	Occasionally:
	Cor pulmonale (signs of cardiomegaly)
	Emphysematous bullae

Because of the decreased lung recoil and air trapping in emphysema, the functional residual capacity increases and the radiographic density of the lungs decreases. Consequently, the resistance to x-ray penetration is not as great, causing areas of translucency or areas that are darker in appearance. Because of the increased functional residual capacity, the diaphragm is depressed or flattened (a hallmark of lung hyperinflation) and the heart often appears long and narrow (Fig. 13.12).

The lateral chest radiograph characteristically shows an increased retrosternal air space (more than 3.0 cm from the anterior surface of the aorta to the back of the sternum measured 3.0 cm below the manubriosternal junction) and flattened diaphragms (Fig. 13.13). Because right ventricular enlargement and cor pulmonale sometimes develop as secondary problems during the advanced stages of emphysema, an enlarged heart may be seen on the chest radiograph (Fig. 13.14).

Occasionally, emphysematous bulla may be seen on the chest radiograph or CT scan. Bullae appear as air-containing cystic spaces whose walls are usually of hairline thickness. They can range in size from 1 to 2 cm in diameter up to an entire hemithorax (Fig. 13.15). These large, radiolucent, air-filled sacs are generally found at the apices or at the bases of the lung. Bullae may become so large that they cause respiratory insufficiency by compressing the remaining relatively normal lung. Fig. 13.16 shows a CT image of emphysematous blebs. Finally, Fig. 13.17 shows a before and after chest radiograph of a 56-year-old woman with severe COPD who qualified for a lung transplant. Before the surgery she was unable to perform the simplest of tasks. After the surgery she was working out regularly at her neighborhood fitness center.

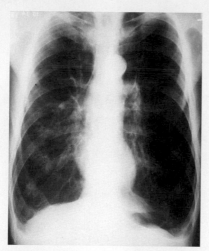

FIGURE 13.12 Chest x-ray film of a patient with emphysema. The heart often appears long and narrow as a result of being drawn downward by the descending diaphragm.

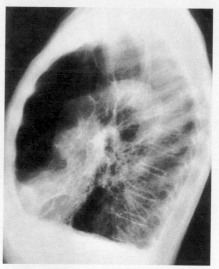

FIGURE 13.13 Emphysema. Lateral chest radiograph demonstrates a characteristically large retrosternal radiolucency with increased separation of the aorta and sternum measuring 4.6 cm, 3 cm below the angle of Louis and extending down to within 3 cm of the diaphragm anteriorly. Both costophrenic angles are obtuse, and both hemidiaphragms are flat. (From Hansel, D. M., Lynch, D., & McAdams, H. P. [2010]. *Imaging of the diseases of the chest* [5th ed.]. Philadelphia, PA: Elsevier.)

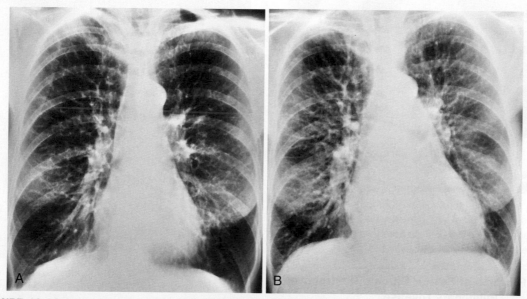

FIGURE 13.14 Cor pulmonale. (A) A 50-year-old man with chronic airflow obstruction. The lungs are large in volume, the diaphragm is flat, and vascular attenuation is evident at the right apex. These features suggest emphysema, and this diagnosis was supported by a low carbon monoxide diffusion capacity. Lung "markings" are increased peripherally, particularly in the left midzone. (B) The patient became chronically hypoxic and, with respiratory infections, hypercapnic. One of these episodes was associated with cor pulmonale when the patient became edematous and the heart and hilar and pulmonary parenchymal vessels became enlarged. The emphysematous right upper zone shows fewer vascular markings and is relatively transient. The diaphragm is less depressed and more curved than before. (From Hansel, D. M., Lynch, D., & McAdams, H. P. [2010]. *Imaging of the diseases of the chest* [5th ed.]. Philadelphia, PA: Elsevier.)

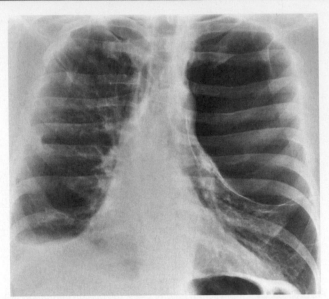

FIGURE 13.15 Giant emphysematous bulla. Air-containing mass fills most of the left hemithorax. (From Eisenberg, R. L., & Johnson, N. M. [2016]. *Comprehensive radiographic pathology* [6th ed.]. St. Louis, MO: Elsevier.)

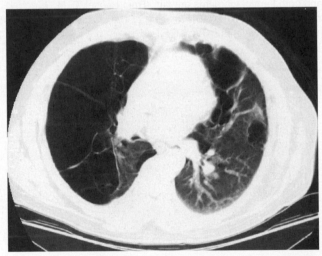

FIGURE 13.16 Emphysematous blebs. Computed tomography image shows the destruction of lung parenchyma. (From Eisenberg, R. L., & Johnson, N. M. [2016]. *Comprehensive radiographic pathology* [6th ed.]. St. Louis, MO: Elsevier.)

Additional Features of Severe Chronic Obstructive Pulmonary Disease

- Fatigue
- Weight loss and anorexia
- Syncope during coughing episodes caused by the rapid increases in intrathoracic pressure changes during prolonged coughing spells.
  - Coughing may cause rib fractures
- Ankle swelling may be the only indicator of cor pulmonale
- Symptoms of depression and/or anxiety, which are associated with an increased risk for exacerbations

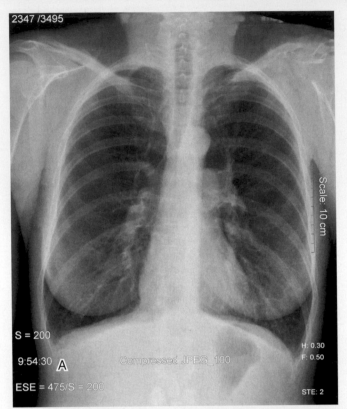

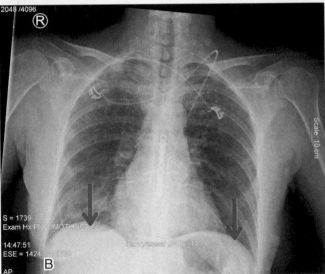

FIGURE 13.17 A before (A) and after (B) chest radiograph of a 56-year-old woman who had severe COPD and qualified for a lung transplantation. Note the domed diaphragmatic leafs, indicating reduced pulmonary hyperexpansion, after the lung transplantation (red arrows). Also note the reduced pulmonary artery enlargement in the left chest after transplantation. (Courtesy Terry Des Jardins.)

General Management of Chronic Obstructive Pulmonary Disease

GOLD provides an outstanding COPD management program that can be easily adapted to local health care systems and resources. An overview of GOLD's management programs for stable COPD and acute COPD exacerbation are presented below.[5]

Overview of GOLD's Management of Stable Chronic Obstructive Pulmonary Disease

After the patient has been diagnosed with COPD and fully assessed (see Combined COPD Assessment Tool, Fig. 13.9), an effective treatment plan should be directed at reducing the current symptoms and preventing future risks for exacerbations (see Fig. 13.6).

GOLD's general management of the COPD patient is to (1) identify and reduce exposure to risk factors, (2) establish a pharmacologic treatment algorithm, and (3) implement various nonpharmacologic treatments, such as education and self-management, physical activity, **pulmonary rehabilitation** programs, exercise training, self-management education, nutritional support, vaccinations, long-term oxygen therapy needs, ventilatory support, and, when needed, **end-of-life and palliative care**. Finally, monitoring and follow-up appointments for COPD outpatient care need to be established.

Reduce Exposure to Risk Factors

The identification and reduction of the patient's exposure to risk factors are very important. For example, cigarette smoking is the most commonly encountered risk factor for COPD. When possible, smokers should be provided with counseling and smoking cessation programs that incorporate behavior change techniques, patient education, and pharmacologic and non-pharmacologic interventions. In addition, efforts to have patients reduce their total exposure to occupational dusts, fumes, gases, and to indoor and outdoor air pollutants should be addressed.

Pharmacologic Treatment Algorithm

Pharmacologic therapies are used to (1) reduce the patient's symptoms and readmissions[6], (2) decrease the risk and severity of exacerbations, and (3) improve the patient's overall health status and exercise tolerance. Table 13.5 provides medications commonly used in the treatment of COPD. According to GOLD, some key points regarding the medications used to treat COPD are shown in Box 13.2.

Applying the Combined Assessment Tool to a Pharmacologic Treatment Algorithm

GOLD recommends using the clinical data obtained from the Combined COPD Assessment Tool—that is, severity of airflow, patient symptoms, and future risk for exacerbation—as the basis for establishing a safe and effective pharmacologic treatment algorithm (see Fig. 13.9). Furthermore, GOLD recommends an *up-regulation and/or down-regulation strategy* for patients placed in Groups A, B, C, and D, as follows:

- *Group A (Low Risk, Fewer Symptoms):* The patients placed in this group should be offered a bronchodilator treatment based on the effects it has on the patient's perceived dyspnea. The bronchodilator can be either a short- or long-acting bronchodilator. Treatment should continue if the patient demonstrates symptomatic benefit (Fig. 13.18).

TABLE 13.5 Medications Commonly Used in the Treatment of Chronic Obstructive Pulmonary Disease (COPD)*

Generic Name	Brand Name
Short-Acting Beta₂ Agents (SABAs)	
Albuterol	Proventil HFA, Ventolin HFA, ProAir HFA
Metaproterenol	Generic only
Levalbuterol	Xopenex, Xopenex HFA, Generic
Long-Acting Beta₂ Agents (LABAs)	
Salmeterol	Serevent Diskus
Formoterol	Perforomist, Foradil Aerolizer
Arformoterol	Brovana
Indacaterol	Arcapta Neohaler
Olodaterol	Striverdi Respimat
Short Acting Antimuscarinic Antagonists (SAMAs)	
Ipratropium	Atrovent HFA
Long-Acting Antimuscarinic Antagonists (LAMAs)	
Tiotropium	Spiriva HandiHaler, Spiriva Respimat
Aclidinium	Tudorza Pressair
Umeclidinium	Incruse Ellipta
Combined SABAs and Anticholinergic Agents	
Ipratropium and albuterol	DuoNeb, Combivent Respimat
Combined LABAs and Anticholinergic Agents	
Umeclidinium and vilanterol	Anoro Ellipta
Combined LABAs and Inhaled Corticosteroids	
Fluticasone and salmeterol	Advair Diskus (250/50 mcg only)
Budesonide and formoterol	Symbicort (60/4.5 mcg only)
Fluticasone and vilanterol	Breo Ellipta
Methylxanthines	
Theophylline	Theochron, Elixophyllin, Theo-24
Aminophylline	Generic
Phosphodiesterase-4 Inhibitor	
Roflumilast	Daliresp

*For the complete listing, doses, and administration of agents approved by the FDA, visit the Drugs@FDA website (http://www.accessdata.fda.gov/scripts/cder/drugsatfda/).

---

[5]To obtain the complete report of the GOLD management program for COPD, go to http://www.goldcopd.org.
[6]Thus, all **cause readmission prevention program (CRPP)** .

BOX 13.2 Key Points Regarding the Medications Used to Treat Chronic Obstructive Pulmonary Disease

Bronchodilators
- Long-acting beta$_2$ agents (LABAs) and long-acting antimuscarinic antagonists (LAMAs) are preferred over short-acting agents—except for the patient with only occasional dyspnea.
- The COPD patient may be started on a single LABA or dual LABAs. For example, in patients with persistent dyspnea, and only on one LABA, the therapy should be up-regulated to two LABAs.
- Inhaled bronchodilators are recommended over oral bronchodilators.
- Theophylline is not recommended unless other long-term bronchodilators are not available or are unaffordable.

Inhaled Corticosteroids (ICS)
- Long-term monotherapy with ICS is not recommended.
- However, long-term therapy with ICS may be used in conjunction with LABAs in the patient with a history of exacerbations.
- Long-term therapy with oral corticosteroids is not recommended.
- In the patient with exacerbations after receiving LABA/ICS or LABA/LAMA/ICS and who has chronic bronchitis and severe to very severe airflow limitations, the addition of a phosphodiesterase-4 inhibitor (PDE-4 inhibitor) can be considered.

Other Pharmacologic Agents
- Mucolytics have not proved beneficial in the treatment of excessive bronchial secretions.

- The patient with severe alpha$_1$-antitrypsin deficiency and diagnosed with COPD may be a candidate for alpha$_1$-antitrypsin deficiency therapy.
- Antitussives are not recommended.
- Vasodilators: Medications for primary pulmonary hypertension are not recommended in patients with pulmonary hypertension secondary to COPD.

Antibiotics (Macrolide)
- Recent studies have shown that the regular use of some antibiotics may reduce the risk for exacerbation in COPD patients. Azithromycin or erythromycin for 1 year in patients prone to exacerbations has shown to reduce exacerbations.

Phosphodiesterase-4 (PDE-4) Inhibitors
- The primary action of PDE-4 inhibitors is to reduce inflammation by preventing the breakdown of intracellular cyclic AMP. Roflumilast is taken once per day with no direct bronchodilator activity. Roflumilast has been shown to reduce moderate and severe exacerbations in patients treated with systemic corticosteroids who have chronic bronchitis, very severe COPD, and a history of exacerbations. Beneficial effects are also seen on lung function when roflumilast is added to long-acting bronchodilators and in patients who are not controlled on fixed-dose LABA/ICS combinations.

- *Group B (Low Risk, More Symptoms):* The initial therapy for patients in this group consists of *a long-acting antimuscarinic antagonist* (LAMA) bronchodilator or a *long-acting beta$_2$-agonist* (LABA) bronchodilator. There is no evidence to support one class of long-acting bronchodilators over another for relief of symptoms. The selection is often based on the patient's perception of symptom relief. However, in the patient with persistent dyspnea while receiving only one long-acting bronchodilator, it is recommended that the therapy be up-regulated to medications contained in a second long-acting bronchodilator classification (LAMA + LABA). For the patient with severe dyspnea, the initial therapy with two long-acting bronchodilators may be considered. If the addition of a second bronchodilator does not improve the patient's symptoms, it is recommended that the therapy be returned to only one bronchodilator. The possibilities of associated comorbidities that affect the patient's conditions should be considered (see Fig. 13.18).
- *Group C (High Risk, Fewer Symptoms):* The patient in this group should be given a single LAMA. LAMAs have been shown to be superior to LABAs and are recommended by GOLD for this group. In patients with persistent exacerbations, a second long-acting bronchodilator (LAMA + LABA), or the combination of a long-acting beta$_2$-agonist and an inhaled corticosteroid (LABA + inhaled

corticosteroid [ICS]) may be considered. Because the administration of ICS agents increases the risk for developing pneumonia in some patients, GOLD's primary recommendation is LABA + LAMA (see Fig. 13.18).
- *Group D (High Risk, More Symptoms):* The patients in this group should be started with a LABA + LAMA combination. Studies have shown superior results when using a LABA + LAMA combination compared with a single medication. Conversely, if a single bronchodilator is preferred to treat an exacerbation episode, a LAMA is recommended. Although a LABA + LAMA combination has been shown to be superior to a LABA + ICS combination, in the patient with a history and/or findings that suggest an asthma and COPD overlap,[7] an initial therapy with LABA + ICS may be the first choice. In addition, a high blood eosinophil count may further support the use of ICS in these patients. However, it should be noted that patients in Group D are at a higher risk for developing pneumonia when receiving ICS treatments.

In the patient who develops further exacerbations on LABA + LAMA, the advancement to a LABA + LAMA + ICS combination should be considered. Finally, if the patient being

---

[7]Asthma and COPD overlap syndrome (ACOS) is discussed in Chapter 14, Asthma.

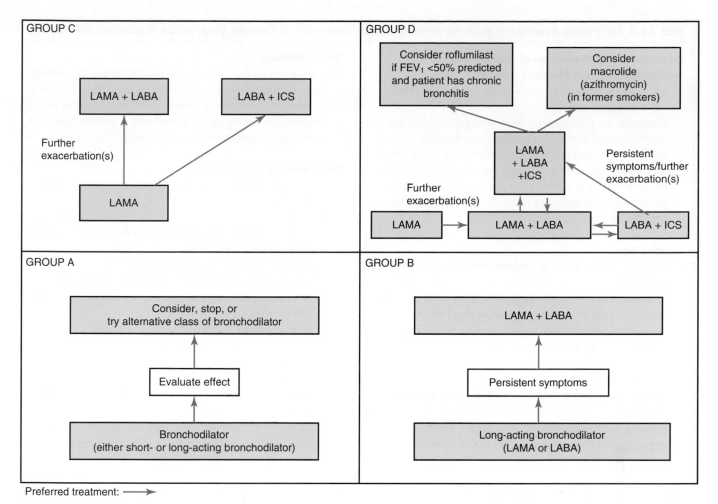

Preferred treatment: ⟶

FIGURE 13.18 Pharmacologic treatment algorithms based on Group A, B, C, or D classifications derived from the Combined COPD Assessment Tool (see Fig. 13.9). *ICI,* Inhaled corticosteroids; *LABA,* long-acting beta$_2$-agonist; *LAMA,* long-acting antimuscarinic antagonist.

treated with a LABA + LAMA + ICS combination continues to have exacerbations, the following options may be considered:

- Add roflumilast if the FEV$_1$ is less than 50% predicted and the patient has chronic bronchitis, especially if the patient has a history of one or more hospitalizations for exacerbation in the past year.
- Add a macrolide antibiotic. GOLD states that the best available evidence exists for the use of azithromycin (see Fig. 13.18).

Nonpharmacologic Treatments

The key points associated with nonpharmacologic treatments for the patient with stable COPD are shown in Box 13.3.

Management of Acute Chronic Obstructive Pulmonary Disease Exacerbations

A COPD exacerbation is defined by GOLD as an acute worsening of the patient's normal baseline respiratory status. An acute exacerbation is associated with increased airway inflammation, increased mucous production, and significant alveolar hyperinflation. These anatomic changes of the lung contribute to the patient's key symptom of an acute exacerbation—increased dyspnea.

Other signs of an acute exacerbation include increased sputum volume and purulence, an increased cough, wheezing, an increased peripheral blood or sputum eosinophil count, and a decline in arterial oxygenation. Because comorbidities are common with COPD patients, exacerbations must be differentiated clinically from other events such as congestive heart failure, pneumonia, or pulmonary embolism. According to GOLD, COPD exacerbations are classified as follows:

- *Mild Exacerbation:* Requires the initial use of inhaled short-acting beta$_2$-agonist (SABAs) with or without a short-acting antimuscarinic bronchodilator.
- *Moderate Exacerbation:* Entails the use of SABAs, plus an antibiotic and/or oral corticosteroids.
- *Severe Exacerbation:* Requires an emergency department visit, hospitalization, or intensive care unit (ICU) admission. A severe exacerbation is associated with acute ventilatory failure.

Acute exacerbations are primarily triggered by respiratory viral infections, although bacterial infections and a variety of environmental factors such as indoor and outdoor pollution and adverse ambient temperatures may cause these events.

BOX 13.3 Key Points Associated With Nonpharmacologic Treatment of Chronic Obstructive Pulmonary Disease

Education, Self-Management, Pulmonary Rehabilitation, and Physical Activity

- Education is required to enhance the patient's understanding of the disease.
- Education to appropriately self-manage routine care is recommended to reduce risk for exacerbations.
- Pulmonary rehabilitation is recommended for all patients with symptoms and/or are high risk for exacerbations.
- Physical activity is a strong predictor of mortality. Patients should be encouraged to increase the level of physical activity.

Vaccination

- Influenza vaccination is recommended for all patients with COPD.
- Pneumococcal vaccination: The PCV13 and PPSV23 are recommended for all patients older than 65 years and in younger patients with significant comorbid conditions (e.g., chronic heart or lung disease).

Nutritional Support

- Nutritional supplementation should be considered in malnourished patients with COPD. Malnourished COPD patients receiving nutritional supplementation have shown significant improvements on their 6-minute walk test, respiratory strength, and overall health status.

Interventional Bronchoscopy and Surgery

- In certain patients with emphysema and significant hyperinflation, **lung volume reduction surgery** or bronchoscopic modes of lung volume reduction (e.g., **endobronchial one-way valves or lung coils**) may be considered.
- Surgical **bullectomy** may be considered in patients with large bulla.
- **Lung transplantation** may be considered in selected patients with very severe COPD who do not have any contradictions.

Comorbidities

- Any symptoms that indicate the worsening and/or development of another comorbid condition, such as obstructive sleep apnea, congestive heart failure, and ischemic heart disease, should be documented and a plan established to manage the problem as indicated.

Monitoring and Follow-Up

- Routine monitoring of COPD patients is essential, including:
  - FEV1
  - Functional capacity as measured by a timed walking test (6-minute walking test)
  - SaO_2 or arterial blood gases
  - Check patient symptoms, including cough, sputum, breathlessness, fatigue, activity limitation, and sleep disturbances
  - Exacerbations, including frequency, severity, type, and likely causes of all exacerbations
  - Sputum volume and presence or absence of sputum purulence should be noted.
  - Imaging—If there is a clear worsening of symptoms, imaging may be considered
  - Smoking status—At each visit, the patients' smoking habits and smoke exposure should be established, followed by appropriate action.

End-of-Life and Palliative Care

- The goal of palliative care is to relive pain and suffering of patients and their families via the comprehensive assessment and treatment of physical, psychosocial, and symptoms presented by the patient.

The symptoms associated with an exacerbation usually last 7 to 10 days. Patients who have had an exacerbation are usually more susceptible to another event. Some patients are especially prone to frequent exacerbations—defined as two or more exacerbations per year. The strongest predictor of a patient's *future* exacerbation history is the number of exacerbations they have had in the past year.

Treatment Options for Acute Exacerbations

According to GOLD, the primary goals of treatment for COPD are to minimize the negative effect of the current exacerbation and prevent the occurrence of future events. Relative to the severity of an exacerbation, the individual's care management may occur in either an outpatient or inpatient setting. At the present time, more than 80% of exacerbations are managed on an outpatient basis with bronchodilators, corticosteroids, and antibiotics.

Box 13.4 provides an overview of the indications of severe exacerbations that require hospitalization. An overview of GOLD's recommended algorithm to manage the patient hospitalized with severe exacerbation is provided in Box 13.5.

Respiratory Care Treatment Protocols
Oxygen Therapy Protocol

Initially, supplemental oxygen should be administered with a target SaO_2 of 88% to 92%. Venturi masks (high-flow devices) offer more precise control of FIO_2 than nasal cannulas.

- According to GOLD, long-term oxygen therapy is indicated in the patient with stable disease who has a:
  - PaO_2 at or below 55 mm Hg or an SaO_2 less than 88%, with or without hypercapnia confirmed two or more times over a 3-week period; or

- PaO_2 between 55 and 60 mm Hg or an SaO_2 of 88% if there is evidence of pulmonary hypertension, peripheral edema suggesting congestive cardiac failure, or polycythemia (hematocrit greater than 55%).
- Once placed on long-term oxygen therapy, the patient should be reevaluated between 60 and 90 days later with repeat ABG or oxygen saturation determinations, while the patient is breathing the prescribed level of oxygen to determine if oxygen is still therapeutic and indicated.

Oxygen therapy is used to treat hypoxemia, decrease the work of breathing, and decrease myocardial work (see Oxygen Therapy Protocol, Protocol 10.1).

Mechanical Ventilation Protocol

Ventilatory support for COPD exacerbations can be provided by either *noninvasive ventilation (NIV)* (e.g., pressure/volume-limited ventilation via a nasal or facial mask) or *invasive ventilation* (e.g., oral-tracheal tube or tracheostomy) (see Box 13.5). When possible, the combination of NIV with long-term oxygen therapy is preferred in patients with stable severe COPD. NIV has shown benefit in patients with significant daytime hypercapnia who have recently been hospitalized. In addition, there are excellent benefits of continuous positive airway pressure (CPAP) in patients who have both COPD and obstructive sleep apnea. The following provides an overview of benefits of NIV, and the indications for invasive mechanical ventilation:

Benefits of Noninvasive Ventilation
- Avoidance of endotracheal intubation
- Reduction of problems associated with intubation

BOX 13.4 Indication for Hospitalization Caused by Acute Exacerbation

- Dyspnea at rest
- High respiratory rate
- Drowsiness
- Confusion
- Impending ventilatory failure—for example:
  - Acute alveolar hyperventilation superimposed on chronic ventilatory failure
    - Typical arterial blood gas values: pH 7.52, $PaCO_2$ 51, HCO_3^- 40, PaO_2 46 (see Table 5.7)
  - Acute ventilatory failure superimposed on chronic ventilatory failure
    - Typical arterial blood gas values: pH 7.28, $PaCO_2$ 99, HCO_3^- 45, PaO_2 34 (see Table 5.8)
  - Decreased arterial oxygen saturation and/or not responding to oxygen therapy
    - Cyanosis or peripheral edema
    - Failure of exacerbation to respond to initial bronchodilator management
    - Presence of comorbidities (e.g. congestive heart failure, arrhythmia, etc.)
    - Insufficient home support

- Comfort of the patient during ventilation
- Reduction of muscle fatigue
- The improvement of alveolar and arterial oxygen and carbon dioxide levels
- The reduction of work of breathing

Indications for Invasive Mechanical Ventilation
- Unable to tolerate NIV
- Respiratory or cardiac arrest
- Massive aspiration
- Severe ventricular arrhythmias
- Severe hypoxemia in patients unable to tolerate NIV

Because acute ventilatory failure superimposed on chronic ventilatory failure is often seen in patients with COPD exacerbation, ventilatory support is justified when the acute ventilatory failure is thought to be reversible; for example, when acute pneumonia exists as a complicating factor (see Mechanical Ventilation Protocol Protocol, 11.1, and Mechanical Ventilation Weaning Protocol Protocol, 11.2).

Aerosolized Medication Therapy Protocol

As outlined earlier by GOLD, pharmacologic therapies are used to (1) reduce the patient's symptoms, (2) decrease the risk and severity of exacerbations, and (3) improve the patient's overall health status and exercise tolerance. GOLD recommends using the clinical data obtained from the Combined COPD Assessment Tool—that is, severity of airflow, patient symptoms, and future risk for exacerbation—as the basis for establishing a safe and effective pharmacologic treatment algorithm (see Figs. 13.9 and 13.18). Furthermore, GOLD recommends an up-regulation and/or down-regulation strategy for patients placed in the Combined COPD Assessment Tool Groups (i.e., Groups A, B, C, and D) (see Fig. 13.18 and Aerosolized Medication Protocol, Protocol 10.4).

Airway Clearance Therapy Protocol

Selected patients who have excessive secretions or an ineffective cough may benefit from a number of techniques used to enhance the mobilization of bronchial secretions, such as postural drainage, positive expiratory pressure therapy, forced expiratory techniques, and flutter valve therapy (see Airway Clearance Therapy Protocol, Protocol 10.2).

Implications of the GOLD Guidelines for Respiratory Care

IMPORTANT: As the GOLD Guidelines for COPD become implemented in care settings where the respiratory therapist is employed, he or she should be aware that the Guidelines set a *standard of care* to an even greater extent than do therapist-driven protocols (TDPs). Thus the GOLD Guidelines almost certainly will be used as the basis for malpractice litigation and reimbursement denial—that is, if and when the Guidelines are violated. The role of the respiratory therapist to guard against this (to the extent that he or she can) cannot be overemphasized.

BOX 13.5 Overview of GOLD's Management Algorithm for Severe Exacerbations

Severe But Not Life-Threatening Exacerbation
- Continually assess the severity of symptoms (e.g., dyspnea, oxygenation, mental status)
- Administer supplement oxygen therapy and bronchodilator
- Increase dose and/or frequency of short-acting beta$_2$-agonoist
- Combine short-acting beta$_2$-agonists and antimuscarinic agents
- Consider use of long-acting bronchodilator once patient becomes stable
- Consider an oral corticosteroid
- Consider oral antibiotics when signs of bacterial infection are present

NOTE: Methylxanthines are not recommended because of increased side effect profiles.

Severe and Life-Threatening Exacerbation
- Severe dyspnea that does not respond adequately to initial therapy
- Signs of respiratory muscle fatigue, increased work of breathing, or both, such as use of respiratory accessory muscles, paradoxical motion of abdomen, or retraction of intercostal spaces.
- Decline in mental status (e.g., confusion, lethargy, coma)
- Persistent decline in PaO$_2$ (e.g., <40 mm Hg), increase in PaCO$_2$, and/or severe/worsening respiratory acidosis (e.g., pH <7.25)

Indications for Mechanical Ventilation

Life-Threatening Exacerbation
- Severe dyspnea that does not respond adequately to initial therapy
- Signs of respiratory muscle fatigue, increased work of breathing, or both, such as use of respiratory accessory muscles, paradoxical motion of abdomen, or retraction of intercostal spaces
- Decline in mental status (e.g., confusion, lethargy, coma)
- Persistent decline in PaO$_2$ (e.g., <40 mm Hg), increase in PaCO$_2$, and/or severe/worsening respiratory acidosis (e.g., pH <7.25)

Consider Mechanical Ventilation
- Initially, the use of noninvasive mechanical ventilation (NIV) is preferred over invasive mechanical ventilation (intubation and positive pressure ventilation)
  - NIV has been shown to improve oxygenation and acute respiratory acidosis, increase pH, decrease PaCO$_2$, and decrease the work of breathing
- Indications for invasive mechanical ventilation
  - Patient unable to receive NIV or NIV failure
  - Postrespiratory or cardiac arrest
  - Diminished consciousness, psychomotor agitation inadequately controlled by sedation
  - Massive aspiration or persistent vomiting
  - Persistent inability to remove airway secretions
  - Severe hemodynamic instability without response to fluids and vasoactive drugs
  - Severe ventricular or supraventricular arrhythmias
  - Life-threatening hypoxemia in patients unable to tolerate NIV

Admitting History and Physical Examination

This 71-year-old man has worked in a cotton mill in South Carolina for the past 37 years. He smoked 40 cigarettes a day for 30 years (60 pack/year), and he also chews tobacco regularly. He sought medical assistance in the chest clinic because of a worsening chronic cough. He described it as a "smoker's cough" and stated that it was present about 4 to 5 months of the year. For the past 3 years, his cough occasionally produced grayish-yellow sputum during the winter months. The sputum was thick and yellow. He stated that he recently was short of breath during moderate exercise. He attributed this to "getting older." The patient stated he had not been taking any pulmonary medications.

On physical examination, the patient was in mild respiratory distress. He was obese (270 lb). He occasionally generated a strong productive cough during the visit. His sputum appeared grayish-yellow. Auscultation of the chest revealed medium bilateral crackles and scattered wheezes. On a 1 L/min nasal cannula, an ABG assessment showed pH 7.36, $PaCO_2$ 87 mm Hg, HCO_3^- 48 mEq/L, PaO_2 64 mm Hg, and SaO_2 91%. The chest radiograph revealed hyperinflation.

PFTs showed a decrease in the FEV_1/FVC (65%) and a decreased FEV_1 (55% of predicted). The patient's mMRC was 1, and he had no reported exacerbations during the past 12 months. Based on the Combined COPD Assessment Tool, the patient would be classified as GOLD Grade 2, Group A (Low Exacerbation Risk, Fewer Symptoms) (see Fig. 13.9).

The respiratory therapist's assessment at this time was documented in the patient's chart as follows.

Respiratory Assessment and Plan

S "Smoker's cough," sputum production, dyspnea.

O Strong productive cough observed. Sputum: Yellow-gray. Breath sounds: Medium bilateral crackles throughout and scattered wheezes. On a 1 L/min nasal cannula ABG: pH 7.36, $PaCO_2$ 87, HCO_3^- 48, PaO_2 64, and SaO_2 91%. X-ray: Hyperinflation. PFTs: FEV_1/FVC ratio 65%, FEV_1 55% of predicted. mMRC 1. Exacerbations 0. GOLD Grade 2, Group A.

A • Combined COPD Assessment: GOLD Grade 2, Group A—Low Exacerbation Risk, Fewer Symptoms
  • Mild acute exacerbation (history, physical examination, Combined COPD Assessment Tool).
  • Bronchospasm (wheezes)
  • Moderate airway secretions (medium crackles)
  • Good ability to mobilize secretions (strong cough and sputum production)
  • Chronic ventilatory failure with mild hypoxemia (ABG)

P Airway Clearance Therapy Protocol (cough and deep breathing, PRN). Patient education on smoking. Refer to Smoking Cessation Clinic. Aerosolized Medication Protocol—inhaled short-acting antimuscarinic antagonist (SAMA)—for example, ipratropium bromide (PRN). Continue Oxygen Therapy Protocol (1 L/min nasal cannula).

At discharge, the patient was advised to stop smoking and seek medical assistance if his sputum became progressively more thick and yellow or his dyspnea became worse. The physician also prescribed PRN use of a long-acting antimuscarinic antagonist (LAMA) and a pneumococcal polysaccharide vaccine. The Smoking Cessation Clinic prescribed slow-release nicotine patches, and the patient attended a week-long smoking cessation program. The patient did well, and at the 6-month follow-up visit he was no longer smoking. At this time, the patient stated that he had not had his "smoker's cough" or produced any sputum in weeks.

Ten Months Later

Emergency Department History and Physical Examination

The patient presented in the emergency department and was clearly *not* doing well. He was back to his three-packs-per-day cigarette smoking habit, and he had been physically inactive and gained 30 lb (to a weight of 300 lb) over the past 10 months. He stated that he frequently coughed, and the cough was more troublesome in the early morning. The patient also reported that his cough was now routinely productive—about 3 to 4 tablespoons of thick yellow and green sputum daily. He complained of dyspnea during light exercise (e.g., stair climbing produced shortness of breath). On some days, his increased work of breathing was more noticeable than on others. He denied hemoptysis, chest pain, orthopnea, fever, chills, or leg edema. In general, he tended to minimize his symptoms.

Despite the patient's history, on observation, his ankles *were* swollen, with pitting edema of 3+. His neck veins were distended. He was cyanotic. Vital signs were blood pressure 165/90, heart rate 116 bpm, and respiratory rate 26 breaths/min. His oral temperature was 98.4°F. Auscultation of the chest revealed bilateral posterior basilar wheezes and coarse crackles, which partially cleared with coughing. Expectorated sputum was copious, purulent, and yellow and green.

A bedside spirometry showed an FEV_1/FVC ratio of 51% and an FEV_1 of 37% of predicted. The patient's mMRC was 2, and he had one exacerbation 10 months earlier, for a total of two per year at this point in time (see previous first SOAP note). Based on the Combined Assessment of COPD Tool, the patient was classified GOLD Grade 3, Group D (High Risk, More Symptoms) (see Fig. 13.9).

On a 1 L/min oxygen nasal cannula, his ABG values were pH 7.51, $PaCO_2$ 51 mm Hg, HCO_3^- 39 mEq/L, PaO_2 41 mm Hg, SaO_2 84%. His resting SpO_2 on room air was 83%. This improved to 89% on 2 L/min oxygen via nasal cannula. His chest x-ray showed diffuse, fibrotic-appearing lung markings and a moderately enlarged right side of the heart. His hemoglobin was 17.8 g%.

At this time, the respiratory therapist recorded the following SOAP note in the patient's chart.

Respiratory Assessment and Plan

S Complains of productive cough and exertional dyspnea (history).

O Bibasilar wheezes and coarse crackles, cyanosis, obesity. Neck veins distended. 3+ leg edema. Vital signs: HR 116, BP 165/90, RR 26/min. Cough: Productive with copious yellow and green sputum. PFT: FEV_1/FVC (51%), FEV_1 (37% of predicted). mMRC 2. Exacerbations 2/yr: GOLD Grade 3, Group D. CXR: Diffuse fibrotic lung markings and cardiomegaly (possible cor pulmonale). ABG on a 1 L/min nasal cannula, pH 7.51, $PaCO_2$ 51, HCO_3^- 39, PaO_2 41, SaO_2 84%. SpO_2 on 2 L/min O_2 89%. Hemoglobin 17.8 g%.

A • Acute exacerbation of chronic bronchitis
  • Combined COPD Assessment: GOLD Grade 3, Group D (High Risk, More Symptoms)
    • Worsening since last assessment 10 months previously
  • Acute exacerbation (history, physical examination, Combined COPD Assessment)
  • Acute alveolar hyperventilation superimposed on chronic ventilatory failure with moderate to severe hypoxemia (ABG, SpO_2)
    • Impending ventilatory failure
  • Bronchospasm (wheezes)
  • Excessive mucous accumulation (sputum, coarse crackles)
  • Infection (yellow and green sputum)
  • Tobacco addiction-worsening (history)

P *Aerosolized Medication Therapy Protocol:* Start on long-acting antimuscarinic antagonist (LAMA) qid. Reassess in 2 hours. If exacerbation persists, change to LAMA plus LABA (long-acting beta$_2$-agonist). Airway Clearance Therapy Protocol (cough and deep breathing under supervision four times daily, cautious trial of chest physiotherapy [CPT] with postural drainage to lower lobes, three times per day). Continue Oxygen Therapy Protocol (1 L/min nasal cannula; monitor SpO_2). Call physician about impending ventilatory failure and chest x-ray report of cardiomegaly.

Over the next 2 weeks and over 60 additional SOAP assessments the patient progressively improved. Mechanical ventilation was not needed in the next 6 months of recorded follow-up. Upon discharge the patient was placed on an LAMA and an inhaled corticosteroid (ICS) regimen and checked off by respiratory care on the appropriate self-administration of the bronchodilator. In addition, he was scheduled for a follow-up appointment for pulmonary rehabilitation and a smoking cessation program.

Discussion

In the first portion of this case study, clearly some of the clinical manifestations caused by excessive bronchial secretions (see Fig. 10.11) were present. These findings were documented in the first SOAP note when the therapist charted the presence of a productive cough, coarse crackle sounds, and pulmonary function findings that indicated airway obstruction. Unfortunately, the first SOAP note (and for that matter the initial admitting history) provided no clue as to the time-course of the patient's complaints. Was his condition stable or worsening? The first part of this case also illustrates a definite role for the modern respiratory therapist. Such a professional may well be working in outpatient settings (e.g., urgent care centers or emergency departments) that necessitate the evaluation and treatment of patients such as this one.

During writing of the first SOAP, the therapist appropriately identified the patient as GOLD Grade 2, Group A on the Combined COPD Assessment Tool. This classification was based on the fact that the patient demonstrated an FEV_1/FVC ratio of 65%, an FEV_1 of 55%, an mMRC of 1, and no recent exacerbations (see Fig. 13.9). In addition, because the patient was placed in Group A (Low Exacerbation Risk, Low Symptoms), the initial Aerosolized Medication Protocol—that is, the inhaled short-acting antimuscarinic antagonist (SAMA)—was appropriate according to the GOLD standard guidelines (see Fig. 13.18).

During the second portion of this case, there were more of the classic clinical manifestations associated with chronic bronchitis. For example, the patient's excessive bronchial secretions (see Fig. 10.11) not only resulted in hypoxia and cyanosis secondary to a decreased $\dot{V}/\dot{Q}$ ratio and pulmonary shunting but also produced increased airway resistance that resulted in coarse crackles and a further worsening of the patient's pulmonary function performance.

The respiratory therapist correctly identified the patient as GOLD Grade 3, Group D (High Exacerbation Risk, More Symptoms) on the Combined COPD Assessment Tool. This was based on these clinical data: FEV_1/FVC 51%, FEV_1 37% of predicted, mMRC 2, and two exacerbations during the past 12 months. Because the patient's airflow limitation was severe (GOLD Grade 3), and because his dyspnea and exacerbation risks placed him in Group D, the Aerosolized Medication Protocol appropriately included a long-acting antimuscarinic antagonist (LAMA) (see Fig. 13.18). In addition, it was noted that if the patient's exacerbation persisted after 2 hours, the treatment plan would be up-regulated to a LAMA plus a LABA (long-acting beta$_2$-agonist) per GOLD's recommendation (see Fig. 13.18).

Regarding the second SOAP, it should be noted that the respiratory therapist was deficient in not fully documenting the new—and serious—chest x-ray findings that strongly suggested pulmonary fibrosis and cor pulmonale. This important clinical information should have been recorded in the patient's assessment and treatment plan. The presence of cor pulmonale places the patient in a 1- to 2-year survival outlook in the less than 50% range. This was a serious assessment oversight, and it should have been recognized by simply recording the abnormal chest x-ray findings in the SOAP.

At discharge, the stable patient was appropriately prescribed a LAMA and ICS regimen. In addition, a prescription for roflumilast might be considered to help reduce the number of flare-ups or exacerbations associated with excessive airway secretions (see Box 13.2). Referral to pulmonary rehabilitation was clearly indicated (see Box 13.3).

It should be noted that this case study started with the patient's persistent smoking, along with increased symptoms and worsening of his obstructive pulmonary disease (dyspnea and productive cough). At the emergency department visit, the findings on the chest radiograph also suggested cor pulmonale, which often occurs in severe bronchitis. His pulmonary function was worsening, and he had acute alveolar hyperventilation superimposed on chronic ventilatory failure with moderate to severe hypoxemia. Impending ventilatory failure was a serious concern.

In addition to treating the acute symptoms with Aerosolized Medication Protocol (see Protocol 10.4) and Airway Clearance Therapy Protocol (see Protocol 10.2), the respiratory therapist does not give up on the longer term and extremely important goal of modifying behavior (smoking cessation) in the patient. A complete pulmonary function test in the near future would further define the patient's disease process, in both its nature and severity. Such data are often helpful to the patient's understanding of just how ill he is and may constitute a "teachable moment" for the physician and therapist. *Complete pulmonary function testing is not, however, recommended during an acute exacerbation.*

CASE STUDY Emphysema

Admitting History and Physical Examination

This 27-year-old man was admitted to the hospital with the chief complaint of dyspnea on exertion. He had a 3-year history of recurrent respiratory problems that had necessitated several hospitalizations of several days' duration in the past. A diagnosis of alpha$_1$-antitrypsin deficiency had been made in the outpatient clinic. This was his third hospitalization in the past 12 months. Recently, his respiratory status had deteriorated to the point where he had to stop working. He had been employed for several years as a cook in a fast-food restaurant, where he was continuously exposed to a smoky environment. He had never smoked. On questioning, the patient related that he had been very short of breath for the past 6 weeks. He further stated that he was unable to walk up one flight of stairs without stopping; his walking tolerance had decreased, and he was walking slower and required more frequent stops when walking at his normal pace.

On physical examination, the patient appeared anxious. He was sweating profusely and was in moderate respiratory distress. He demonstrated a regular heart rate of 120 bpm, blood pressure of 140/70, respiratory rate of 32 breaths/min, and an oral temperature of 100°F. Inspection of the chest revealed suprasternal notch retraction, with some use of the accessory muscles of inspiration. The lungs were hyperresonant to percussion, and breath sounds were diminished. His I/E ratio was 1:4. He had a barrel chest deformity, and his nail beds were moderately cyanotic. The patient was slightly confused and unable to concentrate well.

The chest x-ray showed moderate to severe hyperinflation of the lungs. Some infiltrates were present in the lower lung regions, and possible infiltrates were also noted in the right upper lobe. The radiology report suggested the presence of a pneumonic process superimposed on chronic lung disease.

Bedside spirometry showed an FEV$_1$/FVC ratio of 45% and a FEV$_1$ of 25% of predicted—GOLD Grade 4 (see Box 13.5). The patient's mMRC was 2 (see Table 13.2). He had three exacerbations during the past 12 months. Based on the Combined COPD Assessment Tool, the patient was classified as a GOLD Grade 4, Group D (High Exacerbation Risk, More Symptoms) (see Fig. 13.9).

His ABGs while on 1 L/min O$_2$ via nasal cannula were pH 7.53, PaCO$_2$ 66 mm Hg, HCO$_3^-$ 53 mEq/L, PaO$_2$ 48 mm Hg, SaO$_2$ 87%. Laboratory studies revealed a hemoglobin of 16.5 g/dL and a white blood cell count of 15,000/mm^3. Sputum Gram stains were positive for a variety of pathogenic and nonpathogenic organisms. His serum alpha$_1$-antitrypsin level as an outpatient had recently been 30 mg/dL (normal = 150 to 350 mg/dL).

The respiratory assessment read as follows.

Respiratory Assessment and Plan

S "I'm short of breath with any exercise at all." Cough for past 6 weeks.

O HR 120, BP 140/70, RR 32, and temp 100°F. Use of accessory muscles of inspiration, increased AP diameter, cyanosis. Hyperresonant percussion note and diminished breath sounds. I/E ratio 1:4. Lower lung infiltrates, hyperinflation of lungs on CXR. PFT: FEV$_1$/FVC ratio (45%), FEV$_1$ (25% of predicted). mMRC 3. Exacerbations three/year—GOLD Grade 4, Group D. ABGs on 1 L/min nasal cannula: pH 7.53, PaCO$_2$ 66, HCO$_3^-$ 53, PaO$_2$ 48, SaO$_2$ 87%. Elevated WBC, gram-positive organisms in the sputum. Alpha$_1$-antitrypsin: 30 mg/dL.

A • Panacinar emphysema (history, alpha$_1$-antitrypsin deficiency)
  • Combined COPD Assessment Tool: GOLD Grade 4, Group D—High Risk, More Symptoms)
  • Acute exacerbation (history, physical examination, PFT)
  • Acute alveolar hyperventilation on chronic ventilatory failure with moderate/severe hypoxemia (ABGs)
    • Impending ventilatory failure

- Pulmonary hyperinflation (x-ray, diminished breath sounds, barrel chest)
- Probable pneumonitis (x-ray)

P Notify doctor about acute ventilatory failure stat. Place patient on NIV. Have pressure-limited ventilator on standby. Oxygen Therapy Protocol (Venturi mask at FIO_2 0.28). Monitor and evaluate per ICU standing orders (SpO_2, vital signs). Aerosolized Medication Protocol (e.g., LAMA + LABA). Check ABG in 30 min.

The hospital course was relatively smooth. The Venturi oxygen mask therapy, at an FIO_2 of 0.28, was enough to increase the patient's PaO_2 to an acceptable level. Within an hour the patient's ABGs on an FIO_2 of 0.28 were pH 7.36, $PaCO_2$ 61 mm Hg, HCO_3^- 34 mEq/L, PaO_2 76 mm Hg, and SaO_2 93%. The patient's heart rate, respiratory rate, and blood pressure returned to normal over the next hour.

Blood serology studies suggested *Mycoplasma pneumoniae* infection. Intravenous antibiotics were prescribed. The patient was managed conservatively and improved steadily. When he appeared to have had the maximum benefit from the hospitalization, he was discharged with an oxygen concentrator, a portable "stroller," and an oxygen-conserving device. He was instructed to use O_2 at 1 L/min at rest and 2.5 L/min with exercise for 18 to 24 hours a day. Arrangements were made to have him enroll in an alpha$_1$-antitrypsin therapy trial and attend pulmonary rehabilitation classes. He was urged to secure employment elsewhere, in a clean air environment.

Discussion

This fascinating (but fortunately rare) form of emphysema is one in which "pure" emphysema is the dominant pathology. In patients with alpha$_1$-antitrypsin deficiency, chronic bronchitis may be present, but it is much less common than is the usual, cigarette smoking–induced COPD. In this condition, the patient's deficiency of the protease inhibitor alpha$_1$-antitrypsin resulted in white blood cell–mediated protease destruction of his pulmonary parenchyma. Note the slow, insidious onset of his symptoms.

The respiratory therapist accurately classified the patient as GOLD Grade 4, Group D (High Exacerbation Risk, More Symptoms).

The clinical data that supported this decision were an FEV_1/FVC ratio of 45% and a FEV_1 of 25% of predicted, the GOLD classification of 4, the mMRC of 2, and the fact that the patient had three exacerbations during the past 12 months (see Fig. 13.9).

In this case, because there was no wheezing noted on auscultation, it may not have been absolutely necessary to activate the Aerosolized Medication Protocol to give this patient an inhaled bronchodilator, per GOLD's pharmacologic treatment algorithm guidelines (see Box 13.5). However, given the fact that the ABG findings confirmed acute alveolar hyperventilation on chronic ventilatory failure, which indicates impending ventilatory failure, the administration of LAMA + LABA was justified. Furthermore, because this patient was placed in Group D, a prescription for ICS and a long-acting beta$_2$ agent may be considered at discharge (see Box 13.3).

The patient's emphysema or distal airway and alveolar weakening (see Fig. 10.12) were complicated by additional anatomic alterations of the lungs (i.e., alveolar consolidation) (see Fig. 10.8). The alveolar consolidation was reflected in the patient's immune-inflammatory response (fever and increased white blood cell count), alveolar infiltrates (x-ray), low PaO_2 (caused by a decreased $\dot{V}/\dot{Q}$ ratio and intrapulmonary shunting), and abnormal vital signs (see Fig. 10.8). The effects of distal airway and alveolar weakening were reflected in the patient's increased AP diameter, use of accessory muscles of inspiration, hyperresonant percussion note, diminished breath sounds, PFT results, and the chest x-ray film, which showed *alveolar hyperinflation* and *"probable pneumonitis"* (see Figs. 13.10, 13.12, and 13.13).

The selection of a good program of oxygen supplementation was certainly indicated. Note the selection of a Venturi oxygen mask, which allowed for a safe and precise FIO_2 control regardless of the patient's respiratory rate or tidal volume. Pneumococcal and influenza prophylaxis was certainly indicated in this case. Frequent intravenous administration of alpha$_1$-antitrypsin replacement represents modern therapy in the treatment of this unusual disease, as does counseling the patient that he should not knowingly expose himself to irritants such as those present in the smoky environment of his workplace. Replacement alpha$_1$-antitrypsin therapy does not repair the alveolar damage that has already occurred, but is thought to stabilize the condition.

CASE STUDY Example of Classic Chronic Obstructive Pulmonary Disease

Admitting History and Physical Examination

A 78-year-old man was brought to this Chicago, Illinois, emergency department by his adult son. The son stated that his father had a long history of cardiopulmonary problems with chronic productive cough and had been diagnosed as having COPD about 15 years ago. Over the past 10 years, the patient had been admitted to this hospital on several occasions for COPD exacerbations.

Bedside spirometry showed an FEV_1/FVC ratio of 45% and a FEV_1 of 25% of predicted—GOLD Grade 4. The patient's mMRC was 2. He had three exacerbations during the past 12 months. Based on the Combined COPD

Assessment Tool, the patient was classified as GOLD Grade 4, Group D (High Exacerbation Risk, More Symptoms) (see Fig. 13.9).

At the time of his last hospital discharge (7 months ago), the patient's electronic records showed that his baseline FEV_1/FVC ratio was 55% and his FEV_1 was 35% of predicted—GOLD Grade 3 (see Table 13.1). His DLCO was 60% of predicted. At the time of this hospitalization his mMRC was 3 (see Table 13.2). It was noted that the patient was experiencing his second exacerbation within the past year. Based on the Combined COPD Assessment Tool, the patient was classified as a GOLD Grade 3, Group D patient (High Risk, More Symptoms) (see Fig. 13.9). On a 1 L/min oxygen cannula, his baseline ABG values at his previous hospital discharge had been as follows: pH 7.37, $PaCO_2$ 93 mm Hg, HCO_3^- 52 mEq/L, PaO_2 63 mm Hg, and SaO_2 90%.

The patient had a long history of cigarette smoking, as well as working many long hours in smoke-filled rhythm-and-blues clubs throughout the Chicago area for over 55 years. The patient had been a rhythm-and-blues guitar player since the late 1950s. He had worked with many of the greats—Muddy Waters, Buddy Guy, KoKo Taylor, Lonnie Brooks, and Candy Foster and the Shades of Blue. The patient stated that although he no longer worked in smoke-filled bars, he still smoked two to three packs of cigarettes per day. The patient's son stated that when he had checked in on his father earlier that day, he realized that his father was very confused and disoriented. The son immediately transported his father to the emergency department. The patient had "run out" of previously prescribed medications about 2 months earlier. He also stated that he "could not afford" most of them.

On examination, the patient appeared to be in moderate to severe respiratory distress. He was anxious, confused, and disoriented. The patient stated that he could not take a deep enough breath. His vital signs were as follows: respiratory rate 35 breaths/min, heart rate 145 bpm, blood pressure 145/90, and temperature 98.6°F. The patient was moderately overweight and had a barrel chest. His skin appeared cyanotic. He had a frequent weak cough. He produced a moderate amount of purulent, gray-yellow sputum with each cough. In an upright position, he used accessory muscles of inspiration. Exhalations were prolonged with pursed-lip breathing. He had 3+ pitting edema of his legs, ankles, and feet. His neck veins were distended. The patient had clubbing of his fingers and toes.

Palpation revealed decreased chest expansion. Hyperresonant percussion notes were present over both lung fields. Auscultation revealed diminished heart and breath sounds, with bilateral wheezes and coarse crackles heard over all lung fields. An x-ray taken in the emergency department with a portable film showed lung hyperinflation, depressed diaphragms, increased bronchial vascular markings, and an apparent enlargement of the heart. Bedside spirometry was attempted, but the patient was too weak and confused to generate a good expiratory maneuver. ABG values on a 2 L/min oxygen cannula were pH 7.24, $PaCO_2$ 110 mm Hg, HCO_3^- 46 mEq/L, PaO_2 47 mm Hg, and SaO_2 77%. Laboratory results revealed a hemoglobin level of 19.0 g%.

The respiratory therapist working in the emergency department documented the following assessment.

Respiratory Assessment and Plan

S "I can't take a deep breath."

O Moderate to severe respiratory distress. Vital signs: RR 35, HR 145, BP 145/90, T 98.6°F. Barrel chest, cyanotic, frequent weak cough, moderate amount of purulent, gray-yellow sputum, using accessory muscles of inspiration, prolonged exhalation, pursed-lip breathing, 3+ pitting edema of legs, ankles, and feet. Distended neck veins, digital clubbing. Decreased chest expansion. AUS: Diminished heart and breath sounds. Bilateral wheezes and coarse crackles in all lung fields. PFT baseline (7 months earlier): FEV_1/FVC ratio 55%, FEV 35% of predicted, GOLD 3, DLCO 60% of predicted, mMRC 3. Exacerbations: Two/yr. CXR: hyperinflation, depressed diaphragms, increased bronchial vascular markings, and an enlarged heart. ABG values on 2 L/min O_2: pH 7.24, $PaCO_2$ 110, HCO_3^- 46, PaO_2 47, SaO_2 77%. Hemoglobin 19.0 g%.

A • Combined COPD Assessment Tool: GOLD Grade 3, Group D—High Exacerbation Risk, More Symptoms (GOLD 3, mMRC 3, exacerbations 2/yr.)
 • Acute COPD exacerbation (history, physical examination, PFT)
 • History of poor medication compliance, persistent smoking
 • Acute ventilatory failure superimposed on chronic ventilatory failure with moderate to severe hypoxemia (ABGs)
 • Bronchospasm (wheezing)
 • Excessive airway secretions (COPD history, coarse crackles, purulent, gray-yellow secretions)
 • Pulmonary infection (yellow sputum)
 • Poor ability to mobilize secretions (weak cough effort)
 • Air trapping (hyperresonant percussion notes, hyperinflation on x-ray film, barrel chest)
 • Probable cor pulmonale (swollen feet, ankles, and legs; enlarged heart on x-ray)

P Notify physician stat regarding acute ventilatory failure superimposed on chronic ventilatory failure. Possible cor pulmonale. Recommend noninvasive Mechanical Ventilation Protocol and Oxygen Therapy Protocol. Start Airway Clearance Therapy Protocol (chest physical therapy four times daily, suctioning PRN). Start Aerosolized Medication Protocol (e.g., SABA and antimuscarinic agents) until physician can be reached. If the physician agrees, set up ventilator per noninvasive mechanical ventilation protocol.

Discussion

This case nicely demonstrates the clinical manifestations associated with both chronic bronchitis and emphysema—that is, COPD. The clinical manifestations of chronic bronchitis seen in this case include chronic productive cough, cor pulmonale (swollen lower extremities and distended neck veins), coarse crackles and wheezing on auscultation, digital clubbing, and polycythemia (elevated hemoglobin level).

The clinical indicators that supported that the *patient's bronchitis was also complicated by emphysema* was shown by his DLCO of 60% of predicted, the use of his accessory muscles of inspiration, his hyperresonant percussion note, and the presence of his pursed-lip breathing. The fact that he was in hypoxemic, hypercapnic—and that he required ventilatory support—does not help separate the two diagnoses. These ABG abnormalities can be seen in either condition.

The clinical manifestations (clinical scenarios) in this case are caused by the anatomic alterations of the lungs associated with both chronic bronchitis (see clinical scenarios shown in bronchospasm Fig. 10.10, excessive bronchial secretions Fig. 10.11, and emphysema, see clinical scenario shown in Fig. 10.12 [distal airway and alveolar weakening]).

The respiratory therapist appropriately classified the patient as GOLD Grade 3, Group D—High Exacerbation Risk, More Symptoms via the Combined COPD Assessment Tool. The justification for this was based on the patient's FEV_1/FVC of 55%, FEV_1 of 35% of predicted, GOLD classification of 3, mMRC of 2, and the fact that the patient had two exacerbations during the past 12 months (see Fig. 13.9).

Treatment in this case was first driven by the selection of noninvasive ventilation in the Ventilator Management Protocol—the patient demonstrated hypoxemic, hypercapnic respiratory failure, and clearly required ventilator support (see Chapter 11, Respiratory Insufficiency, Respiratory Failure, and Ventilation Management Protocols). With this in place, the Oxygen Therapy Protocol and elements of the Airway Clearance Therapy and Aerosolized Medication Protocols were begun with standard protocol specifics. Because the patient was evidently in an acute COPD exacerbation, the Aerosolized Medication Protocol appropriately included SABA and antimuscarinic agents per the GOLD COPD acute exacerbation guidelines (see Box 13.5). In addition, the administration of systemic corticosteroids may have been considered in this case to help shorten the patient's recovery time and improve his FEV_1 and PaO_2 level (see Box 13.5). Once the patient is stable, long-term therapy with ICS with LABA should be prescribed (see Box 13.2). In addition, a prescription for roflumilast might be considered to help reduce the number of flare-ups or exacerbations associated with excessive airway secretions (see Box 13.2).

Unfortunately, this patient did not do well and became ventilator-dependent. He died in a skilled nursing facility 3 months later, still "missing his smokes" and listening to rhythm-and-blues on his iPod.

SELF-ASSESSMENT QUESTIONS

1. In chronic bronchitis:
   1. The bronchial walls are narrowed because of vasoconstriction
   2. The bronchial glands are enlarged
   3. The number of goblet cells is decreased
   4. The number of cilia lining the tracheobronchial tree is increased
      a. 1 only
      b. 2 only
      c. 3 only
      d. 3 and 4 only

2. Which of the following bacteria are commonly found in the tracheobronchial tree of patients with chronic bronchitis?
   1. *Staphylococcus*
   2. *Haemophilus influenzae*
   3. *Klebsiella*
   4. *Streptococcus pneumoniae*
      a. 1 only
      b. 2 only
      c. 3 and 4 only
      d. 2 and 4 only

3. In chronic bronchitis, the patient commonly demonstrates which of the following?
   1. Increased FVC
   2. Decreased FEV_1/FVC ratio
   3. Increased VC
   4. Decreased FEV_1
      a. 2 only
      b. 1 and 3 only
      c. 2 and 4 only
      d. 3 and 4 only

4. The patient with severe chronic bronchitis (late stage) commonly has which of the following arterial blood gas values?
   1. Normal pH
   2. Decreased HCO_3^-
   3. Increased $PaCO_2$
   4. Normal PaO_2
      a. 1 only
      b. 1 and 3 only
      c. 2 and 3 only
      d. 3 and 4 only

5. Patients with severe chronic bronchitis may demonstrate which of the following?
   1. Peripheral edema
   2. Distended neck veins
   3. An elevated hemoglobin concentration
   4. An enlarged liver
      a. 3 only
      b. 2 and 4 only
      c. 2, 3, and 4 only
      d. 1, 2, 3, and 4

6. What type of emphysema creates an abnormal enlargement of all structures distal to the terminal bronchioles?
   a. Centrilobular emphysema
   b. Alpha$_1$-protease inhibitor deficiency emphysema
   c. ZZ phenotype emphysema
   d. Panlobular emphysema

7. What is the normal range of alpha$_1$-antitrypsin?
   a. 0 to 150 mg/dL
   b. 150 to 350 mg/dL
   c. 350 to 500 mg/dL
   d. 500 to 750 mg/dL

8. The DLCO of patients with severe emphysema is:
   a. Increased
   b. Decreased
   c. Normal
   d. The DLCO test is not used to assess emphysema patients.

9. Patients with severe emphysema commonly demonstrate which of the following oxygenation indices?
   1. Decreased $S\bar{v}O_2$
   2. Increased O_2ER
   3. Decreased DO_2
   4. Increased $C(a-\bar{v})O_2$
      a. 1 only
      b. 3 only
      c. 4 only
      d. 1, 2, and 3 only

10. Which phenotype is associated with the lowest serum concentration of alpha$_1$-antitrypsin?
    a. MM phenotype
    b. MZ phenotype
    c. ZZ phenotype
    d. M phenotype

11. Which of the following pulmonary function study findings are associated with severe emphysema?
    1. Increased FRC
    2. Decreased PEFR
    3. Increased RV
    4. Decreased FVC
       a. 3 and 4 only
       b. 2 and 3 only
       c. 2, 3, and 4 only
       d. 1, 2, 3, and 4

12. The patient with severe COPD commonly demonstrates which of the following hemodynamic indices?
    1. Decreased CVP
    2. Increased $\overline{PA}$
    3. Decreased RVSWI
    4. Increased PVR
       a. 1 only
       b. 3 only
       c. 2 and 4 only
       d. 1 and 2 only

13. Because acute ventilatory changes are often seen in patients with chronic ventilatory failure (compensated respiratory acidosis), the respiratory therapist must be alert for this problem in patients with severe COPD. Which of the following arterial blood gas values represent(s) acute alveolar hyperventilation superimposed on chronic ventilatory failure?
    1. Increased pH
    2. Increased $PaCO_2$
    3. Increased HCO_3^-
    4. Increased PaO_2
       a. 2 only
       b. 2 and 4 only
       c. 1 and 3 only
       d. 1, 2, and 3 only

14. The lung parenchyma in the chest radiograph of a patient with emphysema appears:
    1. Opaque
    2. White
    3. More translucent than normal
    4. Dark
       a. 2 only
       b. 1 and 3 only
       c. 2 and 3 only
       d. 3 and 4 only

15. What is the single most common etiologic factor in emphysema?
    a. Alpha$_1$-antitrypsin deficiency
    b. Cigarette smoking
    c. Infection
    d. Sulfur dioxide

Chapter Objectives

After reading this chapter, you will be able to:

- Describe the role of the national and international guidelines in the management of asthma.
- Describe the anatomic alterations of the lungs associated with asthma.
- Describe the etiology and epidemiology of asthma.
- List risk factors associated with asthma.
- Describe the cardiopulmonary clinical manifestations associated with asthma.
- Describe the general management of asthma.
- Describe the clinical strategies and rationales of the SOAPs presented in the case study.
- Define key terms and complete self-assessment questions at the end of the chapter and on Evolve.

Key Terms

Allergic Bronchopulmonary Aspergillosis (ABPA)
Allergic or Atopic Asthma
Anaphylactic Hypersensitivity Reaction
Anaphylaxis
Anticholinergic Agents
Aspirin-Induced Asthma (AIA)
Asthma and Chronic Obstructive Pulmonary Disease (COPD) Overlap Syndrome (ACOS)
Asthma Control Action Plan
Asthma Phenotype
Beta$_2$-Agonist
Bronchial Thermoplasty
Charcot-Leyden Crystals
Controller Medications
Cough Variant Asthma
Curschmann Spirals
Difficult-to-Treat Asthma
Dust Mites
Environmental Factors
Eosinophils
Exercise-Induced Bronchoconstriction (EIB)
Extrinsic Asthma (allergic atropic asthma)
Fractional Concentration of Exhaled Nitric Oxide (F$_E$NO)
Gastroesophageal Reflux Disease (GERD)
GINA
Host Factors
Immunologic Mechanism
Immunoglobulin E–Mediated Allergic Reaction
Inhaled Corticosteroids (ICSs)

Instrinsic asthma (nonallergic or nontopic asthma)
Leukotriene Receptor Antagonists (LTRA)
National Asthma Education and Prevention Program (NAEPP)
Nonsteroidal Antiinflammatory Drugs (NSAIDs)
Occupational Asthma
Occupational Sensitizers
Pulsus Paradoxus
Radioallergosorbent Test (RAST)
Refractory Asthma
Reliever (Rescue) Medications
Remodeling
Respiratory Infectious Disease Panel (RIDP)
Respiratory Syncytial Virus (RSV)
Short-Acting Beta$_2$-Agonists (SABAs)
Sick Building Syndrome (SBS)
Specific Immunoglobulin E (sIgE)
Status Asthmaticus
Sublingual Allergen Immunotherapy (SLIT)
Treatment-Resistant Asthma
Valved Holding Chamber (VHC)

Chapter Outline

National Asthma Education and Prevention Program
Global Initiative for Asthma
Anatomic Alterations of the Lungs
Etiology and Epidemiology
  Risk Factors in Asthma
Diagnosis of Asthma
  Other Diagnostic Tests for Asthma
Overview of the Cardiopulmonary Clinical Manifestations Associated With Asthma
General Management of Asthma
  Control-Based Asthma Management Program
  The Stepwise Management Approach to Control Asthma Symptoms and Reduce Risk
  Nonpharmacologic Interventions in the Treatment of Asthma
  Indications for Referral for Expert Evaluation
  Protocol When Asthma Is Controlled
  Management of Asthma Exacerbation
  Management of Asthma With Comorbidities and Special Populations
Respiratory Care Treatment Protocols
Case Study: Asthma
Self-Assessment Questions

Hippocrates first recognized asthma more than 2000 years ago. Today, asthma remains one of the most common diseases encountered in clinical medicine. The burdens associated with asthma in the United States—and worldwide—are enormous. Although the precise annual numbers are not known, it is estimated that asthma is linked to a multitude of lost school days, countless missed work days, numerous doctor visits, frequent hospital outpatient visits, and recurrent emergency department visits and hospitalizations.

Asthma is characterized by chronic airway inflammation and is defined by the history of respiratory symptoms such as wheeze, shortness of breath, chest tightness, and cough that vary over time and in intensity and includes variable expiratory airflow limitation. Both the symptoms and airflow limitation typically vary over time and in intensity. The variations in symptoms and airflow limitation are commonly triggered by factors such as exercise, allergen or irritant exposure, change in weather, or viral respiratory infection. The patient's symptoms and airflow limitation may resolve spontaneously or in response to medications and may be absent for weeks or months at a time. In addition, the patient may experience episodic flare-ups (exacerbation) that may be life-threatening. Asthma episodes are usually associated with airway hyperresponsiveness to direct and indirect stimuli and chronic airway inflammation.

Asthma is also described as a heterogeneous disease that commonly has a set of observable characteristics that result from the interaction of the patient's genotype with the environment—called **asthma phenotype**. The more common asthma phenotypes include the following:

- *Allergic or atopic asthma:* This asthma phenotype is the most easily identified. It typically appears in childhood and is associated with a family history of allergic disorders such as eczema, allergic rhinitis, or food or drug allergies. Before treatment, the sputum of these patients often reveals eosinophilic airway inflammation. Patients with allergic asthma usually respond well to therapy with **inhaled corticosteroids (ICSs)**.
- *Nonallergic asthma:* This asthma phenotype is seen in some adults who do not have allergies. The cellular characteristics of the sputum in these patients may be neutrophilic, eosinophilic, or only a few inflammatory cells. Patients with nonallergic asthma usually do not respond well to ICS therapy
- *Late-onset asthma:* Some adults, especially women, develop asthma for the first time in adult life. These patients are usually nonallergic and typically require higher doses of ICS therapy and are relatively resistant to corticosteroid treatment.
- *Asthma with fixed airflow limitation:* Some patients with a long history of asthma develop a fixed airflow limitation that is believed to be caused by *airway wall remodeling*—that is, airway structural changes that include subepithelial fibrosis, increased smooth muscle mass, enlargement of glands, neovascularization, and epithelial alterations.
- *Asthma with obesity:* Asthma with prominent respiratory symptoms and little eosinophilic airway inflammation is commonly seen in obese patients (body mass index greater

than 30 kg/m²). In addition, asthma is more difficult to control in obese patients.

A relatively new role of the respiratory therapist is that of *asthma educator*.[1] In this function, the therapist's goal is to be sure the patient and the family are cognizant of their role and functions in the care of this usually chronic and often serious condition. The asthma educator must serve as a "change agent," and his/her effect as a convincing, empathetic communicator will be tested. Toward this end, we have greatly expanded this chapter from previous editions.

Fortunately, since 1993 the understanding and treatment of asthma has been updated and continuously refined by the:

1. *National Asthma Education and Prevention Program (NAEPP):* Expert Panel Report 3 (EPR-3), Guidelines for the Diagnosis and Management of Asthma—Full Report, and
2. *Global Initiative for Asthma (GINA):* The information presented in this chapter is consistent with current NAEPP and GINA guidelines.

National Asthma Education and Prevention Program[2]

The first evidence-based asthma guidelines were published in 1991 by NAEPP, which was under the direction of the National Heart, Lung, and Blood Institute (NHLBI) of the National Institutes of Health (NIH). Today, these guidelines are structured around the following four components of care: (1) assessment and monitoring of asthma, (2) patient education, (3) control of factors contributing to asthma severity, and (4) treatment medications. The NAEPP's "stepwise asthma management charts" are used to identify optimal treatment plans for specific age groups—that is, 0 to 4 years, 5 to 11 years, and 12 years and older.[3]

Global Initiative for Asthma[4]

In 1993 the GINA was launched in response to the collaborative work between the NHLBI (see earlier) and the World Health Organization (WHO). Annually, the role of GINA is to collect the most current scientific evidence associated with asthma care and transfer this information into a practical and user-friendly format. When completed, GINA then disseminates the most current standards of asthma care to a large network of health professionals, organizations, and public health officials. Since the inception of GINA, a number of important evidence-based clinical guidelines directed at the education, prevention, diagnosis, and management of asthma

---

[1]The specialty credentialing examination to earn the certified asthma educator (AE-C) credential is available for respiratory therapists and other health care professionals through the National Asthma Educator Certification Board (http://www.naecb.com).
[2]Expert Panel Response 3 (EPR-3): Guidelines for the diagnosis and management of asthma, 2007. http://www.nhlbi.nih.gov/guidelines/asthma/asthgdln .htm. (Last updated April 2012.)
[3]A free download of the EPR-3 summary and the complete guidelines are available at http://www.nhlbi.nih.gov/guidelines/asthma/asthgdln.htm.
[4]See http://www.ginasthma.org.

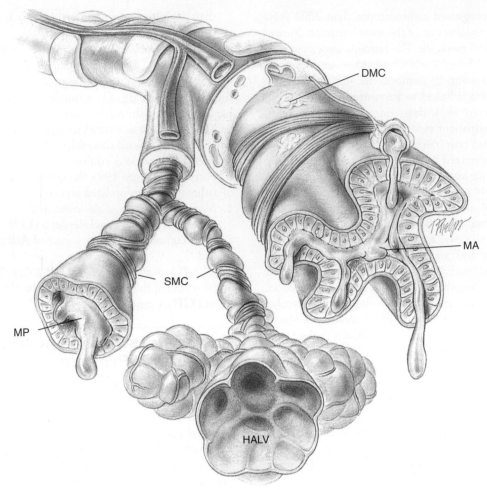

FIGURE 14.1 Asthma. *DMC,* Degranulated mast cell; *HALV,* hyperinflation of alveoli; *MA,* mucous accumulation; *MP,* mucous plug; *SMC,* smooth muscle constriction (bronchospasm).

have been developed, refined, and updated annually. For example, each year GINA provides the following state-of-the-art documents[5]:
- Global Strategy for Asthma Management and Prevention
- At-A-Glance Asthma Management Reference
- Pocket Guide for Asthma Management and Prevention
- GINA teaching slide set

Anatomic Alterations of the Lungs

Asthma is described as a lung disorder characterized by (1) reversible bronchial smooth muscle constriction, (2) airway inflammation, and (3) increased airway responsiveness to an assortment of stimuli. During an asthma attack, the smooth muscles surrounding the small airways constrict. Over time the smooth muscle layers hypertrophy and can increase to three times their normal thickness (Fig. 14.1).

The airway mucosa becomes infiltrated with **eosinophils** and other inflammatory cells, which in turn cause airway inflammation and mucosal edema. Microscopic crystals, called

Charcot-Leyden crystals, are formed from the breakdown of eosinophils in patients with allergic asthma (Fig. 14.2). The crystals are slender and pointed at both ends and have a pair of hexagonal pyramids joined at their bases. They vary in size and may be as large as 50 μm in length. The goblet cells proliferate, and the bronchial mucous glands enlarge. The airways become filled with thick, whitish, tenacious mucus. Extensive mucous plugging and atelectasis may develop.

As a result of smooth muscle constriction, bronchial mucosal edema, and excessive bronchial secretions, air trapping and alveolar hyperinflation develop (see Fig. 14.1). If chronic inflammation develops over time, these anatomic alterations become irreversible, resulting in loss of airway caliber. In addition, the cilia are often damaged, and the basement membrane of the mucosa may become thicker than normal (fibrosis). This whole process is referred to as "**remodeling.**"

A remarkable feature of bronchial asthma, however, is that many of the pathologic anatomic alterations of the lungs that occur during an asthma attack are completely *absent* between asthma episodes and that (at least in mild to moderate cases) remodeling does not occur to any great extent.

In summary, the major pathologic or structural changes observed during an asthma episode are as follows:

---

[5]The GINA global strategy for asthma management and prevention documents are freely available on the GINA website (http://www.ginasthma.org).

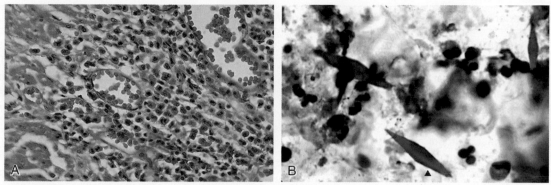

FIGURE 14.2 (A) At high magnification, numerous eosinophils are recognized by their bright red cytoplasmic granules, in this case of bronchial asthma. (B) In another patient with an acute asthma episode, Charcot-Leyden crystals (▲), which are derived from the breakdown of eosinophil granules, are seen microscopically (stained purplish-red). (From Klatt, E. C. [2015]. *Robbins and Cotran atlas of pathology* [3rd ed.]. Philadelphia, PA: Elsevier.)

- Smooth muscle constriction of bronchial airways (bronchospasm)
- Excessive production of thick, whitish bronchial secretions
- Mucous plugging
- Hyperinflation of alveoli (air trapping)
- In severe cases, atelectasis caused by mucous plugging
- Bronchial wall inflammation leading to fibrosis (in severe cases, caused by remodeling)

Etiology and Epidemiology

According to the latest information from the Centers for Disease Control and Prevention (CDC) and the National Center for Health Statistics (NCHS), in the United States about 18.4 million adults (percent of adults: 7.6%), and 6.2 million children (percent of children: 8.4%), have asthma—a total of about 25 million. According to the CDC, about 6.5% of the all physician office visits are asthma related and about 1.9 million visits to the emergency department per year have asthma as the primary diagnosis. Asthma is the cause of about 3651 deaths per year in the United States. Asthma is nearly twice as prevalent in young boys as young girls. In the adult, however, asthma is more common in women than in men.

The WHO[6] estimates that about 235 million people worldwide suffer from asthma. Low-income and middle-income countries account for more than 80% of the mortality. Worldwide, asthma is the most common chronic disease among children. Clearly, the effect of asthma on health, quality of life, and the economy is substantial.

Risk Factors in Asthma

Asthma authorities are not in full agreement as to how the risk factors for certain kinds of asthma should be categorized—for example, should a certain type of asthma be placed under the heading of *extrinsic* versus *intrinsic* asthma, or *allergic* versus *nonallergic* asthma, or *atopic* versus *nonatopic* asthma (Box 14.1).

[6]http://www.who.int/en/.

Regardless of this debate, the experts are—for the most part—in full agreement that the risk factors for asthma can be divided into **host factors**, which are primarily genetic, that result in the development of (intrinsic) asthma, or **environmental factors** that trigger the clinical manifestations of (extrinsic) asthma, or a combination of both (Box 14.2).

Host Factors

Genetics. There are several persistent and intermittent genetic phenotypes of asthma. Although the genetic factors associated with asthma are varied and not fully understood, the search for genetic links to asthma has primarily focused on the following four areas: (1) the production of allergen-specific immunoglobulin E (IgE) antibodies, (2) airway hyperresponsiveness, (3) inflammatory mediators, and (4) T-helper cells (Th1 and Th2), which are an important part of the immune system. The T-helper cells are lymphocytes that recognize foreign pathogens or, in the case of autoimmune disease, normal tissue. Th1 cells are involved in what is called *cell-mediated* immunity, which usually deals with infections caused by viruses and certain bacteria. They are the body's first line of defense against pathogens that invade the body cells. They tend to be inflammatory. Th2 cells are involved in humoral-mediated immunity, which deals with bacteria, toxins, and allergens. They are responsible for stimulating the production of antibodies in response to extracellular pathogens. They tend not to be inflammatory.

Sex. Before the age of 14 years, the prevalence of asthma is nearly two times greater in boys than in girls. Asthma severity in boys generally peaks around age 5 to 7 years and lessens dramatically during puberty. As children become older, the prevalence of asthma narrows between the sexes as many girls experience the onset of asthma during puberty. In adulthood, the prevalence of asthma is greater in women than in men.

Obesity. Asthma is more commonly seen in obese people (body mass index greater than 30 kg/m^2). In addition, asthma is more difficult to control in obese patients. Obese patients also have more problems with lung function and more comorbidities compared with normal weight patients with asthma.

BOX 14.1 Commonly Used Categories for Risk Factors in Asthma

Extrinsic Asthma (Allergic or Atopic Asthma)

When an asthma episode can clearly be linked to exposure to a specific allergen (antigen), the patient is said to have *extrinsic asthma* (also called **allergic or atopic asthma**). Common indoor allergens include house **dust mites**, furred animal dander (e.g., dogs, cats, and mice), cockroach allergen, fungi, molds, and yeast. Outdoor allergens include pollens, fungi, molds, and yeast. In addition, there are a number of occupational substances associated with asthma.

Extrinsic asthma is an immediate (type I) **anaphylactic hypersensitivity reaction**. It occurs in individuals who have atopy, a hypersensitivity condition associated with genetic predisposition, and an excessive amount of IgE antibody production in response to a variety of antigens. From 10% to 20% of the general population are atopic and therefore have a tendency to develop an **immunoglobulin E–mediated allergic reaction** such as asthma, hay fever, allergic rhinitis, and eczema. Such individuals develop a wheal-and-flare reaction to a variety of skin test allergens, called a *positive skin test result*. Extrinsic asthma is family-related and usually appears in children and in adults younger than 30 years old. It often disappears after puberty.

Because extrinsic asthma is associated with an antigen antibody–induced bronchospasm, an *immunologic mechanism* plays an important role. As with other organs, the lungs are protected against injury by certain immunologic mechanisms. Under normal circumstances these mechanisms function without any apparent clinical evidence of their activity. In patients susceptible to extrinsic or allergic asthma, however, the hypersensitive immune response actually creates the disease by causing acute and chronic inflammation.

Immunologic Mechanisms

1. When a susceptible individual is exposed to a certain antigen, lymphoid tissue cells form specific IgE (reaginic) antibodies. The IgE antibodies attach themselves to the surface of mast cells in the bronchial walls (Fig. 14.3A).
2. Reexposure or continued exposure to the same antigen creates an antigen-antibody reaction on the surface of the mast cell, which in turn causes the mast cell to degranulate and release chemical mediators such as histamine, eosinophil chemotactic factor of anaphylaxis (ECF-A), neutrophil chemotactic factors (NCFs), leukotrienes (formerly known as *slow-reacting substances of anaphylaxis [SRS-A]*), *prostaglandins*, and *platelet activating factor (PAF)* (see Fig. 14.3B).
3. *The release of these chemical mediators stimulates parasympathetic nerve endings in the bronchial airways, leading to reflex bronchoconstriction and mucous hypersecretion. Moreover, these chemical mediators increase the permeability of capillaries, which results in the dilation of blood vessels and tissue edema* (see Fig. 14.3C).

The patient with extrinsic asthma may demonstrate an early asthmatic (allergic) response, a late asthmatic response, or a biphasic asthmatic response. The early asthmatic response begins within minutes of exposure to an inhaled antigen and resolves in about 1 hour. A late asthmatic response begins several hours after exposure to an inhaled antigen but lasts much longer. The late asthmatic response may or may not follow an early asthmatic response. An early asthmatic response followed by a late asthmatic response is called a *biphasic response*.

Intrinsic Asthma (Nonallergic or Nonatopic Asthma)

When an asthma episode cannot be directly linked to a specific antigen or extrinsic inciting factor, it is referred to as *intrinsic asthma* (also called *nonallergic* or *nonatopic asthma*) (Fig. 14.4). The etiologic factors responsible for intrinsic asthma are elusive. Individuals with intrinsic asthma are not hypersensitive or atopic to environmental antigens and have a normal serum IgE level. The onset of intrinsic asthma usually occurs after the age of 40 years, and typically there is no strong family history of allergy.

In spite of the general distinctions between extrinsic and intrinsic asthma, a significant overlap exists. Distinguishing between the two is often impossible in a clinical setting. Precipitating factors known to cause intrinsic asthma are referred to as *nonspecific stimuli*. Some of the more common nonspecific stimuli associated with intrinsic asthma are discussed in the main text.

BOX 14.2 Risk Factors for Asthma

Host Factors
- Genetics (e.g., genes predisposing to atopy, airway hyper-responsiveness airway inflammation)
- Obesity
- Sex

Environmental Factors
- Allergens
  - Indoor: Domestic mites, furred animals (e.g., dogs, cats, mice), cockroach allergen, fungi, molds, yeast
  - Outdoor sensitizers and allergens (e.g., flour laboratory rodents, paints)
- Infections (primarily viral)
- Tobacco smoke (passive smoking and active smoking)
- Outdoor/indoor air pollution
- Diet: Especially in the case of food allergies

Other Risk Factors
- Certain drugs (e.g., aspirin) and food additives and preservatives
- Exercise
- Gastroesophageal reflux
- Sleep
- Emotional stress
- Perimenstrual asthma
- Allergic bronchopulmonary aspergillosis

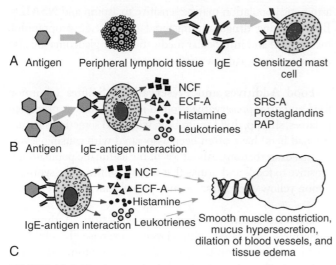

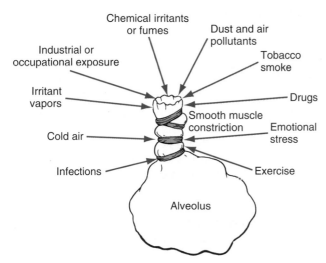

FIGURE 14.3 The immunologic mechanisms in extrinsic asthma (see Box 14.2).

FIGURE 14.4 Some factors known to trigger intrinsic asthma (see Box 14.2).

Environmental Factors

Allergens

Outdoor and Indoor Air Pollution. Outbreaks of asthma exacerbations have been reported in areas of increased levels of air pollution, especially when the environmental air is laden with pollutant particulates less than 5 μm in diameter. The role of outdoor air pollution in causing asthma remains controversial. Similar associations have been reported in relation to indoor pollutants such as smoke and fumes from gas and biomass fuels used for heating and cooling, molds, and cockroach infestation—e.g., in the **sick building syndrome (SBS)**.

Occupational Sensitizers (Occupational Asthma). **Occupational asthma** is defined as asthma caused by exposure to an agent encountered in the work environment. More than 300 different substances have been associated with occupational asthma. Occupational asthma is seen predominantly in adults. It is estimated that **occupational sensitizers** cause about 15% of cases of asthma among adults of working age. High-risk work environments for occupational asthma include farming and agricultural work, painting (including spray painting), cleaning work, and plastic manufacturing. Most occupational asthma is immunologically mediated and has a latency period of months to years after the onset of exposure.

Although the cause is not fully understood, it is known that an IgE-mediated allergic reaction and cell-mediated allergic reactions are often involved. Box 14.3 shows additional agents known to cause occupational asthma. It also should be noted that many leisure-time activities can cause asthma by exposing individuals to harmful particles and fumes. For example, severe asthma episodes have been triggered by hobbies associated with sawdust and sealants (e.g., commonly found in a woodworker's shop) and the various fumes that can be inhaled by car enthusiasts (e.g., car exhaust, paints, polishes, cleaning products, scented air fresheners, etc.).

Infections (Predominantly Viral). Although bacterial infections may cause asthma, viral upper and lower airway infections are more likely to contribute to asthma. For example, several viruses seen during infancy are associated with the activation of the asthma phenotype. Such viruses include the **respiratory syncytial virus (RSV),** human rhinovirus (HRV), and parainfluenza virus. These conditions often produce a pattern of symptoms that parallel many features of childhood asthma. For example, it is estimated that about 40% of children with RSV infection will continue to wheeze or have asthma into later childhood.

Microbiome. The collection of microorganisms and their genetic material, both within the host and the host's surrounding environment, is associated with the development of allergic disorders and asthma. For example, delivery by cesarean section has a higher risk factor for the development of asthma.

Tobacco Smoke. Exposure to tobacco smoke, both prenatally and after birth, is associated with a greater risk for developing asthma-like clinical manifestations in early childhood. Infants of smoking parents are four times more likely to develop wheezing illnesses in the first year of life. In fact, the concern of exposing children to tobacco smoke has resulted in several states enacting legislation that prohibits smoking in motor vehicles when children are passengers.

Outdoor and Indoor Air Pollution. Air pollution causes diminished lung function and increased asthma-related morbidity. Similarly, indoor pollutants (e.g., smoke and fumes from gas or biomass fuels that are used for heating and cooling, molds, and cockroach infestations) are also related to decreased lung function and increased morbidity.

Diet. Research has suggested that infants given formulas of intact cow's milk or soy protein have a higher incidence of wheezing symptoms in early childhood compared with infants given breast milk. Studies have also indicated that certain characteristics of Western diets, such as the following, have been associated with asthma:
- Increased use of processed foods
- Decreased antioxidants (in the form of fruits and vegetables)
- Increased omega-6 polyunsaturated fatty acid (found in margarine, vegetable oil, and eggs)
- Decreased omega-3 polyunsaturated fatty acid (found in fish oil)

Foods that clearly cause an allergy and/or asthma symptoms (usually demonstrated by oral challenges) of course should be avoided.

Other Risk Factors
Drugs. Asthma exacerbations are associated with the ingestion of aspirin and other **nonsteroidal antiinflammatory drugs (NSAIDs).** It is estimated that as much as 20% of the asthmatic population may be sensitive to aspirin and NSAIDs. Beta-blocking drugs administered orally (e.g., propranolol, metoprolol) and intraocular medications for glaucoma are also associated with asthma exacerbations.

Food Additives and Preservatives. Sulfites (common food and drug preservatives found in such foods as processed potatoes, shrimp, dried fruits, beer, wine, and sometimes lettuce in salad bars) have often been associated with causing severe asthma exacerbations. About 5% of the asthmatic population is sensitive to foods and drinks that contain sulfites. The synthetic lemon yellow dye tartrazine may provoke an asthma episode.

Exercise-Induced Bronchoconstriction. Asthma is sometimes associated with vigorous exercise. In children, exercise is a common trigger of asthma symptoms. Research has shown that the drying and cooling of the airways during exercise is the primary trigger mechanism. Running in cold air is the activity that causes the most bronchospasm, whereas swimming in a warm environment causes the fewest asthma symptoms (assuming the water is nonchlorinated and the pool area is well ventilated).

Gastroesophageal Reflux. Gastroesophageal reflux disease (GERD), or regurgitation, appears to significantly contribute to bronchoconstriction in some patients. The precise mechanism of this relationship is not known. The patient may complain of burning, substernal pain, belching, and a bitter, acid taste, particularly when lying down. Incidentally, unrecognized GERD is one of the most common causes of a hard-to-diagnose cough; unrecognized sinusitis is the other most common cause.

Sleep (Nocturnal Asthma). Patients with asthma often have more breathing difficulty late at night or in the early morning as serum cortisol levels drop at night. Precipitating factors associated with nocturnal asthma include gastroesophageal reflux and retained airway secretions (caused by a suppressed cough reflex during sleep). Additional precipitating factors include exposure to irritants or allergens in the bedroom and prolonged time between medication doses. Eradication of nocturnal asthma is one measure of good **asthma control**.

Emotional Stress. In some patients, the exacerbation of asthma appears to correlate with emotional stress and other psychologic factors. This is most likely mediated by histamine release from circulating mast cells.

Perimenstrual Asthma (Catamenial Asthma). Clinical manifestations associated with asthma often worsen in women during the premenstrual and menstrual periods. The symptoms often peak 2 to 3 days before menstruation begins. Premenstrual asthma correlates with the late luteal phase of ovarian activity, the phase during which circulating progesterone and estrogen levels are low.

Allergic Bronchopulmonary Aspergillosis. Allergic **bronchopulmonary aspergillosis (ABPA)** is characterized by an exaggerated response of the immune system—a hypersensitivity response—to the *Aspergillus* fungus (see Chapter 18, Pneumonia, Lung Abscess Formation, and Important Fungal Diseases) in patients with asthma and cystic fibrosis. ABPA can cause airway inflammation and bronchospasm. Patients with ABPA often have symptoms of poorly controlled asthma, such as wheezing, cough, shortness of breath, and reduced exercise tolerance.

Diagnosis of Asthma

The diagnosis of asthma often can be challenging. For example, in early childhood, the diagnosis of asthma frequently is based on the assessment of the child's symptoms and physical findings—and good clinical judgment. For instance, the child has a 5- to 10-fold greater chance of being diagnosed with asthma if the child has what is referred to as either *one major criterion,* such as a parent with asthma or the presence of atopic dermatitis, or *two minor criteria,* such as allergic rhinitis, wheezing apart from colds, or a peripheral eosinophil count greater than 4%.

In the older child and the adult, a complete history and physical examination, along with the demonstration of reversible and variable airflow obstruction, will in most cases confirm the diagnosis of asthma. However, in the elderly patient, asthma is often undiagnosed because of the presence of comorbid diseases that complicate the diagnosis. In addition, the diagnosis of asthma is often missed in the patient who acquires asthma in the workplace. This form of asthma is called occupational asthma (see Box 14.3). Because occupational asthma usually has a slow and insidious onset, the patient's asthma is often misdiagnosed as chronic bronchitis or chronic obstructive pulmonary disease (COPD). As a result, the asthma is either not treated at all or treated inappropriately.

Finally, even though asthma usually can be distinguished from COPD, in some patients—those who have chronic respiratory clinical manifestations and fixed airflow limitations—it is often very difficult to differentiate between the two disorders—that is, asthma or COPD (this problem is discussed further later in this chapter under Asthma and Chronic Obstructive Pulmonary Disease Overlap Syndrome, page 225).

GINA provides an excellent guideline to help in the clinical diagnosis of asthma. GINA's guideline is based on the following two key defining features of asthma:

* A history of variable respiratory symptoms—for example:
  * Wheezing, shortness of breath, chest tightness, and cough that are often worse at night, varying over time and intensity, or triggered by colds, exercise, and allergen exposure.)
  * The patient's physical examination often appears normal, but may demonstrate wheezing on auscultation, especially during a forced expiration.
* The evidence of variable expiratory airflow limitation such as (one or more of the following):
  * FEV_1: >12% (or ≥200 mL) after inhaling a bronchodilator
    * In children: >12% of their predicted
  * PEFR: Daily variability >10%
    * In children: >13%

* FEV_1/FVC ratio is reduced
  * Normal is more than 0.75 to 0.80 in adults
  * Normal is >90% in children
* FEV_1 increases by >12% and (or ≥200 mL) after 4 weeks of antiinflammatory therapy
  * Or peak expiratory flow rate (PEFR) by >20% on the same peak expiratory flowmeter

In addition, the asthma patient needs to be assessed for:

* Control of asthma symptoms over the previous 4 weeks—for example:
  * Daytime or night symptoms
  * Unable to sleep because of asthma symptoms
  * Relievers needed more than twice a week
* Risk factors for more asthma outcomes—for example:
  * Exacerbations for uncontrolled symptoms or poor adherence
  * Fixed airflow limitation for lack of ICS therapy, low initial FEV_1, smoking, or occupational exposures
  * Medication side effects such as frequent use of ICS therapy or long-term high-dose ICS

Every asthma patient should be assessed for inhaler technique, adherence, treatment issues, medication side effects, and any comorbidities (e.g., rhinitis, rhinosinusitis, GERD, obesity, obstructive sleep apnea, depression, and anxiety) and a written action plan.[7]

Other Diagnostic Tests for Asthma

Because patients often have normal lung function between asthma episodes, measurements of airway responsiveness to a *bronchial provocation test, allergy tests,* and an *exhaled nitric oxide test* may be helpful in the diagnosis of asthma.

Bronchial Provocation Test

Because airflow limitation may be absent during the initial assessment in some patients, a bronchial provocation test may be helpful in assessing airway hyperresponsiveness. This is most often done with inhaled methacholine. However, histamine exercise, eucapnic voluntary hyperventilation, or inhaled mannitol may also be used.

Allergy Tests

The presence of allergic asthma can be assessed by skin prick testing or by measuring the level of **specific immunoglobulin E (sIgE), (via radioallergosorbent test [RAST])** in serum. The skin prick test uses common environmental allergens, is inexpensive, has a high sensitivity, and is simple and fast to perform. The measurement of sIgE is more expensive but may be preferred by patients who do not wish to undergo a series of needle pricks, have a widespread skin disease, or have a history of **anaphylaxis.**

Exhaled Nitric Oxide

Clinicians are now able to judge the control of eosinophilic airway inflammation caused by asthma by measuring **fractional concentration of exhaled nitric oxide (F_ENO).** In adults, the

---

[7]For an example of an asthma action plan, see Fig. 14.9, page 235.

normal F_ENO is less than 25 ppb. The normal F_ENO in children is less than 20 ppb. The F_ENO levels rise with eosinophilic airway inflammation; a high F_ENO (greater than 50 ppb) suggests a need to increase the patient's controller medication. A common cause of increased F_ENO is patients' lack of compliance with their prescribed ICS therapy.

Diagnosis of Asthma in Special Populations

GINA describes the challenges associated with diagnosing asthma among special populations, including patients with cough-variant asthma, occupational and work-aggravated asthma, athletes, pregnant women, the elderly, smokers and ex-smokers, patients already taking controller medications, and obese patients.

Cough-Variant Asthma. Some patients have a chronic cough as their primary—if not their only—symptom. It is especially common in children and is most often seen at night. Evaluations during the day are often normal. In these cases, tests directed at the patient's airway hyperresponsiveness, and the search for possible sputum and blood eosinophils, may be helpful in confirming the diagnosis of asthma.

Occupational and Work-Aggravated Asthma. Asthma acquired in the workplace is a frequently missed diagnosis. Because of the insidious onset of occupational asthma, it is often misdiagnosed as chronic bronchitis or COPD and therefore treated inappropriately or not at all. The development of a constant cough, wheezes, and rhinitis should raise suspicion, especially in the nonsmoker. The diagnosis of occupational asthma requires a defined history of occupational exposure to sensitizing agents, the absence of asthma symptoms before beginning employment, and a documented relationship between the asthma symptoms and the workplace—an improvement in the asthma symptoms when away from the workplace and a worsening of the asthma symptoms on return to the workplace.

Athletes. Exercise-induced bronchoconstriction (EIB) should be confirmed by lung function tests, including a bronchial provocation test. Conditions associated with asthma, such as rhinitis, laryngeal disorders, dysfunctional breathing, cardiac conditions, and overtraining, need to be excluded.

Pregnant Women. Women planning a pregnancy should be asked if they have a history of asthma so the appropriate advice can be provided regarding asthma management and medications.

The Elderly. Asthma is often underdiagnosed in the elderly because of their acceptance of dyspnea as being "normal" in old age, lack of fitness, and reduced activity. A careful history and physical examination, combined with an electrocardiogram and chest x-ray, will help in the diagnosis. In addition, a history of smoking or biomass fuel exposure, COPD, and overlapping asthma and COPD (called *asthma-COPD overlap* [ACO], Table 14.1) should be considered.

Smokers and Ex-Smokers. Asthma and COPD may be difficult to distinguish, especially in older patients, smokers and ex-smokers, and patients with ACO. The history and pattern of symptoms and past records can be helpful in distinguishing these patients from patients with asthma.

Confirming the Diagnosis of Asthma in Patients Taking Controller Medications. Between 25% and 35% of the patients with a diagnosis of asthma cannot be confirmed as having asthma. In these patients, a trial of either a lower or higher dose of controller treatment is recommended. If the diagnosis cannot be confirmed, the patient should undergo an expert evaluation and diagnosis.

Obese Patients. Because the respiratory symptoms associated with obesity can mimic asthma, it is important to confirm the diagnosis of asthma with objective measurements of variable airflow limitation.

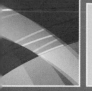

OVERVIEW of the Cardiopulmonary Clinical Manifestations Associated With Asthma

The following clinical manifestations result from the pathophysiologic mechanisms caused (or activated) by bronchospasm (see Fig. 10.10) and excessive bronchial secretions (see Fig. 10.11)—the major anatomic alterations of the lungs associated with an asthma episode (see Fig. 14.1).

CLINICAL DATA OBTAINED AT THE PATIENT'S BEDSIDE

The Physical Examination

Vital Signs

Increased respiratory rate (tachypnea)

Several pathophysiologic mechanisms operating simultaneously may lead to an increased ventilatory rate:

- Stimulation of peripheral chemoreceptors (hypoxemia)
- Decreased lung compliance and increased ventilatory rate relationship
  - When lungs are hyperinflated, the patient must work harder to breathe at the flat portion of the volume-pressure curve (see Fig. 3.2)
  - Anxiety

Increased Heart Rate (Pulse) and Blood Pressure
Use of Accessory Muscles During Inspiration
Use of Accessory Muscles During Expiration
Pursed-Lip Breathing
Substernal Intercostal Retractions

Substernal, supraclavicular, and intercostal retractions during inspiration may be seen, particularly in children.

Increased Anteroposterior Chest Diameter (Barrel Chest)
Cyanosis
Cough and Sputum Production

During an asthma episode the patient may produce an excessive amount of thick, whitish, tenacious mucus. At other times, because of large numbers of eosinophils and other white blood cells, the sputum may be purulent.

Pulsus Paradoxus

When an asthma episode produces severe alveolar air trapping and hyperinflation, **pulsus paradoxus** is a classic clinical manifestation. Pulsus paradoxus is defined as systolic blood pressure that is more than 10 mm Hg lower on inspiration than on expiration. This exaggerated waxing and waning of arterial blood pressure can be detected by using a manual blood pressure cuff or, in severe cases, by palpating the strength of the pulse. Pulsus paradoxus during an asthma attack is believed to be caused by the major intrapleural pressure swings that occur during inspiration and expiration and is associated with a severe life-threatening condition.

Decreased blood pressure during inspiration

During inspiration the patient frequently recruits accessory muscles of inspiration. The accessory muscles help produce an extremely negative intrapleural pressure, which in turn enhances intrapulmonary airflow. The increased negative intrapleural pressure, however, also causes blood vessels in the lungs to dilate and blood to pool. Consequently, the volume of blood returning to the left ventricle decreases. This causes a reduction in cardiac output and arterial blood pressure during inspiration.

Increased blood pressure during expiration

During expiration, the patient often activates the accessory muscles of expiration in an effort to overcome the increased airway resistance. The increased power produced by these muscles generates a greater positive intrapleural pressure. Although increased positive intrapleural pressure may help offset the airway resistance, it also works to narrow or squeeze the blood vessels of the lung. This increased pressure on the pulmonary blood vessels enhances left ventricular filling and results in an increased cardiac output and arterial blood pressure during expiration.

Chest Assessment Findings

- Expiratory prolongation (I/E ratio >1:3)
- Decreased tactile and vocal fremitus
- Hyperresonant percussion note
- Diminished breath sounds
- Diminished heart sounds
- Wheezing
- Crackles

CLINICAL DATA OBTAINED FROM LABORATORY AND SPECIAL PROCEDURES

Pulmonary Function Test Findings
Moderate to Severe Asthma Episode (Obstructive Lung Pathology)

FORCED EXPIRATORY VOLUME AND FLOW RATE FINDINGS

FVC	FEV_T	FEV_1/FVC ratio	$FEF_{25\%-75\%}$
↓	↓	↓	↓

$FEF_{50\%}$	$FEF_{200-1200}$[1]	PEFR	MVV
↓	↓	↓	↓

LUNG VOLUME AND CAPACITY FINDINGS

V_T	IRV	ERV	RV	
N or ↑	N or ↓	N or ↓	↑	

VC	IC	FRC	TLC	RV/TLC ratio
↓	N or ↓	↑	N or ↑	N or ↑

[1]*NOTE:* The $FEF_{200-1200}$ is rarely used in pediatrics.

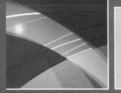
Arterial Blood Gases

MILD TO MODERATE ASTHMA EPISODE

Acute Alveolar Hyperventilation With Hypoxemia[2] (Acute Respiratory Alkalosis)

pH	$PaCO_2$	HCO_3^-	PaO_2	SaO_2 or SpO_2
↑	↓	↓	↓	↓
		(but normal)		

SEVERE ASTHMA EPISODE (STATUS ASTHMATICUS)

Acute Ventilatory Failure With Hypoxemia[3] (Acute Respiratory Acidosis)

pH[4]	$PaCO_2$	HCO_3^-[4]	PaO_2	SaO_2 or SpO_2
↓	↑	↑	↓	↓
		(but normal)		

Oxygenation Indices[5]
Moderate to Severe Stages

$\dot{Q}_S/\dot{Q}_T$	DO_2[6]	$\dot{V}O_2$	$C(a\text{-}\bar{v})O_2$	O_2ER	$S\bar{v}O_2$
↑	↓	N	N	↑	↓

ABNORMAL LABORATORY TESTS AND PROCEDURES
Sputum Examination

- Eosinophils
- Charcot-Leyden crystals
- Casts of mucus from small airways (**Curschmann spirals**)
- IgE level (elevated in extrinsic asthma)

---

[2]See Fig. 5.2 and Table 5.4 and related discussion for the acute pH, $PaCO_2$, and HCO_3^- changes associated with acute alveolar hyperventilation.

[3]See Fig. 5.2 and Table 5.5 and related discussion for the acute pH, $PaCO_2$, and HCO_3^- changes associated with acute ventilatory failure.

[4]When tissue hypoxia is severe enough to produce lactic acid, the pH and HCO_3^- values will be lower than expected for a particular $PaCO_2$ level.

[5]$C(a\text{-}\bar{v})O_2$, Arterial-venous oxygen difference; DO_2, total oxygen delivery; O_2ER, oxygen extraction ratio; $\dot{Q}_S/\dot{Q}_T$, pulmonary shunt fraction; $S\bar{v}O_2$, mixed venous oxygen saturation; $\dot{V}O_2$, oxygen consumption.

[6]The DO_2 may be normal in patients who have compensated to the decreased oxygenation status with (1) an increased cardiac output, (2) an increased hemoglobin level, or (3) a combination of both. When the DO_2 is normal, the O_2ER is usually normal.

ASTHMA-COPD OVERLAP (ACO)

GINA provides an approach to distinguishing among asthma, COPD, and the overlap of asthma and COPD (termed asthma and COPD overlap [ACO]). Rather than attempting to provide a formal definition of ACO, GINA presents the clinical manifestations that identify and characterize ACO, assigning equal weight to features of asthma and COPD. Table 14.1 provides the highlights provided by GINA that distinguish the features of asthma, COPD, and ACO.

RADIOLOGIC FINDINGS
Chest Radiograph (During an Asthma Episode)

- Increased anteroposterior diameter ("barrel chest")
- Translucent (dark) lung fields
- Depressed or flattened diaphragm

As the alveoli become enlarged during an asthma attack, the residual volume and functional residual capacity increase. This condition decreases the radiographic density of the lungs.

Consequently, the chest radiograph shows lung shadows that are translucent or darker than normal in appearance. Because of the increased residual volume, functional residual capacity, and total lung capacity, the diaphragms are depressed and flattened (Fig. 14.5).

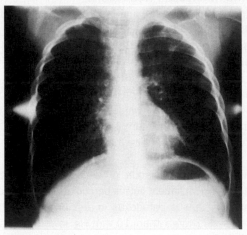

FIGURE 14.5 Chest x-ray film of a 2-year-old patient during an acute asthma attack.

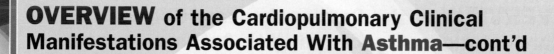
TABLE 14.1 Common Features of Asthma, Chronic Obstructive Pulmonary Disease (COPD), and Asthma and COPD Overlap, Including Features That Favor Asthma or COPD

	Common Features of Asthma, COPD, and Asthma and COPD Overlap			Features That Favor Asthma or COPD	
Feature	Asthma	COPD	Asthma and COPD Overlap	Favors Asthma*	Favors COPD*
Age of onset	Usually childhood onset but can commence at any age	Usually >40 years of age	Usually age >40 years, but may have had symptoms in childhood or early adulthood	Onset before age 20 years	Onset after 40 years
Pattern of respiratory symptoms	Symptoms may vary over time (day to day, or over longer periods), often limiting activity Often triggered by exercise, emotions including laughter, dust, or exposure to allergens	Chronic usually continuous symptoms, particularly during exercise, with better or worse days	Respiratory symptoms including exertional dyspnea are persistent but variability may be prominent	Variation in symptoms over minutes, hours, or days Symptoms worse during the night or early morning Symptoms triggered by exercise, emotions, including laughter, dust, or exposure to allergens	Persistence of symptoms despite treatment Good and bad days but always daily symptoms and exertional dyspnea Chronic cough and sputum preceded onset of dyspnea, unrelated to triggers
Lung function	Current and/or historical variable airflow limitation (e.g., bronchodilator reversibility)	FEV₁ may be improved by therapy, but postbronchodilator FEV₁/FVC <0.7 persists	Airflow limitation not fully reversible, but often with current or historical variability	Record of variable airflow limitation (spirometry, peak flow)	Record of persistent airflow limitation (postbronchodilator FEV_1/FVC <0.7)
Lung function between symptoms	May be normal between symptoms	Persistent airflow limitation	Persistent airflow limitation between symptoms	Lung function normal between symptoms	Lung function abnormal
Past history of family history	Many patients have allergies and a personal history of asthma in childhood, and/or family history of asthma	History of exposure to noxious particles and gases (mainly tobacco smoking and biomass fuels)	Frequently a history of doctor-diagnosed asthma (current or previous), allergies and a family history of asthma, and/or a history of noxious exposures	Previous doctor diagnosis of asthma Family history of asthma, and other allergic conditions (allergic rhinitis or eczema)	Previous doctor diagnosis of COPD, chronic bronchitis or emphysema Heavy exposure to a risk factor: Tobacco smoke, biomass fuels

See directions on next page

Continued

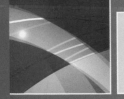

TABLE 14.1 Common Features of Asthma, Chronic Obstructive Pulmonary Disease (COPD), and Asthma and COPD Overlap, Including Features That Favor Asthma or COPD—cont'd

	Common Features of Asthma, COPD, and Asthma and COPD Overlap			Features That Favor Asthma or COPD	
Feature	Asthma	COPD	Asthma and COPD Overlap	Favors Asthma*	Favors COPD*
Time course	Often improves spontaneously or with treatment, but may result in fixed airflow limitation	Generally, slowly progressive over years despite treatment	Symptoms are partly but significantly reduced by treatment. Progression is usual and treatment needs are high	No worsening of symptoms over time; symptoms vary either seasonally, or from year to year. May improve spontaneously or have immediate response to bronchodilator or corticosteroid therapy	Symptoms slowly worsening over time (progressive course over years). Rapid-acting bronchodilator treatment provides only limited relief
Chest x-ray	Usually normal		Similar to COPD	Normal	Severe hyperinflation
Exacerbations	Exacerbations occur, but the risk for exacerbations can be considerably reduced by treatment	Severe hyperinflation and other changes of COPD Exacerbations can be reduced by treatment. If present, comorbidities contribute to impairment	Exacerbations may be more common than in COPD but are reduced by treatment. Comorbidities can contribute to impairment		
Airway inflammation	Eosinophils and/or neutrophils	Neutrophils + eosinophils in sputum, lymphocytes in airways, may have systemic inflammation	Eosinophils and/or neutrophils in sputum		

*Directions: The blue shaded columns list features that, when present, best identify patients with typical asthma and COPD. For a patient, count the number of features in each column. If three or more features are checked for either asthma or COPD, the patient is likely to have that disease. If there are similar numbers of features in each column, the diagnosis of ACO should be considered.

Data from Global Strategy for Asthma Management and Prevention, 2017, GINA (Retrieved from http://www.ginasthma.org).

General Management of Asthma

GINA provides an excellent clinical guideline program for the management and prevention of asthma. The complete GINA guidelines are readily available at http://www.ginasthma.org. An overview of GINA's global strategy for asthma management and prevention are discussed in the following text.

GINA's long-term goals for asthma management are *symptom control* (i.e., obtain control of the respiratory symptoms and maintain normal daily activities) and *risk reduction of future*

exacerbations (e.g., removal of potential risk factors, such as smoking, beta-blockers, or allergen exposure, and checking for correct inhaler technique, adherence, and comorbidities, such as rhinitis, rhinosinusitis, obesity, obstructive sleep apnea, or depression or anxiety). The basic foundation to achieve these two goals is securing a strong partnership between the patient and the health care providers (e.g., good verbal and written communications and, importantly, presented at the patient's basic health literacy level). A good partnership enhances the asthma patient's ability to gain the knowledge, confidence,

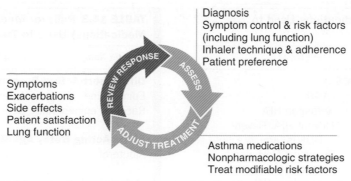

Diagnosis
Symptom control & risk factors
(including lung function)
Inhaler technique & adherence
Patient preference

Symptoms
Exacerbations
Side effects
Patient satisfaction
Lung function

Asthma medications
Nonpharmacologic strategies
Treat modifiable risk factors

FIGURE 14.6 The control-based asthma management cycle. (Modified from Global Strategy for Asthma Management and Prevention, 2017, GINA. http://www.ginasthma.org.)

and skills necessary to self-manage his or her asthma. Along with a strong patient and health care provider partnership, GINA recommends a *control-based asthma management program.*

Control-Based Asthma Management Program

In a control-based asthma management program, the pharmacologic and nonpharmacologic treatment is a continuous cycle that entails the assessment of the patient's condition, treatment selection and/or adjustment (i.e., up-regulate or down-regulate the therapy), and the review of the patient's response (Fig. 14.6). In a control-based management program, both the symptom control and future risk for exacerbations need to be considered when selecting asthma treatment and assessing the patient's response to the therapy. The pharmacologic options for long-term treatment of asthma fall into the following three categories:

- *Controller medications:* These agents are used for regular maintenance treatment. They decrease airway inflammation, control symptoms, and reduce the future risks for exacerbations and decreased lung function. Table 14.2 shows medications commonly used to control the symptoms of asthma.
- *Reliever (rescue) medications:* These agents provide as-needed relief of asthma symptoms, including during worsening asthma or exacerbations. They are also helpful for short-term prevention of exercise-induced bronchoconstriction. Table 14.3 provides common reliever (rescue) medications used to treat the symptoms of asthma.
- *Add-on therapies for patients with severe asthma:* These therapies may be considered when the patient continues to have symptoms and/or exacerbations despite optimized treatment with a high dose of controller medication and the treatment of modifiable risk factors.

The Stepwise Management Approach to Control Asthma Symptoms and Reduce Future Risk

Based on the patient's current level of asthma control and current treatment regimen, GINA recommends one of five possible treatment steps that can be assigned to the patient. The preferred treatment at each step is based on (1) efficacy, (2) effectiveness, (3) safety, and (4) the availability and cost of the treatment. In addition, the patient's asthma characteristics

(phenotype), patient preference (i.e., goals and concerns), and practical issues (e.g., inhaler technique, adherence, and costs) need to be considered at each step.

Fig. 14.7 summarizes GINA's stepwise asthma management approach for adults, adolescents, and children 6 to 11 years.[8] As can be seen, Step 1 through Step 5 progressively increase treatment medication options and intensity. In short, if the patient's asthma symptoms are not controlled on the current treatment program (e.g., Step 2), the treatment should be up-regulated to Step 3, Step 4, or Step 5 until control is achieved. Before considering a step-up, check for common problems such as poor inhaler technique, poor adherence, and environmental exposure to allergic allergens. When the control of the asthma symptoms has been maintained for at least 3 months, the ICS dose should be slowly titrated to the minimum dose that will maintain good symptom control and minimize exacerbation risk and potential side effects.

STEP 1: As-Needed Reliever Inhaler

The preferred option is to start the patient on an as-needed **short-acting beta$_2$-agonist (SABA)**. SABAs are highly effective in controlling asthma symptoms quickly (see Fig. 14.7). A second controller option is a regular low-dose ICS, in addition to as-needed SABA, in patients at risk for exacerbation. Table 14.2 provides common ICS agents used to control asthma symptoms.

STEP 2: Low-Dose Controller Medication Plus Needed Reliever Medication

The preferred option is to place the patient on a regular low-dose ICS, plus an as-needed SABA. ICSs at low doses have been shown to decrease asthma symptoms, improve lung function and quality of life, and reduce the risk for exacerbations and asthma-related hospitalizations and death. A second controller option is **leukotriene receptor antagonists (LTRA)**, although they are considered less effective than ICSs. However, they may be appropriate for some patients who are unable or unwilling to use an ICS, the patient who experiences uncomfortable side effects from ICS, or the patient with concurrent allergic rhinitis. For the adult or adolescent patients, not previously on

---

[8]For the management of asthma in children 5 years and younger, see the Global Strategy for the Diagnosis and Management of Asthma in Children 5 Years and Younger, at http://www.ginasthma.org.

TABLE 14.2 Controller Medications Used to Treat Asthma*

Generic Name	Brand Name
Inhaled Corticosteroids (ICSs)	
Beclomethasone	QVAR
Flunisolide	Aerospan HFA
Fluticasone	Flovent HFA, Flovent Diskus, Arnuity Ellipta
Budesonide	Pulmicort Flexhaler
Mometasone	Asmanex Twisthaler, Asmanex HFA
Ciclesonide	Alvesco
Inhaled Corticosteroids and Long-Acting Beta₂ Agents (Combined)	
Fluticasone and salmeterol	Advair Diskus, Advair HFA
Budesonide and formoterol	Symbicort
Mometasone and formoterol	Dulera
Oral Corticosteroids	
Methylprednisolone	Medrol, Solu-Medrol
Hydrocortisone	Solu-Cortef
Long-Acting Beta₂ Agents (LABAs)	
Salmeterol	Serevent Diskus
Leukotriene Inhibitors (Antileukotrienes)	
Zafirlukast	Accolate
Montelukast	Singulair
Zileuton	Zyflo, Zyflo CR
Long-Acting Antimuscarinic Antagonists (LAMAs)	
Tiotropium	Spiriva HandiHaler, Spiriva Respimat
Aclidinium	Tudorza Pressair
Umeclidinium	Incruse Ellipta
Xanthine Derivatives	
Theophylline	Theochron, Elixophyllin, Theo-24
Oxtriphylline	Choledyl SA
Aminophylline	Generic
Dyphylline	Lufyllin
Agent to Reduce Eosinophilic Inflammation in Allergic Disease	
Anti-interleukin-5	Mepolizumab (subcutaneous), reslizumab (intravenous)
Antiimmunoglobulin E (Anti-IgE)	
Omalizumab	Xolair

*For the complete listing, doses, and administration of agents approved by the US Food and Drug Administration, visit the Drugs@FDA website (http://www.accessdata.fda.gov/scripts/cder/drugsatfda/).

TABLE 14.3 Reliever Medications (Rescue Medications) Used to Treat Asthma*

Generic Name	Brand Name
Ultra-Short-Acting Bronchodilator Agents	
Epinephrine	Adrenalin
Racemic epinephrine	Generic
Short-Acting Beta₂ Agents (SABAs)	
Albuterol	Proventil HFA, Ventolin HFA, ProAir HFA, AccuNeb HFA, Generic
Metaproterenol	Generic
Levalbuterol	Xopenex, Xopenex HFA, Generic

*For the complete listing, doses, and administration of agents approved by the US Food and Drug Administration, visit the Drugs@FDA website (http://www.accessdata.fda.gov/scripts/cder/drugsatfda/).

any controller treatment, a low-dose combination of ICS and **long-acting beta₂-agonists (LABAs)** as the initial treatment has shown to reduce symptoms and improve lung function when compared with a low-dose ICS alone. A low-dose sustained-released theophylline may be considered, although it has only a weak efficacy in asthma (see Fig. 14.7).

STEP 3: One or Two Controllers, Plus As-Needed Reliever Medication

The two preferred options for adults and adolescents are a combination of low-dose ICS/LABA as maintenance treatment, plus an as-needed SABA, or a combination low-dose ICS/formoterol (budesonide or beclomethasone) as both maintenance and reliever treatment. For adult patients with allergic rhinitis and sensitized to house dust mites, with exacerbations despite low- to high-dose ICS, consider adding **sublingual allergen immunotherapy (SLIT)** when the FEV1 is greater than 70% predicted. A second option for adults and adolescents is to increase the ICS to a medium dose or administer a low-dose ICS, along with either an LTRA or a low-dose sustained-release theophylline. The preferred option for children 6 to 11 years is a moderate-dose ICS, plus an as-needed SABA (see Fig. 14.7).

STEP 4: One or Two Controllers Plus As-Needed Reliever Medication

The preferred option for adults and adolescents is a medium/high dose of ICS/LABA, plus an as-needed SABA or low-dose ICS/formoterol. For the adult patients with allergic rhinitis and sensitized to house dust mite, with exacerbations despite low-high dose ICS, consider adding SLIT when the FEV_1 is greater than 70% predicted. A second option for adults and adolescents with a history of exacerbations is tiotropium (long-acting muscarinic antagonist) by mist inhaler, a combination high-dose ICS/LABA, or a sustained-released theophylline. The preferred option for children 6 to 11 years is a referral for expert assessment and advice (see Fig. 14.7).

STEP 5: Higher Level Care and/or Add-On Treatment

The preferred option of Step 5 is referral for specialist investigation and consideration of add-on therapy. Treatment add-on options—if not already tried—include:

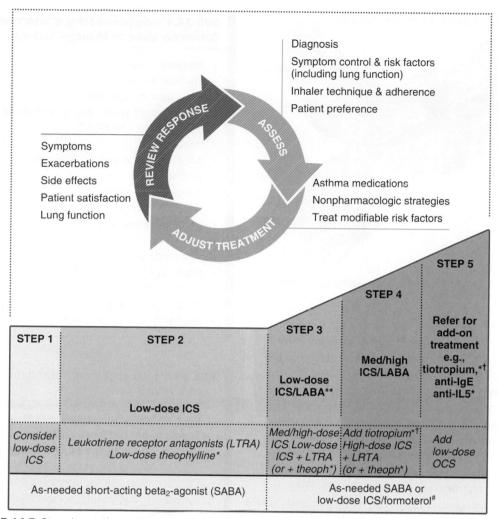

FIGURE 14.7 Stepwise asthma management for adults, adolescents, and children 6 to 11 years. ICS: inhaled corticosteroids; LABA: long-acting beta2-agonists; med: medium dose; OCS: oral cortisosteroids; SLIT: sublingual immunotherapy. (Modified from Global Strategy for Asthma Management and Prevention, 2017, GINA. http://www.ginasthma.org.)

- *Add-on tiotropium* (long-acting muscarinic antagonist) in patients 2 years or older with a history of exacerbation despite Step 4 treatment.
- *Add-on anti–immunoglobulin E (anti-IgE)* (omalizumab) treatment for patients 6 years or older with a history of exacerbation despite Step 4 treatment.
- *Add-on anti–interleukin-5* treatment (subcutaneous mepolizumzab, intravenous reslizumab) for patients 12 years or older with severe eosinophilic asthma that cannot be controlled by Step 4.
- *Sputum-guided treatment* for patients with persisting symptoms and/or exacerbations despite high-dose ICS or ICS/LABA. Treatment may be based on eosinophilia (>3%) in induced sputum.
- *Add-on low-dose oral corticosteroids* (<7.5 mg/day prednisone equivalent) may be helpful for some adults with eosinophilia and/or severe asthma (see Fig. 14.7).
- *Add-on treatment with bronchial thermoplasty* in adults with severe asthma.
  - **Bronchial thermoplasty** involves the use of therapeutic radiofrequency energy applied to the airway walls in patients with severe asthma. The procedure entails the insertion of a standard flexible bronchoscope through the patient's nose or mouth and into the lungs. The tip of the small-diameter catheter, which is threaded through the bronchoscope, is then introduced out into the bronchus and expanded to contact the walls of the targeted airway. As shown in Fig. 14.8 (see arrow), a controlled thermal energy is then applied to the bronchial airways, which in turn heats the airway tissues and shrinks the bronchial smooth muscles that cause the airways to constrict during an asthma episode. This treatment has been shown to cause acute epithelial destruction followed by regeneration in the epithelium, blood vessels, mucosa, and nerves. The bronchial smooth muscles, however, demonstrate no remarkable regeneration and, instead, are replaced by connective tissue.

The full treatment course includes three different bronchial thermoplasty procedures: One treatment for the left lower lung lobe, one treatment for the right lower lung lobe, and one treatment for both the right and left upper lobes. Each procedure is performed at least 3 weeks apart. Side effects include coughing, wheezing, and shortness of breath. Bronchial thermoplasty

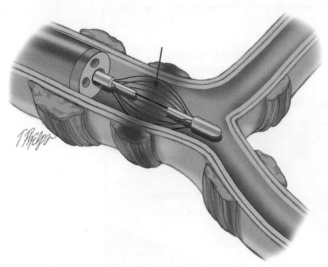

FIGURE 14.8 Bronchial thermoplasty. Arrow points to thermal energy element.

is indicated for patients with severe persistent asthma who are 18 years and older and whose asthma is not well controlled with long-acting beta-agonists and ICSs. Patients who have been treated with bronchial thermoplasty have shown a reduction in severe asthma attacks, fewer visits to the emergency department, a drop in hospitalization for respiratory symptoms, and a decrease in days lost from work or school. Although this treatment has been shown to be safe and effective since it was first approved by the US Food and Drug Administration (FDA) in 2010, further trials are under way to determine the optimal role for bronchial thermoplasty in asthma management as we move forward.

Nonpharmacologic Interventions in the Treatment of Asthma

In addition to the pharmacologic interventions used to manage asthma, a number of other therapies may be helpful in the control of asthma and/or reducing future exacerbation risks. Box 14.4 provides an overview of common nonpharmacologic interventions.

Indications for Referral for Expert Evaluation

Although most patients with asthma usually can be controlled in primary care, some clinical circumstances justify the referral for expert advice regarding the diagnosis and/or management of asthma. Box 14.5 shows common indications for considering referral for expert advice when possible.

Protocol When Asthma Is Controlled

When asthma control has been achieved, regular and ongoing monitoring of the patient's symptom control, risk factors, occurrence of exacerbations, and documentation of responses to any treatment changes is essential to maintain control and determine the lowest step and dose of treatment, which

minimizes cost and maximizes the safety of treatment. It is also important to establish the patient's adherence with medications and other advice and any factors that contribute to poor adherence. It is also essential to ensure the patient has a full understanding of all asthma information associated with the patient's condition.

In addition, it should be confirmed that the patient is adequately trained in guided asthma self-management. Guided self-management may involve varying degrees of independence ranging from patient-directed self-management to doctor-directed self-management. With a doctor-directed self-management plan, the patient has a written action plan but contacts the doctor for most major treatment decisions. With a patient-directed self-management plan, the patient makes changes in accordance with a prior written action plan without needing to first contact the physician. A popular monitoring system is the asthma action plan, using green, yellow, and red zones (Fig. 14.9).

Even when the **asthma action plan** is appropriately designed, the full benefit of any treatment changes may be evident only after 3 to 4 months. It may take much longer in severe cases. Stepping up asthma treatment can be done in the following three ways: (1) sustained step up (which is

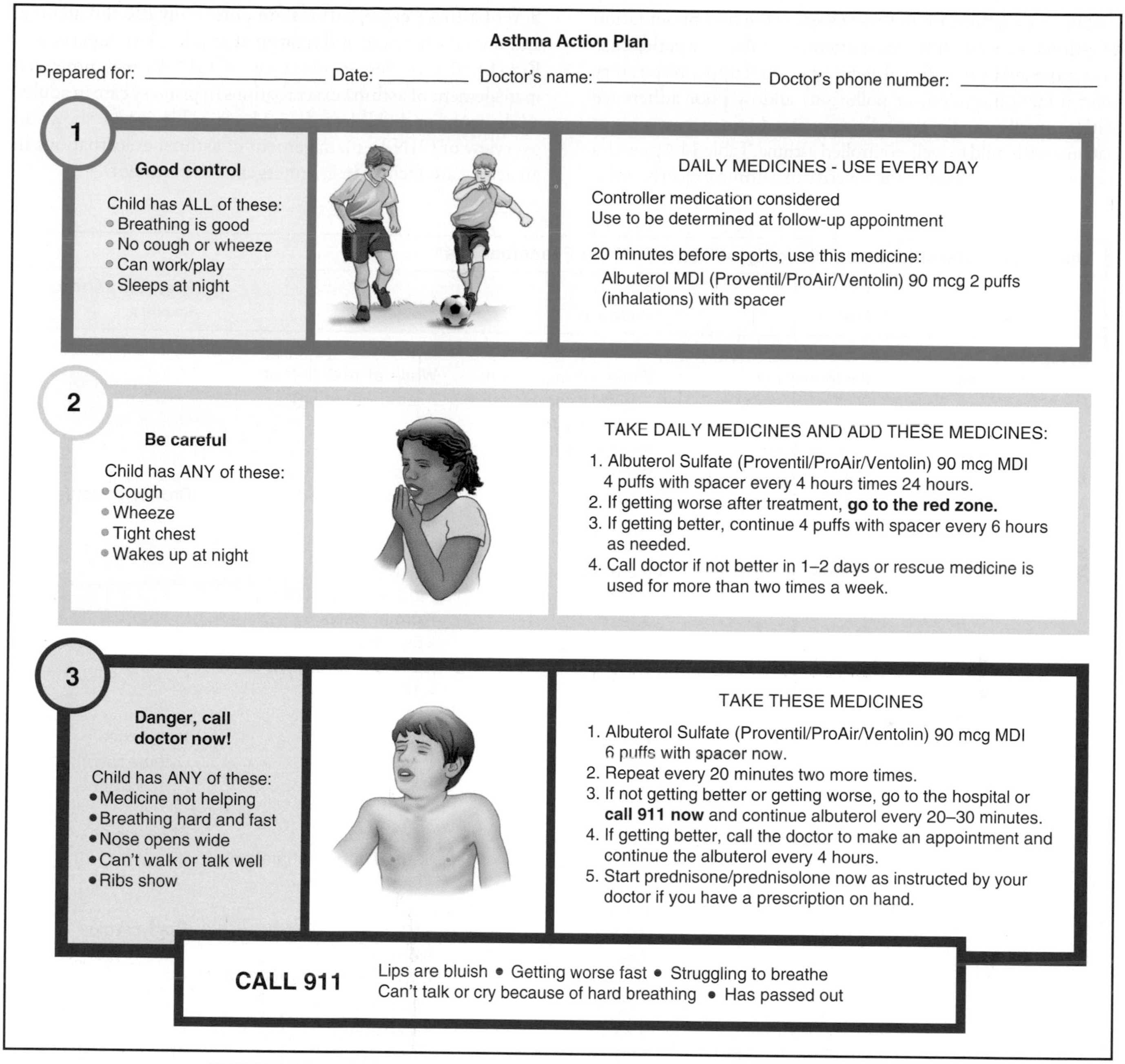

Asthma Action Plan

Prepared for: _____ Date: _____ Doctor's name: _____ Doctor's phone number: _____

1

Good control

Child has ALL of these:
• Breathing is good
• No cough or wheeze
• Can work/play
• Sleeps at night

DAILY MEDICINES - USE EVERY DAY

Controller medication considered
Use to be determined at follow-up appointment

20 minutes before sports, use this medicine:
Albuterol MDI (Proventil/ProAir/Ventolin) 90 mcg 2 puffs (inhalations) with spacer

2

Be careful

Child has ANY of these:
• Cough
• Wheeze
• Tight chest
• Wakes up at night

TAKE DAILY MEDICINES AND ADD THESE MEDICINES:

1. Albuterol Sulfate (Proventil/ProAir/Ventolin) 90 mcg MDI 4 puffs with spacer every 4 hours times 24 hours.
2. If getting worse after treatment, **go to the red zone.**
3. If getting better, continue 4 puffs with spacer every 6 hours as needed.
4. Call doctor if not better in 1–2 days or rescue medicine is used for more than two times a week.

3

Danger, call doctor now!

Child has ANY of these:
• Medicine not helping
• Breathing hard and fast
• Nose opens wide
• Can't walk or talk well
• Ribs show

TAKE THESE MEDICINES

1. Albuterol Sulfate (Proventil/ProAir/Ventolin) 90 mcg MDI 6 puffs with spacer now.
2. Repeat every 20 minutes two more times.
3. If not getting better or getting worse, go to the hospital or **call 911 now** and continue albuterol every 20–30 minutes.
4. If getting better, call the doctor to make an appointment and continue the albuterol every 4 hours.
5. Start prednisone/prednisolone now as instructed by your doctor if you have a prescription on hand.

CALL 911   Lips are bluish • Getting worse fast • Struggling to breathe
Can't talk or cry because of hard breathing • Has passed out

FIGURE 14.9 Asthma action plan. (Courtesy Dayton Children's Hospital Dayton, Ohio.)

designed for 2 to 3 months), (2) short-term step up (which is for 1 to 2 weeks), or (3) day-to-day adjustments. Stepping down treatment may, or should, be considered once good asthma control has been achieved and maintained for 3 months, and lung function has reached a plateau.

The primary goals of stepping down are to find the minimum effective treatment and encourage patients to continue regular controller treatment on their own. Guided asthma self-management education and skills training include:
• Skills training for effective use of inhaler devices
• Patient adherence with medications and related advice
• Asthma information
• Training in guided asthma self-management—for example, self-monitoring of symptoms and/or peak flow, written action plan, and regular review of asthma control, treatment, and skills by a health care provider.

Although the majority of asthma symptoms usually can be managed in primary care, some patients warrant referral for expert advice. Indications for considering a referral for an expert opinion include the following:
• Difficulty confirming the diagnosis of asthma
• Suspected occupational asthma
• Persistent uncontrolled asthma or frequent exacerbations
• Any risk factors for asthma-related death
• Evidence of, or risk for, significant treatment side effects
• Symptoms suggesting complications or subtypes of asthma

Management of Asthma Exacerbation

An asthma exacerbation (also called an *asthma attack* or *asthma episode*) is characterized by a progressive increase in symptoms of shortness of breath, cough, wheezing or chest tightness, and progressive decrease in lung function (e.g., decreased PEFR or FEV_1). Exacerbations may occur in patients with a preexisting diagnosis of asthma or, in some cases, as the first presentation of asthma. Exacerbations most often occur after the patient has been exposed to an external agent (e.g., viral upper respiratory tract infection, pollen, or pollution) and/or poor adherence with controller medications. Severe exacerbations may occur in patients with mild to well-controlled asthma. Table 14.4 provides a clinical scale to classify the severity of asthma exacerbations.

Severe asthma exacerbations are potentially life threatening, and their monitoring and treatment require close supervision. Fig. 14.10 provides an overview of GINA's recommended management of asthma exacerbations in primary care in adults, adolescents, and children 6 to 11 years. Fig. 14.11 shows an overview of GINA's management of asthma exacerbations in an acute care facility (e.g., emergency department).

TABLE 14.4 Classification of Severity of Acute Asthma Exacerbations*

	Mild	Moderate	Severe	Respiratory Arrest Imminent
Symptoms				
Breathlessness	While walking	While talking (infant: softer, shorter cry; difficulty feeding)	While at rest (infant: stops feeding)	
	Can lie down	Prefers sitting	Sits upright	
Talks in	Sentences	Phrases	Words	
Alertness	May be agitated	Usually agitated	Usually agitated	Drowsy or confused
Signs				
Respiratory rate	Increased	Increased	Often >30/min	
		Normal rates of breathing in awake children:		
		Age Normal Rate		
		<2 mo <60/min		
		2–12 mo <50/min		
		1–5 yr <40/min		
		6–8 yr <30/min		
Use of accessory muscles; suprasternal retractions	Usually not	Commonly	Usually	Paradoxical thoracoabdominal movement
Wheeze	Moderate, often only end-expiratory	Loud; throughout exhalation	Usually loud; throughout inhalation and exhalation	Absence of wheeze
		Normal pulse rates in awake children:		
Pulse/min	<100	100–120	>120	Bradycardia
		Age Normal Rate		
		2–12 mo <160/min		
		1–2 yr <120/min		
		2–8 yr <110/min		
Pulsus paradoxus	Absent <10 mm Hg	May be present 10–25 mm Hg	Often present >25 mm Hg (adult) 20–40 mm Hg (child)	Absence suggests respiratory muscle fatigue
Functional Assessment				
PEFR (% predicted or % personal best)	80%	~50%–80%	<50% predicted or personal best or response lasts <2 h	
PaO_2 (on air)	Normal (ABG usually necessary)	>60 mm Hg (ABG usually necessary)	<60 mm Hg: possible cyanosis	
and/or				
$PaCO_2$	<42 mm Hg (ABG usually necessary)	<42 mm Hg (ABG usually necessary)	≥42 mm Hg: possible respiratory failure	
SaO_2 % (on air) at sea level	>95% (ABG usually necessary)	91%–95%	<91%	
	Hypercapnia (hypoventilation) develops more readily in young children than in adults and adolescents			

*The presence of several findings, but not necessarily all, suggests the general classification of the exacerbation. Many of these parameters have not been systematically studied, so they serve only as general guides. From Expert Panel Response 3 (EPR 3): Guidelines for the diagnosis and management of asthma, 2007 (http://www.nhlbi.nih.gov/guidelines/asthma/asthgdln.htm).
PEFR, Peak expiratory flow rate.

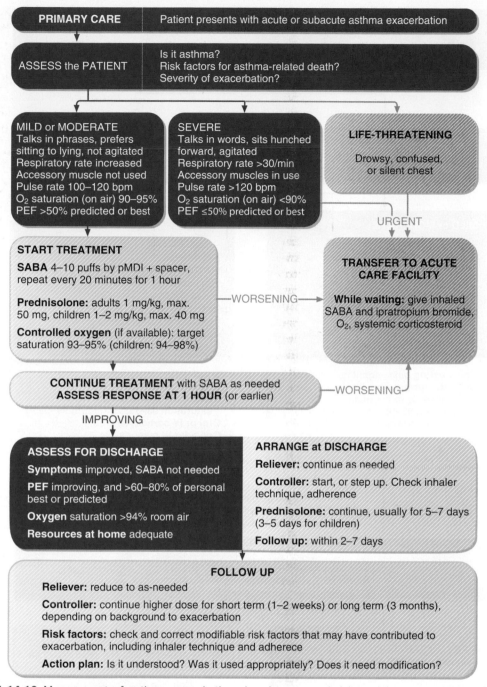

FIGURE 14.10 Management of asthma exacerbations in primary care (adults, adolescents, children 6 to 11 years). (Modified from Global Strategy for Asthma Management and Prevention, 2017, GINA. http://www.ginasthma.org.)

Management of Asthma With Comorbidities and Special Populations

Several comorbidities are often associated with asthma, especially those with **difficult-to-treat asthma** or severe asthma. When possible, the treating of comorbidities is strongly recommended because they often contribute to the patient's symptoms. Common comorbidities associated with asthma include the following:

- *Obesity:* Asthma is more difficult to control in obese patients. Weight loss in the obese patient improves asthma control and lung function and reduces medication needs.

- *Gastroesophageal reflux disease (GERD):* Significant evidence indicates that gastroesophageal reflux is more common in patients with asthma and obstructive sleep apnea than the general population.

- *Anxiety and depression:* Psychiatric disorders, especially depressive and anxiety disorders, are common among people with asthma.

- *Food allergy and anaphylaxis:* Although food allergy as a trigger for asthma symptoms is rare (less than 2% of people with asthma), in patients with confirmed food-induced allergic reaction (anaphylaxis), coexisting asthma is a strong risk factor for more severe and even fatal reactions. Food-induced anaphylaxis often presents as life-threatening asthma.

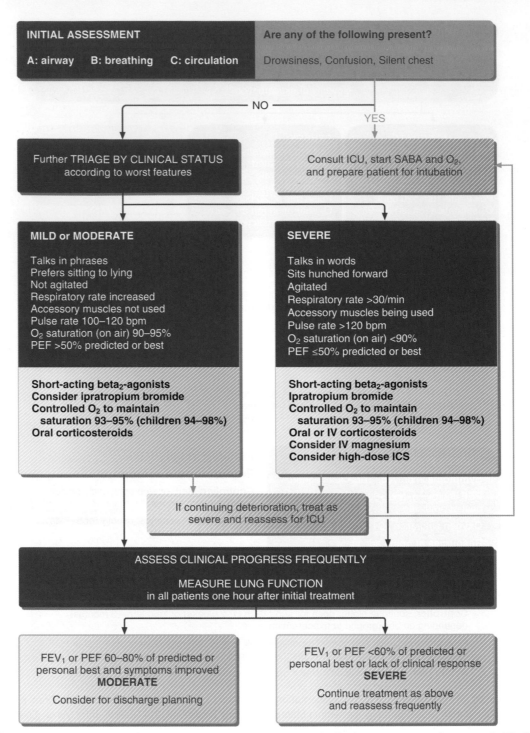

INITIAL ASSESSMENT	Are any of the following present?
A: airway B: breathing C: circulation	Drowsiness, Confusion, Silent chest

NO ———— YES

Further TRIAGE BY CLINICAL STATUS
according to worst features

Consult ICU, start SABA and O_2,
and prepare patient for intubation

MILD or MODERATE

Talks in phrases
Prefers sitting to lying
Not agitated
Respiratory rate increased
Accessory muscles not used
Pulse rate 100–120 bpm
O_2 saturation (on air) 90–95%
PEF >50% predicted or best

Short-acting beta₂-agonists
Consider ipratropium bromide
Controlled O_2 to maintain
  saturation 93–95% (children 94–98%)
Oral corticosteroids

SEVERE

Talks in words
Sits hunched forward
Agitated
Respiratory rate >30/min
Accessory muscles being used
Pulse rate >120 bpm
O_2 saturation (on air) <90%
PEF ≤50% predicted or best

Short-acting beta₂-agonists
Ipratropium bromide
Controlled O_2 to maintain
  saturation 93–95% (children 94–98%)
Oral or IV corticosteroids
Consider IV magnesium
Consider high-dose ICS

If continuing deterioration, treat as
severe and reassess for ICU

ASSESS CLINICAL PROGRESS FREQUENTLY

MEASURE LUNG FUNCTION
in all patients one hour after initial treatment

FEV_1 or PEF 60–80% of predicted or
personal best and symptoms improved
MODERATE

Consider for discharge planning

FEV_1 or PEF <60% of predicted or
personal best or lack of clinical response
SEVERE

Continue treatment as above
and reassess frequently

FIGURE 14.11 Management of asthma exacerbations in acute care facility (e.g., emergency department). (Modified from Global Strategy for Asthma Management and Prevention, 2017, GINA. http://www.ginasthma.org.)

- *Rhinitis, sinusitis, and nasal polyps:* Most patients with asthma, either allergic or nonallergic, have rhinitis. Upper airway disease often adversely influences airway function in some patients with asthma.
- ***Exercise-induced bronchoconstriction (EIB):*** Physical activity is often a stimulus for asthma symptoms in many patients. For example, athletes, especially those competing at a high level, have an increased incidence of asthma symptoms compared with nonathletes.

- *Pregnancy:* Asthma control often worsens in women who have a history of asthma and who are pregnant. Exacerbations are common in pregnancy, especially during the second trimester.
- *Occupational asthma:* Once a diagnosis of occupational asthma has been established, complete avoidance of the relevant exposure is an important component of management.
- *The elderly:* With increasing age, lung function generally decreases because of stiffness of the chest wall, reduced

muscle function, loss of elastic recoil, and airway remodeling. Older patients may not report asthma symptoms and often attribute breathlessness to normal aging or comorbidities such as cardiovascular disease or obesity.

- *Aspirin-exacerbated respiratory disease:* The clinical course of aspirin-exacerbated respiratory disease (AERD, previously called **aspirin-induced asthma**) is well documented. It begins with nasal congestion and anosmia and progresses to chronic rhinosinusitis with nasal polyps that regrow rapidly after surgery. Asthma and hypersensitivity to aspirin develop shortly afterward. After ingestion of aspirin or NSAIDs, an acute asthma episode develops.

- *Difficult-to-treat and severe asthma:* Refers to patients who have ongoing factors such as comorbidities, poor adherence, and allergen exposure that interfere with achieving good asthma control. **Treatment-resistant asthma** refers to the patient with confirmed diagnosis of asthma, but whose symptoms or exacerbations remain poorly controlled in spite of high-dose ICS and second controllers such as LABA. Severe asthma includes patients with **refractory asthma** and those who have not fully responded to treatment of comorbidities.

Respiratory Care Treatment Protocols

Aerosolized Medication Protocol

Inhaled beta$_2$ agents, **anticholinergic agents**, and corticosteroid agents via a metered dose inhaler (pMDI) spacer, dry powder inhaler (DPI), or small volume nebulizer (SVN) are commonly used in the treatment of asthma to induce bronchial smooth muscle relaxation (see Aerosolized Medication Protocol, Protocol 10.4). Continuous nebulization of albuterol is often used in the management of status asthmaticus to prevent acute ventilatory failure.

Oxygen Therapy Protocol

Oxygen therapy may be required to treat hypoxemia, decrease the work of breathing, and decrease myocardial work. The hypoxemia that develops in asthma is usually caused by the ventilation-perfusion mismatch and shunt-like effect associated with bronchospasm and increased airway secretions. Hypoxemia caused by this shunt-like effect can at least partly be corrected by oxygen therapy (see Oxygen Therapy Protocol, Protocol 10.1).

Airway Clearance Therapy Protocol

Because of the excessive mucous production and secretion accumulation associated with asthma, a number of bronchial hygiene treatment modalities may be used to enhance the mobilization of bronchial secretions (see Airway Clearance Therapy Protocol, Protocol 10.2). These modalities should be attempted with patients with acute asthma when they can effectively move enough air to deep breathe and cough.

Mechanical Ventilation Protocol

Because acute ventilatory failure is associated with **status asthmaticus**, continuous mechanical ventilation may be required to maintain an adequate ventilatory status.

Status asthmaticus is defined as a severe asthma episode that does not respond to conventional pharmacologic therapy. When the patient becomes fatigued, the ventilatory rate decreases. Clinically, the patient demonstrates a progressive decrease in PaO$_2$ and pH and a steady increase in PaCO$_2$ (acute ventilatory failure). Noninvasive ventilatory assistance (continuous positive airway pressure [CPAP] or bilevel positive airway pressure [BPAP][9]) may be indicated to provide expiratory resistance, while also providing frequent or continuous aerosolized bronchodilator therapy. If ventilation does not improve and hypercarbia is not reversed, intubation and mechanical ventilation becomes necessary (see Ventilator Initiation and Management Protocol, Protocol 11.1, and Ventilator Weaning Protocol, Protocol 11.2).

---

[9]BPAP should not be confused with BiPAP, which is the brand name of a single manufacturer and is just one of many devices that can be used for BPAP.

CASE STUDY Asthma

A 7-year-old girl was admitted to the emergency department (ED) in severe respiratory distress. Her history of wheezing dated back to age 6 months, when she was hospitalized with viral bronchiolitis. Over the past 3 years she was hospitalized in different hospitals on a number of occasions and was usually managed satisfactorily with aerosolized albuterol and oral steroids. She began coughing and wheezing the night before admission and became progressively worse during the night. Her cough was nonproductive. At 8.00 a.m., she was brought to the ED after she did not get relief from her albuterol MDI at home.

Physical examination revealed an extremely anxious, well-developed female child in acute respiratory distress. She stated in short, terse phrases: "It's hard ... for me ... to breathe." Her vital signs were as follows: blood pressure 128/84, pulse 148 beats/min, and respiratory rate 30 breaths/min. Her temperature was 99.1°F. Her SpO_2 was 88% on room air on arrival. She was actively using her accessory muscles of respiration. On auscultation, her breath sounds were decreased bilaterally with faint expiratory wheezes and coarse crackles.

The ED physician ordered three back-to-back SVN treatments with a combination of albuterol and ipratropium bromide. The patient's level of distress prompted a need to begin bronchodilator treatment with oxygen without attempting serial peak flow measurements. Posttreatment PEFR was less than 70 L/min. (Her personal best was about 200 to 250 L/min.) The patient was then placed on 2 L/min nasal cannula oxygen, and a capillary blood gas (CBG) was drawn: pH 7.27, $PaCO_2$ 52 mm Hg, HCO_3^- 22 mEq/L, PaO_2 76 mm Hg, and SaO_2 91%. A chest x-ray examination was ordered but not performed. The physician ordered a respiratory care consultation and stated that she did not want to commit the patient to a ventilator at this time if possible. The physician asked that aggressive noninvasive pulmonary care be tried first. At this time the respiratory therapist documented the following.

Respiratory Assessment and Plan

S Patient air hungry and stated in chopped phrases, "It's hard for me to breathe"

O Vital signs: On arrival BP 128/84, R 148, RR 30, T 99.1°. SpO_2 88% on room air. Using accessory muscles, subcostal, intercostals, and supraclavicular retractions. Decreased breath sounds bilaterally at bases and faint expiratory wheezes and coarse crackles. PEFR: Less than 70 L/min after three back-to-back albuterol-ipratropium SVN treatments. Oral prednisolone was given. Several fluid boluses are given. CBGs pH 7.27, $PaCO_2$ 52, HCO_3^- 22, PaO_2 76, and SaO_2 91% on 2 L/min posttreatment. No CXR yet.

A • Severe exacerbation (per NAEPP severity scale) of previously partly controlled asthma
  • Respiratory distress (increased heart rate, blood pressure, respiratory rate)
  • Bronchospasm (decreased air entry, wheezing, decreased PEFR, history)
  • Excessive airway secretions (coarse crackles)
  • Acute ventilatory failure (acute respiratory acidosis) with moderate to severe hypoxemia (CBG)
  • Metabolic acidosis also likely (both pH and HCO_3^- are both lower than expected for a $PaCO_2$ of 52). Likely caused by lactic acid because of low SpO_2.

P Oxygen Therapy Protocol. Monitor SpO_2 with oximeter; provide oxygen via continuous medication nebulizer and supplemental cannula as needed. Aerosolized Medication Therapy Protocol (continuous med. neb. with albuterol and ipratropium bromide). Monitor PEFR and breath sounds. Airway Clearance Therapy Protocol (cough and deep breathe as tolerated). Monitor breath sounds. Repeat CBG in 30 minutes. Continuous cardiac monitoring in place. Respiratory Therapy to remain in ED at bedside. Consider noninvasive ventilation if patient does not continue to improve.

In addition to this plan, the patient was treated vigorously with intravenous steroids (Solu-Medrol) and intravenous magnesium sulfate. The chest x-ray results showed depressed diaphragms, hyperinflation bilaterally with patchy atelectasis. A **respiratory infectious disease panel (RIDP)**[10] was ordered to rule out viral infection or mycoplasma pneumonia.

After 3 hours of continuous albuterol aerosol with oxygen, the patient began to slowly improve—that is, bilateral aeration was better and the respiratory distress symptoms began to subside. On a 2 L/min oxygen cannula, the patient's CBG showed pH 7.38, $PaCO_2$ 44 mm Hg, HCO_3^- 24 mEq/L, PaO_2 78 mm Hg, and SpO_2 94%. Asthma scores improved from poor to fair, allowing the patient to be weaned from the continuous albuterol and ipratropium bromide after 6 hours to q2h albuterol medication nebulizer treatments. The RIDP showed the patient was positive for rhinovirus.

Over the next 30 hours the patient was weaned from q2h to q4h, then to q6h albuterol MDI treatments based on the respiratory care asthma protocol. Oxygen requirements subsided after 20 hours of inpatient care. The patient was instructed in proper MDI and **valved holding chamber (VHC)** technique. With each treatment the patient was encouraged to deep breathe and cough. Oral corticosteroids continued daily, and ICSs via MDI and VHC were also ordered as a daily controller for home therapy. Peak flow measurements were now reaching 150 to 180 L/min post-MDI.

The patient was instructed in asthma trigger prevention, and a personalized asthma action plan was reviewed with the patient and family. The parents verbalized their understanding of controller and reliever medications in the prevention and management their child's asthma. Follow-up was scheduled with the primary care physician within 2 days.

Discussion

Asthma is a potentially fatal disease, largely because its severity is often unrecognized in the home or outpatient setting. Even patients with mild asthma can occasionally have a severe, life-threatening attack. Overuse of reliever medications (albuterol), with underutilization of controller medications (ICSs) is also associated with increased severity of attacks. The clinical manifestations presented in this case all can be easily traced back through the Bronchospasm clinical scenario (see Fig. 10.10) and Excessive Bronchial Secretions clinical scenario (see Fig. 10.11). For example, the patient's increased blood pressure, heart rate, and respiratory rate can all be followed back to the hypoxemia caused by the ventilation-perfusion mismatch and pulmonary shunting activated by the bronchospasm and excessive bronchial secretions (see Figs. 10.10 and 10.11). The patient's anxiety and possible previous use of a **beta$_2$-agonist** also may have contributed to her abnormal vital signs (tachycardia). *However, anxiety with an asthma attack always should be attributed to hypoxemia until proved otherwise.*

---

[10]The RIDP includes detection of the following: Adenovirus, coronavirus 229E, coronavirus HKU1, coronavirus NL63, coronavirus OC43, human metapneumovirus, human rhinovirus (1, 2, 3, and 4), enterovirus, influenza A (H1-2009, H1, H3), influenza B, parainfluenza (1, 2, 3, and 4), respiratory syncytial virus, *Bordetella pertussis*, *Chlamydophila pneumoniae*, and *Mycoplasma pneumoniae*.

In addition, the decreased PEFR, use of accessory muscles, diminished breath sounds, and wheezing and coarse crackles reflect the increased airway resistance and air trapping caused by the bronchospasm (see Fig. 10.10) and excessive bronchial secretions (see Fig. 10.11). The fact that the patient's CBG values showed acute ventilatory failure confirmed that the patient was in the severe stages of an asthmatic episode and that mechanical ventilation could be required if the patient failed to respond to the vigorous respiratory care provided.

In the first SOAP presented for this case, the respiratory therapist chose a fairly aggressive approach to both the Oxygen Therapy Protocol (Protocol 10.1) and the Aerosolized Medication Therapy Protocol (Protocol 10.4). Use of a nasal cannula to deliver supplemental oxygen, titrated to an SpO_2 of 92% to 94%, often causes less anxiety than the use of a face mask in children. Frequent monitoring of CBGs and SpO_2 levels was appropriate.

Also note the use of continuous albuterol inhalation in the Aerosolized Medication Therapy Protocol. Because of the severity of the patient's asthma episode, the aggressive administration of albuterol, the short-acting bronchodilator agent, was clearly a correct selection according to GINA guidelines.

Adults may not tolerate aggressive albuterol administration because of coexistent cardiac disease; adults must be monitored closely for development of arrhythmias or myocardial ischemia (ST segment elevation). In an acute asthma attack, albuterol should be nebulized with oxygen to minimize hypoxic cardiac complications. The manner in which any therapy modality is up-regulated may be (1) a different aerosolized drug or procedure, (2) a larger dose of a drug or therapy, or (3) more frequent use of such drugs or therapy. In this case, the continuous larger dose was successful.

Among the lessons to be learned here is that some asthma episodes may initially worsen despite appropriate and vigorous therapy. This patient received optimal emergent treatment of her severe asthma attack, but her recovery required several hours of continuous albuterol and intravenous medications, particularly magnesium sulfate and Solu-Medrol. Intravenous aminophylline in the emergency treatment of acute asthma is controversial and rarely used in children. Care must be taken to avoid theophylline toxicity, and symptoms of toxicity often do not reflect serum concentrations of the drug. Almost continuous assessment by the respiratory therapist is necessary if more invasive therapy (including induced sedation, paralysis, and mechanical ventilation) is to be avoided.

The acutely ill patient with asthma requires almost continuous monitoring and frequent SOAP notes if the patient care team is to be constantly apprised of the patient's progress. (The one such note recorded here is but a small portion of the more than 14 notes that we found on analysis of the patient's medical record from her ED admission alone.) Current best practice would require that the first SOAP assessment would have included a statement about the patient's preadmission asthma control status, which in this case would have been (at best) "partly controlled."

SELF-ASSESSMENT QUESTIONS

1. During an asthma episode, the smooth muscles of the bronchi may hypertrophy as much as:
   a. Two times normal thickness
   b. Three times normal thickness
   c. Four times normal thickness
   d. Five times normal thickness

2. Asthma is associated with which of the following?
   1. Increase in goblet cells
   2. Damage to cilia and reduced mucous clearance
   3. Increase in bronchial gland size
   4. Decrease in eosinophils
      a. 1 and 3 only
      b. 2 and 4 only
      c. 1, 2, and 3 only
      d. 2, 3, and 4 only

3. Which of the following have gained a widespread acceptance for assessing and monitoring a patient's airflow limitation?
   1. PEFR
   2. $FEF_{200-1200}$
   3. FEV_1
   4. FEV_1/FVC ratio
      a. 1 and 3 only
      b. 2 and 4 only
      c. 1, 3, and 4 only
      d. 2, 3, and 4 only

4. A patient clinical history presents the following: Daytime asthma symptoms more than two per week, no limitation in activities, no nocturnal symptoms or awakening, the need for reliever/rescue medications once per week, and a normal PEFR and FEV_1. Which of the following would best classify this patient's level of asthma control?
   a. Controlled
   b. Partly controlled
   c. Uncontrolled
   d. Severe exacerbation

5. Which of the following can be used to help confirm the diagnosis of asthma?
   1. Exercise challenge
   2. Response to inhaled mannitol
   3. Response to inhaled histamine
   4. Response to inhaled methacholine
      a. 1 and 3 only
      b. 2 and 4 only
      c. 2, 3, and 4 only
      d. 1, 2, 3, and 4

6. When pulsus paradoxus appears during an asthma attack:
   1. Left ventricle filling decreases during inspiration
   2. Cardiac output increases during expiration
   3. Left ventricle filling increases during expiration
   4. Cardiac output increases during inspiration
      a. 1 only
      b. 2 only
      c. 3 and 4 only
      d. 1 and 2 only

7. During an asthma episode, which of the following abnormal lung volume and capacity findings are found?
   1. Increased FRC
   2. Decreased ERV
   3. Increased VC
   4. Decreased RV
      a. 1 only
      b. 2 only
      c. 1 and 2 only
      d. 3 and 4 only

8. Which of the following chest assessment findings is/are commonly found during an asthma episode?
   1. Loud heart sounds
   2. Hyperresonant percussion note
   3. Expiratory prolongation
   4. Increased tactile and vocal fremitus
      a. 2 and 3 only
      b. 1 and 4 only
      c. 1, 2, and 4 only
      d. 1, 2, 3, and 4

9. Patients commonly exhibit which of the following arterial blood gas values early during an acute mild to moderate asthma episode?
   1. Increased pH
   2. Increased $PaCO_2$
   3. Decreased HCO_3^-
   4. Decreased PaO_2
      a. 1 and 3 only
      b. 2 and 4 only
      c. 1, 2, and 3 only
      d. 1, 3, and 4 only

10. How long must asthma be controlled before the treatment regimen can be stepped down, with the aim of establishing the lowest step and dose of treatment that maintains control?
    a. At least 2 weeks
    b. At least 1 month
    c. At least 2 months
    d. At least 3 months

CHAPTER
15 | Cystic Fibrosis

Chapter Objectives

After reading this chapter, you will be able to:

- Describe the anatomic alterations of the lungs associated with cystic fibrosis.
- Describe the etiology and epidemiology of cystic fibrosis.
- Describe how the cystic fibrosis gene is inherited.
- Discuss the screening and diagnosis of cystic fibrosis.
- Discuss the cardiopulmonary clinical manifestations associated with cystic fibrosis.
- Describe the general management of cystic fibrosis.
- Describe the clinical strategies and rationales of the SOAPs presented in the case study.
- Define key terms, and complete self-assessment questions at the end of the chapter and on Evolve.

Key Terms

Amniocentesis
Conductance Defect
Cystic Fibrosis Transmembrane Conductance Regulator (CFTR)
Electrical Potential Difference
Fecal fat test
Gating Defect
Genetic Counseling
Genetic Test
Immunoreactive Trypsin Test (IRT)
Inhaled dNASE
Inhaled Tobramycin
Ivacaftor

Lung or Heart-Lung Transplantation
Meconium Ileus
Nasal Potential Difference (NPD)
Pilocarpine
Standard Mendelian Pattern
Sweat Chloride
Sweat Test

Chapter Outline

Anatomic Alterations of the Lungs
Etiology and Epidemiology
    How the Cystic Fibrosis Gene Is Inherited
    Screening and Diagnosis
    Newborn Screening
    Sweat Test
    Molecular Diagnosis (Genetic Testing)
    Nasal Potential Difference
    Prenatal Testing
    Stool Fecal Fat Test
Overview of the Cardiopulmonary Clinical Manifestations Associated With Cystic Fibrosis
General Management of Cystic Fibrosis
    Respiratory Care Treatment Protocols
    Other Medications and Special Procedures Prescribed by the Physician
Lung or Heart-Lung Transplantation
Case Study: Cystic Fibrosis
Self-Assessment Questions

Anatomic Alterations of the Lungs[1]

Although the lungs of patients with cystic fibrosis (CF) appear normal at birth, abnormal structural changes can develop quickly. Initially, the patient has bronchial gland hypertrophy and metaplasia of goblet cells. This condition leads to the excessive production and accumulation of thick, tenacious mucus in the tracheobronchial tree secondary to inadequate hydration of the periciliary fluid layer (sol layer). Because the mucus is thick and inflexible, impairment of the normal mucociliary clearing mechanism ensues and many small bronchi and bronchioles become partially or totally obstructed (mucous

plugging). Partial obstruction leads to overdistention of the alveoli, and complete obstruction leads to patchy areas of atelectasis and in some cases bronchiectasis (see Chapter 16, Bronchiectasis). The anatomic alterations of the lungs associated with CF may result in both restrictive and obstructive lung characteristics, but excessive bronchial secretions, bronchial obstruction, and hyperinflation of the lungs are the predominant features of CF in the advanced stages.

The abundance of stagnant mucus in the tracheobronchial tree also serves as an excellent culture medium for bacteria, particularly *Staphylococcus aureus, Haemophilus influenzae,* and *Pseudomonas aeruginosa.* Some gram-negative bacteria are also commonly associated with CF, such as *Stenotrophomonas maltophilia* and *Burkholderia cepacia* complex. The infection stimulates additional mucous production and further compromises the mucociliary transport system. This condition may lead to secondary bronchial smooth muscle constriction. Finally, as the disease progresses, the patient may develop signs

---

[1]Cystic fibrosis does not affect the lungs exclusively. It also affects the function of exocrine glands in other parts of the body. In addition to being characterized by abnormally viscid secretions in the lungs, the disease is clinically manifested by male impotence, pancreatic insufficiency and high chloride concentrations in the sweat.

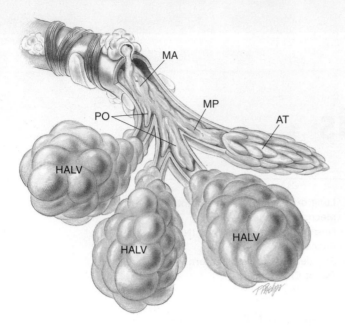

FIGURE 15.1 Cystic fibrosis. *AT,* Atelectasis; *HALV,* hyperinflation of alveoli; *MA,* mucus accumulation; *MP,* mucus plug; *PO,* partial obstruction of the airways.

and symptoms of recurrent pneumonia, chronic bronchitis (Chapter 13, Chronic Obstructive Pulmonary Disease, Chronic Bronchitis, and Emphysema), bronchiectasis (Chapter 16, Bronchiectasis), and lung abscesses (Chapter 18, Pneumonia, Lung Abscess Formation, and Important Fungal Diseases).

As illustrated in Fig. 15.1, the major respiratory pathologic or structural changes associated with CF are as follows:

- Excessive production and accumulation of thick, tenacious mucus in the tracheobronchial tree secondary to inadequate hydration of the periciliary fluid layer.
- Partial bronchial obstruction (mucus plugging)
- Hyperinflation of the alveoli
- Total bronchial obstruction (mucus plugging)
- Atelectasis
- Bronchiectasis (see Chapter 16)

Etiology and Epidemiology

CF is the most common fatal inherited disorder in childhood. CF is an autosomal recessive gene disorder caused by mutations in a pair of genes located on chromosome 7. Under normal conditions, every cell in the body (except the sex cells) has 46 chromosomes—23 pairs (half inherited from the father and the other half from the mother). More than 1700 different mutations in the gene that encodes for the **cystic fibrosis transmembrane conductance regulator (CFTR)** have been described.

The most common genetic defect linked to CF involves the absence of three base pairs in codon 508 (ΔF508) that codes for phenylalanine on chromosome 7 (band q31.2). Because of the loss of these three base pairs, the CFTR protein becomes dysfunctional. This defect accounts for 70% to 75% of the patients with CF tested.

The abnormal expression of the CFTR results in abnormal transport of sodium and chloride ions across many types of epithelial surfaces, including those lining the bronchial airways, intestines, pancreas, liver ducts, and sweat glands (Fig. 15.2). As a result, thick, viscous mucus accumulates in the lungs, and mucus blocks the passageways of the pancreas, preventing enzymes from the pancreas from reaching the intestines.

As shown in Fig. 15.3, six classes of CFTR mutations have been identified. These six different mutations can further be divided into three broad categories affecting either the quantity or function of the CFTR protein. For example, classes I and II can be placed in the "little or no functional CFTR category." Classes III and IV represent the "function of CFTR at the cell surface is affected category." The "reduced quantity of functional CFTR protein category" comprises classes V and VI.

The CFTR mutations are also classified as either a **gating defect** (e.g., class III) in which the channel does not open or a **conductance defect** (e.g., class IV) in which the channel is open but chloride does not move efficiently. Note that with class I mutations, the gene contains a stop signal that prevents CFTR protein from being made. With class II mutations, there is a defect in the CFTR protein processing, and CFTR never reaches the cell membrane. With class III mutations, CFTR protein is made and reaches the cell's surface but is unable to move out of the cell (gating defect). With class IV, the mutations reduce the passage of chloride ions through the channel opening. Class V CFTR is normal but produced in smaller than normal quantities. Class VI mutations are characterized by accelerated turnover.

How the Cystic Fibrosis Gene Is Inherited

Because CF is a recessive gene disorder, the child must inherit two copies of the defective CF gene—one from each parent (cystic fibrosis carriers)—to have the disease. Even though the carrier of the CF gene may be identified through genetic testing, the carrier (heterozygote) does not demonstrate evidence of the disease. However, if both parents carry the CF gene, the possibility of their children having CF (regardless of gender) follows the **standard Mendelian pattern**: there is a 25% chance that each child will have CF, a 25% chance that each child will be completely normal (and not carry the gene), and a 50% chance that each child will be a carrier. Thus when both patients carry a CF gene mutation, there is a one in four chance that the child will have CF (Fig. 15.4). It is estimated that more than 10 million Americans are unknowing, symptomless carriers of a mutant CF gene.

According to the Cystic Fibrosis Foundation, CF affects about 30,000 children and adults in the United States and about 70,000 worldwide. About 1000 new cases of CF are diagnosed each year in the United States. More than 90% of the patients are diagnosed by newborn screening. More than 50% of the patient population with CF are age 18 years or older. The median age of survival for individuals with CF is in the late 30s, but many patients with CF live into their 40s and beyond.[2] CF occurs most often in Caucasians (1:3000). The occurrence in Hispanics is 1:9200, Native Americans

[2]CF Foundation (http://www.cff.org).

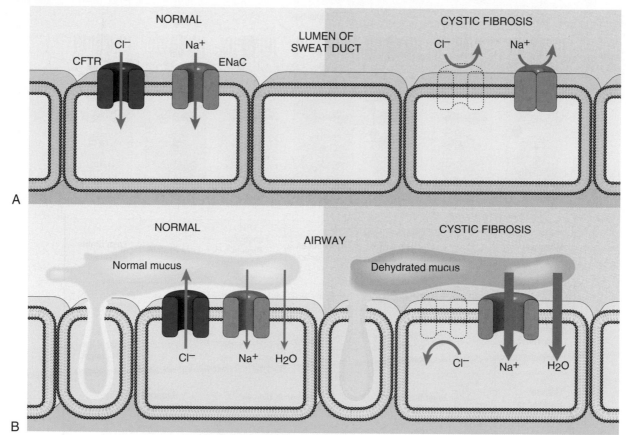

FIGURE 15.2 Abnormalities in the CFTR protein prevent chloride flux in the airway epithelium, resulting in abnormal reabsorption of water creating thick mucus and inadequate mucociliary function. (A) Chloride channel defect in the sweat duct causes increased chloride and sodium concentration in sweat. (B) In the airway, patients with cystic fibrosis have decreased chloride secretion and increased sodium and water reabsorption, leading to dehydration of the mucous layer coating epithelial cells, defective mucociliary action, and mucous plugging of the airways. *CFTR*, Cystic fibrosis transmembrane conductance regulator; *ENaC*, epithelial sodium channel. (Modified from Kumar, V., Abbas, A. K., & Aster, J. C. [2015]. *Robbins and Cotran pathologic basis of disease* [9th ed.]. Philadelphia, PA: Elsevier.)

1:10,900, African-Americans 1:15,000, and Asian-Americans 1:30,000. Death is usually caused by pulmonary complications.

Screening and Diagnosis

The diagnosis of CF is based on the clinical manifestations associated with CF, family history of CF, and laboratory findings.

The following two criteria must be met to diagnose CF:
1. Clinical symptoms consistent with CF in at least one organ system—for example, pulmonary system, sinus disease, pancreatic disease, meconium ileus, biliary disease, and male infertility. Box 15.1 provides common clinical indicators that justify evaluation for CF. A useful mnemonic, "CF PANCREAS" is seen in Box 15.2.
2. Clinical evidence of cystic fibrosis *transmembrane conductance regulator* (CFTR) dysfunction—any of the following:
   - Elevated **sweat chloride** greater than 60 mEq/L (on two occasions)
   - Molecular diagnosis (genetic testing). Presence of two disease-causing mutations in CFTR
   - Abnormal **nasal potential difference**

Newborn Screening

Newborn screening for CF has been a part of the newborn genetic testing protocol in all 50 states since 2011. Most infants with CF have an elevated blood level of immunoreactive trypsin (also called *trypsin-like immunoreactivity* and *serum trypsin*), which can be measured by radioimmunoassay or by an enzyme-linked immunoassay. The **immunoreactive trypsin level (IRT)** is measured from the blood dots collected on all newborn infants on the Guthrie cards.

The CF screening protocol varies among states and will identify more than 90% of infants with CF. The most common protocol is to perform DNA screening for 32 to 85 of the most common CF mutations on 2% to 5% of the samples with the highest IRT levels. Detection of at least one CF mutation is considered a positive screen and is referred to a CF center in most states for further testing.

The diagnosis of CF is established by a positive sweat test and/or genetic analysis for CF mutations. A negative or normal sweat test identifies the newborn as a CF carrier. All families of infants identified through newborn screening programs should receive genetic counseling. These newborn screening programs now identify 95% of infants with CF. It should be remembered that it is always appropriate to sweat test an individual of any age with symptoms consistent with the possible diagnosis of CF.

Sweat Test

The **sweat test** (sometimes called the **sweat chloride test**) is the gold standard diagnostic test for CF. The sweat test

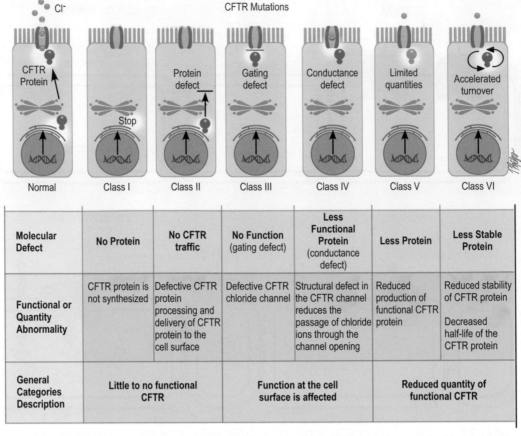

Molecular Defect	No Protein	No CFTR traffic	No Function (gating defect)	Less Functional Protein (conductance defect)	Less Protein	Less Stable Protein
Functional or Quantity Abnormality	CFTR protein is not synthesized	Defective CFTR protein processing and delivery of CFTR protein to the cell surface	Defective CFTR chloride channel	Structural defect in the CFTR channel reduces the passage of chloride ions through the channel opening	Reduced production of functional CFTR protein	Reduced stability of CFTR protein Decreased half-life of the CFTR protein
General Categories Description	Little to no functional CFTR		Function at the cell surface is affected		Reduced quantity of functional CFTR	

FIGURE 15.3 CFTR mutation classifications: A basis for categorizing CFTR mutations. Note: The red ballloon-like icon above represents the CFTR protein.

BOX 15.1 Clinical Indicators Justifying the Initial Evaluation for Cystic Fibrosis

Pulmonary
- Wheezing
- Chronic cough
- Sputum production
- Frequent respiratory infections (*Staphylococcus aureus, Pseudomonas aeruginosa, Haemophilus influenzae*)
- Abnormal chest radiograph and/or computed tomography scan
- Nasal polyps
- Parasinusitis
- Digital clubbing

Gastrointestinal Disorders
- Failure to thrive
- Foul-smelling, greasy stools
- Voracious appetite
- Milk and formula intolerance
- Rectal prolapse

- Meconium ileus
- Meconium peritonitis
- Distal intestinal obstruction syndrome
- Pancreatic insufficiency
- Pancreatitis
- Hepatobiliary disfunction
- Hepatomegaly
- Focal biliary cirrhosis
- Prolonged neonatal jaundice
- Cholelithiasis

Nutritional Deficits
- Fat-soluble vitamin deficiency (vitamins A, D, E, K)
- Hypoproteinemia
- Hypochloremia (metabolic alkalosis)

Infertility (Male)
- Obstructive azoospermia

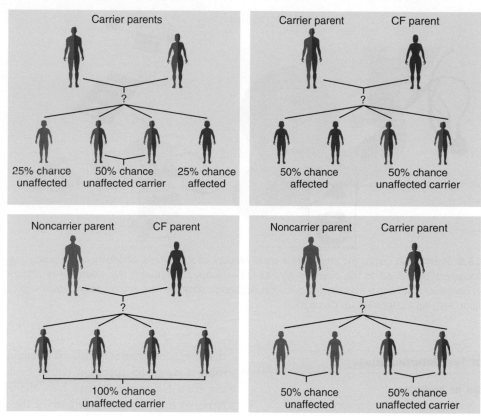

FIGURE 15.4 Standard Mendelian pattern of inheritance of cystic fibrosis.

<table>
<tr><td colspan="2">BOX 15.2 CF Pancreas Mnemonic</td></tr>
<tr><td>C</td><td>Chronic respiratory disease</td></tr>
<tr><td>F</td><td>Failure to thrive</td></tr>
<tr><td>P</td><td>Polyps</td></tr>
<tr><td>A</td><td>Alkalosis, metabolic</td></tr>
<tr><td>N</td><td>Neonatal intestinal obstruction</td></tr>
<tr><td>C</td><td>Clubbing of fingers</td></tr>
<tr><td>R</td><td>Rectal prolapse</td></tr>
<tr><td>E</td><td>Electrolyte increase in sweat</td></tr>
<tr><td>A</td><td>Aspermia/absent vas deferens</td></tr>
<tr><td>S</td><td>Sputum: Staphylococcus aureus, Pseudomonas aeruginosis</td></tr>
</table>

is a reliable test for the identification of about 98% of patients with CF. This test measures the amount of sodium and chloride in the patient's sweat. During the procedure a small amount of a colorless, odorless sweat-producing chemical called **pilocarpine** is applied to the patient's arm or leg—usually the forearm. An electrode is attached to the chemically prepared area, and a mild electric current is applied to stimulate sweat production (Fig. 15.5). The test is usually done twice.

Although the sweat glands of patients with CF are microscopically normal, the glands secrete up to four times the normal amount of sodium and chloride. The actual volume of sweat, however, is no greater than that produced by a normal individual. In both infants and adults, a sweat chloride concentration greater than 60 mEq/L is considered

to be a diagnostic sign of CF. Box 15.3 provides an overview for sweat test interpretations for infants 6 months or younger and infants older than 6 months, children, and adults.

All patients with the following characteristics should undergo a sweat test to help confirm the diagnosis of CF:

- Infants with positive CF newborn screening results (performed after 2 weeks of age and greater than 2 kg if asymptomatic)
- Infants with symptoms suggestive of CF (see Box 15.1)
- Older siblings (including adults) with symptoms suggestive of CF
- Members of the patient's family with confirmed CF

Molecular Diagnosis (Genetic Testing)

With a sample of the patient's blood or cheek cells, a **genetic test** (also called a *genotype test, gene mutation test,* or *mutation analysis*) can be performed to analyze deoxyribonucleic acid (DNA) for the presence of CFTR gene mutations. Intermediate results of sweat chloride testing should be further investigated with a DNA analysis using the *CFTR multimutation method.* The sweat chloride test should also be repeated.

Most of the diagnostic laboratories in the United States are able to screen for at least 30 to 100 of the most common mutations, including gene mutation Delta F508 (ΔF508), which is the most common gene mutation associated with CF. When two CF gene mutations are detected, and the sweat test is intermediate or positive, the diagnosis of CF is confirmed. Although genetic testing for CF is considered a valuable diagnostic tool, it does have its limitations. For example, some

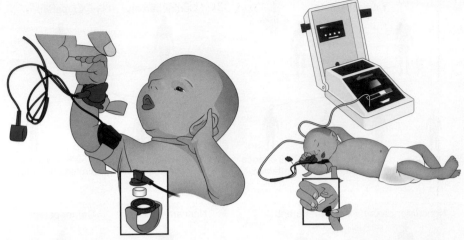

FIGURE 15.5 Sweat test. During the procedure a small amount of a colorless, odorless, sweat-producing chemical called *pilocarpine* is applied to the patient's arm or leg—usually the forearm. An electrode is attached to the chemically prepared area, and a mild electric current is applied to stimulate sweat production. (Used with permission from Wescor, Inc., an ELITech Group Company.)

BOX 15.3 Sweat Test Interpretations

Infants 6 Months or Younger
- ≤29 mmol/L: Normal (cystic fibrosis very unlikely)
- 30 to 59 mmol/L: Intermediate (possible cystic fibrosis)
- ≥60 mmol/L: Abnormal (diagnosis of cystic fibrosis)

Infants Older Than 6 Months, Children, and Adults
- ≤39 mmol/L: Normal (cystic fibrosis very unlikely)
- 40 to 59 mmol/L: Intermediate (possible cystic fibrosis)
- >60 mmol/L: Abnormal (diagnosis of cystic fibrosis)

---

individuals have CFTR mutations but demonstrate no typical clinical manifestations of CF. In addition, some patients may have CFTR mutations, but the mutations cannot be identified without special gene analysis methods. It is estimated that genetic testing can confirm CF in about 90% to 96% of the patients tested.

Nasal Potential Difference

The impaired transport of sodium (Na^+) and chloride (Cl^-) across the epithelial cells lining the airways of the patient with CF can be measured. As the Na^+ and Cl^- ions move across the epithelial cell membrane they generate what is called an **electrical potential difference**—the amount of energy required to move an electrical charge from one point to another. In the nasal passages this electrical potential difference is called the **nasal potential difference (NPD)**. The NPD can be measured with a surface electrode over the nasal epithelial cells lining the inferior turbinate. An increased (i.e., more negative) NPD strongly suggests CF. The NPD is recommended for patients with clinical features of CF who have borderline or normal sweat test values and nondiagnostic CF genotyping.

Prenatal Testing

Both the American College of Obstetrics and Gynecology and the American College of Medical Genetics recommend that pregnant females be offered screening for CF mutations using a 32 to 85 mutation panel. Females who test positive for a CF mutation then have the option of having the father of the fetus tested. If both of the parents test positive for a CF mutation, the fetus has a one in four chance of having CF.

If desired, the fetus can be tested for CF by **amniocentesis** after the first trimester. The amniotic fluid is obtained by ultrasound-guided needle aspiration of amniotic fluid from around the fetus. Fetal cells are tested for the presence of CF mutations and identified as CF affected, CF carrier, or normal. Because most genetic screening only tests for 32 to 85 of more than 2400 mutations associated with CF, a negative or normal result does not entirely rule out the possibility of the person carrying one of the less common CF mutations. Infants have been born with CF when both parents have been normal by genetic screening.

Genetic counseling is very important in all cases of prenatal testing for CF to explain this uncertainty or residual risk to prospective parents. Amniocentesis and genetic analysis of fetal cells can be used to diagnose a large number of genetic disorders and chromosomal abnormalities in the fetus.

Stool Fecal Fat Test

The stool **fecal fat test** measures the amount of fat in the infant's stool and the percentage of dietary fat that is not absorbed by the body. The test is used to evaluate how the liver, gallbladder, pancreas, and intestines are functioning. Fat absorption requires bile from the gallbladder, enzymes from the pancreas, and normal intestines. An elevated stool fecal fat value (i.e., decreased fat absorption) is associated with a variety of disorders, including CF. Fecal elastance is an easier test of pancreatic function because it requires only a small stool sample for analysis. Infants with CF and pancreatic insufficiency will have a fecal elastance of less than 50 μg/g of stool (normal is greater than 300 μg/g of stool).

The following clinical manifestations result from the pathophysiologic mechanisms caused (or activated) by atelectasis (see Fig. 10.7), bronchospasm (see Fig. 10.11), and excessive bronchial secretions (see Fig. 10.11)—the major anatomic alterations of the lungs associated with CF (see Fig. 15.1).

CLINICAL DATA OBTAINED AT THE PATIENT'S BEDSIDE

The Physical Examination

Vital Signs

Increased Respiratory Rate (Tachypnea)

Several pathophysiologic mechanisms operating simultaneously may lead to an increased ventilatory rate:

- Stimulation of peripheral chemoreceptors (hypoxemia)
- Decreased lung compliance–increased ventilatory rate relationship
- Anxiety
- Increased temperature

Increased Heart Rate (Pulse) and Blood Pressure
Use of Accessory Muscles During Inspiration
Use of Accessory Muscles During Expiration
Pursed-Lip Breathing
Increased Anteroposterior Chest Diameter (Barrel Chest)
Cyanosis
Digital Clubbing
Peripheral Edema and Venous Distention

Because polycythemia and cor pulmonale are associated with severe cystic fibrosis, the following may be seen:

- Distended neck veins
- Pitting edema
- Enlarged and tender liver

Cough, Sputum Production, and Hemoptysis
Chest Assessment Findings

- Decreased or increased tactile and vocal fremitus
- Hyperresonant percussion note
- Diminished breath sounds
- Diminished heart sounds
- Bronchial breath sounds (over atelectasis)
- Crackles
- Wheezes

Spontaneous Pneumothorax

Spontaneous pneumothorax is commonly seen in patients with CF. The incidence is greater than 20% in adults with CF. When a patient with CF has a pneumothorax, there is about a 50% chance that it will recur. The respiratory therapist must be alert for the signs and symptoms of this complication (e.g., pleuritic pain, shoulder pain, sudden shortness of breath). Precipitating factors include advanced lung disease, excessive exertion, high altitude, and positive-pressure breathing (see Chapter 23, Pneumothorax).

CLINICAL DATA OBTAINED FROM LABORATORY TESTS AND SPECIAL PROCEDURES

Pulmonary Function Test Findings
Moderate to Severe Cystic Fibrosis (Obstructive Lung Pathophysiology)[1]

FORCED EXPIRATORY VOLUME AND FLOW RATE FINDINGS

FVC	FEV_T	FEV_1/FVC ratio	$FEF_{25\%-75\%}$
↓	↓	↓	↓

$FEF_{50\%}$	$FEF_{200-1200}$	PEFR	MVV
↓	↓	↓	↓

LUNG VOLUME AND CAPACITY FINDINGS

V_T	IRV	ERV	RV
N or ↑	N or ↓	N or ↓	↑

VC	IC	FRC	TLC	RV/TLC ratio
↓	N or ↓	↑	N or ↑	N or ↑

Arterial Blood Gases

MILD TO MODERATE STAGES OF CYSTIC FIBROSIS
Acute Alveolar Hyperventilation With Hypoxemia[2] (Acute Respiratory Alkalosis)

pH	$PaCO_2$	HCO_3^-	PaO_2	SaO_2 or SpO_2
↑	↓	↓ (but normal)	↓	↓

SEVERE STAGE OF CYSTIC FIBROSIS
Chronic Ventilatory Failure With Hypoxemia[3] (Compensated Respiratory Acidosis)

pH	$PaCO_2$	HCO_3^-	PaO_2	SaO_2 or SpO_2
N	↑	↑ (significantly)	↓	↓

Metabolic Alkalosis

In rare cases, hypokalemia and secondary metabolic alkalosis are known complications of CF, especially during warm weather and exercise. Because of the dysfunctional CFTR in the sweat ducts of patients with CF, there can be excessive losses of chloride and sodium. The hypokalemia seen with heat stress is secondary to sweat as well as potassium wasting. The metabolic alkalosis is maintained by the excessive sweat sodium

---

[1]CF is primarily an obstructive lung disorder. However, when extensive total lung obstruction (from mucus plugging) and atelectasis are present throughout the lungs, restrictive pulmonary function testing values will likely appear.
[2]See Fig. 5.2 and Table 5.4 and related discussion for the acute pH, $PaCO_2$, and changes associated with acute alveolar hyperventilation.
[3]See Table 5.6 and discussion for the pH, and related discussion for the pH, $PaCO_2$, and changes associated with chronic ventilatory failure.

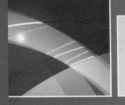

chloride loses, which leads to extracellular fluid (ECF) volume contraction and chloride depletion. Thus the metabolic alkalosis seen in some patients with CF is most likely secondary to hypokalemia with ECF volume contraction.

Acute Ventilatory Changes Superimposed on Chronic Ventilatory Failure[4]

Because acute ventilatory changes are frequently seen in patients with chronic ventilatory failure, the respiratory therapist must be familiar with and alert for the following two dangerous arterial blood gas (ABG) findings:

- Acute alveolar hyperventilation superimposed on chronic ventilatory failure, which should further alert the respiratory therapist to record the following important ABG assessment: possible *impending acute ventilatory failure*
- Acute ventilatory failure (acute hypoventilation) superimposed on chronic ventilatory failure

Oxygenation Indices[5]
Moderate to Severe Stages

$\dot{Q}_S/\dot{Q}_T$	DO_2[6]	$\dot{V}O_2$	$C(a\text{-}\bar{v})O_2$	O_2ER	$S\bar{v}O_2$
↑	↓	N	N	↑	↓

Hemodynamic Indices[7]
Moderate to Severe Stages

CVP	RAP	$\overline{PA}$	PCWP	CO	SV
↑	↑	↑	N	N	N
SVI	CI	RVSWI	LVSWI	PVR	SVR
N	N	↑	N	↑	N

ABNORMAL LABORATORY TESTS AND PROCEDURES
Hematology
- Increased hematocrit and hemoglobin
- Increased white blood cell count

[4]See Table 5.7, Table 5.8, and Table 5.9 and related discussion for the pH, PaCO₂, and changes associated with acute ventilatory changes superimposed on chronic ventilatory failure.
[5]$C(a\text{-}\bar{v})O_2$, Arterial-venous oxygen difference; DO_2, total oxygen delivery; O_2ER, oxygen extraction ratio; $\dot{Q}_S/\dot{Q}_T$, pulmonary shunt fraction; $S\bar{v}O_2$, mixed venous oxygen saturation; $\dot{V}O_2$, oxygen consumption.
[6]The DO₂ may be normal in patients who have compensated to the decreased oxygenation status with an increased cardiac output, an increased hemoglobin level, or a combination of both. When the DO₂ is normal, the O₂ER is usually normal.
[7]CI, Cardiac index; CO, cardiac output; CVP, central venous pressure; LVSWI, left ventricular stroke work index; PCWP, pulmonary capillary wedge pressure; PVR, pulmonary vascular resistance; RAP, right atrial pressure; RVSWI, right ventricular stroke work index; SV, stroke volume; SVI, stroke volume index; SVR, systemic vascular resistance.

Electrolytes
- Hypochloremia (chronic ventilatory failure)
- Increased serum bicarbonate (chronic ventilatory failure)

Sputum Examination
- Increased white blood cells
- Gram-positive bacteria
  - *Staphylococcus aureus*
  - *Haemophilus influenzae*
- Gram-negative bacteria
  - *Pseudomonas aeruginosa*
  - *Stenotrophomonas maltophilia*
  - *Burkholderia cepacia* complex

RADIOLOGIC FINDINGS
Chest Radiograph
- Translucent (dark) lung fields
- Depressed or flattened diaphragms
- Right ventricular enlargement (cor pulmonale)
- Areas of atelectasis and fibrosis
- Tram tracks
- Bronchiectasis (often a secondary complication)
- Pneumothorax (spontaneous)
- Abscess formation (occasionally)

During the late stages of CF the alveoli become hyperinflated, which causes the residual volume and functional residual capacity to increase. Because this condition decreases the density of the lungs and thereby reduces the resistance to x-ray penetration, the chest radiograph appears darker. Tram-track opacities (also called *tram lines*) may be seen on chest x-rays. Tram tracks are parallel or curved opacity lines of varying length caused by bronchial wall thickening. As the patient's residual volume and functional residual capacity increase, the diaphragm moves downward and appears flattened or depressed on the radiograph (Fig. 15.6).

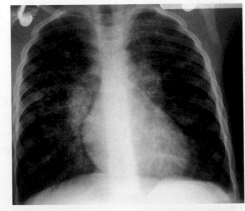

FIGURE 15.6 Chest x-ray of a patient with cystic fibrosis. Note the lung overinflation, the diffuse infiltrates, and the large main pulmonary artery segment, reflecting pulmonary hypertension.

Fig. 15.7 presents four serial chest radiographs of the progression of CF over 26 years. Because right ventricular enlargement and failure often develop as secondary problems during the advanced stages of CF, an enlarged heart may be identified on the radiograph. In some patients, areas of atelectasis, abscess formation, or a pneumothorax may be seen. Finally, computed tomography (CT) and positron emission tomography (PET) scans may be helpful when borderline radiographic findings are present.

COMMON NONRESPIRATORY CLINICAL MANIFESTATIONS

Meconium Ileus

Meconium ileus is an obstruction of the small intestine of the newborn that is caused by the impaction of thick, dry, tenacious meconium, usually at or near the ileocecal valve. This results from a deficiency in pancreatic enzymes and is the earliest manifestation of CF. The disease is suspected in newborns who demonstrate abdominal distention and fail to pass meconium within 12 hours after birth. Meconium ileus may occur in as many as 25% of infants with CF.

Distal Intestinal Obstruction Syndrome

Distal intestinal obstruction syndrome (DIOS) (previously known as *meconium ileus equivalent*) is an intestinal obstruction (similar to meconium ileus in neonates) that occurs in older children and young adults with CF.

Malnutrition and Poor Body Development

In CF, the pancreatic ducts become plugged with mucus, which leads to fibrosis of the pancreas. The pancreatic insufficiency that ensues inhibits the digestion of protein and fat. This condition leads to a deficiency of vitamins A, D, E, and K. Vitamin K deficiency may be the cause of easy bruising and bleeding. About 80% of all patients with CF have vitamin deficiencies and therefore show signs of malnutrition and poor body development throughout life.

NASAL POLYPS AND SINUSITIS

Nasal polyps are seen in between 10% and 30% of patients with CF. The polyps are usually multiple and may cause nasal obstruction; in some cases, they cause distortion of the normal facial features. Between 90% and 100% of patients with CF have sinusitis.

INFERTILITY

About 99% of men with CF are infertile. Women with CF who become pregnant may not be able to carry the infant to term. An infant who is carried to term will either have CF or be a carrier (see Fig. 15.2).

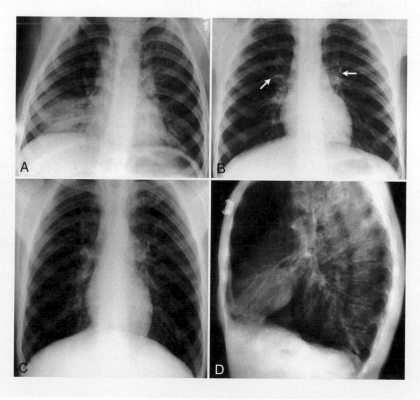

FIGURE 15.7 Cystic fibrosis. Serial chest imaging over a 26-year period showing the progressive changes of cystic fibrosis. (A) At 3 years of age, the patient had right middle lobe pneumonia. (B) Mild hyperinflation and bronchial wall thickening (arrow) manifested at age 7 years. (C) At age 15 years, the patient demonstrated progressive hyperinflation, bronchiectasis, and enlargement of the hila on the chest radiograph. (D) Lateral chest radiograph at 29 years shows typical findings of end-stage cystic fibrosis. Note marked hyperinflation and "barrel chest" deformity, severe bronchiectasis, and tubular opacities consistent with mucous plugs. (From Hansell, D. M., Lynch, D. A., McAdams, H. P., et al. [2010]. *Imaging of diseases of the chest* [5th ed.]. Philadelphia, PA: Elsevier.)

General Management of Cystic Fibrosis

The management of CF entails an interdisciplinary approach. The primary goals are to prevent pulmonary infections, reduce the amount of thick bronchial secretions, improve airflow, and provide adequate nutrition. The patient and the patient's family should be instructed regarding the disease and the way it affects bodily functions. They should be taught home care therapies, the goals of these therapies, and the way to administer medications. Patients with CF commonly are best managed by a pulmonary rehabilitation team. Such teams include a respiratory therapist, a physical therapist, a respiratory nurse specialist, an occupational therapist, a dietitian, a social worker, and a psychologist. A pediatric or adult, pulmonologist, or an internist trained in CF care and respiratory rehabilitation outlines and orchestrates the patient's therapeutic program.

Patients with CF should have regular medical checkups for comparative purposes to determine their general health, weight, height, pulmonary function abilities, and sputum culture results. In addition, oral time-released pancreatic enzymes, such as pancreatic lipase, are prescribed for patients with CF to aid food digestion. Patients are also encouraged to replace body salts either by heavily salting their food or by taking sodium supplements. Supplemental multivitamins and minerals are also important.

Respiratory Care Treatment Protocols

Oxygen Therapy Protocol

Oxygen therapy is used to treat hypoxemia, decrease the work of breathing, and decrease myocardial work in patients with CF with advanced pulmonary disease or during acute exacerbations. The hypoxemia may not respond well to oxygen therapy when true or capillary pulmonary shunting is present (see Oxygen Therapy Protocol, Protocol 10.1).

Airway Clearance Therapy Protocol

Because of the excessive mucus production and accumulation associated with CF, a number of respiratory therapy modalities are used to enhance the mobilization of bronchial secretions. Aggressive and vigorous airway clearance therapy should be performed regularly on patients both while in the hospital and at home. Because many patients with CF require airway clearance therapy at least twice a day for 20 to 30 minutes, manual chest physiotherapy and postural drainage can be overwhelming for the caretaker. Several options for hospital or home care include use of a mechanical percussor with chest physiotherapy and postural drainage, use of a high-frequency chest compression vest, or use of intrapulmonary percussive ventilation to move thick bronchial secretions and improve compliance with prescribed care. Positive expiratory pressure (PEP) and flutter-valve therapy are also effective airway clearance techniques and also can be employed with deep breathing and coughing (Fig. 15.8) (see Airway Clearance Therapy Protocol, Protocol 10.2).

Lung Expansion Therapy Protocol

Lung expansion therapy may be administered to help offset the alveolar atelectasis associated with CF. Deep breathing

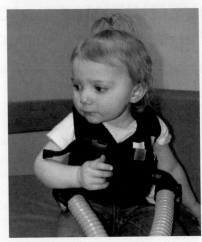

FIGURE 15.8 An 18-month-old female patient with cystic fibrosis wearing a high-frequency chest compression (HFCC) vest (the inCourage System). Today, HFCC is a commonly used bronchopulmonary hygiene treatment for airway clearance in patients with cystic fibrosis.

and effective cough are key to reversing consolidation caused by mucus plugging (see Lung Expansion Therapy Protocol, Protocol 10.3).

Aerosolized Medication Protocol

A variety of bronchodilators (both beta$_2$-adrenergic agonists and anticholinergic drugs) and mucolytic agents are commonly used to induce bronchial smooth muscle relaxation and mucous thinning.

- *Bronchodilators:* Inhaled bronchodilators are routinely administered to all patients with CF, especially during the following situations:
  - Immediately before the patient receives chest physiotherapy or exercise to help mobilize airway secretions.
  - Immediately before the patient receives inhalation of nebulized hypertonic saline, antibiotics and/or DNase (dornase alpha) to offset bronchial constriction that can occur with use of these agents and to help improve the penetration and distribution of the drugs throughout the airways.

Recommended bronchodilators include beta$_2$-adrenergic agonists such as the short-acting agent *albuterol* or long-acting agents such as *salmeterol* or *formoterol*. The anticholinergic agent *ipratropium bromide* and the longer acting *tiotropium* are also used to treat patients with CF.

- *Mucolytic agents*
  - **Inhaled DNase** (dornase alpha) (Pulmozyme) has been shown to be especially helpful in the management of patients with moderate to severe CF. This aerosolized agent is an enzyme that breaks down the DNA of the thick bronchial mucus associated with chronic bacterial infections with CF. Dornase alpha has shown good results in improving the lung function of patients with CF while reducing the frequency and severity of respiratory infections (Fig. 15.9).

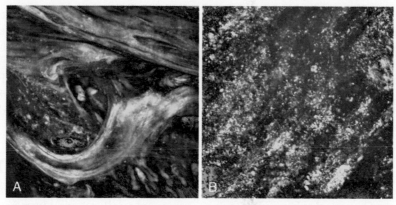

FIGURE 15.9 Dornase alpha (Pulmozyme). Illustration of the mode of action of dornase alpha in reducing DNA polymers in cystic fibrosis sputum. Confocal micrograph showing cystic fibrosis sputum stained (with YOYO-1) for DNA before (A) and after (B) treatment with dornase alpha in vitro. The long DNA polymers are degraded into short units after dornase treatment. (From Gardenhire, D. S. [2016]. *Rau's respiratory care pharmacology* [9th ed.]. St. Louis, MO: Elsevier.)

- Inhaled hypertonic saline may be administered to help hydrate thick mucus in the airways of patients with CF who are 6 years of age or older, have a chronic cough, and have a reduced FEV_1. A typical treatment regimen is, first, the administration of a bronchodilator (e.g., albuterol), followed by 4 mL of a 3% to 7% saline solution, twice a day.
- Inhaled *N*-acetylcysteine has not been clinically proved to be effective in treating patients with CF. In addition, because of its potential to cause airway inflammation and/or bronchospasm and inhibit ciliary function, along with its disagreeable odor and relatively high cost, its use is not recommended (see Protocol 10.4: Aerosolized Medication Protocol, and Appendix II on the Evolve site).

Mechanical Ventilation Protocol

Because acute ventilatory failure superimposed on chronic ventilatory failure is occasionally seen in patients with severe CF, mechanical ventilation may be required to maintain an adequate ventilatory status. Continuous mechanical ventilation is justified when the acute ventilatory failure is thought to be reversible—for example, when pneumonia complicates the condition. Noninvasive ventilation, such as bilevel positive-pressure ventilation by face mask, is generally preferred to intubation when feasible (see Ventilator Initiation and Management Protocol, Protocol 11.1, and Mechanical Ventilation Weaning Protocol, Protocol 11.2).

Other Medications and Special Procedures Prescribed by the Physician

CFTR Modulators

Much of the current research in CF is focused on correcting the cellular defects in CF. Small molecules (medications that work when taken by mouth) that can help CF-mutated cells function more normally are being studied to improve the ability to treat CF. These medications are designed to treat the underlying cellular defects in CF rather than secondary complications of CF, which have been the focus of medical therapy of CF for the past 50 years.

Correctors are drugs that help mutated CFTR reach the epithelial cell surface where the CFTR protein normally functions as a transmembrane regulator of chloride movement out of the cell and sodium transport into the cell. *Potentiators* are drugs that help mutated CFTR function more effectively at the epithelial cell surface transporting chloride out of the cell and inhibiting the movement of sodium into the cell. Correctors are often designed to work on a specific CF mutation or class of mutations (e.g., mutations that alter proper folding of the CFTR protein; ΔF508 is this type of mutation). Potentiators improve the function of mutated CFTR that has reached the epithelial cell surface (gating mutations; G551D is this type of mutation) and are somewhat less mutation specific.

Ivacaftor (Kalydeco) is a new oral potentiator molecule that has been proved effective to improve cell function and clinical status in patients with CF with the G551D mutation. It was approved by the US Food and Drug Administration (FDA) in 2013 for patients over 6 years of age with CF with the G551D mutation. Ivacaftor is the first drug developed that targets the underlying causes of CF, the faulty CF gene *G551D*, and its defective CFTR protein. Ivacaftor appears to be remarkably effective for this mutation, significantly reducing sweat test values and improving lung function and weight gain. Unfortunately, the *G551D* mutation occurs in only 3% to 5% of all patients with CF. All patients with CF should have CFTR genotyping performed to determine if they carry the *G551D* mutation and could benefit from this breakthrough drug. Ivacaftor has now been approved for several other gating mutations.

Lumacaftor/ivacaftor (Orkambi), for patients who are homozygous for delta F508, combines a corrector and potentiator and offers improvement in pulmonary function and pulmonary exacerbations.

Antibiotics

Antibiotics are commonly administered to prevent or combat chronic respiratory tract infections. Antibiotics are administered orally, via inhalation, or intravenously depending on the infecting organism and the severity of the exacerbation. For example, azithromycin is often recommended for patients 6 years and older who are infected with *P. aeruginosa* and have evidence of airway inflammation, such as a chronic cough or a reduction in FEV_1. Inhaled antibiotics widely used to treat *P. aeruginosa* in CF include **inhaled tobramycin** (Bethkis) and inhaled aztreonam. Several other inhaled antibiotics are under study for the treatment of *P. aeruginosa* in CF at this time, such as amikacin, colistin, ciprofloxacin, and levofloxacin.

Unfortunately, a major drawback of long-term use of antibiotics is the development of bacteria that become resistant to antibiotic therapy. Moreover, the long-term use of antibiotics may lead to fungal infections of the mouth, oral pharynx, and tracheobronchial tree (see Appendix II on the Evolve site).

Ibuprofen

High-dose *ibuprofen* is recommended in children and young adolescents with mild CF and who have good lung function (an FEV_1 less than 60% predicted) and no contradictions (e.g., gastrointestinal bleeding or renal impairment). Ibuprofen has been shown to reduce bronchial inflammation without hindering bacterial clearance, reducing the decline in the patient's FEV_1 per year, with no remarkable side effects except painless gastrointestinal bleeding in 1% to 2% of patients. High-dose ibuprofen is thought to work by decreasing neutrophil migration and inflammation in the lungs. The initiation of ibuprofen is not recommended after the age of 13 years. Only a small percentage of US children are being prescribed ibuprofen.

Inhaled Corticosteroids and Systemic Glucocorticoids

In patients with CF, but without airway reactivity or allergic bronchopulmonary aspergillosis, the administration of *inhaled corticosteroids* has not shown any clear benefits and therefore is *not* recommended. However, inhaled corticosteroids may be beneficial in patients with CF who demonstrate airway reactivity. *Systemic glucocorticoids* are *not* recommended in children and adolescents with CF. The benefits of systemic glucocorticoids are outweighed by the adverse effects on growth retardation, glucose metabolism, development of CF-related diabetes, and cataract risks.

Lung or Heart-Lung Transplantation

Several large organ transplant centers are currently performing lung or heart-lung transplantations in selected patients with CF whose general body condition is good. According to the Cystic Fibrosis Foundation, there has been a steady growth in the number of procedures performed annually since 2000, and 4122 adult lung transplants were reported in 2015.

The success of lung transplantation in patients with CF is as good as or better than in patients with other lung diseases (e.g., emphysema). More than 90% of patients with CF are alive 1 year after transplantation, and 80% are alive after 5 years. Lung transplantation does not change the recipient's CF abnormalities of the sinuses, trachea, pancreas, intestines, sweat glands, and reproductive glands. Patients with CF who receive normal lung transplants risk infecting their new lungs with "CF organisms" harbored in their sinuses and trachea. Immunosuppressive drugs required posttransplant may decrease the recipient's ability to fight infections caused by *P. aeruginosa* and *B. cepacia* complex. Many lung transplant centers will not accept CF patients who have *B. cepacia* because of demonstrated lower survival rates.[3]

---

[3]CF Foundation (http://www.cff.org).

Admitting History

A 27-year-old man has a long history of respiratory problems caused by CF. Even though his medical records are incomplete, he reported on admission that his parents told him that he had experienced several episodes of pneumonia during his early years. He is an adopted child and therefore does not know his biologic family history. His parents are actively involved in his general care, which entails the home care suggestions and therapeutic procedures presented by the pulmonary rehabilitation team. He takes supplemental multivitamins and timed-release oral pancreatic enzymes regularly, as prescribed by his doctor.

During his teens he had fewer respiratory symptoms than he has today and was able to lead a relatively normal life. During that time, he took up water-skiing and became proficient in the slalom event. He is known to most of his associates as a "wonder." Although he qualifies for disability income because of his continual shortness of breath, he is able to do various small jobs, which always relate to water-skiing. He is well known throughout the water-skiing circuit as an excellent chief judge at national and regional tournaments. In addition, he is a certified driver for jump-trick and slalom events and recently has become involved in selling water-ski tournament ropes and handles, which provides him with a small additional income.

Over the past 3 years, his cough has become more persistent and increasingly productive, with about a cupful of sputum noted daily. Over the same period, he has noted becoming short of breath when climbing stairs. Even though the man has a normal appetite, he has lost a great deal of weight over the past 2 years. On admission, he reported a history of severe shortness of breath. He denied experiencing any recent changes in bowel habits, despite his weight loss, but said that he has noticed a tendency to pass rather pale stools. Much to the chagrin of his doctor, 3 years ago he began smoking about 10 cigarettes a day, his reason being that the cigarettes "help him cough up the sputum."

Physical Examination

On examination the patient appeared pale, cyanotic, and thin. He had a barrel chest and was using his accessory muscles of respiration. Clubbing of the fingers was present. He demonstrated a frequent, productive cough. His sputum was sweet-smelling, thick, and yellow-green. His neck veins were distended, and he showed mild to moderate peripheral edema. He stated that he had not been this short of breath in a long time.

He had a blood pressure of 142/90, heart rate of 108 beats/min, and respiratory rate of 28 breaths/min. He was afebrile. Palpation of the chest was unremarkable. Expiration was prolonged. Hyperresonant notes were elicited bilaterally during percussion. Auscultation revealed diminished breath sounds and heart sounds. Coarse crackles were heard throughout both lung fields. During his last medical checkup (about 10 months before this admission) a pulmonary function test (PFT) was conducted. Results revealed moderate to severe airway obstruction. Blood gases were not analyzed.

His chest x-ray examination on this admission revealed hyperlucent lung fields, depressed hemidiaphragms, and mild cardiac enlargement (Fig. 15.10). His hemoglobin level was 18 g%. His ABGs on 1.5 L/min oxygen by nasal cannula were pH 7.51, $PaCO_2$ 58 mm Hg, HCO_3^- 43 mEq/L, PaO_2 66 mm Hg, and SaO_2 94%. On the basis of these clinical data, the following SOAP was documented.

Respiratory Assessment and Plan

S "I've not been this short of breath in a long time."

O Known CF patient. Skin: Pale, cyanotic; barrel chest, and use of accessory muscles of respiration; digital clubbing; cough frequent and productive; sputum: sweet-smelling, thick, yellow-green; distended neck veins and peripheral edema; vital signs: BP 142/90, HR 108, RR 28, T° normal; bilateral hyperresonant percussion notes; diminished breath sounds; coarse crackles;

   CXR: Hyperlucency, flattened diaphragms, and mild cardiac enlargement; ABGs (1.5 L/min O_2 by nasal cannula): pH 7.51, $PaCO_2$ 58, HCO_3^- 43, PaO_2 66; and SaO_2 94%.

A • Respiratory distress (general appearance, vital signs)
   • Excessive tracheobronchial tree secretions (productive cough, coarse crackles)
   • Infection likely (yellow-green sputum)
   • Hyperinflated alveoli (barrel chest, use of accessory muscles, CXR)
   • Acute alveolar hyperventilation superimposed on chronic ventilatory failure with mild hypoxia (history, ABGs)
     • Possible impending acute ventilatory failure
   • Cor pulmonale (distended neck veins, peripheral edema, CXR)

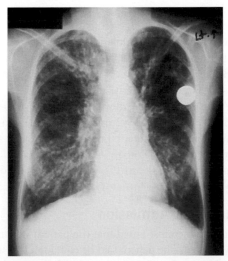

FIGURE 15.10 Chest x-ray film from a 27-year-old man with cystic fibrosis.

P Airway Clearance Therapy Protocol (cough and deep breathe Tx q4 h), sputum culture). Oxygen Therapy Protocol (2 L/min by nasal cannula). Monitor possible impending ventilatory failure closely (pulse oximetry, vital signs, ABGs).

Forty-Eight Hours After Admission

The respiratory therapist from the consult service noted that the patient was still in respiratory distress. The man stated that he could not get enough air to sleep even 10 minutes. He appeared cyanotic and was using his accessory muscles of respiration. His vital signs were blood pressure 147/95, heart rate 117 beats/min, respiratory rate 32 breaths/min, and temperature 37°C (98.6°F).

He coughed frequently, and although his cough was weak, he produced large amounts of thick, green sputum. Hyperresonant notes were produced during percussion over both lung fields. On auscultation, breath sounds and heart sounds were diminished. Coarse crackles and wheezing were heard throughout both lung fields. No recent chest x-ray film was available. A sputum culture obtained at admission suggested the presence of *Pseudomonas aeruginosa*. On a 2 L/min oxygen cannula, his SpO_2 was 92% and his ABGs were pH 7.55, $PaCO_2$ 54 mm Hg, HCO_3^- 45 mEq/L, PaO_2 57 mm Hg, and SaO_2 93%.

On the basis of these clinical data, the following SOAP was documented:

Respiratory Assessment and Plan

S "I can't get enough air to sleep 10 minutes!"

O Cyanosis and use of accessory muscles of respiration; vital signs: BP 147/95, HR 117, RR 32, T 37°C (98.6°F); cough: frequent, weak, and productive of large amounts of thick, green sputum; *Pseudomonas aeruginosa* cultured; bilateral hyperresonant notes and diminished breath sounds; coarse crackles and wheezes; on a 2 L/min oxygen cannula, SpO_2 92%. ABGs: pH 7.55, $PaCO_2$ 54, HCO_3^- 45, PaO_2 57, and SaO_2 93%.

A • Continued respiratory distress (general appearance, vital signs, use of accessory muscles)
  • Excessive bronchial secretions (cough, sputum, coarse crackles)
  • Poor ability to mobilize secretions (weak cough)
  • Acute alveolar hyperventilation superimposed on chronic ventilatory failure with mild to moderate hypoxemia (ABGs)
  • Possible impending ventilatory failure

P Start Aerosolized Medication Protocol (0.5 mL albuterol in 2 mL NS, followed by 2 mL DNase bid). Up-regulate Airway Clearance Therapy per protocol (CPT and PEP therapy q2h). Up-regulate Oxygen Therapy Protocol (Venturi oxygen mask at FIO_2 0.35). Continue to monitor possible impending ventilatory failure closely.

64 Hours After Admission

The respiratory therapist noted that the patient was in obvious respiratory distress. The patient said he could not find a position that allowed him to breathe comfortably. He appeared cyanotic, was using pursed-lip breathing, and was using his accessory muscles of respiration. His vital signs were blood pressure 145/90, heart rate 120 beats/min, respiratory rate 22 breaths/min, and oral temperature 38°C (100.5°F). Chest palpation was normal, but bilateral hyperresonant percussion notes were elicited. Auscultation revealed coarse crackles and wheezing bilaterally. No recent chest radiograph was available. ABGs on an FIO_2 of 0.4 Venturi mask were pH 7.27, $PaCO_2$ 83 mm Hg, HCO_3^- 36 mEq/L, PaO_2 37 mm Hg, and SaO_2 73%.

On the basis of these clinical data, the following SOAP was entered in the patient's chart.

Respiratory Assessment and Plan

S "I can't get into a comfortable position to breathe."

O Cyanosis; pursed-lip breathing and use of accessory muscles of respiration; vital signs BP 145/90, HR 120, RR 22, T 38°C (100.5°F); bilateral hyperresonant percussion notes, coarse crackles, and wheezing; ABGs on FIO_2 of 0.4 were pH 7.27, $PaCO_2$ 83, HCO_3^- 36, PaO_2 37, and SaO_2 73%.

A • Continued respiratory distress (general appearance, vital signs, use of accessory muscles, pursed-lip breathing)
  • Acute ventilatory failure superimposed on chronic ventilatory failure with severe hypoxemia (ABGs, vital signs, worsening)
  • Lactic acidosis likely
  • Excessive bronchial secretions (cough, sputum, breath sounds)

P Contact physician stat. Consider Mechanical Ventilation Protocol. Continue Aerosolized Medication Protocol and Airway Clearance Therapy Protocol (after patient has been placed on ventilator). Up-regulate Oxygen Therapy Protocol (initially, FIO_2 0.50 and reevaluate when patient is placed on ventilator). Monitor closely.

Discussion

The science of respiratory care has advanced over the years, and the prognosis for patients with this multisystem genetic disorder has improved. In this patient's lifetime, the following therapeutic landmarks can be noted:

1. Vigorous use of chest physiotherapy (percussion and postural drainage), including percussion aids
2. The proven benefits of new drugs, such as DNase (Pulmozyme) and ivacaftor (Kalydeco)
3. Positive expiratory pressure (PEP) therapy
4. Lung transplantation (when all else fails)

This patient had received at least three of these treatments and was in the hands of caring parents. His own stubborn nature and interest in athletics were clearly helpful in his prolonged survival. Important to note are the circumstances surrounding his admission, especially the fact that he had experienced hemoptysis, dyspnea, and weight loss during the several years preceding his admission. Note also that he had started smoking cigarettes.

In this case study, the patient's chief complaints purposely have been buried in the admitting history. The reader should have discerned that the patient was coughing productively and had dyspnea and weight loss. The recommended therapeutic strategy arises from recognition of these three presenting complaints. Note also that on admission the patient had neck vein distention and peripheral edema, suggesting cor pulmonale.

If the experience with chronic obstructive pulmonary disease can be extrapolated to patients with CF, this is a bad prognostic sign and one that clearly calls for intensification of the therapeutic regimen, probably from the time of the first assessment and treatment plan selection.

Note that on the initial physical examination, the patient demonstrated excessive bronchial secretions and a productive cough; no baseline ABGs existed with which to compare his current values (see Bronchospasm, Fig. 10.10). Thus the observation of an elevated $PaCO_2$ should initially be taken very, very seriously.

At the time of the second evaluation the patient clearly was not improving. The up-regulation of Airway Clearance Therapy (see Protocol 10.2) and addition of the Aerosolized Medication Protocol at this point were appropriate (the increased chest physical therapy, along with PEP therapy every 2 hours, and Pulmozyme therapy). A repeat chest x-ray study would not be out of order at this time. At that time, more might have been made of the enlargement of pulmonary artery seen in Fig. 15.10. One could argue that the Aerosolized Medication Protocol and more aggressive bronchopulmonary hygiene should have been started earlier, including the use of mucolytics.

The third assessment clearly suggests that the patient was deteriorating despite vigorous noninvasive therapy. At this point, the patient was placed on an FIO_2 of 0.5, and the stat call to the physician regarding the acute ventilatory failure was appropriate. The addition of mechanical ventilation at this time would prevent fatigue, allow deep tracheal suctioning, and facilitate repeat therapeutic bronchoscopy if it were to become necessary.

After this initial downhill course, the patient was placed on a ventilator and slowly improved. Over the next 7 days, he was weaned from noninvasive mechanical ventilation. The therapist should note that despite all the "good" things the patient and family did to treat his illness, the patient's initiation of smoking clearly could be a "last-straw" phenomenon. The patient should be placed on a smoking cessation program. His outpatient program should have been reevaluated, more closely monitored, and possibly up-regulated as to modality selection and frequency. These steps are as important for the long-term prognosis, as is the skill of the practitioner caring for him during this episode of acute ventilatory failure.

SELF-ASSESSMENT QUESTIONS

1. Which of the following organisms is(are) commonly found in the tracheobronchial tree secretions of patients with cystic fibrosis?
   1. *Staphylococcus*
   2. *Haemophilus influenzae*
   3. *Streptococcus*
   4. *Pseudomonas aeruginosa*
      a. 1 only
      b. 2 only
      c. 1 and 4 only
      d. 1, 2, and 4 only

2. When two carriers of cystic fibrosis produce children, there is a:
   1. 75% chance that the baby will be a carrier
   2. 25% chance that the baby will be completely normal
   3. 50% chance that the baby will have cystic fibrosis
   4. 25% chance that the baby will have cystic fibrosis
      a. 1 only
      b. 3 only
      c. 2 and 4 only
      d. 1 and 2 only

3. The cystic fibrosis gene is located on which chromosome?
   a. 5
   b. 6
   c. 7
   d. 8

4. In cystic fibrosis the patient commonly demonstrates which of the following?
   1. Increased FEV_T
   2. Decreased MVV
   3. Increased RV
   4. Decreased FEV_1/FVC ratio
      a. 1 only
      b. 3 only
      c. 3 and 4 only
      d. 2, 3, and 4 only

5. During the advanced stages of cystic fibrosis, the patient generally demonstrates which of the following?
   1. Bronchial breath sounds
   2. Dull percussion notes
   3. Diminished breath sounds
   4. Hyperresonant percussion notes
      a. 1 and 3 only
      b. 2 and 4 only
      c. 1 and 4 only
      d. 1, 3, and 4 only

6. About 80% of all patients with cystic fibrosis demonstrate a deficiency in which of the following vitamins?
   1. A
   2. B
   3. D
   4. E
   5. K
      a. 3 and 4 only
      b. 1, 4, and 5 only
      c. 2, 3, and 4 only
      d. 1, 3, 4, and 5 only

7. Which of the following agents targets the underlying cause of cystic fibrosis, the faulty gene *G551D*, and its defective CFTR protein?
   a. Aztreonam
   b. Ivacafor
   c. Inhaled DNase
   d. *N*-acetylcysteine

8. Which of the following is(are) mucolytic agents?
   1. DNase
   2. Pulmozyme
   3. Tobramycin
   4. Dornase alpha
      a. 1 only
      b. 2 only
      c. 3 and 4 only
      d. 1, 2, and 4 only

9. With regard to the secretion of sodium and chloride, the sweat glands of patients with cystic fibrosis secrete up to:
   a. 2 times the normal amount
   b. 4 times the normal amount
   c. 7 times the normal amount
   d. 10 times the normal amount

10. Which of the following clinical manifestations are associated with severe cystic fibrosis?
    1. Decreased hemoglobin concentration
    2. Increased central venous pressure
    3. Decreased breath sounds
    4. Increased pulmonary vascular resistance
       a. 1 and 3 only
       b. 2 and 3 only
       c. 3 and 4 only
       d. 2, 3, and 4 only

Chapter Objectives

After reading this chapter, you will be able to:

- Describe the anatomic alterations of the lungs associated with bronchiectasis.
- Discuss the etiology and epidemiology of bronchiectasis.
- Identify the common classifications used to group the causes of bronchiectasis and include specific examples under each classification.
- Describe the various diagnostic tests used to identify the presence of bronchiectasis.
- Describe the cardiopulmonary clinical manifestations associated with bronchiectasis.
- Describe the general medical and surgical management of bronchiectasis.
- Describe the respiratory care modalities used in the treatment of bronchiectasis.
- Describe and evaluate the clinical strategies and rationales of the SOAPs presented in the case study.
- Define key terms and complete self-assessment questions at the end of the chapter and on Evolve.

Key Terms

Acquired Bronchial Obstruction
Bronchography
Congenital Anatomic Defects
Cylindrical (Tubular) Bronchiectasis
Cystic (Saccular) Bronchiectasis

High-Frequency Chest Compression Devices
High-Resolution Computed Tomogram (HR-CT)
Kartagener Syndrome
Lung Mapping
Noncystic Fibrosis Bronchiectasis (NCFB)
Pneumovest
Primary Ciliary Dyskinesia
Reid Classification
Varicose (Fusiform) Bronchiectasis

Chapter Outline

Anatomic Alterations of the Lungs
    Varicose Bronchiectasis (Fusiform Bronchiectasis)
    Cylindrical Bronchiectasis (Tubular Bronchiectasis)
    Cystic Bronchiectasis (Saccular Bronchiectasis)
Etiology and Epidemiology
Diagnosis
Overview of the Cardiopulmonary Clinical Manifestations
    Associated With Bronchiectasis
General Management of Bronchiectasis
    Respiratory Care Treatment Protocols
Medications Commonly Prescribed by the Physician
    Expectorants
    Administration of Antibiotics
Case Study Bronchiectasis
Self-Assessment Questions

Anatomic Alterations of the Lungs

Bronchiectasis is an acquired disorder of the major bronchi and bronchioles characterized by chronic dilation and distortion of one or more bronchi, usually as a result of extensive inflammation and destruction of the bronchial wall cartilage, blood vessels, elastic tissue, and smooth muscle components. One or both lungs may be involved. Bronchiectasis is commonly limited to a lobe or segment and is frequently found in the lower lobes. The smaller bronchi, with less supporting cartilage, are predominantly affected.

Because of bronchial wall destruction, normal mucociliary clearance is impaired. This results in the accumulation of copious amounts of bronchial secretions and blood that often become foul-smelling because of secondary colonization with anaerobic organisms. Infection and irritation may lead to secondary bronchial smooth muscle constriction and fibrosis. The small bronchi and bronchioles distal to the affected areas become partially or totally obstructed with secretions. This condition leads to one or both of the following anatomic alterations: (1) hyperinflation of the distal alveoli as a result of expiratory check-valve obstruction or (2) atelectasis, consolidation, and fibrosis as a result of complete bronchial obstruction.

Based on gross anatomic appearance, the long-accepted **Reid classification** subdivides bronchiectasis into the following three patterns:

- Varicose (fusiform)
- Cylindrical (tubular)
- Cystic (saccular)

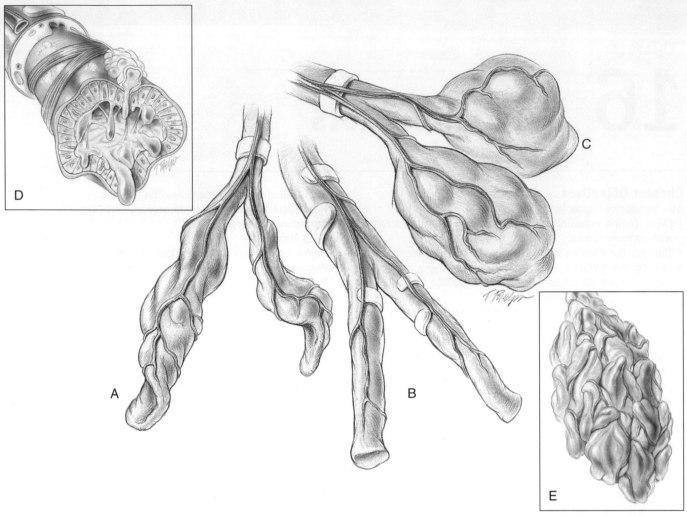

FIGURE 16.1 Bronchiectasis. (A) Varicose bronchiectasis. (B) Cylindrical bronchiectasis. (C) Cystic (saccular) bronchiectasis. Also illustrated are excessive bronchial secretions (D) and atelectasis (E), which are both common anatomic alterations of the lungs in this disease.

Varicose Bronchiectasis (Fusiform Bronchiectasis)

In **varicose (fusiform) bronchiectasis**, the bronchi are dilated and constricted in an irregular fashion similar to varicose veins, ultimately resulting in a distorted, bulbous shape (Fig. 16.1A).

Cylindrical Bronchiectasis (Tubular Bronchiectasis)

In **cylindrical (tubular) bronchiectasis**, the bronchi are dilated and rigid and have regular outlines similar to a tube. X-ray examination shows that the dilated bronchi fail to taper for 6 to 10 generations and then appear to end abruptly because of mucous obstruction (see Fig. 16.1B).

Cystic Bronchiectasis (Saccular Bronchiectasis)

In **cystic (saccular) bronchiectasis**, the bronchi progressively increase in diameter until they end in large, cystlike sacs in the lung parenchyma. This form of bronchiectasis causes the greatest damage to the tracheobronchial tree. The bronchial walls become composed of fibrous tissue alone—cartilage, elastic tissue, and smooth muscle are all absent (see Fig. 16.1C).

The following are the major pathologic or structural changes associated with bronchiectasis:

- Chronic dilation and distortion of bronchial airways
- Excessive production of often foul-smelling sputum (see Fig. 16.1D)
- Bronchospasm
- Hyperinflation of alveoli (air trapping)
- Atelectasis (see Fig. 16.1E)
- Parenchymal consolidation and fibrosis
- Hemoptysis secondary to bronchial arterial erosion

Etiology and Epidemiology

Most causes of bronchiectasis include some combination of bronchial obstruction and infection. In developed countries, cystic fibrosis is the most common cause of bronchiectasis in children. The prevalence of **noncystic fibrosis bronchiectasis (NCFB)** in developed nations is relatively low. For example, in the United States, the incidence of NCFB is about 4.2 per 100,000 young adults. The low incidence of NCFB in developed countries is most often attributed to early medical management (e.g., antibiotic therapy). In other populations, however, such as Polynesia, Alaska, Australia, and New Zealand, the occurrence of NCFB is as high as 15 per 1000 children.

The most common cause of NCFB is pulmonary infection. Although this is not a well-defined entity, it is believed that a possible mechanism for postinfectious NCFB is a significant lung infection during early childhood that causes anatomic alterations of the developing lung that allow persistent bacterial infections. As a result, the continuous bacterial infections lead to bronchiectasis.

Also at risk for chronic pulmonary infection and NCFB are individuals with a mucociliary disorder (**primary ciliary dyskinesia**) or an immunodeficiency disorder involving low levels of immunoglobulin G (IgG), IgM, and IgA. In addition, NCFB is also associated with patients who have rheumatoid arthritis, inflammatory bowel disease (most often in those with chronic ulcerative colitis), and chronic obstructive pulmonary disease (COPD). Finally, other etiologic factors associated with NCFB include foreign-body aspirations, tumors, hilar adenopathy, bronchial airway mucoid impaction, tracheobronchial abnormalities, vascular abnormalities, lymphatic abnormalities, advanced age, malnutrition, socioeconomic disadvantage, and alpha₁-antitrypsin deficiency.

The causes of bronchiectasis are commonly classified into the following categories:

- **Acquired bronchial obstruction**
- **Congenital anatomic defects**
- Immunodeficiency states
- Abnormal secretion clearance
- Miscellaneous disorders (e.g., alpha₁-antitrypsin deficiency)

Table 16.1 provides these common classifications used to group the causes of bronchiectasis, specific examples under each classification, and diagnostic tests used to identify the presence of bronchiectasis.

Diagnosis

A routine chest radiograph may reveal such findings as overinflated lungs or marked volume loss, increased opacities, dilated fluid-filled airways, crowding of the bronchi, and atelectasis. Although bronchoscopy is rarely performed today, bronchograms can confirm cylindrical, cystic, or varicose bronchiectasis, as well as crowding of the bronchi, loss of bronchovascular markings, and, in more severe cases, honeycombing, air-fluid levels, and fluid-filled nodules. Bronchoscopy once was the absolute gold standard for the diagnosis of NCFB.

Today, the **high-resolution computed tomogram (HR-CT)** scan has virtually replaced bronchography (see Computed Tomography Scan later in this chapter) as the best tool for diagnosing NCFB. The diagnosis is made on the basis of the internal diameter of a bronchus that is wider than its adjacent pulmonary artery, a failure of the bronchi to taper, and the visualization of bronchi in the outer 1 to 2 cm of the lung fields. The HR-CT scan is used to better clarify the findings from the chest radiograph and standard CT scans, and allows **lung mapping** of airway abnormalities that cannot be identified on routine films of the chest.

Spirometry testing can be used to determine if the bronchiectasis demonstrates primarily an obstructive or restrictive lung pathophysiology, and arterial blood gas measurements can confirm if the patient has mild, moderate, or severe gas exchange compromise.

TABLE 16.1 Causes of Bronchiectasis

Category	Specific Examples	Diagnostic Tests
Acquired Bronchial Obstruction		
Foreign-body aspiration	Peanuts, chicken bone, teeth	Chest imaging, fiberoptic bronchoscopy
Tumors	Laryngeal papillomatosis, airway adenoma, endobronchial teratoma	Chest imaging, fiberoptic bronchoscopy
Hilar adenopathy	Tuberculosis, histoplasmosis, sarcoidosis	PPD, chest imaging, fiberoptic bronchoscopy
COPD	Chronic bronchitis	Pulmonary function tests
Rheumatic disease	Relapsing polychondritis (RP), tracheobronchial amyloidosis	Clinical syndrome of RP/cartilage biopsy, biopsy for amyloid
Mucoid impaction	Allergic bronchopulmonary aspergillosis, bronchocentric granulomatosis (BG), postoperative mucoid impaction	Total and aspergillus-specific IgE, specific aspergillus IgG, aspergillus skin test, chest imaging, biopsy for BG
Congenital Anatomic Defects That May Cause Bronchial Obstruction		
Tracheobronchial abnormalities	Bronchomalacia, bronchial cyst, cartilage deficiency (Williams-Campbell syndrome), tracheobronchomegaly (Mounier-Kuhn syndrome), ectopic bronchus, tracheoesophageal fistula	Chest CT imaging
Vascular abnormalities	Pulmonary (intralobar) sequestration, pulmonary artery aneurysm	Chest CT imaging
Lymphatic abnormalities	Slow-growing yellowish syndrome	History of dystrophic, slow-growing nails

Continued

TABLE 16.1 Causes of Bronchiectasis—cont'd

Category	Specific Examples	Diagnostic Tests
Immunodeficiency States		
IgG deficiency	Congenital (Bruton's type) agammaglobulinemia, selective deficiency of subclasses (IgG2, IgG4), acquired immune globulin deficiency, common variable hypogammaglobulinemia; Nezelof syndrome, "bare lymphocyte" syndrome	Quantitative immunoglobulin levels, immunoglobulin subclass levels, impaired response to immunization with pneumococcal vaccine
IgA deficiency	Selective IgA deficiency ± ataxia-telangiectasia syndrome	Quantitative immunoglobulin levels
Leukocyte dysfunction	Chronic granulomatous disease (NADPH oxidase dysfunction)	Dihydrorhodamine 123 (DHR) oxidation test, nitroblue tetrazolium test, genetic testing
Other rare humoral immunodeficiencies (CXCR4 mutation, CD40 deficiency, CD40 ligand deficiency, and others)	WHIM syndrome, hypergammaglobulinemia M	Neutrophil count, quantitative immunoglobulin levels
Abnormal Secretion Clearance		
Ciliary defects of airway mucosa	**Kartagener syndrome**, ciliary dyskinesis (formally called *impaired ciliary motility syndrome*)	Chest x-ray showing situs inversus, bronchial biopsy, ciliary motility studies, electron microscopy of sperm or respiratory mucosa
Cystic fibrosis (mucoviscidosis)	Typical early childhood syndrome, later presentation with predominantly sinopulmonary symptoms	Sweat chloride, genetic testing
Young syndrome	Obstructive azoospermia with sinopulmonary infections	Sperm count
Miscellaneous Disorders		
Alpha$_1$-antitrypsin deficiency	Absent or abnormal antitrypsin synthesis and function	Alpha$_1$-antitrypsin level
Recurrent aspiration pneumonia	Alcoholism, neurologic disorders, lipoid pneumonia	History, chest imaging
Rheumatic disease	Associated with rheumatoid arthritis and Sjögren syndrome	Rheumatoid factor, antiSSA/antiSSB, salivary gland MRI or biopsy
Inflammatory bowel disease	Crohn's disease, ulcerative colitis	History, lower gastrointestinal endoscopy, imaging studies, colonic biopsy
Inhalation of toxic fumes and dusts	Ammonia, nitrogen dioxide, or other irritant gases; smoke; talc; silicates	Exposure history, chest imaging
Chronic organ rejection after transplantation	Bone marrow, lung and heart-lung transplantation; associated with obliterative bronchiolitis	History, PFT, chest CT imaging with inspiratory and expiratory views
Childhood infections	Pertussis, measles	History of infection
Bacterial infections	Infections caused by *Staphylococcus aureus*, *Klebsiella*, *Pseudomonas aeruginosa*	History of infection, sputum culture
Viral infections	Infections caused by adenovirus (particularly types 7 and 21), influenza, herpes simplex	History/serologic evidence of infection
Other infections	Fungal (histoplasmosis), *Mycobacterium tuberculosis*, nontuberculous mycobacteria, possibly mycoplasma	Fungal culture, AFB smear and mycobacterial culture

AFB, Acid-fast bacilli; *COPD,* chronic obstructive pulmonary disease; *CT,* computed tomography; *Ig,* immunoglobulin; *MRI,* magnetic resonance imaging; *PFT,* pulmonary function test; *PPD,* percussion and postural drainage.

Modified from Wolters Kluwer Health/UpToDate.com: *Clinical Manifestations and diagnosis of bronchiectasis in adults.* Accessed March 25, 2017.

The following clinical manifestations result from the pathophysiologic mechanisms caused (or activated) by excessive bronchial secretions (see Fig. 10.11), bronchospasm (see Fig. 10.10), atelectasis (see Fig. 10.7), consolidation (see Fig. 10.8), and increased alveolar-capillary membrane thickness (see Fig. 10.9), which are the major anatomic alterations of the lungs associated with bronchiectasis (see Fig. 16.1).

CLINICAL DATA OBTAINED AT THE PATIENT'S BEDSIDE

Depending on the amount of bronchial secretions and the degree of bronchial destruction and fibrosis/atelectasis associated with bronchiectasis, the disease may create an obstructive or a restrictive lung disorder or a combination of both. If the majority of the bronchial airways are only partially obstructed, the bronchiectasis manifests primarily as an obstructive lung disorder. If, by contrast, the majority of the bronchial airways are completely obstructed, the distal alveoli collapse, atelectasis results, and the bronchiectasis manifests primarily as a restrictive disorder. Finally, if the disease is limited to a relatively small portion of the lung—as it often is—the patient may not have any of the following typical clinical manifestations of bronchiectasis.

The Physical Examination
Vital Signs
Increased Respiratory Rate (Tachypnea)

Several pathophysiologic mechanisms operating simultaneously may lead to an increased frequency of breathing (respiratory rate [RR]):

- Stimulation of peripheral chemoreceptors (hypoxemia)
- Decreased lung compliance and increased ventilatory rate relationship
- Anxiety

Increased Heart Rate (Pulse) and Blood Pressure
Use of Accessory Muscles During Inspiration
Use of Accessory Muscles During Expiration
Pursed-Lip Breathing (When Pathology Is Primarily Obstructive in Nature)
Increased Anteroposterior Chest Diameter (Barrel Chest) (When Pathology Is Primarily Obstructive in Nature)
Cyanosis
Digital Clubbing
Peripheral Edema and Venous Distention

Because polycythemia and cor pulmonale are associated with severe bronchiectasis, the following may be seen:

- Distended neck veins
- Pitting edema
- Enlarged and tender liver

Cough, Sputum Production, and Hemoptysis

Chronic cough with production of large quantities of foul-smelling sputum is a hallmark of bronchiectasis. A 24-hour collection of sputum is usually voluminous and tends to settle into several different layers. Streaks of blood are seen frequently in the sputum, presumably originating from necrosis of the bronchial walls and erosion of bronchial blood vessels. Frank hemoptysis also may occur occasionally, but it is rarely life-threatening. Because of the excessive bronchial secretions, secondary bacterial infections are frequent. *Haemophilus influenzae, Streptococcus, Pseudomonas aeruginosa,* and various anaerobic organisms are commonly cultured from the sputum of patients with bronchiectasis.

The productive cough seen in patients with bronchiectasis is triggered by the large amount of secretions that fill the tracheobronchial tree. The stagnant secretions stimulate the subepithelial mechanoreceptors, which in turn produce a vagal reflex that triggers the cough. The subepithelial mechanoreceptors are found in the trachea, bronchi, and bronchioles, but they are predominantly located in the upper airways.

Chest Assessment Findings

When the bronchiectasis pathologic factors are primarily obstructive:

- Decreased tactile and vocal fremitus
- Hyperresonant percussion note
- Diminished breath sounds
- Wheezing
- Crackles

When the bronchiectasis pathologic factors are primarily restrictive (over areas of atelectasis and consolidation):

- Increased tactile and vocal fremitus
- Bronchial breath sounds
- Crackles
- Whispered pectoriloquy
- Dull percussion note

CLINICAL DATA OBTAINED FROM LABORATORY TESTS AND SPECIAL PROCEDURES

Pulmonary Function Test Findings
Moderate to Severe Bronchiectasis
(When Primarily Obstructive Lung Pathophysiology)

FORCED EXPIRATORY VOLUME AND FLOW RATE FINDINGS

FVC	FEV_T	FEV_1/FVC ratio	$FEF_{25\%-75\%}$
↓	↓	↓	↓

$FEF_{50\%}$	$FEF_{200-1200}$	PEFR	MVV
↓	↓	↓	↓

LUNG VOLUME AND CAPACITY FINDINGS

V_T	IRV	ERV	RV
N or ↑	N or ↓	N or ↓	↑

VC	IC	FRC	TLC	RV/TLC ratio
↓	N or ↓	↑	N or ↑	N or ↑

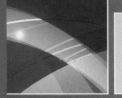
Pulmonary Function Test Findings
Moderate to Severe Bronchiectasis
(When Primarily Restrictive Lung Pathophysiology)

FORCED EXPIRATORY FLOW RATE FINDINGS

FVC	FEV$_T$	FEV$_1$/FVC ratio	FEF$_{25\%-75\%}$
↓	N or ↓	N or ↑	N or ↓

FEF$_{50\%}$	FEF$_{200-1200}$	PEFR	MVV
N or ↓	N or ↓	N or ↓	N or ↓

LUNG VOLUME AND CAPACITY FINDINGS

V$_T$	IRV	ERV	RV
N or ↓	↓	↓	↓

VC	IC	FRC	TLC	RV/TLC ratio
↓	↓	↓	↓	N

Arterial Blood Gases
Bronchiectasis

MILD TO MODERATE STAGES

Acute Alveolar Hyperventilation With Hypoxemia[1]
(Acute Respiratory Alkalosis)

pH	PaCO$_2$	HCO$_3^-$	PaO$_2$	SaO$_2$ or SpO$_2$
↑	↓	↓ (but normal)	↓	↓

SEVERE STAGE

Chronic Ventilatory Failure With Hypoxemia[2] (Compensated Respiratory Acidosis)

pH	PaCO$_2$	HCO$_3^-$	PaO$_2$	SaO$_2$ or SpO$_2$
N	↑	↑ (significantly)	↓	↓

ACUTE VENTILATORY CHANGES SUPERIMPOSED ON CHRONIC VENTILATORY FAILURE[3]

Because acute ventilatory changes are frequently seen in patients with chronic ventilatory failure, the respiratory therapist must be familiar with and alert for the following two dangerous arterial blood gas (ABG) findings:

- Acute alveolar hyperventilation superimposed on chronic ventilatory failure, which should further alert the respiratory therapist to document the following important ABG assessment: possible *impending acute ventilatory failure*
- Acute ventilatory failure (acute hypoventilation) superimposed on chronic ventilatory failure

Oxygenation Indices[4]

BRONCHIECTASIS MODERATE TO SEVERE STAGES

$\dot{Q}_S/\dot{Q}_T$	DO$_2$[5]	$\dot{V}O_2$	C(a-$\bar{v}$)O$_2$	O$_2$ER	S$\bar{v}$O$_2$
↑	↓	N	N	↑	↓

Hemodynamic Indices[6]
Bronchiectasis Moderate to Severe Stages

CVP	RAP	$\overline{PA}$	PCWP	CO	SV
↑	↑	↑	N	N	N

SVI	CI	RVSWI	LVSWI	PVR	SVR
N	N	↑	N	↑	N

ABNORMAL LABORATORY TESTS AND PROCEDURES
Hematology

- Increased hematocrit and hemoglobin
- Elevated white blood count (WBC) if patient is acutely infected

SPUTUM CULTURE RESULTS AND SENSITIVITY

- *Streptococcus pneumoniae*
- *Haemophilus influenzae*
- *Pseudomonas aeruginosa*
- Anaerobic organisms

RADIOLOGIC FINDINGS
Chest Radiograph

When the bronchiectasis is primarily obstructive:

- Translucent (dark) lung fields
- Depressed or flattened diaphragms
- Long and narrow heart (pulled down by diaphragms)
- Enlarged heart (when heart failure is present)
- Tram tracks
- Areas of consolidation and/or atelectasis may or may not be seen

When the pathophysiology of bronchiectasis is primarily obstructive, the lungs become hyperinflated, leading to an increased functional residual capacity and depressed diaphragms. Because right and left ventricular enlargement and

---

[1]See Fig. 5.2 and Table 5.4 and related discussion for the acute pH, PaCO$_2$, and HCO$_3^-$ changes associated with acute alveolar hyperventilation.

[2]See Table 5.6 and related discussion for the pH, PaCO$_2$, and HCO$_3^-$ changes associated with chronic ventilatory failure.

[3]See Table 5.7, Table 5.8, and Table 5.9 and related discussion for the pH, PaCO$_2$, and HCO$_3^-$ changes associated with acute ventilatory changes superimposed on chronic ventilatory failure.

[4]C(a-$\bar{v}$)O$_2$, Arterial-venous oxygen difference; DO$_2$, total oxygen delivery; O$_2$ER, oxygen extraction ratio; $\dot{Q}_S/\dot{Q}_T$, pulmonary shunt fraction; S$\bar{v}$O$_2$, mixed venous oxygen saturation; $\dot{V}O_2$, oxygen consumption.

[5]The DO$_2$ may be normal in patients who have compensated to the decreased oxygenation status with (1) an increased cardiac output, (2) an increased hemoglobin level, or (3) a combination of both. When the DO$_2$ is normal, the O$_2$ER is usually normal.

[6]CI, Cardiac index; CO, cardiac output; CVP, central venous pressure; LVSWI, left ventricular stroke work index; $\overline{PA}$, mean pulmonary artery pressure; PCWP, pulmonary capillary wedge pressure; PVR, pulmonary vascular resistance; RAP, right atrial pressure; RVSWI, right ventricular stroke work index; SV, stroke volume; SVI, stroke volume index; SVR, systemic vascular resistance.

failure may develop as secondary problems during the advanced stages of bronchiectasis, an enlarged heart may be seen on the chest radiograph.

Although the chest radiograph is not as valuable as the computed tomography (CT) scan in identifying a specific type of bronchiectasis (i.e., cystic, varicose, or cylindrical), a careful analysis of chest radiographs usually reveals abnormalities in the majority of cases. For example, tram-track opacities (also called *tram lines*) may be seen in cylindrical bronchiectasis. Tram tracks are parallel or curved opacity lines of varying length caused by bronchial wall thickening. Fig. 16.2 shows the x-ray image of a patient with gross cystic bronchiectasis and over-inflated lungs.

When the bronchiectasis is primarily restrictive:

- Atelectasis and consolidation
- Infiltrates (suggesting pneumonia)
- Increased opacity

In generalized bronchiectasis, such as commonly seen in cystic fibrosis, there is usually overinflation of the lungs. However, when the bronchiectasis is localized, the chest radiograph often reveals restrictive pathologic conditions such as atelectasis, consolidation, or infiltrates. When atelectasis and consolidation develop as a result of bronchiectasis, an increased opacity and reduced lung volume are seen in these areas on the radiograph. For example, Fig. 16.3 illustrates a marked volume loss in a patient with left lower lobe bronchiectasis.

BRONCHOGRAM

In the past, **bronchography** (the injection of an opaque contrast material into the tracheobronchial tree) was routinely performed on patients with bronchiectasis. Fig. 16.4, for example, presents a bronchogram of cylindrical bronchiectasis. Fig. 16.5 shows a bronchogram of cystic (saccular) bronchiectasis. Fig. 16.6 presents a bronchogram of varicose bronchiectasis; the bronchi are dilated and constricted in an irregular fashion and terminate in a distorted, bulbous shape. Today, CT scan of the chest has largely replaced this technique.

COMPUTED TOMOGRAPHY SCAN

With this technique, increased bronchial wall opacity is often seen. The bronchial walls may appear as follows:

- Thick
- Dilated
- Characterized by ring lines or clusters
- Signet ring–shaped
- Flame-shaped

The CT scan changes may include many findings that are similar to those seen on the chest radiograph. The bronchial

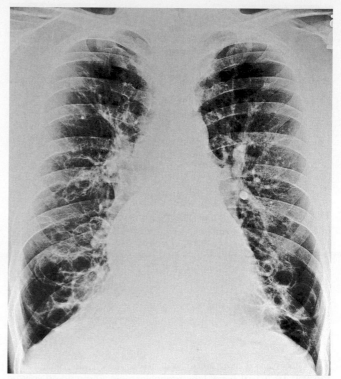

FIGURE 16.2 Gross cystic bronchiectasis. Posteroanterior chest radiograph showing overinflated lungs. There are multiple ring opacities, most obvious at the lung bases, ranging from 3 to 15 mm in diameter. (From Hansell, D. M., Lynch, D. A., McAdams, H. P., et al. [2010]. *Imaging of diseases of the chest* [5th ed.]. Philadelphia, PA: Elsevier.)

walls may appear thick, dilated, or as rings of opacities arranged in lines or clusters. A characteristic appearance in bronchiectasis is the end-on signet ring opacity produced by the ring shadow of a dilated airway with its accompanying artery (Fig. 16.7).

The specific type of bronchiectasis can be confirmed with the CT scan. For example, Fig. 16.8 confirms the presence of cylindrical bronchiectasis. Fig. 16.9 shows varicose bronchiectasis, and Fig. 16.10 shows cystic bronchiectasis. Airways that are filled with secretions produce rounded or flame-shaped opacities that can be identified by following them through adjacent sections to unfilled airways. The CT scan also confirms atelectasis, consolidation, fibrosis, scarring, and hyperinflation.

Finally, it should be mentioned that the CT scan is an excellent tool to use for lung mapping—that is, the ability to map out and determine precisely where chest physiotherapy would be delivered or exactly where surgical resection of lung should be performed.

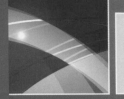

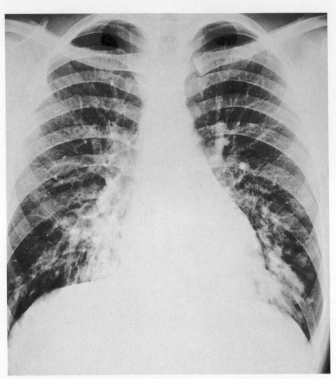

FIGURE 16.3 Left lower lobe bronchiectasis. The marked volume loss of the left lower lobe is indicated by a depressed hilum, vertical left mainstem bronchus, mediastinal shift, and left-sided transradiancy. (From Hansell, D. M., Lynch, D. A., McAdams, H. P., et al. [2010]. *Imaging of diseases of the chest* [5th ed.]. Philadelphia, PA: Elsevier.)

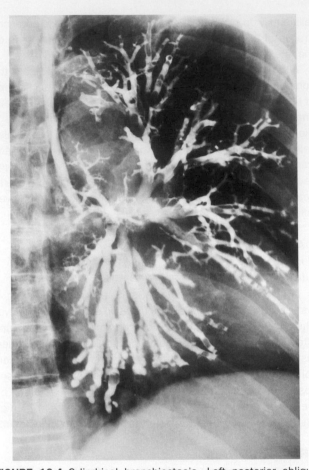

FIGURE 16.4 Cylindrical bronchiectasis. Left posterior oblique projection of a left bronchogram showing cylindrical bronchiectasis affecting the whole of the lower lobe except for the superior segment. Few side branches fill. Basal airways are crowded together, indicating volume loss of the lower lobe, a common finding in bronchiectasis. (From Hansell, D. M., Lynch, D. A., McAdams, H. P., et al. [2010]. *Imaging of diseases of the chest* [5th ed.]. Philadelphia, PA: Elsevier.)

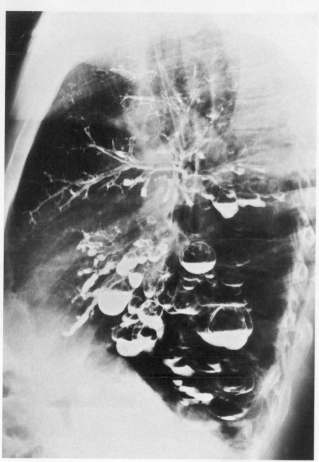

FIGURE 16.5 Cystic (saccular) bronchiectasis. Right lateral bronchogram showing cystic bronchiectasis affecting mainly the lower lobe and posterior segment of the upper lobe. (From Hansell, D. M., Lynch, D. A., McAdams, H. P., et al. [2010]. *Imaging of diseases of the chest* [5th ed.]. Philadelphia, PA: Elsevier.)

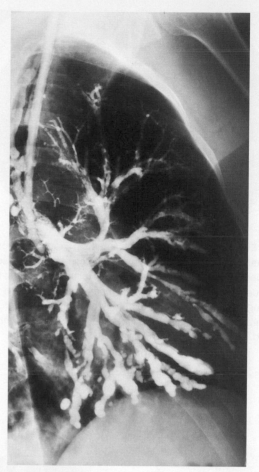

FIGURE 16.6 Varicose bronchiectasis. Left posterior oblique projection of left bronchogram in a patient with the ciliary dyskinesia syndrome. All basal bronchi are affected by varicose bronchiectasis. (From Hansell, D. M., Lynch, D. A., McAdams, H. P., et al. [2010]. *Imaging of diseases of the chest* [5th ed.]. Philadelphia, PA: Elsevier.)

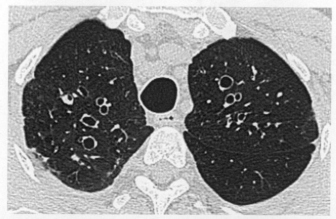

FIGURE 16.7 Signet ring sign in patient with cystic fibrosis. (From Hansell, D. M., Lynch, D. A., McAdams, H. P., et al. [2010]. *Imaging of diseases of the chest* [5th ed.]. Philadelphia, PA: Elsevier.)

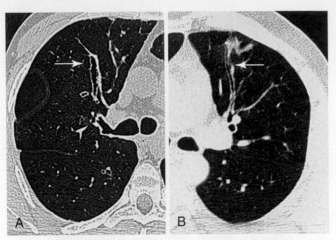

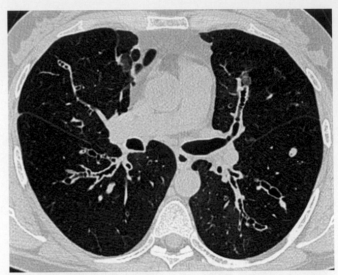

FIGURE 16.8 Cylindrical bronchiectasis. Examples from two patients. Airways parallel to the plane of section in anterior segment of an upper lobe show changes of cylindrical bronchiectasis; bronchi are wider than normal and fail to taper as they proceed toward the lung periphery (arrows). (From Hansell, D. M., Lynch, D. A., McAdams, H. P., et al. [2010]. *Imaging of diseases of the chest* [5th ed.]. Philadelphia, PA: Elsevier.)

FIGURE 16.9 Varicose bronchiectasis. Patient with allergic bronchopulmonary aspergillosis and cystic fibrosis. The bronchiectatic airways have a corrugated, or beaded, appearance. (From Hansell, D. M., Lynch, D. A., McAdams, H. P., et al. [2010]. *Imaging of diseases of the chest* [5th ed.]. Philadelphia, PA: Elsevier.)

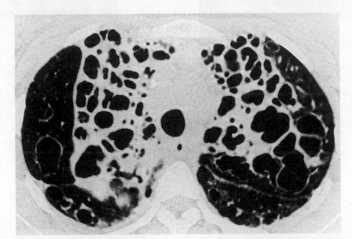

FIGURE 16.10 Cystic bronchiectasis (advanced) in the upper lobes. (From Hansell, D. M., Lynch, D. A., McAdams, H. P., et al. [2010]. *Imaging of diseases of the chest* [5th ed.]. Philadelphia, PA: Elsevier.)

General Management of Bronchiectasis

For most causes of bronchiectasis, the treatment of the underlying disease is not possible. Because exacerbations are commonly caused by acute bacterial infections, the general treatment plan is aimed at controlling pulmonary infections, airway secretions, and airway obstruction and preventing complications. Antibiotics (tailored to the patient's sputum cultures and sensitivities), bronchodilators, and expectorants are often prescribed during periods of exacerbation. Daily chest percussion, postural drainage, and effective coughing exercises to remove bronchial secretions are routine parts of the treatment. Childhood vaccinations and yearly influenza vaccinations help reduce the prevalence of some infections. Avoidance of upper respiratory tract infections, smoking, and polluted environments also helps reduce susceptibility to pneumonia in these patients. Surgical lung resection may be indicated for patients who respond poorly to therapy or demonstrate massive hemoptysis.

Respiratory Care Treatment Protocols

Oxygen Therapy Protocol

Oxygen therapy is used to treat hypoxemia, decrease the work of breathing, and decrease myocardial work. The hypoxemia that develops in bronchiectasis is usually caused by the pulmonary shunting associated with the disorder. The hypoxemia may not respond well to oxygen therapy when true or capillary pulmonary shunting is present (see Oxygen Therapy Protocol, Protocol 10.1).

Airway Clearance Therapy Protocol

A number of airway clearance therapy modalities may be used to enhance the mobilization of bronchial secretions, including the following:

- Directed cough
- Exercise breathing programs
- Autogenic breathing
- Forced expiration
- Chest physiotherapy (CPT) (postural drainage [PD], hand or mechanical chest clapping)
- Suctioning
- Positive expiratory pressure (PEP)
- Oscillatory PEP (e.g., flutter valve acapella device)
- High-frequency chest wall compression

Chest percussion has become more practical and very effective with the advent of **high-frequency chest compression devices** such as the **pneumovest**. However, such compression devices are moderately expensive and chest wall discomfort and claustrophobia may limit their usefulness (see Airway Clearance Therapy Protocol, Protocol 10.2).

Lung Expansion Therapy Protocol

Attempts to keep distal lung units inflated may involve the use of deep breathing and coughing and incentive spirometry (see Lung Expansion Therapy Protocol, Protocol 10.3).

Aerosolized Medication Therapy Protocol

Both sympathomimetic and parasympatholytic agents are commonly used in selected patients with bronchiectasis to induce bronchial smooth muscle relaxation, particularly in patients with spirometrically proved reversible airway obstruction (see Protocol 10.4: Aerosolized Medication Therapy Protocol, and Appendix II on the Evolve site).

The use of corticosteroids is discouraged. There are insufficient data to support the use of nebulized hypertonic saline, inhaled dornaxe (DNase), or acetylcysteine in patients with bronchiectasis. Many centers require use of direct physician order to use them.

Mechanical Ventilation Protocol

Invasive and noninvasive mechanical ventilation may be necessary to provide and temporarily help improve alveolar ventilation and eventually return patients to their baseline condition and/or spontaneous breathing. Because acute ventilatory failure superimposed on chronic ventilatory failure is often seen in patients with severe bronchiectasis, continuous mechanical ventilation is justified when the acute ventilatory failure is thought to be reversible—for example, when acute pneumonia exists as a complicating factor (see Ventilator Initiation and Management Protocol, Protocol 11.1, and Ventilation Weaning Protocol, Protocol 11.2).

Medications Commonly Prescribed by the Physician

Expectorants

Expectorants sometimes are ordered when oral liquids and aerosol therapy alone are not sufficient to facilitate expectoration (see Appendix V on the Evolve site). Their clinical effectiveness is doubtful.

Administration of Antibiotics

Antibiotics are commonly administered to treat associated respiratory tract infections (see Appendix III on the Evolve site).

Admitting History and Physical Examination

A 31-year-old obese male patient consulted his physician regarding an increasingly productive cough. He reported a "bad case" of right lower lobe pneumonia 7 years ago and several episodes of "pulmonary infection" since that time. On those occasions, he usually received an antibiotic, and until 6 months ago the infections responded readily to treatment. However, 6 months ago he noticed that his chronic cough had become increasingly severe and more or less constant and for the first time his cough became productive. Recently, he had produced as much as a cup of thick, tenacious, yellow-white sputum per day. Within the past 2 to 3 days, he noticed a small amount of dark blood mixed with the sputum. He also noticed some dyspnea on exertion, but he was largely sedentary, and this had not been particularly troublesome. His medical history revealed chronic sinusitis since adolescence but was otherwise unremarkable.

Physical examination revealed an obese male adult in no apparent distress. Vital signs were within normal limits. His oral temperature was 98.4°F. He coughed frequently during the examination and produced a moderate amount of thick, yellow, blood-streaked sputum. Coarse crackles were heard over the right lower lung fields posteriorly. His SpO_2 on room air while at rest was 85%.

Laboratory results showed a mild leukocytosis but were otherwise normal. An outpatient sputum culture indicated the presence of *H. influenzae*. An HRCT scan of the chest revealed cystic dilations of the right lower lobe (RLL) bronchus. The respiratory therapist assigned to assess and treat the patient at this time recorded the following in the patient's chart.

Respiratory Assessment and Plan

S Productive cough, hemoptysis, worse in past 6 months. Mild dyspnea on exertion.

O Vital signs: Normal. Afebrile. SpO_2 85%. Observed moderate amount of mucopurulent, blood-streaked sputum. Coarse crackles over RLL. Outpatient sputum culture: *H. influenzae*. HRCT scan suggests saccular dilation of RLL bronchi.

A • Postpneumonic bronchiectasis RLL (history and HRCT scan)
  • Excessive airway secretions and sputum production (coarse crackles and sputum expectoration)
  • Acute bronchial infection and hemoptysis (yellow, blood-streaked sputum, culture results)
  • Moderate hypoxemia (SpO_2)

P Oxygen Therapy Protocol (O_2 via 2 L/min nasal cannula). Airway Clearance Therapy Protocol (CPT and PD, cough and deep breathing, q6h).

The physician prescribed antibiotics and administered pneumococcal vaccine. The patient was discharged from the hospital after 3 days with considerable improvement. However, he was still producing a small amount of thin clear sputum.

He was instructed to seek prompt medical attention for all future pulmonary infections. His wife was instructed in manual chest percussion and postural drainage techniques.

About 6 months later, the patient arrived at the emergency department complaining of a productive cough, pain on the left side of the chest (made worse by deep breathing), shaking chills and fever for 3 days, and noticeable swelling of both ankles. Since his previous visit, he had been doing his manual CPT and PD only one or two times per week. He had gained 30 lb and had taken a new job as a painter's apprentice. He admitted to smoking an occasional cigarette. There had been no known recent infectious disease exposure.

Physical examination revealed a young man in obvious respiratory distress. His vital signs were blood pressure 160/100, heart rate 110 beats/min and regular, respiratory rate 20 breaths/min, and oral temperature 101.5°F. His sputum was foul-smelling (a fecal odor), thick, and yellow-green. His cough was strong. Auscultation revealed coarse crackles over both bases. There was mild clubbing of fingers and toes. The physician wrote "bronchiectasis" in the working diagnosis section of the patient's chart.

Although an HRCT scan was ordered, it had not yet been taken. The patient's WBC was 23,500 mm³, with 80% segmented neutrophils and 10% bands. Room air ABG showed pH 7.51, $PaCO_2$ 28 mm Hg, HCO_3^- 21 mEq/L, PaO_2 45 mm Hg, and SaO_2 87%. His SpO_2 at rest on room air was 86%; it fell to 78% when he got out of bed to go to the bathroom.

The respiratory therapist recorded the following note in the patient's emergency department chart.

Respiratory Assessment and Plan

S Cough, pleuritic left-sided chest pain, chills, fever, leg swelling. 30 lb weight gain. Smoking.

O HR 110; RR 20; BP 160/100; T 101.5°F. Sputum thick, yellow-green, foul-smelling. Coarse crackles both bases. Strong cough. Clubbing of digits. WBC 23,500 (80% neutrophils, 10% bands). Room air ABG pH 7.51; $PaCO_2$ 28; HCO_3^- 21; PaO_2 45, and SaO_2 87%; SpO_2 (room air, rest) 86%, falls to 78% with mild exertion.

A • Bronchiectasis (old chart record)
  • Excessive airway secretions (thick sputum, coarse crackles)
  • Good ability to mobilize secretions (strong cough)
  • Infection likely (fever, yellow-green sputum, leukocytosis)
  • Acute alveolar hyperventilation with moderate hypoxemia (ABG)
  • Possible pneumonia

P Review CXR. Oxygen Therapy Protocol (2 L/min per nasal cannula). Airway Clearance Therapy Protocol (CPT and PD q4h). Obtain sputum for Gram stain and culture. Check I&O. Repeat ABG in a.m. Review deep breathing and cough, flutter valve, and pulmonary rehabilitation strategies with patient and his wife. Train in use of pneumovest chest percussion device. Offer smoking cessation and weight reduction programs.

Discussion

The main challenge facing the respiratory therapist caring for the patient with bronchiectasis is the efficient removal of excessive airway secretions. Over the years, postural drainage and percussion, good systemic hydration, and judicious use of antibiotics have been the hallmarks of therapy. More recently, intermittent (rare) use of mucolytics, percussive ventilation, and the Lung Expansion Therapy Protocol (see Protocol 10.3) has become more common. Pneumococcal prophylaxis is, of course, important, as is prompt attention to parenchymal pulmonary infections such as pneumonia. The clinical distinction between chronic bronchiectasis and cystic fibrosis is a subtle one at the bedside, and the latter condition must always be ruled out in patients with bronchiectasis. The goal of long-term therapy in bronchiectasis is prevention of lung parenchyma–destroying pulmonary infections and avoidance of frequent hospitalizations. Hemoptysis is often a sign of more deep-seated infection requiring antibiotic therapy. At the time of the second admission, severe infection was suspected, and intravenous antibiotic therapy was started.

The clinical manifestations throughout this case were all based on the clinical scenario associated with excessive bronchial secretions and possible infection (see Fig. 10.11). For example, the thick yellow sputum resulted in decreased ventilation-perfusion ratios, venous admixture, and hypoxemia. These pathophysiologic mechanisms caused clinical manifestations of coarse crackles, an increase in blood pressure and heart rate, and acute alveolar hyperventilation with moderate hypoxemia.

Digital clubbing associated with hypoxemia is another clinical manifestation of bronchiectasis. After the first assessment, the Oxygen Therapy Protocol and Airway Clearance Therapy Protocol were administered appropriately (see Protocols 10.1 and 10.2). The therapist's review of the chest x-ray image allowed him to target the postural drainage therapy. Low-flow oxygen per nasal cannula, aerosolized bronchodilators (albuterol), chest percussion, and postural drainage therapy were selected from these protocols and applied with good results.

Finally, during the second admission, patient noncompliance was evident (i.e., weight gain, resumption of smoking, employment in a dusty workplace, failure to continue CPT and PD), which further complicated the patient's respiratory disorder. Note that both of these SOAPs omit the patient's height and weight (although they do suggest that he is obese). This is important because an exercise/weight reduction program would be helpful to his cough efficiency, the idea was not mentioned. In response to the patient's condition, the whole respiratory care regimen was up-regulated by an increase in frequency of treatments, with a strong emphasis on the patient's responsibility for his own care. In addition, in both of these admissions, no note of the patient's state of systemic or secretion hydration was made. This is an important omission, and a factor worth noting.

SELF-ASSESSMENT QUESTIONS

1. **In which of the following forms of bronchiectasis are the bronchi dilated and constricted in an irregular fashion?**
   1. Fusiform
   2. Saccular
   3. Varicose
   4. Cylindrical
      a. 2 only
      b. 3 only
      c. 2 and 4 only
      d. 1 and 3 only

2. **Which of the following is(are) common causes of acquired bronchiectasis?**
   1. Hypogammaglobulinemia
   2. Pulmonary tuberculosis
   3. Kartagener syndrome
   4. Cystic fibrosis
      a. 1 only
      b. 2 only
      c. 3 only
      d. 3 and 4 only

3. **In the primarily obstructive form of bronchiectasis, the patient commonly demonstrates which of the following?**
   1. Decreased FRC
   2. Increased $FEF_{25\%-75\%}$
   3. Decreased PEFR
   4. Increased FEV_T
      a. 1 only
      b. 3 only
      c. 1 and 4 only
      d. 2 and 4 only

4. **Which of the following radiologic findings is(are) associated with bronchiectasis that is primarily obstructive?**
   1. Atelectasis
   2. Depressed or flattened diaphragms
   3. Long and narrow heart
   4. Translucent lung fields
      a. 1 and 2 only
      b. 3 and 4 only
      c. 1 and 4 only
      d. 2, 3, and 4

5. Which of the following is considered the hallmark of bronchiectasis?
   a. Chronic cough and large quantities of foul-smelling sputum
   b. Abnormal bronchogram
   c. Acute ventilatory failure superimposed on chronic ventilatory failure
   d. Presentation as both a restrictive and obstructive pulmonary disorder

6. Which of the following is(are) commonly cultured in the sputum of patients with bronchiectasis?
   1. *Streptococcus pneumoniae*
   2. *Pseudomonas aeruginosa*
   3. *Haemophilus influenzae*
   4. *Klebsiella*
   a. 3 only
   b. 4 only
   c. 1, 2, and 3 only
   d. 1, 2, 3, and 4

7. When the pathophysiology of bronchiectasis is primarily obstructive, the patient demonstrates which of the following clinical manifestations?
   1. Decreased tactile and vocal fremitus
   2. Bronchial breath sounds
   3. Dull percussion note
   4. Rhonchi and wheezing
   a. 2 only
   b. 3 only
   c. 1 and 4 only
   d. 2 and 4 only

8. Which of the following diagnostic procedures is(are) used to positively diagnose bronchiectasis?
   1. Arterial blood gases
   2. Bronchography
   3. Oxygenation indices
   4. Computed tomography
   a. 2 only
   b. 3 only
   c. 1 and 3 only
   d. 2 and 4 only

9. Which of the following causes of bronchiectasis is(are) related to abnormal secretion clearance?
   1. Pertussis
   2. Cystic fibrosis
   3. Kartagener syndrome
   4. Measles
   a. 1 only
   b. 2 only
   c. 3 and 4 only
   d. 2 and 3 only

10. Which of the following hemodynamic indices is(are) associated with bronchiectasis?
   1. Decreased central venous pressure
   2. Increased mean pulmonary artery pressure
   3. Decreased right ventricular stroke work index
   4. Increased right atrial pressure
   a. 2 only
   b. 3 only
   c. 2 and 4 only
   d. 1 and 3 only

11. Which of the following respiratory care protocols may be of importance in the outpatient care of patients with bronchiectasis?
   1. Oxygen Therapy Protocol
   2. Airway Clearance Therapy Protocol
   3. Lung Expansion Therapy Protocol
   4. Aerosolized Medication Therapy Protocol
   a. 2 and 3 only
   b. 2 only
   c. 1 and 2 only
   d. 1, 2, 3, and 4

17 Atelectasis

Chapter Objectives

After reading this chapter, you will be able to:

- List the anatomic alterations of the lungs associated with atelectasis.
- Describe the specific causes of atelectasis.
- List the respiratory disorders associated with atelectasis.
- List the cardiopulmonary clinical manifestations associated with postoperative atelectasis.
- Describe the general management of atelectasis.
- Describe the clinical strategies and rationales of the SOAP presented in the case study.
- Define key terms and complete self-assessment questions at the end of the chapter and on Evolve.

Key Terms

Absorption Atelectasis
Air Bronchograms
Alveolar Degassing
Alveolar Flooding
Incentive Spirometry (IS)
Optimal PEEP Trial
Primary Atelectasis
Primary Lobule
Therapeutic Bronchoscopy

Chapter Outline

Anatomic Alterations of the Lungs
Etiology
Overview of the Cardiopulmonary Clinical Manifestations
   Associated With Postoperative Atelectasis
General Management of Postoperative Atelectasis
   General Considerations
   Respiratory Care Treatment Protocols
Case Study: Postoperative Atelectasis
Self-Assessment Questions

Anatomic Alterations of the Lungs

Atelectasis is an abnormal condition of the lungs characterized by the partial or total collapse of previously expanded alveoli, thus resulting in the prevention of respiratory exchange of carbon dioxide and oxygen in that part of the lung and reduced lung compliance. The failure of the lungs to expand at birth, most commonly seen in premature infants or those narcotized by maternal anesthesia, is known as **primary atelectasis**. Atelectasis may be limited to the smallest lung unit—that is, the alveolus or **primary lobule**,[1] or it may involve an entire lung or a segment or lobe of the lung (Fig. 17.1).

The major pathologic and anatomic alterations associated with atelectasis include partial or total collapse of the following:

- Alveoli of primary lobules (microatelectasis or subsegmental atelectasis)—very common
- Lung segment—fairly common
- Lung lobe—less common
- Entire lung—rare

Etiology

As shown in Box 17.1, there are many respiratory disorders associated with atelectasis. The etiologic factors linked to these disorders, and the subsequent atelectasis that ensues, can be further grouped into pulmonary conditions that (1) reduce alveolar ventilation (e.g., pulmonary edema [**alveolar flooding**], acute respiratory distress syndrome, ventilator-induced lung injury [VILI] or ventilator-associated lung injury [VALI],[2] smoke inhalation, thermal injuries),[3] (2) promote alveolar degassing secondary to airway obstruction (e.g., cystic fibrosis, bronchiectasis, Guillain-Barré syndrome, myasthenia gravis), or (3) compress the lung tissue (e.g., flail chest, pneumothorax, pleural disease).

---

[1]A primary lobule is a cluster of alveoli that originates from a single terminal bronchiole. Each primary lobule is about 3.5 mm in diameter and contains about 2000 alveoli. Each lung contains about 150,000 primary lobules. A primary lobule also is called an *acinus, terminal respiratory unit,* or *functional lung unit.* The lung parenchyma consists of thousands of terminal respiratory units.

[2]See Chapter 11.
[3]See Chapter 45.

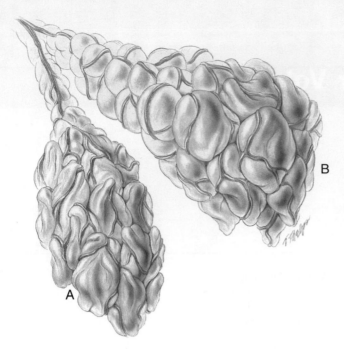

FIGURE 17.1 Alveoli in postoperative atelectasis. (A) Total alveolar collapse. (B) Partial alveolar collapse.

In this chapter, postoperative atelectasis is used as a prototype of the atelectasis process. Postoperative atelectasis is commonly seen after upper abdominal and thoracic surgical procedures. Lung expansion is often decreased after surgery because of postoperative alveolar hypoventilation (anesthesia), external thoracic compression such as from wound dressings, postoperative pain, or development of excessive airway secretions and mucous plugs, which in turn produce distal degassing of lung units (also called **absorption atelectasis**).[4]

Good lung expansion depends on the patient's intact chest cage and the ability to generate an appropriate negative intrapleural pressure. Thoracic and upper abdominal procedures often result in a reduced ability to generate good lung expansion and therefore are considered high-risk factors for subsequent development of postoperative atelectasis. Other precipitating factors of postoperative atelectasis include (1) obesity,

(2) operative and postoperative supine position, (3) advanced age, (4) use of inadequate tidal volumes during mechanical ventilation, (5) malnutrition, (6) free fluid in the abdominal cavity (ascites), or (7) presence of a restrictive lung disorder (e.g., pleural effusion, pneumothorax, acute respiratory distress syndrome, pulmonary edema, interstitial lung disease, or pleural masses).

Finally, postoperative atelectasis is often associated with retained airway secretions and mucous plugs. Precipitating factors for retained secretions include (1) decreased mucociliary transport, (2) excessive secretions, (3) inadequate hydration, (4) weak or absent cough, (5) general anesthesia, (6) smoking history, (7) gastric aspiration, and (8) certain other preexisting conditions (see Box 17.1). When total airway obstruction develops, alveolar oxygen is *absorbed* into the pulmonary circulation and **alveolar degassing** ensues. Breathing high oxygen concentrations favors this pathologic process.

---

[4]In cases in which atelectasis is caused by excessive airway secretions, it is not uncommon to see this condition complicated by bronchospasm and wheezing.

OVERVIEW of the Cardiopulmonary Clinical Manifestations Associated With Postoperative Atelectasis[1]

The following clinical manifestations result from the pathologic mechanisms caused (or activated) by atelectasis (see Fig. 10.7)—the major anatomic alterations of the lungs associated with atelectasis (see Fig. 17.1).

CLINICAL DATA OBTAINED AT THE PATIENT'S BEDSIDE

The Physical Examination

Vital Signs

Increased Respiratory Rate (Tachypnea)

Several pathophysiologic mechanisms operating simultaneously may lead to an increased ventilatory rate:

- Stimulation of peripheral chemoreceptors (hypoxemia)
- Relationship of decreased lung compliance to increased ventilatory rate
- Stimulation of J receptors
- Pain, anxiety, fever

Increased Heart Rate (Pulse) and Blood Pressure

Cyanosis

Chest Assessment Findings

- Increased tactile and vocal fremitus
- Dull percussion note
- Bronchial breath sounds
- Diminished breath sounds (common when atelectasis is caused by mucous plugs)
- Crackles (usually heard initially in the dependent lung regions and during late inspiration)
- Whispered pectoriloquy

CLINICAL DATA OBTAINED FROM LABORATORY TESTS AND SPECIAL PROCEDURES

Pulmonary Function Test Findings
(Primarily Restrictive Lung Pathophysiology)

FORCED EXPIRATORY VOLUME AND FLOW RATE FINDINGS

FVC	FEV_T	FEV_1/FVC ratio	$FEF_{25\%-75\%}$
↓	N or ↓	N or ↑	N or ↓

$FEF_{50\%}$	$FEF_{200-1200}$	PEFR	MVV
N or ↓	N or ↓	N or ↓	N or ↓

LUNG VOLUME AND CAPACITY FINDINGS

V_T	IRV	ERV	RV
N or ↓	↓	↓	↓

VC	IC	FRC	TLC	RV/TLC ratio
↓	↓	↓	↓	N

DECREASED DIFFUSION CAPACITY (DLCO)

Arterial Blood Gases

SMALL OR LOCALIZED ATELECTASIS

Acute Alveolar Hyperventilation With Hypoxemia[2]
(Acute Respiratory Alkalosis)

pH	$PaCO_2$	HCO_3^-	PaO_2	SaO_2 or SpO_2
↑	↓	↓	↓	↓
		(but normal)		

WIDESPREAD ATELECTASIS

Acute Ventilatory Failure With Hypoxemia[3]
(Acute Respiratory Acidosis)

pH[4]	$PaCO_2$	HCO_3^{-}[4]	PaO_2	SaO_2 or SpO_2
↓	↑	↑	↓	↓
		(but normal)		

---

[1]The Overview of Cardiopulmonary Clinical Manifestations presented in this chapter apply to all cases of atelectasis, regardless of the cause (see Box 17.1).

[2]See Fig. 5.2 and Table 5.4 and related discussion for the acute pH, $PaCO_2$, and HCO_3^- changes associated with acute alveolar hyperventilation.
[3]See Fig. 5.2 and Table 5.5 and related discussion for the acute pH, $PaCO_2$, and HCO_3^- changes associated with acute and chronic ventilatory failure.
[4]When tissue hypoxia is severe enough to produce lactic acid, the pH and HCO_3^- values will be lower than expected for a particular $PaCO_2$ level.

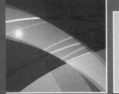

Oxygenation Indices[5]					
$\dot{Q}_S/\dot{Q}_T$	DO_2[6]	$\dot{V}O_2$	$C(a\text{-}\bar{v})O_2$	O_2ER	$S\bar{v}O_2$
↑	↓	N	N	↑	↓

[5]$C(a\text{-}\bar{v})O_2$, Arterial-venous oxygen difference; DO_2, total oxygen delivery; O_2ER, oxygen extraction ratio; $\dot{Q}_S/\dot{Q}_T$, pulmonary shunt fraction; $S\bar{v}O_2$, mixed venous oxygen saturation; $\dot{V}O_2$, oxygen consumption.

[6]The DO_2 may be normal in patients who have compensated to the decreased oxygenation status with (1) an increased cardiac output, (2) an increased hemoglobin level, or (3) a combination of both. When the DO_2 is normal, the O_2ER is usually normal.

RADIOLOGIC FINDINGS
Chest Radiograph
- Increased density in areas of atelectasis
- **Air bronchograms**
- Elevation of the hemidiaphragm on the affected side
- Mediastinal shift toward the affected side

Areas of increased density generally appear initially in dependent lung regions, such as the lower lobes, or posteriorly in patients who must recline in the supine position. Air bronchograms can be seen when large areas of atelectasis are present in the chest film. An elevation of the hemidiaphragm or mediastinal shift toward the affected side is often seen when large areas of atelectasis exist. Fig. 17.2A shows left lung atelectasis caused by a misplaced endotracheal tube in the right mainstem bronchus. Fig. 17.2B shows the same patient 20 minutes after the endotracheal tube was pulled back above the carina.

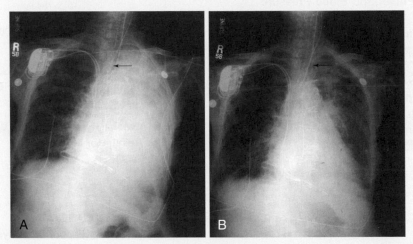

FIGURE 17.2 (A) Endotracheal tube tip misplaced in the right mainstem bronchus (arrow). Note that the left lung has collapsed completely (i.e., white fluffy appearance in the left lung). (B) The same patient 20 minutes after the endotracheal tube was pulled back above the carina (arrow). Note that the left lung is better ventilated (i.e., appears darker). (Used with permission from author Terry Des Jardins.)

General Management of Postoperative Atelectasis

Precipitating factors for postoperative atelectasis should be identified during the preoperative and postoperative assessments (see the previous section on etiology). High-risk patients should be monitored closely and are often treated with preventive measures. Bedside spirometry (vital capacity and inspiratory capacity) is useful in the early detection of atelectasis, and **incentive spirometry** is frequently prescribed to encourage good lung expansion. Preoperative patients with combined obstructive and restrictive pulmonary disease are generally considered extremely high risk for atelectasis. This is especially true if the patient has a condition associated with excessive airway secretions—for example, chronic bronchitis. When postoperative atelectasis has been diagnosed, the following respiratory care procedures may be prescribed.

General Considerations

Whenever possible, treatment of the underlying cause of the postoperative atelectasis should be prescribed immediately (e.g., medication for pain, control/treatment of airway secretions, correction of inadequate tidal volumes during mechanical ventilation, repositioning of an endotracheal tube out of the right mainstem bronchus, or withdrawal of air or fluid from the pleural cavity).

Respiratory Care Treatment Protocols

Oxygen Therapy Protocol

Oxygen therapy is used to treat hypoxemia, decrease the work of breathing, and decrease myocardial work. Because of the hypoxemia that may develop in atelectasis, supplemental oxygen may be required. However, the hypoxemia that develops in postoperative atelectasis is caused by capillary shunting and therefore is often refractory to oxygen therapy (see Oxygen Therapy Protocol, Protocol 10.1).

Airway Clearance Therapy Protocol

When atelectasis is caused by mucus accumulation and mucus plugs, a number of airway clearance therapies may be used to enhance the mobilization of airway secretions (see Airway Clearance Therapy Protocol, Protocol 10.2).

Lung Expansion Therapy Protocol

Lung expansion therapy measures are routinely administered to offset atelectasis and reinflate collapsed lung areas (see Lung Expansion Therapy Protocol, Protocol 10.3).

Mechanical Ventilation Protocol

Short-term mechanical ventilation is often prescribed after major surgery, especially if the patient has one or more high-risk factors for postoperative atelectasis. For example, in patients undergoing cardiac surgery, mechanical ventilation generally is maintained until the cardiopulmonary parameters are stable (see Ventilator Initiation and Management Protocol, Protocol 11.1, and Ventilator Weaning Protocol, Protocol 11.2). An **optimal PEEP trial** should be performed (see Protocol 11.1).

CASE STUDY Postoperative Atelectasis

Admitting History and Physical Examination

A 62-year-old man with a 35-pack-year smoking history and long-standing productive cough had his left lower lobe resected because of small cell lung carcinoma. Anesthesia had been given using a right-sided double-lumen endotracheal tube. At the end of the procedure, the patient was breathing well and the tube was removed.

In the recovery room 30 minutes after arrival, his respiratory rate increased from 22 breaths/min to 34 breaths/min. His pulse increased from 70 to 130 beats/min with regular rhythm, and his blood pressure decreased from 115/85 to 100/60 mm Hg. His SpO_2 dropped from 97% to 85% while he was on 2 L/min O_2 per cannula. Breath sounds were decreased in the left lower posterior chest. A chest radiograph showed atelectasis of the left lower lobe. Arterial blood gas (ABG) values (on 2 L/min O_2 per cannula) were pH 7.29, $PaCO_2$ 63 mm Hg, HCO_3^- 29 mEq/L, PaO_2 55 mm Hg, and SaO_2 84%.

At that time the respiratory therapist recorded the following SOAP note.

Respiratory Assessment and Plan

S N/A. Patient extubated, but still sedated from anesthesia.

O RR 34/min, P 130 and regular, BP 100/60. Breath sounds decreased in left lower chest anteriorly. CXR: Left lower lobe atelectasis. On 2 L/min O_2 per cannula: pH 7.29, $PaCO_2$ 63, HCO_3^- 29, SaO_2 84%.

A • Left lower lobe atelectasis; rule out mucous plugs (CXR and decreased breath sounds)

• Acute ventilatory failure with moderate hypoxemia (ABGs)

P Stat: Contact physician regarding possible reintubation and Mechanical Ventilation Protocol (SIMV mode). Oxygen Therapy Protocol (FIO_2 0.50). Airway Clearance

Therapy Protocol (deep tracheal suction; discuss with physician the possibility of respiratory therapist assistance with therapeutic bronchoscopy). Lung Expansion Therapy Protocol after intubation (Optimal PEEP based on $P(A-a)O_2$ results). Repeat ABGs in 30 minutes and reevaluate. Monitor SpO_2 for next 72 hours. When patient is alert, instruct in cough and deep breathing technique.

The patient was reintubated, ventilated, and oxygenated according to protocol. Optimal PEEP and SIMV were used. On the physician's order, a trial mucolytic (acetylcysteine) was aerosolized and directly instilled into his endotracheal tube. Aggressive tracheobronchial suctioning was performed but produced only small amounts of secretions with little or no benefit to the patient.

In view of this, a fiberoptic bronchoscope was inserted through the endotracheal tube, and a large mucous plug was identified in the orifice of the left lower lobe bronchus. The plug was removed under direct vision. After the bronchoscopy, the patient improved rapidly. A chest radiograph showed full expansion of the left lower lobe. The patient was then extubated, and on the sixth postoperative day he was discharged. The patient was discharged on the sixth postoperative day.

Discussion

Care of a patient with postoperative atelectasis (see Fig. 10.7) is one of the day-to-day responsibilities of the respiratory therapist and was well carried out in this case. Accordingly, the respiratory therapist must be extremely adept in the assessment and management of such patients. The development of immediate postoperative atelectasis is almost always related to excessive bronchial secretions (see Fig. 10.11)—in this case caused by a large mucous plug obstructing the left lower lobe. Because such patients (in the immediate postoperative period) often cannot cough vigorously, particularly after thoracotomy, the decision to initiate **therapeutic bronchoscopy** immediately rather than rely on physiotherapy, suctioning, and mucolytics was certainly in order.

In patients who have undergone abdominal surgery or those who develop atelectasis later, the simpler approaches such as intermittent positive ventilation therapy, should certainly be tried first. Atelectasis has a tendency to recur, and these patients need to be followed for at least 72 hours postoperatively to ensure this has not happened. Therefore the therapist's

suggestion to follow up with pulse oximetry and cough and deep breathing instruction was entirely appropriate.

As important as treatment is, prevention is better. In this regard, the Airway Clearance Therapy Protocol and the Lung Expansion Protocol were very important. Indeed, the application of these simple protocols often prevents the late development of atelectasis in postoperative patients. Unfortunately, no preoperative aggressive respiratory care was reported in this patient's case.

SELF-ASSESSMENT QUESTIONS

1. Which of the following clinical manifestations are associated with postoperative atelectasis?
   1. Frothy, pink sputum
   2. Crackles
   3. Air bronchograms
   4. Increased $S\overline{v}O_2$
      a. 1 and 2 only
      b. 2 and 3 only
      c. 3, and 4 only
      d. 2, 3, and 4 only

2. Which of the following pulmonary function testing values are associated with postoperative atelectasis?
   1. N or ↑ FEV_T
   2. ↑ FVC
   3. ↓RV
   4. N or ↑ FEV_1/FVC ratio
      a. 1 and 2 only
      b. 3 and 4 only
      c. 2, 3, and 4 only
      d. 1, 2, 3, and 4

3. A primary lobule is a cluster of alveoli. About how many alveoli does a primary lobule contain?
   a. 500 alveoli
   b. 1000 alveoli
   c. 1500 alveoli
   d. 2000 alveoli

4. Which of the following are precipitating factors of postoperative atelectasis?
   1. Obesity
   2. Anesthesia
   3. Postoperative pain
   4. Ascites
      a. 1 and 3 only
      b. 2 and 4 only
      c. 2, 3, and 4 only
      d. 1, 2, 3, and 4

5. Which of the following arterial blood gas values are associated with small or localized postoperative atelectasis?
   1. Increased PaO_2
   2. Decreased $PaCO_2$
   3. Increased pH
   4. Decreased HCO_3^- (but normal)
      a. 1 and 3 only
      b. 2 and 4 only
      c. 2, 3, and 4 only
      d. 1, 2, 3, and 4

Pneumonia, Lung Abscess Formation, and Important Fungal Diseases

Chapter Objectives

After reading this chapter, you will be able to:

- List the anatomic alterations of the lungs associated with pneumonia.
- Describe the causes and classifications of pneumonia.
- List the cardiopulmonary clinical manifestations associated with pneumonia.
- Describe the general management of pneumonia.
- Describe the clinical strategies and rationales of the SOAPs presented in the case study.
- Define key terms and complete self-assessment questions at the end of the chapter and on Evolve.

Key Terms

Acute Symptomatic Pulmonary Histoplasmosis
Adenovirus
Allergic Bronchopulmonary Aspergillosis (ABPA)
Anaerobic Gram-Negative Bacilli
Anaerobic Gram-Positive Cocci
Aspergillus
Aspiration Pneumonia
Asymptomatic Histoplasmosis
Atypical Organisms
Avian Influenza A
Bacteroides fragilis
Blastomyces dermatitidis
Blastomycosis
Bronchopneumonia
Candida albicans
Caseous Tubercles
Cavity Formation
Chlamydia pneumoniae
Chlamydia psittaci
Chlamydia trachomatis
Chronic pulmonary histoplasmosis
Cine-videoesophagoscopy
Coccidioides immitis
Coccidioidomycosis
Community-Acquired Pneumonia (CAP)
Consolidation
Coronavirus
Coxiella Burnetii

Cryptococcus neoformans
Croup
Cytomegalovirus
"Desert Arthritis"
Disseminated Histoplasmosis
"Double Pneumonia"
Dysarthria
Dysphagia
Dysphonia
Enterobacter Species
Escherichia coli
Evans Blue Dye Test
Exudate
Fungal Infections
Gastroesophageal Reflux Disease (GERD)
Gram-Negative Organisms
Gram-Positive Organisms
Granulomas
Haemophilus influenzae
Health Care–Associated Pneumonia (HCAP)
Histoplasma capsulatum
Histoplasmin Skin Test
Histoplasmosis
Hospital-Acquired Pneumonia (HAP)
Human Metapneumovirus (hMPV)
Influenza Viruses
Interstitial Pneumonia
Invasive Aspergillosis
Invasive Candidiasis
Klebsiella
Legionella pneumophila
Legionnaire Disease
Lipoid Pneumonitis
Lobar Pneumonia
Lung abscess
Mendelson Syndrome
Moraxella catarrhalis
Multiple Drug–Resistant *Staphylococcus aureus* (MDRSA)
Mycobacterium avium complex (MAC)
Mycoplasma pneumoniae
North American Blastomycosis
Parainfluenza Viruses

Peptococci
Peptostreptococcus
Pneumocystis jiroveci
Prevotella melaninogenica
Pseudomonas aeruginosa
Q Fever
Respiratory Syncytial Virus (RSV)
Rickettsial Infections
Rubella
San Joaquin Valley Fever
Serratia marcescens
Severe Acute Respiratory Syndrome (SARS)
Silent Aspiration
Staphylococcus
Staphylococcus aureus
Streptococcus
Swallowing Mechanics
Thrush
Tracheoesophageal Fistula
Tuberculosis
Varicella
Ventilator-Associated Pneumonia
"Walking Pneumonia"

Pneumonia: Anatomic Alterations of the Lungs

Pneumonia,[1] or pneumonitis with consolidation, is the result of an inflammatory process that primarily affects the gas exchange area of the lung. In response to the inflammation, fluid (serum) and some red blood cells (RBCs) from adjacent pulmonary capillaries pour into the alveoli. This process of fluid transfer is called *effusion*. Polymorphonuclear leukocytes move into the infected area to engulf and kill invading bacteria on the alveolar walls. This process has been termed *surface phagocytosis*. Increased numbers of macrophages also appear in the infected area to remove cellular and bacterial debris. If the infection is overwhelming, the alveoli become filled with fluid, RBCs, polymorphonuclear leukocytes, and macrophages. When this occurs, the lungs are said to be **consolidation** (Fig. 18.1). Fig. 18.2 provides a microscopic view of bacterial pneumonia. Atelectasis is often associated with patients who have **aspiration pneumonia**.

The major pathologic or structural changes associated with pneumonia are as follows:
- Inflammation of the alveoli
- Alveolar consolidation
- Atelectasis (e.g., in aspiration pneumonia)

---

[1]As of this writing, pneumonia is one of several conditions in which readmission to the hospital for any cause will result in possible significant financial penalties to the hospital for patients on Medicare (for more on this, see Chapter 13, Chronic Obstructive Pulmonary Disease, Chronic Bronchitis, and Emphysema). Accordingly, careful evaluation of all such patients, particularly the elderly, should be done for comorbid conditions, especially those with chronic heart and lung disease, swallowing difficulties, and problems with cognition.

Etiology and Epidemiology

Taken together, pneumonia and influenza combined are the eighth leading cause of death among Americans and the sixth leading cause of death over the age of 65 years. It is estimated that about 50,000 Americans die of pneumonia each year. Pneumonia and influenza are especially life-threatening in individuals whose lungs are already damaged by chronic obstructive pulmonary disease (COPD), asthma, or smoking. The risk for death from pneumonia or influenza is also higher among people with heart disease, diabetes, or a weakened immune system.

Pneumonia is the leading cause of morbidity and mortality in children beyond the neonatal period. It accounts for an estimated 900,000 deaths worldwide, and its effect on outpatient visit rate is extremely high. The chest x-ray, which is often used as a clinical reference standard to guide management, does not differentiate viral from bacterial disease or predict clinical course, particularly in children.

Causes of pneumonia include bacteria, viruses, fungi, protozoa, parasites, tuberculosis, anaerobic organisms, aspiration, and the inhalation of irritating chemicals such as chlorine. Pneumonia is an insidious disease because its symptoms vary greatly, depending on the patient's specific underlying condition and the type of organism causing the pneumonia. Pneumonia often mimics a common cold or the flu. For example, the patient may suddenly experience chills, shivering, high fever, sweating, chest pain (pleurisy), and a dry and nonproductive cough. Often what initially appears to be a cold or the flu, however, can in fact be a much more serious pulmonary infection. The early recognition and treatment of pneumonia provide the best chance for a full recovery.

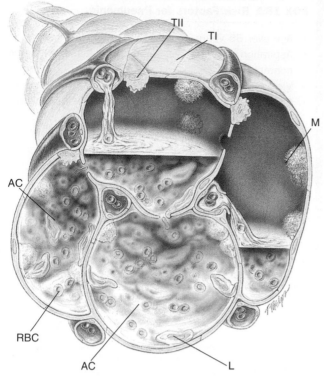

FIGURE 18.1 Cross-sectional view of alveolar consolidation in pneumonia. *AC,* Alveolar consolidation; *L,* leukocyte; *M,* macrophage; *RBC,* red blood cell; *TI,* type I cell.

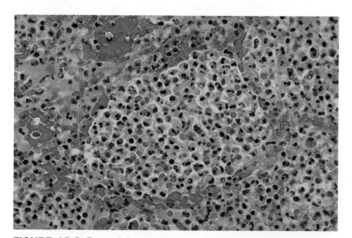

FIGURE 18.2 Bacterial pneumonia, microscopic. These alveolar exudates are mainly composed of neutrophils. The surrounding alveolar walls have capillaries that are congested (dilated and filled with red blood cells). Such an exudative process is typical of bacterial infection. This exudate gives rise to the productive cough of purulent yellow sputum seen with bacterial pneumonias. The alveolar structure is still maintained, which is why even an extensive pneumonia often resolves with minimal residual destruction or damage to the pulmonary parenchyma. In patients with compromised lung function from underlying obstructive or restrictive lung disease or cardiac disease, however, even limited pneumonic consolidation can be life threatening. (From Klatt, E. [2015], *Robbins and Cotran atlas of pathology* [3rd ed.]. Philadelphia, PA: Elsevier.)

The terms *bronchopneumonia, lobar pneumonia,* and *interstitial pneumonia* refer to the anatomic location of the inflammation (Fig. 18.3). **Bronchopneumonia** is characterized by a patchy pattern of infection that is limited to the segmental bronchi and surrounding lung parenchyma. Bronchopneumonia usually

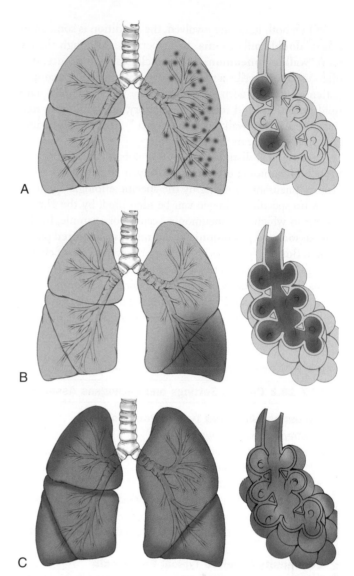

FIGURE 18.3 (A) Bronchopneumonia is limited to the segmental bronchi and surrounding lung parenchyma. (B) Lobar pneumonia is a widespread or diffuse alveolar inflammation and consolidation. Lobar pneumonia is often the end result of severe bronchopneumonia in which the infection spreads from one lung segment to another until the entire lung lobe is involved. (C) Interstitial pneumonia is usually diffuse and is commonly associated with infections with *Mycoplasma pneumoniae* or viruses.

involves both lungs and is seen more often in the lower lobes of the lung. **Lobar pneumonia** is a widespread or diffuse alveolar inflammation and consolidation confined to one or more lobes of the lung. Lobar pneumonia is typically the end result of a severe or long-term bronchopneumonia in which the infection has spread from one lung segment to another until the entire lung lobe is involved. **Interstitial pneumonia** is usually a diffuse and often bilateral inflammation that primarily involves the alveolar septa and interstitial spaces. In contrast to alveolar pneumonia caused by bacteria, the polymorphonuclear leukocytes do not migrate into the alveoli—they remain in the alveolar interstitial spaces. Typically, *Mycoplasma pneumoniae* and some viruses cause interstitial pneumonias. Fortunately, most interstitial pneumonias cause only minor permanent alveolar damage and usually resolve without consequences.

When both lungs are involved, the condition is sometimes called "double pneumonia" by laypersons. Although the lay term "walking pneumonia" has no clinical significance, it is often used to describe a mild case of pneumonia. For example, patients infected with *M. pneumoniae*, who generally have mild symptoms and remain ambulatory, are sometimes told that they have "walking pneumonia." Box 18.1 provides common risk factors for pneumonia.

Because the distinction between lobar pneumonia and bronchopneumonia often can be hazy, it is generally best to classify pneumonias either by the specific etiologic agent or, when no specific pathogen can be identified, by the clinical setting in which the pneumonia occurs; for example, **health care–associated pneumonia** or **community-acquired pneumonia**. Box 18.2 provides an overview of seven different clinical settings and the respective pathogens associated with pneumonia. The importance of promptly obtaining a sputum sample for a Gram stain and culture analysis early in the course of the clinical illness cannot be overemphasized. A more in-depth

---

BOX 18.1 Risk Factors for Pneumonia

- Age over 65 years
- Aspiration of oropharyngeal secretions and/or gastric contents
- Viral respiratory infections
- Chronic illness and debilitation (e.g., diabetes mellitus, uremia)
- Chronic respiratory disease (COPD, asthma, cystic fibrosis)
- Cancer (especially lung cancer)
- Prolonged bed rest
- Tracheostomy or endotracheal tube
- Abdominal or thoracic surgery
- Rib fractures
- Immunosuppressive therapy
- AIDS

BOX 18.2 Clinical Settings and Pathogens Associated With Pneumonia

Community-Acquired Typical Pneumonia

- *Streptococcus pneumoniae*
- *Staphylococcus aureus* (also hospital-acquired pneumonia)
- *Haemophilus influenzae*
- *Legionella pneumophila*
- Enterobacteriaceae (*Klebsiella* pneumonia)
- *Moraxella catarrhalis*
- *Pseudomonas aeruginosa* (also hospital-acquired pneumonia)

Community-Acquired Typical Pneumonia

- *Mycoplasma pneumoniae*
- **Coxiella burnetii**
- *Chlamydia* spp.—*C. pneumonia, C. psittaci, C. trachomatis,* and *C. burnetii* (**Q fever**)
- Viruses: Respiratory syncytial virus, parainfluenza virus (children); influenza A and B (adults); adenovirus (military recruits), human metapneumovirus

Hospital-Acquired, Health Care–Associated, and Ventilator-Associated Pneumonia

- Hospital-acquired pneumonia (HAP): *P. aeruginosa,* methicillin-sensitive *S. aureus,* and methicillin-resistant *S. aureus* (MRSA). Other important pathogens include enteric gram-negative bacteria (mainly *Enterobacter* spp., *Klebsiella pneumoniae, Escherichia coli, Serratia marcescens, Proteus* spp., and *Acinetobacter* spp.). Between 4 to 7 days of hospitalization, methicillin-sensitive *S. aureus, Streptococcus pneumoniae,* and *H. influenzae.*
- Health care–associated pneumonia (HCAP): Mixed aerobic and anaerobic mouth flora, *S. aureus,* enteric gram-negative bacillis, influenza, and *M. tuberculosis.*
- Ventilator-associated pneumonia (VAP): *P. aeruginosa, Enterobacter, Klebsiella, Acinetobacter* spp., *Stenotrophomonas maltophilia,* and *S. aureus.*

Aspiration Pneumonia

- Anaerobic oral flora: Gram-positive cocci—peptostreptococci, peptococci; and gram-negative bacilli—*Bacteroides fragilis, Prevotella melaninogenica,* and *Fusobacterium* spp.).
- Anaerobic bacteria mixed with aerobic bacteria such as *Klebsiella, Staphylococcus, Mycobacterium tuberculosis* tuberculosis (including the **atypical organisms** *Mycobacterium kansasii* and *Mycobacterium avium*), *Histoplasma capsulatum, Coccidioides immitis, Blastomyces,* and *Aspergillus fumigatus.*

Chronic Pneumonia

- Granulomatous: *M. tuberculosis* and atypical mycobacteria, *H. capsulatum, C. immitis, Blastomyces dermatitidis*
- *Candida albicans, Cryptococcus neoformans,* and *Aspergillus*
- *Nocardia*
- *Actinomyces*

Pneumonia in the Immunocompromised Host

- Cytomegalovirus
- *Pneumocystis jiroveci*
- *Mycobacterium avium* complex (MAC)
- Invasive aspergillosis
- Invasive candidiasis
- "Usual" bacterial, viral, and fungal organisms (listed above)

Necrotizing Pneumonia and Lung Abscess

- Anaerobic bacteria (extremely common), with or without mixed aerobic infection from *S. aureus, K. pneumoniae, Streptococcus pyogenes,* and type three pneumococcus (uncommon)

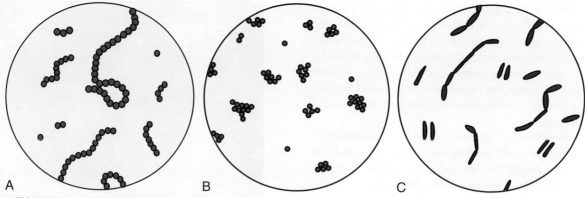

FIGURE 18.4 Microscopic presentation of common causes of pneumonia. (A) The *Streptococcus* organism is a gram-positive, nonmotile bacterium that occurs singly, in pairs, and in short chains. (B) The *Staphylococcus* organism is a gram-positive, nonmotile coccus that is found singly, in pairs, and in irregular clusters. (C) Bacilli are rod-shaped microorganisms and are the major gram-negative organisms responsible for pneumonia.

discussion of these pathogens is presented in the following sections.[2]

Community-Acquired Typical Pneumonia

Community-acquired pneumonia (CAP) refers to a pneumonia acquired from normal social contact (i.e., in the community) as opposed to being acquired while in hospitals or extended-care facilities (e.g., nursing homes). Common causes of a CAP are discussed as follows.

Streptococcus pneumoniae pneumonia (commonly called *pneumococcal pneumonia*) accounts for more than 80% of all the bacterial pneumonias (Fig. 18.4A). ***Streptococcus*** is a **gram-positive organism**, nonmotile coccus that is found singly, in pairs (called *diplococci*), and in short chains. The cocci are enclosed in a smooth, thick polysaccharide capsule that is essential for virulence. There are more than 80 different types of *S. pneumoniae*. Serotype 3 organisms are the most virulent. Streptococci are generally transmitted by aerosol from a cough or sneeze of an infected individual. Most strains of *S. pneumoniae* are sensitive to penicillin and its derivatives. *S. pneumoniae* is also commonly cultured from the sputum of patients having an acute exacerbation of chronic bronchitis.

There are two major groups of ***Staphylococcus:*** (1) ***Staphylococcus aureus***, which is responsible for most "staph" infections in humans, and (2) *Staphylococcus albus* and *Staphylococcus epidermidis*, which are part of the normal skin flora. The staphylococci are gram-positive cocci found singly, in pairs,

and in irregular clusters (see Fig. 18.4B). Staphylococcal pneumonia often follows a predisposing virus infection and is seen most often in children and immunosuppressed adults. *S. aureus* is commonly transmitted by air from a cough or sneeze of an infected individual and indirectly via contact with contaminated floors, bedding, clothes, and the like. Staphylococci are a common cause of **hospital-acquired pneumonia**, or *nosocomial pneumonia* (discussed later in this chapter), and are becoming increasingly antibiotic resistant—thus the term **multiple drug–resistant S. aureus (MDRSA)** organisms (some centers shorten this acronym to *MRSA*).

Haemophilus influenzae is a common inhabitant of human pharyngeal flora. *H. influenzae* is one of the smallest gram-negative bacilli, measuring about 1.5 mm in length and 0.3 mm in width (see Fig. 18.4C). It appears as coccobacilli on Gram stain. There are six types of *H. influenzae*, designated A to F, but only type B is commonly pathogenic. Pneumonia caused by *H. influenzae* type B is seen most often in children 1 month to 6 years old. *H. influenzae* type B is almost always the cause of acute epiglottitis. The organism is transmitted via aerosol or contact with contaminated objects. It is sensitive to cold and does not survive long after expectoration. *H. influenzae* is commonly cultured from the sputum of patients having an acute exacerbation of chronic bronchitis. Additional risk factors for *H. influenzae* infection include COPD, defects in B-cell function, functional and anatomic asplenia, and human immunodeficiency virus (HIV) infection.

In July 1976 a severe pneumonia-like disease outbreak occurred at an American Legion convention in Philadelphia. The causative agent eluded identification for many months, despite the concerted efforts of the nation's top epidemiologic experts. When the organism finally was recovered from a patient, it was found to be an unusual and fastidious gram-negative bacillus with atypical concentrations of certain branched-chain lipids. The initial isolate was designated as ***Legionella pneumophila***. More than 20 *Legionella* spp. have now been identified, and the pneumonia associated with them is termed **Legionnaire's disease**.

Most of the species are free-living in soil and water, where they act as decomposer organisms. The organism also multiplies in standing water such as contaminated mud puddles, large air-conditioning systems, and water tanks. The organism is

---

[2]It is important to note that the infective causes of pneumonia described in this chapter include all those grouped by the Centers for Medicare and Medicaid Services (CMS) in its Specifications Manual for National Inpatient Quality Measures Discharges (2013–2014). Pneumonia is one of three conditions that the CMS is monitoring for excessive readmissions as an indicator of inappropriate, resource-wasteful care. At present, the other two conditions are COPD and congestive heart failure (CHF). The penalties for excessive all-cause readmissions of patients with these conditions has increased to around 4% of the hospital's yearly total Medicare/Medicaid income for the year in question, by 2016. Accordingly, all caregivers must practice meticulous, evidence-based respiratory care if hospitals are to survive economically. Particularly crucial will be the use of the transitional care specialist, in this connection.

transmitted when it becomes airborne and enters the patient's lungs as an aerosol. No convincing evidence suggests that the organism is transmitted from person to person. The organism can be detected in pleural fluid, sputum, or lung tissue by direct fluorescent antibody microscopy. Although it is rarely found outside the lungs, the organism may be found in other tissues. The disease is most commonly seen in middle-aged men who smoke.

Klebsiella pneumoniae (Friedländer bacillus) (Enterobacteriaceae family) organisms have long been associated with lobar pneumonia, particularly in men older than 40 years and in chronic alcoholics of both genders. ***Klebsiella*** is a gram-negative bacillus that is found singly, in pairs, and in chains of varying lengths. It is a normal inhabitant of the human gastrointestinal tract. The organism can be transmitted directly by aerosol or indirectly by contact with freshly contaminated articles. *K. pneumoniae* is a common nosocomial, or hospital-acquired, disease. It is typically transmitted by routes such as clothing, intravenous solutions, foods, and the hands of health care workers. The mortality of patients with *K. pneumoniae* is very high because septicemia is a frequent complication.

Moraxella catarrhalis is a gram-negative diplococcus that commonly colonizes the upper respiratory tract, particularly in children. Research has established that *M. catarrhalis* is an important and common human respiratory tract pathogen. It is often found as a cause of acute otitis media in children and also is associated with exacerbations in adults with COPD.

Pseudomonas aeruginosa is a highly mobile, gram-negative bacillus. It is often found in the gastrointestinal tract, burns, and catheterized urinary tract and is a contaminant in many aqueous solutions. *P. aeruginosa* is frequently cultured from the respiratory tract of patients who are chronically ill and tracheostomized and is a leading cause of health care–associated pneumonia (see page 282). This makes *P. aeruginosa* a particular problem for the respiratory therapist. Risk factors include neutropenia, HIV infection, preexisting lung disease, endotracheal intubation, and previous antibiotic use. Because the *Pseudomonas* organism thrives in dampness, it is often cultured from contaminated respiratory therapy equipment. The organism is commonly transmitted by aerosol or by direct contact with freshly contaminated articles. *P. aeruginosa* grows in a very mucoid colonial form, and the sputum from patients with *Pseudomonas* infection is frequently green and sweet smelling (Fig. 18.5).

Community-Acquired Atypical Pneumonia

The clinical presentation of the patient with community-acquired atypical pneumonia is often subacute. The patient typically presents with a variety of both pulmonary and extrapulmonary findings (e.g., respiratory symptoms such as cough *plus* headache, general fatigue, or diarrhea). Common causes of community-acquired atypical pneumonia are described as follows.

The mycoplasma organism is the most common cause of an acquired atypical pneumonia. The mycoplasma are tiny, cell wall–deficient organisms (Fig. 18.6). They are smaller than bacteria but larger than viruses. The pneumonia caused

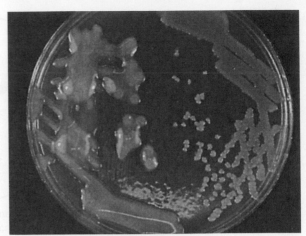

FIGURE 18.5 *Pseudomonas aeruginosa* isolated from the sputum of patients with cystic fibrosis characteristically grows in a very mucoid colonial form (left), with the normal colonial form (right) for comparison. (From Goering, R., Dockrell, H. M., Zuckerman, M., et al. [2013]. *Mims' medical microbiology* [5th ed.]. Philadelphia, PA: Elsevier.)

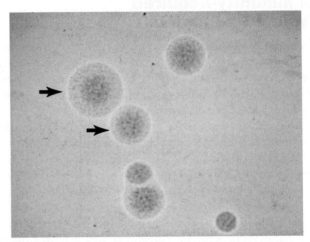

FIGURE 18.6 *Mycoplasma pneumoniae. M. pneumoniae* is a small bacterium that lacks a cell wall. (Courtesy Clinical Microbiology Laboratory, SUNY Upstate Medical University, Syracuse, New York. In Tille, P. M. [2017]. *Bailey and Scott's diagnostic microbiology* [14th ed.]. St. Louis, MO: Elsevier.)

by the mycoplasmal organism is commonly described as a *primary atypical pneumonia.* The term *atypical* refers to the fact that (1) the organism escapes identification by standard bacteriologic tests, (2) there is generally only a moderate amount of expectorated sputum, (3) there is an absence of alveolar consolidation, (4) there is only a moderate elevation of white cell count, and (5) there is a lack of alveolar **exudate**.

The mycoplasma organism causes symptoms similar to those of both bacterial and viral pneumonia, although the symptoms develop more gradually and are often milder. Chills and fever are early symptoms. The patient typically presents with a mild fever and patchy inflammatory changes in the lungs that are mostly confined to the alveolar septa and pulmonary interstitium. A common symptom of mycoplasma pneumonia is a cough that tends to come in violent attacks, producing only a small amount of white mucus. Some patients experience nausea or vomiting. In some cases, the patients may experience a profound weakness that lasts for a long time. Mycoplasma pneumonia is commonly seen among children and young adults. This type of pneumonia spreads easily in areas where people congregate, such as child-care centers, schools, and homeless shelters. Patients with *M. pneumoniae* often are said to have "walking pneumonia" because the condition is mild (i.e., slight fever, fatigue, and a characteristic dry, hacking cough) and the patient is usually ambulatory.

Coxiella burnetii is a gram-negative bacterium that causes **Q fever** in humans. It is more resistant than other rickettsiae and may be passed from infected human aerosols and in living animals such as cattle, sheep, and goats. Acute pneumonia and chronic endocarditis are also associated with this species.

Chlamydia spp. pneumonia (***Chlamydia pneumoniae***, ***Chlamydia psittaci***, ***Chlamydia trachomatis***) and *C. burnetii* (Q fever) closely resemble the clinical manifestations of those caused by *M. pneumoniae*. *Chlamydia* is a type of bacterium that may be found in the cervix, urethra, rectum, throat, and respiratory tract. Chlamydia is also found in the feces of a variety of birds (e.g., parrots, parakeets, lorikeets, cockatoos, chickens, pigeons, ducks, pheasants, turkeys). The clinical manifestations of *C. psittaci* closely resemble those caused by *M. pneumoniae*.

Viruses account for about 50% of all pneumonias, and several are associated with a community-acquired atypical pneumonia. Although most viruses attack the upper airways, some can produce pneumonia. Most of these pneumonias are not life-threatening and last only a short time. Viral pneumonia tends to start with flulike signs and symptoms. The early symptoms are a dry (nonproductive) cough, headache, fever, muscle pain, and fatigue. As the disease progresses, the patient may become short of breath, cough, and produce a small amount of clear or white sputum. *Viral pneumonia always carries the risk for development of a secondary bacterial pneumonia.*

Viruses are minute organisms not visible by ordinary light microscopy. They are parasitic and depend on nutrients inside cells for their metabolic and reproductive needs. About 90% of acute upper respiratory tract infections are caused by viruses. Respiratory viruses are the most common cause of pneumonia in young children, peaking between the ages of 2 and 3 years. By school age, *M. pneumoniae* pneumonia becomes more prevalent (see previous section).

Common viruses associated with community-acquired atypical pneumonia include *respiratory syncytial virus, parainfluenza virus* (children), *influenza A and B* (adults), *adenovirus* (military recruits), and *human metapneumovirus*. These viruses are discussed in more detail as follows.

The **respiratory syncytial virus (RSV)** (see Chapter 39, Respiratory Syncytial Virus [Bronchiolitis]) is a member of the paramyxovirus group. Parainfluenza, mumps, and **rubella** viruses also belong to this group. RSV is most often seen in children younger than 12 months of age and in older adults with underlying heart or pulmonary disease. Almost all children will be infected with RSV by their second birthday. The infection is rarely fatal in infants. RSV often goes unrecognized but may play an important role as a forerunner to bacterial infections. Early attempts to develop an RSV vaccine have been unsuccessful. The virus is transmitted by the aerosol route and by direct contact with infected individuals. RSV infections are most commonly seen in patients during the late fall, winter, or early spring months. Many times the virus is misdiagnosed in older children, who are given antibiotics that do not produce improvement.

The **parainfluenza viruses** are also members of the paramyxovirus group and therefore are related to mumps, rubella, and RSV. There are five types of parainfluenza viruses: types 1, 2, 3, 4A, and 4B. Types 1, 2, and 3 are the major causes of infections in humans. Type 1 is considered a **croup** type of virus. Types 2 and 3 are associated with severe infections. Although type 3 is seen in persons of all ages, it usually is seen in infants younger than 2 months of age; types 1 and 2 are seen most often in children between the ages of 6 months and 5 years. Types 1 and 2 typically occur in the fall, whereas type 3 infection most often is seen in the late spring and summer. Parainfluenza viruses are transmitted by aerosol droplets and by direct person-to-person contact. The parainfluenza viruses are known for their ability to spread rapidly among members of the same family.

The **influenza viruses** A and B are the most common causes of viral respiratory tract infections. In the United States, influenza A and B commonly occur in epidemics during the winter months. Children, young adults, and older individuals are most at risk. Influenza is transmitted from person to person by aerosol droplets. Often the first sign of an epidemic is an increase in school absenteeism. The virus survives well in conditions of low temperatures and low humidity. It also has been found in horses, swine, and birds. Influenza viruses have an incubation period of 1 to 3 days and usually cause upper respiratory tract infections. Epidemiologists fear a pandemic of influenza, stating it is an issue of "when" and "where" rather than "if." The 2013 epidemic of H1 avian influenza is a case in point.

The **adenovirus** serotypes 4, 7, 14, and 21 cause viral infections and pneumonia in all age groups. Serotype 7 has been related to fatal cases of pneumonia in children. Adenoviruses are transmitted by aerosol. Pneumonia caused by adenoviruses generally occurs during the fall, winter, and spring.

The **human metapneumovirus (hMPV)** is a negative single-stranded RNA virus associated with a family of viruses that also includes RSV virus and parainfluenza virus. After RSV, hMPV is the second most common cause of lower respiratory tract infections in young children. In comparison to RSV, the hMPV tends to occur in older children and is less severe. Most patients with hMPV infection have mild symptoms, including cough, runny nose or nasal congestion, sore throat, and fever. More severe cases demonstrate wheezing, difficulty breathing, hoarseness, cough, and pneumonia.

Hospital-Acquired, Health Care–Associated, and Ventilator-Associated Pneumonia

Hospital-acquired pneumonia (HAP) (also called *hospital-associated* and *nosocomial pneumonia*) is defined as pneumonia that occurs 48 hours or more after hospital admission and that was not present at the time of admission. In general, the most important pathogens are *P. aeruginosa*, methicillin-sensitive *Staphylococcus aureus*, and methicillin-resistant *S.*

aureus (MRSA). Other important pathogens include enteric gram-negative bacteria (mainly ***Enterobacter* spp.**, *K. pneumoniae*, ***Escherichia coli*, *Serratia marcescens*, *Proteus* spp., and *Acinetobacter* spp. In the patient who develops pneumonia between 4 and 7 days of hospitalization, the most common pathogens are MRSA, *S. pneumoniae,* and *H. influenza*. In patients hospitalized longer than 7 days, *P. aeruginosa*, MRSA, and enteric **gram-negative organisms** are common causes of pneumonia.

Health care–associated pneumonia (HCAP) refers to patients who have recently been hospitalized in an acute-care hospital within 90 days of the infection, who have resided in a nursing home or long-term care facility, or who have received parenteral antimicrobial therapy, chemotherapy, or wound care within 30 days of pneumonia. Common pathogens include mixed aerobic and anaerobic mouth flora, *S. aureus*, enteric gram-negative bacillis, influenza, and *M. tuberculosis*.

Ventilator-associated pneumonia (VAP) (also called *ventilator-acquired pneumonia*) can also be included under the nosocomial pneumonia category. A VAP is defined as a pneumonia of infectious disease origin that develops more than 48 to 72 hours after endotracheal intubation. Common ventilator-associated infection agents include *P. aeruginosa, Enterobacter, Klebsiella, Acinetobacter* spp., *Stenotrophomonas maltophilia*, and *S. aureus*. Concern that the occurrence of VAP is preventable lies as the root of possible reimbursement penalties for hospitals in which it occurs.

Aspiration Pneumonia

Common pathogenic agents associated with *aspiration pneumonia* include anaerobic oral flora (***Peptostreptococcus*, peptococci, *Bacteroides fragilis*, *Prevotella melaninogenica***, and *Fusobacterium* spp.), admixed with aerobic bacteria such as *Klebsiella, Staphylococcus*, and *Mycobacterium tuberculosis*.

Aspiration of gastric fluid with a pH of 2.5 or less causes a serious and often fatal form of pneumonia. Aspiration of oropharyngeal secretions and gastric fluids are the major causes of anaerobic lung infections (see discussion of anaerobic bacterial infections earlier). Aspiration pneumonitis is commonly missed because acute inflammatory reactions may not begin until several hours after observed aspiration of the gastric fluid. The inflammatory reaction generally increases in severity for 12 to 26 hours and may progress to acute respiratory distress syndrome (ARDS), which includes interstitial and intraalveolar edema, intraalveolar hyaline membrane formation, and atelectasis. In the absence of a secondary bacterial infection, the inflammation usually becomes clinically insignificant in approximately 72 hours. In 1946, Mendelson first described the clinical manifestations of tachycardia, dyspnea, and cyanosis associated with the aspiration of acid stomach contents. The clinical picture he described is now known as **Mendelson syndrome** and is usually confined to aspiration pneumonitis in pregnant women.

Aspiration pneumonia is broadly defined as the pulmonary result of the entry of material from the stomach or upper respiratory tract into the lower airways. There are at least three distinctive forms of aspiration pneumonia, classified according to the nature of the aspirate, the clinical presentation, and management guidelines, as follows:

1. Toxic injury to the lung (such as that caused by gastric acid)
2. Obstruction (by foreign bodies or fluids)
3. Infection

Aspiration is presumed to be the cause of nearly all cases of anaerobic pulmonary infections. Studies suggest that anaerobic bacteria are also the most common causative agents of lung abscesses; they are also commonly isolated in cases of empyema.

There is a difference between the aspiration of gastric contents and the aspiration of food. Aspiration of gastric contents causes initial hypoxemia regardless of the pH level of the aspirate. *Consequently, oximetry is a good measurement if aspiration is suspected*. If the pH of the aspirate is relatively high (greater than 5.9), the initial injury is rapidly reversible. Such aspiration occurs in patients who receive antacids or proton pump inhibitors (PPIs). If the pH is low (pH of unbuffered gastric contents normally ranges from 1 to 1.5), parenchymal damage may occur, with inflammation, edema, and hemorrhage. When food is aspirated, obliterative bronchiolitis with subsequent granuloma formation occurs.

Gastroesophageal reflux disease (GERD) is the regurgitation of stomach contents into the esophagus. GERD causes disruption in nerve-mediated reflexes in the distal esophagus, resulting in alteration of the primary and secondary esophageal peristaltic wave and reflux. Therefore "to-and-fro" peristalsis can result from spasticity at the distal esophageal sphincter and retropulsion of middle and upper esophageal contents. This may result in aspiration, although not necessarily.

GERD is three times more prevalent in patients with asthma than in other patients. In other words, GERD is a frequently unrecognized cause of asthma. Presumably, acid reflux into the esophagus causes vagal stimulation, resulting in a reflexive increase in bronchial tone in patients with asthma. Recent literature suggests that asymptomatic reflux does not contribute to worsening lung function, although it and chronic sinusitis are the two most unrecognized causes of chronic cough. GERD causes chronic cough in 10% to 20% of patients.

Normal **swallowing mechanics** has four phases, as follows:
1. Oral preparatory
2. Oral
3. Pharyngeal
4. Esophageal

The first two phases are considered voluntary stages (cerebral). These phases occur as the food or liquid is prepared for entry to the pharynx and esophagus. The airway is open while food is prepared in the oral cavity. Adequate tongue function is important for the manipulation and propulsion of the prepared food or liquid (called a *bolus*) into the pharynx. Spillage of liquid into the pharynx during the chewing of food is usually not a problem in patients with good airway protection.

The pharyngeal phase (involuntary brain stem function) of swallowing involves numerous physiologic actions that direct the bolus into the esophagus:
- Elevation and retraction of the velopharyngeal port (velum closure)
- Pharyngeal muscle contraction

- Elevation and forward excursion of the larynx (epiglottic closure)
- Closure of the laryngeal vestibule, false vocal folds, and true vocal folds (laryngeal closure)
- Relaxation of the upper esophageal sphincter (UES)

Airway closure progresses inferiorly to superiorly in the larynx as the food bolus is directed laterally around the airway and into the esophagus.

Respiration is halted during the pharyngeal phase for approximately 1 second, although duration varies with bolus volume and viscosity. Bolus transit in the esophageal phase (under both brain stem and intrinsic neural control) lasts 8 to 20 seconds. In this phase, the UES relaxes to receive the bolus with a peristaltic wave from the pharyngeal superior constrictor muscles, forcing the bolus through the relaxed UES. The primary peristalsis propels the bolus through the esophagus and lower esophageal sphincter and into the stomach.

Six cranial nerves carry motor signals generated by cerebral and brain stem swallowing centers:

- V (trigeminal)
- VII (facial)
- IX (glossopharyngeal)
- X (vagus)
- XI (spinal accessory [minor involvement])
- XII (hypoglossal)

The relationship between respiration and swallowing is not random. Expiration before and after the pharyngeal phase in normal swallowing is believed to serve as an inherent closure and clearance mechanism against penetration of food or liquids into the airway entrance.

Dysphagia is the result of an abnormal swallow that can involve the oral, pharyngeal, and esophageal phases. Penetration into the laryngeal vestibule occurs when food or liquid (or both) enters the larynx but does not pass through the vocal cords into the trachea. Aspiration is the passage of food or liquid into the trachea via the vocal cords.

Diagnostic tests for dysphagia include the modified barium swallow, video fluoroscopy, video-fiberoptic endoscopy, and the modified Evans blue dye tests. The **Evans blue dye test** involves instilling a deep blue dye into the gastrointestinal tract and seeing if it can be suctioned from the trachea. If it can, it suggests a communication between the two structures, such as a **tracheoesophageal fistula**. The modified barium swallow and **cine-videofluoroscopy** tests are most definitive for identification of the particular phase of the swallow that is dysfunctional. The modified Evans blue dye test can be unreliable (as much as 40% of the time) as a test suggesting aspiration in a patient who is tracheostomized. In it, both false-positive and false-negative test results occur.

A compromised respiratory system can cause dysphagia and, conversely, dysphagia may cause respiratory complications. COPD can result in a slowed oral and pharyngeal transit time, reduced coordination and strength of the oral and pharyngeal musculature, and reduced airway clearance by coughing.

Treatment of dysphagia is specific to the nature of the disorder. Varied methods of presentation of foods and liquids, bolus volumes and consistency, postural movements, and food temperature can affect the dynamics of the relation between respiration and swallowing. Large volumes of liquid requiring uninterrupted swallowing can be difficult for patients who are short of breath. Small-volume bites and swallows make sense in this setting.

Unilateral cerebrovascular accidents (strokes) and hemorrhage tend to cause hypopharyngeal hemiparesis. Difficulty in swallowing (with impairment of the oral phase) and aspiration of thin fluids therefore may follow. The facial and tongue weakness associated with such conditions can result in poor bolus control in the oral cavity.

Silent aspiration is defined as aspiration that does not evoke clinically observable adverse symptoms such as overt coughing, choking, and immediate respiratory distress. Some patients have silent aspiration after a stroke (see Chapter 31, Respiratory Insufficiency in the Patient With Neurorespiratory Disease). Evidence also suggests that some sequelae of stroke include laryngopharyngeal sensory deficits with *no* subjective or objective evidence of dysphagia, such as choking, gagging, or cough.

Some patients with severe and bilateral sensory deficits develop aspiration pneumonia. The clinical findings of **dysphonia**, **dysarthria**, abnormal gag reflex, abnormal volitional cough, cough after swallow, and voice change after swallow all significantly relate to aspiration and are predictors of silent aspiration. Conversely, a normal reflex cough after a stroke indicates an intact laryngeal cough reflex, a protected airway, and low risk for developing aspiration pneumonia with oral feeding. The cough reflex is significantly reduced in older patients.

Patients with a tracheostomy are at high risk for silent aspiration. *It is estimated that 55% to 70% of intubated or tracheostomy patients aspirate.* A tracheostomy tube has a direct effect on the pharyngeal phase of a swallow because of the alteration of normal respiratory function (exhalation timing) and the anatomic alteration and the physical resistance imposed by the tracheostomy tube itself. Normal laryngeal elevation during swallowing is reduced, particularly with the cuff inflated, which leads to inadequate airway closure and increased pharyngeal residue.

Poor sensory response to material entering the larynx contributes to the slowing of an uncoordinated laryngeal closure. The protective cough may be lessened because of the impaired laryngeal sensation. Subglottic air pressure (coordinated exhalation with swallow) helps prevent entry of material into the trachea and is reduced in patients with a tracheostomy. An inflated cuffed tracheostomy can cause complications that can anchor the larynx to the anterior wall of the neck and desensitize the pharynx. Delayed triggering of the swallowing response and increased pharyngeal residue are prevalent.

Recommendations for oral feeding include considerations of dietary consistency, specifically defined for solids and liquids, skilled supervision with oral intake, safe swallowing strategies, positioning requirements, cuff deflation, and tracheal occlusion issues. It may be necessary to coordinate mealtime with ventilator weaning attempts to optimize more positive pressure generation to aid in expelling laryngeal residue and creating subglottic pressure.

The dynamic changes a patient may experience clinically necessitate a coordinated team approach, including physical,

Chronic Pneumonia

Chronic pneumonia is typically a localized lesion in patients with a normal immune system, with or without regional lymph node involvement. Patients with chronic pneumonia usually have granulomatous inflammation. **Granulomas** associated with chronic pneumonia are commonly seen in patients with tuberculosis and fungal diseases of the lung. In patients whose immune system is compromised (e.g., patients with HIV), the dissemination of the causative organism throughout the body is the usual presentation. **Tuberculosis** is by far the most important organism within the category of chronic pneumonias and will be fully presented in Chapter 19, Tuberculosis.

Fungal Diseases: Anatomic Alterations of the Lungs

Because most fungi are aerobes, the lung is a prime site for **fungal infections**. When fungal spores are inhaled, they may reach the lungs and germinate. When this happens, the spores produce a frothy, yeastlike substance that leads to an inflammatory response. Polymorphonuclear leukocytes and macrophages move into the infected area and engulf the fungal spores. The pulmonary capillaries dilate, the interstitium fills with fluid, and the alveolar epithelium swells with edema fluid. Regional lymph node involvement commonly occurs during this period. Because of the inflammatory reaction, the alveoli in the infected area eventually become consolidated (Fig. 18.7).

In severe cases, tissue necrosis, granulomas, and **cavity formation** may be seen. During the healing process, fibrosis and calcification of the lung parenchyma ultimately replace the granulomas. In response to the fibrosis and occasional calcification, the lung tissue retracts and becomes firm. The apical and posterior segments of the upper lobes are most commonly involved. The anatomic changes of the lungs caused by fungal diseases are similar to those seen in tuberculosis.

Fungal diseases of the lung cause a chronic restrictive pulmonary disorder. The major pathologic or structural changes of the lungs associated with fungal diseases of the lungs are as follows:
- Alveolar consolidation
- Alveolar-capillary destruction
- **Caseous tubercles** or granulomas
- Cavity formation
- Fibrosis and secondary calcification of the lung parenchyma
Fungal spores of various types are widely distributed throughout the air, soil, fomites, and animals and even exist in the normal flora of humans. As many as 300 fungal species may be linked to disease in animals. In plants, fungal disease is the most common cause of death and destruction. In humans, most exposures to fungal pathogens do *not* lead to overt infection because humans have a relatively high resistance to

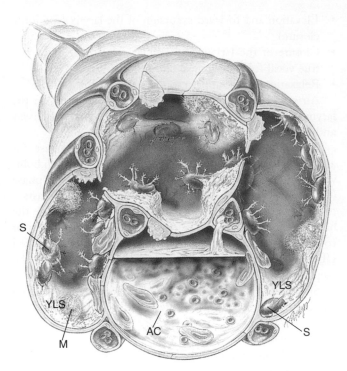

FIGURE 18.7 Fungal disease of the lung. Cross-sectional view of alveoli infected with *Histoplasma capsulatum. AC,* Alveolar consolidation; *M,* alveolar macrophage; *S,* fungal spore; *YLS,* yeastlike substance.

them. Human fungal disease (also called *mycotic disease* or *mycosis*) can be caused by primary or "true" fungal pathogens that exhibit some degree of virulence or by opportunistic or secondary pathogens that take advantage of a weakened immune defense system (e.g., in acquired immunodeficiency syndrome and HIV infection).

Primary Pathogens

Histoplasmosis

Histoplasmosis is the most common fungal infection in the United States. It is caused by the dimorphic fungus *Histoplasma capsulatum.* In the United States, the prevalence of histoplasmosis is especially high along the major river valleys of the Midwest and South (e.g., in Ohio, Michigan, Illinois, Mississippi, Missouri, Kentucky, Tennessee, Georgia, and Arkansas). On the basis of skin test surveys it is estimated that 80% to 90% of the population throughout these areas shows signs of previous infection. Histoplasmosis is often called "Ohio Valley Fever."

H. capsulatum is commonly found in soils enriched with bird excreta, such as the soil near chicken houses, pigeon lofts, barns, and trees where starlings and blackbirds roost. The birds themselves, however, do not carry the organism, although the *H. capsulatum* spore may be carried by bats. Generally, an individual acquires the infection by inhaling the fungal spores that are released when the soil from an infected area is disturbed (e.g., children playing in dirt).

When the *H. capsulatum* organism reaches the alveoli at body temperature, it converts from its mycelial form (mold) to a parasitic yeast form. The clinical manifestations of histoplasmosis are strikingly similar to those of tuberculosis. The incubation period for the infection is approximately 17 days. Only about 40% of those infected demonstrate symptoms, and only about 10% of these patients are ill enough to consult a physician. Depending on the individual's immune system, the disease may take one of the following forms: asymptomatic primary histoplasmosis, acute symptomatic pulmonary histoplasmosis, chronic histoplasmosis, or disseminated histoplasmosis.

Asymptomatic histoplasmosis is the most common form of histoplasmosis. Normally it produces no signs or symptoms in otherwise healthy individuals who become infected. The only residual sign of infection may be a small, healed lesion of the lung parenchyma or calcified hilar lymph nodes. The patient will have a positive **histoplasmin skin test** result, much like that for tuberculosis described in Chapter 19, Tuberculosis.

Acute symptomatic pulmonary histoplasmosis tends to occur in otherwise healthy individuals who have had an intense exposure to *H. capsulatum*. Depending on the number of spores inhaled, the individual signs and symptoms may range from mild to serious illness. Mild signs and symptoms include fever, muscle and joint pain, headache, dry hacking cough, chills, chest pain, weight loss, and sweats. People who have inhaled a large number of spores may develop a severe acute pulmonary syndrome, a potentially life-threatening condition in which the individual becomes extremely short of breath. This is often referred to as *spelunker lung* because it frequently develops after excessive exposure to bat excrement stirred up by individuals exploring caves. During this phase of the disease, the patient's chest radiograph generally shows single or multiple infection sites resembling those associated with pneumonia.

Chronic pulmonary histoplasmosis is characterized by infiltration and cavity formation in the upper lobes of one or both lungs. This type of histoplasmosis often affects people with an underlying lung disease such as emphysema. It is most commonly seen in middle-aged white men who smoke. Signs and symptoms include fatigue, fever, night sweats, weight loss, productive cough, and hemoptysis—similar to signs and symptoms of tuberculosis. Often the infection is self-limiting. In some patients, however, progressive destruction of lung tissue and dissemination of the infection may occur.

Disseminated histoplasmosis may follow either self-limited histoplasmosis or chronic histoplasmosis. It is most often seen in very young or very old patients with compromised immune systems (e.g., patients with HIV infection). Even though the macrophages can remove the fungi from the bloodstream, they are unable to kill the fungal organisms. As a result, disseminated histoplasmosis can affect nearly any part of the body, including eyes, liver, bone marrow, skin, adrenal glands, and intestinal tract. Depending on which body organs are affected, the patient may develop anemia, pneumonia, pericarditis, meningitis, or adrenal insufficiency and ulcers of the mouth, tongue, or intestinal tract. If untreated, disseminated histoplasmosis is usually fatal.

Screening and Diagnosis

Fungal Culture. The fungal culture test is considered the gold standard for detecting histoplasmosis. A small amount

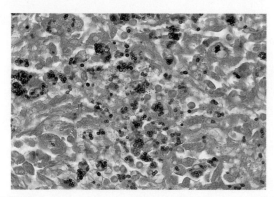

FIGURE 18.8 *Histoplasma capsulatum.* This is a micrograph of tissue infected with *H. capsulatum*, a fungus whose yeast cell stage causes histoplasmosis. (From Tille, P. M. [2017]. *Bailey and Scott's diagnostic microbiology* [14th ed.]. St. Louis, MO: Elsevier.)

of blood, sputum, or tissue from a lymph node, lung, or bone marrow is cultured. The disadvantage of this test is that it takes time for the fungus to grow—4 weeks or longer. For this reason, it is not the test of choice in cases of disseminated histoplasmosis. Treatment delays in patients may prove fatal.

Fungal Stain. In the fungal stain test a sample, which may be obtained from sputum or tissues such as bone marrow, lungs, or a skin lesion, is stained with dye and examined under a microscope for *H. capsulatum* (Fig. 18.8). A positive test result is 100% accurate. The disadvantage of this test is that obtaining a sputum sample can be difficult, and obtaining a sample from other sites requires invasive procedures.

Serology. A blood serology test checks blood serum for antigens and antibodies. When an individual is exposed to histoplasmosis spores (antigens), the body's immune system produces antibodies (proteins) to react to the histoplasmosis antigens. Tests that check for histoplasmosis antigen and antibody reactions are relatively fast and fairly accurate. False-negative results, however, may occur in people who have compromised immune systems or who are infected with other types of fungi.

Coccidioidomycosis

Coccidioidomycosis is caused by inhalation of the spores of *Coccidioides immitis*, which are spherical fungi carried by wind-borne dust particles. The disease is endemic in hot, dry regions. In the United States, coccidioidomycosis is especially prevalent in California, Arizona, Nevada, New Mexico, Texas, and Utah. About 80% of the people in the San Joaquin Valley have positive coccidioidin skin-test results. Because the prevalence of coccidioidomycosis is high in these regions, the disease is also known as "California fever," "desert rheumatism," **San Joaquin Valley Fever**, and "Valley Fever." The fungus has been isolated in these regions from soils, plants, and a large number of vertebrates (e.g., mammals, birds, reptiles, and amphibians).

When *C. immitis* spores are inhaled, they settle in the lungs, begin to germinate, and form round, thin-walled cells called *spherules*. The spherules, in turn, contain endospores that make more spherules (the spherule-endospore phase). The disease usually takes the form of an acute, primary, self-limiting

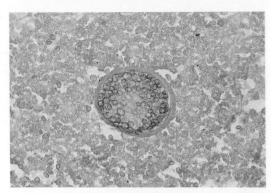

FIGURE 18.9 *Coccidioides immitis.* This is a micrograph of *C. immitis,* a dimorphic fungus that causes coccidioidomycosis. The numerous small spherules are seen within the large, encircling outer capsule. (From Tille, P. M. [2017]. *Bailey and Scott's diagnostic microbiology* [14th ed.]. St. Louis, MO: Elsevier.)

pulmonary infection with or without systemic involvement. Some cases, however, progress to disseminated disease.

Clinical manifestations are absent in about 60% of the people who have a positive skin-test result. In the remaining 40%, cold-like symptoms such as fever, chest pain, cough, headaches, and malaise are often present. In uncomplicated cases, patients generally recover completely and enjoy lifelong immunity. In approximately 1 in 200 cases, however, the primary infection does not resolve and progresses with varied clinical manifestations. Chronic progressive pulmonary disease is characterized by nodular growths called *fungomas* and cavity formation in the lungs. Disseminated coccidioidomycosis occurs in about 1 in 6000 exposed persons. When this condition exists, the lymph nodes, meninges, spleen, liver, kidney, skin, and adrenals may be involved. The skin lesions (e.g., bumps on the face and chest) are commonly accompanied by arthralgia or arthritis, especially in the ankles and knees. This condition is commonly called "desert bumps," "**desert arthritis**," or "desert rheumatism."

Screening and Diagnosis

The diagnosis of coccidioidomycosis can be made by direct visualization of distinctive spherules in microscopy of the patient's sputum, tissue exudates, biopsy samples, or spinal fluid (Fig. 18.9). The diagnosis can be further supported by blood tests that detect antibodies to the fungus or from a culture of the organism from infected fluid or tissue.

Blastomycosis

Blastomycosis (also called "Chicago disease," Gilchrist disease, and **North American blastomycosis**) is caused by *Blastomyces dermatitidis.* Blastomycosis occurs in people living in the south-central and midwestern United States and in Canada. The infection occurs in 1 to 2 of every 100,000 people in these areas. Cases also have been reported in Central America, South America, Africa, and the Middle East. *B. dermatitidis* inhabits areas high in organic matter, such as forest soil, decaying wood, animal manure, and abandoned buildings. Blastomycosis is most common among pregnant women and middle-aged African-American men. The disease also is found in dogs, cats, and horses.

The primary portal of entry of *B. dermatitidis* is the lungs. The acute clinical manifestations resemble those of acute histoplasmosis, including fever, cough, hoarseness, joint and muscle aches, and, in some cases, pleuritic pain. Unlike in histoplasmosis infection, however, the cough is frequently productive and the sputum is purulent. Acute pulmonary infections may be self-limiting or progressive. When the condition is progressive, nodules and abscesses develop in the lungs. Extrapulmonary lesions commonly involve the skin, bones, reproductive tract, spleen, liver, kidney, or prostate gland. The skin lesions may, in fact, be the first signs of the disease. It often begins on the face, hands, wrists, or legs as subcutaneous nodules that erode to the skin surface. Yeast dissemination also may cause arthritis and osteomyelitis, and involvement of the central nervous system causes headache, seizures, coma, and mental confusion. Standardized serologic testing procedures for blastomycosis are not available, and neither is an accurate blastomycin skin test. The diagnosis of blastomycosis can be made from direct visualization of the yeast in sputum smears, or the fungus can be cultured.

Opportunistic Pathogens

Opportunistic yeast pathogens such as *Candida albicans, Cryptococcus neoformans,* and *Aspergillus* also are associated with lung infections in certain patients.

C. albicans occurs as normal flora in the oral cavity, genitalia, and large intestine. *C. albicans* infection of the mouth, or **thrush**, is characterized by a white, adherent, patchy infection of the mouth, gums, cheeks, and throat. In patients with HIV infection, *C. albicans* often causes infection of the mouth, pharynx, vagina, skin, and lungs.

C. neoformans proliferates in the high nitrogen content of pigeon droppings and is readily scattered into the air and dust. Today, *Cryptococcus* is most often seen in patients with HIV infection and persons undergoing steroid therapy.

Aspergillus may be the most pervasive of all fungi (Fig. 18.10). *Aspergillus* is found in soil, vegetation, leaf detritus, food, and compost heaps. Persons breathing the air of granaries, barns, and silos are at greatest risk. *Aspergillus* infection usually occurs in the lungs, where it may present in the form of **allergic bronchopulmonary aspergillosis (ABPA)**, a form of asthma (see Chapter 14, Asthma). It is almost always an opportunistic infection and poses a serious threat to patients with HIV infection.

Pneumonia in the Immunocompromised Host

Cytomegalovirus (CMV), a member of the herpesvirus family, is the most common viral pulmonary complication of AIDS. CMV infection commonly coexists with *Pneumocystis jiroveci* infection.

Pneumocystis jiroveci (also formerly known as *Pneumocystis carinii*) pneumonia is an opportunistic, often fatal, form of pneumonia seen in patients who are profoundly immunosuppressed. Although the *Pneumocystis* organism has been identified as a protozoan, recent information suggests that it is more closely related to fungi. *Pneumocystis* can normally be found in the lungs of humans, but it does not cause disease in healthy hosts, only

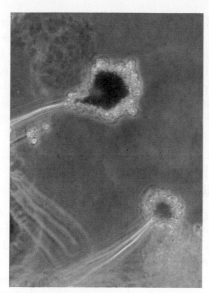

FIGURE 18.10 *Aspergillus* spp. This is a micrograph of *Aspergillus,* an opportunistic fungal pathogen that can cause a variety of diseases collectively called *aspergillosis.* (From VanMeter, K. C., Hubert, R. J. [2016]. *Microbiology for the healthcare professional.* St. Louis, MO: Elsevier.)

in individuals whose immune systems are critically impaired. Currently, *Pneumocystis* pneumonia is the major pulmonary infection seen in patients with AIDS and HIV infection.

In vulnerable hosts the disease spreads rapidly throughout the lungs. Before AIDS, *P. jiroveci* pneumonia was seen primarily in patients with malignancy, in organ transplant recipients, and in patients with diseases requiring treatment with large doses of immunosuppressive agents. Today, most cases of *P. jiroveci* pneumonia are seen in patients with AIDS. The early clinical manifestations of *Pneumocystis* in patients with AIDS are indistinguishable from those of any other pneumonia. Typical signs and symptoms include progressive exertional dyspnea, a dry cough that may or may not produce mucoid sputum, difficulty in taking a deep breath (not caused by pleurisy), and fever with or without sweats. The therapist may hear normal breath sounds on auscultation or end-inspiratory crackles. The chest x-ray film may be normal at first; later it will show bilateral interstitial infiltrates, which may progress to alveolar filling and "white out" of the chest x-ray film.

Mycobacterium avium **complex (MAC)** is a serious opportunistic infection that is caused by two similar bacteria: *Mycobacterium avium* and *Mycobacterium intercellulare.* MAC is found in the soil and dust particles. MAC is commonly found in patients with AIDS. The mode of infection is usually inhalation or ingestion. MAC can spread through the bloodstream to infect lymph nodes, bone marrow, the liver, the spleen, spinal fluid, the lungs, and the intestinal tract. Typical symptoms of MAC include fever, night sweats, weight loss, fatigue, anemia, diarrhea, and enlarged spleen.

Invasive aspergillosis is a general term used for a wide variety of infections caused by the fungi of the genus *Aspergillus.* The most common forms are allergic bronchopulmonary aspergillosis, pulmonary aspergilloma, and invasive aspergillosis. Most humans inhale *Aspergillus* spores every day. However, in individuals who are immunocompromised, an aspergillosis pneumonia may develop.

Invasive candidiasis is a general term describing fungal infections caused by a variety of species of the genus *Candida,* most often by *Candida albicans,* a yeastlike fungus. These fungi are normally found in the mouth, vagina, and intestines of healthy individuals. Under normal circumstances, the normal bacteria in these areas keep the amount of *Candida* spp. in balance. However, in patients with a weakened immune system (such as people with HIV/AIDS), the fungi can invade tissue that normally would be resistant to infection—thus, producing an opportunistic infection. *Candida* infections can involve any part of the body. In some cases, the fungus enters the bloodstream and causes invasive disease affecting internal body organs such as the kidneys, spleen, lungs, liver, eyes, meninges, brain, and heart valves.

Other Causes

Rickettsiae

Rickettsiae are small, pleomorphic coccobacilli. Most rickettsiae are intracellular parasites possessing both ribonucleic acid (RNA) and deoxyribonucleic acid (DNA). There are several members of the *Rickettsia* family that cause **rickettsial infections**: *Rickettsia rickettsii* (Rocky Mountain spotted fever), *Rickettsia akari* (rickettsialpox), *Rickettsia prowazekii* (typhus), and *Rickettsia burnetii,* also called *Coxiella burnetii* (Q fever).

All species of the genus *Rickettsia* are unstable outside of cells except for *R. burnetii* (Q fever), which is extremely resistant to heat and light. Q fever can cause pneumonia and a prolonged febrile illness, an influenza-like illness, and endocarditis. The organism is commonly transmitted by arthropods (lice, fleas, ticks, mites). It also may be transmitted by cattle, sheep, goats, and possibly in raw milk.

Varicella (Chickenpox)

The **varicella** virus usually causes a benign disease in children aged 2 to 8 years, and complications of varicella are not common. In some cases, however, varicella has been noted to spread to the lungs and cause a serious secondary pneumonitis. The mortality rate of varicella pneumonia is about 20%.

Rubella (Measles)

Measles virus spreads from person to person by the respiratory route. Respiratory complications are often encountered in measles because of the widespread involvement of the mucosa of the respiratory tract (e.g., excessive bronchial secretions and infection).

Severe Acute Respiratory Syndrome

In 2002, China reported the first case of **severe acute respiratory syndrome (SARS)**. Shortly after this report, the disease was documented in numerous countries, including Vietnam, Singapore, and Indonesia. Both the United States and Canada have reported imported cases. Health officials believe that the cause of SARS is a newly recognized virus strain called a **coronavirus**. Other viruses, however, are still under investigation as potential causes. Coronaviruses are a group of viruses that have a halo-like or corona-like appearance when observed under an electron microscope. Known forms of coronavirus cause common colds and upper respiratory tract infections. SARS is highly contagious on close personal contact with infected individuals. It spreads through droplet transmission by coughing and sneezing. SARS might be transmitted through the air or from objects that have become contaminated.

The incubation period for SARS is typically 2 to 7 days. Initially, the patient usually develops a fever (>100.4°F [>38.0°C]), followed by chills, headaches, general feeling of discomfort, and body aches. Toward the end of the incubation period, the patient with SARS usually develops a dry, nonproductive cough, shortness of breath, and malaise. In severe cases, hypoxemia develops. According to the Centers for Disease Control and Prevention (CDC), 10% to 20% of patients with SARS require mechanical ventilation. In spite of this fact, death from SARS is rare. No specific treatment recommendations exist at this time. The CDC, however, recommends that patients with SARS receive the same treatment used for any patient with serious community-acquired atypical pneumonia of unknown cause.

Lipoid Pneumonitis

The aspiration of mineral oil, used medically as a lubricant, has been known to cause pneumonitis—**lipoid pneumonitis**. The severity of the pneumonia depends on the type of oil aspirated. Oils from animal fats cause the most serious reaction, whereas oils of vegetable origin are relatively inert. When mineral oil is inhaled in an aerosolized form, an intense pulmonary tissue reaction occurs.

Avian Influenza A

Avian influenza A (also called *bird flu* and *H5N1*) is a subtype of the A strain virus and is highly contagious in birds. Historically, bird flu has not been known to infect humans. However, in Hong Kong in 1997 the first avian influenza virus to infect humans directly was reported. This outbreak was linked to chickens and classified as avian influenza A (H5N1). Since

the Hong Kong outbreak, the bird flu virus has been reported in parts of Europe, Turkey, Romania, the Near East, and Africa. Many of the infected patients have died. Experts are concerned that if the avian flu virus continues to spread, a worldwide pandemic outbreak could occur. People with bird flu may develop life-threatening complications, such as viral pneumonia and ARDS (the most common cause of bird flu–related deaths).

Necrotizing Pneumonia and Lung Abscess

Necrotizing pneumonia refers to a pneumonia that causes the death of lung tissue cells within the infected pulmonary parenchyma. It is often characterized as a localized area of pus and tissue necrosis. In severe cases, necrotizing pneumonia can result in a **lung abscess**. A *lung abscess* (also known as *necrotizing pneumonia* or *lung gangrene*) is characterized as a localized air- and fluid-filled cavity, which is a collection of purulent exudate that is composed of liquefied white blood cell remains, proteins, and tissue debris. The air- and fluid-filled cavity is encapsulated in a so-called *pyogenic membrane* that consists of a layer of fibrin, inflammatory cells, and granulation tissue.

During the early stages of a lung abscess, the pathologic findings are indistinguishable from those of any acute pneumonia. Polymorphonuclear leukocytes and macrophages move into the infected area to engulf any invading organisms. This action causes the pulmonary capillaries to dilate, the interstitial space to fill with fluid, and the alveolar epithelium to swell from the edema fluid. In response to this inflammatory reaction, the alveoli in the infected area become consolidated (Fig. 18.11).

As the inflammatory process progresses, tissue necrosis occurs. In severe cases the tissue necrosis can rupture into adjacent bronchi, which in turn allows a partial or total drainage

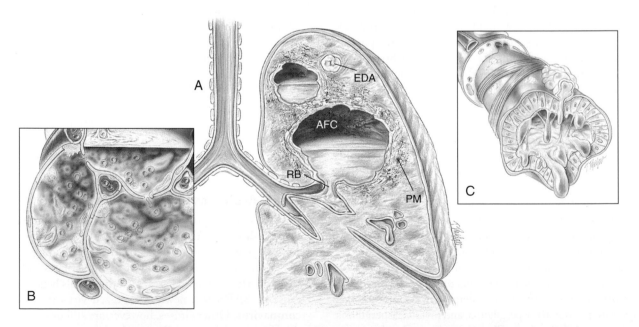

FIGURE 18.11 Lung abscess. (A) Cross-sectional view of lung abscess. (B) Consolidation. (C) Excessive bronchial secretions are common secondary anatomic alterations of the lungs. *AFC,* Air-fluid cavity; *EDA,* early development of abscess; *PM,* pyogenic membrane; *RB,* ruptured bronchus (and drainage of the liquefied contents of the cavity).

BOX 18.3 Organisms Known to Cause Lung Abscess

Common Organisms Associated With Aspiration
- Anaerobic gram-positive cocci
  - Peptostreptococci
  - Peptococci
- Anaerobic gram-negative bacilli
  - *Bacteroides fragilis*
  - *Prevotella melaninogenica*
  - *Fusobacterium* spp.

Less Common Organisms
- *Klebsiella*
- Staphylococci
- *Mycobacterium tuberculosis* (plus atypical organisms *Mycobacterium kansasii* and *Mycobacterium avium*)

- *Histoplasma capsulatum*
- *Coccidioides immitis*
- *Blastomyces*
- *Aspergillus fumigatus*

Parasites
- *Paragonimus westermani*
- *Echinococcus*
- *Entamoeba histolytica*

Rare Causes
- *Streptococcus pneumoniae*
- *Pseudomonas aeruginosa*
- *Legionella pneumophila*

---

of the liquefied contents from the cavity to flow into the bronchi. In addition, an air- and fluid-filled cavity also may rupture into the intrapleural space and cause pleural effusion and empyema (see Chapter 24, Pleural Effusion and Empyema). This may lead to inflammation of the parietal pleura, pleuritic chest pain, decreased chest expansion, and atelectasis. After a time, fibrosis and calcification of the tissues around the cavity encapsulate the abscess (see Fig. 18.11).

The major pathologic or structural changes associated with a lung abscess are as follows:
- Alveolar consolidation
- Alveolar-capillary tissue and bronchial wall destruction
- Tissue necrosis
- Cavity formation
- Fibrosis and calcification of the lung parenchyma
- Bronchopleural fistulas and empyema
- Atelectasis
- Excessive airway secretions

Lung abscesses most commonly occur as a complication of aspiration pneumonia—that is, the pathologic events that follow shortly after aspirating either (1) acidic gastric fluids or (2) a variety of organisms (both anaerobic and aerobic) that are normally found in oropharyngeal secretions. The aspiration of acidic gastric fluids is associated with immediate injury to the tracheobronchial tree and lung parenchyma—often likened

to a flash burn. Box 18.3 provides a summary of organisms known to cause lung abscess. Such organisms commonly colonize and multiply in the small grooves, gingival crevices, and spaces between the teeth and gums in patients with poor oral hygiene. For example, anaerobic organisms are frequently found in patients with gingivitis and dead or abscessed teeth.

Aspiration often occurs in the patient with a decreased level of consciousness. Predisposing factors include (1) alcohol abuse, (2) seizure disorders, (3) general anesthesia, (4) head trauma, (5) cerebrovascular accidents, and (6) swallowing disorders. Anatomically, lung abscesses most commonly develop in lung regions that are dependent in the recumbent position (e.g., the posterior segments of the upper lobes or the superior segments of the lower lobes). The right lung is more commonly involved than the left.

Finally, a lung abscess may also develop as a result of (1) bronchial obstruction with secondary cavitating infection (e.g., distal to bronchogenic carcinoma or an aspirated foreign body), (2) vascular obstruction with tissue infarction (e.g., septic embolism, vasculitis), (3) interstitial lung disease with cavity formation (e.g., pneumoconiosis [silicosis], Wegener granulomatosis, and rheumatoid nodules), (4) bullae or cysts that become infected (e.g., congenital or bronchogenic cysts), or (5) penetrating chest wounds that lead to an infection (e.g., bullet wound).

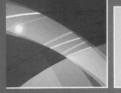
The following clinical manifestations result from the pathologic mechanisms caused (or activated) by alveolar consolidation (see Fig. 10.8), increased alveolar-capillary membrane thickness (see Fig. 10.9), and atelectasis (see Fig. 10.7)—the major anatomic alterations of the lungs associated with pneumonia (see Fig. 18.1).

During the resolution stage of pneumonia, excessive bronchial secretions (see Fig. 10.11) may also play a part in the clinical presentation.

CLINICAL DATA OBTAINED AT THE PATIENT'S BEDSIDE

The Physical Examination

Vital Signs

Increased Respiratory Rate (Tachypnea)

Several pathophysiologic mechanisms operating simultaneously may lead to an increased ventilatory rate:

- Stimulation of peripheral chemoreceptors (hypoxemia)
- Relationship of lung compliance to increased ventilatory rate
- Stimulation of J receptors
- Pain, anxiety, fever

Increased Temperature (Bacterial >101°F and Viral <101°F)

Increased Heart Rate (Pulse) and Blood Pressure

Chest Pain (Pleuritic) and Decreased Chest Expansion

Cyanosis

Cough, Sputum Production, and Hemoptysis

Initially the patient with pneumonia usually has a nonproductive barking or hacking cough. As the disease progresses, however, the cough becomes productive. When the disease progresses to this point, the patient often expectorates small amounts of purulent, blood-streaked, or rusty sputum. This is caused by fluid moving from the pulmonary capillaries into the alveoli in response to the inflammatory process. As fluid crosses into the alveoli, some RBCs may also move into the alveoli and produce the blood-streaked or rusty appearance of the fluid (see Fig. 18.1). Some of the fluid that moves in the alveoli also may work its way into the bronchioles and bronchi. As the fluid accumulates in the bronchial tree, the subepithelial receptors in the trachea, bronchi, and bronchioles are stimulated and initiate a cough reflex. Because the bronchioles and the smaller bronchi are deep in the lung parenchyma, the patient with pneumonia initially has a dry, hacking cough, and fluid cannot be easily expectorated until secretions reach the larger bronchi.

Chest Assessment Findings

- Increased tactile and vocal fremitus
- Dull percussion note
- Bronchial breath sounds
- Crackles
- Pleural friction rub (if process extends to pleural surface)
- Whispered pectoriloquy

CLINICAL DATA OBTAINED FROM LABORATORY TESTS AND SPECIAL PROCEDURES

Pulmonary Function Test Findings
(Restrictive Lung Pathophysiology)[1]

FORCED EXPIRATORY VOLUME AND FLOW RATE FINDINGS[2]

FVC	FEV_T	FEV_1/FVC ratio	$FEF_{25\%-75\%}$
↓	N or ↓	N or ↑	N or ↓

$FEF_{50\%}$	$FEF_{200-1200}$	PEFR	MVV
N or ↓	N or ↓	N or ↓	N or ↓

LUNG VOLUME AND CAPACITY FINDINGS

V_T	IRV	ERV	RV
N or ↓	↓	↓	↓

VC	IC	FRC	TLC	RV/TLC ratio
↓	↓	↓	↓	N

Arterial Blood Gases

MILD TO MODERATE STAGES

Acute Alveolar Hyperventilation With Hypoxemia[3] (Acute Respiratory Alkalosis)

pH	$PaCO_2$	HCO_3^-	PaO_2	SaO_2 or SpO_2
↑	↓	↓	↓	↓
		(but normal)		

SEVERE STAGE

Acute Ventilatory Failure With Hypoxemia[4] (Acute Respiratory Acidosis)

pH[5]	$PaCO_2$	HCO_3^-[5]	PaO_2	SaO_2 or SpO_2
↓	↑	↑	↓	↓
		(but normal)		

Oxygenation Indices[6]

$\dot{Q}_S/\dot{Q}_T$	DO_2[7]	$\dot{V}O_2$[8]	$C(a-\bar{v})O_2$[8]	O_2ER	$S\bar{v}O_2$
↑	↓	N	N	↑	↓

---

[1]The pulmonary function tests (PFTs) here are for a typical case of interstitial or alveolar-filling pneumonia, not complicated with excessive airway secretions, bronchospasm, etc.

[2]The decreased forced expiratory volumes and flow rate findings are primarily caused by the low vital capacity associated with the disorder.

[3]See Fig. 5.2 and Table 5.4 and related discussion for the acute pH, $PaCO_2$, and HCO_3^- changes associated with acute alveolar hyperventilation.

[4]See Fig. 5.2 and Table 5.5 and related discussion for the acute pH, $PaCO_2$, and HCO_3^- changes associated with acute ventilatory failure.

[5]When tissue hypoxia is severe enough to produce lactic acid, the pH and HCO_3^- values will be lower than expected for a particular $PaCO_2$ level.

[6]$C(a-\bar{v})O_2$, Arterial-venous oxygen difference; DO_2, total oxygen delivery; O_2ER, oxygen extraction ratio; $\dot{Q}_S/\dot{Q}_T$, pulmonary shunt fraction; $S\bar{v}O_2$, mixed venous oxygen saturation; $\dot{V}O_2$, oxygen consumption.

[7]The DO_2 may be normal in patients who have compensated to the decreased oxygenation status with (1) an increased cardiac output, (2) an increased hemoglobin level, or (3) a combination of both. When the DO_2 is normal, the O_2ER is usually normal.

[8]May be increased in the patient with a fever caused by bacterial pneumonia.

ABNORMAL LABORATORY TEST AND PROCEDURE RESULTS

Sputum examination findings (see discussion of etiology in this chapter, Box 18.2)

RADIOLOGIC FINDINGS

Chest Radiograph

- Increased density (from consolidation and atelectasis)
- Air bronchograms
- Lung abscess and/or air- and fluid-filled cavity
- Pleural effusions/empyema

The radiographic signs vary considerably depending on the causative agent and the stage of the pneumonia process. In general, pneumonia (alveolar consolidation) appears as an area of increased density that may involve a small lung segment, a lobe, or one or both lungs (Figs. 18.3 and 18.12). The process may appear patchy or uniform throughout the area. As the alveolar consolidation intensifies, alveolar density increases and air bronchograms may be seen (Fig. 18.13). A lung abscess—or air- and fluid-filled cavity—appears on the radiograph as a circular radiolucency that contains an air-fluid level, surrounded by a dense wall of lung parenchyma (Fig. 18.14).

During the early stages of many pulmonary fungal infections, localized infiltration and consolidation with or without lymph node involvement are commonly seen (Fig. 18.15). Single or numerous spherical nodules may be seen (Fig. 18.16). During the advanced stages, bilateral cavities in the apical and posterior segments of the upper lobes are often seen (Fig. 18.17). A pleural effusion may be identified on the chest radiograph (see Chapter 24, Pleural Effusion and Empyema).

COMPUTED TOMOGRAPHY SCAN

Alveolar consolidation and air bronchograms can also be seen on the computed tomography (CT) scan (Fig. 18.18).

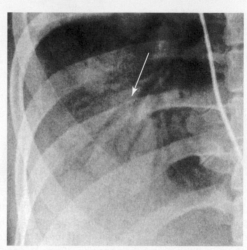

FIGURE 18.13 Air bronchogram (shown in chest radiograph). The branching linear lucencies within the consolidation in the right lower lobe are particularly well demonstrated (arrow) in this example of staphylococcal pneumonia. (From Hansell, D. M., Lynch, D. A., McAdams, H. P., et al. [2010]. *Imaging of diseases of the chest* [5th ed.]. Philadelphia, PA: Elsevier.)

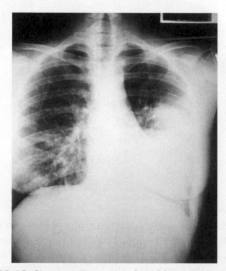

FIGURE 18.12 Chest radiograph of a 20-year-old woman with severe pneumonia of the left lung and patchy pneumonia in the right middle and lower lobes.

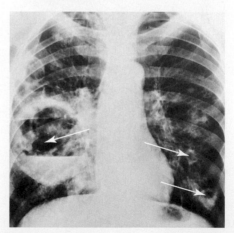

FIGURE 18.14 A large cavitary lesion containing an air-fluid level in the right lower lobe (see arrow). Smaller cavitary lesions are also seen in other lobes (see arrows). (From Hansell, D. M., Armstrong, P., Lynch, D. A., McAdams, H. P. [Eds.]. [2005]. *Imaging of diseases of the chest* [4th ed.]. Philadelphia, PA: Elsevier.)

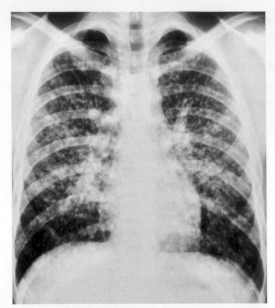

FIGURE 18.15 Acute inhalational histoplasmosis in an otherwise healthy patient. This young man developed fever and cough after tearing down an old barn. The radiograph shows bilateral hilar adenopathy and diffuse nodular opacities. (From Hansell, D. M., Lynch, D. A., McAdams, H. P., et al. [2010]. *Imaging of diseases of the chest* [5th ed.]. Philadelphia, PA: Elsevier.)

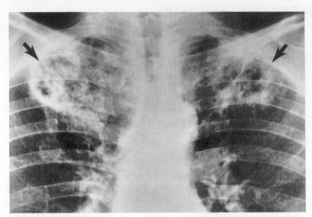

FIGURE 18.17 Chronic cavitary histoplasmosis. Note the striking upper zone predominance of the shadows resembling tuberculosis (arrows). Numerous large cavities are seen. (From Hansell, D. M., Armstrong, P., Lynch, D. A., McAdams, H. P. [Eds.]. [2005]. *Imaging of diseases of the chest* [4th ed.]. Philadelphia, PA: Elsevier.)

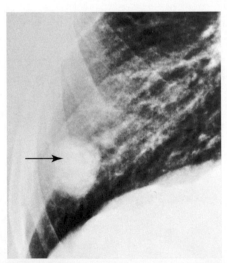

FIGURE 18.16 A histoplasmoma, showing a well-defined spherical nodule (arrow). The central portion of the nodule shows calcification. (From Hansell, D. M., Armstrong, P., Lynch, D. A., McAdams, H. P. [Eds.]. [2005]. *Imaging of diseases of the chest* [4th ed.]. Philadelphia, PA: Elsevier.)

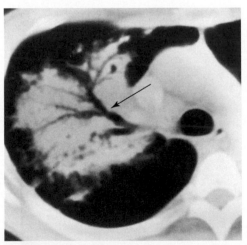

FIGURE 18.18 Air bronchograms (see arrow) shown by computed tomography in a patient with pneumonia. (From Hansell, D. M., Armstrong, P., Lynch, D. A., McAdams, H. P. [Eds.]. [2005]. *Imaging of diseases of the chest* [4th ed.]. Philadelphia, PA: Elsevier.)

General Management of Pneumonia

The treatment of pneumonia is based on the specific cause of the pneumonia and the severity of symptoms demonstrated by the patient. For bacterial pneumonia, the first line of defense is usually an antibiotic prescribed by the attending physician (see Appendix III on the Evolve site). For fungal disorders, antifungal agents are administered (see Appendix IV on the Evolve site).

Although there are a few *viral pneumonias* that may be treated with antiviral medications, the recommended treatment is usually the same as for the flu—bed rest and plenty of fluids. In addition, over-the-counter medications are often helpful to reduce fever, treat aches and pains, and depress the dry cough associated with pneumonia. In severe pneumonia, hospitalization may be required. The following is an overview of the treatments used for pneumonia.

The general management of *lung abscess* varies based on the severity of the pneumonia and the severity of the lung abscess. Treatment includes appropriate (usually intravenous) antimicrobial therapy coupled with prompt drainage and surgical debridement. When it is treated properly, most patients with a lung abscess show improvement. In acute cases, the size of the abscess quickly decreases and eventually closes altogether. In severe or chronic cases, the patient's improvement may be slow or insignificant, even with appropriate therapy.

The standard treatment for a lung abscess caused by an anaerobic pathogen is *clindamycin*. Other drugs that may be used are any combination of *beta-lactam–beta-lactamase inhibitors* (e.g., ampicillin-sulbactam), *penicillin* plus *metronidazole*, or a *carbapenem*. When the lung abscess is caused by MRSA, *linezolid* is recommended. An alternative to linezolid is *vancomycin;* followed by *ceftaroline, trimethoprim-sulfamethoxazole,* and *telavancin.*

Respiratory Care Treatment Protocols

Oxygen Therapy Protocol

Oxygen therapy is used to treat hypoxemia, decrease the work of breathing, and decrease myocardial work. Because of the hypoxemia associated with pneumonia, supplemental oxygen may be required. The hypoxemia that develops in pneumonia is most commonly caused by alveolar consolidation and capillary shunting associated with the disorder. Hypoxemia caused by capillary shunting is often at least partially refractory to oxygen therapy (see Oxygen Therapy Protocol, Protocol 10.1).

Lung Expansion Therapy Protocol

Lung expansion therapy may be administered to attempt to offset the atelectasis associated with some pneumonias, but its effects are not consistently good (see Lung Expansion Therapy Protocol, Protocol 10.3).

Airway Clearance Therapy Protocol

Because secretion accumulation is associated with severe pneumonias and lung abscess, a number of airway clearance therapies may be used to enhance the mobilization of bronchial secretions (see Airway Clearance Therapy Protocol, Protocol 10.2). A 1- or 2-day trial of chest physiotherapy modalities is not contraindicated in the otherwise stable patient.

Thoracentesis

Diagnostic and therapeutically, thoracentesis may be used if a pleural effusion is present (see Chapter 24). From a diagnostic standpoint, fluid samples may be examined for the following:

- Color
- Odor
- RBC count
- Protein
- Glucose
- Lactic dehydrogenase (LDH)
- Amylase
- pH
- Wright, Gram, and acid-fast bacillus (AFB) stains
- Aerobic, anaerobic, tuberculosis, and fungal cultures
- Cytology

Therapeutic thoracentesis may be used to encourage lung reexpansion when atelectasis is part of the clinical presentation.

CASE STUDY Pneumonia

Admitting History and Physical Examination

A 47-year-old man spent a week deer hunting in northern Michigan with some friends. They spent considerable time outdoors in inclement weather and indulged freely in alcoholic beverages during the afternoons and evenings. Previously the man had been essentially healthy. He smoked one pack of cigarettes a day.

Returning home, he felt listless and thought that he was "coming down with a cold." That night, he noticed a mild, nonproductive cough. He had a headache and some pain in the right side of his chest on deep inspiration and noticed that he was somewhat short of breath when he climbed one flight of stairs. During the night, he woke up and felt very chilled, then very warm. His wife put her hand on his forehead and was certain that he had a "high fever." Because he felt miserable, they went to the emergency department of the nearest hospital.

On physical examination, his vital signs were blood pressure 150/88, pulse 116 beats/min, respiratory rate 28 breaths/min, and temperature (oral) 39.9°C. He was in moderate respiratory distress. Percussion of the chest revealed dullness on the right lower side, and on inspiration there were fine crackles heard in that area. The breath sounds were described as "bronchial." The chest radiograph showed pneumonic consolidation of the right lower lung field. On room air, his arterial blood gas (ABG) values were pH 7.53, $PaCO_2$ 27 mm Hg, HCO_3^- 21 mEq/L, PaO_2 62 mm Hg, and SaO_2 93%.

The respiratory therapist assigned to assess and treat the patient recorded the following SOAP note.

Respiratory Assessment and Plan

S Mild dyspnea (patient stated he was "short of breath")

O Alert, cooperative, acutely ill. Mild nonproductive cough. Vital signs T 39.9°C, BP 150/88, P 116, RR 28. Dull to percussion over RLL, along with crackles and bronchial breath sounds. CXR: Pneumonic consolidation RLL. ABG on room air pH 7.53, $PaCO_2$ 27, HCO_3^- 21, PaO_2 62, and SaO_2 93%.

A • RLL consolidation (pneumonia presumed)
   • Acute alveolar hyperventilation with mild hypoxemia (ABG)

P Oxygen Therapy Protocol: Monitor SpO_2. (Titrate O_2 per NC as needed to keep SpO_2 >90%.)

The patient was started on oxygen (2 L/min) via a nasal cannula. The physician prescribed intravenous antibiotic therapy. Over the next 72 hours, the patient steadily improved, although he felt nauseated and vomited three times. On the fourth hospital day, however, the patient complained of increased shortness of breath. He started to cough up large amounts (3 to 4 tablespoons every 2 hours) of foul-smelling, greenish-yellow sputum. He also complained of choking on his secretions, a bitter taste in his mouth, belching (aspiration likely), mild substernal discomfort, and chills.

On physical examination, the patient appeared anxious. His vital signs were blood pressure 120/82, pulse 140 bpm, respiratory rate 20 breaths/min, and oral temperature 40°C. His sputum was thick, yellow-green, and foul-smelling. His cough was strong. He had bronchial breath sounds and coarse, nonclearing, crackles over the right midportion of the anterior chest and over both lower lobes posteriorly. There was mild cyanosis of the nail beds. The abdominal examination was unremarkable. There was no peripheral edema. A chest x-ray examination showed new infiltrates in the right middle lung field and left lower lobe. The opaque infiltrate obstructed the view of the heart and was described by the radiologist as "consolidation." On 2 L/min O_2 nasal cannula, his ABGs were pH 7.50, $PaCO_2$ 29 mm Hg, HCO_3^- 21 mEq/L, PaO_2 36 mm Hg, and SaO_2 81%.

At this time the respiratory therapist charted the following SOAP progress note.

Respiratory Assessment and Plan

S Dyspnea (patient complained of increased shortness of breath), worsening

O Anxious appearance. BP 120/82, HR 140, RR 20, T 40°C. Cyanotic. Strong productive cough (foul-smelling, yellow-green sputum). Bronchial breath sounds, coarse crackles, persistent crackles in right middle anterior chest and both

bases. CXR: RML and LLL infiltrate and consolidation. ABGs (on 2 L/min) pH 7.50, $PaCO_2$ 29, HCO_3^- 21, PaO_2 36, and SaO_2 81%.

A • Aspiration complicating community-acquired pneumonia, involving RML and LLL (history, CXR)
   • Alveolar consolidation (CXR)
   • Excessive airway secretions (thick, yellow-green sputum)
   • Good ability to mobilize secretions (strong cough)
   • Acute alveolar hyperventilation with severe hypoxemia (ABG)

P Oxygen Therapy Protocol: Increase FIO_2 to 0.60 via Venturi mask. Airway Clearance Therapy Protocol: Deep breathe and cough instructions; PRN oropharyngeal suctioning. Trial P&D to lower lobes and RML q shift as tolerated. ABG in 1 hour.

Discussion

A history of cold exposure in conjunction with the use of alcoholic beverages before the onset of pneumonia is not uncommon. The first part of this case begins with a classic presentation for community-acquired pneumonia with alveolar **consolidation** (see Fig. 10.8). For example, the fever and tachycardia represent a normal functioning immune response, and the tachycardia and tachypnea reflect the body's response to shunt-induced hypoxemia. The auscultation of crackles and bronchial breath sounds also reflects the patient's pulmonary consolidation. An attempt at improving his oxygenation, although not successful, was certainly in order. It was hoped that by providing an oxygen-enriched gas to both normal and partially consolidated alveoli, the effects of pulmonary shunting would be at least partially offset.

The second SOAP presents the complication of the patient's community-acquired pneumonia with probable aspiration pneumonitis. Alcoholics frequently have gastritis or esophagitis, and the patient's eructation (belching) and pyrosis (heartburn) were clues to the development of that complication. At this time, there were new clinical manifestations associated with excessive bronchial secretions (see Fig. 10.11). For example, the patient demonstrated a cough, sputum production, and coarse crackles. The selection of modalities from the Airway Clearance Therapy Protocol (deep breathe and cough, suctioning, and percussion and drainage [P&D]) was appropriate. A trial of lung expansion therapy (see Protocol 10.3) was not given in this case. However, atelectasis (see Fig. 10.7) often complicates aspiration pneumonia, and such a trial would not have been inappropriate.

In cases of pneumonia, the respiratory therapist is often tempted to do too much. Typically, volume expansion therapy, bronchodilator aerosol therapy, and bland aerosol therapy have all been ordered for affected patients, even in the acute, consolidative stage of their pneumonia. Often, however, all that is needed is the appropriate selection of antibiotics, rest, fluids, and supplementary oxygen. When the pneumonia "breaks up" (resolution stage) or is complicated by aspiration (as in this case), excessive bronchial secretions (see Fig. 10.11) and even bronchospasm (see Fig. 10.10) may appear. When this happens, use of other protocol modalities is necessary.

SELF-ASSESSMENT QUESTIONS

1. Which of the following is also known as Friedländer bacillus?
   a. *Haemophilus influenzae*
   b. *Pseudomonas aeruginosa*
   c. *Legionella pneumophila*
   d. *Klebsiella*

2. Which of the following accounts for more than 80% of all the bacterial pneumonias?
   a. *Klebsiella* pneumonia
   b. Streptococcal pneumonia
   c. *Chlamydia* pneumonia
   d. Staphylococcal pneumonia

3. Which of the following is associated with Q fever?
   a. *Mycoplasma pneumoniae*
   b. *Rickettsia*
   c. Ornithosis
   d. *Varicella*

4. Mendelson syndrome is associated with which of the following?
   a. Lipoid pneumonitis
   b. Rubella
   c. Varicella
   d. Aspiration pneumonia

5. Which of the following is the most common viral pulmonary complication of AIDS?
   a. *Aspergillus*
   b. *Cryptococcus*
   c. *Pneumocystis jirovecii*\
   d. *Cytomegalovirus*

6. Which of the following infects almost all children by age 2?
   a. *Klebsiella*
   b. *Haemophilus influenzae* type B
   c. Respiratory syncytial virus
   d. *Pseudomonas aeruginosa*

7. Which of the following is almost always the cause of acute epiglottitis?
   a. *Haemophilus influenzae* type B
   b. *Klebsiella*
   c. *Streptococcus*
   d. *Mycoplasma pneumoniae*

8. Which of the following is related to mumps, rubella, and RSV?
   a. *Streptococcus*
   b. Parainfluenza virus
   c. *Mycoplasma pneumoniae*
   d. Adenovirus

9. In the absence of a secondary bacterial infection, lung inflammation caused by the aspiration of gastric fluids usually becomes insignificant in approximately how many days?
   a. 2 days
   b. 3 days
   c. 5 days
   d. 7 days

10. Which of the following findings is/are associated with pneumonia?
    1. Decreased tactile and vocal fremitus
    2. Increased $C(a-\bar{v})O_2$
    3. Decreased functional residual capacity
    4. Increased vital capacity
       a. 1 only
       b. 3 only
       c. 2 and 4 only
       d. 1 and 3 only

11. Which of the following is the most common fungal infection in the United States?
    a. Coccidioidomycosis
    b. Histoplasmosis
    c. San Joaquin Valley disease
    d. Blastomycosis

12. Which of the following is(are) anaerobic organisms?
    1. *Blastomyces*
    2. *Peptococcus*
    3. *Coccidioides immitis*
    4. *Bacteroides*
       a. 1 and 2 only
       b. 2 and 4 only
       c. 3 and 4 only
       d. 2, 3, and 4 only

13. Anatomically, a lung abscess most commonly forms in which part(s) of the lung?
    1. Posterior segment of the upper lobe
    2. Lateral basal segment of the lower lobe
    3. Anterior segment of the upper lobe
    4. Superior segment of the lower lobe
       a. 1 only
       b. 3 only
       c. 1 and 4 only
       d. 2 and 3 only

14. Incidence of histoplasmosis is especially high in which of the following area(s)?
    1. Arizona
    2. Mississippi
    3. Nevada
    4. Texas
       a. 2 only
       b. 4 only
       c. 2 and 4 only
       d. 2 and 3 only

15. The condition called "desert bumps," "desert arthritis," or "desert rheumatism" is associated with which fungal disorder?
    a. Histoplasmosis
    b. Blastomycosis
    c. Coccidioidomycosis
    d. Aspergillosis

Chapter Objectives

After reading this chapter, you will be able to:

- List the anatomic alterations of the lungs associated with tuberculosis.
- Describe the causes of tuberculosis.
- List the cardiopulmonary clinical manifestations associated with tuberculosis.
- Describe the general management of tuberculosis.
- Describe the clinical strategies and rationales of the SOAP presented in the case study.
- Define key terms and complete self-assessment questions at the end of the chapter and on Evolve.

Key Terms

Acid-Fast Bacilli
Acid-Fast Bacteria
Caseous Granuloma
Caseous Lesion
Centers for Disease Control and Prevention (CDC)
Directly Observed Therapy (DOT)
Disseminated Tuberculosis
Dormant Tuberculosis (Latent Tuberculosis)
Ethambutol
Exposure Risk in Health Care Workers
Fluorescent Acid-Fast Stain
Ghon Complex
Ghon Nodules
Granuloma
Hemoptysis
Induration
Infection Control Measures
Isolation Procedures
Isoniazid (INH)
Mantoux Tuberculin Skin Test
Maliary Tuberculosis
Multidrug-Resistant Tuberculosis (MDR-TB)
Mycobacterium avium
Mycobacterium kansasii
Mycobacterium tuberculosis

Nontuberculous Acid-Fast Mycobacteria
Occupational Safety and Health Administration (OSHA)
Postprimary Tuberculosis
Primary Tuberculosis
Prophylactic Use of Isoniazid
Purified Protein Derivative (PPD)
Pyrazinamide (PZA)
Respiratory Isolation
Respiratory Patient Isolation Procedures
Respiratory Protection Devices
Rifampin
Sputum Smear
Streptomycin
Transmission of Tuberculosis
Treatment Noncompliance
Tubercle
Ziehl-Neelsen Stain

Chapter Outline

Anatomic Alterations of the Lungs
    Primary Tuberculosis
    Reactivation Tuberculosis
    Disseminated Tuberculosis
Etiology and Epidemiology
Tuberculosis Among Health Care Workers
Diagnosis
    Mantoux Tuberculin Skin Test
    Acid-Fast Staining
    Sputum Culture
    QuantiFERON-TB Gold Test
    Xpert MTB/RIF Assay
Overview of the Cardiopulmonary Clinical Manifestations
    Associated With Tuberculosis
General Management of Tuberculosis
    Pharmacologic Agents Used to Treat Tuberculosis
    Respiratory Care Treatment Protocols
Case Study: Tuberculosis
Self-Assessment Questions

Anatomic Alterations of the Lungs

Tuberculosis (TB) is a contagious chronic bacterial infection that primarily affects the lungs, although it may involve almost any part of the body. Clinically, TB is classified as primary TB, reactivation TB, or disseminated TB.

Primary Tuberculosis

Primary tuberculosis (also called the *primary infection stage*) follows the patient's first exposure to the TB pathogen, *Mycobacterium tuberculosis*—a rod-shaped bacterium with a waxy capsule. Primary TB begins when the inhaled bacilli implant in the alveoli. As the bacilli multiply over a 3- to 4-week period, the initial response of the lungs is an inflammatory reaction that is similar to acute pneumonia (Fig. 19.1). In other words, a large influx of polymorphonuclear leukocytes and macrophages moves into the infected area to engulf, but not fully kill, the bacilli. This action also causes the pulmonary capillaries to dilate, the interstitium to fill with fluid, and the alveolar epithelium to swell from the edema fluid. Eventually the alveoli become consolidated (i.e., filled with fluid, polymorphonuclear leukocytes, and macrophages). Clinically, this phase of TB coincides with a positive tuberculin reaction—a positive purified protein derivative (PPD) skin test result (see discussion of diagnosis later in this chapter).

Unlike in pneumonia, however, the lung tissue that surrounds the infected area slowly produces a protective cell wall called a **tubercle**, or **granuloma**. In essence, the tubercles work to encapsulate, or trap, the TB bacilli in a nutshell-like structure (see Fig. 19.1A). Although the initial lung lesions may be difficult to identify on a chest radiograph, the lesions may be seen as small, sharply defined opacities. When detected on a chest radiograph, these initial lung lesions are called **Ghon nodules**. As the disease progresses, the combination of tubercles and the involvement of the lymph nodes in the hilar region is known as the **Ghon complex** (Fig. 19.2).

Structurally, a tubercle consists of a central core containing caseous necrosis and TB bacilli (also called **caseous lesion** or **caseous granuloma**). The central core is surrounded by enlarged epithelioid macrophages, lymphocytes, and multinucleated giant cells. A tubercle takes about 2 to 10 weeks to form. The function of the tubercle is to contain the TB bacilli, thus preventing the further spread of infectious TB organisms. Unfortunately, the tubercle has the potential to break down occasionally, especially in a patient with a depressed immune system. The patient is potentially contagious at this stage. In most cases however, the TB bacilli are effectively contained within the tubercles.

Once the bacilli are controlled—either by the patient's immunologic defense system (which contains the TB bacilli in a tubercle) or by antituberculosis drugs—the healing process begins. Tissue fibrosis and calcification of the lung parenchyma slowly replace the tubercle. This tissue fibrosis and calcification cause lung tissue retraction and scarring. In some cases, the calcification and fibrosis cause the bronchi to distort and dilate—that is, to develop bronchiectasis.

Finally, when the bacilli are isolated within tubercles and immunity develops, the TB bacilli may remain dormant for months, years, or life. Individuals with **dormant TB** (also called **latent TB**) do not feel sick or have any TB-related symptoms. They are still infected with TB but do not have clinically active TB. The only indication of a TB infection is

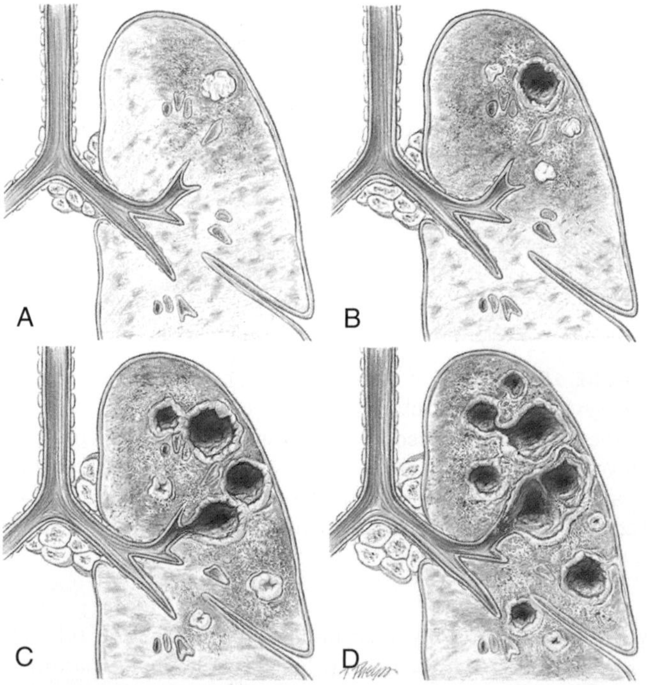

FIGURE 19.1 Tuberculosis. (A) Early primary infection. (B) Cavitation of a caseous tubercle and new primary lesions developing. (C) Further progression and development of cavitations and new primary infections. Note the subpleural location of some of these lesions. (D) Severe lung destruction caused by tuberculosis.

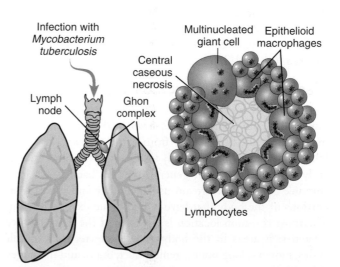

FIGURE 19.2 Ghon complex, typical of pulmonary tuberculosis, consists of a parenchymal focus and hilar lymph node lesions. The detailed section of the diagram (right) shows the typical features of tuberculous granuloma: central caseous necrosis surrounded by epithelioid cells, multinucleated giant cells, and lymphocytes. (From Damjanov, I. [2017]. *Pathology for the health professions* [5th ed.]. St. Louis, MO: Elsevier.)

a positive reaction to the tuberculin skin test (Mantoux test, discussed later), or TB blood test, and the finding of possible residual scarring on the chest radiograph. Individuals with dormant (latent) TB are not infectious and cannot spread the TB bacilli to others.

Reactivation Tuberculosis

Reactivation tuberculosis (also called **postprimary tuberculosis**, *reinfection tuberculosis*, or *secondary tuberculosis*) is a term used to describe the reappearance (i.e., signs and symptoms) of TB months or even years after the initial infection has been controlled. Even though most patients with primary TB recover completely from a clinical standpoint, it is important to note that live tubercle bacilli can remain dormant for decades. A positive tuberculin reaction generally persists even after the primary infection stage has been controlled. At any time, TB may become reactivated, especially in patients with depressed immune systems. Most reactivation TB cases are associated with the following risk factors:

• Malnourished individuals
• People in institutional housing (e.g., nursing homes, prisons, homeless shelters)
• People living in overcrowded conditions
• Immunosuppressed patients (e.g., organ transplant patients, cancer patients)
• Human immunodeficiency virus (HIV) patients (TB is a leading cause of death in HIV patients)
• Alcohol abuse

If the TB infection is uncontrolled, further growth of the caseous granuloma tubercle develops. The patient progressively experiences more severe symptoms, including violent coughing episodes, greenish or bloody sputum (possibly mixed with TB bacilli), low-grade fever, anorexia, weight loss, extreme fatigue, night sweats, and chest pain. It is this gradual wasting of the body that provided the basis for an earlier name for TB—*consumption*. The patient is highly contagious at this stage. In severe cases a tubercle cavity may rupture and allow air and infected material to flow into the pleural space or the tracheobronchial tree. Pleural complications are common in TB (see Fig. 19.1C).

Disseminated Tuberculosis

Disseminated tuberculosis (also called *extrapulmonary TB*, **miliary TB**, and *tuberculosis—disseminated*) refers to infection from TB bacilli that escape from a tubercle and travel to other sites throughout the body by means of the bloodstream or lymphatic system. In general, the TB bacilli that gain entrance to the bloodstream usually gather and multiply in portions of the body that have a high tissue oxygen tension. The most common location is the apex of the lungs. Other oxygen-rich areas in the body include the regional lymph nodes, kidneys, long bones, genital tract, brain, and meninges (Fig. 19.3).

Genital TB in males damages the prostate gland, epididymis, seminal vesicles, and testes and in females, the fallopian tubes, ovaries, and uterus. The spine is a frequent site of TB infection, although the hip, knee, wrist, and elbow also can be involved. Tubercular meningitis is caused by an active brain lesion seeding TB bacilli into the meninges. *Endobronchial TB* may develop

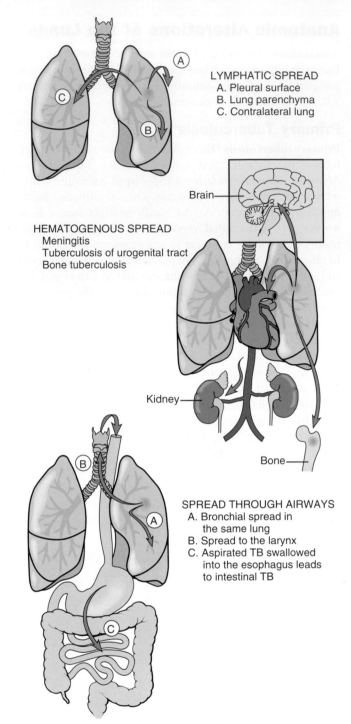

FIGURE 19.3 Spread of tuberculosis (TB). TB bacilli can spread through the lymphatics, blood vessels, or bronchi. TB bacillis spread by the blood usually accounts for TB in distal sites, such as the urogenital tract, bone, or the brain. Expectorated bacilli may be swallowed and cause intestinal TB. (From Damjanov, I. [2017]. *Pathology for the health professions* [5th ed.]. St. Louis, MO: Elsevier.)

via direct extension to the bronchi from an adjacent tubercle cavity or the spread of the TB bacilli via infected sputum.

TB *complications* include massive **hemoptysis**, pneumothorax, bronchiectasis, extensive pulmonary destruction, malignancy, and chronic pulmonary aspergillosis. Over time, the TB infection may cause mental deterioration, intelletual disability, blindness, and deafness.

When a large number of bacilli are freed into the bloodstream, the result can be the presence of numerous small tubercles—about the size of a pinhead (1 to 5 mm)—scattered throughout the body. This form of TB is termed *miliary TB*. Miliary TB may be seen in the lungs, liver, and spleen.

Tuberculosis primarily results in a chronic restrictive pulmonary disorder. The major pathologic or structural changes of the lungs associated with TB (moderate to severe reactivation TB) are as follows:

- Alveolar consolidation
- Alveolar-capillary membrane destruction
- Caseous tubercles or granulomas
- Cavity formation
- Fibrosis and secondary calcification of the lung parenchyma
- Distortion and dilation of the bronchi
- Increased bronchial secretions

Etiology and Epidemiology

TB is one of the oldest diseases known and remains one of the most widespread diseases in the world. Unmistakable evidence has been provided from mummies dating back to the Stone Age, ancient Egypt, and ancient Peru that TB is a long-lived human disease. In early writings, the disease was variously called "consumption," "Captain of the Men of Death," and "white plague." In the nineteenth century, the disease was named *tuberculosis,* a term that derives mainly from the tubercle formations found during postmortem examinations of victims of the disease.

According to the **Centers for Disease Control and Prevention (CDC),** there were 9093 (a rate of 2.8 cases per 100,000 persons) new cases of TB were provisionally reported in the United States in 2017. This provisional TB case count was the lowest in the United States since national TB surveillance began in 1953. In 2015, the most recent CDC data available, 470 deaths were attributed to TB. Minority populations continue to disproportionately bear the burden to TB disease. For example, the incidence rates for racial/ethnic groups in 2016 were:

- American Indians or Alaska Natives: 4.7 TB cases per 100,000 persons
- Asians: 18.0 TB cases per 100,000 persons
- Blacks or African Americans: 4.9 cases per 100,000 persons
- Native Hawaiilans and other Pacific Islanders: 13.9 TB cases per 100,000 persons
- Hispanics or Latinos: 4.5 TB cases per 100.000 persons
- Whites: 0.6 TB cases per 100,000 persons

TB is still very prevalent globally. According to the World Health Organization (WHO) 2017 report, TB is one of the top 10 causes of death worldwide. In 2017, 10 million people fell ill with TB, and 1.6 million died from the disease (including 0.3 million among people with HIV). In 2017, an estimated 1 million children became ill with TB and 230 000 children died of TB (including children with HIV associated TB). TB is a leading killer of HIV-positive people. Multidrug-resistant TB (MDR-TB) remains a public health crisis and a health security threat.

WHO estimates that there were 558 000 new cases with resistance to rifampicin – the most effective first-line drug,

of which – 82% had MDR-TB (see General Management of Tuberculosis, page 308). Globally, TB incidence is falling at about 2% per year. This needs to accelerate to a 4–5% annual decline to reach the 2020 milestones of the End TB Strategy. An estimated 54 million lives were saved through TB diagnosis and treatment between 2000 and 2017. Ending the TB epidemic by 2030 is among the health targets of the Sustainable Development Goals.

In humans, TB is primarily caused by the bacterium *Mycobacterium tuberculosis.* The mycobacteria are long, slender, straight, or curved rods. The **transmission of tuberculosis** is almost exclusively caused by aerosol droplets produced by coughing, sneezing, or laughing of an individual with active TB. This accounts for the use of strict **isolation procedures** in acutely ill patients hospitalized and suspected of having active TB. In fact, it has been shown that in very fine aerosolized spray droplets (0.5 to 1.0 µm), the TB bacilli can remain suspended in the air for several hours after a cough or sneeze. When inhaled, some of the bacilli may be trapped in the mucus of the nasal passages and removed. The smaller bacilli, however, can easily be inhaled into the bronchioles and alveoli. The TB bacilli are highly aerobic organisms and thrive best in areas of the body with high oxygen tension, especially in the apex of the lung.

Patients with **treatment noncompliance** are a significant reservoir for the transmission of tuberculosis.

People living in closed small rooms with limited access to sunlight and fresh air are especially at risk. Other possible ways of contracting TB include the ingestion of unpasteurized milk from cattle infected with the TB pathogen (usually *Mycobacterium bovis*) or, in rare cases, direct inoculation through the skin (e.g., a laboratory accident during a postmortem examination).

Tuberculosis Among Health Care Workers

The CDC and **Occupational Safety and Health Administration (OSHA)** carefully monitor the **exposure risk in health care workers** and the incidence. The CDC and OSHA periodically issue guidelines for **respiratory protective devices** and **patient isolation procedures**. The risk for TB, without question, is elevated in health care workers and those who work in chronic institutionalized environments such as jails, homeless shelters, and nursing homes. The respiratory therapist who assists in *bronchoscopy* and performs *secretion suctioning* or other procedures dealing with the patient who has a tracheotomy has an increased risk for TB exposure.

Diagnosis

Symptoms vary with the severity and the extent of the disease. They can be very misleading. They include persistent cough, hemoptysis, loss of appetite and weight loss, pleuritic chest pain, nights sweats, low-grade fever, and chills. Along with chest radiology, commonly used diagnostic methods for TB include the **Mantoux tuberculin skin test**, acid-fast bacilli (AFB) sputum cultures, the QuantiFERON-TB Gold (QFT-G) test, and the rapid Xpert MTB/RI assay.

Mantoux Tuberculin Skin Test

The most widely used tuberculin test is the Mantoux test, which consists of an intradermal injection of a small amount of a **purified protein derivative (PPD)** of the tuberculin bacillus (Fig. 19.4). The skin is then observed for **induration** (a wheal) after 48 hours and 72 hours, with results interpreted as follows:

- An induration less than 5 mm is a negative result.
- An induration of 5 to 9 mm is considered suspicious, and retesting is required.
- An induration of 10 mm or greater is considered a positive result. A positive reaction is fairly sound evidence of recent or past infection or of active disease.

It should be stressed, however, that a positive reaction does not necessarily confirm that a patient has active TB, but only that the patient has been exposed to the bacillus and has developed cell-mediated immunity to it (i.e., latent TB).

Acid-Fast Staining

Because the *M. tuberculosis* organism has an unusual, waxy coating on the cell surface, which makes the cells impervious to staining, an **acid-fast bacteria** test (also called a **sputum smear**) is performed instead. Several variations of the acid-fast stain are currently in use. The frequently used **Ziehl-Neelsen stain** reveals bright red **acid-fast bacilli (AFB)** against a blue background (Fig. 19.5A). Another popular technique involves a **fluorescent acid-fast stain** that reveals luminescent yellow-green bacilli against a dark brown background. The fluorescent acid-fast stain is becoming the acid-fast test of choice because it is easier to read; the stained organism provides a striking contrast to the background material (see Fig. 19.5B).

Sputum Culture

Because a variety of nontuberculous strains of *Mycobacterium* can appear on an AFB smear, a sputum culture is often necessary to differentiate *M. tuberculosis* from other acid-fast organisms. For example, common **nontuberculous acid-fast mycobacteria** associated with chronic obstructive pulmonary disease (COPD) are *Mycobacterium avium* and *Mycobacterium kansasii*. Sputum cultures can also identify drug-resistant bacilli and their sensitivity to antibiotic therapy. *M. tuberculosis* grows

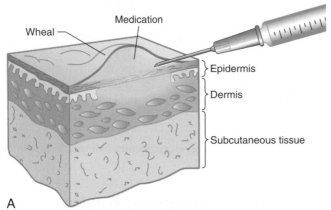
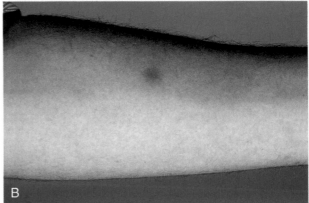

FIGURE 19.4 (A) Intradermal injections are used to administer the Mantoux skin test, which consists of an intradermal injection of a small amount of a purified protein derivative (PPD) of the tuberculin bacillus. An induration of 10 mm or greater is considered positive. A positive reaction is fairly sound evidence of recent or past infection or disease. (B) Positive tuberculin skin test. (A, From Bonewit-West, K., Hunt, S., & Applegate, E. [2016]. *Today's medical assistant* [3rd ed.]. St. Louis, MO: Elsevier. B, From Helbert, M. [2017]. *Immunology for medical students* [3rd ed.]. Philadelphia, PA: Elsevier.)

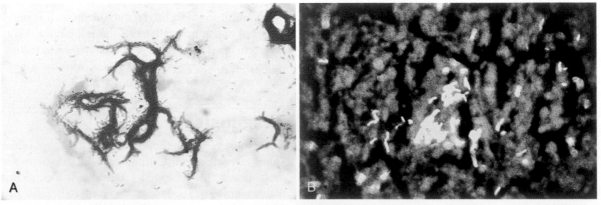

FIGURE 19.5 Acid-fast staining techniques. (A) Ziehl-Neelsen staining of *Mycobacterium tuberculosis* from sputum. The red rods are *M. tuberculosis*. (B) A fluorescent acid-fast stain of *M. tuberculosis* from sputum. Organisms appear yellow (fluorescent). (From Murray, P. R., Rosenthal, K. S., Pfaller, M. A. [2016]. *Medical microbiology* [8th ed.]. Philadelphia, PA: Elsevier.)

very slowly. It takes up to 6 weeks for colonies to appear in culture. When the TB bacterium was first studied, it was given the misleading prefix *Myco,* which gave the impression that the TB pathogen was fungal. The bacterium growing in agars appeared as colonies and was similar to fungal colonies (Fig. 19.6). However, they are unrelated; TB is caused by a bacterium and not a fungus.

QuantiFERON-TB Gold Test

In 2005 the US Food and Drug Administration (FDA) approved the QFT-G test. The QFT-G test is a whole-blood test used for diagnosing *M. tuberculosis* infection, including latent TB infection. Samples of the patient's blood are mixed with antigens (substances that can generate an immune response) and controls. The QFT-G test contains synthetic antigens that represent two *M. tuberculosis* proteins (ESAT-6 and CFP-10). The mixture is then allowed to incubate for 16 to 24 hours. After this period, the mixture is measured for the presence of interferon-gamma (IFN-gamma). In patients infected with *M. tuberculosis*, the white blood cells will release IFN-gamma when in contact with the TB antigens. An elevated IFN-gamma level is diagnostic of TB. Additional clinical evaluations, such as AFB stain of the sputum smear and the chest radiograph, are recommended to further support a positive QFT-G finding.

Xpert MTB/RIF Assay

The Xpert MTB/RIF assay simultaneously detects *Mycobacterium tuberculosis* and **rifampin (RIF)** resistance directly from the patient's sputum. The test results are back quickly (in under 2 hours), and minimal technical training is required to

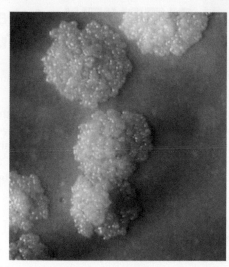

FIGURE 19.6 Cultural appearance of *Mycobacterium tuberculosis.* From Centers for Disease Control and Prevention, Office of the Associate Director for Communications, Division of Public Affairs, Public Health Image Library. Retrieved from https://phil.cdc.gov/Details.aspx?pid=4428.

run the test. In 2010 the WHO recommended Xpert MTB/RIF for use in TB-endemic countries and is monitoring and helping in the coordination of the global roll-out of the technology of this assay.

More than 100 countries are already using the test, and 6.2 million Xpert MTB/RIF cartridges were attained globally in 2015.

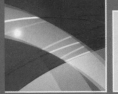

OVERVIEW of the Cardiopulmonary Clinical Manifestations Associated With Tuberculosis

The following clinical manifestations result from the pathophysiologic mechanisms caused (or activated) by alveolar consolidation (see Fig. 10.8) and increased alveolar-capillary membrane thickness (see Fig. 10.9)—the major anatomic alterations of the lungs associated with tuberculosis (see Fig. 19.1).

CLINICAL DATA OBTAINED AT THE PATIENT'S BEDSIDE

The Physical Examination

Vital Signs

Increased Respiratory Rate (Tachypnea)

Several pathophysiologic mechanisms operating simultaneously may lead to an increased ventilatory rate:

- Stimulation of peripheral chemoreceptors
- Relationship of decreased lung compliance to increased ventilatory rate
- Pain, anxiety, fever

Increased Heart Rate (Pulse) and Blood Pressure

Chest Pain, Decreased Chest Expansion

Cyanosis

Digital Clubbing

Peripheral Edema and Venous Distention

Because polycythemia and cor pulmonale are associated with severe tuberculosis (TB), the following may be seen:

- Distended neck veins
- Pitting edema
- Enlarged and tender liver

Cough, Sputum Production, and Hemoptysis

Chest Assessment Findings

- Increased tactile and vocal fremitus
- Dull percussion note
- Bronchial breath sounds
- Crackles, wheezing
- Pleural friction rub (if process extends to pleural surface)
- Whispered pectoriloquy

CLINICAL DATA OBTAINED FROM LABORATORY TESTS AND SPECIAL PROCEDURES

Pulmonary Function Test Findings[1]
Severe and Extensive Cases (Restrictive Lung Pathology)

FORCED EXPIRATORY VOLUME AND FLOW RATE FINDINGS

FVC	FEV_T	FEV_1/FVC ratio	$FEF_{25\%-75\%}$
↓	N or ↓	N or ↑	N or ↓

$FEF_{50\%}$	$FEF_{200-1200}$	PEFR	MVV
N or ↓	N or ↓	N or ↓	N or ↓

LUNG VOLUME AND CAPACITY FINDINGS

V_T	IRV	ERV	RV	
N or ↓	↓	↓	↓	
VC	IC	FRC	TLC	RV/TLC ratio
↓	↓	↓	↓	N

Arterial Blood Gases

MODERATE TUBERCULOSIS
Acute Alveolar Hyperventilation With Hypoxemia[2]
(Acute Respiratory Alkalosis)

pH	$PaCO_2$	HCO_3^-	PaO_2	SaO_2 or SpO_2
↑	↓	↓	↓	↓
		(but normal)		

EXTENSIVE TUBERCULOSIS WITH PULMONARY FIBROSIS
Chronic Ventilatory Failure With Hypoxemia[3]
(Compensated Respiratory Acidosis)

pH	$PaCO_2$	HCO_3^-	PaO_2	SaO_2 or SpO_2
N	↑	↑	↓	↓↓
		(significantly)		

ACUTE VENTILATORY CHANGES SUPERIMPOSED ON CHRONIC VENTILATORY FAILURE[4]

Because acute ventilatory changes are frequently seen in patients with chronic ventilatory failure, the respiratory therapist must be familiar with and alert for the following two dangerous arterial blood gas findings:

- Acute alveolar hyperventilation superimposed on chronic ventilatory failure, which should further alert the respiratory therapist to record the following important ABG assessment: possible *impending acute ventilatory failure*
- Acute ventilatory failure (acute hypoventilation) superimposed on chronic ventilatory failure

---

Oxygenation Indices[5]
Moderate to Severe Stages

$\dot{Q}_S/\dot{Q}_T$	DO_2[6]	$\dot{V}O_2$	$C(a-\bar{v})O_2$	O_2ER	$S\bar{v}O_2$
↑	↓	N or ↑[7]	N or ↑[7]	↑	↓

---

[2]See Fig. 5.2 and Table 5.4 and related discussion for the acute pH, $PaCO_2$, and HCO_3^- changes associated with acute alveolar hyperventilation.

[3]See Table 5.6 and related discussion for the acute pH, $PaCO_2$, and HCO_3^- changes associated with acute ventilatory failure.

[4]See Table 5.7, Table 5.8, and Table 5.9 and related discussion for the pH, $PaCO_2$, and HCO_3^- changes associated with acute ventilatory changes superimposed on chronic ventilatory failure.

[5]$C(a-\bar{v})O_2$, Arterial-venous oxygen difference; DO_2, total oxygen delivery; O_2ER, oxygen extraction ratio; $\dot{Q}_S/\dot{Q}_T$, pulmonary shunt fraction; $S\bar{v}O_2$, mixed venous oxygen saturation; $\dot{V}O_2$, oxygen consumption.

[6]The DO_2 may be normal in patients who have compensated to the decreased oxygenation status with (1) an increased cardiac output, (2) an increased hemoglobin level, or (3) a combination of both. When the DO_2 is normal, the O_2ER is usually normal.

[7]Increased if febrile.

---

[1]Pulmonary function test (PFT) findings are usually normal in most cases of TB.

Hemodynamic Indices[8]
Severe Tuberculosis

CVP	RAP	$\overline{PA}$	PCWP	CO	SV
↑	↑	↑	N	N	N

SVI	CI	RVSWI	LVSWI	PVR	SVR
N	N	↑	N	↑	N

ABNORMAL LABORATORY TEST AND PROCEDURE RESULTS

- Positive tuberculosis skin test (PPD)
- Positive sputum acid-fast bacillus (AFB) stain test
- Positive ABF sputum culture
- Positive QuantiFERON-TB Gold Test

RADIOLOGIC FINDINGS
Chest Radiograph

- Increased opacity
- Ghon nodule
- Ghon complex
- Cavity formation
- Cavitary lesion containing an air-fluid level (see Fig. 18.11 and Fig. 18.14)

- Pleural effusion
- Calcification and fibrosis
- Retraction of lung segments or lobe
- Right ventricular enlargement

Chest radiography is most valuable in the diagnosis of pulmonary TB. During the initial primary infection stage, peripheral pneumonic infiltrates (Ghon nodules) can be identified. As the disease progresses, the combination of tubercles and involvement of the lymph nodes in the hilar region (the Ghon complex) can be seen. In severe cases, cavity formation and pleural effusion are seen (Fig. 19.7). Healed lesions appear fibrotic or calcified. Retraction of the healed lesions or segments also is revealed on chest radiographs. In patients with postprimary TB of the lungs, lesions involving the apical and posterior segments of the upper lobes are often seen. In disseminated **maliary tuberculosis**, the lungs may show myriad 2- to 3-mm granulomatous foci. The radiographic result is widespread fine nodules that are uniformly distributed and equal in size (Fig. 19.8). Finally, because right-sided heart failure (cor pulmonale) may develop as a secondary problem during the advanced stages of TB, an enlarged heart may be seen on the chest radiograph.

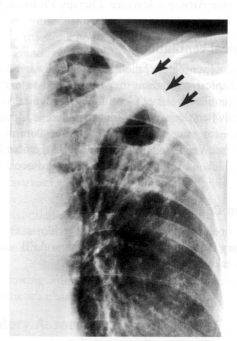

FIGURE 19.7 Cavitary reactivation tuberculosis showing a left upper lobe cavity and localized pleural thickening (arrows). (From Hansell, D. M., Lynch, D. A., McAdams, H. P., et al. [2010]. *Imaging of diseases of the chest* [5th ed.]. Philadelphia, PA: Elsevier.)

[8]*CO,* Cardiac output; *CVP,* central venous pressure; *LVSWI,* left ventricular stroke work index; $\overline{PA}$, mean pulmonary artery pressure; *PCWP,* pulmonary capillary wedge pressure; *PVR,* pulmonary vascular resistance; *RAP,* right atrial pressure; *RVSWI,* right ventricular stroke work index; *SV,* stroke volume; *SVI,* stroke volume index; *SVR,* systemic vascular resistance.

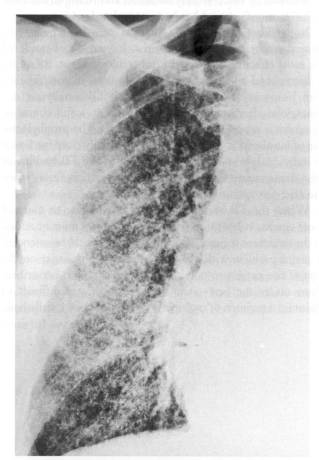

FIGURE 19.8 Miliary tuberculosis showing widespread uniformly distributed fine nodulation of the lung. (From Hansell, D. M., Lynch, D. A., McAdams, H. P., et al. [2010]. *Imaging of diseases of the chest* [5th ed.]. Philadelphia, PA: Elsevier.)

SELF-ASSESSMENT QUESTIONS

1. Which of the following are known as the first stage of tuberculosis?
   1. Reinfection tuberculosis
   2. Primary tuberculosis
   3. Secondary tuberculosis
   4. Primary infection stage
      a. 2 only
      b. 3 only
      c. 1 and 3 only
      d. 2 and 4 only

2. What is the name of the protective wall that surrounds and encases lung tissue infected with tuberculosis?
   1. Miliary tuberculosis
   2. Reinfection tuberculosis
   3. Granuloma
   4. Tubercle
      a. 1 only
      b. 3 only
      c. 4 only
      d. 3 and 4 only

3. The tubercle bacillus is:
   1. Highly aerobic
   2. Acid-fast
   3. Capable of surviving for months outside of the body
   4. Rod-shaped
      a. 2 only
      b. 4 only
      c. 2 and 3 only
      d. 1, 2, 3, and 4

4. At which size wheal is a tuberculin skin test considered to be positive?
   a. Greater than 4 mm
   b. Greater than 6 mm
   c. Greater than 8 mm
   d. Greater than 10 mm

5. Which of the following is often prescribed as a prophylactic daily dose for 1 year in individuals who have been exposed to tuberculosis bacilli?
   a. Streptomycin
   b. Ethambutol
   c. Isoniazid
   d. Rifampin

Chapter Objectives

After reading this chapter, you will be able to:

- List the anatomic alterations of the lungs associated with pulmonary edema.
- Describe the causes of pulmonary edema.
- List the cardiopulmonary clinical manifestations associated with cardiogenic and noncardiogenic pulmonary edema.
- Describe the general management of pulmonary edema.
- Describe the clinical strategies and rationales of the SOAPs presented in the case study.
- Define key terms and complete self-assessment questions at the end of the chapter and on Evolve.

Key Terms

Afterload Reduction
Albumin
Angiotensin-Converting Enzyme (ACE) Inhibitors
Antidysrhythmic Agents
Brain Natriuretic Peptide (BNP)
Captopril
Cardiogenic Pulmonary Edema
Cardiomegaly
Cephalogenic Pulmonary Edema
Cheyne-Stokes Respiration
Congestive Heart Failure (CHF)
Decompression Pulmonary Edema
Digitalis
Dobutamine
Dopamine
Echocardiogram
Enalapril
Furosemide (lasix)
High-Altitude Pulmonary Edema
Increased Capillary Permeability

Kerley A and B Lines
Left Ventricular Ejection Fraction (LVEF)
Loop Diuretics
Lymphangitic Carcinomatosis
Lung Transplantation
Mask Continuous Positive Airway Pressure (CPAP)
Metoprolol
Morphine Sulfate
Nifedipine
Nitroglycerin
Nitroprusside
Noncardiogenic Pulmonary Edema
Norepinephrine
Oncotic Pressure
Orthopnea
Paroxysmal Nocturnal Dyspnea (PND)
Positive Inotropic Agent
Procainamide
Starling Equation
Transudate

Chapter Outline

Anatomic Alterations of the Lungs
Etiology and Epidemiology
    Cardiogenic Pulmonary Edema
    Noncardiogenic Pulmonary Edema
Overview of the Cardiopulmonary Clinical Manifestations
    Associated With Pulmonary Edema
General Management of Pulmonary Edema
    Noncardiogenic Pulmonary Edema
    Cardiogenic Pulmonary Edema
    Respiratory Care Treatment Protocols
Case Study: Pulmonary Edema
Self-Assessment Questions

Anatomic Alterations of the Lungs

Pulmonary edema results from excessive movement of fluid from the pulmonary vascular system to the extravascular system and air spaces of the lungs. Fluid first seeps into the perivascular and peribronchial interstitial spaces; depending on the degree of severity, fluid may progressively move into the alveoli, bronchioles, and bronchi (Fig. 20.1).

As a consequence of this fluid movement, the alveolar walls and interstitial spaces swell. As the swelling intensifies, the alveolar surface tension increases and causes alveolar shrinkage and atelectasis. Moreover, much of the fluid that accumulates in the tracheobronchial tree is churned into a frothy white (sometimes blood-tinged or pink) sputum as a result of air moving in and out of the lungs. The abundance of fluid in the interstitial spaces causes the lymphatic vessels to widen and the lymph flow to increase.

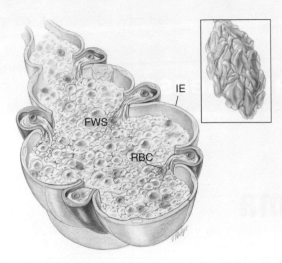

FIGURE 20.1 Pulmonary edema. Cross-sectional view of alveoli and alveolar duct in pulmonary edema. *FWS,* Frothy white secretions; *IE,* interstitial edema; *RBC,* red blood cell. *Inset,* Atelectasis, a common secondary anatomic alteration of the lungs.

Pulmonary edema produces a restrictive pulmonary disorder. The major pathologic or structural changes of the lungs associated with pulmonary edema are as follows:

- Interstitial edema, including fluid engorgement of the perivascular and peribronchial spaces and the alveolar wall interstitium
- Alveolar flooding
- Increased surface tension of alveolar fluids
- Alveolar shrinkage and atelectasis
- Frothy white (or pink) secretions throughout the tracheo-bronchial tree

Etiology and Epidemiology

The causes of pulmonary edema can be divided into two major categories: *cardiogenic* and *noncardiogenic.*

Cardiogenic Pulmonary Edema

According to the American Heart Association (AHA) 2018 Heart Disease and Stroke Statistic Update, Heart Disease (including Coronary Heart Disease, Hypertension, and Stroke) remains the No. 1 cause of death in the US. Coronary heart disease accounts for 1 in 7 deaths in the US, killing over 366,800 people a year. The overall prevalence for a myocardial infarction in the US is about 7.9 million, or 3 percent, in US adults. In 2015, heart attacks claimed 114,023 lives in the US The estimated annual incidence of heart attack in the US is 720,000 new attacks and 335,000 recurrent attacks. Average age at the first heart attack is 65.6 years for males and 72.0 years for females. Approximately every 40 seconds, an American will have a heart attack. From 2005 to 2015, the annual death rate attributable to coronary heart disease declined 34.4 percent and the actual number of deaths declined 17.7% – but the burden and risk factors remain alarmingly high. The estimated direct and indirect cost of heart disease in 2013 to 2014 (average annual) was $204.8 billion. Heart attacks ($12.1 billion) and Coronary Heart Disease ($9.0 billion) were 2 of the 10 most expensive conditions treated in US hospitals in 2013. Between 2013 and 2030, medical costs of Coronary Heart Disease are projected to increase by about 100 percent.

Cardiac pulmonary edema occurs when the left ventricle is unable to pump out a sufficient amount of blood during each ventricular contraction. The ability of the left ventricle to pump blood can be determined by means of the **left ventricular ejection fraction (LVEF)** with a noninvasive cardiac imaging procedure **echocardiogram** that reflects the patient's left ventricular *systolic* cardiac contractility. Poor ventricular function also may be caused by an increased ventricular stiffness or impaired myocardial relaxation. This condition is called *diastolic* dysfunction and is associated with a relatively normal LVEF. Normal values for the LVEF range between 55% and 70%. An LVEF less than 40% may confirm heart failure; an LVEF less than 35% is life-threatening, and cardiac arrhythmias are likely.

When the patient's LVEF is low, the blood pressure inside the pulmonary veins and capillaries increases as a result. This action literally causes fluid to be pushed through the capillary walls and into the alveoli in the form of a **transudate**. The basic pathophysiologic mechanism for this action is described in the following sections.

Ordinarily, hydrostatic pressure of about 10 to 15 mm Hg tends to move fluid *out* of the pulmonary capillaries into the interstitial space. This force is normally offset by colloid osmotic forces of about 25 to 30 mm Hg that tend to keep fluid *in* the pulmonary capillaries. The colloid osmotic pressure is referred to as **oncotic pressure** and is produced by the albumin and globulin in the blood. The stability of fluid within the pulmonary capillaries is determined by the balance between hydrostatic and oncotic pressures. This relationship also maintains fluid stability in the interstitial compartments of the lung.

Movement of fluid in and out of the capillaries is expressed by the **Starling equation**:

$$J = K(Pc - Pi) - (\pi c - \pi i)$$

where J is the net fluid movement out of the capillary, K is the capillary permeability factor, Pc and Pi are the hydrostatic pressures in the capillary and interstitial space, and πc and πi are the oncotic pressures in the capillary and interstitial space.

Although conceptually valuable, this equation has limited practical use. Of the four pressures, only the oncotic and hydrostatic pressures of blood in the pulmonary capillaries can be measured with any certainty. The oncotic and hydrostatic pressures within the interstitial compartments cannot be readily determined.

When the hydrostatic pressure within the pulmonary capillaries rises to more than 25 to 30 mm Hg, the oncotic pressure loses its holding force over the fluid within the vessels. Consequently, fluid starts to spill into the interstitial spaces and alveoli of the lungs (see Fig. 20.1).

Clinically, the patient with left ventricular failure often has activity intolerance, weight gain, anxiety, delirium, dyspnea, orthopnea, paroxysmal nocturnal dyspnea, cough, fatigue, cardiac arrhythmias (particularly atrial fibrillation), and adventitious breath sounds. Because of poor peripheral circulation, such patients often have cool skin, diaphoresis, cyanosis of the digits, and peripheral pallor. Major organ failure of the brain and kidney may be the result of hypoperfusion. Increased pulmonary capillary hydrostatic pressure is the most common cause of pulmonary edema. Box 20.1 provides common causes of **cardiogenic pulmonary edema**. Box 20.2 provides common risk factors for coronary heart disease (CHD).

Noncardiogenic Pulmonary Edema

Noncardiogenic pulmonary edema is less common and develops as a result of damage to the lungs. In these conditions, the lung tissue becomes inflamed and swollen and fluid can readily leak from the pulmonary capillaries into the alveoli. The more common causes of noncardiogenic pulmonary edema include the following:

Increased Capillary Permeability

Pulmonary edema may develop as a result of **increased capillary permeability** stemming from infectious, inflammatory, and other processes. The following are some other causes of increased capillary permeability:

- Alveolar hypoxia (e.g. high altitude)
- Acute respiratory distress syndrome (ARDS)
- Inhalation of toxic agents such as chlorine, sulfur dioxide, nitrogen dioxides, ammonia, and phosgene
- Pulmonary infections (e.g., certain pneumonias)
- Therapeutic radiation of the lungs
- Acute head injury (also known as **cephalogenic pulmonary edema**)

Lymphatic Insufficiency

Should the normal lymphatic drainage of the lungs be decreased, intravascular and extravascular fluid begins to pool and pulmonary edema ensues. Lymphatic drainage may be slowed because of obliteration or distortion of lymphatic vessels. The lymphatic vessels may be obstructed by tumor cells in **lymphangitic carcinomatosis**. Because the lymphatic vessels empty into systemic veins, increased systemic venous pressure may slow lymphatic drainage. Lymphatic insufficiency also has been observed after **lung transplantation**.

Decreased Intrapleural Pressure

Reduced intrapleural pressure may cause pulmonary edema. With severe airway obstruction, for example, the negative intrapulmonary pressure exerted by the patient during inspiration may create a suction effect on the pulmonary capillaries and cause fluid to move into the alveoli. Furthermore, the increased negative intrapleural pressure promotes filling of the right side of the heart and hinders blood flow in the left side of the heart. This condition may cause pooling of the blood in the lungs and subsequently an elevated hydrostatic pressure and pulmonary edema. A related kind of pulmonary edema is caused by the sudden removal of a pleural effusion. Clinically, this condition is called **decompression pulmonary edema.**

High-Altitude Pulmonary Edema

High-altitude pulmonary edema (HAPE) can occur in people who exercise at altitudes above 8000 feet without having first acclimated to the high altitude. HAPE often affects recreational hikers and skiers.

Decreased Oncotic Pressure

Although this condition is rare, if the oncotic pressure is reduced from its normal 25 to 30 mm Hg and falls below the patient's normal hydrostatic pressure of 10 to 15 mm Hg, fluid may begin to seep into the interstitial and air spaces of the lungs. Decreased oncotic pressure may be caused by the following:

- Overtransfusion and/or rapid transfusion of hypotonic or normotonic intravenous fluids
- Uremia
- Hypoproteinemia (e.g., severe malnutrition)
- Acute nephritis
- Polyarteritis nodosa

Although the exact mechanisms are not known, Box 20.3 provides other causes of conditions associated with **noncardiogenic pulmonary edema.**

General Management of Pulmonary Edema

The treatment for pulmonary edema is based on the cause—that is, noncardiogenic versus cardiogenic pulmonary edema—and the severity.

Noncardiogenic Pulmonary Edema

The treatment for noncardiogenic pulmonary edema is largely supportive and aimed at ensuring adequate ventilation and oxygenation. Unfortunately, there are no specific treatments to correct an underlying alveolar-capillary membrane permeability problem or to control the pulmonary inflammatory events that ensue once they are triggered—for example, by inhaled toxic agents or a drug overdose—beyond mechanical ventilation and supportive care. Occasionally, the specific cause of the noncardiogenic pulmonary edema can be identified and treated. For example, noncardiogenic pulmonary edema caused by a severe infection, such as sepsis, is treated with antibiotics, and high altitude pulmonary edema (HAPE) by returning the patient to a lower elevation or by supplemental oxygen and positive-pressure ventilation.

Cardiogenic Pulmonary Edema

For cardiogenic pulmonary edema, the initial management is directed at the use of **digitalis** (if indicated), supplemental oxygen, assisted ventilation if necessary, and a **loop diuretics** for volume overload.

The therapeutic intervention to address the patient's circulatory systems has the following three main goals: (1) reduction of pulmonary venous return (preload reduction), (2) reduction of systemic vascular resistance (**afterload reduction**), and (3) inotropic support (treatment of reduced cardiac contractility).

Reduction of the preload decreases pulmonary capillary hydrostatic pressure and reduces fluid transudation into the pulmonary interstitium and alveoli. Reduction of afterload increases cardiac output and improves renal perfusion, which in turn allows for diuresis in the patient with fluid overload. Inotropic agents are used to treat hypotension or signs of organ hypoperfusion. While the patient's circulatory problem(s)

is/are treated, intubation and mechanical ventilation may be necessary to achieve adequate ventilation, oxygenation, and airway management. Common medications used to treat cardiogenic pulmonary edema are discussed as follows.

Preload Reducers

Reduced pulmonary venous return decreases pulmonary capillary hydrostatic pressure and reduces fluid transudation into the pulmonary interstitium and alveoli. Preload reducers include:

- *Nitroglycerin (Nitro-Bid, Minitran, Nitrostat):* A very effective, predictable, and rapid-acting medication for preload.
- *Loop diuretics (e.g., furosemide):* Considered a cornerstone in the treatment of cardiogenic pulmonary edema. Loop diuretics are presumed to decrease preload through diuresis and direct vasodilation.
- *Morphine sulfate:* May be used in some cases to reduce preload. However, the adverse effects (e.g., nausea and vomiting or respiratory depression) may outweigh the potential benefit, especially with the availability of nitroglycerin, which is a more effective preload reducing agent.

Afterload Reducers

Reduced systemic vascular resistance increases cardiac output and improves renal perfusion, allowing for diuresis. Afterload reducers include:

- *Captopril:* Prevents the conversion of angiotensin I to angiotensin II. It is a potent vasodilator. Afterload and cardiac output usually improve in 10 to 15 minutes.
- *Enalapril (Vasotec):* Is a competitive **angiotensin-converting enzyme (ACE) inhibitor** and reduces angiotensin II levels.
- *Nitroprusside (Nitropress):* Is a potent, direct smooth muscle-relaxing agent that primarily reduces afterload. It can also mildly reduce preload.

Positive Inotropic Agents

These agents are used for their vasodilation effects and to increase myocardial contraction and cardiac output. **Positive inotropic agents** include the following:

- *Dobutamine:* Is a synthetic catecholamine that mainly has $beta_1$-receptor activity but also has some $beta_2$-receptor and alpha-receptor activity. Commonly used for patients with mild hypotension (e.g., systolic blood pressure 90 to 100 mm Hg).
- *Dopamine:* Is a naturally occurring catecholamine that acts as a precursor to norepinephrine. Dopamine hemodynamic effect is dose dependent. A low dose is associated with dilation in the renal and splanchnic vasculature, enhancing diuresis. A moderate dose enhances cardiac contractility and heart rate. A high dose increases afterload because of peripheral vasoconstriction and must be used with care in patients with normal blood pressure (i.e., normotensive). Dopamine is generally reserved for patients with moderate hypotension (e.g., systolic blood pressure 70 to 90 mm Hg).
- *Norepinephrine:* Is a naturally occurring catecholamine with potent alpha-receptor and mild beat-receptor activity. It simulates $beta_1$-adrenergic and alpha-adrenergic receptors, increasing myocardial contractility, heart rate, and vasoconstriction. Norepinephrine increases blood pressure and

The following clinical manifestations result from the pathologic mechanisms caused (or activated) by atelectasis (see Fig. 10.7), increased alveolar-capillary membrane thickness (see Fig. 10.9), and, in severe cases, excessive bronchial secretions (see Fig. 10.11)—the major anatomic alterations of the lungs associated with pulmonary edema (see Fig. 20.1).

CLINICAL DATA OBTAINED AT THE PATIENT'S BEDSIDE

The Physical Examination

Vital Signs

Increased Respiratory Rate (Tachypnea)

Several pathophysiologic mechanisms operating simultaneously may lead to an increased ventilatory rate:

- Stimulation of peripheral chemoreceptors (hypoxemia)
- Relationship of decreased lung compliance to increased ventilatory rate
- Stimulation of J receptors and baroreceptors
- Anxiety

Increased Heart Rate (Pulse) and Blood Pressure

Cheyne-Stokes Respiration

Cheyne-Stokes respiration may be seen in patients with severe left-sided heart failure and pulmonary edema. Some authorities have suggested that the cause of Cheyne-Stokes respiration in these patients may be related to the prolonged circulation time between the lungs and the central chemoreceptors. Cheyne-Stokes respiration is a classic clinical manifestation in central sleep apnea (see Chapter 32, Sleep Apnea).

Paroxysmal Nocturnal Dyspnea and Orthopnea

Patients with pulmonary edema often awaken with severe dyspnea after several hours of sleep. This condition is called **paroxysmal nocturnal dyspnea (PND)**. This condition is particularly prevalent in patients with cardiogenic pulmonary edema. While the patient is awake, more time is spent in the erect position and, as a result, excess fluids tend to accumulate in the dependent portions of the body. When the patient lies down, however, the excess fluids from the dependent parts of the body move into the bloodstream and cause an increase in venous return to the lungs. This action raises the pulmonary hydrostatic pressure and promotes pulmonary edema. The pulmonary edema in turn produces pulmonary shunting, venous admixture, and hypoxemia. When the hypoxemia becomes severe, the peripheral chemoreceptors are stimulated and initiate an increased ventilatory rate (see Figs. 3.5 and 3.6). The decreased lung compliance, J receptor stimulation, and anxiety may also contribute to the paroxysmal nocturnal dyspnea commonly seen in this disorder at night. A patient is said to have **orthopnea** when dyspnea increases while the patient is lying in a recumbent position.

Cyanosis

Cough and Sputum (Frothy and Pink in Appearance)

Chest Assessment Findings

- Increased tactile and vocal fremitus
- Crackles and wheezing

CLINICAL DATA OBTAINED FROM LABORATORY TESTS AND SPECIAL PROCEDURES

Pulmonary Function Test Findings
Moderate to Severe Pulmonary Edema (Restrictive Lung Pathology)

FORCED EXPIRATORY VOLUME AND FLOW RATE FINDINGS[1]

FVC	FEV_T	FEV_1/FVC ratio	$FEF_{25\%-75\%}$
↓	N or ↓	N or ↑	N or ↓

$FEF_{50\%}$	$FEF_{200-1200}$	PEFR	MVV
N or ↓	N or ↓	N or ↓	N or ↓

LUNG VOLUME AND CAPACITY FINDINGS

V_T	IRV	ERV	RV	
N or ↓	↓	↓	↓	

VC	IC	FRC	TLC	RV/TLC ratio
↓	↓	↓	↓	N

Arterial Blood Gases

MILD TO MODERATE PULMONARY EDEMA

Acute Alveolar Hyperventilation With Hypoxemia[2] (Acute Respiratory Alkalosis)

pH	$PaCO_2$	HCO_3^-	PaO_2	SaO_2 or SpO_2
↑	↓	↓ (but normal)	↓	↓

SEVERE PULMONARY EDEMA

Acute Ventilatory Failure With Hypoxemia[3] (Acute Respiratory Acidosis)

pH[4]	$PaCO_2$	HCO_3^-[4]	PaO_2	SaO_2 or SpO_2
↓	↑	↑ (but normal)	↓	↓

---

[1]The decreased forced expiratory volumes and flow rate findings are primarily caused by the low vital capacity associated with the restrictive pulmonary disorder.

[2]See Fig. 5.2 and Table 5.4 and related discussion for the acute pH, $PaCO_2$, and HCO_3^- changes associated with acute alveolar hyperventilation.

[3]See Fig. 5.2 and Table 5.5 and related discussion for the acute pH, $PaCO_2$, and HCO_3^- changes associated with acute and chronic ventilatory failure.

[4]When tissue hypoxia is severe enough to produce lactic acid, the pH and HCO_3^- values will be lower than expected for a particular $PaCO_2$ level (metabolic acidosis). This is particularly common when systemic hypotension is present.

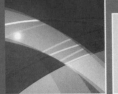

Oxygenation Indices[5]					
$\dot{Q}_S/\dot{Q}_T$	DO_2[6]	$\dot{V}O_2$	$C(a\text{-}\bar{v})O_2$	O_2ER	$S\bar{v}O_2$
↑	↓	N	N	↑	↓

Hemodynamic Indices[7] Cardiogenic Pulmonary Edema (Moderate to Severe)					
CVP	RAP	$\overline{PA}$	PCWP	CO	SV
↑	↑	↑	↑	↓	↓
SVI	CI	RVSWI	LVSWI[8]	PVR	SVR
↓	↓	↑	↓	↑	↑

Other Important Hemodynamic Indices:
Left Ventricular Ejection Fraction (LVEF)

ABNORMAL LABORATORY TEST AND PROCEDURE RESULTS

- Serum potassium: Low
- Serum sodium: Low
- Serum chloride: Low
- Brain natriuretic peptide (BNP): Elevated

Hypokalemia, hyponatremia, and hypochloremia are often seen in patients with left-sided heart failure and may result from diuretic therapy or excessive fluid retention. The **brain natriuretic peptide (BNP)**, also known as B-type natriuretic peptide or ventricular natriuretic peptide (still BNP) is an important biomarker used to help establish the diagnosis of congestive heart failure (CHF). The BNP hormone is produced by the heart and reflects how well the heart is functioning. Normally, only a low amount of BNP (<100 pg/mL) is found in blood. However, when the heart is working harder than normal over a long period, the heart releases more of the substance, increasing the blood level of BNP. The following provides various BNP levels and the cardiac status associated with these levels:

- BNP levels below 100 pg/mL indicate no heart failure.
- BNP levels of 100 to 300 pg/mL suggest heart failure may be present.
- BNP levels above 300 pg/mL indicate mild heart failure.
- BNP levels above 600 pg/mL indicate moderate heart failure.
- BNP levels above 900 pg/mL indicate severe heart failure.

[5]$C(a\text{-}\bar{v})O_2$, Arterial-venous oxygen difference; DO_2, total oxygen delivery; O_2ER, oxygen extraction ratio; $\dot{Q}_S/\dot{Q}_T$, pulmonary shunt fraction; $S\bar{v}O_2$, mixed venous oxygen saturation; $\dot{V}O_2$, oxygen consumption.
[6]The DO_2 may be normal in patients who have compensated to the decreased oxygenation status with (1) an increased cardiac output, (2) an increased hemoglobin level, or (3) a combination of both. When the DO_2 is normal, the O_2ER is usually normal.
[7]CO, Cardiac output; CVP, central venous pressure; $LVSWI$, left ventricular stroke work index; HCO_3^-, mean pulmonary artery pressure; $PCWP$, pulmonary capillary wedge pressure; PVR, pulmonary vascular resistance; RAP, right atrial pressure; $RVSWI$, right ventricular stroke work index; SV, stroke volume; SVI, stroke volume index; SVR, systemic vascular resistance; $LVEF$, left ventricular ejection fraction.
[8]Decreased LVEF when cardiogenic pulmonary edema is present. May be normal in noncardiogenic pulmonary edema.

RADIOLOGIC FINDINGS
Chest Radiograph

- Bilateral fluffy opacities with a predominantly central position in the chest
- Dilated pulmonary arteries
- Left ventricular hypertrophy (cardiomegaly)
- Kerley A and B lines
- "Bat's wing" or "butterfly" pattern
- Pleural effusion (transudate)—see Chapter 24, Pleural Effusion and Empyema

Cardiogenic Pulmonary Edema

The radiographic findings associated with left heart failure are commonly described as follows:

- Mild left-sided heart failure: Pulmonary venous congestion with dilated pulmonary arteries is present.
- Moderate left-sided heart failure: **Cardiomegaly**, engorgement of the pulmonary arteries, and **Kerley A and B lines** are present. When cardiomegaly is present, the heart is greater than half the diameter of the thorax in a posteroanterior chest radiograph (Fig. 20.2). Because radiographic densities primarily reflect alveolar filling and not early interstitial edema, by the time abnormal findings are encountered, the pathologic changes associated with pulmonary edema are advanced. Chest x-ray films typically reveal dense, fluffy opacities that spread outward from the hilar areas to the peripheral borders of the lungs (Figs. 20.2 and 20.4).
- Kerley A lines, which represent deep interstitial edema, radiate out from the hilum into the central portions of the lungs. Kerley A lines do not reach the pleura and are most prevalent in the middle and upper lung regions. Kerley B lines are short, thin, horizontal lines of interstitial edema, usually less than 1 cm in length, that extend inward from the pleural

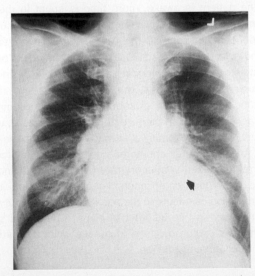

FIGURE 20.2 Cardiomegaly (arrow), hilar prominence, and pulmonary edema in congestive heart failure. Note that the heart diameter is greater than half the diameter of the thorax.

surface. They appear peripherally in contact with the pleura and are parallel to one another at right angles to the pleura. Although they may be seen in any lung region, they are most commonly seen in the lung bases (Fig. 20.3).

- Severe left-sided heart failure: During this stage, the patient's chest radiograph shows cardiomegaly; pulmonary artery engorgement; interstitial pulmonary edema; fluffy, patchy areas of alveolar edema; and often the appearance of the "bat's wing pattern" (also called the *butterfly pattern*). The peripheral portion of the lungs often remains clear, and this produces what is described as a "butterfly" or "bat's wing" distribution (see Fig. 20.4). Pleural effusion also may be seen.

Noncardiogenic Pulmonary Edema

In noncardiogenic pulmonary edema the chest radiograph commonly shows areas of fluffy densities that are usually more dense near the hilum. The infiltrates may be unilateral or bilateral. Pleural effusion is usually not present and (most important) the cardiac silhouette is not enlarged.

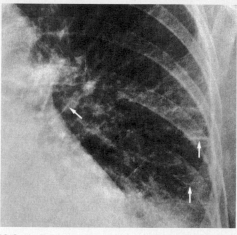

FIGURE 20.3 Kerley lines. Septal lines caused by pulmonary edema. Kerley B lines are short horizontal lines at the lung periphery (vertical arrows). Kerley A lines are lines radiating from the hila (oblique arrow). (From Hansell, D. M., Lynch, D. A., McAdams, H. P., et al. [2010]. *Imaging of diseases of the chest* [5th ed.]. Philadelphia, PA: Elsevier.)

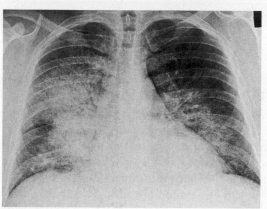

FIGURE 20.4 Bat's wing or butterfly pattern caused by pulmonary edema. This example is typical in that it is bilateral but not symmetric. The shadowing is maximal in the central (perihilar) portions of the lung, and the outer portions of the lungs are relatively clear. (From Hansell, D. M., Lynch, D. A., McAdams, H. P., et al. [2010]. *Imaging of diseases of the chest* [5th ed.]. Philadelphia, PA: Elsevier.)

afterload. Norepinephrine is generally reserved for patients with severe hypotension (e.g., systolic blood pressure less than 70 mm Hg).

- *Milrinone:* Is a positive inotropic agent and vasodilator. It reduces afterload and preload and increases cardiac output.

Other Agents

- *Antidysrhythmic agents:* Such as drugs to control bradycardia (e.g., atropine) or tachycardia (e.g., **digitalis, procainamide** or **metoprolol**) may be administered.
- *Albumin:* Is sometimes administered to increase the patient's oncotic pressure in an effort to offset the increased hydrostatic forces of cardiogenic pulmonary edema, if the patient's osmotic pressure is extremely low.

Respiratory Care Treatment Protocols

Oxygen Therapy Protocol

Oxygen therapy is used to treat hypoxemia, decrease the work of breathing, and decrease myocardial work. The hypoxemia that develops in pulmonary edema is most commonly caused by the interstitial and alveolar fluid, atelectasis, and capillary shunting associated with the disorder. Hypoxemia caused by capillary shunting is at least partially refractory to oxygen therapy (see Oxygen Therapy Protocol, Protocol 10.1).

Lung Expansion Therapy Protocol

Lung expansion therapy is commonly used to offset the fluid accumulation and atelectasis associated with cardiogenic pulmonary edema. High-flow mask continuous positive airway pressure (CPAP) has been shown to produce a significant and rapid improvement in oxygenation and ventilatory status in patients with pulmonary edema. **Mask continuous positive airway pressure** improves decreased lung compliance, reduces the work of breathing, enhances gas exchange, and decreases vascular congestion in patients with pulmonary edema. In fact, mask CPAP is initially prescribed (at least for a trial period) for patients with pulmonary edema who have arterial blood gas (ABG) values that indicate impending ventilatory failure or acute ventilatory failure—the hallmark clinical manifestations for mechanical ventilation. Often, mask CPAP dramatically improves oxygenation and ventilatory status in these patients and eliminates the need for mechanical ventilation (see Lung Expansion Therapy Protocol, Protocol 10.3).

Mechanical Ventilation Protocol

Mechanical ventilation may be necessary to provide and support alveolar gas exchange and eventually return the patient to spontaneous breathing. Because acute ventilatory failure is occasionally seen in patients with severe cardiogenic and noncardiogenic pulmonary edema, continuous mechanical ventilation may be required. Continuous mechanical ventilation is justified when the acute ventilatory failure is thought to be reversible (see Ventilator Initiation and Management Protocol, Protocol 11.1, and Ventilator Weaning Protocol, Protocol 11.2).

CASE STUDY Pulmonary Edema

Admitting History and Physical Examination

This 76-year-old man was admitted to the emergency department (ED) in obvious respiratory distress. His wife reported that her husband had gone to bed feeling well. He woke up with chest pain at about 2:30 a.m., very short of breath. She became concerned and called an ambulance. Neither the patient nor the wife was a good historian, but they did report that the patient had been under a physician's care for some time for "heart trouble" and that he was taking "little white pills" on a daily basis. For the previous 3 days, he had not taken any medication.

On admission to the ED, the patient was mildly disoriented and slightly cyanotic. He repeatedly tried to take the oxygen mask from his face. He complained of a feeling of suffocation. His neck veins were distended, and the skin of his extremities was mottled. On auscultation, there were coarse crackles in both lower lung fields and some crackles in the middle and upper lung fields.

His cough was productive of pinkish, frothy sputum. His vital signs were blood pressure 105/50, heart rate 124 beats/min, and respiratory rate 28 breaths/min. He was afebrile. An electrocardiogram (ECG) showed evidence of an old myocardial infarct, sinus tachycardia, and an occasional premature ventricular contraction. Chest x-ray films taken in the ED with the patient in a sitting position revealed bilateral fluffy infiltrates, more marked in the lower lung fields. The heart was enlarged. All other laboratory findings were within normal limits. Blood gases on an FIO_2 of 0.30 were pH 7.11, $PaCO_2$ 72 mm Hg, HCO_3^- 22 mEq/L, PaO_2 56 mm Hg, and SaO_2 75%.

The respiratory therapist working in the ED during the night shift recorded the following SOAP note.

Respiratory Assessment and Plan

S Patient states "a feeling of suffocation."

O Cyanosis, disorientation. Distended neck veins and mottled extremities. BP 105/50, HR 124, RR 28. ECG: Sinus tachycardia and occasional PVCs. Coarse crackles bilaterally. Frothy pink sputum. CXR: Bilateral fluffy infiltrates and an enlarged heart. ABGs: pH 7.11, $PaCO_2$ 72, HCO_3^- 22, PaO_2 56, and SaO_2 75% (FIO_2 0.30).

A • Myocardial infarction (old)
• Acute pulmonary edema (CXR)
• Acute ventilatory failure with moderate hypoxemia (ABG)
• Lactic acidosis likely
• Large and small airway secretions (coarse crackles)

P Oxygen Therapy Protocol: Increase FIO_2 to 0.60 via continuous CPAP mask at 25 cm H_2O per Lung Expansion Therapy Protocol. Remain on standby for emergency endotracheal intubation and ventilator support. Continue ECG and oximetry monitoring, and repeat ABG in 30 minutes.

The patient was admitted on the cardiology service with a diagnosis of pulmonary edema–cardiogenic congestive heart failure (CHF). ECG monitoring and continuous oximetry were followed. Treatment consisted of intravenous furosemide, dopamine, nitroprusside, and mask CPAP at 25 cm H_2O pressure with an FIO_2 of 0.60. A Foley catheter was placed.

Two hours later, the patient's condition was very much improved and he was no longer cyanotic. Vital signs were blood pressure 126/70, heart rate 96 beats/min, and respiratory rate 18 breaths/min. The ECG revealed no ectopic beats. Auscultation showed considerable improvement. There were still some basilar crackles, but the upper lung fields were clear. Cough was much reduced and no longer productive. Repeat chest x-ray examination at the bedside showed considerable improvement. Urine output was in excess of 600 mL/h. The patient was calm and rational, stating that he was less short of breath and had no pain. Repeat ABGs revealed pH 7.35, $PaCO_2$ 46 mm Hg, HCO_3^- 24 mEq/L, PaO_2 120 mm Hg, SaO_2 97% on an FIO_2 of 0.60 and CPAP of 25 cm H_2O. His LVEF was 47%.

The following respiratory therapy SOAP note was made at the time.

Respiratory Assessment and Plan

S Patient states, "I'm less short of breath. No pain."

O Not cyanotic. BP 126/70, HR 96, RR 18. ECG: Mild sinus tachycardia without ectopic beats. Fewer crackles; no sputum production; CXR: Improved. ABGs: pH 7.35, $PaCO_2$ 46, HCO_3^- 24, PaO_2 120, and SaO_2 97% (FIO_2 0.60 and CPAP of 25 cm H_2O).

A
- Decreased pulmonary edema (overall impression from the data)
- No longer in acute ventilatory failure (ABG)
- Acceptable acid-base status with mild overcorrected hypoxemia (ABG)
- Secretions controlled (no sputum and fewer crackles)
- Congestive heart failure with resolving pulmonary edema

P Reduce O_2 per Oxygen Therapy Protocol to 2 L/min by nasal cannula. Discontinue CPAP per Lung Expansion Therapy Protocol. Continue ECG and oximetry monitoring. Repeat ABG in 60 minutes.

Discussion

Acute pulmonary edema is a classic finding in severe CHF. Several clinical manifestations associated with increased alveolar-capillary membrane thickness (see Fig. 10.9) were present in this case. For example, the patient's decreased lung compliance was manifested in his tachycardia and tachypnea, whereas his hypoxemia reflected diffusion blockade and intrapulmonary shunting associated with classic pulmonary edema. His lung compliance was so reduced that he had progressed to acute ventilatory failure—that is, the severe stage of pulmonary edema. Frank pulmonary edema caused by left ventricular failure typically improves markedly when treated with CPAP. Some atelectasis (see Fig. 10.7) was doubtless also present and provided further rationale for CPAP therapy.

Often, the first-line management of pulmonary edema consists only of improving myocardial efficiency, decreasing the cardiovascular afterload, decreasing the hypervolemia, providing CPAP, and improving oxygenation. Furosemide (Lasix) is a potent loop diuretic, dopamine has direct inotropic effects, and nitroprusside is a potent peripheral vasodilator. In this case, the combination of all these therapies resulted in a marked improvement of the patient's condition.

In short, this patient had an acute respiratory problem but the basic cause was cardiac. After the cardiac condition was treated, the respiratory symptoms rapidly disappeared. CPAP and an increased FIO_2 were adequate, and this patient was spared the trauma and risk associated with intubation and mechanical ventilation. No evidence of acute myocardial infarction was found. He was discharged after 48 hours, with his condition much improved. He was instructed to take his cardiac medication and diuretics without fail and to return to his family physician in 3 days.

SELF-ASSESSMENT QUESTIONS

1. **Which of the following is an afterload reducer?**
   a. Procainamide
   b. Dopamine
   c. Furosemide
   d. Nitroprusside

2. **What is the normal hydrostatic pressure in the pulmonary capillaries?**
   a. 5 to 10 mm Hg
   b. 10 to 15 mm Hg
   c. 15 to 20 mm Hg
   d. 20 to 25 mm Hg

3. **What is the normal oncotic pressure of the blood?**
   a. 10 to 15 mm Hg
   b. 15 to 20 mm Hg
   c. 20 to 25 mm Hg
   d. 25 to 30 mm Hg

4. **Which of the following are causes of cardiogenic pulmonary edema?**
   1. Excessive fluid administration
   2. Right ventricular failure
   3. Mitral valve disease
   4. Pulmonary embolus
      a. 1 and 2 only
      b. 1, 2, and 3 only
      c. 2, 3, and 4 only
      d. 1, 3, and 4 only

5. **As a result of pulmonary edema, the patient's:**
   1. RV is decreased
   2. FRC is increased
   3. VC is increased
   4. TLC is increased
      a. 1 only
      b. 1 and 4 only
      c. 2 and 3 only
      d. 3 and 4 only

6. **The left ventricular ejection fraction:**
   1. Normally is greater than 75%
   2. Is a good measure of alveolar ventilation
   3. Correlates well with the brain natriuretic peptide values
   4. Provides a noninvasive measurement of cardiac contractility
      a. 1 and 2 only
      b. 2 and 4 only
      c. 3 and 4 only
      d. 2, 3, and 4 only

Pulmonary Vascular Disease

PULMONARY EMBOLISM AND PULMONARY HYPERTENSION

Chapter Objectives

After reading this chapter, you will be able to:

- List the anatomic alterations of the lungs associated with pulmonary embolism.
- Describe the causes of pulmonary embolism.
- List the cardiopulmonary clinical manifestations associated with pulmonary embolism.
- Describe the general management of pulmonary embolism.
- Define pulmonary hypertension.
- Differentiate the five clinical classifications of pulmonary hypertension.
- Identify the common signs and symptoms associated with pulmonary hypertension.
- Describe the tests and procedures used to diagnose pulmonary hypertension.
- Describe the pulmonary hypertension severity rating.
- Differentiate the signs and symptoms between right-sided heart failure and left-sided heart failure.
- Describe the role of the respiratory therapist in pulmonary vascular disorders.
- Discuss the treatment selections used to manage acute pulmonary embolism, pulmonary infarction, and pulmonary hypertension.
- Describe the clinical strategies and rationales of the SOAPs presented in the case study.
- Define key terms and complete self-assessment questions at the end of the chapter and on Evolve.

Key Terms

Alteplase
Biventricular Failure
Calcium Channel Blockers
Chronic Thromboembolic Pulmonary Hypertension
Computed Tomography Pulmonary Angiogram (CTPA)
Cor pulmonale
D-Dimer Blood Test
Deep Venous Thrombosis (DVT)
Echocardiography
Embolus/Embolism
High-Molecular-Weight Heparins
Inferior Vena Cava Vein Filter (Greenfield Filter)
Inhaled Nitric Oxide (iNO) Therapy
Left-Sided Heart Failure
Low-Molecular-Weight Heparins

Phosphodiesterase-5 Inhibitors
Physiologic Dead Space (Wasted Ventilation)
P-Pulmonale (ECG Finding)
Prostanoids
Pulmonary Angiogram
Pulmonary Artery Pressure
Pulmonary Embolectomy
Pulmonary Embolism (PE)
Pulmonary Hypertension (PH)
Pulmonary Infarction
Pulmonary Veno-occlusive Disease
Reteplase
Right-Sided Heart Failure
Saddle Embolus
Streptokinase
Thrombolytic Agents
Thrombus
Ultrasonography
Urokinase
Venous Thrombosis
Ventilation-Perfusion Lung Scan (V̇/Q̇ Scan)
Virchow's Triad
Warfarin (Coumadin)
Wells Clinical Prediction Rule for Deep Venous Thrombosis
Westermark Sign

Chapter Outline

Pulmonary Embolism
Anatomic Alterations of the Lungs
Etiology and Epidemiology
Diagnosis and Screening
    Common Tests for Suspected Pulmonary Embolism
Overview of the Cardiopulmonary Clinical Manifestations
    Associated With Pulmonary Embolism
General Management of Pulmonary Embolism
    Thrombolytic Agents
    Preventive Measures
    Respiratory Care Treatment Protocols
Pulmonary Hypertension
    Diagnosis
    Management of Pulmonary Hypertension
The Emerging Role of the Respiratory Therapist in Pulmonary
    Vascular Disorders
Case Study: Pulmonary Embolism
Self-Assessment Questions

PULMONARY EMBOLISM

Anatomic Alterations of the Lungs

A blood clot that forms and remains in a vein is called a **thrombus**. A blood clot that becomes dislodged and travels to another part of the body is called an **embolus (embolism).** In some cases, when the embolus significantly disrupts pulmonary arterial blood flow, **pulmonary infarction** may develop, which in turn may cause alveolar atelectasis, consolidation, and tissue necrosis. Bronchial smooth muscle constriction occasionally accompanies pulmonary embolism. Although the precise mechanism is not known, it is believed that the embolism causes the release of cellular mediators such as serotonin, histamine, and prostaglandins from platelets, which in turn leads to bronchoconstriction. Local areas of alveolar hypocapnia and hypoxemia may also contribute to the bronchoconstriction associated with pulmonary embolism.

An embolus may originate from one large thrombus or occur as a shower of small thrombi and may or may not interfere with the right ventricle's ability to perfuse the lungs adequately. When a large embolus detaches from a thrombus and passes through the right side of the heart, it may lodge in the bifurcation of the pulmonary artery, where it forms what is known as a **saddle embolus**. A large saddle embolus is often quickly fatal, because it can significantly block pulmonary blood from returning to the left ventricle and being pumped out to the systemic circulation (partially shown in Fig. 21.1A).

The major pathologic or structural changes of the lungs and heart associated with pulmonary embolism are as follows:
* Blockage of the pulmonary vascular system
  * Pulmonary hypertension
  * Right-heart failure (**cor pulmonale**)
* Pulmonary infarction (when severe)
* Alveolar atelectasis
* Alveolar consolidation
* Bronchial smooth muscle constriction (bronchospasm)

Etiology and Epidemiology

Deep vein thrombosis (DVT) and **pulmonary embolism (PE)** are often clinically insidious disorders. If the pulmonary embolus is relatively small, the early signs and symptoms of its presence are often vague and nonspecific. By contrast, sudden death is often the first symptom in about 25% of people who have a large pulmonary embolus. A massive pulmonary embolism is one of the most common causes of sudden and unexpected death in all age groups. Many cases of pulmonary emboli are undiagnosed and therefore untreated. In fact, because of the subtle and misleading clinical manifestations associated with a pulmonary embolus, the possibility of a blood clot lodged in the lung is often not considered *until autopsy* in about 70% to 80% of cases.

In the United States, about 100,000 individuals die each year from a pulmonary embolism. Pulmonary embolism is slightly more common in males than females, and the incidence increases with age. The experienced health care practitioner actively works to confirm the diagnosis of a pulmonary embolism as *soon as the suspicion arises*. This is especially true as the origin of the signs and symptoms of pulmonary embolic disease often cannot be readily identified.

Although there are many possible sources of pulmonary emboli (e.g., fat, air, amniotic fluid, bone marrow, tumor fragments), blood clots are by far the most common. Most pulmonary blood clots originate—or break away from—sites of deep **venous thrombosis** in the lower part of the body (i.e., the leg and pelvic veins and the inferior vena cava). When a thrombus or a piece of a thrombus breaks loose in a deep vein, the blood clot (now called an *embolus*) is carried

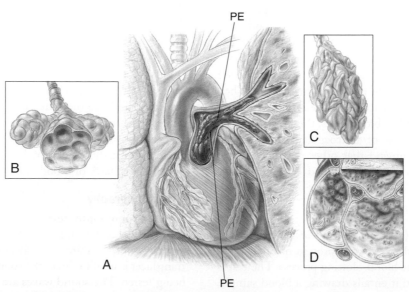

FIGURE 21.1 (A) Pulmonary embolism (PE). (B) Bronchial smooth muscle constriction; (C) atelectasis; and (D) alveolar consolidation are common secondary anatomic alterations of the lungs.

through the venous system to the right atrium and ventricle of the heart and ultimately lodges in the pulmonary arteries or arterioles. There are three primary factors (known as the **Virchow triad**) associated with the formation of DVT. The Virchow triad includes (1) venous stasis (i.e., slowing or stagnation of blood flow through the veins), (2) hypercoagulability (i.e., the increased tendency of blood to form clots), and (3) injury to the endothelial cells that line the vessels. Box 21.1 provides common risk factors for pulmonary embolism.

Diagnosis and Screening

The diagnosis of a pulmonary embolism is primarily based on the clinical manifestations that support the possibility of pulmonary embolism, followed by the results of a variety of possible blood tests, venous ultrasonography, and one or more lung imaging techniques to secure a definitive diagnosis. Depending on how much of the lung is involved, the size of the embolism, and the overall health of the patient, the signs and symptoms of a pulmonary embolism can vary greatly. Box 21.2 provides common signs and symptoms associated with a suspected pulmonary embolism. As shown in Table 21.1, when a pulmonary embolism is possible, the most commonly used tool to predict its clinical probability is the modified Wells Scoring System. Table 21.2 provides the **Wells Clinical Prediction Rule for Deep Venous Thrombosis**.

Common Tests for Suspected Pulmonary Embolism

Blood Tests

Once it has been established that there is a likely probability of a pulmonary embolism, an array of blood tests may be performed to exclude important secondary causes of pulmonary embolism, including a full blood count, clotting status evaluation, and some screening tests (e.g., erythrocyte sedimentation rate, renal function, liver enzymes, electrolytes). Should any of these tests be abnormal, further investigation is justified.

In individuals who (1) have a family history of blood clots, (2) have had more than one episode of blood clots, or (3) have experienced blood clots for no known reason, the doctor may prescribe a series of blood tests to determine if there are any inherited abnormalities in the blood-clotting system. When genetic abnormalities (e.g., factor V [Leiden] deficiency) are found or there is a history of blood clots, the physician may recommend a lifelong course of anticoagulant therapy. The physician also may recommend that other members of the family receive a screening series of blood tests and other pertinent evaluations.

D-Dimer Blood Test

The **D-dimer blood test** (also called the *fibrinogen test*) is used to check for an increased level of the protein fibrinogen, an integral component of the blood-clotting process. The test is relatively simple and fast; it entails drawing a blood sample, and the results can be available in less than 1 hour. D-Dimer values higher than 500 ng/mL are considered positive, which

may suggest the possibility of blood clots. However, it should be emphasized that there are many conditions that can increase an individual's D-dimer level, including recent surgery. Thus an elevated D-dimer value is usually used to supplement other clinical information. A normal D-dimer level essentially rules out the possibility of blood clots.

Ultrasonography

An **ultrasonography** test uses high-frequency sound waves to detect blood clots in the thigh veins. The test is noninvasive and takes only 30 minutes or less to perform. A wand-shaped transducer is used to direct the sound waves to the thigh veins being tested. The sound waves are then reflected back to the transducer and converted to a moving image on a computer screen. The test is very accurate for the diagnosis of blood

BOX 21.2 Signs and Symptoms Commonly Associated With Pulmonary Embolism

- Sudden shortness of breath
- Cardiac arrhythmias
  - Sinus tachycardia
  - Atrial arrhythmias
  - Atrial tachycardia
  - Atrial flutter
  - Atrial fibrillation
  - Acute right ventricular strain pattern and right bundle branch block
  - P pulmonale (peaked P waves)
- Weak pulse
- Lightheadedness or fainting
- Anxiety
- Excessive sweating
- Cyanosis
- Cool or clammy skin to the touch
- Chest pain that resembles a heart attack—that is, chest pain that may radiate to the shoulder, arm, neck, or jaw. The pain is often described as sharp, stabbing, aching, or dull. The pain often intensifies when the patient inhales deeply, coughs, eats, or bends over. The pain often intensifies during exertion but may not go completely away during rest.
- Cough
- Blood-streaked sputum
- Wheezing
- Leg swelling

TABLE 21.1 Wells Clinical Prediction Rule for Pulmonary Embolism

Clinical Feature	Points
Clinical symptoms of DVT	3
Other diagnosis less likely than PE	3
Heart rate greater than 100 beats per minute	1.5
Immobilization or surgery within past 4 weeks	1.5
Previous deep vein thrombosis or pulmonary embolism	1.5
Hemoptysis	1
Malignancy	1
Total points	

Clinical Probability of Pulmonary Embolism
- High: >6 points
- Moderate: 2–6
- Low: <2

Modified from Wells PS, Hirsh J, Anderson DR, Lensing AW, Foster G, Kearon C, Weitz J, D'Ovidio R, Cogo A, Prandoni P, Lancet. 1995;345(8961):1326.

TABLE 21.2 Wells Clinical Prediction Rule for Deep Venous Thrombosis

Clinical Feature	Points
Active cancer (treatment within 6 months, or palliation)	1
Paralysis, paresis, or immobilization of lower extremity	1
Bedridden for more than 3 days because of surgery (within 4 weeks)	1
Localized tenderness along distribution of deep veins	1
Entire leg swollen	1
Unilateral calf swelling of greater than 3 cm (below tibial tuberosity)	1
Unilateral pitting edema	1
Collateral superficial veins	1
Alternative diagnosis as likely as or more likely than deep vein thrombosis	−2
Total points	

Clinical Probability of Deep Venous Thrombosis
- High: >3
- Moderate: 1–2
- Low: <1

Modified from Wells PS, Hirsh J, Anderson DR, Lensing AW, Foster G, Kearon C, Weitz J, D'Ovidio R, Cogo A, Prandoni P, Lancet. 1995;345(8961):1326.

---

clots behind the knee or thigh. Although it is relatively sensitive in detecting DVT above the knee, it is insensitive in detecting DVT below the knee

Chest X-Ray

Although the chest x-ray result is often normal in the patient with a pulmonary embolism, it can be used to rule out conditions that mimic a pulmonary embolism, such as pneumonia and pneumothorax. In addition, infiltrates or atelectasis will be seen in about 50% of pulmonary embolism/infarction cases, and an elevated hemidiaphragm occurs in as many as 40% of cases.

Computed Tomography Pulmonary Angiogram

The spiral (helical) volumetric **computed tomography pulmonary angiogram (CTPA)** (also called *CT pulmonary angiography*) with intravenous contrast is fast becoming the first-line test for diagnosing suspected pulmonary embolism. The CTPA is increasingly being preferred to the previous gold standards for diagnosing a pulmonary embolism— ventilation-perfusion ($\dot{V}/\dot{Q}$) scanning or direct pulmonary angiography—because (1) the scan requires only an intravenous line, (2) the image resolution is very good, (3) the volumetric scanning allows the contrast material to be administered more economically and timed more precisely, and (4) the entire chest can be scanned in a single breath hold, or in several

successive short breath holds. (See CTPA scan in Radiologic Findings, page 311.)

Ventilation-Perfusion Scan

The $\dot{V}/\dot{Q}$ scan is rarely used today to identify a pulmonary embolus. A $\dot{V}/\dot{Q}$ scan is reliable only at the extremes of interpretation (i.e., the test confirms that the lungs are normal or that there is a high probability of a pulmonary embolism). The V̇/Q̇ scan often raises more questions than it answers. This test is quickly being replaced by more sensitive and rapid tests, such as spiral CTPA scans (see earlier discussion).

Pulmonary Angiogram

A **pulmonary angiogram** provides a clear image of the blood flow in the lung's arteries. It is an extremely accurate test for diagnosis of pulmonary embolism. However, because it is invasive (catheter insertion and dye injection), is time-consuming (about 1 hour), and requires a high degree of skill to administer, it is usually performed only when other tests have failed to provide a definitive diagnosis. More contrast dye is used in this study than in the pulmonary embolism CTPA scan (see Pulmonary Angiogram in Radiologic Findings, page 311).

Magnetic Resonance Imaging

A magnetic resonance imaging (MRI) scan of the chest may be used for individuals whose kidneys may be harmed by dyes used in x-ray tests and for women who are pregnant.

Magnetic Resonance Angiography

Magnetic resonance angiography (MRA) may be used to differentiate among blood (usual), thromboemboli, and tumor emboli in patients with malignancy.

General Management of Pulmonary Embolism

Pulmonary embolism/infarction is a life-threatening condition. On admission to hospital, immediate transfer to an intensive care unit is mandatory. The treatment of pulmonary embolism usually begins with treating the symptoms. Oxygen is administered per the Oxygen Therapy Protocol (Protocol 10.1). The physician provides analgesics for pain and fluids and cardiovascular agents to correct blood pressure and cardiac rhythm disturbances if present.

Fast-acting anticoagulants, such as heparin, are given to prevent existing blood clots from growing and prevent the formation of new ones. Heparin is administered intravenously to achieve a rapid effect. **High-molecular-weight heparin** (unfractionated heparin) has, until recently, been the mainstay of treatment for patients with acute pulmonary embolism. The unfractionated heparin dosing must be governed by frequent monitoring of the activated partial thromboplastin time (APTT). This is because bleeding from unfractionated heparin can develop. Recently, **low-molecular-weight heparins** have become available (e.g., enoxaparin, dalteparin, and tinzaparin) and have been shown to be safer and more effective than unfractionated heparin for prophylaxis of DVT or pulmonary emboli. They are also more cost-effective and do not necessitate APTT monitoring. Doctors strive to achieve a full anticoagulant effect within the first 24 hours of treatment.

This is typically followed by the administration of slow-acting, oral anticoagulant **warfarin** (**Coumadin**, Panwarfarin). Heparin and warfarin are given together for 5 to 7 days, until blood tests show that the warfarin is effectively preventing clotting. Then the heparin is discontinued. How long anticoagulants are given varies, based on each patient's condition. For example, if the pulmonary embolism is caused by a temporary risk factor, such as surgery, treatment is given for 2 to 3 months. If the cause is from some long-term condition, such as prolonged bed rest, the treatment is usually given for 3 to 6 months. Some patients may need to take anticoagulants indefinitely. For example, patients who have recurrent pulmonary embolism because of a hereditary clotting disorder may need to take anticoagulants for life. Patients taking warfarin need to have their blood tested periodically to determine if the dose needs to be adjusted.

Because many drugs can adversely interact with warfarin, the patient needs to be careful—that is, check with the physician—before taking any other drugs. Drugs that alter the blood's ability to clot include over-the-counter acetaminophens, ibuprofens, herbal preparations, and dietary supplements. In addition, foods that are high in vitamin K (which affects blood clotting), such as broccoli, spinach, and other leafy green vegetables, liver, grapefruit and grapefruit juice, and green tea, may need to be avoided.

Thrombolytic Agents

Fibrinolytic agents such as **streptokinase** (Streptase), **urokinase** (Abbokinase), **alteplase** (Activase), and **reteplase** (Retavase) actually dissolve blood clots. These systemic agents (commonly referred to as *clot-busters*) have proved beneficial in treating acute pulmonary embolism. These **thrombolytic agents** are sometimes used in conjunction with heparin. Their effect in patients with hemodynamic instability may be dramatic. Because of the excessive risk for bleeding, however, the use of fibrinolytic agents in treating pulmonary embolism is somewhat limited.

Preventive Measures

Directions to patients at high risk for developing thromboembolic disease include the following:

- *Walking:* If possible, the patient is encouraged to walk frequently. When riding in a car, the patient should be instructed to stop often to walk around or perform a few deep knee bends. When flying in an airplane, the patient should move around the cabin every hour or so.
- *Exercise while seated:* When sitting, the patient should be encouraged to flex, extend, and rotate his/her ankles or press his/her feet against the seat in front him/her. Rising up and down on the toes is a good alternative.
- *Drink fluids:* Drinking plenty of water to avoid dehydration, which can contribute to the formation of blood clots, should be encouraged. Patients should avoid alcohol, which also contributes to fluid loss.
- *Wear graduated compression stockings:* Patients should be encouraged to wear tight-fitting elastic stockings that squeeze the legs, thus helping the veins and leg muscles move blood more efficiently. Compression stockings provide a safe, simple, and inexpensive way to keep blood from stagnating. Research has shown that compression stockings used in combination with heparin are much more effective than heparin alone.

Cont. on page 330

OVERVIEW of the Cardiopulmonary Clinical Manifestations Associated With Pulmonary Embolism[1]

The following clinical manifestations result from the pathologic mechanisms caused (or activated) by atelectasis (see Fig. 10.7)—the major anatomic alteration of the lungs associated with a pulmonary infarction (see Fig. 21.1). Bronchospasm (see Fig. 10.10) also may explain some of the following findings. It occurs rarely and is of little clinical significance compared with the atelectasis caused by pulmonary infarction and hypoxemia resulting from the increased physiologic dead space.

CLINICAL DATA OBTAINED AT THE PATIENT'S BEDSIDE

The Physical Examination

Vital Signs

Increased Respiratory Rate (Tachypnea)

Several unique mechanisms probably work simultaneously to increase the rate of breathing in patients with pulmonary embolism.

Increased Physiologic (Alveolar) Dead Space

Pulmonary embolic disease is the classic example of this type of pathophysiology. For example, when an embolus lodges in the pulmonary vascular system, blood flow is reduced or completely absent distal to the obstruction. Consequently, the alveolar ventilation beyond the obstruction is wasted, or dead space, ventilation, and no carbon dioxide–oxygen exchange occur. The ventilation-perfusion ($\dot{V}/\dot{Q}$) ratio distal to the pulmonary embolus is high and may even be infinite if there is no perfusion at all (Fig. 21.2).

Although portions of the lungs have a high $\dot{V}/\dot{Q}$ ratio at the onset of a pulmonary embolism, this condition is quickly reversed and a decrease in the $\dot{V}/\dot{Q}$ ratio occurs. The pathophysiologic mechanisms responsible for the decreased $\dot{V}/\dot{Q}$ ratio are as follows. In some cases of pulmonary embolus, pulmonary infarction may develop and cause alveolar atelectasis, consolidation, and pulmonary parenchymal necrosis. In addition, the

embolus is thought to activate the release of humoral agents such as serotonin, histamine, and prostaglandins into the pulmonary circulation, causing bronchial constriction. Collectively, the alveolar atelectasis, consolidation, tissue necrosis, and bronchial constriction lead to decreased alveolar ventilation relative to the alveolar perfusion (decreased $\dot{V}/\dot{Q}$ ratio). As a result of the decreased $\dot{V}/\dot{Q}$ ratio, pulmonary shunting and venous admixture ensue.

Stimulation of Peripheral Chemoreceptors Producing Hypoxemia

The result of the venous admixture is a decrease in the patient's PaO_2 and CaO_2 (Fig. 21.3). It should be emphasized that it is not the pulmonary embolism but rather the decreased $\dot{V}/\dot{Q}$ ratio that develops from the pulmonary infarction (atelectasis and consolidation) and bronchial constriction (release of cellular mediators) that actually causes the reduced PaO_2. As this condition intensifies, the patient's oxygen level may decline to a point low enough to stimulate the peripheral chemoreceptors, which in turn initiates an increased ventilatory rate.

Reflexes From the Aortic and Carotid Sinus Baroreceptors

If obstruction of the pulmonary vascular system is severe, left ventricular output will diminish and cause the systemic blood pressure to drop. The decreased systemic blood pressure reduces the tension of the walls of the aorta and carotid artery,

[1]In an uncomplicated pulmonary embolism, none of the clinical scenarios presented in Figs. 10.7 through 10.12 is activated. In these patients, increased alveolar **physiologic dead space (wasted ventilation)** is the primary pathophysiologic mechanism (i.e., the ventilation of embolized [nonperfused] pulmonary subsegments, segments, or lobes).

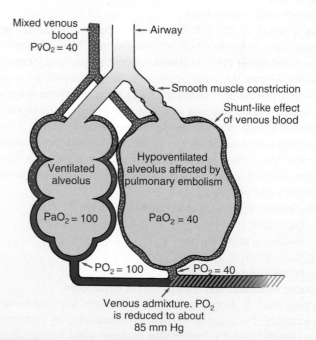

FIGURE 21.3 Venous admixture may develop in pulmonary embolism as a result of bronchial smooth muscle constriction (shunt-like effect). Venous admixture also may occur when an embolus leads to pulmonary infarction and causes alveolar atelectasis and consolidation (true capillary shunt). Alveolar atelectasis and consolidation are not shown in this illustration.

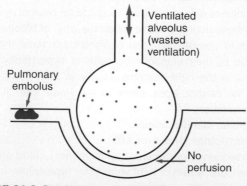

FIGURE 21.2 Dead-space ventilation in pulmonary embolism.

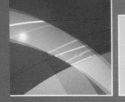

which activates the baroreceptors. Activation of the baroreceptors in turn initiates an increased heart and ventilatory rate.

Other pathophysiologic mechanisms that may increase the patient's dyspnea and ventilatory rate include stimulation of the J receptors, anxiety, and pain.

Increased Heart Rate

The two major mechanisms responsible for the increased heart rate associated with pulmonary embolism are reflexes from the aortic and carotid sinus baroreceptors and stimulation of the pulmonary reflex mechanism.

For a discussion of reflexes from the aortic and carotid sinus baroreceptors, see the previous section on increased respiratory rate. The increased heart rate also may reflect an indirect response to hypoxic stimulation of the peripheral chemoreceptors, mainly the carotid bodies. When the carotid bodies are stimulated in this manner, the patient's ventilatory rate increases. As a result of the increased rate of lung inflation, the pulmonary reflex mechanism is activated; this mechanism triggers tachycardia.

Systemic Hypotension (Decreased Blood Pressure)

When significant pulmonary hypertension develops in pulmonary embolic disease, it is nearly always present because of the decrease in the cross-sectional area of the pulmonary vascular system, which reduces cardiac return and causes a decrease in *left* ventricular output and systemic hypotension. This is an ominous sign.

Cyanosis

Cough and Hemoptysis

As a result of the pulmonary hypertension, the pulmonary hydrostatic pressure, which is normally about 15 mm Hg, often becomes higher than the pulmonary oncotic pressure (normally about 25 mm Hg). This increase in the hydrostatic pressure permits plasma and red blood cells to move across the alveolar-capillary membrane and into alveolar spaces in a process similar to that seen in **cardiogenic pulmonary edema**. If this process continues, the subepithelial mechanoreceptors located in the bronchioles, bronchi, and trachea are stimulated. Such stimulation initiates a cough reflex and the expectoration of blood-tinged sputum.

Peripheral Edema and Venous Distention

- Distended neck veins
- Swollen and tender liver
- Ankle and feet swelling
- Pitting edema

Chest Pain and Decreased Chest Expansion

Chest pain is frequently noted in patients with pulmonary embolism. The origin of the pain is obscure. It may be cardiac or pleuritic, but it is one of the common early findings in all forms of pulmonary embolism, even in the absence of clinically obvious cor pulmonale or pleural involvement. If the patient has systemic hypotension, perfusion of the coronary arteries decreases and classic angina-like chest pain (and electrocardiographic [ECG] findings) may result.

Syncope, Lightheadedness, and Confusion

If the left ventricular output and systemic blood pressure decrease substantially, blood flow to the brain may also diminish significantly. This may cause periods of lightheadedness, confusion, and even syncope.

Abnormal Heart Sounds

- Increased second heart sound (S_2)
- Increased splitting of the second heart sound (S_2)
- Third heart sound (or ventricular gallop) (S_3)

Increased Second Heart Sound (S_2)

As a result of pulmonary embolization, abnormally high blood pressure develops in the pulmonary artery. This condition causes the pulmonic valve to close more forcefully. As a result, the sound produced by the pulmonic valve (P_2) is often louder than the aortic sound (A_2). This finding may be noted in the patient's chart as "$P_2 > A_2$," which reflects that S_2 is louder when the area over the pulmonic valve in the second intercostal, left of the sternal notch, as compared with the intensity of sound to the right of the sternal notch. (The aortic second heart sound [A_2], is normally widely heard over the entire anterior left chest.)

Increased Splitting of the Second Heart Sound (S_2)

Two major mechanisms either individually or together may contribute to the increased splitting of S_2 sometimes noted in pulmonary embolism: increased pulmonary hypertension and incomplete right bundle branch block.

The incomplete right bundle branch block (RBBB) that sometimes accompanies pulmonary embolism also may contribute to the increased splitting of S_2. In incomplete heart block, the electrical activity through the right side of the heart is delayed; this delayed activity in turn slows right ventricular contraction. The blood pressure in the pulmonic valve area remains higher than normal for a longer time during right ventricular contraction. As a result, the closure of the pulmonic valve is delayed, which may further widen the S_2 split.

Splitting of the second heart sound is usually best heard in the second left intercostal space, close to the upper sternal border with a diaphragm of the stethoscope.

Third Heart Sound (S_3, Ventricular Gallop)

A third heart sound (S_3), or ventricular gallop, is sometimes heard in patients with pulmonary embolism. It occurs early in diastole, about 0.12 to 0.16 seconds after S_2. Although its precise origin is unknown, S_3 is thought to be created by cardiac wall vibrations during diastole, when the rush of blood into the ventricles is abruptly stopped by ventricular walls that have lost some of their elasticity because of hypertrophy. An S_3 generated in the right ventricle usually is best heard to the right of the cardiac apex, close to the lower sternal border during inspiration.

Other Cardiac Manifestations

Right Ventricular Heave or Lift

As a consequence of the elevated pulmonary blood pressure, right ventricular strain or right ventricular hypertrophy (or both) often develops. When this occurs, a sustained outward lift of

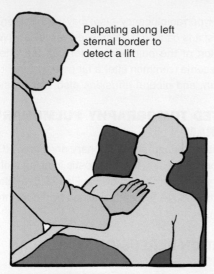

Palpating along left sternal border to detect a lift

FIGURE 21.4 A right ventricular lift can be detected in patients with a pulmonary embolism if significant pulmonary hypertension is present.

the chest wall can be felt at the lower left side of the sternum during systole (Fig. 21.4), because the right ventricle lies directly beneath the sternum.

Chest Assessment Findings

- Crackles
- Wheezes
- Pleural friction rub (especially when pulmonary infarction involves the pleura)

CLINICAL DATA OBTAINED FROM LABORATORY TESTS AND SPECIAL PROCEDURES

Arterial Blood Gases

MILD TO MODERATE STAGES

Acute Alveolar Hyperventilation With Hypoxemia[2] (Acute Respiratory Alkalosis)

pH	$PaCO_2$	HCO_3^-	PaO_2[3]	SaO_2 or SpO_2[3]
↑	↓	↓ (but normal)	↓	↓

SEVERE STAGE

Acute Ventilatory Failure With Hypoxemia[4] (Acute Respiratory Acidosis)

pH[4]	$PaCO_2$	HCO_3^{-}[4]	PaO_2[3]	SaO_2 or SpO_2[3]
↓	↑	↑ (but normal)	↓↓	↓↓

[2]See Fig. 5.2 and Table 5.4 and related discussion for the acute pH, $PaCO_2$, and HCO_3^- changes associated with acute alveolar hyperventilation.
[3]NOTE: A large saddle embolus can cause a sudden and dramatic drop in PaO_2, SaO_2, or SpO_2 values.
[4]See Fig. 5.2 and Table 5.5 and related discussion for the acute pH, $PaCO_2$, and HCO_3^- changes associated with acute and chronic ventilatory failure.
[5]When tissue hypoxia is severe enough to produce lactic acid, the pH and HCO_3^- values will be lower than expected for a particular $PaCO_2$ level.

Oxygenation Indices[6]

$\dot{Q}_S/\dot{Q}_T$	DO_2[7]	$\dot{V}O_2$	$C(a-\bar{v})O_2$	O_2ER	$S\bar{v}O_2$
↑	↓	N	N	↑	↓

Hemodynamic Indices[8]

EXTENSIVE PULMONARY EMBOLISM

CVP	RAP	$\overline{PA}$	PCWP	CO	SV
↑	↑	↑	↓ or N	↓	↓

SVI	CI	RVSWI	LVSWI	PVR	SVR
↓	↓	↑	↓	↑	N

Normally the **pulmonary artery pressure** is no greater than 25/10 mm Hg, with a mean pulmonary artery pressure of about 15 mm Hg. Most patients with a pulmonary embolism, however, have a mean pulmonary artery pressure in excess of 20 mm Hg. Three major mechanisms may contribute to this: (1) decreased cross-sectional area of the pulmonary vascular system because of the embolism, (2) vasoconstriction induced by humoral agents, and (3) vasoconstriction induced by alveolar hypoxia.

Decreased Cross-Sectional Area of the Pulmonary Vascular System Because of the Embolus

The cross-sectional area of the pulmonary vascular system will decrease significantly if a large embolus becomes lodged in a major artery or if many small emboli become lodged in numerous small pulmonary vessels.

Vasoconstriction Induced by Humoral Agents

One of the consequences of pulmonary embolism is the release of certain humoral agents, primarily serotonin and prostaglandin. These agents induce smooth muscle constriction of both the tracheobronchial tree and the pulmonary vascular system. Such smooth muscle vasoconstriction may further reduce the total cross-sectional area of the pulmonary vascular system and cause the pulmonary artery pressure to rise further.

Vasoconstriction Induced by Alveolar Hypoxia

In response to the humoral agents liberated in pulmonary embolism, the smooth muscles of the tracheobronchial tree constrict and cause the $\dot{V}/\dot{Q}$ ratio to decrease and the PaO_2

[6]$C(a-\bar{v})O_2$, Arterial-venous oxygen difference; DO_2, total oxygen delivery; O_2ER, oxygen extraction ratio; $\dot{Q}_S/\dot{Q}_T$, pulmonary shunt fraction; $S\bar{v}O_2$, mixed venous oxygen saturation; $\dot{V}O_2$, oxygen consumption.
[7]The DO_2 may be normal in patients who have compensated to the decreased oxygenation status with (1) an increased cardiac output, (2) an increased hemoglobin level, or (3) a combination of both. When the DO_2 is normal, the O_2ER is usually normal.
[8]CO, Cardiac output; CI, cardiac index; CVP, central venous pressure; LVSWI, left ventricular stroke work index; $\overline{PA}$, mean pulmonary artery pressure; PCWP, pulmonary capillary wedge pressure; PVR, pulmonary vascular resistance; RAP, right atrial pressure; RVSWI, right ventricular stroke work index; SV, stroke volume; SVI, stroke volume index; SVR, systemic vascular resistance.

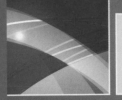
to decline. Although the precise mechanism is unclear, when the PaO_2 and $PaCO_2$ decrease, pulmonary vasoconstriction routinely ensues. This action appears to be a normal compensatory mechanism that offsets the shunt produced by underventilated alveoli. When the number and/or extent of hypoxic areas becomes significant, however, generalized pulmonary vasoconstriction may develop and further contribute to the increase in pulmonary blood pressure. When the pulmonary embolism is severe, right-sided heart strain and cor pulmonale may ensue. Cor pulmonale leads to an increased central venous pressure, distended neck veins, and a swollen and tender liver.

ABNORMAL ELECTROCARDIOGRAPHIC PATTERNS

- Sinus tachycardia
- Atrial arrhythmias
- Trial tachycardia
- Atrial flutter
- Atrial fibrillation
- Acute right ventricular strain pattern and right bundle branch block
- **P pulmonale** (peaked P waves)

In some cases, the obstruction of pulmonary blood flow produced by pulmonary emboli leads to abnormal ECG patterns. However, there is no single ECG pattern diagnostic of pulmonary embolism. Abnormal patterns merely suggest the possibility of pulmonary embolic disease. *Sinus tachycardia is the most common arrhythmia seen.* The sinus tachycardia and atrial arrhythmias sometimes noted are also thought to be related to the increased right-sided heart strain and cor pulmonale. In about 15% to 25% of patients with a pulmonary embolism, an $S_1Q_3T_3$ pattern may be seen, which is a large S wave in lead I, plus a large Q wave and an inverted T wave in lead III.

RADIOLOGIC FINDINGS

Chest Radiograph

- Increased density (in infarcted areas)
- Hyperradiolucency distal to the embolus (in noninfarcted areas)
- Dilation of the pulmonary arteries
- Pulmonary edema
- Right ventricular cardiomegaly (cor pulmonale)
- Pleural effusion (usually small)

Patients with a pulmonary embolus often demonstrate no radiographic signs. However, a density with an appearance similar to that of pneumonia may be seen if infarction has occurred. Hyperradiolucency also may be apparent distal to the embolus; it is caused by decreased vascularity (**Westermark sign**). Dilation of the pulmonary artery on the affected side, pulmonary edema (common after a fat embolus), right ventricular cardiomegaly, and pleural effusions also may be seen.

COMPUTED TOMOGRAPHY PULMONARY ANGIOGRAM

The computed tomography pulmonary angiogram (CTPA) scan is fast becoming the first-line diagnostic imaging tool to confirm a pulmonary embolism. As shown in Fig. 21.5, a relatively dark area—the thrombus—is clearly outlined by the brighter contrast (blood flow).

VENTILATION-PERFUSION LUNG SCAN FINDINGS

Although the **ventilation-perfusion ($\dot{V}/\dot{Q}$) lung scan** has largely been replaced by the CTPA scan (see previous section), Fig. 21.6 provides a nice example of how one or more pulmonary emboli might appear on the $\dot{V}/\dot{Q}$ lung scan. In this case, Fig. 21.6 (V) shows how the radioactive gas xenon-133, confirmed normal lung ventilation—that is, a black appearance throughout both lungs. By contrast, Fig. 21.6 (P) shows how the intravenous radiolabeled particles (a gamma-emitting isotope, usually iodine or technetium) confirmed multiple peripheral subsegmental pulmonary emboli—that is, the white areas interspersed throughout the black areas of the lungs.

PULMONARY ANGIOGRAPHY

Because pulmonary angiography is invasive (catheter insertion and dye injection), is time-consuming (about 1 hour), and requires a high degree of skill to administer, it is rarely performed today. The procedure requires a catheter to be advanced through the right side of the heart and into the pulmonary artery. A radiopaque dye is then rapidly injected into the pulmonary artery while serial x-ray images are taken. Pulmonary embolism is confirmed by abnormal filling within the artery or a cutoff of the artery. A dark area appears on the angiogram distal to the embolization because the radiopaque material is prevented from flowing past the obstruction (Fig. 21.7). The procedure generally poses no risk to the patient unless there is severe pulmonary hypertension (mean pulmonary artery pressure greater than 45 mm Hg) or the patient is in shock or is allergic to the contrast medium. Pulmonary angiography has primarily been replaced by the high-resolution CT scan (see earlier discussion).

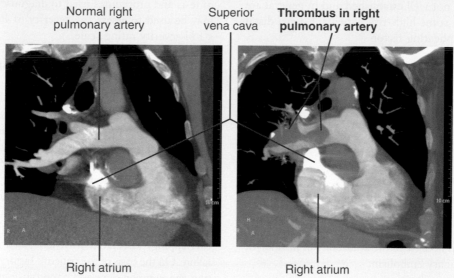

Normal right pulmonary artery   Superior vena cava   **Thrombus in right pulmonary artery**

Right atrium   Right atrium

FIGURE 21.5 Oblique coronal projections from a computed tomography pulmonary angiogram (CTPA). Intravenous contrast material is very bright in the visible portions of the superior vena cava and in the superior portion of the right atrium because the contrast material was injected into an antecubital vein. The contrast material mixes in the right atrium with darker blood (without contrast) from the inferior vena cava, resulting in moderate brightness in that chamber, the right ventricle, and the pulmonary artery. The relatively dark area (thrombus) in the right pulmonary artery is clearly outlined by the brighter area (blood flow). CTPA is the best imaging procedure when pulmonary embolus is suspected. (From Vilensky, J. A., Weber, E. C., Carmichael, S. W., & Sarosi, T. E. [2010]. *Medical imaging of normal and pathologic anatomy*. Philadelphia, PA: Elsevier.)

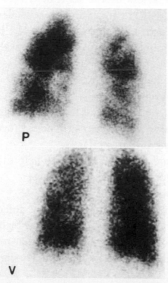

P

V

FIGURE 21.6 Fat embolism in a patient with dyspnea and hypoxemia after a recent orthopedic procedure. Perfusion (P) and ventilation (V) radionuclide scans show multiple peripheral subsegmental perfusion defects suggestive of fat embolism. (From Hansell, D. M., Lynch, D. A., McAdams, H. P., et al. [2010]. *Imaging of diseases of the chest* [5th ed.]. Philadelphia, PA: Elsevier.)

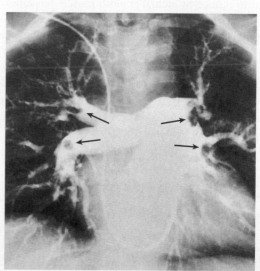

FIGURE 21.7 Pulmonary emboli. Pulmonary angiogram shows numerous filling defects. Trailing ends of the occluding thromboemboli are particularly well shown (arrows). (From Hansell, D. M., Lynch, D. A., McAdams, H. P., et al. [2010]. *Imaging of diseases of the chest* [5th ed.]. Philadelphia, PA: Elsevier.)

Inferior Vena Cava Filter

An **inferior vena cava (Greenfield) vein filter** may be surgically placed in the inferior vena cava to prevent clots being carried into the pulmonary circulation. Their effectiveness and the safety of the filter are not well established and in general are recommended only in some high-risk patients. Edema distal to the filters is a complicating factor.

Pneumatic Compression

This treatment uses thigh-high cuffs that automatically inflate every few minutes to massage and compress the veins in a patient's legs. Studies show that this procedure can significantly decrease the risk for blood clots, especially in patients who undergo hip replacement surgery.

Pulmonary Embolectomy

Surgical removal of blood clots from the pulmonary circulation (**pulmonary embolectomy**) is generally a last resort in treating pulmonary embolism because of the mortality rate associated with the procedure and because of the availability of fibrinolytic agents to treat pulmonary embolism.

Respiratory Care Treatment Protocols

Oxygen Therapy Protocol

Oxygen therapy is used to treat hypoxemia, decrease the work of breathing, and decrease myocardial work (see Oxygen Therapy Protocol, Protocol 10.1).

Aerosolized Medication Protocol

Both sympathomimetic and parasympatholytic agents may be used to induce bronchial smooth muscle relaxation when wheezing is present (see Protocol 10.4: Aerosolized Medication Therapy Protocol, and Appendix V on the Evolve site).

Lung Expansion Therapy Protocol

Patients who present with or develop significant atelectasis may benefit from a trial of lung hyperinflation, certainly if mechanical ventilation is instituted (see Lung Expansion Therapy Protocol, Protocol 10.3).

PULMONARY HYPERTENSION

Pulmonary hypertension (PH) is defined as an increase in mean pulmonary artery pressure greater than 25 mm Hg (normal range 10 to 20 mm Hg) at rest. PH is a frequent complication of chronic pulmonary disease (e.g., chronic obstructive pulmonary disease [COPD] and interstitial lung disease) and is more common among women than among men at a ratio of 3:1. The World Health Organization divides PH into five different group classifications based on the cause and treatment options (Box 21.3).

Diagnosis

PH can be very insidious. The patient may have mild to moderate PH for years with no remarkable signs or symptoms. Box 21.4 provides signs and symptoms associated with PH.

The diagnosis of PH is based on the patient's medical and family histories, physical examination, and the results from a variety of tests and procedures. Tests such as **echocardiography**, chest x-ray, electrocardiograms, and right-heart catheterization may be used to diagnose PH. Table 21.3 provides an overview of tests and procedures used to diagnose PH. Exercise testing may be used to assess the severity of PH. Table 21.4 shows a PH severity rating scale.

Left-Sided Heart Failure Versus Right-Sided Heart Failure

Although there are several clinical conditions that can cause **right-sided heart failure** and cor pulmonale (e.g., COPD, coronary artery disease, pulmonary embolic disease, pulmonic stenosis, tricuspid stenosis, and tricuspid regurgitation), **left-sided heart failure** (congestive heart failure) is more commonly the cause of PH. Because the respiratory therapist frequently encounters patients in left-sided or right-sided failure or a combination of both (**biventricular failure**) it is important to differentiate and identify the major signs and symptoms (although sometimes overlapping) associated with left-sided and right-sided heart failure. On the basis of the patient's history and physical examination, the common signs and symptoms caused by either left-sided or right-sided heart failure are presented in Box 21.5.

Management of Pulmonary Hypertension

Although, in general, pulmonary hypertension has no cure, treatment may help reduce the symptoms and slow the progress of the disease depending on the cause of the condition. The management of PH includes medicines, procedures, and other therapies. The precise treatment selection depends on what type of PH the patient has and its severity. Table 21.5 provides an overview of the treatment selections currently used to manage PH. In addition, several different treatments may be used to manage all types of PH. For example, therapies commonly used to treat all types of PH include the following:

- *Diuretics:* To help decrease fluid buildup, including swelling in ankles and feet.
- *Phosphodiesterase inhibitors:* Especially in group I patients.
- *Blood-thinning medications:* To help prevent blood clots from forming or getting larger.
- *Cardiac glycosides (digoxin, etc.):* To help the heart to pump stronger or to control the heart rate.
- *Oxygen therapy:* To treat hypoxemia.
- *Physical activity:* To improve exercise tolerance.
- *Inhaled nitric oxide (iNO) therapy:* May be helpful in groups 1 and 4 (Box 21.3). An oral agent that mimics the effect of the inhaled gas is now available (riociguat).

The Emerging Role of the Respiratory Therapist in Pulmonary Vascular Disorders

In the future, the role of the respiratory therapist will, undoubtedly, expand in the diagnosis and management areas of patients with pulmonary vascular disease. For example, at the patient

Cont. on page 335

BOX 21.3 Clinical Classification of Pulmonary Hypertension*

Group 1 Pulmonary Arterial Hypertension (PAH)
- Idiopathic
- Heritable
- Drugs and toxins induced (including methamphetamines and other diet medications)
- PAH associated with:
  - Connective tissue disease
  - Human immunodeficiency virus (HIV)
  - Portal hypertension
  - Congenital heart disease
  - Schistosomiasis
- Pulmonary veno-occlusive disease and/or pulmonary capillary hemangiomatosis
  - Idiopathic
  - Heritable
  - Drugs, toxins, and radiation induced
  - Associated with connective tissue disease and HIV infection
- Persistent pulmonary hypertension of the newborn (see Chapter 33, The Newborn Disorders)

Group 2 Pulmonary Hypertension Because of Left Heart Disease
- PH because of left heart disease—systolic and diastolic dysfunction
- Valvular disease
- Congenital/acquired left heart inflow/outflow tract obstruction and congenital cardiomyopathies
- Congenital/acquired pulmonary venous stenosis

Group 3 Pulmonary Hypertension Because of Lung Disease and/or Hypoxia
- Chronic obstructive pulmonary disease (COPD)
- Interstitial lung disease (ILD)
- Sleep-disordered breathing (e.g., sleep apnea)
- Alveolar hypoventilation disorders
- Chronic exposure to high altitude

Group 4 Chronic Thromboembolic Pulmonary Hypertension and Other Pulmonary Artery Obstructions

Group 5 Pulmonary Hypertension With Unclear and/or Multifactorial Mechanisms
- Polycythemia
- S/P splenectomy
- Essential thrombocythemia
- Sarcoidosis (10% of all patients)
- Lymphangioleiomyomatosis
- Vasculitis, including certain connective tissue disorders
- Myeloproliferative disorders
- Metabolic disorders
  - Glycogen storage disease
  - Gaucher disease
  - Thyroid disorders
- Other conditions
  - Chronic renal failure
  - Fibrosing mediastinitis

*The World Health Organization first defined the classifications of PH in Evian, France, in 1973, and the classifications have been revised over the years. The most recent update reflects the 2015 European Society of Cardiology (ESC)/European Respiratory Society (ERS) Guidelines on the Diagnosis and Management of Pulmonary Hypertension (PH), which divides PH into five main groups according to shared pathophysiology, clinical features, and therapeutic approaches.

BOX 21.4 Common Signs and Symptoms Associated With Pulmonary Hypertension

General Findings
- Dyspnea (during routine activity)
- Lightheaded, dizziness, confusion
- Fatigue
- Nonproductive cough
- Hemoptysis
- Hoarseness
- Fainting or syncope
- Chest pain and decreased chest expansion
- A racing heartbeat
- Pain on the upper right side of the abdomen
- Decreased appetite
- Peripheral edema and venous distention
  - Distended neck veins
  - Swollen and tender liver
  - Ankle and feet swelling
  - Pitting edema
- Cyanosis

- Raynaud's phenomenon (blanching of the fingers on exposure to cold)
- Fluid in the abdomen.

Test and Procedure Findings
- Abnormal heart sounds
  - Loud second heart sound (S_2)
  - Increased splitting (time delay) of the second heart sound (S_2)
  - Third heart sound (or ventricular gallop) (S_3)
- Palpable right ventricular heave or lift
- Abnormal electrocardiographic (ECG) findings
  - Sinus tachycardia
  - Atrial arrhythmias
    - Atrial tachycardia
    - Atrial flutter
    - Atrial fibrillation

Cont. on page 332

- Acute right ventricular strain pattern and right bundle branch block
- P pulmonale (peaked P waves)
- Radiologic findings
  - Enlargement of the pulmonary arteries
  - Pulmonary edema
  - Narrowing of the peripheral arteries
  - Enlargement of the right ventricle and atrium (cor pulmonale)
  - Pleural effusion
- Echocardiography
  - Enlarged heart chambers
- Right-heart catheterization
  - High pulmonary artery pressure, confirming pulmonary hypertension

TABLE 21.3 Tests and Procedures Used to Diagnose Pulmonary Hypertension

Test or Procedure	Description
Echocardiography	The echocardiogram can be used to show the size and thickness of the right ventricle and right atrium and tricuspid regurgitation. It also can be used to estimate the pressure in the pulmonary arteries (Fig. 21.8).
Chest x-ray	A chest x-ray image can show whether the pulmonary arteries and right ventricle are enlarged. The chest x-ray image also shows signs of an underlying lung disease causing or contributing to pulmonary hypertension (PH).
Electrocardiogram (ECG)	Used to establish whether cardiac rhythm is steady or irregular. ECG findings often reveal right-axis deviation, right ventricular hypertrophy, and ventricular strain.
Right-heart catheterization (Swan-Ganz catheter)	Used to confirm the diagnosis of PH and to establish the degree of hemodynamic damage, the presence of vasoreactivity (via a vasoreactivity test), and prognosis (Fig. 21.9). A vasoreactivity test is recommended for patients in group 1 pulmonary arterial hypertension (PAH) (because they are most likely to respond favorably). This involves the administration of a short-acting vasodilator and then the measurement of the hemodynamic response using a right-heart catheter. Agents commonly used for vasoreactivity testing include epoprostenol, adenosine, and inhaled nitric oxide. The purpose of vasoreactivity testing is to identify the small minority of patients with a positive test result who may benefit from an oral **calcium channel blocker** with a dihydropyridine or diltiazem. In contrast, patients with a negative vasoreactivity test require advanced therapy with a prostanoid, endothelin receptor antagonist, or phosphodiesterase-5 inhibitor (see Table 21.5).
Chest high-resolution computed tomography (CT) scan	Used to rule out underlying causes or condition(s) that may be causing PH.
Chest MRI	Chest magnetic resonance imaging, or chest MRI, can help detect signs of PH or an underlying condition causing PH. The chest MRI shows how the right ventricle is working and how blood is moving through the lungs.
Pulmonary function tests	Used to rule out the presence of significant restrictive or obstructive pulmonary disease—for example, chronic obstructive pulmonary disease (COPD) versus interstitial lung disease (ILD). Patients with idiopathic pulmonary arterial hypertension (IPAH) commonly have a decreased pulmonary diffusion capacity (DLCO). The 6-minute walk test is helpful as a screening tool but nonspecific.
Polysomnogram (PSG)	Used to help determine apneas and low oxygen levels during sleep, which are common in PH (see Chapter 31, Respiratory Insufficiency in the Patient With Neurorespiratory Disease).
Ventilation/perfusion ($\dot{V}/\dot{Q}$) scan	Used to help detect blood clots in the lungs. Is largely being replaced by high-resolution CT scan.
Blood tests	Used to rule out other diseases, such as HIV, liver disease, and autoimmune diseases (e.g., rheumatoid arthritis).

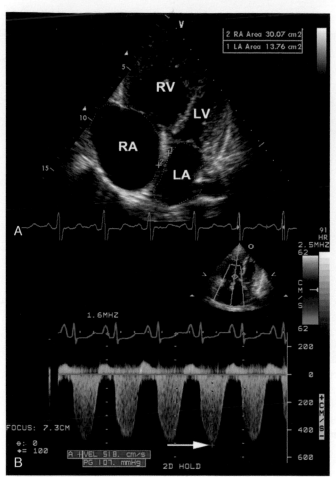

FIGURE 21.8 Echocardiography in pulmonary hypertension. (A) Apical four-chamber view of the heart reveals enlarged right atrium and ventricle compressing the left cardiac chambers. (B) Doppler echocardiography shows tricuspid insufficiency jet (arrow) used to estimate the right ventricular systolic pressure, in this case 107 mm Hg. *LA,* Left atrium; *LV,* left ventricle; *RA,* right atrium; *RV,* right ventricle. (From Kacmarek, R. M., Stoller, J. K., & Heuer, A. J. [2017]. *Egan's fundamentals of respiratory care* [11th ed.]. St. Louis, MO: Elsevier.)

TABLE 21.4 Pulmonary Hypertension Severity Rating Based on Exercise Testing*

Class	Description
Class 1	No remarkable limits. The patient performs regular physical activities (e.g., walking or climbing stairs) without causing pulmonary hypertension (PH) symptoms (e.g., tiredness, shortness of breath, or chest pain).
Class 2	Slight or mild limits. The patient is comfortable while resting, but regular physical activity (e.g., walking or climbing stairs) causes PH symptoms.
Class 3	Marked or noticeable limits. Comfortable while resting. However, regular physical activity (e.g., walking or climbing stairs) causes PH symptoms.
Class 4	Severe limits. Patient unable to do any physical activity without discomfort. PH symptoms may be present at rest.

*Exercise testing typically entails either (1) a 6-minute walk test, which measures the distance the patient can quickly walk in 6 minutes, or (2) a cardiopulmonary exercise test (CPET), which measures, in detail, how well the cardiopulmonary system functions while exercising on a treadmill or bicycle.

BOX 21.5 Signs and Symptoms: Left-Sided Heart Failure Versus Right-Sided Heart Failure

Right-Sided Heart Failure
- Shortness of breath
- Irregular fast heart rate
- Distended neck veins
- Peripheral edema and venous distention
- Distended neck veins
- Swollen and tender liver
- Ankle and feet swelling
- Pitting edema
- Heart palpitations
- Abdominal distention (bloating)—ascites
- Abdominal pain
- Urinating more frequently at night
- Anorexia
- Nausea
- Fatigue, weakness, faintness
- Weight gain

Left-Sided Heart Failure
- Shortness of breath
- Lightheadedness or fainting
- Frothy, blood-tinged sputum
- Crackles
- Cough and hemoptysis
- Orthopnea
- Paroxysmal nocturnal dyspnea
- Weak pulse
- Hypotension
- Decreased urine production
- Activity intolerance
- Fatigue, weakness, faintness
- Weight gain and fluid retention
- Heart palpitations
- Anxiety
- Excessive sweating
- Cyanosis
- Cool or clammy skin to touch

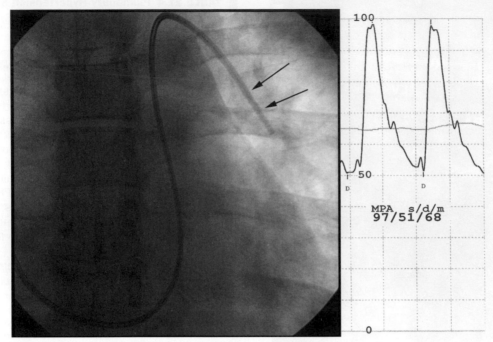

FIGURE 21.9 Right-heart catheterization in pulmonary hypertension. In the left panel, a pulmonary artery catheter is observed in the left pulmonary artery (arrows). In the right panel, the corresponding pulmonary artery pressure tracing is shown, confirming the diagnosis of pulmonary hypertension. In this case, the pulmonary artery systolic, diastolic, and mean pressures were 97 mm Hg, 51 mm Hg, and 68 mm Hg. (From Kacmarek, R. M., Stoller, J. K., & Heuer, A. J. [2017]. *Egan's fundamentals of respiratory care* [11th ed.]. St. Louis, MO: Elsevier.)

TABLE 21.5 Treatment Selections Used to Manage Pulmonary Hypertension

Group 1 Pulmonary arterial hypertension (PAH)	Treatments for Group 1 PH include the following medications and medical procedures: Medications Positive vasoreactivity test: Separates various types of pulmonary hypertension from each other Oral calcium channel blocker (CCB) with a dihydropyridine or diltiazem Negative vasoreactivity test (advanced therapy) Prostanoids (e.g., treprostinil, iloprost, and epoprostenol) Endothelin receptor antagonists (e.g., bosentan and ambrisentan) Phosphodiesterase-5 inhibitors (e.g., sildenafil) Surgical procedures Lung transplant Heart transplant
Group 2 Pulmonary hypertension (PH)	Treating the underlying condition (e.g., mitral valve disease in left-side heart failure) can help Group 2 PH. Management includes lifestyle changes, medications, and surgery.
Group 3 Pulmonary hypertension (PH)	Oxygen therapy is the primary treatment selection in Group 3 when the PH is caused by hypoxemia resulting from chronic obstructive pulmonary disease (COPD), chronic interstitial lung disease (ILD), and sleep apnea.
Group 4 Pulmonary hypertension (PH)	Blood-thinning medications are used to treat blood clots in the lungs or blood-clotting disorders associated with Group 4 PH. Potentially curative pulmonary thromboendarterectomy surgery must be considered.
Group 5 Pulmonary hypertension (PH)	Because various different diseases or conditions, such as thyroid disease and sarcoidosis, can cause Group 5 PH, treatment is directed at the cause of the PH.

As many as 25%–30% of patients with **chronic thromboembolic pulmonary hypertension** may never have had a diagnosed pulmonary embolism or even a history suggestive of pulmonary embolism, and 45%–55% may never have had a history of deep vein thrombus.

bedside, the perceptive respiratory therapist may likely be the first to recognize and report important signs and symptoms associated with left-sided heart failure or right-sided heart failure and, importantly, identify key signs and symptoms of deep venous thrombosis, pulmonary embolism, or pulmonary hypertension itself. Such information-gathering and timely communication may be lifesaving. In addition, the role of the respiratory therapist in the management of pulmonary vascular diseases will further broaden as inhaled gas (e.g., inhaled nitric oxide [iNO]) and various aerosolized medications (e.g., iloprost and treprostinil) continue to demonstrate long-term therapeutic benefits.[2] Excellent patient education materials on this topic are available from the Pulmonary Hypertension Association website (https://phassociation.org).

[2]See more on the role of the respiratory therapist in administering iNO in treating persistent pulmonary hypertension of the newborn, Chapter 33, The Newborn Disorders.

CASE STUDY Pulmonary Embolism

Admitting History

A 32-year-old motorcycle enthusiast who smoked one pack of cigarettes per day fell from his bike while riding with a group of Harley "hogs" to the annual Sturgis Rally in North Dakota. Although his motorcycle sustained extensive damage, the man was conscious when the ambulance arrived. Before he was transported to the local hospital, he was treated in the field; splints and an immobilizer were applied. His injuries were thought to include a fractured pelvis, left tibia, and left knee.

En route to the hospital, a nonrebreathing oxygen mask was placed over the man's face. An intravenous infusion was started with 5% glucose solution. The patient was alert and able to answer questions. His vital signs were blood pressure 150/90 mm Hg, heart rate 105 beats/min, and respiratory rate 20 breaths/min. Various small lacerations and scrapes on his face and left shoulder were treated. Each time the man was moved slightly or when the ambulance suddenly bounced or turned sharply as it moved over the highway, he complained of abdominal and bilateral chest pain. The emergency medical technician (EMT) crew all thought his helmet and his youth had saved his life.

In the emergency department, a laboratory technician drew the patient's blood; several x-ray films were taken, and the man was given morphine for the pain. Within an hour the patient was taken to surgery to have the broken bones in his left leg repaired. He was transferred 4 hours later to the intensive care unit (ICU) with his left leg in a cast. Thrombosis and embolism prophylaxis had been started with low-dose heparin. Busy with another surgery, the physician ordered a respiratory care consultation for the patient.

Physical Examination

The respiratory therapist found the patient lying in bed with his left leg suspended about 25 cm (10 inches) above the bed surface. He had a partial rebreathing oxygen mask on his face and was alert. His wife and twin boys, who were 10 years of age and wearing black motorcycle jackets, were at the man's bedside. The patient stated that he was feeling much better and that his breathing was "OK."

His vital signs were blood pressure 115/75 mm Hg, heart rate 75 beats/min, and respiratory rate 12 breaths/min. He was afebrile and his skin color appeared good. No remarkable breathing problems were noted. Palpation revealed mild tenderness over the left shoulder and left anterior chest area. Chest percussion was unremarkable, and auscultation revealed normal vesicular breath sounds. The chest x-ray film taken earlier that morning in the emergency department was normal. His arterial blood gas values (ABGs) on a nonrebreathing oxygen mask were pH 7.40, $PaCO_2$ 41 mm Hg, HCO_3^- 24 mEq/L, PaO_2 504 mm Hg, and SaO_2 97%. On the basis of these clinical data, the following SOAP was documented.

Respiratory Assessment and Plan

S "My breathing is OK."

O No remarkable respiratory distress noted. Vital signs: BP 115/75, HR 75, RR 12; afebrile; tenderness over left shoulder and left anterior chest area; normal vesicular breath sounds; CXR: Normal; ABGs (partial rebreathing mask) pH 7.40, $PaCO_2$ 41, HCO_3^- 24, PaO_2 504 mm Hg, and SaO_2 97%.

A • No remarkable respiratory problems
  • Normal acid-base status with overoxygenation

P Reduce FIO_2 per protocol (2 L/min by nasal cannula). Recheck SpO_2.

Three Days After Admission

On the second hospital day, he was transferred out of the ICU. The man's general course of recovery was uneventful until the third day after his admission, when the nurses noticed swelling of the left calf while giving him a bath. Venous ultrasonography revealed a large left femoral vein deep venous thrombosis (DVT). The physician was informed, and anticoagulant therapy was started. Five hours later, the patient became short of breath and agitated. A spontaneous cough was noted, with production of a small amount of blood-tinged sputum. Concerned, the nurse called the physician and respiratory care.

When the therapist walked into the patient's room, the man appeared cyanotic, extremely short of breath, and stated that he felt awful. The patient also said that he had precordial chest pain, felt lightheaded, and had a feeling of impending doom. His vital signs were blood pressure 90/45 mm Hg, heart rate 125 beats/min, respiratory rate 30 breaths/min, and oral temperature 37.2°C (99°F). Palpation and percussion of the chest were unremarkable. Auscultation revealed faint wheezing throughout both lung fields. A pleural friction rub was audible anteriorly over the right middle lobe. The patient's electrocardiogram (ECG) pattern alternated between a normal sinus rhythm, sinus tachycardia, and atrial flutter.

The chest x-ray showed increased density in the right middle lobe consistent with atelectasis and consolidation. On an FIO_2 of 0.50, the ABGs were pH 7.53, $PaCO_2$ 26 mm Hg, HCO_3^- 21 mEq/L, PaO_2 53, and SaO_2 91%. Because a pulmonary embolism was suspected, a modified Wells Scoring System was administered and produced a score of 7, which revealed a high probability that the patient had developed a pulmonary embolism. At this time, the physician started the patient on intravenous streptokinase, ordered a CTPA, and requested that the respiratory care staff see the patient again. On the basis of these clinical data, the following SOAP was documented.

Respiratory Assessment and Plan

S "I feel awful. I'm short of breath and lightheaded."

O Cyanosis; agitation; dyspnea; cough productive of small amount of blood-tinged sputum; vital signs: BP 90/45, HR 125, RR 30, T 37.2°C (99°F), slight wheezing throughout both lung fields; pleural friction rub, right mid-lung; ECG: Varies among normal sinus rhythm, sinus tachycardia, atrial flutter. CXR: Atelectasis and consolidation in the right middle lobe. On FIO_2 = 0.5, ABGs pH 7.53, $PaCO_2$ 26, HCO_3^- 21, PaO_2 53, SaO_2 91%. Wells Score: 7.

A • High probability of a pulmonary embolism (Wells score of 7)
• Hypotension (BP)
• Tachycardia, atrial flutter (ECG)
• Respiratory distress (cyanosis, heart rate, respiratory rate, ABGs)
• Pulmonary embolism and infarction likely (history, vital signs, CXR, ECG, blood-tinged sputum, wheezing, pleural friction rub)
• Bronchospasm, probably secondary to pulmonary embolism or infarction (wheezing)
• Alveolar atelectasis and consolidation (CXR)
• Acute alveolar hyperventilation with moderate hypoxemia (ABGs)

P Contact physician and transfer to ICU. Increase oxygen therapy per Protocol. Begin Aerosolized Medication Protocol (med. neb. with 2 mL albuterol premix qid). Monitor and reevaluate in 30 minutes (e.g., ABG). Remain on standby with mechanical ventilator available.

Two Hours Later

The CTPA scan showed no blood flow to the right middle lobe. The patient's eyes were closed, and he no longer was responsive to questions. His skin appeared cyanotic, and his cough was productive of a small amount of blood-tinged sputum. His vital signs were blood pressure 70/35 mm Hg, heart rate 160 beats/min, respiratory rate 25 breaths/min and shallow, and rectal temperature 37.5°C (99.2°F). Findings on palpation of the chest were normal. Dull percussion notes were elicited over the right mid-lung. Wheezing was heard throughout both lung fields, and a pleural friction rub was audible over the right middle lobe.

The patient's ECG pattern alternated between a normal sinus rhythm, sinus tachycardia, and atrial flutter. The patient's ABGs on 100% oxygen were pH 7.25, $PaCO_2$ 69 mm Hg, HCO_3^- 27 mEq/L, PaO_2 37 mm Hg, and SaO_2 59%.

On the basis of these clinical data, the following SOAP was documented.

Respiratory Assessment and Plan

S N/A (patient not responsive)

O CTPA scan: No blood flow to right middle lobe; cyanosis; cough: small amount of blood-tinged sputum; vital signs BP 70/35, HR 160, RR 25 and shallow, T 37.5°C (99.2°F); palpation negative; dull percussion notes over right middle lobe; wheezing over both lungs; pleural friction rub over right middle lobe; ECG: Alternating among normal sinus rhythm, sinus tachycardia, and atrial flutter; ABGs on 100% O_2 pH 7.25, $PaCO_2$ 69, HCO_3^- 27, PaO_2 37, and SaO_2 59%.

A • Acute ventilatory failure with severe hypoxemia (ABGs)
• Pulmonary embolism and infarction (CTPA scan)
• Bronchospasm (wheezing)

P Contact physician stat. Discuss acute ventilatory failure and need for intubation and Mechanical Ventilation Protocol. Manually ventilate until physician arrives. Continue Oxygen Therapy Protocol via manual resuscitation at an FIO_2 of 1.0—add continuous positive airway pressure (CPAP) at 10 cm H_2O. Increase Aerosolized Medication Protocol (continue med. neb. with 2 mL albuterol premix qid).

Discussion

Risk factors for development of a fatal pulmonary embolism include pelvis and long bone fractures, immobilization, malignant disease, and a history of thrombotic disease (including venous thrombosis), congestive heart failure, and chronic lung disease. Only about 10% of patients with pulmonary emboli do not have at least one of these risk factors. The symptoms of ultimately fatal pulmonary embolism include dyspnea (in about 60% of patients), syncope (in about 25% of patients), altered mental status, apprehension, nonpleuritic chest pain, sweating, cough, and hemoptysis (in a smaller percentage of patients).

The signs of acute pulmonary embolism and infarction include tachypnea, tachycardia, crackles, low-grade fever, lower extremity edema, hypotension, cyanosis, gallop rhythm, diaphoresis, and clinically evident phlebitis (in a small percentage of patients).

It is interesting to note that in surgical patients, at least half of the deaths caused by pulmonary embolism occur within the first week after the surgical procedure, most commonly on the third to seventh day after the operation. The remainder of the deaths, however, divide equally among the second, third, and fourth postoperative weeks. The current patient certainly had one of the obvious causes for pulmonary embolism—pelvis and long bone fractures and immobilization of the left leg, which was put in a cast after surgery.

At the time of the first assessment, the patient was not in any respiratory distress. His chest physical examination was basically unremarkable, as were the chest x-ray and ABGs. The patient might well have been placed on hyperexpansion therapy, such as incentive spirometry or even mask CPAP therapy, to be proactive in preventing atelectasis. This fact was particularly important for this patient, who was on morphine and might have been prone to hypoventilate because of his left shoulder and left anterior chest pain and tenderness.

By the time of the second assessment, however, things had changed dramatically; the patient demonstrated many of the signs and symptoms associated with a pulmonary embolism and infarction. The assessing therapist should have recognized the seriousness of the situation from the patient's complaints, history, physical findings, Wells score of 7, and ABGs. The patient's wheezing most likely was a result of pulmonary embolism and infarction, as was the atelectasis. However, a trial of aerosolized bronchodilation was not inappropriate given the patient's smoking history. The data were abnormal enough to prompt the therapist to suggest that the patient be transferred to the ICU and to prepare for ventilator support because acute ventilatory failure might not have been far off.

Indeed, in the last assessment, things had progressed to the point at which the patient was in severe respiratory acidosis with severe hypoxemia, and mechanical ventilation became necessary. Much more lung tissue than just the right middle lobe must have been embolized, and a repeat CTPA later in the patient's clinical course was almost certainly indicated and might have justified even more aggressive therapy. The treating therapist should recognize that the therapeutic options in such cases are limited by the amount of ventilation "wasted" in these patients because of their embolic disease. High minute volume ventilation may be necessary to improve (even slightly) the ABGs in such patients. Some centers would have considered an attempt at pulmonary embolectomy at this juncture.

One final note: The outlook for this patient was extremely poor. Indeed, he died during the fifth week of his hospitalization. He remained on ventilator support until the time of his death.

SELF-ASSESSMENT QUESTIONS

1. Most pulmonary emboli originate from thrombi in the:
   a. Lungs
   b. Right side of the heart
   c. Leg and pelvic veins
   d. Pulmonary veins

2. The aortic and carotid sinus baroreceptors initiate which of the following in response to a decreased systemic blood pressure?
   1. Increased heart rate
   2. Increased ventilatory rate
   3. Decreased heart rate
   4. Decreased ventilatory rate
   5. Ventilatory rate is not affected by the aortic and carotid sinus baroreceptors.
      a. 1 and 5 only
      b. 2 and 3 only
      c. 3 and 4 only
      d. 1 and 2 only

3. What is the upper limit of the normal mean pulmonary artery pressure?
   a. 5 mm Hg
   b. 10 mm Hg
   c. 15 mm Hg
   d. 20 mm Hg

4. Pulmonary hypertension develops in pulmonary embolism because of which of the following?
   1. Increased cross-sectional area of the pulmonary vascular system
   2. Vasoconstriction caused by humoral agent release
   3. Vasoconstriction induced by decreased arterial oxygen pressure (PaO_2)
   4. Vasoconstriction induced by decreased alveolar oxygen pressure (PaO_2)
      a. 1 and 3 only
      b. 2 and 4 only
      c. 1, 2, and 3 only
      d. 2, 3, and 4 only

5. In severe pulmonary embolism, which of the following hemodynamic indices is(are) commonly seen?
   1. Decreased pulmonary vascular resistance
   2. Increased mean pulmonary artery pressure
   3. Decreased central venous pressure
   4. Increased pulmonary capillary wedge pressure
      a. 2 only
      b. 3 only
      c. 4 only
      d. 1 and 2 only

6. When humoral agents such as serotonin are released into the pulmonary circulation, which of the following occur?
   1. The bronchial smooth muscles dilate
   2. The ventilation-perfusion ratio decreases
   3. The bronchial smooth muscles constrict
   4. The ventilation-perfusion ratio increases
      a. 1 only
      b. 2 only
      c. 4 only
      d. 2 and 3 only

7. Which of the following is(are) thrombolytic agents?
   1. Urokinase
   2. Heparin
   3. Warfarin
   4. Streptokinase
      a. 1 only
      b. 4 only
      c. 2 and 3 only
      d. 1 and 4 only

8. Which of the following is the most prominent source of pulmonary emboli?
   a. Fat
   b. Blood clots
   c. Bone marrow
   d. Air

9. Pulmonary hypertension is defined as an increase in mean pulmonary pressure greater than:
   a. 15 mm Hg
   b. 20 mm Hg
   c. 25 mm Hg
   d. 30 mm Hg

10. An oral calcium channel blocker may be used to help manage some patients who have which of the following classifications of pulmonary hypertension?
    a. Group 1 pulmonary arterial hypertension
    b. Group 3 pulmonary hypertension
    c. Group 4 pulmonary hypertension
    d. Group 5 pulmonary hypertension

CHAPTER

22 Flail Chest

Chapter Objectives

After reading this chapter, you will be able to:
- List the anatomic alterations of the lungs associated with a flail chest.
- Describe the causes of a flail chest.
- Describe the cardiopulmonary clinical manifestations associated with a flail chest.
- Describe the general management of a flail chest.
- Describe the clinical strategies and rationales of the SOAPs presented in the case study.
- Define key terms and complete self-assessment questions at the end of the chapter and on Evolve.

Key Terms

Double Fractures
Fractured Ribs
Flail Chest

Flail Chest Wall Motion
Paradoxical Movement of the Chest Wall
Pendelluft
Positive End-Expiratory Pressure (PEEP)
Pulmonary Contusion
Venous Admixture
Ventilator Settings in Flail Chest

Chapter Outline

Anatomic Alterations of the Lungs
Etiology and Epidemiology
Overview of the Cardiopulmonary Clinical Manifestations
   Associated With Flail Chest
General Management of Flail Chest
   Respiratory Care Treatment Protocols
Case Study: Flail Chest
Self-Assessment Questions

Anatomic Alterations of the Lungs

Flail chest wall motion is the result of **double fractures** of at least three or more adjacent ribs, which causes the thoracic cage to become unstable—to flail, which is defined as to wave, swing, or have abnormal movement (Fig. 22.1). The affected ribs paradoxically cave in (**flail**) during inspiration as a result of the generated subatmospheric intrapleural pressure. This compresses and restricts the underlying lung and promotes a number of pathologic conditions, including atelectasis and lung collapse. There may be **pulmonary contusion** (i.e., alveolar hemorrhage and parenchymal damage) under the **fractured ribs**. Sharp rib fragments may damage underlying tissue such as the diaphragm, spleen, liver, and large blood vessels.

A flail chest causes a restrictive lung disorder, is often life-threatening in severe cases, and requires immediate medical intervention. The major pathologic or structural changes of the lungs that may result from a flail chest are as follows:

- Double fracture of numerous adjacent ribs
- Rib instability
- Lung volume restriction
- Atelectasis
- Lung collapse (pneumothorax)
- Pulmonary contusion (e.g., from trauma)
- Secondary pneumonia (e.g., from weak cough because of pain)

Etiology and Epidemiology

A blunt or crushing injury to the chest is usually the cause of flail chest. Such trauma may result from the following:
- Motor vehicle accidents
- Falls
- Blast injury
- Direct compression (trauma) by a heavy object
- Occupational and industrial accident

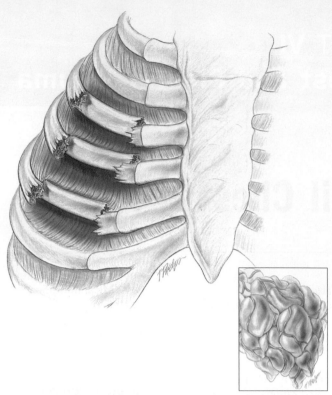

FIGURE 22.1 Flail chest. Double fractures of three or more adjacent ribs produce instability of the chest wall and paradoxical motion of the thorax. Inset, Atelectasis, a common secondary anatomic alteration of the lungs.

General Management of Flail Chest

In mild cases, analgesia and routine airway clearance therapies may be the only actions needed. In more severe cases, however, stabilization of the chest is usually required to allow bone healing and prevent atelectasis. Today, continuous mechanical ventilation, accompanied by **positive end-expiratory pressure (PEEP)**, is commonly used to stabilize a flail chest. The use of pharmacologic paralytics may be required in severe flail chest for ventilatory control. Generally, mechanical ventilation for 5 to 10 days is adequate for sufficient bone healing to occur.[1]

Respiratory Care Treatment Protocols

Oxygen Therapy Protocol

Oxygen therapy is used to treat hypoxia, decrease the work of breathing, and decrease myocardial work. It should be noted, however, that the hypoxemia that develops in flail chest is most commonly caused by the alveolar atelectasis and capillary shunting associated with the disorder. Hypoxemia caused by capillary shunting is often refractory to oxygen therapy (see Oxygen Therapy Protocol, Protocol 10.1).

Lung Expansion Therapy Protocol

Lung expansion techniques are commonly administered to offset and prevent the alveolar consolidation and atelectasis associated with flail chest (see Lung Expansion Therapy Protocol, Protocol 10.3). Mild analgesia may be helpful if the pulmonary expansion technique used causes excessive pain.

Mechanical Ventilation Protocol

Because acute ventilatory failure is associated with flail chest, continuous mechanical ventilation, often with PEEP, is often required to maintain an adequate ventilatory status (see Ventilator Initiation and Management Protocol, Protocol 11.1, and Ventilator Weaning Protocol, Protocol 11.2).

---

[1]Before mechanical ventilation with PEEP, external fixation and stabilization was the common treatment for large flail chest injuries.

The following clinical manifestations result from the pathologic mechanisms caused (or activated) by atelectasis (see Fig. 10.7) and consolidation (see Fig. 10.8)—the major anatomic alterations of the lungs associated with flail chest (see Fig. 22.1).

CLINICAL DATA OBTAINED AT THE PATIENT'S BEDSIDE

The Physical Examination

Vital Signs

Increased Respiratory Rate (Tachypnea)

Several pathophysiologic mechanisms operating simultaneously may lead to an increased ventilatory rate. These include the following:

- Stimulation of peripheral chemoreceptors (hypoxemia)
- Paradoxical movement of the chest wall

Paradoxical Movement of the Chest Wall

When double fractures exist in at least three or more adjacent ribs, a **paradoxical movement of the chest wall** is seen. During inspiration the fractured ribs are pushed inward by the atmospheric pressure surrounding the chest and negative intrapleural pressure. During expiration (and particularly during forced exhalation), the flail area bulges outward when the intrapleural pressure becomes greater than the atmospheric pressure.

As a result of the paradoxical movement of the chest wall, the lung area directly beneath the broken ribs is compressed during inspiration and is pushed outward with the flail segment during expiration. This abnormal chest and lung movement causes gas to be shunted from one lung to another during a ventilatory cycle.

When the lung on the affected side is compressed during inspiration, gas moves into the lung on the unaffected side. During expiration, however, gas from the unaffected lung moves into the affected lung. The shunting of gas from one lung to another is known as **pendelluft** (Fig. 22.2). As a consequence of the pendelluft, the patient rebreathes dead-space gas and hypoventilates. In addition to the hypoventilation produced by the pendelluft, alveolar ventilation also may be decreased by the lung compression and atelectasis associated with the unstable chest wall.

As a result of the pendelluft, lung compression, and atelectasis, the ventilation-perfusion ratio decreases. This leads to intrapulmonary shunting and **venous admixture** (Fig. 22.3). Because of the venous admixture, the patient's PaO_2 and CaO_2 decrease. As this condition intensifies, the patient's oxygen level may decline to a point low enough to stimulate the peripheral chemoreceptors, which in turn initiate an increased ventilatory rate.

Other Possible Mechanisms

- Relationship of decreased lung compliance to increased ventilatory rate
- Activation of the deflation receptors
- Activation of the irritant receptors

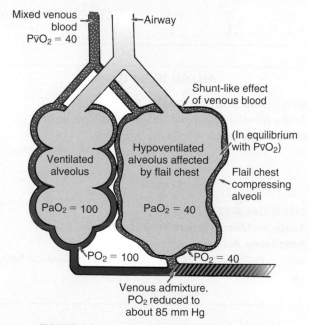

Mixed venous blood $P\bar{v}O_2 = 40$

Airway

Shunt-like effect of venous blood

(In equilibrium with PvO_2)

Ventilated alveolus

Hypoventilated alveolus affected by flail chest

Flail chest compressing alveoli

$PaO_2 = 100$

$PaO_2 = 40$

$PO_2 = 100$

$PO_2 = 40$

Venous admixture. PO_2 reduced to about 85 mm Hg

FIGURE 22.3 Venous admixture in flail chest.

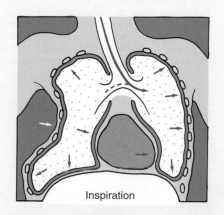
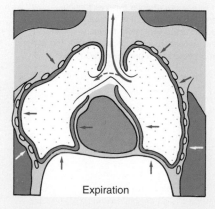

Inspiration

Expiration

FIGURE 22.2 Lateral flail chest with accompanying pendelluft.

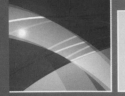
- Stimulation of the J receptors
- Pain, anxiety

Increased Heart Rate (Pulse) and Blood Pressure (e.g., caused by hypoxemia and paisn)

Cyanosis

Chest Assessment Findings

- Diminished breath sounds, on both the affected and the unaffected sides

CLINICAL DATA OBTAINED FROM LABORATORY TESTS AND SPECIAL PROCEDURES

Pulmonary Function Test Findings
(Restrictive Lung Pathology)

LUNG VOLUME AND CAPACITY FINDINGS

V_T	IRV	ERV	RV
N or ↓	↓	↓	↓

VC	IC	FRC	TLC	RV/TLC ratio
↓	↓	↓	↓	N

Arterial Blood Gases

MILD TO MODERATE FLAIL CHEST

Acute Alveolar Hyperventilation With Hypoxemia[1]
(Acute Respiratory Alkalosis)

pH	$PaCO_2$	HCO_3^-	PaO_2	SaO_2 or SpO_2
↑	↓	↓	↓	↓
		(but normal)		

SEVERE FLAIL CHEST

Acute Ventilatory Failure With Hypoxemia[2] (Acute Respiratory Acidosis)

pH[3]	$PaCO_2$	HCO_3^-[3]	PaO_2	SaO_2 or SpO_2
↓	↑	↑	↓	↓
		(but normal)		

[1]See Fig. 5.2 and Table 5.4 and related discussion for the acute pH, $PaCO_2$, and HCO_3^- changes associated with acute alveolar hyperventilation.

[2]See Fig. 5.2 and Table 5.5 and related discussion for the acute pH, $PaCO_2$, and HCO_3^- changes associated with acute ventilatory failure.

[3]When tissue hypoxia is severe enough to produce lactic acid, the pH and HCO_3^- values will be lower than expected for a particular $PaCO_2$ level.

Oxygenation Indices[4]

$\dot{Q}_S/\dot{Q}_T$	DO_2[5]	$\dot{V}O_2$	$C(a-\bar{v})O_2$	O_2ER	$S\bar{v}O_2$
↑	↓	N	↑	↑	↓
		(severe)			

Hemodynamic Indices[6]
Severe Flail Chest Disorder

CVP	RAP	$\overline{PA}$	PCWP	CO	SV
↑	↑	↑	↓	↓	↓

SVI	CI	RVSWI	LVSWI	PVR	SVR
↓	↓	↑	↓	↑	↓

RADIOLOGIC FINDINGS
Chest Radiograph

- Increased opacity (in atelectatic areas or areas with post-flail pneumonia).
- Rib fractures may need a special radiologic technique (rib series) to demonstrate.
- Because of the lung compression and atelectasis associated with flail chest, the density of the lung on the affected side increases. The increase in lung density is revealed on the chest radiograph as increased opacity (i.e., whiter in appearance). The chest radiograph may also show the rib fractures (Fig. 22.4).

[4]$C(a-\bar{v})O_2$, Arterial-venous oxygen difference; DO_2, total oxygen delivery; O_2ER, oxygen extraction ratio; $\dot{Q}_S/\dot{Q}_T$, pulmonary shunt fraction; $S\bar{v}O_2$, mixed venous oxygen saturation; $\dot{V}O_2$, oxygen consumption.

[5]The DO_2 may be normal in patients who have compensated to the decreased oxygenation status with (1) an increased cardiac output, (2) an increased hemoglobin level, or (3) a combination of both. When the DO_2 is normal, the O_2ER is usually normal.

[6]CO, Cardiac output; CI, cardiac index; CVP, central venous pressure; LVSWI, left ventricular stroke work index; $\overline{PA}$, mean pulmonary artery pressure; PCWP, pulmonary capillary wedge pressure; PVR, pulmonary vascular resistance; RAP, right atrial pressure; RVSWI, right ventricular stroke work index; SV, stroke volume; SVI, stroke volume index; SVR, systemic vascular resistance.

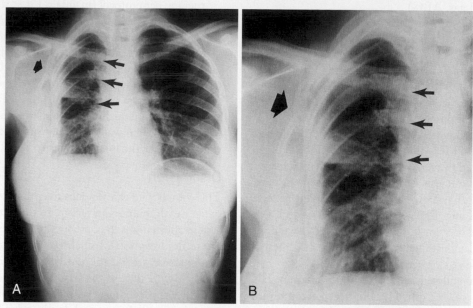

FIGURE 22.4 (A) Chest x-ray of a 20-year-old woman with a severe right-sided flail chest. (B) Close-up of the same x-ray film, demonstrating rib fractures (arrows).

CASE STUDY Flail Chest

Admitting History and Physical Examination

A 40-year-old obese male truck driver was involved in a major four-vehicle accident and was taken to the emergency department of a nearby medical center, where he was found to be markedly agitated and uncooperative. He was conscious and in obvious respiratory distress. His vital signs were blood pressure 80/62 mm Hg, pulse 90 beats/min, respiration rate 42 breaths/min and shallow. Paradoxical movement of the right chest wall was evident.

He had a laceration of the right eyelid and deep lacerations of the right thigh with rupture of the patellar tendon. Pain and tenderness were present on palpation of the right antero-lateral chest wall. The ribs moved paradoxically inward with inspiration. The anteroposterior (AP) diameter of the chest was increased. Breath sounds were decreased bilaterally, and expiration was prolonged.

Chest radiographs revealed double fractures of ribs 2 through 10 on the patient's right anterolateral chest. He had 4+ hematuria, but his other laboratory findings were within normal limits.

The patient was intubated in the emergency department and placed on a mechanical ventilator with 5 cm H_2O PEEP, a V_T of 8 mL/kg, and ventilatory rate of 12. An arterial line was placed, and the patient was taken to the operating room, where surgical repair of the eyelid and thigh was performed. In the operating room, with an FIO_2 of 1.0, the patient's blood gas values were pH 7.48, $PaCO_2$ 30 mm Hg, HCO_3^- 23 mEq/L, PaO_2 360 mm Hg, and SaO_2 98%. His blood pressure was 110/70 mm Hg, and his heart rate was 100 beats/min. The patient was transferred to the surgical intensive care unit, where the respiratory therapist on duty made the following assessment.

Respiratory Assessment and Plan

S N/A—patient is intubated on a mechanical ventilator, sedated, and pharmacologically paralyzed (vecuronium bromide).

O No spontaneous respirations. No paradoxical movement of chest wall on ventilator. BP 110/70, HR 100 regular, RR 12 on vent. On FIO_2 1.0, pH 7.48, $PaCO_2$ 30,

HCO_3^- 23, PaO_2 360, SaO_2 98%. Double fractures of ribs 2 through 10 on the patient's right anterolateral chest: No pneumothorax, no hemothorax.

A • Flail chest (history, paradoxical chest movement, CXR)
• Acute alveolar hyperventilation with overoxygenation (arterial blood gas, ABG)

P Mechanical Ventilation Protocol: Decrease V_T to correct acute alveolar hyperventilation and maintain patient on controlled ventilation and PEEP per protocol until chest wall is stable. Wean oxygen per Ventilator Protocol (decreased to FIO_2 0.40). Routine ABG monitoring. Careful chest assessment and auscultation to monitor for secondary pneumothorax and pneumonia.

Over the next 72 hours, the patient was kept intubated and ventilated with an FIO_2 of 0.40 and a mechanical ventilation rate of 12/min. However, his hospital course was stormy. Aggressive fluid volume resuscitation with intravenous fluids at the rate of 100 mL/h was given. His sputum rapidly became thick and yellow. Lung Expansion Therapy Protocol was increased to a PEEP of 8 cm H_2O. On the second day, a right pneumothorax was demonstrated and a chest tube was inserted. A persistent air leak was present.

The next day, his pulse increased to 160 beats/min. His blood pressure was 142/82 mm Hg. His rectal temperature was 99.2°F. His ventilator rate was 12 breaths/min, with a PEEP of 10 cm H_2O. Auscultation revealed bilateral crackles. On an FIO_2 of 0.70, his ABG values were pH 7.37, $PaCO_2$ 38 mm Hg, HCO_3^- 23 mEq/L, PaO_2 58 mm Hg, and SaO_2 90%. Rapid diuresis was initiated, and his cardiac function improved dramatically. Over the next few days, the chest radiograph showed dense infiltrates in both lungs, and it was difficult to maintain adequate oxygenation, even with high inspired oxygen concentrations. His sputum was yellow and thick. At this time, the respiratory assessment was as follows:

Respiratory Assessment and Plan

S N/A—intubated, sedated, and paralyzed.

O Afebrile. HR 160 regular, BP 142/82, RR 12 (on vent). Right chest tube shows air leak. Crackles bilaterally. CXR: Fractures appear in line; bilateral dense infiltrates. ABG on an FIO_2 of 0.70 are pH 7.37, $PaCO_2$ 38, HCO_3^- 23, PaO_2 58, and SaO_2 90%. Sputum thick, yellow.

A • Persistent right-sided flail chest (if allowed to breathe on his own) (CXR)
• Bilateral dense infiltrates suggest atelectasis versus pulmonary edema versus acute respiratory distress syndrome (ARDS) versus pneumonia (CXR)
• Adequate alveolar ventilation with moderate hypoxemia on present ventilator settings; oxygenation continues to worsen (ABG)

• Thick, yellow bronchial secretions (sputum)
• Pneumonia possible (despite normal temperature)
• Bronchopleural fistula on right side (chest tube bubbles)

P Mechanical Ventilation Protocol and Lung Expansion Therapy Protocol. Increase PEEP to 12 cm H_2O. Oxygen therapy per protocol (maintain FIO_2 of 0.70). Start Airway Clearance Therapy Protocol (suction PRN; obtain sputum for Gram stain and culture). Continue SaO_2 monitoring.

During the patient's first week of hospitalization, his blood urea nitrogen (BUN) increased to 60 mg/dL and his creatinine to 1.9 mg/dL, thought to be related to trauma. Liver function values remained within normal limits. The abnormal BUN and creatinine gradually returned to normal during the second week. The patient was slowly but successfully weaned off the ventilator over the next 2 weeks.

Discussion

This complicated case demonstrates the care of the traumatized patient with multiorgan failure. In this case, the second organ system affected was the cardiovascular system, probably secondary to fluid overload. Initial therapy included chest wall rest and internal stabilization with mechanical ventilation and PEEP. By the time of the second assessment, the more classic clinical manifestations of pulmonary parenchymal change secondary to flail chest had developed. The clinical scenarios of atelectasis (see Fig. 10.7) and/or alveolar consolidation (see Fig. 10.8) were well established, with oxygen-refractory pulmonary capillary shunting clearly in evidence.

Later, when what appeared to be acute respiratory distress syndrome (ARDS) supervened, additional PEEP was added, both for its effect on the ARDS and to stabilize the chest wall. Although these problems were dramatic enough, the therapist alertly noted the thick yellow bronchial secretions and suctioned as needed. The ordering of a sputum Gram stain and culture was appropriate. As the patient was being slowly weaned off the ventilator, pain control for the nonintubated patient was considered.

Clearly, a patient this ill should be assessed at least once—possibly more—per shift. Because this patient was hospitalized for 40 days, more than 120 such assessments were found in his chart. As we reviewed his case, this certainly did not seem to be excessive.

It is strongly suggested that notation of the **ventilator settings in flail chest** be a part of the "objective" recordings in the patient's SOAP notes—just as the FIO_2 must accompany the patient's ABG values.

SELF-ASSESSMENT QUESTIONS

1. In flail chest, which of the following occur?
   1. Tidal volume (V_T) increases
   2. Atelectasis often occurs
   3. Intrapulmonary shunting occurs
   4. Pneumothorax is rare
      a. 1, 2, and 4 only
      b. 1 and 3 only
      c. 2 and 3 only
      d. 2 and 4 only

2. When a patient has a severe flail chest, which of the following occurs?
   a. Venous return increases
   b. Cardiac output increases
   c. Systemic blood pressure increases
   d. Central venous pressure increases

3. A flail chest consists of a double fracture of at least:
   a. Two adjacent ribs
   b. Three adjacent ribs
   c. Four adjacent ribs
   d. Five adjacent ribs

4. Which of the following respiratory care technique(s) is(are) commonly used in the treatment of severe flail chest?
   1. Cough and deep breathe
   2. Intubation with continuous mandatory ventilation
   3. Negative pressure ventilation (cuirass)
   4. Positive end-expiratory pressure/continuous positive airway pressure (PEEP/CPAP)
      a. 1 only
      b. 3 only
      c. 2 and 4 only
      d. 2, 3, and 4 only

5. When mechanical ventilation is used to stabilize a flail chest, how much time generally is needed for adequate bone healing to occur?
   a. 5 to 10 days
   b. 10 to 15 days
   c. 15 to 20 days
   d. 20 to 25 days

Chapter Objectives

After reading this chapter, you will be able to:

- List the anatomic alterations of the lungs associated with a pneumothorax.
- Describe the causes of a pneumothorax.
- List the cardiopulmonary clinical manifestations associated with a pneumothorax.
- Describe the general management of a pneumothorax.
- Describe the clinical strategies and rationales of the SOAPs presented in the case study.
- Define key terms and complete self-assessment questions at the end of the chapter and on Evolve.

Key Terms

Bleomycin Sulfate
Closed Pneumothorax
Iatrogenic Pneumothorax
Open Pneumothorax
Pendelluft
Pleurisy
Pleurodesis
Sclerosant Agents
Spontaneous Pneumothorax

Sucking Chest Wound
Talc Pleurodesis
Tension Pneumothorax
Tetracycline Pleurodesis
Thoracic Free Air
Thoracostomy Chest Tube
Tracheal Shift
Traumatic Pneumothorax

Chapter Outline

Anatomic Alterations of the Lungs
Etiology, Epidemiology, and Symptoms
   Traumatic Pneumothorax
   Spontaneous Pneumothorax
   Iatrogenic Pneumothorax
   Symptoms
Overview of the Cardiopulmonary Clinical Manifestations
   Associated With Pneumothorax
General Management of Pneumothorax
   Respiratory Care Treatment Protocols
   Pleurodesis
Case Study: Spontaneous Pneumothorax
Self-Assessment Questions

Anatomic Alterations of the Lungs

A pneumothorax exists when gas (sometimes called **thoracic free air**) accumulates in the pleural space (Fig. 23.1). When gas enters the pleural space, the visceral and parietal pleura separate. This enhances the natural tendency of the lung to recoil, or collapse, and the natural tendency of the chest wall to move outward, or expand. As the lung collapses, the alveoli are compressed and atelectasis ensues. In severe cases, the great veins may be compressed and cause the venous return to the heart to diminish.

A pneumothorax produces a restrictive lung disorder. The major pathologic or structural changes associated with a pneumothorax are as follows:

- Lung collapse
- Atelectasis
- Chest wall expansion (in tension pneumothorax)
- Compression of the great veins and decreased cardiac venous return

Etiology, Epidemiology, and Symptoms

Gas can gain entrance to the pleural space in the following three ways:

1. From the lungs through a perforation of the visceral pleura
2. From the surrounding atmosphere through a perforation of the chest wall and parietal pleura or, rarely, through an esophageal fistula or a perforated abdominal viscus
3. From gas-forming microorganisms in an empyema in the pleural space (rare)

A pneumothorax may be classified as either closed or open according to the way gas gains entrance to the pleural space. In a **closed pneumothorax**, gas in the pleural space is not in direct contact with the atmosphere. An **open pneumothorax**, however, is a condition in which the pleural space is in direct contact with the atmosphere such that gas can move freely in and out. A pneumothorax in which the intrapleural pressure exceeds the intraalveolar (or atmospheric) pressure is known

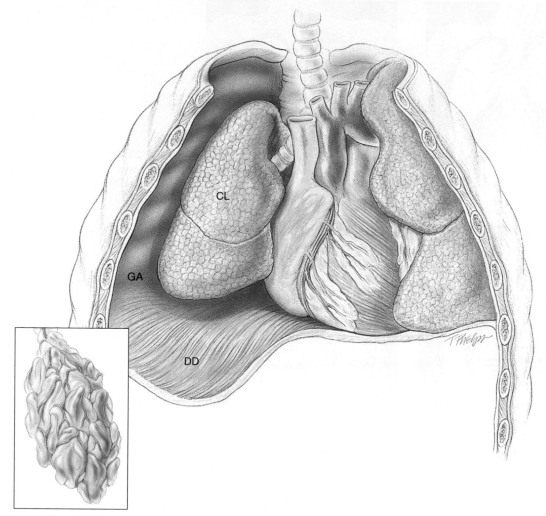

FIGURE 23.1 A right tension pneumothorax. *CL,* Collapsed lung; *DD,* depressed diaphragm; *GA,* gas accumulation in the pleural cavity. Inset, atelectasis, a common secondary anatomic alteration of the lungs.

as a **tension pneumothorax**. Some forms of pneumothorax are identified on the basis of origin, as follows:

- Traumatic pneumothorax
- Spontaneous pneumothorax
- Iatrogenic pneumothorax

Traumatic Pneumothorax

Penetrating wounds to the chest wall from a knife, a bullet, or an impaling object in an automobile or industrial accident are common causes of traumatic pneumothorax. When this type of trauma occurs, the pleural space is in direct contact with the atmosphere, and gas can move into and out of the pleural cavity. This condition is known as a **sucking chest wound** and is classified as an *open pneumothorax* (Fig. 23.2).

A piercing chest wound also may result in a closed (valvular), or tension, pneumothorax through a one-way valve-like action of the ruptured parietal pleura. In this form of pneumothorax, gas enters the pleural space during inspiration but cannot leave during expiration because the parietal pleura (or more infrequently, the chest wall itself) acts as a check valve. This condition may cause the intrapleural pressure to exceed the atmospheric pressure in the affected area. Technically this

form of pneumothorax is classified as a *tension pneumothorax* (Fig. 23.3). This form of pneumothorax is the most serious of all because gas continues to accumulate in the intrapleural space and progressively increases the compressing pressures on the lungs and mediastinal structures of the affected area.

When a crushing chest injury occurs, the pleural space may not be in direct contact with the atmosphere, but the sharp end of a fractured rib may pierce or tear the visceral pleura. This may permit gas to leak into the pleural space from the lungs. Technically, this form of pneumothorax is classified as a *closed pneumothorax.*

Spontaneous Pneumothorax

When a pneumothorax occurs suddenly and without any obvious underlying cause, it is referred to as a *spontaneous pneumothorax.* A spontaneous pneumothorax is secondary to certain underlying pathologic processes such as pneumonia, tuberculosis, and chronic obstructive pulmonary disease (COPD). A spontaneous pneumothorax is sometimes caused by the rupture of a small bleb or bulla on the surface of the lung. This type of pneumothorax often occurs in tall, thin people aged 15 to 35 years. It may result from the high negative

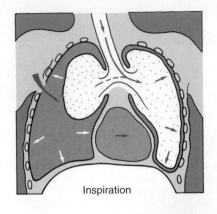
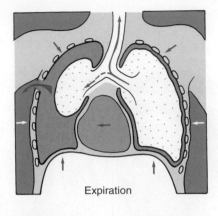

Inspiration | Expiration

FIGURE 23.2 Sucking chest wound with accompanying pendelluft in an open right pneumothorax. The large arrow illustrates the chest wall injury.

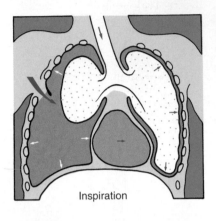
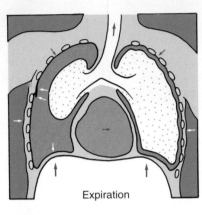

Inspiration | Expiration

FIGURE 23.3 Closed (tension) pneumothorax produced by a right chest wall wound. The large arrow illustrates the chest wall injury and the parietal pleural "valve."

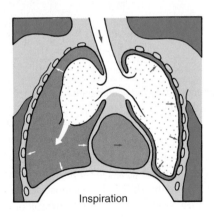
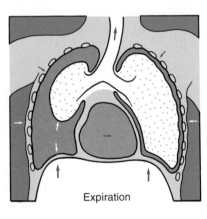

Inspiration | Expiration

FIGURE 23.4 Right pneumothorax produced by a rupture in the visceral pleura that functions as a check valve. Progressive enlargement of the pneumothorax occurs, producing atelectasis on the affected side.

intrathoracic pressure and mechanical stresses that take place in the upper zone of the upright lung (Fig. 23.4).

A spontaneous pneumothorax also may behave as a tension pneumothorax. Air from the lung parenchyma may enter the pleural space via a tear in the visceral pleura during inspiration, but is unable to leave during expiration because the visceral tear functions as a check valve (see Fig. 23.4). This condition may cause the intrapleural pressure to exceed the intraalveolar pressure. This form of pneumothorax is classified as both a *closed pneumothorax* and a *tension pneumothorax*.

Iatrogenic Pneumothorax

An **iatrogenic pneumothorax** sometimes occurs during specific diagnostic or therapeutic procedures. For example, a pleural or liver biopsy may cause a pneumothorax, as may a transthoracic needle biopsy of the lung itself. Thoracentesis, intercostal nerve block, cannulation of a subclavian vein,

and tracheostomy are other possible causes of an iatrogenic pneumothorax. Rarely, bronchoscopy (particularly with lung biopsy) may produce an iatrogenic pneumothorax as well.

An iatrogenic pneumothorax is always a hazard during positive-pressure mechanical ventilation, particularly when high tidal volumes or high system pressures are used. This is particularly common in COPD and in human immunodeficiency virus (HIV)–related acute respiratory distress syndrome (ARDS).

Symptoms

The classic presentation of a pneumothorax is that of sudden crisis onset (see Fig. 3.9), with severe dyspneic pleuritic chest pain, cough, and cardiovascular collapse. Hemoptysis may occur, but it is usually not life-threatening. Occasionally, a pneumothorax may develop more slowly, but this is unusual.

The following clinical manifestations result from the pathologic mechanisms caused (or activated) by atelectasis (see Fig. 10.7)—the major anatomic alteration of the lungs associated with pneumothorax (see Fig. 23.1).

CLINICAL DATA OBTAINED AT THE PATIENT'S BEDSIDE

The Physical Examination

Vital Signs

Increased Respiratory Rate (Tachypnea)

Several pathophysiologic mechanisms operating simultaneously may lead to an increased ventilatory rate.

Stimulation of Peripheral Chemoreceptors (Hypoxemia)

As gas moves into the pleural space, the visceral and parietal pleura separate and the lung on the affected side begins to collapse. As the lung collapses, atelectasis develops, and alveolar ventilation decreases.

If the patient has a pneumothorax as a result of a sucking chest wound, an additional mechanism also may promote hypoventilation. In other words, when a patient with this type of pneumothorax inhales, the intrapleural pressure on the unaffected side decreases. As a result the mediastinum often moves to the unaffected side, where the pressure is lower, and compresses the normal lung. The intrapleural pressure on the affected side also may decrease, and some air may enter through the chest wound and further shift the mediastinum toward the normal lung. During expiration the intrapleural pressure on the affected side rises above atmospheric pressure, and gas escapes from the pleural space through the chest wound. As gas leaves the pleural space, the mediastinum moves back toward the affected side. Because of this back-and-forth movement of the mediastinum, some gas from the normal lung may enter the collapsed lung during expiration and cause it to expand slightly. During inspiration, however, some of this "rebreathed dead space gas" may move back into the normal lung. This paradoxical movement of gas within the lungs is known as **pendelluft**. As a result of the pendelluft, the patient hypoventilates (see Fig. 23.2).

Therefore when a patient has a pneumothorax, alveolar ventilation is reduced because of lung collapse and atelectasis. If the pneumothorax is accompanied by a sucking chest wound, alveolar ventilation may be further decreased by pendelluft.

As a result of the reduced alveolar ventilation, the patient's ventilation-perfusion ratio decreases. This leads to intrapulmonary shunting and venous admixture (Fig. 23.5). Because of the venous admixture, the PaO_2 and CaO_2 decrease. As this condition intensifies, the patient's arterial oxygen level may decline to a point low enough to stimulate the peripheral chemoreceptors. Stimulation of the peripheral chemoreceptors in turn initiates an increased ventilatory rate.

Other Possible Mechanisms

- Relationship of decreased lung compliance to increased ventilatory rate
- Activation of the deflation receptors

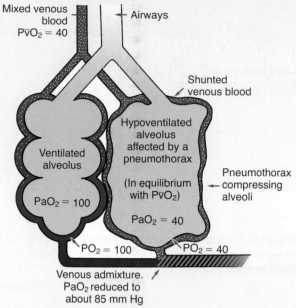

FIGURE 23.5 Venous admixture in pneumothorax.

- Activation of the irritant receptors
- Stimulation of the J receptors
- Pain, anxiety

Increased Heart Rate (Pulse) and Blood Pressure (Small Pneumothorax)

Cyanosis

Chest Assessment Findings

- Hyperresonant percussion note over the pneumothorax
- Diminished breath sounds over the pneumothorax
- **Tracheal shift** (away from the affected side in a tension pneumothorax)
- Displaced heart sounds
- Increased thoracic volume on the affected side (particularly in tension pneumothorax)

As gas accumulates in the pleural space, the ratio of air to solid tissue increases. Percussion notes resonate more freely throughout the gas in the pleural space and in the air spaces within the lung (Fig. 23.6). When this area is auscultated, however, the breath sounds are diminished (Fig. 23.7). When intrapleural gas accumulates and intrathoracic pressure is excessively high, the mediastinum may be forced to the unaffected side. If this is the case, there will be a tracheal shift and the heart sounds will be displaced during auscultation.

Finally, the gas that accumulates in the pleural space enhances not only the natural tendency of the lungs to collapse, but also the natural tendency of the chest wall to expand. Therefore in a large pneumothorax the chest often appears larger on the affected side. This is especially true in patients with a severe tension pneumothorax (Fig. 23.8).

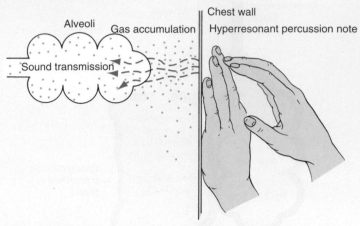

FIGURE 23.6 Because the ratio of extrapulmonary gas to solid tissue increases in a pneumothorax, hyperresonant percussion notes are produced over the affected area.

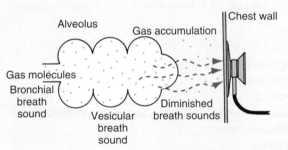

FIGURE 23.7 Breath sounds diminish as gas accumulates in the intrapleural space.

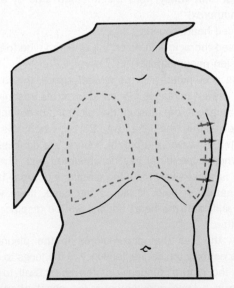

FIGURE 23.8 As gas accumulates in the intrapleural space, the chest diameter increases on the affected side in a tension pneumothorax.

CLINICAL DATA OBTAINED FROM LABORATORY TESTS AND SPECIAL PROCEDURES

Pulmonary Function Test Findings (Restrictive Lung Pathology)

LUNG VOLUME AND CAPACITY FINDINGS

V_T	IRV	ERV	RV	
N or ↓	↓	↓	↓	
VC	IC	FRC	TLC	RV/TLC ratio
↓	↓	↓	↓	N

Arterial Blood Gases

SMALL PNEUMOTHORAX

Acute Alveolar Hyperventilation With Hypoxemia[1] (Acute Respiratory Alkalosis)

pH	$PaCO_2$	HCO_3^-	PaO_2	SaO_2 or SpO_2
↑	↓	↓	↓	↓
		(but normal)		

LARGE PNEUMOTHORAX

Acute Ventilatory Failure With Hypoxemia[2] (Acute Respiratory Acidosis)

pH[3]	$PaCO_2$	HCO_3^{-}[3]	PaO_2	SaO_2 or SpO_2
↓	↑	↑	↓	↓
		(but normal)		

Oxygenation Indices[4]

$\dot{Q}_S/\dot{Q}_T$	DO_2[5]	$\dot{V}O_2$	$C(a-\bar{v})O_2$	O_2ER	$S\bar{v}O_2$
↑	↓	N	↑	↑	↓
			(severe)		

[1]See Fig. 5.2 and Table 5.4 and related discussion for the acute pH, $PaCO_2$, and HCO_3^- changes associated with acute alveolar hyperventilation.

[2]See Fig. 5.2 and Table 5.5 and related discussion for the acute pH, $PaCO_2$, and HCO_3^- changes associated with acute ventilatory failure.

[3]When tissue hypoxia is severe enough to produce lactic acid, the pH and HCO_3^- values will be lower than expected for a particular $PaCO_2$ level.

[4]$C(a-\bar{v})O_2$, Arterial-venous oxygen difference; DO_2, total oxygen delivery; O_2ER, oxygen extraction ratio; $\dot{Q}_S/\dot{Q}_T$, pulmonary shunt fraction; $S\bar{v}O_2$, mixed venous oxygen saturation; $\dot{V}O_2$, oxygen consumption.

[5]The DO_2 may be normal in patients who have compensated to the decreased oxygenation status with (1) an increased cardiac output, (2) an increased hemoglobin level, or (3) a combination of both. When the DO_2 is normal, the O_2ER is usually normal.

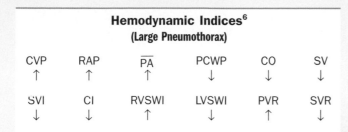

Hemodynamic Indices[6]
(Large Pneumothorax)

CVP	RAP	$\overline{PA}$	PCWP	CO	SV
↑	↑	↑	↓	↓	↓
SVI	CI	RVSWI	LVSWI	PVR	SVR
↓	↓	↑	↓	↑	↓

RADIOLOGIC FINDINGS
Chest Radiograph

- Increased translucency (darker lung fields) on the side of pneumothorax
- Mediastinal shift to unaffected side in tension pneumothorax
- Depressed diaphragm on the affected side
- Lung collapse
- Atelectasis

Ordinarily, the presence of a pneumothorax is easily identified on the chest radiograph in the upright posteroanterior view. A small collection of air is often visible if the exposure is made at the end of maximal expiration because the translucency of the pneumothorax is more obvious when contrasted with the density of a partially deflated lung. The pneumothorax is usually seen in the upper part of the pleural cavity when the film is exposed, while the patient is in the upright position. Severe adhesions, however, may limit the collection of gas to a specific portion of the pleural space. Fig. 23.9A shows the development of a tension pneumothorax in the lower part of the right lung. Fig. 23.9B shows progression of the same pneumothorax 30 minutes later. Fig. 23.10 shows the classic body shape of a 19-year-old man who is 6 feet 5 inches tall and who experienced a spontaneous left-sided pneumothorax while playing a round of golf.

Fig. 23.11 shows a pneumothorax caused by a gunshot wound to the upper left chest/shoulder area.

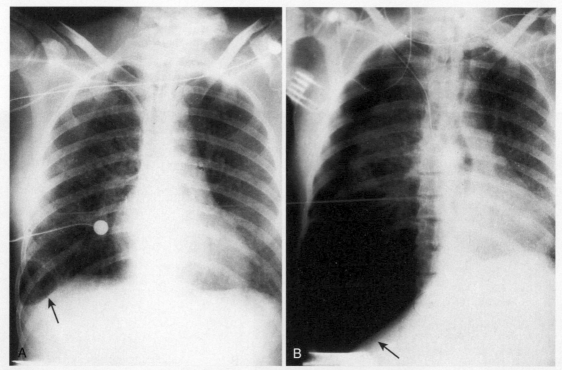

FIGURE 23.9 (A) Development of a small tension pneumothorax in the lower part of the right lung (arrow). (B) The same pneumothorax 30 minutes later. Note the shift of the heart and mediastinum to the left away from the tension pneumothorax. Also note the depression of the right hemidiaphragm (arrow).

[6]CO, Cardiac output; CI, cardiac index; CVP, central venous pressure; LVSWI, left ventricular stroke work index; $\overline{PA}$, mean pulmonary artery pressure; PCWP, pulmonary capillary wedge pressure; PVR, pulmonary vascular resistance; RAP, right atrial pressure; RVSWI, right ventricular stroke work index; SV, stroke volume; SVI, stroke volume index; SVR, systemic vascular resistance.

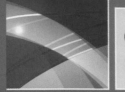

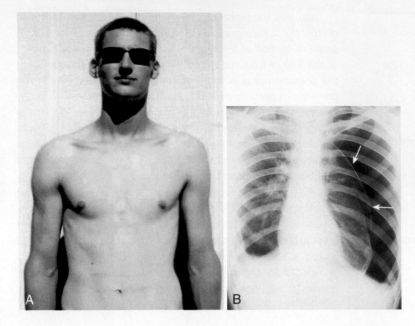

FIGURE 23.10 (A) A 19-year-old male patient, 6 feet 5 inches tall, who experienced a sudden spontaneous left-sided pneumothorax while playing a round of golf. A spontaneous pneumothorax is not uncommon in people who are tall and thin. (B) Chest radiograph of the same patient 45 minutes later in the emergency department. Note the slight shift of the heart and mediastinum to the right (toward the unaffected side), away from the tension pneumothorax, and the markedly depressed diaphragm on the patient's left side.

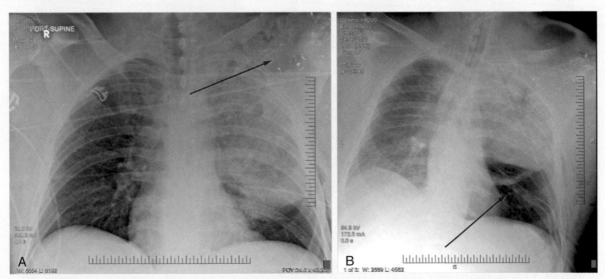

FIGURE 23.11 (A) Fragments of a bullet faintly seen (white dots) in the upper left chest/shoulder area (see red arrow). (B) Four hours later, the patient clearly revealed a left pneumothorax (see red arrow). Note the increased radiodensity of the left upper lung suggesting the presence of compression atelectasis of the left upper lobe. (Radiographs courtesy Dr. Willam E. Faught and Dr. Mark Faught.)

General Management of Pneumothorax

The management of pneumothorax depends on the degree of lung collapse. When the pneumothorax is relatively small (15% to 20%), the patient may need only bed rest or limited physical activity. In such cases, reabsorption of intrapleural gas usually occurs within 30 days.

When the pneumothorax is larger than 20%, it should be evacuated. In less severe cases, air may simply be withdrawn from the pleural cavity by needle aspiration. In more serious cases, a **thoracostomy chest tube** attached to an underwater seal is inserted into the patient's pleural cavity. Because air rises, the tube is usually placed anteriorly near the lung's apex, above the rib to avoid injury to the vessels and nerves that run under the ribs in the costal grooves. Typically, a no. 28 to 36 gauge French thoracostomy tube is used for adults, with smaller sizes used for children. The tube permits evacuation of air and enhances the reexpansion and pleural adherence of the affected lung. The chest tube may or may not be attached to gentle suction. When suction is used, the negative pressure need not exceed -12 cm H_2O; -5 cm H_2O is generally all that is needed. After the lung has reexpanded and bubbling from the chest tube has ceased, the tube is clamped and left in place without suction for another 24 to 48 hours.

Respiratory Care Treatment Protocols

Oxygen Therapy Protocol

Oxygen therapy is used to treat hypoxemia, decrease the work of breathing, and decrease myocardial work. It should be noted, however, that the hypoxemia that develops in a pneumothorax is most commonly caused by the alveolar atelectasis and capillary shunting associated with the disorder. Hypoxemia caused by capillary shunting is often refractory to oxygen therapy (see Oxygen Therapy Protocol, Protocol 10.1).

Lung Expansion Therapy Protocol

With caution, lung expansion techniques are commonly administered to offset the atelectasis associated with a pneumothorax (see Lung Expansion Therapy Protocol, Protocol 10.3) in patients with chest tubes.

Mechanical Ventilation Protocol

Because acute ventilatory failure may develop with severe pneumothorax, continuous monitoring and use of mechanical ventilation with positive end-expiratory pressure (PEEP) may be required to maintain adequate ventilatory status (see Ventilator Initiation and Management Protocol, Protocol 11.1, and Ventilator Weaning Protocol, Protocol 11.2). When mechanical ventilation is needed, a tube thoracotomy (preventive thoracotomy) is required to offset the possible development of a tension pneumothorax.

Pleurodesis

On occasion, a thoracentesis may be performed before a procedure called **pleurodesis**. During the pleurodesis procedure a **sclerosant agent** (**talc, tetracycline,** or **bleomycin sulfate**) is injected into the chest cavity. The chemical substance or medication causes an intense inflammatory reaction over the outer surface of the lung and inside of the chest cavity. This procedure is performed to cause the surface of the lung to adhere to the chest cavity, thus preventing or reducing recurrent pneumothorax or recurrent pleural effusions. An intense pleuritis is produced, which may be quite painful (**pleurisy**).

CASE STUDY   Spontaneous Pneumothorax

Admitting History and Physical Examination

This patient was a 20-year-old man, a university student who was in excellent health until 5 hours before admission. He was sitting quietly in his dorm room studying for an examination when he suddenly developed a sharp pain in his left lower thoracic region. It was most acute in the anterior axillary line. The pain was exacerbated by deep inspiration and radiated anteriorly, almost to the midline. It did not radiate into the shoulder or neck. The patient became mildly dyspneic and had episodes of nonproductive cough that seemed to increase the chest pain. These symptoms worsened, and at 1 a.m. his roommate drove him to the university hospital emergency department (ED).

On examination, the patient was a tall, thin, well-nourished young man in moderately acute distress. His trachea was shifted to the right of the midline. His blood pressure was 150/82 mm Hg, pulse 96 beats/min, and respirations 28 breaths/min and shallow. On room air, his SpO_2 was 90%. The left side of the chest was hyperresonant to percussion, and the breath sounds were described as "distant." The patient was not cyanotic. The ED physician was momentarily busy with another patient and asked the respiratory therapist on duty to assess the patient's respiratory status.

The respiratory therapist assigned to the ED during the night shift made the following assessments and plans.

Respiratory Assessment and Plan

S Sudden left chest pain worsened by cough; shortness of breath

O Normal vital signs. Left chest hyperresonant. Trachea shifted to the right. Breath sounds on left "distant." Room air SpO_2 90%.

A Probable left spontaneous tension pneumothorax (history and objective indicators)

P Notify physician (who was in the next room). Request stat CXR and ABG. Oxygen Therapy Protocol (partial rebreathing mask). Obtain supplies for tube thoracostomy and place at the patient's bedside.

The patient stated that he was more comfortable on the oxygen mask, but that some left-sided chest pain was still present. His physical findings were unchanged from his initial evaluation. The chest radiograph confirmed the diagnosis of a 50% left-sided pneumothorax, lung collapse, and mediastinal shift to the right. The arterial blood gas values on a partial rebreathing mask were pH 7.53, $PaCO_2$ 29 mm Hg, HCO_3^- 21 mEq/L, PaO_2 56 mm Hg, and SaO_2 92%. The physician was still busy with the patient in the next room.

With this new information, the respiratory therapist charted the following.

Respiratory Assessment and Plan

S "This oxygen mask helps a little."

O Persistent symptoms and physical findings as in SOAP-1 above. CXR: 50% left tension pneumothorax. Mediastinum shifted to right. ABGs pH 7.53, $PaCO_2$ 29, HCO_3^- 21, PaO_2 56, and SaO_2 92% (on partial rebreathing mask).

A • 50% left pneumothorax with mediastinal shift—lung collapse and atelectasis (CXR)

   • Acute alveolar hyperventilation with moderate hypoxemia (ABG)

P Inform physician of previous and current assessment. Up-regulate Oxygen Therapy Protocol (increase FIO_2 via a nonrebreathing mask). Stay at patient's bedside until physician arrives. Assist in placement of chest tube.

Approximately 15 minutes later, the attending physician entered the room and quickly reviewed the clinical data and assessments. Moments later, she performed a needle decompression and thoracentesis, followed by the placement of a chest tube. A small about of bloody fluid was aspirated. To help enhance lung expansion, the respiratory therapist placed a continuous positive airway pressure (CPAP) mask on the patient's face at 5 cm H_2O. The FIO_2 on the mask was adjusted to 0.40. Over the next 30 minutes, the lung expanded well and the patient's ventilatory and oxygenation status quickly improved. The chest tube was removed after 48 hours. Follow up examination after 2 weeks revealed full expansion of the left lung. There was no evidence of blebs or bullae. A tuberculin skin test result was negative, and the cause of the pneumothorax was never found.

Discussion

The spontaneous pneumothorax described in this case study is often seen in tall, thin people between the ages of 15 and 35 years (see Fig. 23.10). It also can develop in hospitalized patients as a complication of ventilator management, as is mentioned in Chapter 11, Respiratory Insufficiency, Respiratory Failure, and Ventilator Management Protocols. Few respiratory conditions persist with a "crisis" onset, and this is one of them. In short, a spontaneous pneumothorax is an emergency that requires immediate attention; the respiratory therapist should aggressively work to help stabilize the patient's condition as soon as possible.

This case nicely demonstrates the signs and symptoms of atelectasis and oxygen-refractory intrapulmonary shunting (see Fig. 10.7). The physician and respiratory therapist could not hear crackles, however, presumably because the atelectatic segments were separated (distant) from the chest wall and the examiner's stethoscope.

The results of the thoracentesis may have been important but were not yet available when this note was written.

Although the respiratory care administered in this case (oxygen therapy) was fairly routine and ordinary, the therapist's assistance in the assessment of this patient and his presence at bedside made a great difference in the speed and ease with which the patient was treated. The value of an assessing and treating therapist in this situation cannot be overestimated.

SELF-ASSESSMENT QUESTIONS

1. When gas moves between the pleural space and the atmosphere during a ventilatory cycle, the patient is said to have a(n):
   a. Closed pneumothorax
   b. Iatrogenic pneumothorax
   c. Valvular pneumothorax
   d. Sucking chest wound

2. When gas enters the pleural space during inspiration but is unable to leave during expiration, the patient is said to have a(n):
   1. Iatrogenic pneumothorax
   2. Valvular pneumothorax
   3. Tension pneumothorax
   4. Open pneumothorax
      a. 1 only
      b. 3 only
      c. 2 and 3 only
      d. 3 and 4 only

3. Which of the following may cause a pneumothorax?
   1. Pneumonia
   2. Tuberculosis
   3. Chronic obstructive pulmonary disease
   4. Blebs
      a. 1 and 2 only
      b. 2 and 3 only
      c. 2, 3, and 4 only
      d. 1, 2, 3, and 4

4. When a patient has a pneumothorax because of a sucking chest wound, which of the following occurs?
   1. Intrapleural pressure on the unaffected side increases during inspiration.
   2. The mediastinum often moves to the unaffected side during inspiration.
   3. Intrapleural pressure on the affected side often rises above the atmospheric pressure during expiration.
   4. The mediastinum often moves to the affected side during expiration.
      a. 1 and 4 only
      b. 1 and 3 only
      c. 2 and 3 only
      d. 2, 3, and 4 only

5. The increased ventilatory rate commonly manifested in patients with pneumothorax may result from which of the following?
   1. Stimulation of the J receptors
   2. Increased lung compliance
   3. Increased stimulation of the Hering-Breuer reflex
   4. Stimulation of the irritant reflex
      a. 1 and 4 only
      b. 2 and 3 only
      c. 3 and 4 only
      d. 2, 3, and 4 only

6. The physician usually elects to evacuate the intrathoracic gas when the pneumothorax is greater than:
   a. 5%
   b. 10%
   c. 15%
   d. 20%

7. During treatment of a pneumothorax with a chest tube and suction, the negative (suction) pressure usually need not exceed:
   a. -6 cm H_2O
   b. -8 cm H_2O
   c. -10 cm H_2O
   d. -12 cm H_2O

8. A patient with a severe tension pneumothorax demonstrates which of the following on the affected side?
   1. Diminished breath sounds
   2. Hyperresonant percussion note
   3. Dull percussion notes
   4. Whispered pectoriloquy
      a. 2 only
      b. 1 and 2 only
      c. 3 and 4 only
      d. 1, 2, and 4 only

9. When a patient has a large tension pneumothorax, which of the following occur(s)?
   a. pH increases
   b. $PaCO_2$ increases
   c. HCO_3^- decreases
   d. $PaCO_2$ decreases

10. When a patient has a large tension pneumothorax, which of the following occur(s)?
    a. PVR decreases
    b. PA increases
    c. CVP decreases
    d. CO increases

24 Pleural Effusion and Empyema

Chapter Objectives

After reading this chapter, you will be able to:

- List the anatomic alterations of the lungs associated with pleural diseases.
- Describe the causes of pleural diseases.
- Describe the use of thoracentesis and pleural fluid examination in the etiology of pleural diseases.
- List the cardiopulmonary clinical manifestations associated with pleural diseases.
- Describe the general management of pleural diseases.
- Describe the clinical strategies and rationales of the SOAPs presented in the case study.
- Define key terms and complete self-assessment questions at the end of the chapter and on Evolve.

Key Terms

Chylothorax
Congestive Heart Failure
Decortication
Empyema
Exudative Pleural Effusion
Fungal Diseases
Hemothorax
Hepatic Hydrothorax
Lateral Decubitus Radiograph
Left-Sided Heart Failure
Light Criteria
Loculated Pleural Effusion
Malignant Mesothelioma
Meniscus Sign
Nephrotic Syndrome
Parapneumonic Pleural Effusion

Peritoneal Dialysis
Pigtail Catheter
Pleural Effusion
Pleurisy
Pleurodesis
Point-of-Care Chest Ultrasonography
Postpneumonic Pleural Effusion
Pulmonary Infarction
Pulmonary Emboli
Reexpansion Pulmonary Edema
Right-Sided Heart Failure
Sclerosant
Thoracentesis
Transudative Pleural Effusion
Tuberculosis
Video-Assisted Thoracic Surgery (VATS)

Chapter Outline

Anatomic Alterations of the Lungs

A number of pleural diseases can cause fluid to accumulate in the pleural space; this fluid is called a **pleural effusion** or, if infected, an **empyema** (Fig. 24.1). Similar to free air in the pleural space, fluid accumulation separates the visceral and parietal pleura and compresses the lungs. In severe cases, atelectasis will develop, the great veins may be compressed, and cardiac venous return may be diminished. Pleural effusion and empyema produce a restrictive lung disorder.

The major pathologic or structural changes associated with significant pleural effusion are lung compression, atelectasis, and compression of the great veins and decreased cardiac venous return.

Pleural Anatomy and Pathophysiology

Approximately 0.26 mL of fluid per kilogram of body weight is estimated to be contained in each pleural cavity. It is produced and absorbed primarily on the parietal (chest wall) surface. As illustrated in Fig. 24.2, under normal circumstances the amount of fluid in the pleural space depends on the balance of *hydrostatic* and *oncotic pressures* between the parietal and visceral pleura and the pleural space. Fluid in the pleural space

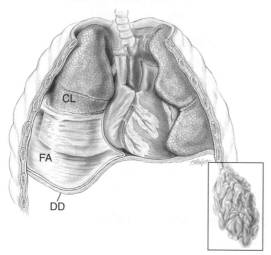

FIGURE 24.1 Right-sided pleural effusion. *CL,* Collapsed lung (partially collapsed); *DD,* depressed diaphragm; *FA,* fluid accumulation. Inset, Atelectasis, a common secondary anatomic alteration of the lungs.

is primarily produced from the parietal pleura because the hydrostatic pressures are higher on the parietal pleura than on the visceral pleura and the oncotic pressures are equal. The hydrostatic pressure is a function of the arterial circulation. The oncotic pressure reflects largely the protein concentration in the blood and lymphatic vessels. The lymphatic vessels in the parietal (chest wall) pleura are responsible for fluid resorption. They have a tremendous capability (up to 20-fold) to respond to increased pleural fluid formation. This is another "sinister" bit of pathophysiology referred to initially in Chapter 1, The Patient Interview (see Fig. 1.1).

Evaluation of pleural effusions is of key importance in the diagnosis of potentially significant conditions. The use of **point-of-care ultrasonography** now joins portable chest radiology as a tremendous aid to evaluation of these patients in critical care units. The technique can be used to localize the effusion, and thus there are fewer complications compared with "blind" needle aspiration. A chest physician is usually involved in this procedure to help the timely evaluation of the effusion, to decrease the likelihood of possible complications, and to ensure appropriate follow-up.

Etiology and Epidemiology

Pleural effusion affects more than 1.5 million people each year in the United States. Congestive heart failure, cancer, and pneumonia account for the majority of cases. Early signs and symptoms include pleuritic chest pain, "chest pressure," dyspnea, and cough. Chest *pain* can occur early when there is intense inflammation of the pleural surfaces. Chest pressure does not usually develop until the effusion reaches the moderate

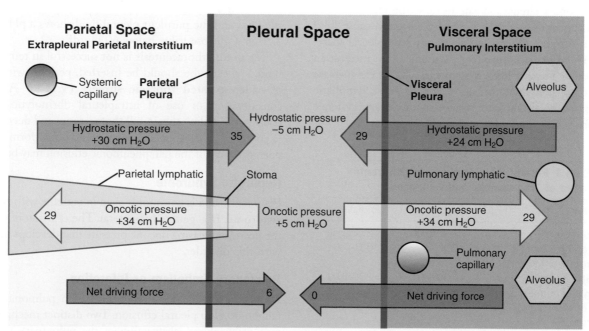

FIGURE 24.2 Balance of forces regulating pleural fluid formation. The amount of fluid in the pleural pace depends on the balance of hydrostatic and oncotic pressures between the parietal and visceral pleura and the pleural space. Because hydrostatic pressures are higher on the parietal pleura than on the visceral pleura and the oncotic pressures are equivalent, pleural fluid is primarily produced from the parietal pleura. Likewise, the lymphatic vessels on the parietal pleura are responsible for the majority of pleural fluid resorption.

(500 to 1500 mL) to large (more than 1500 mL) category. Dyspnea rarely occurs in small effusions unless significant **pleurisy** is present. A cough is usually directly related to the degree of atelectasis caused by the effusion.

A pleural effusion can be classified by (1) the origin of the fluid—that is, serous fluid (hydrothorax), blood (hemothorax), chyle (chylothorax), pus (pyothorax or empyema), or urine (urinothorax)—or (2) by the pathophysiology of the pleural effusion—that is, **transudative pleural effusion** or **exudative pleural effusion**. A *transudate* develops when fluid from the pulmonary capillaries moves into the pleural space. The fluid is thin and watery, containing a few blood cells and little protein. The pleural surfaces are not involved in producing the transudate. In contrast, an *exudate* develops when the pleural surfaces are diseased. The fluid has a high protein content and a great deal of cellular debris. Exudate is usually caused by inflammation, infection, or malignancy.

Table 24.1 contains the criteria for differential diagnosis of transudates and exudates that largely rely on the **Light criteria**. Careful, systematic analysis of pleural fluid will reveal the diagnosis as one or the other in about 75% of the patients and give good evidence of its causes (with additional Gram stain and cultures) and with microscopic examination for abnormal (e.g., malignant) cell types.

Common Causes of Transudative Pleural Effusion

Congestive Heart Failure

Congestive heart failure is the most common cause of pleural effusion. Both right- and left-sided heart failure can result in pleural effusion. In general, left-sided heart failure is more likely to produce pleural effusion than right-sided heart failure. In **left-sided heart failure**, an increase in hydrostatic pressure in the pulmonary circulation can decrease the rate of pleural fluid absorption through the visceral pleura and cause fluid movement through the visceral pleura into the pleural space. In **right-sided heart failure** (cor pulmonale), an increase in the hydrostatic pressure in the systemic circulation can increase the rate of pleural fluid formation and decrease lymphatic drainage from the pleural space because of the elevated systemic venous pressure.

TABLE 24.1 Pleural Fluid Analysis in Differential Diagnoses of Transudates and Exudates

Parameter	Transudates	Exudates
Total protein (TP)	<3.0 g/dL	>3.0 g/dL
Ratio of TP (fluid)/TP (serum)*	<0.5	>0.5
Pleural fluid lactate dehydrogenase (LDH)*	<200 IU/L	>200 IU/L
Ratio of LDH (fluid)/LDH (serum)*	<0.6	>0.6
Fluid cholesterol	<60 mg/dL	>60 mg/dL

*Based on the original Light criteria for diagnosis of exudates from Feller-Kopman, D., & Light, R. W. (2018). Pleural disease: A review article. *The New England Journal of Medicine, 378*(8), 740-751; Light, R. W. (2006). Parapneumonic effusions and empyema. *Proceedings of the American Thoracic Society, 3*, 75-80.

Hepatic Hydrothorax

Hepatic hydrothorax is defined as a pleural effusion, usually greater than 500 mL, in patients with cirrhosis (particularly when ascitic fluid is present in the abdomen) and without primary cardiac, pulmonary, or pleural disease. It develops most likely because of diaphragmatic defects that have been opened by increased peritoneal pressure—thus allowing the passage of fluid from the peritoneal space to the pleural space. Hepatic hydrothorax may be difficult to manage in end-stage liver failure and often fails to respond to therapy. Because of the location of the liver, the pleural effusion in these patients is generally right-sided.

Peritoneal Dialysis

As in the pleural effusion that occurs as a result of abdominal ascites (see above), on rare occasions a pleural effusion may develop as a complication of **peritoneal dialysis** in the treatment of severe chronic kidney disease. Peritoneal dialysis uses the patient's peritoneum in the abdomen as a membrane across which fluids and dissolved substances (electrolytes, urea, glucose, albumin, and other small molecules) are exchanged with the blood. When the peritoneal dialysis is stopped, the pleural effusion usually disappears rapidly.

Parapneumonic Pleural Effusions

Effusions that occur as a result of underlying pulmonary infection are termed **parapneumonic effusions** (e.g., those following a pneumococcal or staphylococcal pneumonia) abutting up to the visceral pleural surface. In patients with these effusions an invasive procedure more than a simple diagnostic thoracentesis may be necessary. This is true when the effusion occupies more than 50% of the hemithorax and presents as a **loculated pleural effusion** (bound down to the pleural surfaces) or shows a positive Gram stain or culture of the fluid and the purulent pleural fluid shows a pH less than 7.20 or a glucose value below 60 mg/dL.

If a needle thoracentesis is not successful in removing the fluid, a chest tube should be inserted, perhaps with the use of **video-assisted thoracic surgery (VATS)**. After this, consideration of use of intrapleural fibrinolytics may be considered. Failing that, a full thoracotomy and **decortication** (a so-called "pleural peel") may need to be performed and/or open drainage of the parapneumonic effusion may be required.

Nephrotic Syndrome

Pleural effusion is commonly seen in patients with **nephrotic syndrome**. It is generally bilateral. The effusion is a result of the decreased plasma oncotic pressure that develops in patients with this disorder.

Pulmonary Embolism or Infarction

Between 30% and 50% of patients with pulmonary arterial emboli develop pleural effusion. Two distinct mechanisms are responsible. First, obstruction of the pulmonary vasculature can lead to right-sided heart failure, which in turn can lead to pleural effusion. Second, increased permeability of the capillaries **pulmonary infarction** in the visceral pleura develops in response to the ischemic infarction caused by the **pulmonary emboli**.

Common Causes of Exudative Pleural Effusion

Empyema

The accumulation of pus in the pleural cavity is called **empyema**. Empyema commonly develops as a result of inflammation. Thoracentesis may confirm the diagnosis and determine the specific causative organism. The pus is usually removed by thoracostomy tube drainage. Open thoracotomy drainage may occasionally be necessary.

Malignant Pleural Effusions

About two-thirds of malignant pleural effusions occur in women. Malignant pleural effusions are highly associated with breast cancer. The pleural effusion is usually caused by a disturbance of the normal Starling forces regulating reabsorption of fluid in the pleural space, secondary to obstruction of mediastinal lymph nodes draining the parietal pleura. Tumors that metastasize frequently to these nodes (e.g., lung cancer, breast cancer, and lymphoma) cause most malignant effusions.

Malignant mesothelioma arises from the mesothelial cells that line the pleural cavities. Individuals who have had chronic exposure to asbestos have a much greater risk for developing mesothelioma. The pleural fluid is exudative and generally contains a mixture of normal mesothelial cells, differentiated and undifferentiated malignant mesothelial cells, and a varying number of lymphocytes and polymorphonuclear leukocytes.

Bacterial Pneumonias

Up to 40% of patients with bacterial pneumonia have an accompanying pleural effusion. Most pleural effusions associated with pneumonia resolve without any specific therapy. Approximately 10%, however, require some sort of therapeutic intervention. If appropriate antibiotic therapy is not instituted, bacteria invade the pleural fluid from the lung parenchyma. Eventually, pus will accumulate in the pleural cavity (empyema). Pleural effusion also can be produced by viruses, *Mycoplasma pneumoniae* and *Rickettsia*, although the pleural effusions are usually small.

Tuberculosis

Pleural effusion may develop from extension of a caseous tubercle into the pleural cavity. It also is possible that the inflammatory reaction that develops in **tuberculosis** obstructs the lymphatic pores in the parietal pleura. This in turn leads to an accumulation of protein and fluid in the pleural space. Pleural effusion caused by tuberculosis is generally unilateral and small to moderate in size (see Chapter 19, Tuberculosis).

Fungal Diseases

Patients with **fungal diseases** occasionally have secondary pleural effusions. Common fungal diseases that may produce pleural effusions are histoplasmosis, coccidioidomycosis, and blastomycosis (see Chapter 18, Pneumonia, Lung Abscess Formation, and Important Fungal Diseases).

Pleural Effusion Resulting From Diseases of the Gastrointestinal Tract

Pleural effusion is sometimes associated with diseases of the gastrointestinal tract such as pancreatitis, subphrenic abscess, intrahepatic abscess, esophageal perforation, abdominal operations, and diaphragmatic hernia.

Pleural Effusion Resulting From Collagen Vascular Diseases

Pleural effusion occasionally develops as a complication of collagen vascular diseases. Such diseases include rheumatoid pleuritis, systemic lupus erythematosus, Sjögren syndrome, familial Mediterranean fever, and Wegener granulomatosis.

Other Pathologic Fluids That Separate the Parietal From the Visceral Pleura

In addition to transudates and exudates, other pathologic fluids can separate the parietal pleura from the visceral pleura.

Chylothorax

Chylothorax is the presence of chyle in the pleural cavity. Chyle is a milky liquid produced from the food in the small intestine during digestion. It consists mainly of fat particles in a stable emulsion. Chyle normally is taken up by fingerlike intestinal lymphatics called *lacteals* and transported by the thoracic duct to the neck. From the thoracic duct the chyle moves into the venous circulation and mixes with blood. The presence of chyle in the pleural cavity is usually caused by trauma to the neck or thorax or by cancer occluding the thoracic duct.

Hemothorax

The presence of blood in the pleural space is known as a **hemothorax**. Most of these are caused by penetrating or blunt chest trauma. An iatrogenic hemothorax may develop from trauma caused by the insertion of a central venous or pulmonary artery catheter.

Blood can gain entrance into the pleural space from trauma to the chest wall, diaphragm, lung, or mediastinum. A hematocrit of the pleural fluid always should be obtained if the pleural fluid looks like blood. A hemothorax is said to be present only when the hematocrit of the pleural fluid is at least 50%.

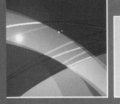

OVERVIEW of the Cardiopulmonary Clinical Manifestations Associated With Pleural Effusion and Empyema

The following clinical manifestations result from the pathologic mechanisms caused (or activated) by atelectasis (see Fig. 10.7)—the major anatomic alteration of the lungs associated with pleural effusion (see Fig. 24.1).

CLINICAL DATA OBTAINED AT THE PATIENT'S BEDSIDE

The Physical Examination

Vital Signs

Increased Respiratory Rate (Tachypnea)

Several pathophysiologic mechanisms operating simultaneously may lead to an increased ventilatory rate:

- Stimulation of peripheral chemoreceptors (hypoxemia)
- Relationship of decreased lung compliance to increased ventilatory rate
- Activation of the deflation receptors
- Activation of the irritant receptors
- Stimulation of J receptors
- Pain, anxiety

Increased Heart Rate (Pulse) and Blood Pressure

Chest Pain (Often Pleuritic)

Decreased Chest Expansion

Cyanosis

Cough (Dry, Nonproductive)

Chest Assessment Findings

- Tracheal shift
- Decreased tactile and vocal fremitus
- Dull percussion note
- Diminished breath sounds
- Displaced heart sounds
- Pleural friction rub (occasionally)

CLINICAL DATA OBTAINED FROM LABORATORY TESTS AND SPECIAL PROCEDURES

Pulmonary Function Test Findings
(Restrictive Lung Pathology)

LUNG VOLUME AND CAPACITY FINDINGS

V_T	IRV	ERV	RV
N or ↓	↓	↓	↓

VC	IC	FRC	TLC	RV/TLC ratio
↓	↓	↓	↓	N

Arterial Blood Gases

SMALL PLEURAL EFFUSION

Acute Alveolar Hyperventilation With Hypoxemia[1]
(Acute Respiratory Alkalosis)

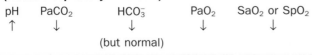

pH	$PaCO_2$	HCO_3^-	PaO_2	SaO_2 or SpO_2
↑	↓	↓	↓	↓
		(but normal)		

[1]See Fig. 5.2 and Table 5.4 and related discussion for the acute pH, $PaCO_2$, and HCO_3^- changes associated with acute alveolar hyperventilation.

LARGE PLEURAL EFFUSION

Acute Ventilatory Failure With Hypoxemia[2]
(Acute Respiratory Acidosis)

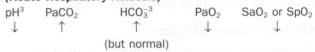

pH[3]	$PaCO_2$	HCO_3^-[3]	PaO_2	SaO_2 or SpO_2
↓	↑	↑	↓	↓
		(but normal)		

Oxygenation Indices[4]
(Large Pleural Effusion)

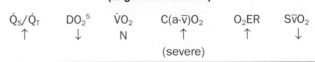

$\dot{Q}_S/\dot{Q}_T$	DO_2[5]	$\dot{V}O_2$	$C(a-\bar{v})O_2$	O_2ER	$S\bar{v}O_2$
↑	↓	N	↑	↑	↓
			(severe)		

Hemodynamic Indices[6]
(Large Pleural Effusion)

CVP	RAP	$\overline{PA}$	PCWP	CO	SV
↑	↑	↑	↓	↓	↓

SVI	CI	RVSWI	LVSWI	PVR	SVR
↓	↓	↑	↓	↑	↓

RADIOLOGIC FINDINGS

Chest Radiograph

- Blunting of the costophrenic angle
- Fluid level on the affected side (Fig. 24.3)
- Depressed diaphragm
- Mediastinal shift (possibly) to unaffected side
- Atelectasis
- **Meniscus sign**

The diagnosis of a pleural effusion is generally based on the chest radiograph. A pleural effusion of less than 300 mL usually cannot be seen on a chest radiograph in an upright patient. In a moderate pleural effusion (greater than 1000 mL) in the upright position, an increased density usually appears at the costophrenic angle. The fluid first accumulates posteriorly in the most dependent part of the thoracic cavity between the inferior surface of the lower lobe and the diaphragm. As the

[2]See Fig. 5.3 and Table 5.5 and related discussion for the acute pH, $PaCO_2$, and HCO_3^- changes associated with acute and chronic ventilatory failure.
[3]When tissue hypoxia is severe enough to produce lactic acid, the pH and HCO_3^- values will be lower than expected for a particular $PaCO_2$ level.
[4]$C(a-\bar{v})O_2$, Arterial-venous oxygen difference; DO_2, total oxygen delivery; O_2ER, oxygen extraction ratio; $\dot{Q}_S/\dot{Q}_T$, pulmonary shunt fraction; $S\bar{v}O_2$, mixed venous oxygen saturation; $\dot{V}O_2$, oxygen consumption.
[5]The DO_2 may be normal in patients who have compensated to the decreased oxygenation status with (1) an increased cardiac output, (2) an increased hemoglobin level, or (3) a combination of both. When the DO_2 is normal, the O_2ER is usually normal.
[6]CO, Cardiac output; CVP, central venous pressure; LVSWI, left ventricular stroke work index; $\overline{PA}$, mean pulmonary artery pressure; PCWP, pulmonary capillary wedge pressure; PVR, pulmonary vascular resistance; RAP, right atrial pressure; RVSWI, right ventricular stroke work index; SV, stroke volume; SVI, stroke volume index; SVR, systemic vascular resistance.

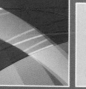
fluid volume increases, it extends upward around the anterior, lateral, and posterior thoracic walls in the **meniscus sign** (Fig. 24.4). Interlobar fissures are sometimes highlighted as a result of fluid filling.

As nicely illustrated in the upright chest radiograph of a pleural effusion shown in Fig. 24.3, the lateral costophrenic angle is usually obliterated, and the outline of the diaphragm on the affected side is lost. In severe cases the weight of the fluid may cause the diaphragm to become inverted (concave). Clinically this inversion is seen only in left-sided pleural effusions; the gastric air bubble is pushed downward, and the superior border of the left diaphragmatic leaf is concave. In addition, the mediastinum may be shifted to the unaffected side, and the intercostal spaces may appear widened.

Pleural effusion, atelectasis, and parenchymal infiltrates can obliterate one or both diaphragms. Therefore when a posteroanterior or lateral chest radiograph suggests pleural effusion, additional radiographic studies are generally necessary to document the presence of pleural fluid or other pathology. The **lateral decubitus radiograph** is recommended because free fluid gravitates to the most dependent part of the pleural space and layers out there (see Fig. 24.4).

FIGURE 24.3 Right-sided pleural effusion (black arrow) complicated by a pneumothorax (white arrow). Note that the lateral costophrenic angle on the right side is obliterated, and the outline of the diaphragm on the affected side is lost.

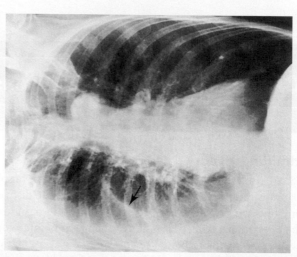

FIGURE 24.4 Subpulmonic pleural effusion. Right lateral decubitus view. Subdiaphragmatic fluid has run up the lateral chest wall, producing a band of soft tissue or water density (meniscus sign). The medial curvilinear shadow (arrow) indicates fluid in the major fissure.

General Management of Pleural Effusion

The management of each patient with a pleural effusion must be individualized. Questions to be asked include the following: Should a **thoracentesis** be performed? Can the underlying cause be treated? What is the appropriate antibiotic? Should a chest tube be inserted? When it is determined that a chest tube should be inserted, it is normally placed in the fourth or fifth intercostal space at the midaxillary line. Typically, a no. 28 to 36 French thoracostomy tube is used for adults, with a smaller size for children. A **pigtail catheter** may be used in draining fluids or air from the pleural spaces.

The best way to resolve a pleural effusion is to direct the treatment at what is causing it, rather than treating the effusion itself. For example, if the heart failure is reversed or the lung infection is cured by antibiotics, the effusion usually resolves. When the cause of the pleural effusion is not readily evident, microscopic and chemical examination of pleural fluid may determine whether the effusion is a transudate or an exudate. If the fluid is a transudate, treatment is directed to the underlying problem (e.g., congestive heart failure, cirrhosis, nephrosis).

When an exudate is present, a cytologic examination may identify a malignancy. The fluid must be examined for its biochemical makeup (e.g., protein, sugar, various enzymes) and for the presence of bacteria. Examination of the effusion may reveal blood after trauma or surgery, pus in empyema, or milky fluid in chylothorax. The presence of blood in the pleural fluid in the absence of trauma or surgery suggests malignant disease, pulmonary embolization or infarction.

Respiratory Care Treatment Protocols

Oxygen Therapy Protocol

Oxygen therapy is used to treat hypoxemia, decrease the work of breathing, and decrease myocardial work. The hypoxemia that develops in pleural effusion is mostly caused by the atelectasis and pulmonary shunting associated with the disorder. Hypoxemia caused by capillary shunting is often refractory to oxygen therapy (see Oxygen Therapy Protocol, Protocol 10.1).

Lung Expansion Therapy Protocol

Lung expansion techniques are often administered to offset the atelectasis associated with pleural effusions and are particularly helpful once the pleural fluid has been removed by thoracentesis or thoracostomy (see Lung Expansion Therapy Protocol, Protocol 10.3).

Mechanical Ventilation Protocol

Because acute ventilatory failure and hypoxemia may be seen in severe pleural effusions, continuous mechanical ventilation may be required to maintain an adequate ventilatory status. Continuous mechanical ventilation is justified when the acute ventilatory failure is thought to be reversible (see Ventilator Initiation and Management Protocol, Protocol 11.1, and Ventilator Weaning Protocol, Protocol 11.2).

Pleurodesis

A **pleurodesis** may be performed to cause irritation and inflammation (pleuritis) between the parietal and visceral layers of the pleural. During the pleurodesis procedure a **sclerosant** (talc, tetracycline, or bleomycin sulfate) is injected into the chest cavity. The chemical substance or medication causes an intense inflammatory reaction over the outer surface of the lung and inside the chest cavity. This procedure is performed to cause the surface of the lung to adhere to the chest wall, thus preventing or reducing recurrent pneumothorax or recurrent pleural effusions. An intense pleuritis is produced, which may be quite painful (pleurisy).

CASE STUDY Pleural Disease

Admitting History

A 38-year-old woman had discharged herself from the hospital against medical advice 2 months before the admission discussed here. She had originally been admitted for severe right lower lobe pneumonia. After 5 days of treatment, she became angry because she was not allowed to smoke. She was a longtime, three-pack-per-day smoker. When a nurse found her smoking in her hospital bed while on a 2 L/min oxygen nasal cannula, the nurse quickly confiscated her cigarettes and matches.

The woman became upset. She told her doctor that this was the last straw and that she was going to leave the hospital on her own. Her doctor wanted her to remain so that a thorough follow-up could be performed for what was described as a "spot" on her lower right lung. The woman promised that she would make an appointment at the doctor's office the next week. She then got dressed and left. However, 2 days later, she felt so much better that she decided the spot on her lung was not an issue for concern. The woman told her friends that smoking one pack of cigarettes made her feel better than 5 days' worth of nurses, doctors, and hospitals.

On the day of the admission discussed here, the woman appeared at her doctor's office without an appointment. She told the receptionist that something was very wrong. She thought that she had the flu and that it had been getting progressively worse over the previous 4 days. At the time of the office visit, she could speak in short sentences only and was unable to inhale deeply. Seeing that the woman was in obvious respiratory distress, the physician was notified. The doctor had the woman transported and admitted to the hospital a few blocks away.

Physical Examination

The woman appeared malnourished, exhibited poor personal hygiene, and had yellow tobacco stains around her fingers. She appeared to be in moderate to severe respiratory distress. Her nails and mucous membranes were cyanotic, and her shirt was wet from perspiration. She demonstrated an occasional hacking, nonproductive cough. She stated that she could not take a deep breath and that maybe the problem stemmed from "that spot" on her lung.

Her vital signs were blood pressure 130/60 mm Hg, heart rate 112 beats/min, and respiratory rate 36 breaths/min with shallow respirations. She was slightly febrile, with an oral temperature of 37.7°C (99.8°F). Palpation showed that the trachea was shifted slightly to the left. Dull percussion notes were found over the right middle and right lower lobes. Auscultation revealed normal vesicular breath sounds over the left lung fields and upper right lobe. No breath sounds could be heard over the right middle and right lower lobes.

The patient's chest radiograph showed a large, right-sided pleural effusion. The right costophrenic angle demonstrated severe blunting, the right hemidiaphragm was depressed, and the right middle and lower lung lobes were partially collapsed and showed changes consistent with pneumonia. The patient was immediately placed on a nonrebreathing mask, and an arterial blood gas (ABG) sample was drawn. The results were pH 7.48, PaCO$_2$ 24 mm Hg, HCO$_3^-$ 17 mEq/L, PaO$_2$ 37 mm Hg, and SaO$_2$ 73%. The doctor, assisted by the respiratory therapist, performed a thoracentesis, and slightly more than 2 L of yellow fluid was withdrawn.[1] The patient then was started on intravenous antibiotics. A portable radiograph of the chest was ordered, and a respiratory therapy consultation was requested. On the basis of these clinical data, the following SOAP was documented.

Respiratory Assessment and Plan

S "I can't take a deep breath."

O Malnourished appearance with poor personal hygiene; cyanosis with an occasional hacking, nonproductive cough; vital signs BP 130/60, HR 112, RR 36 and shallow, temperature 37.7°C (99.8°F); trachea slightly shifted to the left; dull percussion notes over the right middle and right lower lobes; normal vesicular breath sounds over the left lung fields and right upper lobe; no breath sounds over the right middle and right lower lobes; chest x-ray (CXR): large, right-sided pleural effusion, right middle and right lower lobes partially collapsed and consolidated; about 2 L of yellow fluid obtained via thoracentesis. ABGs (on 3 L/min O$_2$ by nasal cannula) before thoracentesis: pH 7.48, PaCO$_2$ 24, HCO$_3^-$ 17, PaO$_2$ 37, SaO$_2$ 73%.

A • Right-sided pneumonia and pleural effusion (CXR)
• Partially collapsed right middle and lower lobes (CXR)
• Respiratory distress (vital signs, ABGs)
• Acute alveolar hyperventilation with severe hypoxemia (ABGs)
• Metabolic (lactic) acidosis likely (ABGs compared with PCO$_2$/HCO$_3^-$/pH relationship nomogram)

P Begin Lung Expansion Therapy Protocol (e.g., positive expiratory pressure [PEP] or continuous positive airway pressure [CPAP] therapy q2h) and Oxygen Therapy Protocol (FIO$_2$ 0.50 per Venturi mask). Monitor vital signs carefully and reevaluate.

Three Hours After Admission

At this time the patient was sitting up in bed. She stated that although she was feeling better, she did not feel great. She still had an occasional dry-sounding, nonproductive cough. Her skin appeared pale. She was still cyanotic. She was no longer perspiring, as she was when she was first admitted. Her vital signs were blood pressure 135/85 mm Hg, heart rate 100 beats/min, respiratory rate 24 breaths/min, and temperature normal. Her respiratory efforts, however, no longer appeared shallow. Palpation of the chest was not remarkable. Dull percussion notes were found over the right middle and right lower lobes. Normal vesicular breath sounds were heard over the left lung and upper right lung. Loud bronchial breath sounds were audible over the right middle and right lower lobes.

The patient's chest radiograph showed a moderate, right-sided pleural effusion. Increased opacity was still present in the right middle and lower lung, consistent with pneumonia. The patient's trachea and mediastinum were in their normal positions. On an FIO$_2$ of 0.50, her ABGs were pH 7.52,

PaCO$_2$ 29 mm Hg, HCO$_3^-$ 23 mEq/L, PaO$_2$ 57 mm Hg, SaO$_2$ 92%. At this time, the following SOAP was charted.

Respiratory Assessment and Plan

S "I'm feeling better but not great yet."

O Cyanotic and pale appearance; occasional dry, nonproductive cough; vital signs BP 135/85, HR 100, RR 24, temperature normal; dull percussion notes over right middle and right lower lobes; normal vesicular breath sounds over left lung and over right upper lobe; bronchial breath sounds over right middle and lower lobes; CXR: moderate right-sided pleural effusion; right middle and right lower lobe consolidation; ABGs pH 7.52, PaCO$_2$ 29, HCO$_3^-$ 23, PaO$_2$ 57; SaO$_2$ 92% on an FIO$_2$ of 0.50.

A • Small right-sided pneumonia and pleural effusion, greatly improved (CXR)
• Atelectasis and consolidation in right middle and lower lung lobes (CXR)
• Continued respiratory distress, but improving (vital signs, ABGs)
• Acute alveolar hyperventilation with moderate hypoxemia, improved (ABGs)

P Up-regulate Lung Expansion Therapy Protocol (CPAP mask at 10 cm H$_2$O q2h for 15 minutes). Up-regulate Oxygen Therapy Protocol (FIO$_2$ 0.60 per Venturi mask). Monitor and reevaluate.

Five Hours After Admission

The patient was sitting in the semi-Fowler position. She appeared relaxed and alert. She stated that she had finally caught her breath. Although she still appeared pale, she did not look cyanotic. No spontaneous cough was observed at this time.

Her vital signs were blood pressure 128/79 mm Hg, heart rate 88/min, respiratory rate 16/min, and temperature normal. Palpation of the chest was unremarkable. Dull percussion notes were found over the right middle and right lower lobes. Normal vesicular breath sounds were heard over the left lung and right upper lobe. Bronchial breath sounds were audible over the right middle and right lower lobes. No current chest radiograph was available. The patient's ABG values on an FIO$_2$ of 0.60 were pH 7.45, PaCO$_2$ 36 mm Hg, HCO$_3^-$ 24 mEq/L, PaO$_2$ 77 mm Hg, and SaO$_2$ 95%.

On the basis of these clinical data, the following SOAP was documented.

Respiratory Assessment and Plan

S "I've finally caught my breath."

O Relaxed, alert appearance, in semi-Fowler position; pale but not cyanotic; no spontaneous cough; vital signs BP 128/79, HR 88, RR 16, temperature normal; dull percussion notes in right middle and right lower lung lobes; normal vesicular breath sounds over left lung and right upper lobe; bronchial breath sounds over right middle and right lower lobes; ABGs pH 7.45, PaCO$_2$ 36, HCO$_3^-$ 24, PaO$_2$ 77; SaO$_2$ 95%.

A • Small, right-sided pneumonia and pleural effusion, greatly improved (previous CXR)
• Atelectasis and consolidation in right middle and right lower lung lobes (previous CXR)
• Normal acid-base status with mild hypoxemia (ABGs)

---

[1]See *reexpansion pulmonary edema* in discussion section of this case.

P Maintain present level of Lung Expansion Therapy Protocol and Oxygen Therapy Protocols. Monitor and reevaluate each shift. Provide patient with smoking cessation materials and suggest pulmonary function testing as an outpatient.

Discussion

This case illustrates a patient with **postpneumonic pleural effusion**, one of the pleural diseases that generally can be improved with appropriate therapy—in this case, the removal of a large amount of yellow fluid via a thoracentesis. This portion of the case study provides a good opportunity to introduce the concept of **reexpansion pulmonary edema**. It is a rare complication resulting from rapid emptying of air or liquid from the pleural cavity performed by either thoracentesis or chest drainage. The condition usually appears unexpectedly—and dramatically—within the first few minutes to an hour after the fluid or air removal. The radiographic evidence of reexpansion pulmonary edema is a unilateral alveolar filling pattern, seen within a few hours of reexpansion of the lung. The edema may progress for 24 to 48 hours and persist for 4 to 5 days.

During the first assessment, the respiratory therapist recognized that the patient had significant respiratory morbidity. Indeed, the patient had an extensive right-sided pneumonia and pleural effusion and partially collapsed right middle and lower lobes. Clearly the patient was in respiratory distress. The patient's acute alveolar hyperventilation and severe hypoxemia were a direct result of the partial collapse of the lung lobes. Because of the extremely low PaO_2 noted on the initial ABG sample, the presence of lactic acid was very likely. In fact, this was confirmed by the respiratory therapist with the $PCO_2/HCO_3^-/pH$ nomogram. Understanding that atelectasis was the main pathophysiologic mechanism in this case (see Fig. 10.7), the therapist correctly assessesed the situation as one that required careful monitoring and began the Lung Expansion Therapy Protocol (Protocol 10.3) (e.g.,

PEP or CPAP therapy) and the Oxygen Therapy Protocol (Protocol 10.1) (with a high concentration of oxygen).

Given the patient's history, the respiratory therapist also would be interested in the results of the cytologic studies for malignancy in both the sputum and thoracentesis fluid. Frequently, blood gas values do not improve immediately after a thoracentesis, despite the fluid removal, because the atelectasis under the pleural effusion takes some time (hours or days) to dissipate. For this reason, the Lung Expansion Therapy Protocol, after thoracentesis, was appropriate.

At the time of the second assessment, the patient was beginning to improve, although she still had signs of right middle and lower lobe consolidation (see Fig. 10.8). Good breath sounds were heard over the left lung and upper right lung, although bronchial breath sounds reflecting consolidation were still noted on the right. The respiratory therapist was appropriately concerned that atelectasis was still present, and in such a case the therapist should increase the Lung Expansion Therapy Protocol (Protocol 10.3). In this case, the therapist selected a CPAP mask at 10 cm H_2O every 2 hours for 15 minutes. The therapist could have also intensified use of incentive spirometry, carefully used intermittent positive-pressure breathing, or extended the amount of time the patient was using the CPAP mask.

In the last assessment the patient continued to do fairly well, although she was far from returning to baseline values. The pneumonia, atelectasis, and mild hypoxemia, which persisted despite supplemental oxygen therapy, suggested the need for continued significant (though unchanged) therapy. This case demonstrates that in-place therapy often does not need to be changed at each assessment. Indeed, this guide may apply to as many as 50% to 60% of accurately performed serial assessments. For pedagogic reasons, this option has not been exercised often in this text. However, this third assessment (in a patient with pleural effusion and underlying atelectasis and pneumonia) is a good case in point.

SELF-ASSESSMENT QUESTIONS

1. Which of the following is(are) associated with exudative effusion?
   1. Few blood cells
   2. Inflammation
   3. Thin and watery fluid
   4. Disease of the pleural surfaces
      a. 2 only
      b. 4 only
      c. 1 and 3 only
      d. 2 and 4 only

2. Which of the following is probably the most common cause of a transudative pleural effusion?
   a. Pulmonary embolus
   b. Congestive heart failure
   c. Hepatic hydrothorax
   d. Nephrotic syndrome

3. A hemothorax is said to be present when the hematocrit of the pleural fluid is at least:
   a. 20%
   b. 30%
   c. 40%
   d. 50%

4. What percentage of patients with pulmonary emboli develop pleural effusion?
   a. 0% to 20%
   b. 20% to 30%
   c. 30% to 50%
   d. 50% to 60%

5. Which of the following is(are) associated with pleural effusion?
   a. Increased RV
   b. Decreased RV/TLC ratio
   c. Increased V_T
   d. Decreased VC

25 Kyphoscoliosis

Chapter Objectives

After reading this chapter, you will be able to:

- List the anatomic alterations of the lungs associated with kyphoscoliosis.
- Describe the causes of kyphoscoliosis.
- List the cardiopulmonary clinical manifestations associated with kyphoscoliosis.
- Describe the general management of kyphoscoliosis.
- Describe the clinical strategies and rationales of the SOAPs presented in the case study.
- Define key terms and complete self-assessment questions at the end of the chapter and on Evolve.

Key Terms

Adolescent Scoliosis
Boston Brace
Cervicothoracolumbosacral Orthosis (CTLSO)
Charleston Bending Brace
Cobb Angle
Cor Pulmonale
Congenital Scoliosis
Cotrel-Dubousset Technique
"Dizzy Gillespie Pouch"
Harrington Rod
Idiopathic Scoliosis
Infantile Scoliosis
Juvenile Scoliosis
Kyphoscoliosis
Kyphosis
Milwaukee Brace
Neuromuscular Scoliosis
Nonstructural Scoliosis

Pulmonary Hypertension
Rod Instrumentation
Scoliosis
Scheuermann Disease
Spinal Fusion
SpineCor
Structural Scoliosis
Therapeutic Bronchoscopy
Thoracolumbosacral Orthosis (TLSO)

Chapter Outline

Anatomic Alterations of the Lungs
Etiology and Epidemiology
Scoliosis
   Congenital Scoliosis
   Neuromuscular Scoliosis
   Idiopathic Scoliosis
   Diagnosis of Scoliosis
Kyphosis
Overview of the Cardiopulmonary Clinical Manifestations
   Associated With Kyphoscoliosis
General Management of Scoliosis
   Conservative Treatment
   Braces
   Surgery
   Other Approaches
Respiratory Care Treatment Protocols
   Oxygen Therapy Protocol
   Airway Clearance Therapy Protocol
   Lung Expansion Therapy Protocol
Case Study: Kyphoscoliosis
Self-Assessment Questions

Anatomic Alterations of the Lungs

Kyphoscoliosis is a combination of two different thoracic deformities that commonly appear together. In **kyphosis**, there is a posterior curvature of the spine (humpback or hunchback). In **scoliosis**, the spine is curved to one side, typically appearing as an S or C shape. Its appearance is most obvious in the anteroposterior plane.

When these two disorders appear together as kyphoscoliosis, the deformity of the thorax can—in severe cases—compress the lungs and restrict alveolar expansion. This condition in turn can lead to alveolar hypoventilation and atelectasis. In addition, the patient's ability to cough and mobilize secretions also may be impaired, further causing atelectasis as secretions accumulate throughout the tracheobronchial tree. Because kyphoscoliosis involves both the posterior and the lateral curvature of the spine, the thoracic contents generally twist in such a way as to cause a mediastinal shift in the same direction as the lateral curvature of the spine. Severe kyphoscoliosis causes a chronic restrictive lung disorder that makes

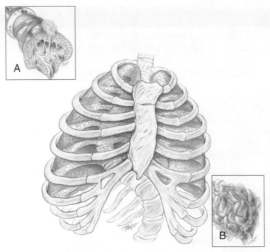

FIGURE 25.1 Kyphoscoliosis. Posterior and lateral curvature of the spine causing lung compression. (A) Excessive bronchial secretions and (B) atelectasis are common secondary anatomic alterations of the lungs.

it more difficult to clear airway secretions. Fig. 25.1 illustrates the lung and chest wall abnormalities in a typical case of kyphoscoliosis.

The major pathologic or structural changes of the lungs associated with kyphoscoliosis are as follows:

- Lung restriction and compression as a result of the thoracic deformity
- Mediastinal shift
- Mucous accumulation throughout the tracheobronchial tree
- Atelectasis

Etiology and Epidemiology

Kyphoscoliosis affects approximately 1% to 2% of people in the United States—mostly young children who are going through a growth spurt. The precise reason why scoliosis and kyphosis often appear together as the combined disorder kyphoscoliosis is often unclear. However, some of the known causes, classifications, and risk factors associated with both scoliosis and kyphosis are as follows.

Scoliosis

In most cases of scoliosis, the cause is unknown. However, in some cases, the scoliosis can be placed in one of the following categories:

Congenital Scoliosis

- A condition resulting from a formation of the spine or fused ribs during fetal development.

Neuromuscular Scoliosis

- A condition caused by poor muscle control, muscle weakness, or paralysis because of diseases such as cerebral palsy, muscular dystrophy, spina bifida, or poliomyelitis.

Idiopathic Scoliosis

- Scoliosis from an unknown cause that appears in a previously straight spine. When kyphoscoliosis arises without a known cause (80% to 85% of cases), it is referred to as *idiopathic kyphoscoliosis.*

Other possible causes include hormonal imbalance, trauma, extraspinal contractures, infections involving the vertebrae, metabolic bone disorders (e.g., rickets, osteoporosis, osteogenesis imperfecta), dwarfism, joint disease, and tumors.

Depending on the child's age at the time of onset, idiopathic scoliosis is classified as infantile, juvenile, or adolescent. In **infantile scoliosis** the curvature of the spine develops during the first 3 years of life. In **juvenile scoliosis** the curvature occurs at 4 years of age to the onset of adolescence. In **adolescent scoliosis** the spinal curvature develops after the age of 10 years. Adolescent scoliosis is the most common. Early signs of scoliosis (i.e., appearing when a child is approximately 8 years of age) include uneven shoulder height, prominent shoulder blade(s), uneven waist height, elevated hips, and leaning to one side.

Risk factors include the following:

- *Gender:* Girls are more likely to develop curvature of the spine than boys.
- *Age:* The younger the child is when the diagnosis is first made, the greater the chance of curve progression.
- *Angle of the curve:* The greater the initial curvature of the spine, the greater the risk that the curve progression will worsen.
- *Location:* Curves in the middle to lower spine are less likely to progress than those in the upper spine.
- *Height:* Taller people have a greater chance of curve progression.
- *Spinal problems at birth:* Children with scoliosis at birth (**congenital scoliosis**) have a greater risk for worsening of the curve with aging.

Diagnosis of Scoliosis

Scoliosis is diagnosed by the patient's medical history, physical examination, x-ray evaluation, and curve measurement. Clinically, scoliosis is commonly defined according to the following factors related to the curvature of the spine:

- *Shape* (**nonstructural scoliosis** and **structural scoliosis**): Nonstructural scoliosis is a curve that develops side-to-side as a C- or S-shaped curve. This form of scoliosis results from a cause other than the spine itself (e.g., poor posture, leg length discrepancy, pain). A structural scoliosis is a curvature of the spine associated with vertebral rotation. Structural scoliosis involves the twisting of the spine and appears in three dimensions.
- *Location:* The curve of the spine may develop in the upper back area where the ribs are located (thoracic), the lower back area (lumbar), or in both areas (thoracolumbar).
- *Direction:* Scoliosis can bend the spine left or right.
- *Angle:* A normal spine viewed from the back is zero degrees—a straight line. Scoliosis is defined as a spinal curvature of greater than 10 degrees (i.e., bending toward the ground when in the upright position). The degree of

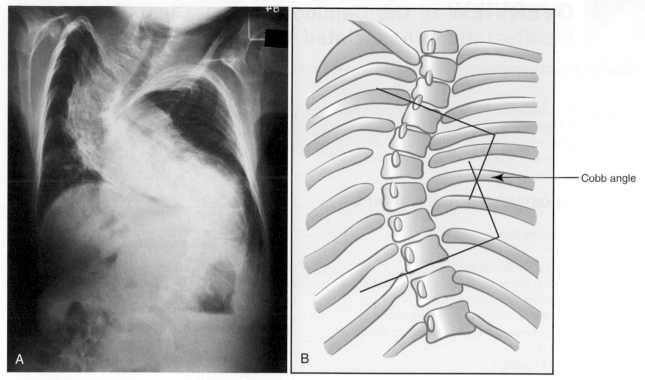

FIGURE 25.2 (A) Chest radiograph of a patient with kyphoscoliosis. (B) Method of calculating the Cobb angle. Scoliosis is defined as a spinal curvature of 10 degrees or greater. Because the Cobb angle reflects curvature only in a single plane, it may fail to fully identify the severity of the scoliosis, especially when the patient has vertebral rotation and three-dimensional spinal deformity.

the lateral curvature is expressed by the **Cobb angle**, which is calculated from a radiograph as shown in Fig. 25.2.

Kyphosis

Kyphosis can occur at any age, although it is rare at birth. Known causes of kyphosis are (1) degenerative diseases of the spine (such as arthritis or disk degeneration), (2) fractures caused by osteoporosis (osteoporotic compression fractures),

and (3) slipping of one vertebra forward on another (spondylolisthesis). Other disorders associated with the cause of kyphosis include certain endocrine diseases, connective tissue disorders, infections (e.g., tuberculosis), muscular dystrophy, neurofibromatosis, Paget disease, polio, spina bifida, and tumors. Kyphosis also may be caused by **Scheuermann disease**, which is the wedging together of several bones of the vertebrae in a row. The precise cause of Scheuermann disease is unknown.

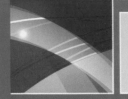

OVERVIEW of the Cardiopulmonary Clinical Manifestations Associated With Kyphoscoliosis[1]

The following clinical manifestations result from the pathophysiologic mechanisms caused (or activated) by atelectasis (see Fig. 10.7) and excessive airway secretions (see Fig. 10.11)—the major anatomic alterations of the lungs associated with kyphoscoliosis (see Fig. 25.1).

CLINICAL DATA OBTAINED AT THE PATIENT'S BEDSIDE

The Physical Examination

Vital Signs

Increased Respiratory Rate (Tachypnea)

Several pathophysiologic mechanisms operating simultaneously may lead to an increased ventilatory rate:

- Stimulation of peripheral chemoreceptors (hypoxemia)
- Relationship of decreased lung compliance to increased ventilatory rate
- Stimulation of the J receptors
- Pain, anxiety

Increased Heart Rate (Pulse) and Blood Pressure

Cyanosis

Digital Clubbing

Peripheral Edema and Venous Distention

Because polycythemia and cor pulmonale are late findings associated with kyphoscoliosis, the following may be seen:

- Distended neck veins
- Pitting edema
- Enlarged and tender liver

Cough and Sputum Production

Chest Assessment Findings

- Limited thoracic expansion
- Obvious thoracic deformity
- Tracheal shift
- Increased tactile and vocal fremitus
- Dull percussion note
- Bronchial breath sounds
- Whispered pectoriloquy
- Crackles and wheezing

CLINICAL DATA OBTAINED FROM LABORATORY TESTS AND SPECIAL PROCEDURES

Pulmonary Function Test Findings
Moderate to Severe Kyphoscoliosis (Restrictive Lung Pathology)

FORCED EXPIRATORY VOLUME AND FLOW RATE FINDINGS

FVC	FEV_T	FEV_1/FVC ratio	$FEF_{25\%-75\%}$
↓	N or ↓	N or ↑	N or ↓

$FEF_{50\%}$	$FEF_{200-1200}$	PEFR	MVV
N or ↓	N or ↓	N or ↓	N or ↓

[1]It is important to note that kyphoscoliosis is a progressive disease and thus changes in the clinical manifestations associated with this disorder will occur over time as the patient ages and the disease progresses.

LUNG VOLUME AND CAPACITY FINDINGS

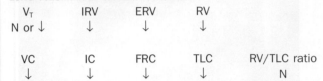

V_T	IRV	ERV	RV	
N or ↓	↓	↓	↓	

VC	IC	FRC	TLC	RV/TLC ratio
↓	↓	↓	↓	N

Arterial Blood Gases

MODERATE KYPHOSCOLIOSIS
Acute Alveolar Hyperventilation With Hypoxemia[2]
(Acute Respiratory Alkalosis)

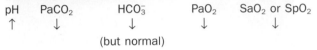

pH	$PaCO_2$	HCO_3^-	PaO_2	SaO_2 or SpO_2
↑	↓	↓ (but normal)	↓	↓

SEVERE KYPHOSCOLIOSIS
Chronic Ventilatory Failure With Hypoxemia[3]
(Compensated Respiratory Acidosis)

pH	$PaCO_2$	HCO_3^-	PaO_2	SaO_2 or SpO_2
N	↑	↑ (significantly)	↓	↓

ACUTE VENTILATORY CHANGES SUPERIMPOSED ON CHRONIC VENTILATORY FAILURE[4]

Because acute ventilatory changes are frequently seen in patients with chronic ventilatory failure, the respiratory therapist must be familiar with—and alert for—the following two dangerous arterial blood gas (ABG) findings:

- Acute alveolar hyperventilation superimposed on chronic ventilatory failure, which should further alert the respiratory therapist to record the following important ABG assessment: possible *impending acute ventilatory failure*
- Acute ventilatory failure (acute hypoventilation) superimposed on chronic ventilatory failure

Oxygenation Indices[5]
Moderate to Severe Kyphoscoliosis

$\dot{Q}_S/\dot{Q}_T$	DO_2[6]	$\dot{V}O_2$	$C(a-\bar{v})O_2$	O_2ER	$S\bar{v}O_2$
↑	↓	N	N	↑	↓

[2]See Fig. 5.2 and Table 5.4 and related discussion for the acute pH, $PaCO_2$, and HCO_3^- changes associated with acute alveolar hyperventilation.

[3]See Table 5.6 and related discussion for the pH, $PaCO_2$, and HCO_3^- changes associated with chronic ventilatory failure.

[4]See Table 5.7, Table 5.8, and Table 5.9 and related discussion for the pH, $PaCO_2$, and HCO_3^- changes associated with acute ventilatory changes superimposed on chronic ventilatory failure

[5]$C(a-\bar{v})O_2$, Arterial-venous oxygen difference; DO_2, total oxygen delivery; O_2ER, oxygen extraction ratio; $\dot{Q}_S/\dot{Q}_T$, pulmonary shunt fraction; $S\bar{v}O_2$, mixed venous oxygen saturation; $\dot{V}O_2$, oxygen consumption.

[6]The DO_2 may be normal in patients who have compensated to the decreased oxygenation status with (1) an increased cardiac output, (2) an increased hemoglobin level, or (3) a combination of both. When the DO_2 is normal, the O_2ER is usually normal.

Hemodynamic Indices[7] Moderate to Severe Kyphoscoliosis					
CVP	RAP	$\overline{PA}$	PCWP	CO	SV
↑	↑	↑	N	N	N
SVI	CI	RVSWI	LVSWI	PVR	SVR
N	N	↑	N	↑	N

LABORATORY FINDINGS

Severe and/or late-stage kyphoscoliosis (if the patient is chronically hypoxemic)

- Increased hematocrit and hemoglobin (polycythemia)
- Hypochloremia (Cl^-)
- Hypernatremia (Na^+)

RADIOLOGIC FINDINGS

Chest Radiograph

- Thoracic deformity
- Mediastinal shift
- Increased lung opacity
- Atelectasis in areas of compressed (atelectatic) lungs
- Enlarged heart (**cor pulmonale**)

The extent of the thoracic deformity in kyphoscoliosis is demonstrated in anteroposterior and lateral radiographs. When

[7]CO, Cardiac output; CI, cardiac index; CVP, central venous pressure; LVSWI, left ventricular stroke work index; $\overline{PA}$, mean pulmonary artery pressure; PCWP, pulmonary capillary wedge pressure; PVR, pulmonary vascular resistance; RAP, right atrial pressure; RVSWI, right ventricular stroke work index; SV, stroke volume; SVI, stroke volume index; SVR, systemic vascular resistance.

present, a mediastinal shift is best shown on an anteroposterior chest radiograph. As the alveoli collapse, the density of the lung increases and is revealed on the chest radiograph as increased opacity (Fig. 25.3). In severe cases, cor pulmonale may be seen.

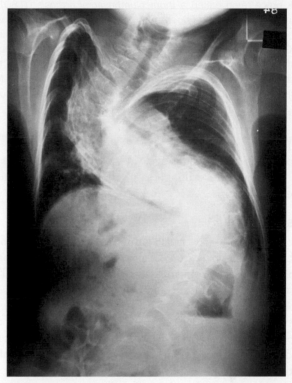

FIGURE 25.3 Severe kyphoscoliosis in a 14-year-old male patient.

General Management of Scoliosis

Conservative Treatment

The treatment of scoliosis largely depends on the cause of the scoliosis, the size and location of the curve, and how much more growing the patient is expected to do. In most cases of scoliosis (less than 20 degrees), the degree of abnormal spine curvature is relatively small and requires only observation to ensure that the curve does not worsen. Observation is usually recommended in patients with a spine curvature of less than 20 degrees. In young children who are still growing, observation checkups are usually scheduled at 3- to 6-month intervals. When the curve is determined to be progressing to a more serious degree (more than 25 to 30 degrees in a child who is still growing), the following treatment options are available.

Braces

A brace device is usually recommended as the first line of defense for growing children who have a spinal curvature of 25 to 45 degrees. Bracing is the primary treatment for adolescent **idiopathic scoliosis**. The mechanical objective of the brace is to hyperextend the spine and limit forward flexion. It does not reverse the curve. Although a brace does not cure scoliosis (or even improve the condition), it has been shown to prevent the curve progression in more than 90% of patients who wear it. Bracing is not effective in congenital or **neuromuscular scoliosis**. The therapeutic effects of bracing are also less helpful in infantile and juvenile idiopathic scoliosis. Today a number of braces are available, including the **Boston brace**, **Charleston bending brace**, and **Milwaukee brace** (Fig. 25.4). A soft brace, called **SpineCor**, is also available in the United States, Canada, and Europe. The type of brace is selected

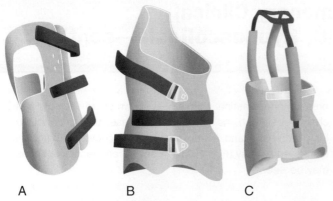

FIGURE 25.4 Common types of braces for scoliosis. (A) Boston back brace (also called a *thoracolumbosacral orthosis [TLSO]*, a *low-profile brace*, or an *underarm brace*). Typically used for curves in the lumbar (low-back) or thoracolumbar sections of the spine. (B) Charleston bending brace (also known as a *part-time brace*). Commonly used for spinal curves of 20 to 35 degrees, with the apex of the curve below the level of the shoulder blade. (C) Milwaukee brace (also called *cervicothoracolumbosacral orthosis [CTLSO]*) is used for high thoracic (mid-back) curves.

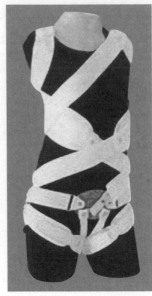

FIGURE 25.5 The SpineCor brace is composed of soft, elastic corrective bands that wrap around the patient's body and resist the body's movement back to the abnormal position.

according to the patient's age, the specific characteristics of the curve, and the willingness of the patient to tolerate a specific brace.

Boston Brace

The Boston brace (also called a **thoracolumbosacral orthosis [TLSO]**, a *low-profile brace*, or an *underarm brace*) is composed of plastic that is custom-molded to fit the patient's body. The Boston brace is the most commonly used brace for adolescent idiopathic scoliosis. The brace extends from below the breast to the top of the pelvic area in front and from below the scapula to the coccyx in the back. The Boston brace is typically used for curves in the lumbar (low-back) or thoracolumbar sections of the spine. The Boston brace is worn about 23 hours a day but can be taken off to shower, swim, or engage in sports (see Fig. 25.4A).

Charleston Bending Brace

The Charleston bending brace (also known as a *part-time brace*) is worn for only 8 to 10 hours at night, when the human growth hormone level is at its highest. The Charleston bending brace is molded to conform to the patient's body when the patient bends toward the convexity—or outward bulge—of the curve. This brace works to overcorrect the curve while the patient is asleep. For the Charleston brace to be effective, the patient's curve must be in the 20- to 40-degree range and the apex of the curve needs to be below the level of the scapula. The Charleston bending brace works on the principle that the spine should be bent to grow in the correct direction during the time of day that most growing occurs. Many studies have shown that the Charleston nighttime brace is as effective as the braces that need to be worn for 23 hours (see Fig. 25.4B).

Milwaukee Brace

The Milwaukee brace (also known as a **cervicothoracolumbosacral orthosis [CTLSO]**) is used for high thoracic

(mid-back) curves. The Milwaukee brace is a full-torso brace with a neck ring that serves as a rest for the chin and for the back of the head. It extends from the neck to the pelvis. It consists of a specially contoured plastic pelvic girdle and a neck ring that is connected by metal bars in the front and back of the brace. The metal bars work to extend the length of the torso, and the neck ring keeps the head centered over the pelvis. The Milwaukee brace is used less frequently now that more form-fitting plastic braces are available (see Fig. 25.4C).

SpineCor Brace

The SpineCor brace is a soft and dynamic brace designed to provide a progressive correction of idiopathic scoliosis from 15 degrees Cobb angle and above. It is comfortably worn under clothing. The brace is composed of soft, elastic corrective bands that wrap around the patient's body and resist and compress the body's movement back toward the abnormal position (Fig. 25.5). The corrective movements of the SpineCor brace are able to put the patient's body through countless repetitions each day, as opposed to the 10 to 50 repetitions that are the typical routine with other rehabilitation techniques. The SpineCor brace is designed to generate a constant correction and relaxation action that gently guides the patient's posture and spinal alignment in an optimal direction. The brace works well to preserve normal body movements and growth and better allows for normal daily living activities. The brace is usually worn 20 hours a day. The patient should not have it off for more than 2 hours at a time.

Surgery

In general, surgery is performed to correct unacceptable deformity and prevent further curvature. Surgery is usually recommended in patients who have curvatures of the spine greater than 40 to 50 degrees. As a general rule, the surgery

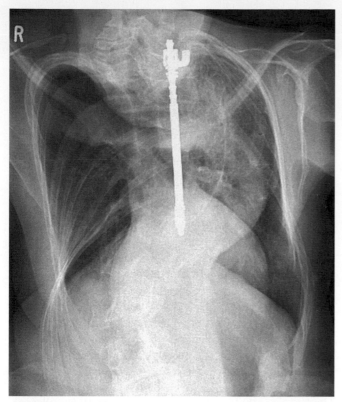

FIGURE 25.6 Radiograph of patient with scoliosis treated with a Harrington rod. (From Spiro, S. G., Silvestri, G. A., Agusti, A. [2012]. *Clinical respiratory medicine* [4th ed.]. Philadelphia, PA: Elsevier.)

is extensive and invasive; even the best surgical techniques do not completely straighten the patient's spine. Also, surgery often does not improve ventilatory function. Surgical procedures include the following.

Spinal Fusion

Spinal fusion is the most widely performed surgery for scoliosis. A spinal fusion, followed by casting, involves placing pieces of bone between two or more vertebrae. The bone sections are taken from the patient's pelvis or rib. Eventually the bone pieces and the vertebrae fuse together. This procedure has now been largely replaced by **rod instrumentation**.

Rod Instrumentation

In 1962, Paul Harrington introduced a metal spinal system that involved the insertion of a metal rod (the **Harrington rod**) after a fusion procedure, hooks, screws, and wires to prevent the curve from moving for 3 to 12 months and to allow the fusion to become solid (Fig. 25.6). The system

provides disruption to the concave side of the spine and compression to the convex side. This action enhances stabilization, reduces any rotational tendency, and applies force to the spine to correct the curvature. Although the Harrington rod improved up to 50% of the curvature in patients who elected to have the procedure, it is now obsolete. Its major shortcomings were that it failed to produce a posture that allowed the skull to be in proper alignment with the pelvis and it did not address rotational deformity. Currently, the Cotrel-Dubousset system is the most common technique for this procedure. The Cotrel-Dubousset technique has been shown to work well in improving pelvic area sagittal imbalance and rotational defects. The **Cotrel-Dubousset technique** has shown relatively good success (e.g., it reduces or prevents the rib hump) and exhibits low rates of infection. The long-term success of this technique is still being studied.

Other Approaches

Some physicians may try electrical stimulation of muscles, chiropractic manipulation, and exercise to treat scoliosis. There is no evidence that any of these procedures will stop the progression of spine curvature. Exercise, however, may improve the patient's overall health and well-being.

Respiratory Care Treatment Protocols

Oxygen Therapy Protocol

Oxygen therapy is used to treat hypoxemia, decrease the work of breathing, and decrease myocardial work. The hypoxemia that develops in kyphoscoliosis is commonly caused by atelectasis and pulmonary shunting. Hypoxemia caused by capillary shunting is often refractory to oxygen therapy (see Oxygen Therapy Protocol, Protocol 10.1).

Airway Clearance Therapy Protocol

A number of airway clearance therapies may be used to enhance the mobilization of the excessive bronchial secretions associated with kyphoscoliosis (see Airway Clearance Therapy Protocol, Protocol 10.2). Prophylactic deep breathing and coughing exercises are also taught. Their long-term effect is debatable. Use of prophylactic therapies such as chest vibrating belts or vests also have not been systematically studied in this regard to date.

Lung Expansion Therapy Protocol

Lung expansion therapy is often used to offset atelectasis (see Lung Expansion Therapy Protocol, Protocol 10.3).

Admitting History

A 62-year-old woman began to develop kyphoscoliosis when she was 6 years old. She lived in the mountains of Virginia all her life, first with her parents and later with her two older sisters. Although she wore various types of body braces until she was 17 years old, her disorder was classified as severe by the time she was 15 years old. Her doctors, who were few and far between, always told her that she would have to learn to live with her condition the best she could, and as a general rule she did.

She finished high school with no other remarkable physical or personal problems. She was well liked by her classmates and was actively involved in the school newspaper and art club. After graduation, she continued to live with her parents for a few more years. At 21 years of age, she moved in to live with her two older sisters, who were buying a large farmhouse near a small but popular tourist town. All three sisters made various arts and crafts, which they sold at local tourist shops. The woman's physical disability and general health were relatively stable until she was about 40 years old. At that time, she started to experience frequent episodes of dyspnea, coughing, and sputum production. As the years progressed, her baseline condition was marked by increasingly severe and chronic dyspnea, marked by frequent exacerbations of productive cough.

Because the sisters rarely ventured into the city, the woman's medical resources were poor until she was introduced to a social worker at a nearby church. The church had just become part of an outreach program based in a large city nearby. The social worker was charmed by the patient and fascinated by the beauty of the colorful quilts she made.

The social worker, however, was also concerned by the woman's limited ability to move about because of her dyspnea that was related to her severe chest deformity. In addition, the social worker thought that the woman's cough "sounded serious." She noted that the woman appeared grayish-blue, weak, and ill. The sisters told the social worker that their sibling had had a bad "cold" for about 6 months. After much urging, the social worker persuaded the woman to travel to the city, accompanied by her sisters, to see a physician at a large hospital associated with the church outreach program. On arrival there, the patient was immediately admitted to the hospital. The sisters stayed in a nearby hotel room provided by the hospital.

Physical Examination

Although chronically ill, the patient appeared to be well nourished; the lateral curvature of her spine was twisted significantly to the left. She also demonstrated forward (anterior) bending of the thoracic spine. She appeared older than her stated age, and she was in obvious respiratory distress. The patient stated that she was having trouble breathing. Her skin was cyanotic. She had digital clubbing, and her neck veins were distended, especially on the right side. The woman demonstrated a frequent and strong cough. During each coughing episode, she expectorated a moderate amount of thick, yellow nonodorous sputum.

When the patient generated a strong cough, a large unilateral bulge appeared at the right anterolateral base of her neck, directly posterior to the clavicle. The patient referred to the bulge as her "Dizzy Gillespie pouch[1]." The physician thought the bulge was a result of her severe kyphoscoliosis, which had in turn stretched and weakened the suprapleural membrane that normally restricts and contains the parietal pleura at the apex of the lung. Because of the weakening of the suprapleural membrane, any time the woman performed a Valsalva maneuver for any reason (e.g., for coughing), the increased intrapleural pressure herniated the suprapleural membrane outward. Despite the odd appearance of the bulge, the doctor did not consider it a serious concern.

The patient's vital signs were blood pressure 160/100 mm Hg, heart rate 90 beats/min, respiratory rate 18 breaths/min, and oral temperature 36.3°C (97.3°F). Palpation revealed a trachea deviated to the right and 2+ cervical venous distention, more on the right. Dull percussion notes were produced over both lungs; coarse crackles were also heard bilaterally. There was 2+ pitting edema below both knees. A pulmonary function test (PFT) conducted that morning showed vital capacity (VC), functional residual capacity (FRC), and residual volume (RV) were all 45% to 50% of predicted values.

Although the patient's electrolyte levels were all normal, her hematocrit was 58% and her hemoglobin level was 18 g%. A chest radiograph examination revealed a severe thoracic spinal deformity, a mediastinal shift, an enlarged heart with prominent pulmonary artery segments bilaterally, and bilateral infiltrates in the lung bases consistent with pneumonia and atelectasis. The patient's arterial blood gas values (ABGs) on room air were pH 7.52, $PaCO_2$ 58 mm Hg, HCO_3^- 46 mEq/L, PaO_2 49 mm Hg, and SaO_2 88%. The physician requested a respiratory care consultation and stated that mechanical ventilation was probably not an option and would not be his choice at this time per the patient's request and his knowledge of the case.

---

[1]The **"Dizzy Gillespie pouch"** refers to the condition in which the cheeks of the mouth expand greatly with pressure, similar to that demonstrated by the famous bebop trumpet player Dizzy Gillespie. Dizzy played his horn incorrectly for some 50 years, letting his cheeks expand when he played, instead of keeping them taut, as is considered correct. This was mostly a result of his general lack of early musical education. Although Mr. Gillespie was able to create a surprisingly good sound using this form, over time it left his cheeks saggy and loose. A physician who wanted to use his image in a textbook named the condition after him. With Gillespie pouches, the cheeks inflate to look almost like balloons. Besides brass players, Gillespie pouches may be found among some balloon artists, who regularly apply great pressure to their cheeks while inflating balloons.

On the basis of these clinical data, the following SOAP was documented.

Respiratory Assessment and Plan

S "I'm having trouble breathing."

O Well-nourished appearance; severe anterior and left lateral curvature of the spine; cyanosis, digital clubbing, and distended neck veins—especially on the right side; strong cough: frequent, adequate, and productive of moderate amounts of thick yellow sputum; 2+ pitting edema below both knees; vital signs BP 160/100, HR 90, RR 18, T 36.3°C (97.3°F); trachea deviated to the right; both lungs: dull percussion notes, coarse crackles; PFT: VC, FRC, and RV 45% to 50% of predicted; Hct 58%, Hb 18 g%; CXR: Severe thoracic and spinous deformity, mediastinal shift, cardiomegaly, and bilateral infiltrates in the lung bases consistent with pneumonia or atelectasis; ABGs (room air) pH 7.52, $PaCO_2$ 58, HCO_3^- 46, PaO_2 49; SaO_2 88%.

A • Severe kyphoscoliosis (history, CXR, physical examination)
   • Atelectasis and consolidation (CXR)
   • Acute alveolar hyperventilation superimposed on chronic ventilatory failure with moderate hypoxemia (ABGs)
     • Impending ventilatory failure
   • Increased work of breathing (elevated blood pressure, heart rate, and respiratory rate)
   • Cor pulmonale (CXR and physical examination)
   • Excessive bronchial secretions (sputum, coarse crackles)
   • Infection likely (thick, yellow sputum)
   • Good ability to mobilize secretions (strong cough)

P Initiate Oxygen Therapy Protocol (Venturi mask at FIO_2 0.28). Airway Clearance Therapy Protocol (obtain sputum for culture; DB&C instructions and oral suction PRN). Lung Expansion Therapy Protocol (incentive spirometry qid and PRN). Notify physician of admitting ABGs and impending ventilatory failure. Monitor closely.

10 Hours After Admission

The patient's condition had not improved, and she was transferred to the intensive care unit. The physician had trouble titrating the cardiac drugs and decided to insert a pulmonary artery catheter, a central venous catheter, and an arterial line. Because of the woman's cardiac problems, several medical students, respiratory therapists, nurses, and doctors were constantly in and out of her room, performing and assisting in various procedures. As a result, working with the patient for any length of time was difficult, and the intensity of respiratory care was less than desirable. Eventually, the patient's cardiac status stabilized, and the physician requested an update on the woman's pulmonary condition.

The respiratory therapist working on the pulmonary consultation team found the patient in extreme respiratory distress. She was sitting up in bed, appeared frightened, and stated that she was extremely short of breath. A pulmonary artery catheter (Swan-Ganz) had been inserted previously. Both of her sisters were in the room; one sister was putting cold towels on the patient's face while the other sister was holding the patient's hands. Both sisters were crying softly. The woman's skin appeared cyanotic, and perspiration was visible on her face. Her neck veins were still distended. She demonstrated a weak, spontaneous cough. Although no sputum was noted, she sounded congested when she coughed. Dull percussion notes and coarse crackles were still present throughout both lungs. Her vital signs were blood pressure 180/120 mm Hg, heart rate 130 beats/min, respiratory rate 26 breaths/min, and rectal temperature 37.8°C (100°F).

Several of the patient's hemodynamic indices were elevated: CVP, RAP, PA, RVSWI, and PVR.[2] Her oxygenation indices were increased $\dot{Q}_s/\dot{Q}_T$ and O_2ER. Decreased DO_2 and $S\bar{v}O_2$. Her $\dot{V}O_2$ and $C(a-\bar{v})O_2$ were normal.[3] No recent chest radiograph was available. Her ABGs on an FIO_2 of 0.28 were pH 7.57, $PaCO_2$ 49 mm Hg, HCO_3^- 43 mEq/L, PaO_2 43 mm Hg, and SaO_2 87%. On the basis of these clinical data, the following SOAP was documented.

Respiratory Assessment and Plan

S Severe dyspnea; "I'm extremely short of breath."

O Extreme respiratory distress; cyanosis and perspiration noted; distended neck veins; weak, spontaneous cough; sounds of pulmonary congestion but no sputum produced; bilateral dull percussion notes, coarse crackles; vital signs BP 180/120, HR 130, RR 26, T 37.8°C (100°F); hemodynamics: increased CVP, RAP, PA, RVSWI, and PVR; oxygenation indices: increased $\dot{Q}_s/\dot{Q}_T$, and O_2ER and decreased DO_2 and $S\bar{v}O_2$. $\dot{V}O_2$ and $C(a-\bar{v})O_2$ normal. ABGs worse on FIO_2 0.28: pH 7.57, $PaCO_2$ 49, HCO_3^- 43, PaO_2 43; SaO_2 87%.

A • ABGs worse: on FIO_2 of 0.35
   • Acute alveolar hyperventilation superimposed on chronic ventilatory failure with moderate to severe hypoxemia (ABGs and history)
     • Impending ventilatory failure
   • Severe kyphoscoliosis (history, physical examination, CXR)
   • Increased work of breathing, worsening (increased blood pressure, heart rate, and respiratory rate)
   • Excessive bronchial secretions (coarse crackles, congested cough)
   • Atelectasis and consolidation (previous CXR)
   • **Pulmonary hypertension** (hemodynamic indices)
   • Continued critically ill status but chances of avoiding ventilatory failure improving

P Up-regulate Oxygen Therapy Protocol (Venturi oxygen mask at 0.35). Up-regulate Airway Clearance Therapy Protocol (add chest physical therapy [CPT] and postural drainage [PD] qid). Contact physician regarding impending ventilatory failure. Discuss possibility of noninvasive mechanical ventilation and **therapeutic bronchoscopy** with physician. Monitor and reevaluate in 30 minutes.

---

[2]*CVP*, Central venous pressure; *PA*, mean pulmonary artery pressure; *PVR*, pulmonary vascular resistance; *RAP*, right atrial pressure; *RVSWI*, right ventricular stroke work index.
[3] $C(a-\bar{v})O_2$, Arterial-venous oxygen difference; DO_2, total oxygen delivery; O_2ER, oxygen extraction ratio; $\dot{Q}_s/\dot{Q}_T$, pulmonary shunt fraction; $S\bar{v}O_2$, mixed venous oxygen saturation; $\dot{V}O_2$, oxygen consumption.

24 Hours After Admission

At this time the respiratory therapist found the patient watching the morning news on television with her two sisters. The woman was situated in a semi-Fowler's position eating the last few bites of her breakfast. The patient stated that she felt "so much better" and that "finally I have enough wind to eat some food."

Although her skin still appeared cyanotic, she did not look as ill as she had the day before. On request, she produced a strong cough and expectorated a small amount of white sputum. Her vital signs were blood pressure 140/85 mm Hg, heart rate 83 beats/min, respiratory rate 14 breaths/min, and temperature normal. Chest assessment findings demonstrated coarse crackles and dull percussion notes over both lung fields. The coarse crackles were less intense, however, than they had been the day before.

Although the patient's hemodynamic and oxygenation indices were better than they had been the day before, she still had room for improvement. Her hemodynamic parameters, still abnormal, revealed an elevated CVP, RAP, PA, RVSWI, and PVR. All other hemodynamic indices were normal. Her oxygenation indices still showed an increased $\dot{Q}_s/\dot{Q}_T$ and O_2ER and a decreased DO_2 and $S\bar{v}O_2$. Her $\dot{V}O_2$ and $C(a-\bar{v})O_2$ were normal. The patient's chest radiograph, taken earlier that morning, showed some clearing of the pneumonia and atelectasis described on admission. Her ABGs on an FIO_2 of 0.35 were pH 7.45, $PaCO_2$ 73 mm Hg, HCO_3^- 49 mEq/L, PaO_2 68 mm Hg, and SaO_2 94%. On the basis of these clinical data, the following SOAP was recorded.

Respiratory Assessment and Plan

S "I feel so much better. I finally have enough wind to eat some food."

O Cyanotic appearance; cough: strong, small amount of white sputum; vital signs: BP 140/85, HR 83, RR 14, T normal; coarse crackles, and dull percussion notes over both lung fields; coarse crackles improving; hemodynamic and oxygenation indices improving, but still an elevated CVP, RAP, PA, RVSWI, and PVR and still an increased $\dot{Q}_s/\dot{Q}_T$ and O_2ER and a decreased DO_2 and $S\bar{v}O_2$. CXR: Improvement of the bilateral pneumonia and atelectasis. ABGs worse on FIO_2 0.35: pH 7.45, $PaCO_2$ 73, HCO_3^- 49, PaO_2 68; SaO_2 94%.

A • Generally slightly improved overall status (history, CXR, hemodynamic and oxygenation indices, ABGs)
• ABGs worse on FIO_2 0.35 (likely close to the patient's normal baseline values)
• Significant improvement in problem with excessive bronchial secretions (coarse crackles, cough)
• Improvement in atelectasis and consolidation (CXR)
• Chronic ventilatory failure with mild hypoxemia (ABGs)
• Persistent pulmonary hypertension (hemodynamic indices)

P Down-regulate Oxygen Therapy Protocol and Airway Clearance Therapy Protocol. Continue to monitor closely and reevaluate ABGs on reduced FIO_2. Recommend pulmonary rehabilitation and patient and family education (noninvasive positive pressure ventilation cuirass ventilation, possibly rocking bed, bilevel positive airway pressure, or positive expiratory pressure).

Discussion

This case contains an excessive amount of extraneous historical and personal material. This was done to demonstrate, in part, how the respiratory therapist must cut through to the core of the case in the SOAP note, no matter how interesting the other information may be. Care of the patient with symptomatic advanced kyphoscoliosis consists of treatment of the conditions that can complicate it (e.g., bronchitis, pneumonia, atelectasis, pleural effusion) and treatment of the underlying condition itself.

In the first assessment, the SOAP documented excessive bronchial secretions and a likely infection because of the thick yellow sputum and recent history. The patient exhibited good ability to mobilize the secretions as charted by a strong cough. The chest radiograph confirmed atelectasis and consolidation, although the report did not precisely identify its location in the chest itself. Although acute alveolar hyperventilation on top of chronic ventilatory failure was present, the possibility of impending ventilatory failure was real. The therapist's decisions to oxygenate the patient with a low FIO_2 (0.28), administer airway clearance therapy, and be prepared for ventilator support were all appropriate (see the second SOAP note). The patient's cor pulmonale, but not her polycythemia, would have been expected to improve rapidly as overall oxygenation improved. Improvement in her polycythemia would take some time. The digital clubbing and cor pulmonale suggested that the hypoxemia was long-standing.

At the time of the second assessment, the intensity of the patient's respiratory distress was increasing. This was verified by the continued observation of the high pulse and respiratory rate, excessive airway secretions, dull percussion notes, acute alveolar hyperventilation on top of chronic ventilatory failure with moderate to severe hypoxemia, atelectasis on the chest x-ray, and poor response to oxygen therapy. Undoubtedly, impending ventilatory failure was more likely.

Atelectasis is often refractory to oxygen therapy, suggesting that therapeutic bronchoscopy might have been worthwhile. At that point in time, the up-regulation of the Oxygen Therapy Protocol (Protocol 10.1) and Airway Clearance Therapy Protocol (Protocol 10.2) were all justified by the clinical indicators. Note that use of any prognostication is discouraged in SOAP notes, and the therapist's recording that "chances of avoiding respiratory failure were improving" (at the end of the second SOAP note) is in general not appropriate.

In the last assessment, the clinical manifestations associated with the patient's disorder had all improved substantially, except for the increased $PaCO_2$, thought (again) to be related to "a return to baseline values" may have represented wishful thinking, and his decision to monitor it closely was appropriate. The down-regulation of the Oxygen Therapy Protocol and Airway Clearance Therapy Protocol was appropriate. The recommendation of pulmonary rehabilitation and family education was appropriately considered.

It is correct that the patient's ABGs were most likely at the patient's baseline level, because the pH was in the normal range. In fact, according to the pH (normal, but on the alkalotic side of normal) the patient's usual $PaCO_2$ was most likely somewhat higher than the last assessment value. This case nicely demonstrates how a patient with a severe, chronic restrictive lung disorder—in this case, kyphoscoliosis—can, over time, demonstrate ABGs with very high $PaCO_2$ levels, a normal pH (which has been corrected by an increased HCO_3^- level provided by kidney compensation), and a low PaO_2 level. In other words, the patient with severe kyphoscoliosis may demonstrate ABG findings that reflect chronic ventilatory failure (compensated respiratory acidosis) with hypoxemia, very similar to the patient with severe chronic obstructive pulmonary disease (i.e., emphysema and chronic bronchitis) who displays chronic ventilatory failure ABGs.

Comparison with baseline values (if available) would have been appropriate at such a time, and consideration of cuirass ventilation, a rocking bed, or positive expiratory pressure to assist nocturnal ventilation might be in order. Oxygenation can easily be assessed by oximetry at home. This case is an excellent example of the value of hemodynamic monitoring (specifically the normal PCWP) in differentiating left-sided from right-sided cardiac failure.

SELF-ASSESSMENT QUESTIONS

1. What kind of curvature of the spine is manifested in kyphosis?
   a. Posterior
   b. Anterior
   c. Lateral
   d. Medial

2. Kyphoscoliosis affects approximately what percentage of the US population?
   a. 2%
   b. 5%
   c. 10%
   d. 15%

3. Which of the following is associated with kyphoscoliosis?
   a. Decreased RV/TLC ratio
   b. Increased V_T
   c. Decreased RV
   d. Increased TLC

4. Which of the following is associated with kyphoscoliosis?
   a. Bronchial breath sounds
   b. Hyperresonant percussion note
   c. Decreased tactile and vocal fremitus
   d. Diminished breath sounds

5. During the advanced stages of kyphoscoliosis, the patient commonly demonstrates which of the following arterial blood gas values?
   1. Increased HCO_3^-
   2. Decreased pH
   3. Increased $PaCO_2$
   4. Normal pH
      a. 2 only
      b. 3 and 4 only
      c. 1 and 4 only
      d. 1, 3, and 4 only

CHAPTER

26 | Cancer of the Lung

Chapter Objectives

After reading this chapter, you will be able to:

- List the anatomic alterations of the lungs associated with lung cancer.
- Describe the causes of lung cancer.
- List the cardiopulmonary clinical manifestations associated with lung cancer.
- Describe the general management of lung cancer.
- Describe the clinical strategies and rationales of the SOAPs presented in the case study.
- Define key terms and complete self-assessment questions at the end of the chapter and on Evolve.

Key Terms

Adenocarcinoma
Aerosolized Morphine
Benign Tumors
Brachytherapy
Bronchogenic Carcinoma
Chemotherapy
Cigarette Smoking
Coin Lesion
End-of-Life Directives
Endobronchial Ultrasound (EBUS)
External Beam Radiation Therapy (EBRT)
Five-Year Survival Rate
Large Cell Carcinoma (Undifferentiated)
Lobectomy
Malignant Tumors
Malignant Pleural Effusion
Mediastinoscopy
Mesothelioma
Metastatic Cancer of the Lungs
Navigational Bronchoscopy
Neoplasm
Non–Small Cell Lung Carcinoma (NSCLC)

Pack-Years
PET/CT Imaging
Pneumonectomy
Positron Emission Tomography (PET) Lung Scan
Radiation Therapy
Radiofrequency Ablation (RFA)
Segmentectomy
Sleeve Resection
Small Cell (Oat Cell) Carcinoma
Small Cell Lung Carcinoma (SCLC)
Smoking Cessation Education
Squamous Cell (Epidermoid) Carcinoma
Staging of Lung Cancer
Stereotactic Body Radiation Therapy (SBRT)
Stereotactic Radiosurgery (SRS)
Video-Assisted Thoracic Surgery (VATS)
Wedge Resection

Chapter Outline

Anatomic Alterations of the Lungs
Etiology and Epidemiology
    Types of Cancers
    Non–Small Cell Lung Carcinoma
    Small Cell Lung Carcinoma
    Other Types of Lung Tumors
Screening and Diagnosis
    Staging of Non–Small Cell Lung Carcinoma
    Staging of Small Cell Lung Carcinoma
Overview of Cardiopulmonary Clinical Manifestations
    Associated With Cancer of the Lung
General Management of Lung Cancer
    Treatment Options for Non–Small Cell Lung Cancer
    Treatment Options for Small Cell Lung Cancer
Case Study: Cancer of the Lung
Self-Assessment Questions

Anatomic Alterations of the Lungs

Cancer is a general term that refers to abnormal new tissue growth characterized by the progressive, uncontrolled multiplication of cells. This abnormal growth of new cells is called a **neoplasm** or *tumor*. A tumor may be localized or invasive, benign or malignant.

Benign tumors do not endanger life unless they interfere with the normal functions of other organs or affect a vital organ. They grow slowly and push aside normal tissue but do not invade it. Benign tumors are usually encapsulated, well-demarcated growths. They are not invasive or metastatic; that is, tumor cells do not travel by way of the bloodstream or lymphatics and invade or form secondary tumors in other organs.

Malignant tumors are composed of embryonic, primitive, or poorly differentiated cells. They grow in a disorganized manner and so rapidly that nutrition of the cells becomes a problem. For this reason, necrosis, ulceration, and cavity formation are commonly associated with malignant tumors. They also invade surrounding tissues and may be metastatic. Although malignant changes may develop in any portion of the lung, they most commonly originate in the epithelium of the tracheobronchial tree.

A tumor that originates in the bronchial mucosa is called **bronchogenic carcinoma**. The terms *lung cancer* and *bronchogenic carcinoma* are used interchangeably. As a tumor enlarges, the surrounding bronchial airways and alveoli become irritated, inflamed, and swollen. The adjacent alveoli may fill with fluid or become consolidated or collapse. In addition, as the tumor protrudes into the tracheobronchial tree, excessive mucus production and airway obstruction develop. As the surrounding blood vessels erode, blood enters the tracheobronchial tree causing hemoptysis. Peripheral tumors may also invade the pleural space and impinge on the mediastinum, chest wall, ribs, or diaphragm. A secondary pleural effusion is often seen in lung cancer. A pleural effusion further compresses the lung and causes atelectasis.

The major pathologic or structural changes associated with bronchogenic carcinoma are as follows:

- Inflammation, swelling, and destruction of the bronchial airways and alveoli
- Excessive mucus production
- Tracheobronchial mucus accumulation and plugging
- Airway obstruction (from blood, mucus accumulation, or a tumor projecting into a bronchus)
- Atelectasis
- Alveolar consolidation
- Cavity formation
- Pleural effusion (when a tumor invades the parietal pleura and mediastinum)

Etiology and Epidemiology

Lung cancer is the second most common cause of cancer in both men (prostate is first in men) and women (breast cancer is first in women). About 14% of all new cancers are lung cancer. In 2017 the American Cancer Society (ACS) reported that there were about 222,500 new cases of lung cancer (116,990 in men and 105,510 in women) and about 155,870 deaths from lung cancer (84,590 in men and 71,280 in women). Lung cancer is the leading cause of cancer deaths, accounting for about 1 in 4 cancer deaths. More people die from lung cancer deaths each year than from colon, breast, and prostate cancers combined. About 2 in 3 people diagnosed with lung cancer are 65 years or older. The average age at the time of diagnosis is about 70 years. Black men are about 20% more likely to develop lung cancer than white men. The rate is about 10% lower in black women than in white women. Risk factors for lung cancer include the following:

- **Cigarette smoking**[1] is the most common cause of lung cancer. Although various studies and professional organizations report slightly different numbers, all figures are grim. Heavy smokers are 64 times more likely to develop lung cancer. According to the ACS, about 80% of lung cancer deaths are thought to be caused by smoking. The longer one smokes and the more packs a day (**pack-years**)[2], the greater the risk is for developing lung cancer. Smoking low-tar or "light" cigarettes generates the same risk for lung cancer as regular cigarettes. In addition, smoking menthol cigarettes likely increases the risk for lung cancer even more because the menthol allows the smoker to inhale more deeply. Cigar smoking and pipe smoking are almost as likely to cause lung cancer. They are also commonly associated with cancer of the lip, mouth, and throat. Secondhand smoke can increase the risk for developing lung cancer. According to the ACS, secondhand smoke is thought to cause more than 7000 deaths from lung cancer each year.
- *Radon exposure* is the second leading cause of lung cancer in this country according to the US Environmental Protection Agency (EPA). Radon is a naturally occurring radioactive gas that is produced from the breakdown of uranium in the soil and rocks. Breathing radon increases the risk for lung cancer. Outdoors, radon is not likely to be dangerous. Indoors, however, radon can be more concentrated and, therefore, the risk for lung cancer increases.
- Exposure to other cancer-causing agents:
  - *Asbestos* (e.g., in mines, mills, textile plants, insulation, and shipyards) exposure constitutes risk for developing **mesothelioma,** a cancer that starts in the pleura
  - *Radioactive ores* (such as uranium)
  - *Inhaled chemicals or minerals* (e.g., arsenic, beryllium, cadmium, silica, vinyl chloride, nickel compounds, chromium compounds, coal products, mustard gas, and chloromethyl ethers)
  - *Diesel exhaust*

---

[1]The role of the respiratory therapist as a patient educator is becoming increasingly important and nowhere more so than in the field of **smoking cessation education**. This function occurs best in outpatient and inpatient settings as part of well-organized pulmonary rehabilitation programs, in the public domain (e.g., lectures to high school students), and on an individual basis with patients. The role of smoking cessation education has been discussed elsewhere (see Chapter 13, Chronic Obstructive Pulmonary Disease, Chronic Bronchitis, and Emphysema) as part of evidence-based practice in chronic obstructive pulmonary disease (COPD). *Documentation of efforts and patient adherence and compliance to smoking cessation efforts has become increasingly complex and important for reimbursement purposes. The effect of smoking cessation on established lung cancer is, unfortunately, not particularly successful.*

[2]Pack-years = packs per day × years smoked; e.g., one pack of cigarettes smoked per day × 20 years = 20 pack-years.

- *Air pollution* (especially near heavily trafficked roads)
- *Arsenic* in drinking water
- *Radiation therapy to lungs* (e.g., individuals who have had radiation therapy to the chest for other cancers, such as radiation after a mastectomy for breast cancer, are at higher risk for lung cancer)
- *Personal or family history of lung cancer*

Types of Cancers

As shown in Fig. 26.1, bronchogenic carcinomas can be divided into the following two major categories: **non–small cell lung carcinoma (NSCLC)** and **small cell lung carcinoma (SCLC)**.

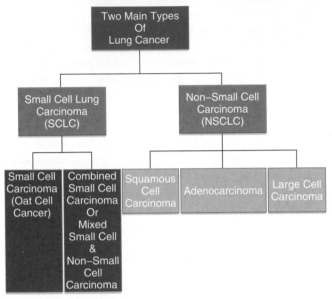

FIGURE 26.1 Types of lung cancer.

The NSCLC category is further subdivided into the following three types of lung cancer: (1) squamous cell carcinoma, (2) adenocarcinoma (including bronchial alveolar cell carcinoma), and (3) large cell carcinoma. The SCLC category is composed of small cell carcinoma (also called *oat cell carcinoma*), or combined small cell carcinoma, or a mixture of SCLC and NSCLC.

Each type of lung cancer grows and spreads in a different way. For example, SCLC spreads aggressively and responds best to **chemotherapy** and **radiation therapy**. SCLC occurs almost exclusively in smokers and accounts for 15% to 20% of all lung cancers in the United States. NSCLCs are more common and account for 75% to 85% of all lung cancers in the United States. When confined to a small area and identified early, NSCLCs often can be removed surgically. Table 26.1 provides general characteristics of these cancer cell types, including growth rates, metastasis, and means of diagnosis. A more in-depth description of each cancer cell type follows.

Non–Small Cell Lung Carcinoma

According to the ACS, non–small cell cancer is the most common type of lung cancer. About 85% of all lung cancers are non–small cell cancers. Subtypes of NSCLC are squamous cell carcinoma, adenocarcinoma, and large cell carcinoma (see Fig. 26.1).

Squamous Cell Carcinoma

Squamous cell (epidermoid) carcinoma constitutes about 25% to 30% of the bronchogenic carcinomas. The incidence of this type of cancer has sharply declined over the past two decades. This type of tumor is commonly located near a central bronchus or hilus and projects into the large bronchi. Squamous

TABLE 26.1 Characteristics of Lung Cancers

Tumor Type	Growth Rate	Metastasis	Means of Diagnosis	Clinical Manifestations and Treatment
Non–Small Cell Lung Carcinoma (NSCLC)				
Squamous cell carcinoma	Slow	Late; mostly to hilar lymph nodes	Biopsy, sputum analysis, bronchoscopy, electron microscopy, immunohistochemistry	Cough, sputum production, airway obstruction; treated surgically, chemotherapy adjunctive
Adenocarcinoma	Moderate	Early	Radiography, fiberoptic bronchoscopy, electron microscopy	Pleural effusion; treated surgically, chemotherapy adjunctive
Large cell carcinoma	Rapid	Early and widespread	Sputum analysis, bronchoscopy, electron microscopy (by exclusion of other cell types)	Chest wall pain, pleural effusion, cough, sputum production, hemoptysis, airway obstruction resulting in pneumonia (if airways involved); treated surgically
Small Cell Lung Carcinoma (SCLC)				
Small cell (oat cell) carcinoma	Very rapid	Very early; to mediastinum or distally in lung	Radiography, sputum analysis, bronchoscopy, electron microscopy, immunohistochemistry, and clinical manifestations (cough, chest pain, dyspnea, hemoptysis, localized wheezing)	Airway obstruction, signs and symptoms of excessive hormone secretion; treated by chemotherapy and ionizing radiation to thorax and central nervous system

cell tumors are often seen projecting into the bronchi during bronchoscopy. The tumor originates from the basal cells of the bronchial epithelium and grows through the epithelium before invading the surrounding tissues.

The tumor has a slow growth rate and a late metastatic tendency (mostly to hilar lymph nodes). These tumors generally remain fairly well localized and tend not to metastasize until late in the course of lung cancer. Cavitation and necrosis within the center of the cancer are common findings. Surgical resection is the preferred treatment if metastasis has not taken place. Chemotherapy has limited effectiveness. In about one-third of cases, squamous cell carcinoma originates in the periphery. Because of the location in the central bronchi, obstructive manifestations are generally nonspecific and include a nonproductive cough and hemoptysis. Pneumonia and atelectasis are often secondary complications of squamous cell carcinoma. Cavity formation with or without an air-fluid interface is seen in 10% to 20% of cases (Fig. 26.2A).

Adenocarcinoma

Adenocarcinoma (previously called *bronchioloalveolar carcinoma*) arises from the mucous glands of the tracheobronchial tree. In fact, the glandular configuration and mucous production caused by this type of cancer are the pathologic features that distinguish adenocarcinoma from the other types of bronchogenic carcinoma. Adenocarcinoma accounts for about 40% of all bronchogenic carcinomas. It has the weakest association with smoking. Among people who have never smoked, adenocarcinoma is the most common form of lung cancer.

Adenocarcinoma tumors are usually smaller than 4 cm and are most commonly found in the peripheral regions of the lung parenchyma. The growth rate is moderate, and the metastatic tendency is early. Secondary cavity formation and pleural effusion are common (see Fig. 26.2B). When the cancer is discovered early, surgical resection is possible in a high percentage of cases. These tumors typically arise from the terminal bronchioles and alveoli. They have a slow growth rate, and their metastasis pattern is unpredictable.

Large Cell Carcinoma (Undifferentiated)

Large cell carcinoma (undifferentiated) accounts for about 10% to 15% of all bronchogenic carcinoma cases. Because this tumor has lost all evidence of differentiation, it is commonly referred to as *undifferentiated large cell anaplastic cancer*. Although these tumors commonly arise peripherally, they also may be found centrally and often distort the trachea and large airways. Large cell carcinoma has a rapid growth rate and early and widespread metastasis. Common secondary complications include chest wall pain, pleural effusion, pneumonia, hemoptysis, and cavity formation (see Fig. 26.2C).

Small Cell Lung Carcinoma

Small cell (oat cell) carcinoma accounts for about 10% to 15% of all bronchogenic carcinomas. Most of these tumors arise centrally near the hilar region. They tend to arise in the larger airways (primary and secondary bronchi). Cell size ranges from 6 to 8 μm. The tumor grows very rapidly, becoming very large, and metastasizes early. Because the tumor cells are often compressed into an oval shape, this form of cancer is commonly referred to as *oat cell carcinoma*. Small cell carcinoma has the poorest prognosis. The average survival time for untreated small cell carcinoma is about 1 to 3 months. About 90% of patients respond to treatment (e.g., chemotherapy, radiation, or both), but nearly all relapse within 24 months. Small cell carcinoma has the strongest correlation with cigarette smoking and is associated with the worst prognosis (see Fig. 26.2D).

Other Types of Lung Tumors

In addition to the two main types of lung cancer discussed previously (i.e., SCLC and NSCLC), the following types of lung cancer can occur:

- *Lung carcinoid tumor* (also called *lung carcinoids*): A type of cancer that starts in the lungs. Lung carcinoid tumors are uncommon and tend to grow slower than other types of lung cancers. Lung carcinoid tumors are made up of special types of cells called *neuroendocrine cells*. Lung carcinoids account for about 1% to 2% of all lung cancers. Most carcinoid tumors originate in the digestive tract; only about 30% of all carcinoid tumors start in the lungs. There are four types of neuroendocrine lung tumors:
- *Small cell lung cancer:* The fastest growing and spreading of all cancers.
- *Large cell neuroendocrine carcinoma:* A rare cancer and a subtype of NSCLC.
- *Typical carcinoids:* Tend to grow slowly and rarely spread beyond the lungs. About 90% of lung carcinoids are typical carcinoids.
- *Atypical carcinoids:* Grow a little faster and are likely to spread outside of the lungs.

Carcinoids also may be classified based on where they are found in the lungs. For example:

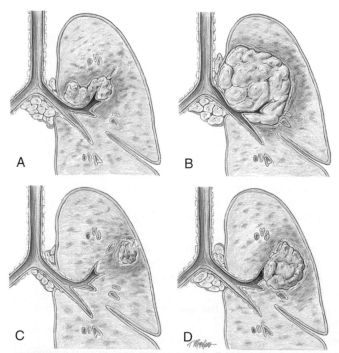

FIGURE 26.2 Cancer of the lung. (A) Squamous cell carcinoma. (B) Adenocarcinoma. (C) Large cell carcinoma. (D) Small cell (oat cell) carcinoma.

- *Central carcinoids* are found in the walls of large bronchi near the center of the lungs. The majority of lung carcinoid tumors are central carcinoids and are also typical carcinoids.
- *Peripheral carcinoids* are found in the smaller bronchioles toward the periphery of lungs. Most peripheral carcinoids are typical carcinoids, although they are more likely than central carcinoids to be atypical.
- *Additional lung tumors:* For example, adenoid cystic carcinoma, lymphoma, sarcoma, and benign lung tumors (e.g., hamartomas) are rare.
- *Cancers that spread to the lungs:* Cancer that begins in other parts of the body, such as breast, pancreas, kidney, or skin, can metastasize to the lungs. However, it is important to point out that cancers that start in other organs and spread to the lungs are not lung cancer. For example, cancer that starts in the breast and metastasizes to the lungs is still breast cancer. The treatment for **metastatic cancer of the lungs** is based on where the cancer originated—that is, the primary cancer site.

Screening and Diagnosis

Unfortunately, most lung cancers are not diagnosed until after the patient presents with symptoms that suggest lung cancer. Symptoms associated with lung cancer include (1) a progressively worsening cough that often includes bloody or rust-colored sputum; (2) chest pain, especially with deep breathing, coughing, or laughing; (3) hoarse voice; (4) poor appetite and weight loss; (5) shortness of breath; (6) fatigue; (7) frequent bronchial infections or pneumonia episodes; and (8) the sudden onset of wheezing.

When lung cancer spreads to other parts of the body, the patient may have other symptoms of cancer that include bone pain (e.g., back or hips), neurologic problems (e.g., headache, arm and leg weakness or numbness, dizziness or balance problems, seizures), jaundice, and enlarged lymph nodes (e.g., mediastinum, neck, or axillae). In addition, the patient may demonstrate a group of very specific syndromes associated with lung cancer, such as the following:

- *Horner syndrome:* Caused by a tumor near the apex of the lung that damages the nerve that passes from the upper chest to the neck; causing drooping or weakness of one eyelid, small pupil in the same eye, and reduced or no perspiration on the same side of the face.
- *Superior vena cava syndrome:* Caused by a tumor near the upper portion of the right lung that compresses the superior vena cava and obstructs venous blood flow. This condition causes headaches, dizziness, and swelling in the face, neck, arms, and upper chest, sometimes with a bluish-red skin color.
- *Paraneoplastic syndromes:* These are the indirect effects of a variety of tumors that occur distant to the tumor or metastatic site. These tumors produce active proteins, polypeptides, or hormone-like substances that enter the bloodstream and cause problems distant from the tumor. Common paraneoplastic syndromes caused by NSCLC include (1) high blood calcium levels (hypercalcemia), (2) excess growth of certain bones (e.g., fingertips), and (3) blood clots.

When symptoms are present that suggest lung cancer, a full medical history and physical examination, along with a check for risk factors, are indicated. When the results of these activities further support the possibility of lung cancer, additional diagnostic tests are ordered—for example, imaging tests and tissue sampling techniques.

Table 26.2 provides an overview of the common screening and diagnostic tests for lung cancer. The primary goal of these diagnostic procedures is to (1) confirm the presence of a lung

TABLE 26.2 Screening and Diagnostic Tests for Lung Cancer

Technique	Description
Imaging for Lung Cancer Imaging is performed to (1) identify suspicious areas of the lungs that might be cancerous, (2) determine if and where the cancer may have spread, (3) evaluate the effectiveness of treatment, and (4) assess signs that a cancer has returned after a treatment program.	
Chest radiograph	The chest x-ray is often the first test used to determine if there are any masses or spots on the lungs. If any suspicious areas are identified, one or more of the following imaging methods are ordered.
Computed tomography (CT) scan	The CT scan better identifies a lung tumor than a routine chest x-ray. It also provides excellent information about the size, shape, and location of the tumor. It can help identify enlarged lymph nodes that might contain cancer cells.
Positron emission tomography (PET) scan	The PET scan is used to help determine if an abnormal area on the chest x-ray film or CT scan might be cancer. It helps assess if the cancer has spread to nearby lymph nodes or other areas of the body, which helps determine if surgery is an option.
Magnetic resonance imaging (MRI) scan	The MRI scan may be used to determine if the cancer cells have spread from the lungs to the brain or spinal cord.
Bone scan	The bone scan can help determine if the cancer has spread to the bones. Because the PET scan can usually identify if cancer has spread to the bones, the bone scan is now primarily ordered only when the patient has bone pain symptoms.

TABLE 26.2 Screening and Diagnostic Tests for Lung Cancer—cont'd

Technique	Description
Diagnostic Tests for Lung Cancer	
Identifying cancer cells under a microscope makes the actual diagnosis of lung cancer. The cells can be obtained from sputum samples, taken from a suspicious area (biopsy), or removed from pleural fluid (thoracentesis).	
Sputum cytology	A sputum sample is obtained and viewed under the microscope to determine if it contains any cancer cells.

Bronchoscopy
  Needle biopsy
  Bronchial brushing
  Bronchial washing
	A bronchoscope is commonly used to visually evaluate the tracheobronchial tree of the patient. In addition, small instruments can easily be passed down the bronchoscope to obtain tissue biopsies via needle aspiration, bronchial brushing, or bronchial washing. The tissue and cell samples are then evaluated under a microscope.

Navigational bronchoscopy (also called electromagnetic navigation bronchoscopy)	**Navigational bronchoscopy** is a diagnostic and treatment procedure that combines electromagnetic navigation with real-time virtual three-dimensional (3-D) CT imaging that allows the physician to reach distal tumors, take a biopsy sample, and administer treatment (see Fig. 9.5).
Endobronchial ultrasound (EBUS)	EBUS may be performed during a bronchoscopy to view lymph nodes and other structures in the mediastinum area. EBUS also may be used for a needle biopsy. Tissue samples are viewed under the microscope. EBUS may provide sufficient information to stage a cancer without other more invasive procedures such as **mediastinoscopy**, thoracoscopy, or thoracotomy.
Endoscopic esophageal ultrasound	Similar to EBUS, the endoscopic esophageal ultrasound can be passed into the esophagus and directed to view lymph nodes and other structures in the chest that appear suspicious for cancer. When enlarged lymph nodes are identified, a biopsy needle can pass through the endoscope to obtain a tissue sample.
Mediastinoscopy and mediastinotomy	These procedures are performed to view a suspicious area more directly and obtain a tissue sample. They are performed in the operating room while the patient is under general anesthesia. *Mediastinoscopy* entails a small incision in the front of the neck, which allows a thin, hollow, lighted tube to be inserted behind the sternum and in front of the trachea. Tissue samples can be obtained from the lymph nodes along the trachea and major bronchi. *Mediastinotomy* entails a slightly larger incision (about 2 inches) between the left second and third ribs adjacent to the sternum. This permits the surgeon to reach some lymph nodes that cannot be reached by mediastinoscopy.
Thoracentesis	Thoracentesis is used to obtain fluid that accumulates (pleural effusion) between the chest wall and the lungs. Thoracentesis entails the insertion of a needle between the ribs to aspirate the fluid (and possible cancer cells) for microscopic study.
Video-assisted thoracic surgery (VATS)	VATS may be performed to determine if the cancer has spread to the intrapleural space. It also can be used to obtain tissue biopsy samples on the outer surface of the lungs, nearby lymph nodes, and fluid. It may help assess if a tumor is growing into nearby organs or tissues. Because VATS is performed in the operating room under general anesthesia, it is not often done just to diagnose cancer unless other procedures have been unsuccessful in obtaining a tissue sample.
Analysis of Tissue Biopsy Samples	
The tissue samples obtained from one of the above procedures may be used for additional tests to help better classify the cancer.	
Immunohistochemistry	This test entails treating the tissue sample with certain antibodies designed to attach only to specific substances found in certain cancer cells.
Molecular tests	In some cases, the identification of specific gene changes in the cancer cells may help pinpoint certain targeted drugs that might be effective in treating the cancer.
Complete blood count (CBC)	Although blood tests are not used to diagnose lung cancer, they are useful in assessing the overall health of the patient and, in some cases, to determine if the patient is healthy enough for surgery. In addition, a CBC is repeated regularly in patients being treated with chemotherapy, which often affects blood-forming cells of the bone marrow. Also, when a cancer has spread to the liver and bones, it may cause abnormal levels of certain chemicals in the blood (e.g., higher than normal level of lactate dehydrogenase).

carcinoma, (2) establish the cancer cell type, and (3) confirm the stage of the cancer. The definitive diagnosis of lung cancer is made by a microscopic examination of a tissue sample (biopsy).

The treatment and prognosis of any cancer depend, to a large extent, on the stage of the cancer. The **staging** of NSCLC and small cell lung carcinoma is discussed in more detail as follows.

Staging of Non–Small Cell Lung Carcinoma

The most commonly used classification tool to stage NSCLC is the American Joint Committee on Cancer (AJCC) TNM system (Table 26.3). The **staging of lung cancer** is determined by a combination of all of the following factors:

- **T:** Represents the size and location of the primary tumor
- **N:** Denotes the regional lymph node involvement
- **M:** Signifies the extent of metastasis (e.g., common sites are the brain, bones, adrenal glands, liver, kidneys, and other lung)

The numbers and letters after the T, N, and M classification provide more information about each of these factors. Higher numbers represent increased severity. Once the T, N, and M categories have been established, the information is grouped together to determine the overall stage grouping of the patient's lung cancer (see explanation later).

Stage Grouping for Lung Cancer

Stages 0, I, II, III, and IV are used to identify the overall stage of the lung cancer, with stage 0 and stage I being the least advanced and stage IV the most advanced. Some stages are subdivided into A and B. This process is called *stage grouping*. The lower the stage the better the prognosis. Table 26.4 provides an overview of the stage grouping for lung cancer.

Staging of Small Cell Lung Carcinoma

SCLC is staged differently from non–small cell cancer. For treatment reasons, SCLC is usually classified as a limited stage or an extensive stage:

- *Limited stage:* The cancer is confined to only one lung and to its neighboring lymph nodes. It can be treated with a

---

TABLE 26.3 The American Joint Committee on Cancer Tumor, Node, Metastasis Staging System for Lung Cancer

TNM Category	Description
Primary Tumor (T)	
TX	The main (primary) tumor cannot be assessed, or cancer cells were seen on sputum cytology or bronchial washing but no tumor can be found.
T0	There is no evidence of a primary tumor.
Tis	The cancer is found only in the top layers of cells lining the air passages. It has not invaded into deeper lung tissues. This is also known as *carcinoma in situ*.
T1	The tumor is no larger than 3 cm—slightly less than 1.25 inches—across, has not reached the membranes that surround the lungs (visceral pleura), and does not affect the main branches of the bronchi. If the tumor is 2 cm (about 0.8 of an inch) or less across, it is called T1a. If the tumor is larger than 2 cm but not larger than 3 cm across, it is called T1b.
T2	The tumor has one or more of the following features: • It is larger than 3 cm across but not larger than 7 cm. • It involves a main bronchus, but is not closer than 2 cm (about 0.75 of an inch) to the carina (the point where the windpipe splits into the left and right main bronchi). • It has grown into the membranes that surround the lungs (visceral pleura). The tumor partially clogs the airways, but this has not caused the entire lung to collapse or develop pneumonia.
T2a	Tumor >3 cm but ≤5 cm
T2b	Tumor >5 cm but ≤7 cm
T3	The tumor has one or more of the following features: • It is larger than 7 cm across. • It has grown into the chest wall, the breathing muscle that separates the chest from the abdomen (diaphragm), the membranes surrounding the space between the two lungs (mediastinal pleura), or membranes of the sac surrounding the heart (parietal pericardium). • It invades a main bronchus and is closer than 2 cm (about 0.75 of an inch) to the carina, but it does not involve the carina itself. • It has grown into the airways enough to cause an entire lung to collapse or to cause pneumonia in the entire lung. • Two or more separate tumor nodules are present in the same lobe of a lung.
T4	The cancer has one or more of the following features: • A tumor of any size has grown into the space between the lungs (mediastinum), the heart, the large blood vessels near the heart (e.g., the aorta), the windpipe (trachea), the tube connecting the throat to the stomach (esophagus), the spine, or the carina. • Two or more separate tumor nodules are present in different lobes of the same lung.

TNM Category	Description
Regional Lymph Nodes (N)	
NX	Nearby lymph nodes cannot be assessed.
N0	There is no spread to nearby lymph nodes.
N1	The cancer has spread to lymph nodes within the lung and/or around the area where the bronchus enters the lung (hilar lymph nodes). Affected lymph nodes are on the same side as the primary tumor.
N2	The cancer has spread to lymph nodes around the carina (the point where the windpipe splits into the left and right bronchi) or in the space between the lungs (mediastinum). Affected lymph nodes are on the same side as the primary tumor.
N3	The cancer has spread to lymph nodes near the clavicle on either side, and/or spread to hilar or mediastinal lymph nodes on the side opposite the primary tumor.
Distant Metastasis (M)	
M0	No spread to distant organs or areas. This includes the other lung, lymph nodes further away than those mentioned in the N stages above, and other organs or tissues such as the liver, bones, or brain.
M1a	Any of the following: • The cancer has spread to the other lung. • Cancer cells are found in the pleural fluid (called *malignant pleural effusion*). • Cancer cells are found in the fluid around the heart (called *malignant pericardial effusion*).
M1b	The cancer has spread to distant lymph nodes or to other organs such as the liver, bones, or brain.

Modified from the American Cancer Society, http://www.cancer.org.

TABLE 26.4 Stage Groupings: Tumor, Node, Metastasis Subsets

After the T, N, and M categories have been established, the information is merged together to assign an overall stage of 0, I, II, III, or IV.

Stage Grouping	TNM Subsets	Description
Occult (hidden) cancer	TX, N0, M0	Cancer cells are found in sputum or other lung fluids, but the cancer is not identified in other tests; thus the location cannot be established.
Stage 0	Tis, N0, M0	Cancer found only in the top layers of cells lining the airways. It has not invaded deeper into other lung tissue and has not spread to lymph nodes or distant sites.
Stage IA	T1a-T1b, N0, M0	The cancer is no larger than 3 cm across, has not reached the membranes that surround the lungs, and does not affect the main branches of the bronchi. It has not spread to lymph nodes or distant sites.
Stage IB	T2a, N0, M0	The cancer has one or more of the following features: • The main tumor is larger than 3 cm across but not larger than 5 cm. • The tumor has grown into a main bronchus, but is not within 2 cm of the carina (and it is not larger than 5 cm). • The tumor has grown into the visceral pleura (the membranes surrounding the lungs) and is not larger than 5 cm. • The tumor is partially obstructing the airways (and is not larger than 5 cm). The cancer has not spread to lymph nodes or distant sites.
Stage IIA (Three main combinations of categories make up this stage.)	T1a/T1b, N1, M0	The cancer is no larger than 3 cm across, has not grown into the membranes that surround the lungs, and does not affect the main branches of the bronchi. It has spread to lymph nodes within the lung and/or around the area where the bronchus enters the lung (hilar lymph nodes). These lymph nodes are on the same side as the cancer. It has not spread to distant sites.
	T2a, N1, M0	The cancer has one or more of the following features: • The main tumor is larger than 3 cm across but not larger than 5 cm. • The tumor has grown into a main bronchus but is not within 2 cm of the carina (and it is not larger than 5 cm). • The tumor has grown into the visceral pleura (the membranes surrounding the lungs) and is not larger than 5 cm. • The tumor is partially obstructing the airways (and is not larger than 5 cm). The cancer has also spread to lymph nodes within the lung and/or around the area where the bronchus enters the lung (hilar lymph nodes). These lymph nodes are on the same side as the cancer. It has not spread to distant sites.

Continued

TABLE 26.4 Stage Groupings: Tumor, Node, Metastasis Subsets—cont'd

	T2b, N0, M0	The cancer has one or more of the following features: • The main tumor is larger than 5 cm across but not larger than 7 cm. • The tumor has grown into a main bronchus, but is not within 2 cm of the carina (and it is between 5 and 7 cm across). • The tumor has grown into the visceral pleura (the membranes surrounding the lungs) and is between 5 and 7 cm across. • The tumor is partially obstructing the airways (and is between 5 and 7 cm across). The cancer has not spread to lymph nodes or distant sites.
Stage IIB (Two combinations of categories make up this stage.)	T2b, N1, M0	The cancer has one or more of the following features: • The main tumor is larger than 5 cm across but not larger than 7 cm. • The tumor has grown into a main bronchus, but is not within 2 cm of the carina (and it is between 5 and 7 cm across). • The tumor has grown into the visceral pleura (the membranes surrounding the lungs) and is between 5 and 7 cm across. • The cancer is partially obstructing the airways (and is between 5 and 7 cm across). It has also spread to lymph nodes within the lung and/or around the area where the bronchus enters the lung (hilar lymph nodes). These lymph nodes are on the same side as the cancer. It has not spread to distant sites.
	T3, N0, M0	The main tumor has one or more of the following features: • It is larger than 7 cm across. • It has grown into the chest wall, the breathing muscle that separates the chest from the abdomen (diaphragm), the membranes surrounding the space between the lungs (mediastinal pleura), or membranes of the sac surrounding the heart (parietal pericardium). • It invades a main bronchus and is closer than 2 cm (about 0.75 of an inch) to the carina, but it does not involve the carina itself. • It has grown into the airways enough to cause an entire lung to collapse or to cause pneumonia in the entire lung. • Two or more separate tumor nodules are present in the same lobe of a lung. The cancer has not spread to lymph nodes or distant sites.
Stage IIIA (Three main combinations of categories make up this stage.)	T1 to T3, N2, M0	The main tumor can be any size. It has not grown into the space between the lungs (mediastinum), the heart, the large blood vessels near the heart (such as the aorta), the windpipe (trachea), the tube connecting the throat to the stomach (esophagus), the spine, or the carina. It has not spread to different lobes of the same lung. The cancer has spread to lymph nodes around the carina (the point where the windpipe splits into the left and right bronchi) or in the space between the lungs (mediastinum). These lymph nodes are on the same side as the main lung tumor. The cancer has not spread to distant sites.
	T3, N1, M0	The cancer has one or more of the following features: • It is larger than 7 cm across. • It has grown into the chest wall, the diaphragm, the membranes surrounding the space between the lungs (mediastinal pleura), or membranes of the sac surrounding the heart (parietal pericardium). • It invades a main bronchus and is closer than 2 cm to the carina, but it does not involve the carina itself. • Two or more separate tumor nodules are present in the same lobe. • It has grown into the airways enough to cause an entire lung to collapse or to cause pneumonia in the entire lung. It has also spread to lymph nodes within the lung and/or around the area where the bronchus enters the lung (hilar lymph nodes). These lymph nodes are on the same side as the cancer. It has not spread to distant sites.
	T4, N0 or N1, M0	The cancer has one or more of the following features: • A tumor of any size has grown into the space between the lungs (mediastinum), the heart, the large blood vessels near the heart (such as the aorta), the trachea, the tube connecting the throat to the stomach (esophagus), the spine, or the carina. • Two or more separate tumor nodules are present in different lobes of the same lung. It may or may not have spread to lymph nodes within the lung and/or around the area where the bronchus enters the lung (hilar lymph nodes). Any affected lymph nodes are on the same side as the cancer. It has not spread to distant sites.

TABLE 26.4 Stage Groupings: Tumor, Node, Metastasis Subsets—cont'd

Stage IIIB (Two combinations of categories make up this stage.)	Any T, N3, M0	The cancer can be of any size. It may or may not have grown into nearby structures or caused pneumonia or lung collapse. It has spread to lymph nodes near the clavicle on either side, and/or has spread to hilar or mediastinal lymph nodes on the side opposite the primary tumor. The cancer has not spread to distant sites.
	T4, N2, M0	The cancer has one or more of the following features: • A tumor of any size has grown into the space between the lungs (mediastinum), the heart, the large blood vessels near the heart (such as the aorta), the trachea, the tube connecting the throat to the stomach (esophagus), the backbone, or the carina. • Two or more separate tumor nodules are present in different lobes of the same lung. The cancer has also spread to lymph nodes around the carina (the point where the windpipe splits into the left and right bronchi) or in the space between the lungs (mediastinum). Affected lymph nodes are on the same side as the main lung tumor. It has not spread to distant sites.
Stage IV (Two combinations of categories make up this stage.)	Any T, any N, M1a	The cancer can be any size and may or may not have grown into nearby structures or reached nearby lymph nodes. In addition, any of the following is true: • The cancer has spread to the other lung. • Cancer cells are found in the pleural fluid (called a *malignant pleural effusion*). Cancer cells are found in the fluid around the heart (called a *malignant pericardial effusion*).
	Any T, any N, M1b	The cancer can be any size and may or may not have grown into nearby structures or reached nearby lymph nodes. It has spread to distant lymph nodes or to other organs such as the liver, bones, or brain.

Modified from the American Cancer Society, http://www.cancer.org.

single radiation field. In some cases, the lymph nodes at the center of the chest (mediastinal lymph nodes) may be included, even when the cancer is close to the other lung. Lymph nodes above the clavicle (supraclavicular nodes) can be included in limited stage as long as they are on the same side of the chest as the cancer. About 30% of the patients with SCLC have limited stage SCLC.

• *Extensive stage:* The cancer has spread beyond one lung and nearby lymph nodes. It may have invaded lung tissue, more remote lymph nodes, and other distant organs (including bone marrow). SCLC that has spread to the intrapleural space around the lung also may be considered an extensive stage. About 65% of the patients with SCLC have extensive stage SCLC.

SCLC is commonly staged this way to help identify which patients might benefit more from aggressive treatments—for example, chemotherapy combined with radiation therapy is commonly used to treat limited stage SCLC, compared with treating the patient with only chemotherapy, which would be the better option for extensive stage SCLC.

Five-Year Survival Rate

The percentage of people who are still alive 5 years after the cancer has been discovered (**5-year survival rate**) depends on the type and stage of the lung cancer. NSCLC generally grows and spreads more slowly than SCLC. The survival rates for both decrease when the stage of cancer involves the patient's lymph nodes, pleura, bone marrow, or other body organs. According to the ACS, the general 5-year survival

TABLE 26.5 Five-Year Survival Rate for Non–Small Cell Lung Carcinoma

Stage	Average Percent Survival at Five Years (%)
IA	~49
IB	~45
IIA	~30
IIB	~31
IIIA	~14
IIIB	~5
IV	~1

TABLE 26.6 Five-Year Survival Rate for Small Cell Lung Carcinoma

Stage	Average Percent Survival at Five Years (%)
I	<31
II	<19
III	<8
IV	<2

rates for NSCLC are shown in Table 26.5. Although SCLC is less common than NSCLC, it generally grows very fast and is more likely to spread to other organs. Table 26.6 provides a general overview of the 5-year survival rates for SCLC.

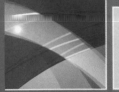

OVERVIEW of the Cardiopulmonary Clinical Manifestations Associated With Cancer of the Lung

The following clinical manifestations result from the pathologic mechanisms caused (or activated) by atelectasis (see Fig. 10.7), alveolar consolidation (see Fig. 10.8), and excessive bronchial secretions (see Fig. 10.11)—the major anatomic alterations of the lungs associated with cancer of the lung (see Fig. 26.2).

CLINICAL DATA OBTAINED AT THE PATIENT'S BEDSIDE

The Physical Examination

Vital Signs

Increased Respiratory Rate (Tachypnea)

Several pathophysiologic mechanisms operating simultaneously may lead to an increased ventilatory rate:

- Stimulation of peripheral chemoreceptors (hypoxemia)
- Relationship of decreased lung compliance to increased ventilatory rate
- Stimulation of J receptors
- Pain, anxiety

Increased Heart Rate (Pulse) and Blood Pressure

Cyanosis

Cough, Sputum Production, and Hemoptysis

Chest Assessment Findings

- Crackles and wheezing

CLINICAL DATA OBTAINED FROM LABORATORY TESTS AND SPECIAL PROCEDURES

Pulmonary Function Test Findings

Depending on where the malignancy originates, the pulmonary function test (PFT) results may show either obstructive or restrictive values. For example, when the malignancy obstructs major airways, the PFT values may show pathologic obstruction, especially when chronic obstructive pulmonary disease (COPD) is present. However, when large amounts of pulmonary tissue, chest wall, and/or diaphragm are involved (extensive adenocarcinoma), testing may show restrictive PFT values.

Arterial Blood Gases

LOCALIZED (e.g., LOBAR) LUNG CANCER

Acute Alveolar Hyperventilation With Hypoxemia[1]
(Acute Respiratory Alkalosis)

pH	$PaCO_2$	HCO_3^-	PaO_2	SaO_2 or SpO_2
↑	↓	↓	↓	↓
		(but normal)		

EXTENSIVE OR WIDESPREAD LUNG CANCER

Acute Ventilatory Failure With Hypoxemia[2]
(Acute Respiratory Acidosis)

pH[3]	$PaCO_2$	HCO_3^-[3]	PaO_2	SaO_2 or SpO_2
↓	↑	↑	↓	↓
		(but normal)		

Oxygenation Indices[4]

$\dot{Q}_S/\dot{Q}_T$	DO_2[5]	$\dot{V}O_2$	$C(a-\bar{v})O_2$	O_2ER	$S\bar{v}O_2$
↑	↓	N	N	↑	↓

Hemodynamic Indices[6]

When hypoxemia and acidemia are present, or when a tumor invades the mediastinum and compresses the superior vena cava, the following may be expected.

CVP	RAP	$\overline{PA}$	PCWP	CO	SV
↑	↑	↓	↓ or N	↓ or N	↓ or N

SVI	CI	RVSWI	LVSWI	PVR	SVR
↓ or N	↓ or N	↑	↓ or N	↑	N

RADIOLOGIC FINDINGS

Chest Radiograph

- Small oval or coin lesion
- Large irregular mass
- Alveolar consolidation
- Atelectasis
- Pleural effusion (see Chapter 24, Pleural Effusion and Empyema)
- Involvement of the mediastinum or diaphragm

A routine chest radiograph often provides the first indication or suspicion of lung cancer. Depending on how long the tumor has been growing, the chest radiograph may show a small radiodense nodule (called a **coin lesion**) or a large irregular radiodense mass. Unfortunately, by the time a tumor is identified

---

[1]See Fig. 5.2 and Table 5.4 and related discussion for the acute pH, $PaCO_2$, and HCO_3 changes associated with acute alveolar hyperventilation.

[2]See Fig. 5.3 and Table 5.5 and related discussion for the acute pH, $PaCO_2$, and HCO_3^- changes associated with acute and chronic ventilatory failure.
[3]When tissue hypoxia is severe enough to produce lactic acid, the pH and HCO_3^- values will be lower than expected for a particular $PaCO_2$ level.
[4]$C(a-\bar{v})O_2$, Arterial-venous oxygen difference; DO_2, total oxygen delivery; O_2ER, oxygen extraction ratio; $\dot{Q}_S/\dot{Q}_T$, pulmonary shunt fraction; $S\bar{v}O_2$, mixed venous oxygen saturation; $\dot{V}O_2$, oxygen consumption.
[5]The DO_2 may be normal in patients who have compensated to the decreased oxygenation status with (1) an increased cardiac output, (2) an increased hemoglobin level, or (3) a combination of both. When the DO_2 is normal, the O_2ER is usually normal.
[6]CO, Cardiac output; CVP, central venous pressure; LVSWI, left ventricular stroke work index; $\overline{PA}$, mean pulmonary artery pressure; PCWP, pulmonary capillary wedge pressure; PVR, pulmonary vascular resistance; RAP, right atrial pressure; RVSWI, right ventricular stroke work index; SV, stroke volume; SVI, stroke volume index; SVR, systemic vascular resistance.

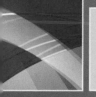
radiographically, regardless of its size, it is usually in the invasive stage and thus difficult to treat. Another common radiographic presentation of lung cancer is that of volume loss involving a single lobe or an individual segment within a lobe.

Because there are four major forms of lung cancer, chest radiograph findings are variable. In general, squamous cell and small cell carcinoma usually appear as a white mass near the hilar region; adenocarcinoma appears in the peripheral portions of the lung; and large cell carcinoma may appear in either the peripheral or the central portion of the lung. Fig. 26.3 is a representative example of a large bronchogenic carcinoma in the right lung. Common secondary chest radiograph findings caused by bronchial obstruction include alveolar consolidation, atelectasis, pleural effusion, and mediastinal or diaphragmatic involvement. The radiograph appearance of cavity formation within a bronchogenic carcinoma is similar regardless of the type of cancer.

Clinically, a **positron emission tomography (PET) scan** is an excellent test to rule out a possible cancerous area identified on either a chest radiograph or a computed tomography (CT) scan. For example, Fig. 26.4 shows a chest radiograph that identifies two suspicious findings—one small nodule in the right upper lung lobe and a larger density in the left lower lung lobe, just behind the heart. Fig. 26.5 shows two CT scans that also identify the two suspicious findings and their precise location. Figs. 26.6, 26.7, and 26.8 show PET scans that all confirm a "hot spot" (likely cancer) in the lower left lobe.

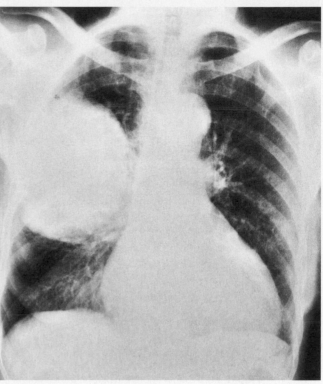

FIGURE 26.3 Right lung squamous cell carcinoma of the bronchus illustrating the huge size these tumors may attain before discovery. (From Hansell, D. M., Lynch, D. A., McAdams, H. P., et al. [2010]. *Imaging of diseases of the chest* [5th ed.]. Philadelphia, PA: Elsevier.)

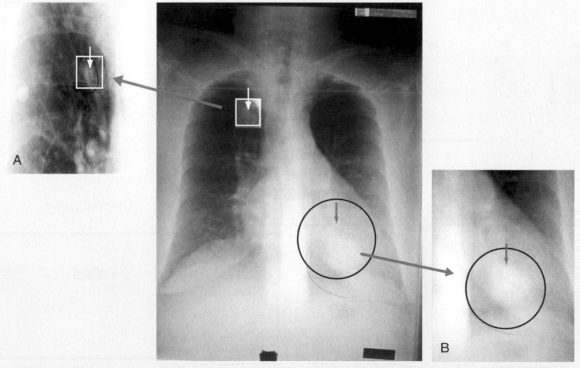

FIGURE 26.4 Chest radiograph identifying two suspicious findings: (A) in the right upper lobe (white arrow) and (B) in the left lower lobe, just behind the heart (blue arrows).

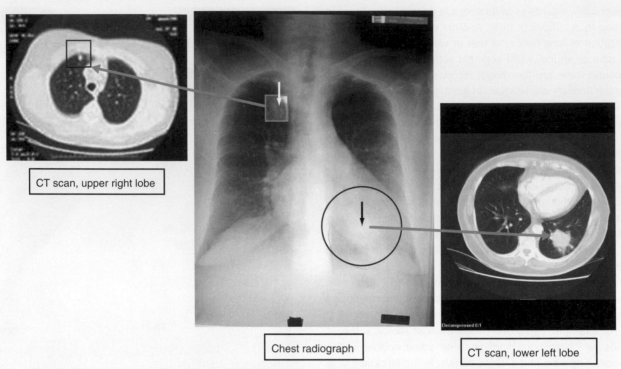

CT scan, upper right lobe

Chest radiograph

CT scan, lower left lobe

FIGURE 26.5 Same chest radiograph as shown in Fig. 26.4 (see blue arrows). Note that the computed tomography (CT) scan also identifies the suspicious nodules and their precise location.

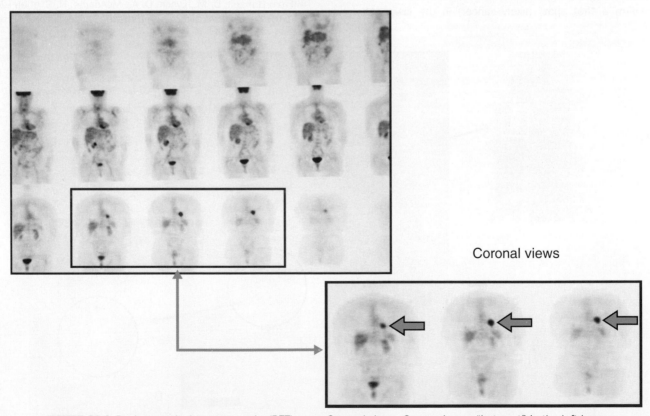

Coronal views

FIGURE 26.6 Positron emission tomography (PET) scan: Coronal views. Scans show a "hot spot" in the left lower lobe.

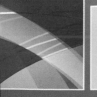
However, the PET scan shown in Fig. 26.9 confirms that the nodule in the right upper lobe is benign (i.e., no "hot spot" is noted).

Finally, the **PET/CT image** provides an image of excellent quality and high sensitivity and specificity in detecting malignant lesions in the chest. Fig. 26.10 shows a CT/PET scan alongside a CT scan and a PET scan; all of the images show the same malignant nodule in the right upper lobe.

BRONCHOSCOPIC FINDINGS

· Bronchial tumor or mass lesion

The fiberoptic bronchoscope may permit direct visualization of a bronchial tumor for further inspection, biopsy, and assessment of the extent of the disease (Fig. 26.11A; see Fig. 9.1).

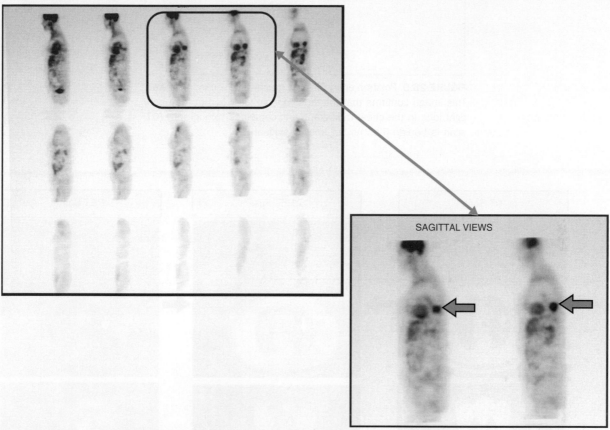

SAGITTAL VIEWS

FIGURE 26.7 Positron emission tomography (PET) scan: Sagittal views. The encircled images show a "hot spot" in the lower left lobe.

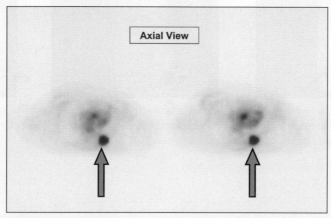

Axial View

FIGURE 26.8 Positron emission tomography (PET) scan: Axial view. A "hot spot" is further confirmed in left lower lobe.

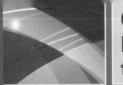

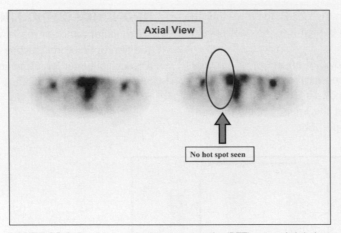

FIGURE 26.9 Positron emission tomography (PET) scan: Axial view. This image confirms that the small nodule identified in the upper right lobe in the chest radiograph and computed tomography (CT) scan is benign (i.e., no hot spot is evident).

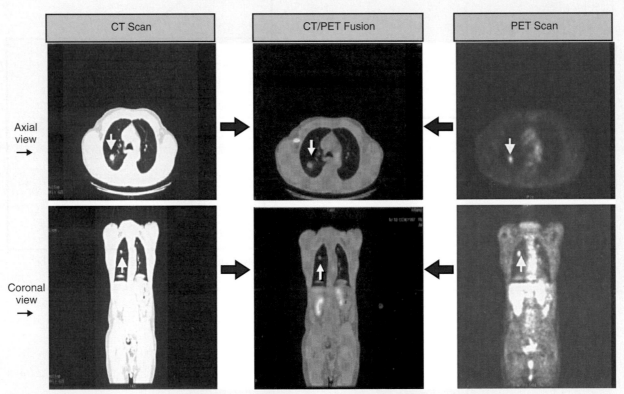

FIGURE 26.10 Computed tomography/positron emission tomography (CT/PET) scan (center). CT scan, CT/PET fusion, and PET scan, all showing the same malignant nodule in right upper lobe (white arrow). Note: CT/PET fusion is normally presented in color (e.g., red, blue, yellow).

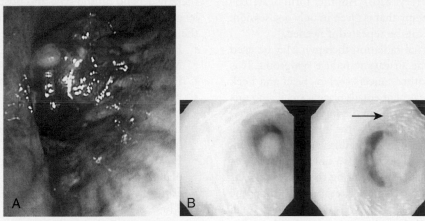

FIGURE 26.11 (A) Bronchoscopic view of a small cell carcinoma tumor protruding into the right mainstem bronchus. (B) A wire stent is in place to help hold the airway open (black arrow).

General Management of Lung Cancer[3]

Treatment Options for Non–Small Cell Lung Cancer

Depending on the stage of the lung cancer and other factors (e.g., the patient's general health conditions), treatment options for NSCLC include the following.

Surgery

Surgery may be an option for early stage NSCLC. Surgery provides the best chance to cure NSCLC. Common surgical procedures include the following:
- **Pneumonectomy:** The entire lung is removed in this surgery.
- **Lobectomy:** An entire section (lobe) of a lung is removed in this surgery.
- **Segmentectomy** or **wedge resection:** A part of a lobe is removed in this surgery.
- **Sleeve resection:** Entails removal of some tumors in the large airways. The airway is completely cut above and below the tumor, and the shortened airway is reattached.
- **Video-assisted thoracic surgery (VATS):** May be used to treat early-stage lung cancers that are located in the pleura and peripheral parts of the lungs. VATS requires a smaller incision than a thoracotomy.

Radiofrequency Ablation

Radiofrequency ablation (RFA) may be used for some small lung tumors near the outer edge of the lungs. RFA entails the use of high-energy radio waves to heat the tumor. A thin, needle-like probe is inserted into the tumor, and, once it is in place, an electric current is passed through the probe, which heats the tumor and destroys the cancer cells.

Radiation Therapy

Radiation therapy uses high-intensity rays (e.g., x-rays) to kill cancer cells. The two primary types of radiation therapy are external beam radiation therapy and brachytherapy (internal radiation therapy).
- **External beam radiation therapy (EBRT):** Directs radiation from outside the body to the cancer cells. EBRT is the most common form of radiation used to treat primary lung cancer or its spread to other organs. As a general rule, EBRT to the lungs is administered 5 days a week for 5 to 7 weeks. Newer EBRT techniques, which treat the lung cancer more accurately while lowering the radiation exposure, offer better success rates and fewer side effects, including the following:
- *Three-dimensional conformal radiation therapy (3D-CRT):* Uses special computers to precisely map the location of the tumor(s). Radiation beams are directed at the tumor(s) from several directions. This technique is less likely to damage surrounding normal tissues.
- *Intensity modulated radiation therapy (IMRT):* A more advanced type of 3D-CRT. IMRT uses a computer-driven device that moves around the patient while it delivers radiation beams. The intensity (strength) of the beams can be adjusted to limit the dose reaching the more sensitive normal tissues. IMRT is most commonly used to treat tumors near important structures such as the spinal cord.
- *Stereotactic body radiation therapy (SBRT), also known as stereotactic ablative radiotherapy (SABR):* Can be used to treat very early stage lung cancers when surgery is not an option (e.g., because of issues with the patient's

---

[3]Modified from the American Cancer Society, http://www.cancer.org.

health or in patients who do not want surgery). SBRT applies very focused beams of high-dose radiation in fewer (1 to 5) treatments. The success rate for smaller tumors has been very promising and appears to have a low risk for complications.

- *Stereotactic radiosurgery (SRS):* Another form of stereotactic radiation therapy that is given in only one session. These treatments can be repeated if needed.
- **Brachytherapy** (internal radiation therapy): May be used to shrink tumors in the airways to reduce symptoms. It is used more often for other cancers such as head and neck cancer. This type of treatment entails placing small amounts of radioactive material (usually in the form of small pellets) via a bronchoscope directly into the tumor or into the airway near the cancer. This procedure also may be performed during surgery. The radiation only travels a short distance from the source, thus limiting the adverse effects on surrounding healthy tissue. After a short time the radiation source is usually removed. Occasionally, small radioactive "seeds" are left in place permanently. The radiation from the seeds decreases over several weeks. Common side effects depend on where the radiation is aimed and can include:
  - Sunburn-like skin problems
  - Hair loss where the radiation enters the body
  - Fatigue
  - Nausea and vomiting
  - Loss of appetite and weight loss

Chemotherapy

Chemotherapy uses anticancer agents that can be injected into a vein or taken orally. Depending on the stage of the NSCLC, chemotherapy may be used (1) before surgery—sometimes along with radiation therapy—to help shrink a tumor; (2) after surgery—sometimes along with radiation therapy—to kill any cancer cells that may still be present after the surgery (called *adjuvant therapy*); (3) along with radiation therapy (concurrent therapy) for tumors that cannot be removed by chemotherapy alone; and (4) as the primary therapy—sometimes along with radiation therapy—for the more advanced cancers or in patients too ill for surgery. Box 26.1 lists chemotherapeutic agents currently used to treat NSCLC. The

---

BOX 26.1 Current Drugs Used to Treat Non–Small Cell Lung Carcinoma

- Cisplatin
- Carboplatin
- Paclitaxel (Taxol)
- Albumin-bound paclitaxel (nab-paclitaxel, Abraxane)
- Docetaxel (Taxotere)
- Gemcitabine (Gemzar)
- Vinorelbine (Navelbine)
- Irinotecan (Camptosar)
- Etoposide (VP-16)
- Velban
- Pemetrexed (Alimta)

---

treatment for NSCLC typically uses a combination of two different chemotherapy drugs—for example, cisplatin or carboplatin plus one other drug.

Possible Side Effects. The possible side effects of chemotherapy depend on the type and dose of drugs given and the length of time they are taken. Common side effects include the following:

- Hair loss
- Mouth sores
- Loss of appetite
- Nausea and vomiting
- Diarrhea or constipation
- Increased chance of infection (from having too few white blood cells)
- Easy bruising or bleeding (from having too few blood platelets)
- Fatigue (from having too few red blood cells)

These side effects are generally short-lived and resolve after treatment is finished.

Targeted Therapy Drugs for Non–Small Cell Lung Cancer

Researchers have had some success with newer drugs that *specifically target the blood vessels that nourish the tumor.* Classifications of targeted therapy drugs for NSCLC are as follows.

Agents That Target Tumor Blood Vessel-Supplying Growth (Angiogenesis). Some targeted drugs, called *angiogenesis inhibitors,* are used to obstruct the new vessels supplying blood to the tumors. These agents include bevacizumab (Avastin) and ramucirumab (Cyramza). Common side effects of these agents include the following:

- Hypertension
- Fatigue
- Bleeding
- Low white blood cell count
- Headaches
- Mouth sores
- Loss of appetite
- Diarrhea

Agents That Target Tumor Cells With Epidermal Growth Factor Receptor Changes. A protein on the surface of cells, epidermal growth factor receptor (EGFR), normally helps the cell grow and divide. Some NSCLC cancer cells have too much EGFR, which makes them grow faster. Agents called EGFR inhibitors may be used to block the cell growth signal. EGFR inhibitors include erlotinib (Tarceva), afatinib (Gilotrif), and gefitinib (Iressa). Necitumumab (Portrazza) is used along with chemotherapy as the first treatment in patients with advanced squamous cell NSCLC.

Agents That Target Cells With *ALK* Gene Changes. Some NSCLC cancer cells have a rearrangement in the gene *ALK*. The condition is most often seen in the nonsmoker who has the adenocarcinoma subtype of NSCLC. The *ALK* gene encodes the development of an abnormal ALK protein that stimulates the cells to grow and spread. Agents that target cells with abnormal ALK protein and help shrink tumors include crizotinib (Xalkori), ceritinib (Zykadia), Alectinib (Alecensa), and brigatinib (Alunbrig).

Agents That Target Cells With *BRAF* Gene Changes. In some NSCLC cases, the tumor cells demonstrate changes in the *BRAF* gene, which helps the cells grow. Agents used to offset this problem include dabrafenib (Tafinlar) and trametinib (Mekinist).

Treatment Options for Small Cell Lung Cancer

Depending on the stage of the lung cancer and other factors (e.g., the patient's general health condition), treatment options for SCLC include chemotherapy, radiation therapy, and surgery.

Chemotherapy

Chemotherapy for SCLC is typically given along with other treatments such as surgery or radiation therapy. For example, for patients with limited stage SCLC, chemotherapy is often administered along with radiation therapy—called *chemoradiation therapy*). For patients with extensive stage SCLC, chemotherapy alone is the typical therapy regimen. However, sometimes radiation therapy also will be given. Common drug combinations used for chemotherapy include the following:

- Cisplatin and etoposide
- Carboplatin and etoposide
- Cisplatin and irinotecan
- Carboplatin and irinotecan

Chemotherapy is given in cycles—for example, a 1- to 3-day period of chemotherapy, followed by a rest period to allow the body to recover. Each cycle lasts about 3 to 4 weeks. The initial treatment usually requires four to six cycles. If the cancer worsens during the treatment or returns after the initial treatment cycles, another treatment cycle may be given with the same chemotherapeutic drugs or other agents may be tried.

Radiation Therapy

Similar to NSCLC, external beam radiation therapy (EBRT) is the most common type of radiation used to treat SCLC. Newer EBRT techniques that are helpful in the treatment of SCLC, while lowering the radiation exposure to nearby healthy tissues, include three-dimensional conformal radiation therapy (3D-CRT) and intensity modulated radiation therapy (IMRT) (see earlier description of these techniques).

Surgery

Surgery is rarely a treatment option for SCLC. Occasionally, surgery may be an option for early stage cancers when a single lung tumor is found, with no lymph node or other organ involvement. Surgery is usually followed by chemotherapy and radiation therapy. Although the surgery options are the same as for NSCLC (i.e., pneumonectomy, lobectomy, segmentectomy or wedge resection, or sleeve resection), a lobectomy is generally the preferred choice for SCLC, if it can be done. This is because a lobectomy offers a better chance of removing all the cancer compared with a segmentectomy or wedge resection.

Respiratory Care Treatment Protocols

Oxygen Therapy Protocol. Oxygen therapy is used to treat hypoxemia, decrease the work of breathing, and decrease myocardial work. Because hypoxemia is associated with lung cancer, supplemental oxygen may be required. However, capillary shunting is common because of the alveolar compression and consolidation often produced by lung cancer. Hypoxemia caused by capillary shunting is often refractory to oxygen therapy (Oxygen Therapy Protocol, Protocol 10.1).

Airway Clearance Therapy Protocol. Because of the excessive mucous production and accumulation associated with lung cancer and some of its treatments, a number of airway clearance therapies may be used to enhance the mobilization of bronchial secretions (Airway Clearance Therapy Protocol, Protocol 10.2).

Lung Expansion Therapy Protocol. Lung expansion techniques are used to offset (at least temporarily) the alveolar compression and consolidation associated with lung cancer (Lung Expansion Therapy Protocol, Protocol 10.3).

Aerosolized Medication Protocol. Aerosolized bronchodilators are often indicated, particularly when COPD and bronchospasm coexist (Aerosolized Medication Protocol, Protocol 10.4).

CASE STUDY Cancer of the Lung

Admitting History

A 66-year-old retired man lives with his wife in a small, two-bedroom ranch house in Peoria, Illinois, during the summer months. During the rest of the year, they live in a 22-foot trailer in a retirement park just outside Las Vegas, Nevada. The trailer park is located conveniently on the casinos' shuttle-bus route; a bus comes by at the top of every hour.

Both the man and his wife are described by their children as addicted gamblers. They gamble almost every day of the year. During the summer months, they play keno and blackjack on the Par-A-Dice Riverboat Casino, which is docked along the shores of the Illinois River in downtown East Peoria. While in Las Vegas, they play bingo, blackjack, and the slot machines at several different casinos. They dress in matching warm-up suits, ride the bus to one of the casinos, and gamble until 10:00 or 11:00 p.m. every day.

Their children, adults with their own families, homes, and jobs in the Peoria area, have been very concerned about their parents' gambling. They have tried to no avail to get their parents to see a compulsive-gambling therapist, who actually is provided by the Par-A-Dice Riverboat Casino. Their children's concern is justified. Their parents are always gambling on a shoestring budget. Although they still own their trailer and small home in Peoria, within the past 2 years they have gambled away most of their life savings, which included stocks, bonds, and mutual funds. Because they let their health insurance premium lapse, their policy was recently cancelled. They still receive a small monthly pension check, and some Social Security income.

Before he retired, the man worked for 17 years as a boiler tender for Methodist Hospital in Peoria. He also was a part-time firefighter. For more than 52 years, he smoked two and a half to three packs of unfiltered cigarettes daily. While in Las Vegas, the man began experiencing periods of dyspnea, coughing, and weakness. His cough was productive of small amounts of clear secretions. Also around this time, his wife first noticed that his voice sounded hoarse.

Although he missed several days of gambling and remained in bed because of weakness, he did not seek medical attention. He hated doctors and thought that he merely had a bad cold and the flu. When he returned to Peoria for the summer, however, the children became concerned and insisted that he see a doctor. Despite the man's lack of health insurance, two medical students from the University of Illinois (who were working in the physician's office as a team) ordered a full diagnostic workup.

A pulmonary function test showed that the man had a combined restrictive and obstructive pulmonary disorder. Lung CT scanning revealed several masses, ranging from 2 to 5 cm in diameter, in the right and left mediastinum at the level of the hilar region. The masses, especially on the right side, also could be seen clearly on the posteroanterior chest radiograph. Both the CT scan and the chest x-ray showed increased opacity consistent with atelectasis of the medial basal segments of the left lower lobe as well.

A bronchoscopic examination was conducted by the pulmonary physician, with the assistance of a respiratory care practitioner trained in special procedures. It showed several large, protruding bronchial masses in the second- and third-generation bronchi of the right lung and in the second-, third-, and fourth-generation bronchi of the left lung. During the bronchoscopy, several mucus plugs were suctioned. Biopsy of three of the larger tumors was positive for squamous cell bronchogenic carcinoma, and the man was admitted to the hospital.

The physician told the patient that he had cancer and that his prognosis was poor. Treatment, at best, would be palliative. The patient asked what the odds were on his life expectancy. The physician stated that the patient had only about a 50%

chance of living longer than 6 to 8 weeks. Surgery was out of the question. In the interim, however, the physician promised to do what was possible to make the man comfortable. The physician outlined a treatment plan of radiation therapy and chemotherapy and requested a respiratory care consultation.

Physical Examination

The respiratory care practitioner reviewed the admitting history information in the patient's chart and found the man sitting up in bed in obvious respiratory distress. He appeared weak. His skin appeared cyanotic, and his face, arms, and chest were damp with perspiration. Wheezing was audible without the aid of a stethoscope. He stated in a hoarse voice that he had coughed up a cup of sputum since breakfast 2 hours earlier. He demonstrated a weak cough every few minutes or so. His cough was productive of large amounts of blood-streaked sputum. The viscosity of the sputum was thin. After each coughing episode, he stated that he wanted a cigarette and then laughed.

His vital signs were blood pressure 155/85 mm Hg, heart rate 90 beats/min, respiratory rate 22 breaths/min, and temperature normal. Palpation was unremarkable. Percussion produced dull notes over the left lower lobe. On auscultation, wheezing and coarse crackles could be heard throughout both lung fields. His arterial blood gas values on 2 L/min oxygen nasal cannula were pH 7.51, $PaCO_2$ 29 mm Hg, HCO_3^- 23 mEq/L, PaO_2 66 mm Hg, and SaO_2 94%. On the basis of these clinical data, the following SOAP was documented.

Respiratory Assessment and Plan

S "I've coughed up a cup of sputum since breakfast."

O Vital signs: BP 155/85, HR 90, RR 22, T normal; perspiring and weak and cyanotic appearance; voice hoarse-sounding; weak cough; large amounts of blood-streaked sputum; dull percussion notes over left lower lobe; wheezing and coarse crackles throughout both lung fields; recent PFTs: restrictive and obstructive pulmonary disorder; CT scan and CXR: 2- to 5-cm masses in right and left mediastinum in hilar regions and atelectasis of left lower lobe. Bronchoscopy: Protruding tumors in both left and right large airways, mucus plugging. Biopsy: Squamous cell bronchogenic carcinoma. ABGs (2 L/min O_2 by nasal cannula): pH 7.51, $PaCO_2$ 29, HCO_3^- 23, PaO_2 66, SaO_2 94%.

A
- Bronchogenic carcinoma (CT scan and biopsy)
- Respiratory distress (vital signs, ABGs)
- Bronchospasm (wheezing)
- Excessive bloody bronchial secretions (sputum, coarse crackles)
- Mucus plugging (bronchoscopy)
- Poor ability to mobilize secretions (weak cough)
- Atelectasis of left lower lobe (CXR)
- Acute alveolar hyperventilation with mild hypoxemia (ABGs)

P Up-regulate Oxygen Therapy Protocol (4 L nasal cannula and titration by oximetry). Also begin Aerosolized Medication Protocol (0.5 mL albuterol in 2 mL NS q6h), followed by Airway Clearance Therapy Protocol (DB&C). Begin Lung Expansion Therapy Protocol (incentive spirometry q2 h and prn). Closely monitor and reevaluate.

Three Days After Admission

A respiratory therapist evaluated the patient during morning rounds. After reviewing the patient's chart, the practitioner went to the patient's bedside and discovered that the man was not tolerating the chemotherapy well. He had been vomiting intermittently for the past 10 hours and was still in obvious respiratory distress. He appeared cyanotic and tired, and his hospital gown was wet from perspiration. His cough was still weak and productive of large amounts of moderately thick, clear, and white sputum. He stated in a hoarse voice that he was still not breathing very well.

His vital signs were blood pressure 166/90 mm Hg, heart rate 95 beats/min, respiratory rate 28 breaths/min, and temperature normal. Dull percussion notes were elicited over both the right and left lower lobes. Wheezing and coarse crackles were auscultated throughout both lung fields. His ABG values on a 4.0 L/min cannula were pH 7.55, $PaCO_2$ 25 mm Hg, HCO_3^- 21 mEq/L/min, PaO_2 53 mm Hg, and SaO_2 92%.

On the basis of these clinical data, the following SOAP was documented.

Respiratory Assessment and Plan

S "I'm still not breathing very well."

O Vital signs: BP 166/90, HR 95, RR 28, T normal; vomiting over past 10 hours; cyanosis, tiredness, and dampness from perspiration; cough: weak and productive of moderately thick, clear, and white sputum; dull percussion notes over both right and left lower lobes; wheezing and coarse crackles over both lung fields; ABGs on a 4 L/min cannula pH 7.55, $PaCO_2$ 25, HCO_3^- 21, PaO_2 53, SaO_2 92%.

A • Bronchogenic carcinoma (previous CT scan and biopsy)
  • Not tolerating chemotherapy well (excessive vomiting)
  • Continued respiratory distress
  • Bronchospasm (wheezing)
  • Excessive bronchial secretions (sputum, coarse crackles)
  • Mucus plugging still likely (previous bronchoscopy, secretions becoming thicker)
  • Poor ability to mobilize secretions (weak cough)
  • Atelectasis of left lower lobes; atelectasis likely in right lower lobe now (CXR, dull percussion notes)
  • Acute alveolar hyperventilation with moderate hypoxemia, worsening (ABGs)
  • Possible impending ventilatory failure (ABGs, weak cough, worsening vital signs)

P Up-regulate Oxygen Therapy Protocol (simple oxygen mask). Up-regulate Aerosolized Medication Protocol (increasing treatment frequency to q3h; consider adding acetylcysteine q6h). Up-regulate Airway Clearance Therapy Protocol (CPT and PD q3h). Up-regulate Lung Expansion Therapy Protocol (change incentive spirometry to +5 to +10 cm H_2O CPAP mask, qid). Contact physician about possible ventilatory failure. Discuss therapeutic bronchoscopy. Closely monitor and reevaluate.

Sixteen Days After Admission

Although the physician's original intention and hope were to discharge the patient soon, stabilizing the man for any length of time proved difficult. Over the next 2 weeks, the patient had continued to be nauseated on a daily basis. He did, however, have occasional periods of relief during which he could breathe easier, but he generally was in respiratory distress. On day 16 the respiratory therapist observed and collected the following clinical data.

The patient was lying in bed in the supine position. His eyes were closed, and he was unresponsive to the therapist's questions. The patient was in obvious respiratory distress. He appeared pale, cyanotic, and diaphoretic. No cough was observed at this time, but coarse crackles could easily be heard from across the patient's room. The nurse in the patient's room stated that the doctor had called the coarse crackles a "death rattle." The patient's vital signs were blood pressure 170/105 mm Hg, heart rate 110 beats/min, respiratory rate 12 breaths/min and shallow, and rectal temperature normal. Percussion was not performed. Wheezing and coarse crackles were heard throughout both lung fields. On an FIO_2 of 0.60, his ABG values were pH 7.28, $PaCO_2$ 63 mm Hg, HCO_3^- 28 mEq/L, PaO_2 66 mm Hg, and SaO_2 89%.

At that time, the following SOAP was recorded.

Respiratory Assessment and Plan

S N/A (patient comatose)

O Unresponsive; pale, cyanotic, and perspiring appearance; no cough noted; coarse crackles heard without stethoscope; vital signs BP 170/105, HR 110, RR 12 and shallow, T normal; wheezing and coarse crackles over both lung fields; ABGs are pH 7.28, $PaCO_2$ 63, HCO_3^- 28, PaO_2 66, SaO_2 89%.

A • Bronchogenic carcinoma (previous CT scan and biopsy)
  • Bronchospasm (wheezing)
  • Excessive bronchial secretions (coarse crackles)
  • Mucus plugging still likely (previous bronchoscopy, coarse crackles)
  • Poor ability to mobilize secretions (no cough)
  • Atelectasis (CXR)
  • Acute ventilatory failure with moderate hypoxemia (ABGs)—worsening

P Contact physician about acute ventilatory failure, and discuss code status; and the need to up-regulate Oxygen Therapy Protocol, Airway Clearance Therapy Protocol, and Aerosolized Medication Therapy Protocol. Monitor and reevaluate.

Discussion

This case demonstrates the few specific treatments that a respiratory therapist can bring to the care of patients with lung cancer. Specifically, it illustrates that most of the patients who have concomitant obstructive pulmonary disease have a need for a good Airway Clearance Therapy Protocol (Protocol 10.2). Comfort of the patient must be kept in mind at all times.

The first assessment was performed soon after bronchoscopy and diagnosis. The patient's blood-stained sputum could have reflected the primary tumor or, as likely, bleeding from the bronchoscopy sites. In such cases the practitioner must monitor this sputum as the days go along. No improvement in the patient's wheezing can be expected if a bronchial tumor is the cause, but it may improve if bronchospasm (from cigarette smoking) is the causative factor.

The wheezing and coarse crackles indicated the need for vigorous airway clearance therapy. The atelectasis in the left lower lobe suggested that a trial of careful Lung Expansion Therapy Protocol (Protocol 10.3) and Aerosolized Medication Therapy Protocol (Protocol 10.4) were in order. The ABG values assessed with the patient on 2 L/min oxygen showed acute alveolar hyperventilation with moderate hypoxemia. At this time, the patient's oxygen therapy was up-regulated to a 4 L/min nasal cannula. Certainly, a trial of oxygen therapy via an air-entrainment mask (or nonrebreathing mask) also would have been appropriate. Patient anxiety may be alleviated with appropriate treatment of the hypoxemia.

The second assessment revealed that the patient may have developed atelectasis in both the right and left lower lobes (where the tumor masses had been noted previously). This case may present a setting in which therapeutic bronchoscopy or laser-assisted endobronchial resection of the tumor masses may be helpful. The patient continued to be hypoxemic, despite alveolar hyperventilation. A higher FIO_2 (e.g., through a Venturi oxygen mask) was indicated.

Vigorous suctioning was appropriate. Because of the impending ventilatory failure, ordering at least one cycle of ventilator support, perhaps in the form of noninvasive positive pressure ventilation (see Chapter 11, Respiratory Insufficiency, Respiratory Failure, and Ventilatory Management Protocols), for such a patient would not be surprising given that he had just recently received radiation and chemotherapy. The patient's wishes in this respect should have been checked against his Living Will or Durable Power of Attorney for Health Care (**end-of-life directives**), if such a document existed.

The last assessment indicates that the patient had slipped into acute ventilatory failure. All health care personnel had agreed that the patient was close to death. The practitioner may be excused for not suggesting the use of chest physical therapy and postural drainage at this time, because of the patient's wishes. **Aerosolized morphine** is now being used to relieve dyspnea in terminally ill cancer patients. If, however, aggressive therapy was still in order, formal evaluation and treatment of superimposed atelectasis or pneumonia, or both, would be in order.

SELF-ASSESSMENT QUESTIONS

1. Which of the following is commonly located near a central bronchus or hilus and projects into the large bronchi?
   a. Squamous cell carcinoma
   b. Oat cell carcinoma
   c. Large cell carcinoma
   d. Adenocarcinoma

2. Which of the following arises from the mucous glands of the tracheobronchial tree?
   a. Small cell carcinoma
   b. Adenocarcinoma
   c. Squamous cell carcinoma
   d. Oat cell carcinoma

3. Which of the following carcinomas has the strongest correlation with cigarette smoking?
   a. Adenocarcinoma
   b. Small cell carcinoma
   c. Large cell carcinoma
   d. Squamous cell carcinoma

4. Which of the following has the fastest growth (doubling) rate?
   a. Large cell carcinoma
   b. Small cell carcinoma
   c. Adenocarcinoma
   d. Squamous cell carcinoma

5. Which of the following is(are) associated with bronchogenic carcinoma?
   1. Alveolar consolidation
   2. Pleural effusion
   3. Alveolar hyperinflation
   4. Atelectasis
   a. 2 and 3 only
   b. 1 and 4 only
   c. 2 and 3 only
   d. 1, 2, and 4 only

CHAPTER

27 Interstitial Lung Diseases

Chapter Objectives

After reading this chapter, you will be able to:

- List the anatomic alterations of the lungs associated with chronic interstitial lung disease.
- Describe the causes of chronic interstitial lung disease.
- List the cardiopulmonary clinical manifestations associated with chronic interstitial lung disease.
- Describe the general management of chronic interstitial lung disease.
- Describe the clinical strategies and rationales of the SOAPs presented in the case study.
- Define key terms and complete self-assessment questions at the end of the chapter and on Evolve

Key Terms

Allergic Alveolitis
Angiotensin Converting Enzyme (ACE Test)
Asbestos
Asbestosis
Beryllium
Berylliosis
Black Lung
Bronchial Lavage
Bronchiolitis Obliterans Organizing Pneumonia (BOOP)
Caplan Syndrome
Chronic Eosinophilic Pneumonia
Churg-Strauss Syndrome
Coal Miner Lung
Coal Worker Pneumoconiosis (CWP)
Connective Tissue (Collagen Vascular) Disorders
Cryptogenic Organizing Pneumonia (COP)
Desquamative Interstitial Pneumonia (DIP)
Extrinsic Allergic Alveolitis
Farmer Lung
Focal Emphysema
Glomerular Basement Membrane
Goodpasture Syndrome
Hemoptysis
Honeycombing
Hypersensitivity Pneumonitis
Idiopathic Pulmonary Fibrosis (IPF)
Idiopathic Pulmonary Hemosiderosis
Interstitial Lung Disease (ILD)
Late Fibrotic Phase

Lymphangioleiomyomatosis (LAM)
Lymphocytic Interstitial Pneumonia (LIP)
Lymphomatoid Granulomatosis
Mononeuritus Multiplex
Plasmapheresis
Pleural Calcifications
Pneumoconiosis
Polymyositis-Dermatomyositis
Progressive Massive Fibrosis (PMF)
Progressive Systemic Sclerosis (PSS)
Pulmonary Alveolar Proteinosis
Pulmonary Langerhans Cell Histiocytosis (PLCH)
Pulmonary Vasculitides
Quartz Silicosis (Grinder Disease)
Rheumatoid Pneumoconiosis
Sarcoidosis
Scleroderma
Silica
Silicosis
Sjögren Syndrome
Systemic Lupus Erythematosus (SLE)
Usual Interstitial Pneumonia (UIP)
Wegener Granulomatosis

Chapter Outline

Anatomic Alterations of the Lungs
Etiology and Epidemiology
   Interstitial Lung Diseases of Known Causes or
      Associations
   Systemic Diseases
   Idiopathic Interstitial Pneumonias
   Specific Pathology
   Miscellaneous Diffuse Interstitial Lung Diseases
Overview of the Cardiopulmonary Clinical Manifestations
   Associated With Chronic Interstitial Lung Diseases
General Management of Interstitial Lung Disease
   Medications and Procedures Commonly Prescribed by
      the Physician
   Respiratory Care Treatment Protocols
   Other Treatment
Case Study: Interstitial Lung Disease
Self-Assessment Questions

The term **interstitial lung disease (ILD)** (also called *diffuse interstitial lung disease, fibrotic interstitial lung disease,* and *pulmonary fibrosis*) refers to a broad group of inflammatory lung disorders. More than 180 disease entities are characterized by acute, subacute, or chronic inflammatory infiltration of alveolar walls by cells, fluid, and connective tissue. If left untreated, the inflammatory process can progress to irreversible pulmonary fibrosis. The ILD group consists of a wide range of illnesses with varied causes, treatments, and prognoses. However, because the ILDs all reflect similar anatomic alterations of the lungs and therefore cardiopulmonary clinical manifestations, they are presented as a group in this chapter.

Anatomic Alterations of the Lungs

The anatomic alterations of ILD may involve the bronchi, alveolar walls, and adjacent alveolar spaces. In severe cases the extensive inflammation leads to pulmonary fibrosis, granulomas, **honeycombing**, and cavitation. During the acute stage of any ILD, the general inflammatory condition is characterized by edema and the infiltration of a variety of white blood cells (e.g., neutrophils, eosinophils, basophils, monocytes, macrophages, and lymphocytes) in the alveolar walls and interstitial spaces (Fig. 27.1A). Bronchial inflammation and thickening and increasing airway secretions also may be present.

During the chronic stage, the general inflammatory response is also characterized by the infiltration of large numbers of various white blood cells (especially monocytes, macrophages, and lymphocytes) and some fibroblasts may be present in the alveolar walls and interstitial spaces. This stage may be followed

by further interstitial thickening, fibrosis, granulomas, and, in some cases, honeycombing and cavity formation. Pleural effusion may be present. In the chronic stages the basic pathologic features of interstitial fibrosis are identical in any interstitial lung disorder (so-called *end-stage pulmonary fibrosis*).

As a general rule the interstitial lung disorders produce restrictive lung conditions. However, because bronchial inflammation and excessive airway secretions can develop in the small airways, the clinical manifestations associated with an obstructive lung disorder also may be seen. Therefore the patient with ILD may demonstrate a restrictive disorder, an obstructive disorder, or a combination of both.

The major pathologic or structural changes associated with chronic ILDs are as follows:
- Destruction of the alveoli and adjacent pulmonary capillaries
- Fibrotic thickening of the respiratory bronchioles, alveolar ducts, and alveoli
- Granulomas
- Honeycombing and cavity formation
- Fibrocalcific pleural plaques (particularly in asbestosis)
- Bronchospasm
- Excessive bronchial secretions (caused by inflammation of airways)

Etiology and Epidemiology

Because there are more than 180 different pulmonary disorders classified as ILD, it is helpful to group them according to their occupational or environmental exposure, disease associations, and specific pathology. Table 27.1 provides an overview

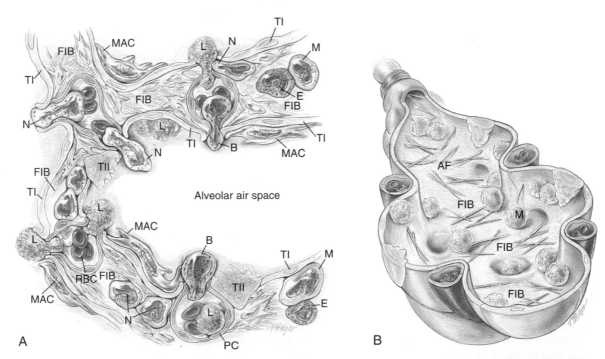

FIGURE 27.1 (A) Interstitial lung disease. Cross-sectional microscopic view of alveolar-capillary unit. *B,* Basophil; *E,* eosinophil; *FIB,* fibroblast (fibrosis); *L,* lymphocyte; *M,* monocyte; *MAC,* macrophage; *N,* neutrophil; *PC,* pulmonary capillary; *RBC,* red blood cell; *TI,* type I alveolar cell; *TII,* type II alveolar cell. (B) Asbestosis (close-up of one alveolar unit). *AF,* Asbestos fiber; *FIB,* fibrosis; *M,* macrophage.

TABLE 27.1 Overview of Interstitial Lung Diseases

Occupational, Environmental, and Therapeutic Exposures	Systemic Diseases	Idiopathic Interstitial Pneumonia	Specific Pathology	Miscellaneous ILDs
Occupation/Environmental	**Connective Tissue Disease**	• Idiopathic pulmonary fibrosis	• Lymphangioleiomyomatosis (LAM)	• Goodpasture syndrome
Inorganic Substance Exposure	• Scleroderma	• Nonspecific cryptogenic organizing pneumonia (BOOP)	• Pulmonary Langerhans cell histiocytosis	• Idiopathic pulmonary hemosiderosis
• Asbestosis	• Rheumatoid arthritis	• Lymphocytic interstitial pneumonia (LIP)	• Pulmonary alveolar proteinosis	• Chronic eosinophilic pneumonia
• Coal dust	• Sjögren syndrome		• The pulmonary vasculitides	
• Silica	• Polymyositis or dermatomyositis		• Wegener granulomatosis	
• Beryllium	• Systemic lupus erythematosus		• Churg-Strauss syndrome	
• Aluminum			• Lymphomatoid granulomatosis	
• Barium	**Sarcoidosis**			
• Clay				
• Iron				
• Certain talcs				
Organic Exposure				
• Hypersensitivity pneumonitis				
• Moldy hay				
• Silage				
• Moldy sugar cane				
• Mushroom compost				
• Barley				
• Cheese				
• Wood pulp, bark, dust				
• Cork dust				
• Bird droppings				
• Paints				
Medications and Illicit Drugs				
• Antibiotics				
• Antiinflammatory agents				
• Cardiovascular agents				
• Chemotherapeutic agents				
• Drug-induced systemic lupus erythematosus				
• Illicit drugs				
Radiation Therapy				
Irritant Gases				

of common ILD groups. A discussion of the more common ILDs follows.

Interstitial Lung Diseases of Known Causes or Associations (Pneumoconioses)

Occupational, Environmental, and Therapeutic Exposures

Inorganic Particulate (Dust) Exposure

Asbestos. Exposure to **asbestos** may cause **asbestosis**, a common form of ILD. Asbestos fibers are a mixture of fibrous minerals composed of hydrous silicates of magnesium, sodium, and iron in various proportions. There are two primary types: the amphiboles (crocidolite, amosite, and anthophyllite) and chrysotile (most commonly used in industry). Asbestos fibers typically range from 50 to 100 μm in length and are about 0.5 μm in diameter. The chrysotiles have the longest and strongest fibers. Box 27.1 lists common sources associated with asbestos fibers.

As shown in Fig. 27.1B, asbestos fibers can be seen by microscope within the thickened septa as brown or orange batonlike structures. The fibers characteristically stain for iron with Perls stain. The pathologic process may affect only one lung, a lobe, or a segment of a lobe, although multilobe involvement is the most common. The lower lobes are most commonly affected. **Pleural calcification** is common and diagnostic in patients with an asbestos exposure history (see Fig. 27.5).

Coal Dust. The pulmonary deposition and accumulation of large amounts of coal dust cause **coal worker pneumoconiosis (CWP)** (Fig. 27.2). CWP is also known as **coal miner lung** and **black lung**. Miners who use cutting machines at the coalface have the greatest exposure, but even relatively minor exposures may result in the disease. Indeed, cases have been reported in which coal miners' wives developed the disease, presumably from shaking the dust from their husbands' work clothes.

Simple CWP is characterized by the presence of pinpoint nodules called *coal macules (black spots)* throughout the lungs.

The coal macules often develop around the first- and second-generation respiratory bronchioles and cause the adjacent alveoli to retract. This condition is called **focal emphysema**.

Complicated CWP or **progressive massive fibrosis (PMF)** is characterized by areas of fibrotic nodules greater than 1 cm in diameter. The fibrotic nodules generally appear in the peripheral regions of upper lobes and extend toward the hilum with growth. The nodules are composed of dense collagenous tissue with black pigmentation. Coal dust by itself is chemically inert. The fibrotic changes in CWP are usually caused by **silica**.

Silica. **Silicosis** (also called **quartz silicosis or grinder disease**) is caused by the chronic inhalation of crystalline, free silica, or silicon dioxide particles. Silica is the main component of more than 95% of the rocks of the earth. It is found in sandstone, quartz (beach sand is mostly quartz), flint, granite, many hard rocks, and some clays.

Simple silicosis is characterized by small rounded nodules scattered throughout the lungs. No single nodule is greater than 9 mm in diameter. Patients with simple silicosis are usually symptom-free.

Complicated silicosis is characterized by nodules that coalesce and form large masses of fibrous tissue, usually in the upper lobes and perihilar regions. In severe cases the fibrotic regions may undergo tissue necrosis and cavitate. Box 27.2 lists common occupations associated with silica exposure.

Beryllium. **Beryllium** is a steel-gray, lightweight metal found in certain plastics and ceramics, rocket fuels, and x-ray tubes. As a raw ore, beryllium is not hazardous. When it is processed into the pure metal or one of its salts, however, it may cause a tissue reaction when inhaled into the lungs or implanted into the skin. The acute inhalation of beryllium fumes or particles may cause a toxic or allergic pneumonitis

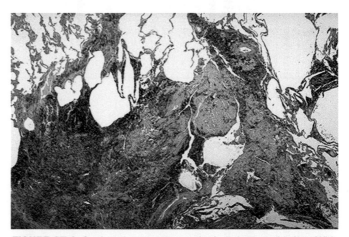

FIGURE 27.2 Coal worker pneumoconiosis, microscopic view. With massive amounts of inhaled particles (as in black lung disease in coal miners), a fibrogenic response can be elicited to produce the coal worker's pneumoconiosis with the coal macule seen here. Progressive massive fibrosis results. (From Klatt, E. [2010]. *Robbins and Cotran atlas of pathology* [2nd ed.]. Philadelphia, PA: Elsevier.)

BOX 27.1 Common Sources Associated With Asbestos Fibers

- Acoustic products
- Automobile undercoating
- Brake lining
- Cements
- Clutch casings
- Floor tiles
- Fire-fighting suits
- Fireproof paints
- Insulation
- Roofing materials
- Ropes
- Steam pipe material

BOX 27.2 Common Occupations Associated With Silica Exposure

- Tunneling
- Hard-rock mining
- Sandblasting
- Quarrying
- Stonecutting
- Foundry work
- Ceramics work
- Abrasives work
- Brick making
- Paint making
- Polishing
- Stone drilling
- Well drilling

BOX 27.3 Additional Inorganic Causes of Interstitial Lung Disease

- Aluminum
  - Ammunition workers
- Baritosis (barium)
  - Barite millers and miners
  - Ceramic workers
- Kalonosis (clay)
  - Brickmakers and potters
  - Ceramics workers
- Siderosis (iron)
  - Welders
- Talcosis (certain talcs)
  - Ceramics workers
  - Papermakers
  - Plastics and rubber workers

sometimes accompanied by rhinitis, pharyngitis, and tracheobronchitis. The more complex form of **berylliosis** is characterized by the development of granulomas and a diffuse interstitial inflammatory reaction.

Other Inorganic Causes. Box 27.3 lists other inorganic causes of ILD.

Organic Materials Exposure

Hypersensitivity Pneumonitis. Hypersensitivity pneumonitis (also called **allergic alveolitis** or **extrinsic allergic alveolitis**) is a cell-mediated immune response of the lungs caused by the inhalation of a variety of offending agents or antigens. Such antigens include grains, silage, bird droppings or feathers, wood dust (especially redwood and maple), cork dust, animal pelts, coffee beans, fish meal, mushroom compost, and molds that grow on sugar cane, barley, and straw. The immune response to these allergens results in the production of antibodies and an inflammatory response. The lung inflammation, or pneumonitis, develops after repeated and prolonged exposure to the allergen. The term *hypersensitivity pneumonitis* (or *allergic alveolitis*) is often renamed according to the type of exposure that caused the lung disorder. For example, the hypersensitivity pneumonitis caused by the inhalation of moldy hay is called **farmer lung**. Table 27.2 provides common causes, exposure sources, and disease syndromes associated with hypersensitivity pneumonitis.

Medications and Illicit Drugs. As the list of medications and illicit drugs continues to grow, so does the list of possible side effects (Box 27.4). Unfortunately, the lungs are a major target organ affected by these side effects. Although it is impossible to discuss in detail the various lung-related side effects of every drug, it is possible to describe some of the general concerns related to drug-induced lung disease and to list some of the pharmacologic agents that may be responsible.

The chemotherapeutics (anticancer agents) are by far the largest group of agents associated with ILD. Bleomycin, mitomycin, busulfan, cyclophosphamide, methotrexate, and carmustine (BCNU) are the major offenders. Nitrofurantoin

(an antibacterial drug used in the treatment of urinary tract infections) is also associated with ILD. Gold and penicillamine for the treatment of rheumatoid arthritis also have been shown to cause ILD. The excessive long-term administration of oxygen (oxygen toxicity) is known to cause diffuse pulmonary injury and fibrosis (see Chapter 11, Respiratory Insufficiency, Respiratory Failure, and Ventilatory Management Protocols). As a general rule, the risk for these drugs causing an interstitial lung disorder is directly related to the cumulative dosage. However, drug-induced interstitial disease may be seen as early as 1 month to as late as several years after exposure to these agents.

The precise cause of drug-induced ILD is not known. Diagnosis is confirmed by an open lung biopsy. When interstitial fibrosis is found with no infectious organisms or known industrial exposure, a drug-induced interstitial process must be suspected.

Radiation Therapy. Radiation therapy in the management of cancer may cause ILD. Radiation-induced lung disease is commonly divided into two major phases: the **acute pneumonitic phase** and the **late fibrotic phase**. Acute pneumonitis is rarely seen in patients who receive a total radiation dose of less than 3500 rad. By contrast, doses in excess of 6000 rad over 6 weeks almost always cause ILD in and near the radiated areas. The acute pneumonitic phase develops about 2 to 3 months after exposure. Chronic radiation fibrosis is seen in all patients who develop acute pneumonitis.

The late phase of fibrosis may develop (1) immediately after the development of acute pneumonitis, (2) without an acute pneumonitic period, or (3) after a symptom-free latent period. When fibrosis does develop, it generally does so 6 to 12 months after radiation exposure. Pleural effusion is often associated with the late fibrotic phase.

The precise cause of radiation-induced lung disease is not known. The establishment of a diagnosis is similar to that for drug-induced interstitial disease (i.e., by obtaining a history of recent radiation therapy and confirming the diagnosis with an open lung biopsy).

TABLE 27.2 Causes of Hypersensitivity Pneumonitis

Antigen	Exposure Source	Disease Syndrome
Bacteria, Thermophilic		
Saccharopolyspora rectivirgula	Moldy hay, silage	Farmer lung
Thermoactinomyces vulgaris	Moldy sugarcane	Bagassosis
Thermoactinomyces sacchari	Mushroom compost	Mushroom worker lung
Thermoactinomyces candidus	Heated water reservoirs	Air conditioner lung
Bacteria, Nonthermophilic		
Bacillus subtilis, Bacillus cereus	Water, detergent	Humidifier lung, washing powder lung
Fungi		
Aspergillus sp.	Moldy hay	Farmer lung
	Water	Ventilation pneumonitis
Aspergillus clavatus	Barley	Malt worker lung
Penicillium casiei, P. roqueforti	Cheese	Cheese washer lung
Alternaria sp.	Wood pulp	Woodworker lung
Cryptostroma corticale	Wood bark	Maple bark stripper lung
Graphium, Aureobasidium pullulans	Wood dust	Sequoiosis
Merulius lacrymans	Rotten wood	Dry root lung
Penicillium frequentans	Cork dust	Suberosis
Aureobasidium pullulans	Water	Humidifier lung
Cladosporium sp.	Hot tub mist	Hot tub HP*
Trichosporon cutaneum	Damp wood and mats	Japanese summer-type HP*
Amoebae		
Naegleria gruberi	Contaminated water	Humidifier lung
Acanthamoeba polyphaga	Contaminated water	Humidifier lung
Acanthamoeba castellanii	Contaminated water	Humidifier lung
Animal Proteins		
Avian proteins	Bird droppings, feathers	Bird-breeder lung
Urine, serum, pelts	Rats, gerbils	Animal handler lung
Chemicals		
Isocyanates, trimellitic anhydride	Paints, resins, plastics	Chemical worker lung
Copper sulfate	Bordeaux mixture	Vineyard sprayer lung
Phthalic anhydride	Heated epoxy resin	Epoxy resin lung
Sodium diazobenzene sulfate	Chromatography reagent	Pauli reagent alveolitis
Pyrethrum	Pesticide	Pyrethrum HP*

From Selman, M. (2003). Hypersensitivity pneumonitis. In Schwarz, M. I., & Kin, T. E. (Eds.), *Interstitial lung disease* (4th ed.). Hamilton, Ontario, Canada: BC Decker.
*HP, Hypersensitivity pneumonitis.

Irritant Gases. The inhalation of irritant gases may cause acute chemical pneumonitis and, in severe cases, ILD. Most exposures occur in an industrial setting. Table 27.3 lists some of the more common irritant gases and the industrial settings where they may be found.

Systemic Diseases

Connective Tissue (Collagen Vascular) Diseases

Scleroderma. **Scleroderma** is characterized by chronic hardening and thickening of the skin caused by new collagen formation. It may occur in a localized form or as a systemic disorder (called *systemic sclerosis*). **Progressive systemic sclerosis (PSS)** is a relatively rare autoimmune disorder that affects the blood vessels and connective tissue. It causes fibrous degeneration of the connective tissue of the skin, lungs,

TABLE 27.3 Common Irritant Gases Associated With Interstitial Lung Disease

Gas	Industrial Setting
Chlorine	Chemical and plastic industries; water disinfection
Ammonia	Commercial refrigeration; smelting of sulfide ores
Ozone	Welding
Nitrogen dioxide	May be liberated after exposure of nitric acid to air
Phosgene	Used in the production of aniline dyes

- Antibiotics
  - Nitrofurantoin
  - Sulfasalazine
- Antiinflammatory agents
  - Aspirin
  - Gold
  - Penicillamine
  - Methotrexate
  - Etanercept
  - Infliximab
- Cardiovascular agents
  - Amiodarone
  - Tocainide
- Chemotherapeutic agents
  - Bleomycin
  - Mitomycin-C
  - Busulfan
  - Cyclophosphamide
  - Chlorambucil
  - Melphalan
  - Azathioprine
  - Cytosine arabinoside
  - Methotrexate
  - Procarbazine
  - Zinostatin
  - Etoposide
  - Vinblastine
  - Imatinib
  - Flutamide
- Drug-induced systemic lupus erythematosus
  - Procainamide
  - Isoniazid
  - Hydralazine
  - Hydantoins
  - Penicillamine
- Illicit drugs (controlled substances)
  - Heroin
  - Methadone
  - Propoxyphene
  - Talc as an intravenous contaminant
- Miscellaneous agents
  - Oxygen
  - Drugs inducing pulmonary infiltrates and eosinophilia: L-tryptophan
  - Hydrochlorothiazide
  - Radiation

From Camus, P. (2003). Drug-induced infiltrative lung diseases. In Schwarz, M. I., & King, T. E. (Eds.), *Interstitial lung disease* (4th ed.). Hamilton, Ontario, Canada: BC Decker.

and internal organs, especially the esophagus, digestive tract, and kidney.

Scleroderma of the lung appears in the form of ILD and fibrosis. Of all the **collagen vascular disorders**, scleroderma is the one in which pulmonary involvement is most severe and most likely to cause significant scarring of the lung parenchyma

(see Fig. 27.3). The pulmonary complications include diffuse interstitial fibrosis, severe pulmonary hypertension, pleural disease, and aspiration pneumonitis (secondary to esophageal involvement). Scleroderma also may involve the small pulmonary blood vessels and appears to be independent of the fibrotic process involving the alveolar walls. The disease is most commonly seen in women 30 to 50 years of age.

Rheumatoid Arthritis. Rheumatoid arthritis is primarily an inflammatory joint disease. It may, however, involve the lungs in the form of (1) pleurisy, with or without effusion; (2) interstitial pneumonitis; (3) necrobiotic nodules, with or without cavities; (4) Caplan syndrome; and (5) pulmonary hypertension secondary to pulmonary vasculitis.

Pleurisy with or without effusion is the most common pulmonary complication associated with rheumatoid arthritis. When present, the effusion is generally unilateral (often on the right side) (see Fig. 27.9). Men appear to develop rheumatoid pleural complications more often than women. Rheumatoid interstitial pneumonitis is characterized by alveolar wall fibrosis, interstitial and intraalveolar mononuclear cell infiltration, and lymphoid nodules. In severe cases, extensive fibrosing alveolitis and honeycombing may develop. Rheumatoid interstitial pneumonitis is also more common in male patients. Necrobiotic nodules are characterized by the gradual degeneration and swelling of lung tissue.

The pulmonary nodules generally appear as well-circumscribed masses that often progress to cavitation. The nodules usually develop in the periphery of the lungs and are more common in men. Histologically, the pulmonary nodules are identical to the subcutaneous nodules that develop in rheumatoid arthritis.

Caplan syndrome (also called **rheumatoid pneumoconiosis**) is a progressive pulmonary fibrosis of the lung commonly seen in coal miners. Caplan syndrome is characterized by rounded densities in the lung periphery that often undergo cavity formation and, in some cases, calcification. Pulmonary hypertension is a common secondary complication caused by the progression of fibrosing alveolitis and pulmonary vasculitis.

Sjögren Syndrome. **Sjögren syndrome** is a lymphocytic infiltration that primarily involves the salivary and lacrimal glands and manifests by dry mucous membranes, usually of the mouth and eyes. Pulmonary involvement frequently occurs in Sjögren syndrome and includes (1) pleurisy with or without effusion, (2) interstitial fibrosis that is indistinguishable from that of other collagen vascular disorders, and (3) infiltration of lymphocytes of the tracheobronchial mucous glands, which in turn causes atrophy of the mucous glands, mucous plugging, atelectasis, and secondary infections. Sjögren syndrome occurs most often in women (90%) and is commonly associated with rheumatoid arthritis (50% of patients with Sjögren syndrome).

Polymyositis-Dermatomyositis. *Polymyositis* is a diffuse inflammatory disorder of the striated muscles that primarily weakens the limbs, neck, and pharynx. *Dermatomyositis* is the term used when an erythematous skin rash accompanies the muscle weakness. Pulmonary involvement develops in response to (1) recurrent episodes of aspiration pneumonia caused by esophageal weakness and atrophy, (2) hypostatic pneumonia secondary to a weakened diaphragm, and (3) drug-induced interstitial pneumonitis.

Polymyositis-dermatomyositis is seen more often in women than men, at about a 2:1 ratio. The disease occurs primarily in two age groups: before the age of 10 years and from 40 to 50 years of age. In about 40% of the patients, the pulmonary manifestations are seen 1 to 24 months before the striated muscle or skin shows signs or symptoms.

Systemic lupus erythematosus (SLE) is a multisystem disorder that mainly involves the joints and skin. It also may cause serious problems in numerous other organs, including the kidneys, lungs, nervous system, and heart. Involvement of the lungs appears in about 50% to 70% of cases. Pulmonary manifestations are characterized by (1) pleurisy with or without effusion, (2) atelectasis, (3) diffuse infiltrates and pneumonitis, (4) diffuse ILD, (5) uremic pulmonary edema, (6) diaphragmatic dysfunction, and (7) infections.

Pleurisy with or without effusion is the most common pulmonary complication of SLE. The effusions are usually exudates with high protein concentration and are frequently bilateral. Atelectasis commonly develops in response to the pleurisy, effusion, and diaphragmatic elevation associated with SLE. Diffuse noninfectious pulmonary infiltrates and pneumonitis are common. In severe cases, chronic interstitial pneumonitis may develop. Because SLE frequently impairs the renal system, uremic pulmonary edema may occur. SLE also has been found to be associated with diaphragmatic dysfunction and reduced lung volumes. Some research suggests that a diffuse myopathy affecting the diaphragm is the source of this problem. About 50% of cases have a complicating pulmonary infection.

Sarcoidosis. **Sarcoidosis** is a relatively common chronic disorder of unknown origin characterized by the formation of tubercles of nonnecrotizing epithelioid tissue (noncaseating granulomas). Common sites are the eyes, lungs, spleen, liver, skin, mucous membranes, and lacrimal and salivary glands, usually with the involvement of the lymph glands. The lung is the most frequently affected organ, with manifestations generally including ILD, enlargement of the mediastinal lymph nodes, or a combination of both (see Fig. 27.7). One of the clinical laboratory hallmarks of sarcoidosis is an increase in all three major immunoglobulins (IgM, IgG, and IgA). Also common is an elevation of the **angiotensin converting enzyme (ACE test)**. The disease is more common among African-Americans and appears most frequently in patients 10 to 40 years of age, with the highest incidence at age 20 to 30. Women are affected more often than men, especially among African-Americans.

Idiopathic Interstitial Pneumonias

Some patients with ILD do not have a readily identified specific exposure, a systemic disorder, or an underlying genetic cause. Such conditions are commonly placed in the idiopathic interstitial pneumonia (ILD) group or the group with other specific pathology.

Idiopathic Pulmonary Fibrosis

Idiopathic pulmonary fibrosis (IPF) is a progressive inflammatory disease with varying degrees of fibrosis and, in severe cases, honeycombing. The precise cause is unknown. Although *idiopathic pulmonary fibrosis* is the term most frequently used for this disorder, numerous other names appear in the literature, such as *acute interstitial fibrosis of the lung, cryptogenic fibrosing alveolitis, Hamman-Rich syndrome, honeycomb lung, interstitial fibrosis,* and *interstitial pneumonitis.*

IPF is commonly separated into the following two major disease entities according to it's predominant histologic appearance: **desquamative interstitial pneumonia (DIP)** and **usual interstitial pneumonia (UIP)**. In DIP the most prominent features are hyperplasia and desquamation of the alveolar type II cells. The alveolar spaces are packed with macrophages, and there is an even distribution of the interstitial mononuclear infiltrate.

In UIP the most prominent features are interstitial and alveolar wall thickening caused by chronic inflammatory cells and fibrosis. In severe cases, fibrotic connective tissue replaces the alveolar walls, the alveolar architecture becomes distorted, and eventually honeycombing develops. When honeycombing is present, the inflammatory infiltrate is significantly reduced. The prognosis for patients with DIP is significantly better than that for patients with UIP.

Some experts think DIP and UIP are two distinct ILD entities. Others, however, think DIP and UIP are different stages of the same disease process. IPF is most commonly seen in men 40 to 70 years of age. Diagnosis is generally confirmed by an open lung biopsy. Most patients diagnosed with IPF have a more chronic progressive course, and death usually occurs in 4 to 10 years. Death usually is the result of progressive acute ventilatory failure, complicated by pulmonary infection.

Cryptogenic Organizing Pneumonia

Cryptogenic organizing pneumonia (COP) (also known as **bronchiolitis obliterans organizing pneumonia [BOOP]**) is characterized by connective tissue plugs in the small airways (hence the term *bronchiolitis obliterans*) and mononuclear cell infiltration of the surrounding parenchyma (hence the term *organizing pneumonia*). Although most cases have no identifiable cause and therefore are considered idiopathic, COP has been associated with various connective tissue diseases, toxic gas inhalation, and infection. The chest radiograph commonly shows patchy infiltrates of alveolar rather than interstitial involvement. Diagnosis may require a surgical biopsy when the clinical and radiographic data are uncertain. COP is one of the ILDs in which both restrictive and obstructive pathophysiologic findings are present.

Lymphocytic Interstitial Pneumonia

Lymphocytic interstitial pneumonia (LIP) is a diffuse pulmonary disorder characterized by fibrosis and accumulation of lymphocytes in the lungs. It is commonly associated with lymphoma. The diagnosis usually requires a surgical lung biopsy.

Specific Pathology

Lymphangioleiomyomatosis

Lymphangioleiomyomatosis (LAM) is a rare lung disease involving the smooth muscles of the airways and affects women of childbearing age. It is characterized by the proliferation of disorderly smooth muscle proliferation throughout the bronchioles, alveolar septa, perivascular spaces, and lymphatics. LAM causes the obstruction of small airways and lymphatics. Common clinical features associated with LAM are recurrent pneumothorax and chylothorax. The diagnosis of LAM is confirmed with an open lung biopsy. The prognosis is poor; the disease slowly progresses over 2 to 10 years, ending in death resulting from ventilatory failure.

Pulmonary Langerhans Cell Histiocytosis

Pulmonary Langerhans cell histiocytosis (PLCH) is a smoking-related ILD characterized by midlung zone star-shaped nodules with adjacent thin-walled cysts. It was once considered a benign condition in adults, but long-term complications such as pulmonary hypertension are becoming increasingly recognized. Diagnosis is confirmed histologically by tissue biopsy.

Pulmonary Alveolar Proteinosis

Pulmonary alveolar proteinosis is a condition of unknown cause in which the alveoli become filled with protein and lipids. The lipoprotein material is similar to the pulmonary surfactant produced by type II cells. In addition, the alveolar macrophages are generally dysfunctional in this disorder. The disease is most commonly seen in adults 20 to 50 years of age. Men are affected twice as often as women. The chest radiograph typically reveals bilateral infiltrates that are most prominent in the perihilar regions (butterfly pattern). It is often indistinguishable from pulmonary edema. Air bronchograms are commonly seen. The diagnosis is confirmed by transbronchial or open lung biopsy or by analysis of fluid removed during **bronchial lavage**.

Pulmonary Vasculitides

The **pulmonary vasculitides** (also called *granulomatous vasculitides*) consist of a heterogeneous group of pulmonary disorders characterized by inflammation and destruction of the pulmonary vessels. The major disorders in this category include Wegener granulomatosis, Churg-Strauss syndrome, and lymphomatoid granulomatosis.

Wegener Granulomatosis. **Wegener granulomatosis** is a multisystem disorder characterized by (1) a necrotizing, granulomatous vasculitis, (2) focal and segmental glomerulo-nephritis, and (3) variable degrees of systemic vasculitis of the small veins and arteries. In the lungs, numerous 1- to 9-cm-diameter nodules are commonly seen in the upper lobes, and cavity formation is often associated with larger lesions (see Fig. 27.8).

Wegener granulomatosis is considered an aggressive and fatal disorder, although the prognosis has significantly improved with the use of cytotoxic agents (e.g., cyclophosphamide). This disorder is most commonly seen in men older than 50 years of age. Diagnosis is confirmed by an open lung biopsy. Histologic examination reveals lesions with marked central necrosis of the pulmonary parenchyma. The area surrounding the necrotizing lesion contains numerous inflammatory white blood cells with some fibroblasts. Inflammatory cell infiltrate and necrotizing vasculitis are seen in the adjacent blood vessels.

Churg-Strauss Syndrome. **Churg-Strauss syndrome** is a necrotizing vasculitis that predominantly involves the small vessels of the lungs. The granulomatous lesions are characterized by a heavy infiltrate of *eosinophils,* central necrosis, and peripheral eosinophilia. Cavity formation is rare in this disorder. *Clinically, symptoms of asthma usually precede the onset of vasculitis.* In recent years, rapid tapering of oral steroids with substitution of leukotriene inhibitors such as montelukast (Singulair) and zafirlukast (Accolate) have been associated with deaths from fulminant Churg-Strauss syndrome reactions. Neurologic disorders such as **mononeuritis multiplex**, a simultaneous disease of several peripheral nerves, are frequently associated with this disorder. Diagnosis is usually confirmed with an open lung biopsy, and the disease is often rapidly fatal.

Lymphomatoid Granulomatosis. **Lymphomatoid granulomatosis** is a rare necrotizing vasculitis that primarily involves the lungs, although neurologic and cutaneous lesions are sometimes seen. The lesions are usually in the lower lobes, and cavities develop in more than one-third of cases. Pleural effusion is common.

Although the clinical presentation is similar to that of Wegener granulomatosis, there are some distinct differences. For example, more mature lymphoreticular cells are involved in the formation of the granulomatous lesions and no glomerulonephritis is seen. Histologically, the lesions simulate malignant lymphoma. This disorder is most commonly seen in men 50 to 70 years of age. Diagnosis is confirmed by open lung biopsy.

Miscellaneous Diffuse Interstitial Lung Diseases

Goodpasture Syndrome

Goodpasture syndrome is a disease of unknown cause that involves two organ systems: the lungs and the kidneys. In the lungs there are recurrent episodes of pulmonary hemorrhage and **hemoptysis** and in some cases pulmonary fibrosis, presumably as a consequence of episodes of pulmonary bleeding. In the kidneys there is a glomerulonephritis characterized by the infiltration of antibodies within the **glomerular basement membrane (GBM)**. These circulating antibodies function against the patient's own GBM. They are commonly abbreviated as *anti-GBM antibodies*. It is thought that the anti-GBM antibodies cross-react with the basement membrane of the alveolar wall and that their deposition in the kidneys and lungs is responsible for producing the pathophysiologic processes of the disease.

Goodpasture syndrome is usually seen in young adults. With appropriate treatment, the 5-year survival rate is almost 80%. An interesting feature of Goodpasture syndrome is that the patient frequently demonstrates an increased pulmonary

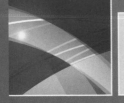

OVERVIEW of the Cardiopulmonary Clinical Manifestations Associated With Chronic Interstitial Lung Diseases

The following clinical manifestations result from the pathophysiologic mechanisms caused (or activated) by an increased alveolar-capillary membrane thickness (see Fig. 10.9) and excessive bronchial secretions (see Fig. 10.11)—the major anatomic alterations of the lungs associated with chronic interstitial lung disease (ILD) (see Fig. 27.1).

CLINICAL DATA OBTAINED AT THE PATIENT'S BEDSIDE

The Physical Examination

Vital Signs

Increased Respiratory Rate (Tachypnea)

Several pathophysiologic mechanisms operating simultaneously may lead to an increased ventilatory rate:

- Stimulation of peripheral chemoreceptors (hypoxemia)
- Relationship of decreased lung compliance to increased ventilatory rate
- Stimulation of the J receptors
- Pain, anxiety

Increased Heart Rate (Pulse) and Blood Pressure

Cyanosis

Digital Clubbing

Peripheral Edema and Venous Distention

Because polycythemia and cor pulmonale are associated with chronic ILD, the following may be seen:

- Distended neck veins
- Pitting edema
- Enlarged and tender liver

Nonproductive Cough

Chest Assessment Findings

- Increased tactile and vocal fremitus
- Dull percussion note
- Bronchial breath sounds
- Crackles
- Pleural friction rub
- Whispered pectoriloquy

CLINICAL DATA OBTAINED FROM LABORATORY TESTS AND SPECIAL PROCEDURES

Pulmonary Function Test Findings
Moderate to Severe Interstitial Lung Disease
(Restrictive Lung Pathology)

FORCED EXPIRATORY VOLUME AND FLOW RATE FINDINGS

FVC	FEV_T	FEV_1/FVC ratio	$FEF_{25\%-75\%}$
↓	N or ↓	N or ↑	N or ↓

$FEF_{50\%}$	$FEF_{200-1200}$	PEFR	MVV
N or ↓	N or ↓	N or ↓	N or ↓

LUNG VOLUME AND CAPACITY FINDINGS

V_T	IRV	ERV	RV	
N or ↓	↓	↓	↓	

VC	IC	FRC	TLC	RV/TLC ratio
↓	↓	↓	↓	N

DECREASED DIFFUSION CAPACITY

There is an exception to the expected decreased diffusion capacity in the two ILDs Goodpasture syndrome and idiopathic pulmonary hemosiderosis. The DLCO is often elevated in response to the increased amount of hemoglobin retained in the alveolar spaces that is associated with these two disorders.

Arterial Blood Gases

MILD TO MODERATE INTERSTITIAL LUNG DISEASE

Acute Alveolar Hyperventilation With Hypoxemia[1]
(Acute Respiratory Alkalosis)

pH	$PaCO_2$	HCO_3^-	PaO_2	SaO_2 or SpO_2
↑	↓	↓	↓	↓
		(but normal)		

SEVERE CHRONIC INTERSTITIAL LUNG DISEASE

Chronic Ventilatory Failure With Hypoxemia[2]
(Compensated Respiratory Acidosis)

pH	$PaCO_2$	HCO_3^-	PaO_2	SaO_2 or SpO_2
N	↑	↑	↓	↓
		(significantly)		

ACUTE VENTILATORY CHANGES SUPERIMPOSED ON CHRONIC VENTILATORY FAILURE[3]

Because acute ventilatory changes are frequently seen in patients with chronic ventilatory failure, the respiratory therapist must be familiar with—and alert for—the following two dangerous arterial blood gas (ABG) findings:

- Acute alveolar hyperventilation superimposed on chronic ventilatory failure, which should further alert the respiratory therapist to record the following important ABG assessment: possible *impending acute ventilatory failure*
- Acute ventilatory failure (acute hypoventilation) superimposed on chronic ventilatory failure

---

[1]See Fig. 5.2 and Table 5.4 and related discussions for the acute pH, $PaCO_2$, and HCO_3^- changes associated with acute alveolar hyperventilation.
[2]See Table 5.7, Table 5.8, and Table 5.9 and related discussion for the pH, $PaCO_2$, and HCO_3^- changes associated with chronic ventilatory failure.
[3]See Table 5.7, Table 5.8, and Table 5.9 and related discussion for the pH, $PaCO_2$, and HCO_3^- changes associated with acute ventilatory changes superimposed on chronic ventilatory failure.

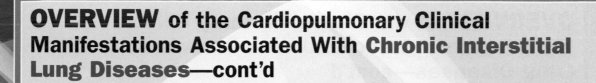
Oxygenation Indices[4]
Moderate to Severe Stage Interstitial Lung Disease

$\dot{Q}_S/\dot{Q}_T$	DO_2[5]	$\dot{V}O_2$	$C(a\text{-}\bar{v})O_2$	O_2ER	$S\bar{v}O_2$
↑	↓	N	N	↑	↓

Hemodynamic Indices[6]
(Severe Interstitial Lung Disease)

CVP	RAP	$\overline{PA}$	PCWP	CO	SV
↑	↑	↑	N	N	N
SVI	CI	RVSWI	LVSWI	PVR	SVR
N	N	↑	N	↑	N

LABORATORY FINDINGS

· Increased hematocrit and hemoglobin (polycythemia)

RADIOLOGIC FINDINGS

Radiologic findings vary according to the cause.

Chest Radiograph

· Bilateral reticulonodular pattern
· Irregularly shaped opacities
· Granulomas
· Cavity formation
· Honeycombing
· Pleural effusion (see Chapter 24, Pleural Effusion and Empyema)
· Pleural Thickening

   As shown in Fig. 27.3, in a patient with severe scleroderma, a bilateral reticulonodular pattern is commonly seen on the radiographs. In patients with asbestosis the opacity is often described as cloudy or as having a ground-glass appearance or pleural thickening and is especially apparent in the lower lobes (Fig. 27.4). Calcified pleural plaques may be seen on the superior border of the diaphragm or along the chest wall (Fig. 27.5). The inflammatory response elicited by the asbestos fibers may produce a fuzziness and irregularity of the cardiac and diaphragmatic borders.

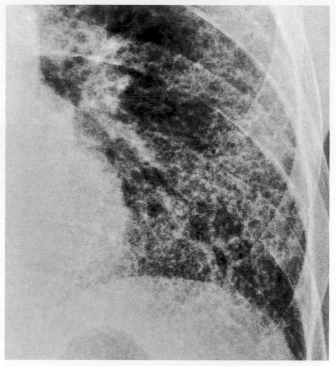

FIGURE 27.3 Reticulonodular pattern of interstitial pulmonary fibrosis in a patient with scleroderma. (From Hansell, D. M., Lynch, D. A., McAdams, H. P., et al. [2010]. *Imaging of diseases of the chest* [5th ed.]. Philadelphia, PA: Elsevier.)

[4]*C(a-v̄)O₂*, Arterial-venous oxygen difference; *DO₂*, total oxygen delivery; *O₂ER*, oxygen extraction ratio; *Q̇ₛ/Q̇ₜ*, pulmonary shunt fraction; *Sv̄O₂*, mixed venous oxygen saturation; *V̇O₂*, oxygen consumption.

[5]The DO₂ may be normal in patients who have compensated to the decreased oxygenation status with (1) an increased cardiac output, (2) an increased hemoglobin level, or (3) a combination of both. When the DO₂ is normal, the O₂ER is usually normal.

[6]*CO*, Cardiac output; *CVP*, central venous pressure; *LVSWI*, left ventricular stroke work index; *PA*, mean pulmonary artery pressure; *PCWP*, pulmonary capillary wedge pressure; *PVR*, pulmonary vascular resistance; *RAP*, right atrial pressure; *RVSWI*, right ventricular stroke work index; *SV*, stroke volume; *SVI*, stroke volume index; *SVR*, systemic vascular resistance.

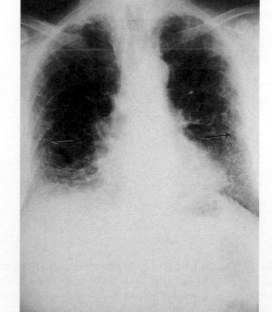

FIGURE 27.4 Chest x-ray film of a patient with asbestosis. See red arrow for pleural thickening.

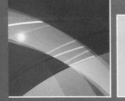
Fig. 27.6 shows a diffuse parenchymal ground-glass pattern with some areas of consolidation in a patient with acute farmer lung. The severity of parenchymal opacification in this case is rare.

In Fig. 27.7 the honeycomb appearance is nicely illustrated in a computed tomography (CT) scan of a patient with sarcoidosis. Fig. 27.8 shows a patient with Wegener granulomatosis with numerous nodules with a large cavitary lesion adjacent to the right hilus. Fig. 27.9 shows a pleural effusion in a patient with rheumatoid disease.

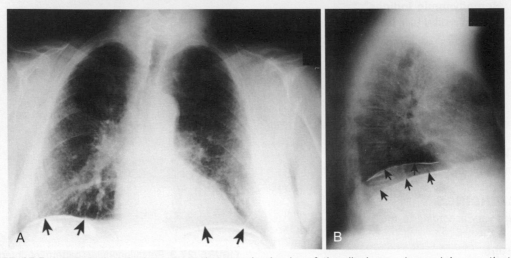

FIGURE 27.5 Calcified pleural plaques on the superior border of the diaphragm (arrows) in a patient with asbestosis. Thickening of the pleural margins is also seen along the lower lateral borders of the chest. (A) Anteroposterior view. (B) Lateral view.

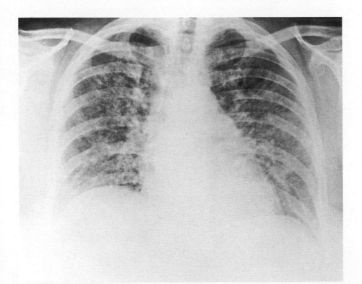

FIGURE 27.6 Acute farmer lung. Chest radiograph shows diffuse parenchymal ground-glass pattern with some areas of consolidation. The severity of parenchymal opacification in this case is unusual. (From Hansell, D. M., Lynch, D. A., McAdams, H. P., et al. [2010]. *Imaging of diseases of the chest* [5th ed.]. Philadelphia, PA: Elsevier.)

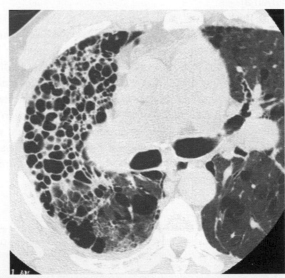

FIGURE 27.7 Honeycomb cysts in sarcoidosis. High-resolution computed tomography (HRCT) through the right midlung shows perfuse clustered honeycomb cysts. The cysts are larger than the typical honeycomb cysts seen in usual interstitial pneumonia. Cysts are much less extensive in the left lung. (From Hansell, D. M., Lynch, D. A., McAdams, H. P., et al. [2010]. *Imaging of diseases of the chest* [5th ed.]. Philadelphia, PA: Elsevier.)

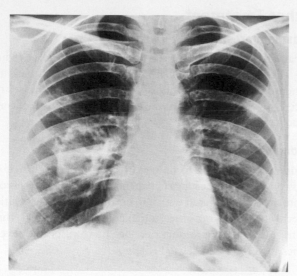

FIGURE 27.8 Wegener granulomatosis. Numerous nodules with a large (6-cm) cavitary lesion adjacent to the right hilus. Its walls are thick and irregular. (From Hansell, D. M., Lynch, D. A., McAdams, H. P., et al. [2010]. *Imaging of diseases of the chest* [5th ed.]. Philadelphia, PA: Elsevier.)

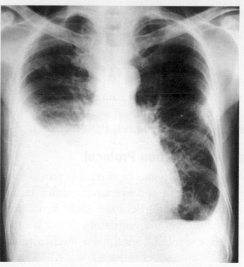

FIGURE 27.9 Pleural effusion in rheumatoid disease. Bilateral pleural effusions are present with mild changes of fibrosing alveolitis. The effusions were painless, and the one on the right had been present, more or less unchanged, for 5 months. Note the bilateral meniscus signs. (From Hansell, D. M., Lynch, D. A., McAdams, H. P., et al. [2010]. *Imaging of diseases of the chest* [5th ed.]. Philadelphia, PA: Elsevier.)

diffusion capacity (DLCO), which is in direct contrast to most interstitial lung disorders. The increased carbon monoxide uptake commonly seen in this disorder is thought to be caused by the increased amount of retained hemoglobin in the pulmonary tissue.

Idiopathic Pulmonary Hemosiderosis

Idiopathic pulmonary hemosiderosis is an entity of unknown cause that is characterized by recurrent episodes of pulmonary hemorrhage similar to that seen in Goodpasture syndrome. Histologic examination reveals an alveolar hemorrhage with hemosiderin-laden macrophages and hyperplasia of the alveolar epithelium. Unlike in Goodpasture syndrome, however, there is no evidence of circulating anti-GBM antibodies attacking the alveoli or GBMs, and this disorder is not associated with renal disease.

Idiopathic pulmonary hemosiderosis is most often seen in children. As in Goodpasture syndrome, patients commonly demonstrate an increased DLCO, which is in direct contrast to most interstitial lung disorders. Again, the increased uptake of carbon monoxide is thought to be caused by the increased amount of hemoglobin retained in the lungs.

Chronic Eosinophilic Pneumonia

Chronic eosinophilic pneumonia is characterized by infiltration of eosinophils and, to a lesser extent, macrophages into the alveolar and interstitial spaces. Clinically, a unique feature

of this disorder is often seen on the chest radiograph, consisting of a peripheral distribution of pulmonary infiltrates. This radiographic pattern is commonly referred to as a *photographic negative of pulmonary edema*. This is because of the dense peripheral infiltration, with the sparing of the perihilar areas, seen in chronic eosinophilic pneumonia compared with the central pulmonary infiltration with the sparing of the lung periphery seen in pulmonary edema. An increased number of eosinophils is also commonly seen in the peripheral blood. Histologic diagnosis is made by means of an open lung biopsy.

General Management of Interstitial Lung Disease

Medications and Procedures Commonly Prescribed by the Physician

The management of interstitial lung disorders is directed at the inflammation associated with the various disorders.

Corticosteroids

In general, corticosteroids are commonly administered in this group of illnesses with reasonably good results, but the benefit varies remarkably from one patient and condition (cause) to another (see Appendix II on the Evolve site).

Immunosuppressive Agents

Like steroids, these agents are helpful in many ILDs. Though effective, side effects are common.

Respiratory Care Treatment Protocols

Oxygen Therapy Protocol

Oxygen therapy is used to treat hypoxemia, decrease the work of breathing, and decrease myocardial work. Because of the hypoxemia associated with ILDs, supplemental oxygen is often required. The hypoxemia that develops in an interstitial lung disorder is most commonly caused by alveolar thickening, fibrosis, and capillary shunting associated with the disorder (see Oxygen Therapy Protocol, Protocol 10.1).

Mechanical Ventilation Protocol

Mechanical ventilation may be needed to provide and support alveolar gas exchange and eventually return the patient to spontaneous breathing. Because acute ventilatory failure superimposed on chronic ventilatory failure is often seen in patients with severe ILD, continuous mechanical ventilation may be required. Continuous mechanical ventilation is justified when the acute ventilatory failure is thought to be reversible (see Ventilator Initiation and Management Protocol, Protocol 11.1, and Ventilator Weaning Protocol, Protocol 11.2).

Other Treatment

Plasmapheresis

Treatment for Goodpasture syndrome is directed at reducing the circulating anti-GBM antibodies that attack the patient's GBM. **Plasmapheresis**, which directly removes the anti-GBM antibodies from the circulation, has been of some benefit.

Bronchial Lavage

Bronchial lavage is a technique involving therapeutic bronchoscopy, wherein the lungs of patients with pulmonary alveolar proteinosis are irrigated with a neutral solution. The solution effectively "washes out" the protein containing material which is discarded. This procedure may need to be repeated several times to achieve the desired results.

CASE STUDY Interstitial Lung Disease

Admitting History

An 89-year-old man is well known to the treating-hospital staff members, having received care there for more than 12 years. While in the US Navy during World War II, he worked on the East Coast in the ship construction industry. After his discharge in 1945, he returned to his home in Mississippi for about 6 months; he then moved to Detroit, Michigan, and worked for an automobile manufacturer. His primary job for the next 20 years was undercoating automobiles.

In the early 1970s the man was transferred to a nearby automotive plant, where he worked on an assembly line fastening bumpers and chrome trim to cars. He was popular with his fellow workers and considered a hard worker by the management. When he retired in 1980, he was one of four supervisors in charge of the chrome trim assembly line.

Although the man smoked two packs a day for more than 40 years, his health was essentially unremarkable until about 4 years before he retired. At that time he started to experience periods of coughing, dyspnea, and weakness. A complete examination including a chest x-ray provided by the company concluded that the man had moderate interstitial lung disease (ILD).

On the basis of the man's work history, the doctor speculated that the ILD was caused by asbestos fibers. This theory was confirmed later with the finding of asbestos fibers in a Perls stain of sputum, and the diagnosis of asbestosis was recorded in the patient's chart. Just before the man retired, his pulmonary function test (PFT) results showed a mild to moderate combined restrictive and obstructive disorder.

Although the man was able to enjoy a couple of relatively good years of retirement with his wife, his health declined rapidly. His cough and dyspnea quickly became a daily problem. Despite his deteriorating health, the man continued to smoke. When he was 72 years old, he was hospitalized for 8 days for treatment of pneumonia and severe respiratory distress. When he was discharged at that time, his PFTs still showed a moderate to severe restrictive disorder. He started using oxygen at home regularly.

Approximately 10 months before the current admission, the man was hospitalized because of congestive heart failure. He was treated aggressively and sent home within 5 days. At the time of discharge, his PFTs showed that he had a worsening restrictive respiratory disorder. His arterial blood gas (ABG) values on 2 L/min oxygen by nasal cannula were pH 7.38, $PaCO_2$ 86 mm Hg, HCO_3^- 49 mEq/L, PaO_2 63 mm Hg, and SaO_2 91%.

Approximately 3 hours before the current admission, the man awoke from an afternoon nap extremely short of breath. His wife stated that he coughed almost continuously and had difficulty speaking. She measured his oral temperature, which read 38°C (100°F). Concerned, she drove her husband to the hospital emergency department (ED).

Physical Examination

As the man was wheeled into the ED, he appeared nervous, weak, and in obvious respiratory distress. He was on 1.5 L/min oxygen by nasal cannula, which was connected to an E-tank attached to the wheelchair. His skin felt damp and clammy. He appeared pale and cyanotic. His neck veins were distended, and his fingers and toes were clubbed. He demonstrated a frequent but weak cough productive of a moderate amount of thick, whitish-yellow secretions. He had 3+ peripheral edema of the ankles and feet. He said this was the worst his breathing had ever been.

The patient's vital signs were blood pressure 180/96 mm Hg, heart rate 108 beats/min, respiratory rate 32 breaths/min, and oral temperature 38.3°C (100.8°F). Palpation of the chest was negative. Percussion produced bilateral dull notes in the lung bases. Coarse crackles were auscultated throughout both lungs. A pleural friction rub could be heard over the right middle lobe between the sixth and seventh ribs, between the anterior axillary line and midaxillary line.

The patient's lower lobes had a diffuse, ground-glass appearance on the chest radiograph. Irregularly shaped opacities in the right and left lower pleural spaces were identified by the radiologist as calcified pleural plaques. A possible infiltrate consistent with pneumonia was also visible in the right middle lobe. In addition, the chest x-ray suggested that the right side of the heart was moderately enlarged. His ABGs on a 1.5 L/min oxygen nasal cannula were pH 7.56, $PaCO_2$ 51 mm Hg, HCO_3^- 43 mEq/L, PaO_2 47 mm Hg, and SaO_2 86%.

The physician started the patient on intravenous furosemide (Lasix) to treat the man's cor pulmonale and began administering an antibiotic to treat suspected pneumonia. A respiratory therapist was called to obtain a sputum culture, perform a respiratory care evaluation, and outline further respiratory therapy. The physician said that she did not want to commit the patient to a ventilator unless absolutely necessary. On the basis of this information, the following SOAP was recorded.

Respiratory Assessment and Plan

S "This is the worst my breathing has ever been."

O Vital signs: BP 180/96, HR 108, RR 32, T 38.3°C (100.8°F); weak appearance; skin: cyanotic, damp, and clammy; distended neck veins and digital clubbing; cough: frequent, weak, moderate amount of thick, whitish-yellow secretions; peripheral edema 3+ of ankles and feet. Bilateral dull percussion notes in lung bases. Over both lungs: coarse crackles; pleural friction rub over right middle lobe between sixth and seventh ribs, between anterior axillary line and midaxillary line; CXR: ground-glass appearance in lower lobes; calcified pleural plaques in right and left lower pleural spaces; consolidation in right middle lung lobe; right heart enlargement; ABGs (1.5 L/min O_2 by nasal cannula) pH 7.56, $PaCO_2$ 51, HCO_3^- 43, PaO_2 47, SaO_2 86%.

A • Respiratory distress (general appearance, vital signs, ABGs, history of congestive heart failure)

• Pulmonary fibrosis (history, diagnosis of asbestosis, CXR)
• Alveolar consolidation in right middle lobe (CXR)
• Pleurisy (asbestosis or pneumonitis) in area of right middle lobe (pleural friction rub)
• Excessive bronchial secretions (coarse crackles, sputum production)
• Chest infection likely (yellow sputum, fever)
• Acute alveolar hyperventilation superimposed on chronic ventilatory failure with moderate to severe hypoxemia (history, ABGs)
• Impending ventilatory failure (ABGs)

P Up regulate Oxygen Therapy Protocol (air entrainment mask at FIO_2 0.35). Airway Clearance Therapy Protocol (DB&C q4h; obtain sputum for Gram stain and culture). Initiate Lung Expansion Therapy Protocol (incentive spirometry followed by C&DB). Monitor with pulse oximeter, set SpO_2 alarm at 85%.

The Next Morning

Throughout the night the patient's condition remained unstable. He continued to cough frequently but could not expectorate secretions adequately on his own. When the therapist assisted the patient during coughing episodes, a moderate amount of thick, white and yellow sputum was produced. Even though he was conscious, alert, and able to follow simple directions, he did not answer any of the respiratory therapist's specific questions about his breathing.

His skin was cold and damp to the touch, and he appeared short of breath. His color was improved, but he still appeared pale and cyanotic. His neck veins were still distended, although not so severely as they had been on admission, and edema of his ankles and feet could still be seen. The patient's vital signs were blood pressure 192/108 mm Hg, heart rate 113 beats/min, respiratory rate 34 breaths/min, and oral temperature 38°C (100.4°F). Palpation of the chest was negative.

Dull percussion notes were elicited over the lung bases. Coarse crackles continued to be auscultated throughout both lungs. A pleural friction rub could still be heard over the right middle lung between the sixth and seventh ribs, between the anterior axillary line and midaxillary line. No recent chest radiograph was available. His ABGs (FIO_2 0.35) were pH 7.57, $PaCO_2$ 47 mm Hg, HCO_3^- 41 mEq/L, PaO_2 40 mm Hg, and SaO_2 83%.

On the basis of these clinical data, the following SOAP was documented.

Respiratory Assessment and Plan

S N/A (patient too dyspneic to reply)

O Condition unstable; cough: frequent, weak, productive of thick, white and yellow secretions; skin: cyanotic, pale, cool, and damp; distended neck veins and peripheral edema, but improving; vital signs BP 192/108, HR 113, RR 34, T 38°C (100.4°F); dull percussion notes over both lung bases; coarse crackles throughout both lungs; pleural friction rub over right middle lobe between sixth and seventh ribs, between anterior axillary line and midaxillary line; ABGs (FIO_2 0.35) pH 7.57, $PaCO_2$ 47, HCO_3^- 41, PaO_2 40, SaO_2 83%.

A • Continued respiratory distress (general appearance, vital signs, ABGs)
   • Pulmonary fibrosis in lower lobes (history, diagnosis of asbestosis, recent CXR)
   • Alveolar consolidation in right middle lobe (CXR, pneumonia)
   • Pleurisy or pneumonia that has extended into pleural space over right middle lobe (pleural friction rub)
   • Excessive bronchial secretions (coarse crackles, sputum production)
   • Infection likely (yellow sputum)
   • Acute alveolar hyperventilation superimposed on chronic ventilatory failure with severe hypoxemia, worsening (history, ABGs)
   • Impending ventilatory failure (ABGs: Increased alveolar hyperventilation and worsening PaO_2)

P Up-regulate Oxygen Therapy Protocol (nonrebreather oxygen mask). Airway Clearance Therapy Protocol (adding intensive nasotracheal suctioning q2h). Start Aerosolized Medication Protocol (nebulize albuterol unit dose qid). Continue Lung Expansion Therapy Protocol (continuing to coach and monitor incentive spirometry; if FVC falls below 15 mL/kg, administer CPAP mask at +10 cm H_2O for 20 minutes qid). Continue to monitor closely and observe for improvement.

Twenty Hours Later

At 6:15 a.m. the alarm on the patient's cardiac monitor sounded. The electrocardiogram strip showed frequent premature ventricular contractions followed by ventricular flutter and fibrillation. The head nurse called for a Code Blue. Cardiopulmonary resuscitation was started immediately. Epinephrine and dopamine were administered through the patient's intravenous line. Approximately 12 minutes into the code, the patient exhibited a normal sinus rhythm and spontaneous respirations.

The patient was intubated, transferred to the intensive care unit (ICU), and placed on a pressure-cycled mechanical ventilator. Based on the patient's weight of 183 lb (83 kg), he was started on a low tidal volume of 500 mL (6 mL/kg = 498). Other ventilatory settings were 12 breaths/min, FIO_2 1.0, pressure support 7 cm H_2O, and 5 cm H_2O positive end-expiratory pressure (PEEP). His cardiopulmonary status remained unstable. Premature ventricular contractions were frequently seen on the electrocardiographic monitor. A pulmonary artery catheter and arterial line were inserted.

The patient's skin was pale, cyanotic, and clammy. His neck veins were still distended, and his ankles and feet were swollen. Vital signs were blood pressure 135/90 mm Hg, heart rate 84 beats/min, and rectal temperature 38.3°C (100.8°F). Palpation of the chest wall was negative. Dull percussion notes were noted over the lung bases. Coarse crackles continued to be auscultated throughout both lungs. Thick, greenish-yellow sputum was frequently suctioned from the patient's endotracheal tube.

A pleural friction rub could still be heard over the right middle lung lobe between the sixth and seventh ribs, between the anterior axillary line and midaxillary line. A chest radiograph had been taken but had not yet been interpreted by the radiologist. His ABGs on FIO_2 1.0 were pH 7.53, $PaCO_2$ 56 mm Hg, HCO_3^- 45 mEq/L, PaO_2 246 mm Hg, and SaO_2 98%.

At this time, the following SOAP note was charted.

Respiratory Assessment and Plan

S N/A (patient intubated on ventilator)

O Vital signs: BP 135/90 on vasopressors, HR 84, T 38.3°C (100.8°F); frequent premature ventricular contractions; skin: pale, cyanotic, and clammy; distended neck veins; peripheral edema of ankles and feet; dull percussion notes over lung bases; coarse crackles throughout both lungs; thick, greenish-yellow sputum frequently suctioned; pleural friction rub over right middle lung lobe between sixth and seventh ribs and between anterior axillary line and midaxillary line; ABGs (FIO_2 1.0) pH 7.53, $PaCO_2$ 56, HCO_3^- 45, PaO_2 246, SaO_2 98%.

A • Pulmonary fibrosis, lower lung lobes (history, diagnosis of asbestosis, recent CXR)
   • Alveolar consolidation, right middle lobe (recent CXR showing pneumonia)
   • Pneumonia possibly extended into pleural space over right middle lobe (pleural friction rub)
   • Excessive bronchial secretions (coarse crackles, sputum production)
   • Infection likely (fever, greenish-yellow sputum, possible new organism)
   • Acute alveolar hyperventilation superimposed on chronic ventilatory failure and overly corrected hypoxemia (ABGs)
   • Alveolar hyperventilation and overoxygenation caused by mechanical ventilator and FIO_2 setting

P Down-regulate Oxygen Therapy Protocol (reduce FIO_2 to 0.50). Down-regulate Mechanical Ventilation Protocol (e.g., decrease the tidal volume to increase the $PaCO_2$ to patient's baseline—e.g., 80 to 90 mm Hg). Continue Airway Clearance Therapy Protocol and Aerosolized Medication Protocol. Continue Lung Expansion Therapy Protocol (10 cm H_2O PEEP, but monitor mean airway pressure). Continue to closely monitor and reevaluate.

Discussion

The admitting history revealed that the patient had been diagnosed with moderate **pneumoconiosis** (probable asbestosis). Not surprisingly, pulmonary function tests in the past had shown mild to moderate restrictive pulmonary disorders.

Significant new findings were the recent history suggesting congestive heart failure and the ABG values on his discharge from the hospital 10 months before the admission under discussion, which demonstrated chronic ventilatory failure. The patient's recent fever and cough and purulent sputum production both before and in his ED admission suggested an infectious cause for his symptoms. His cyanosis, neck-vein distention, and digital clubbing suggested chronic hypoxemia. The sputum purulence confirmed that infection may indeed have been present and that the assessing therapist's desire to obtain a sputum culture was appropriate. *This was not followed up in subsequent SOAP notes.* The pleural rub demonstrated by this patient could have been related to his asbestosis or to a pneumonic infiltrate extending to the pleural surface.

In the initial assessment the patient's severe hypertension and his fever were noted. Both deserved vigorous therapy if his pulmonary function were to improve at all. The patient's severe hypoxemia reflected common clinical indicators caused by alveolar-capillary membrane thickening (see Fig. 10.9) and excessive bronchial secretions (see Fig. 10.11). Although there is no therapy available to reverse the increased alveolar membrane thickening, which reflects the alveolitis from his almost certain asbestosis, the excessive bronchial secretions can be effectively treated in most cases.

The patient was hyperventilating with respect to his earlier outpatient blood gases. During such an assessment the patient's underlying pulmonary conditions (chronic pulmonary fibrosis, bronchitis, and congestive heart failure) should be recorded, but the assessment should really zero in on the treatable issues, specifically in this case the pulmonary infection, as suggested by the patient's fever, sputum purulence, and chest radiograph.

At the time of the second evaluation, the patient's hypoxemia had worsened despite oxygen therapy. If not already being used, Venturi oxygen mask therapy was indicated there, and aggressive endotracheal suctioning also could be indicated. A trial of Lung Expansion Therapy Protocol (Protocol 10.3) was appropriate to attempt to offset the pathologic effects of the alveolar consolidation and, possibly, atelectasis. The physician may have ordered a trial of diuretic therapy to reduce the fluid retention and also a course of antibiotic therapy. *It was not clear whether appropriate (culture-based) antibiotic therapy was selected in this case.*

The last assessment revealed ventricular arrhythmias. The change in the patient's sputum from thick and white to greenish-yellow suggests superinfection with another organism, and reculture of the sputum was appropriate. The respiratory therapist responded quickly and appropriately to readjust the mechanical ventilator. The FIO_2 was decreased to 0.50 to correct the patient's overoxygenation (PaO_2 246), and the tidal volume was reduced to increase the $PaCO_2$ to the baseline—80 to 90 mm Hg, according to the ABG history. Ventilator parameters should be adjusted to provide good pulmonary expansion while avoiding high mean airway pressures. A cautious trial of PEEP would have been in order.

Despite all that was done for this patient, he died 4 days later as a result of left-sided congestive heart failure and pneumonia complicating his pulmonary asbestosis.

SELF-ASSESSMENT QUESTIONS

1. Which of the following is another name for hypersensitivity pneumonitis?
   a. Sarcoidosis
   b. Extrinsic allergic alveolitis
   c. Alveolar proteinosis
   d. Idiopathic pulmonary hemosiderosis

2. Which of the following is(are) considered pulmonary vasculitides?
   1. Rheumatoid arthritis
   2. Wegener granulomatosis
   3. Lymphomatoid granulomatosis
   4. Churg-Strauss syndrome
      a. 1 only
      b. 3 only
      c. 2, 3, and 4 only
      d. 1, 2, and 3 only

3. Which of the following disorders is associated with desquamative interstitial pneumonia and usual interstitial pneumonia?
   a. Idiopathic pulmonary fibrosis
   b. Eosinophilic granuloma
   c. Rheumatoid arthritis
   d. Sarcoidosis

4. Which of the following is(are) systemic connective tissue diseases?
   1. Pulmonary Langerhans cell histiocytosis
   2. Rheumatoid arthritis
   3. Sjögren syndrome

4. Alveolar proteinosis
   a. 3 only
   b. 2 and 4 only
   c. 1 and 4 only
   d. 2 and 3 only

5. Which of the following pulmonary function study findings is(are) are associated with chronic interstitial lung disease?
   1. Increased FRC
   2. Decreased FEVT
   3. Increased RV
   4. Decreased FVC
      a. 1 only
      b. 3 only
      c. 2 and 4 only
      d. 3 and 4 only

6. Which of the following hemodynamic indices is(are) associated with advanced or severe interstitial lung disease?
   1. Increased CVP
   2. Decreased PCWP
   3. Increased PA
   4. Decreased RAP
      a. 1 only
      b. 4 only
      c. 1 and 3 only
      d. 2 and 4 only

7. Which of the following chest assessment findings is associated with interstitial lung disease?
   a. Diminished breath sounds
   b. Hyperresonant percussion note
   c. Decreased tactile fremitus
   d. Bronchial breath sounds

8. Which of the following oxygenation indices is(are) associated with the pneumoconioses?
   1. Decreased $C(a-\bar{v})O_2$
   2. Increased O_2ER
   3. Decreased $S\bar{v}O_2$
   4. Increased $S\bar{v}O_2$
      a. 1 only
      b. 3 only
      c. 2 and 3 only
      d. 1 and 4 only

9. The fibrotic changes that develop in coal worker pneumoconiosis usually result from which of the following?
   a. Barium
   b. Silica
   c. Iron
   d. Coal dust

10. Which of the following are associated with interstitial lung disease?
    1. Pleural friction rub
    2. Dull percussion note
    3. Cor pulmonale
    4. Elevated $\overline{PA}$
       a. 2 and 4 only
       b. 3 and 4 only
       c. 2, 3, and 4 only
       d. 1, 2, 3, and 4

CHAPTER
28

Acute Respiratory Distress Syndrome

Chapter Objectives

After reading this chapter, you will be able to:

- List the anatomic alterations of the lungs associated with acute respiratory distress syndrome.
- Describe the causes of acute respiratory distress syndrome.
- List the cardiopulmonary clinical manifestations associated with acute respiratory distress syndrome.
- Describe the general management of acute respiratory distress syndrome.
- Describe and justify the clinical strategies and rationales of the SOAPs presented in the case study.
- Define key terms and complete self-assessment questions at the end of the chapter and on Evolve.

Key Terms

ARDSNet Ventilation Protocol
Barotrauma
Berlin Definition of ARDS
ECMO
Ground-Glass Appearance
Hyaline Membrane

Inhaled Nitric Oxide (iNO)
Low Tidal Volume Ventilation (LTVV)
Oxygen Toxicity
Permissive Hypercapnia
Prone Ventilation
SpO_2/FIO_2 Ratio
Volutrauma

Chapter Outline

Anatomic Alterations of the Lungs
Etiology and Epidemiology
Diagnostic Criteria for Acute Respiratory Distress Syndrome
Overview of the Cardiopulmonary Clinical Manifestations
    Associated With Acute Respiratory Distress Syndrome
General Management of Acute Respiratory Distress
    Syndrome
    Corticosteroids
    Respiratory Care Treatment Protocols
    Ventilation Strategy
Case Study: Acute Respiratory Distress Syndrome
Self-Assessment Questions

Anatomic Alterations of the Lungs

The lungs of patients affected by acute respiratory distress syndrome (ARDS) undergo similar anatomic changes, regardless of the cause of the disease. In response to injury, the pulmonary capillaries become engorged and the permeability of the alveolar-capillary membrane increases. Interstitial and intraalveolar edema and hemorrhage ensue as well as scattered areas of hemorrhagic alveolar consolidation. These processes result in a decrease in alveolar surfactant and in alveolar collapse, or atelectasis.

As the disease progresses, the intraalveolar walls become lined with a thick, rippled **hyaline membrane** similar to the hyaline membrane seen in newborns with respiratory distress syndrome (hyaline membrane disease) (see Chapter 37,

Respiratory Distress Syndrome). The membrane contains fibrin and cellular debris. In severe cases, hyperplasia and swelling of the type II cells occur. Fibrin and exudate develop and lead to intraalveolar fibrosis.

In gross appearance the lungs of patients with ARDS are heavy and "red," "beefy," or "liverlike." The anatomic alterations that develop in ARDS create a restrictive lung disorder (Fig. 28.1).

The major pathologic or structural changes associated with ARDS are as follows:

- Interstitial and intraalveolar edema and hemorrhage
- Alveolar consolidation
- Intraalveolar hyaline membrane formation
- Pulmonary surfactant deficiency or qualitative abnormality
- Atelectasis

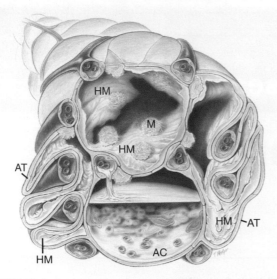

FIGURE 28.1 Cross-sectional view of alveoli in acute respiratory distress syndrome. *AC,* Alveolar consolidation; *AT,* atelectasis; *HM,* hyaline membrane; *M,* macrophage.

Historically, ARDS was first referred to as the "shock lung syndrome" when the disease was first identified in combat casualties during World War II. Since that time the disease has appeared in the medical literature under many different names, all based on the conditions believed to be responsible for the disease. In 1967 the disease was first described as a specific entity, and the term *acute respiratory distress syndrome* was suggested. This term is predominantly used today. Box 28.1 provides some of the other names that have appeared in the medical journals to identify ARDS.

Etiology and Epidemiology

ARDS accounts for 10% to 15% of all intensive care unit admissions and about 25% of patients on mechanical ventilation. A multitude of causative factors may produce ARDS. Although more than 60 possible pulmonary insults have been identified to cause ARDS, only a few common causes account for most cases of ARDS. Box 28.2 provides some of the better-known causes. The clinical manifestations associated with ARDS usually appear within 6 to 72 hours of an inciting event and worsen rapidly. The patient typically presents with dyspnea, cyanosis, bilateral crackles, tachypnea, tachycardia, diaphoresis, and use of accessory muscles of inspiration. Systemic hypotension is frequently an early event, and the dyspnea is often out of proportion to the extent of the radiologic abnormality. A cough and

chest pain also may be present. The general clinical course is characterized by several days of hypoxemia that requires moderate to high concentrations of inspired oxygen. The bilateral alveolar infiltrates and diffuse crackles worsen during this period, and the patient's overall health status is often fragile as a result of severe hypoxemia. Between 12% and 35% of patients die within the first 72 hours. Most patients who survive this initial clinical course begin to show oxygenation improvements and decreasing alveolar infiltrates over the next several days.

Diagnostic Criteria for Acute Respiratory Distress Syndrome

As shown in Box 28.3, the **Berlin Definition of ARDS** is used as the diagnostic criteria for ARDS. Note that the Berlin Definition of ARDS requires that all the elements listed in Box 28.3 must be present to diagnose ARDS. For the most part, ARDS is a diagnosis of exclusion—that is, excluding other possible causes of acute hypoxemic respiratory failure with bilateral alveolar infiltrates. *Cardiogenic pulmonary edema is the primary alternative that needs to be ruled out.* Other possible alternative causes of acute hypoxemic respiratory failure with bilateral alveolar infiltrates include diffuse alveolar hemorrhage, idiopathic acute exacerbation of preexisting interstitial lung disease, acute eosinophilic pneumonia, cryptogenic organizing pneumonia, acute interstitial pneumonia, and rapidly disseminating (metastatic) malignancy.

BOX 28.2 Causes of Acute Respiratory Distress Syndrome

Most Common

- *Sepsis:* The most common cause of ARDS. It should be the first cause considered whenever ARDS develops in an adult patient.
  - The risk factors are especially high in patients with sepsis who also have a history of alcoholism.
- *Aspiration* (e.g., of gastric contents). ARDS occurs in about one-third of patients who have a recognized episode of aspiration of gastric contents.
- *Pneumonia:* Community-acquired pneumonia is one of the most common causes of ARDS that develops outside of the hospital. Common pathogens include *Streptococcus pneumoniae, Legionella pneumophila, Pneumocystis jiroveci* (formerly called *Pneumocystis carinii*), *Staphylococcus aureus,* enteric gram-negative organisms, and a variety of respiratory viruses.
- *Severe trauma:* ARDS is a common complication of severe trauma. Such trauma often includes the following:
  - *Bilateral lung contusion caused by blunt trauma* (e.g., steering wheel smashed into the chest during a car accident).
  - *Fat embolism from a long-bone fracture* (e.g., ARDS symptoms typically appear 12 to 48 hours after the trauma).
  - *Sepsis:* Perhaps the most common cause of ARDS that develops several days after severe trauma.
  - *Massive traumatic tissue injury:* Predisposes the patient to ARDS.

- *Massive blood transfusion* (in stored blood the quantity of aggregated white blood cells, red blood cells, platelets, and fibrin increases; these blood components may in turn occlude or damage small blood vessels).
- *Lung and hematopoietic stem cell transplantation:* Patients are at risk for ARDS resulting from a variety of infectious and noninfectious causes.
- *Drug abuse* (e.g., heroin, barbiturates, morphine, methadone).

Other Causes

- *Central nervous system (CNS) disease* (particularly when complicated by increased intracranial pressure)
- *Cardiopulmonary bypass* (especially when the bypass is prolonged).
- *Disseminated intravascular coagulation* (seen in patients with shock; it is a condition of paradoxical simultaneous clotting and bleeding that produces microthrombi in the lungs).
- *Inhalation of toxins and irritants* (e.g., chlorine gas, nitrogen dioxide, smoke, ozone; oxygen may also be included in this category of irritants).
- *Immunologic reactions* (e.g., allergic alveolar reaction to inhaled material or Goodpasture syndrome).
- *Oxygen toxicity* (e.g., prolonged exposure to FIO_2 >0.60).

BOX 28.3 Berlin Definition of Acute Respiratory Disease Syndrome: Diagnostic Criteria

- Respiratory symptoms associated with ARDS have manifested within 1 week of a known clinical event or new or worsening symptoms over the past 7 days.
- Bilateral opacities similar to pulmonary edema appear on the chest radiograph or computed tomography scan. The opacities cannot be fully explained by pleural effusion, lobar or lung collapse, or pulmonary nodules.
- The patient's respiratory failure cannot be fully explained by heart failure or fluid overload. An objective assessment to rule out hydrostatic pulmonary edema is required if risk factors for ARDS are not present.
- A moderate to severe impairment of oxygenation must be present, as defined by the ratio of arterial oxygen tension to fraction of inspired oxygen ratio (PaO_2/FIO_2 ratio). The severity of the hypoxemia defines the severity of the ARDS*:

- *Mild ARDS:* The PaO_2/FIO_2 is >200, but ≤300, on ventilator settings that include positive end-expiratory pressure (PEEP) or continuous positive airway pressure (CPAP) ≥5 cm H_2O.
- *Moderate ARDS:* The PaO_2/FIO_2 is >100, but ≤200, on ventilator settings that include PEEP ≥5 cm H_2O.
- *Severe ARDS:* The PaO_2/FIO_2 is ≤100 on ventilator settings that include PEEP ≥5 cm H_2O.

Modified from ARDS Definition Task Force. (2012). Acute respiratory distress syndrome: The Berlin Definition. *Journal of the American Medical Association 307*(23), 2526-2533.

*To determine the PaO_2/FIO_2 ratio, the PaO_2 is measured in mm Hg and the FIO_2 is expressed as a decimal fraction between 0.21 and 1. For example, if a patient has a PaO_2 of 60 mm Hg while receiving 85% oxygen, then the PaO_2/FIO_2 is 60/0.85 = 70. *The normal PaO_2/FIO_2 ratio is between 350 and 450.*

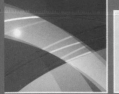

OVERVIEW of the Cardiopulmonary Clinical Manifestations Associated With Acute Respiratory Distress Syndrome

The following clinical manifestations result from the pathologic mechanisms caused (or activated) by atelectasis (see Fig. 10.7), alveolar consolidation (see Fig. 10.8), and increased alveolar-capillary membrane thickness (see Fig. 10.9)—the major anatomic alterations of the lungs associated with ARDS (see Fig. 28.1).

CLINICAL DATA OBTAINED AT THE PATIENT'S BEDSIDE

The Physical Examination

Vital Signs

Increased Respiratory Rate (Tachypnea)

Several pathophysiologic mechanisms operating simultaneously may lead to an increased ventilatory rate:

- Stimulation of peripheral chemoreceptors (hypoxemia)
- Relationship of decreased lung compliance to increased ventilatory rate
- Stimulation of J receptors
- Anxiety

Increased Heart Rate (Pulse) and Blood Pressure

Substernal or Intercostal Retractions

Cyanosis

Chest Assessment Findings

- Dull percussion note
- Bronchial breath sounds
- Crackles

CLINICAL DATA OBTAINED FROM LABORATORY TESTS AND SPECIAL PROCEDURES

Pulmonary Function Test Findings
(Restrictive Lung Pathophysiology)

FORCED EXPIRATORY VOLUME AND FLOW RATE FINDINGS

FVC	FEV_T	FEV_1/FVC ratio	$FEF_{25\%-75\%}$
↓	N or ↓	N or ↑	N or ↓

$FEF_{50\%}$	$FEF_{200-1200}$	PEFR	MVV
N or ↓	N or ↓	N or ↓	N or ↓

LUNG VOLUME AND CAPACITY FINDINGS

V_T	IRV	ERV	RV
N or ↓	↓	↓	↓

VC	IC	FRC	TLC	RV/TLC ratio
↓	↓	↓	↓	N

DECREASED DIFFUSION CAPACITY (DLCO)

Arterial Blood Gases[1]

MILD TO MODERATE ACUTE RESPIRATORY DISTRESS SYNDROME

Acute Alveolar Hyperventilation With Hypoxemia[2]
(Acute Respiratory Alkalosis)

pH	$PaCO_2$	HCO_3^-	PaO_2	SaO_2 or SpO_2
↑	↓	↓ (but normal)	↓	↓

SEVERE ACUTE RESPIRATORY DISTRESS SYNDROME

Acute Ventilatory Failure With Hypoxemia[3]
(Acute Respiratory Acidosis)

pH[4]	$PaCO_2$	HCO_3^-[4]	PaO_2	SaO_2 or SpO_2
↓	↑	↑ (but normal)	↓	↓

Oxygenation Indices[5]

$\dot{Q}_S/\dot{Q}_T$	DO_2[6]	$\dot{V}O_2$	$C(a-\bar{v})O_2$	O_2ER	$S\bar{v}O_2$
↑	↓	N	N	↑	↓

Hemodynamic Indices[7]
Severe ARDS

CVP	RAP	$\overline{PA}$	PCWP	CO	SV
↑	↑	↑	N[8] or ↓	N or ↑[9]	N or ↑[9]

SVI	CI	RVSWI	LVSWI	PVR	SVR
N or ↑[9]	N or ↑[9]	↑	↓	↑	N or ↓[9]

[1]*NOTE:* The use of the **SpO₂/FIO₂ ratio** (which does not require ABG analysis) has simplified the monitoring, diagnosis, and treatment of ARDS compared with the PaO_2/F_iO_2 difference, which does require an arterial blood gas stick (see Chapter 6, Assessment of Oxygenation).
[2]See Fig. 5.2 and Table 5.4 and related discussion for the acute pH, $PaCO_2$, and HCO_3^- changes associated with acute alveolar hyperventilation.
[3]See Fig. 5.3 and Table 5.5 and related discussion for the acute pH, $PaCO_2$, and HCO_3^- changes associated with acute and chronic ventilatory failure.
[4]When tissue hypoxia is severe enough to produce lactic acid, the pH and HCO_3^- values will be lower than expected for a particular $PaCO_2$ level.
[5]$C(a-\bar{v})O_2$, Arterial-venous oxygen difference; DO_2, total oxygen delivery; O_2ER, oxygen extraction ratio; $\dot{Q}_S/\dot{Q}_T$, pulmonary shunt fraction; $S\bar{v}O_2$, mixed venous oxygen saturation; $\dot{V}O_2$, oxygen consumption.
[6]The DO_2 may be normal in patients who have compensated to the decreased oxygenation status with (1) an increased cardiac output, (2) an increased hemoglobin level (rare), or (3) a combination of both. When the DO_2 is normal, the O_2ER is usually normal.
[7]CO, Cardiac output; CI, cardiac index; CVP, central venous pressure; LVSWI, left ventricular stroke work index; $\overline{PA}$, mean pulmonary artery pressure; PCWP, pulmonary capillary wedge pressure; PVR, pulmonary vascular resistance; RAP, right atrial pressure; RVSWI, right ventricular stroke work index; SV, stroke volume; SVI, stroke volume index; SVR, systemic vascular resistance.
[8]A normal PCWP (<18 mm Hg) is the hallmark of ARDS, distinguishing it from cardiogenic pulmonary edema, in which the PCWP is elevated.
[9]If sepsis with systemic hypotension is present.

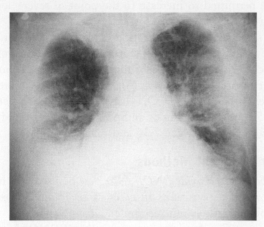

FIGURE 28.2 Chest radiograph of a patient with moderately severe acute respiratory distress syndrome.

RADIOLOGIC FINDINGS

Chest Radiograph

- Increased opacity, diffusely throughout lungs

Because of the bilateral alveolar infiltrates that develop in ARDS, an increased radiodensity is seen on the chest radiograph. The increased lung density resists x-ray penetration and is revealed on the radiograph as increased opacity. Therefore the more severe the ARDS, the denser the lungs become and the "whiter" the radiograph (Fig. 28.2). Ultimately, the lungs may have a **ground-glass appearance**. This is in contrast to cardiogenic pulmonary edema, where the infiltrates appear more *central*.

OTHER CLINICAL MANIFESTATIONS ASSOCIATED WITH ACUTE RESPIRATORY DISTRESS SYNDROME COMPLICATIONS

Patients with ARDS are at high risk for complications. Some of the complications are related to the patient who requires mechanical ventilation (e.g., pulmonary barotrauma and hospital-acquired pneumonia), whereas others are associated with the patient's underlying critical illness and/or being under intensive care—for example, delirium, deep venous thrombosis, gastrointestinal bleeding caused by stress ulceration, and catheter-related infections. Common complications include the following:

- *Barotrauma:* The patient with ARDS is often susceptible to pulmonary **barotrauma** resulting from the physical tension of high positive-pressure mechanical ventilation (plateau airway pressure greater than 30 cm H_2O) on acutely damaged alveoli. It is most likely that the areas of the lungs affected by barotrauma are, in fact, the healthy alveoli, which are interspersed with the pathologically altered alveoli. This is because the relatively high pressures required to manage patients with ARDS not only help recruit collapsed alveoli but also may work to overdistend the healthier alveoli, thus resulting in the overexpansion of the alveoli, tearing ("popping"), and collapse (called **volutrauma** and/or barotrauma). This complication is less common now that the **low tidal volume ventilation (LTVV)** and high respiratory rate strategy for providing ventilator support for ARDS has become widespread (see Ventilator Initiation and Management Protocol, Protocol 11.1, and Ventilator Weaning Protocol, Protocol 11.2). This ventilator strategy works to reduce the overall plateau airway pressure (less than 30 cm H_2O).
- *Delirium:* ARDS and other forms of acute ventilatory failure are often complicated by delirium. Deep sedation and neuromuscular blocking agents are used to treat agitated delirium and self-extubation, but their use is discouraged in the current literature.
- *Deep venous thrombosis (DVT):* Prolonged bed rest and/or immobilization are commonly associated with a DVT.
- *Gastrointestinal bleeding attributable to stress ulceration:* The incidence of overt gastrointestinal bleeding caused by stress ulceration ranges from 1.5% to 8.5% among all patients in the intensive care unit.
- *Pneumonia: Streptococcus pneumoniae* is commonly associated with ARDS. Antibiotic treatment is usually a combination of seftriaxone, levofloxacin, and azithromycin.

General Management of Acute Respiratory Distress Syndrome

Corticosteroids

Intravenous corticosteroids significantly reduce the rate of treatment failure both early (first 72 hours) and late (72 to 120 hours) based on radiographic progression and late septic shock.

Respiratory Care Treatment Protocols

Oxygen Therapy Protocol

Oxygen therapy is used to treat hypoxemia, decrease the work of breathing, and decrease myocardial work. Because of the hypoxemia associated with ARDS, supplemental oxygen is often required. The hypoxemia that develops in ARDS is most commonly caused by widespread alveolar consolidation, atelectasis, and increased alveolar capillary thickening.

Hypoxemia caused by capillary shunting is often refractory to oxygen therapy (see Oxygen Therapy Protocol, Protocol 10.1).

Lung Expansion Therapy Protocol

Lung expansion measures (e.g., positive end-expiratory pressure [PEEP] or continuous positive airway pressure [CPAP]) are key to attempt to offset the alveolar consolidation and atelectasis associated with mild ARDS (see Lung Expansion Protocol, Protocol 10.3).

Mechanical Ventilation Protocol

Mechanical ventilation is usually needed to provide and support alveolar gas exchange and eventually return the patient to spontaneous breathing. Continuous mechanical ventilation is justified when the acute ventilatory failure is thought to be reversible (see Ventilator Initiation and Management Protocol, Protocol 11.1, and Ventilation Weaning Protocol, Protocol 11.2).

Ventilation Strategy

For most patients in acute ventilatory failure caused by ARDS, it is recommended that the patient be immediately placed on invasive mechanical ventilation, rather than doing an initial trial of noninvasive positive pressure ventilation. In addition, a full support mode of mechanical ventilation is recommended, rather than a partially supported mode of ventilation. Either volume-limited or pressure-limited modes of ventilation are acceptable.

According to the National Institutes of Health (NIH); National Heart, Lung, and Blood Institute (NHLBI); and Acute Respiratory Distress Syndrome (ARDS) Network (ARDSnet) the recommended ventilatory strategy for ARDS is low tidal volume ventilation (LTVV) and high respiratory rates. The initial tidal volume is usually set at 8 mL/kg predicted body weight (PBW), with the ability to drop down, at 1 mL/kg intervals, to 6 mL/kg PBW, if needed to maintain a low plateau pressure (Pplat). Ideally, the Pplat should be maintained between 25 and 30 cm H_2O. The initial ventilatory rate is set to approximate the patient's baseline minute ventilation (not greater than 35 breaths/min). If the Pplat drops below 25 cm H_2O, the most common protocol is to increase the tidal volume (V_T). An overview of the recommended mechanical **ARDSnet Ventilation Protocol** is provided in Protocol 28.1.[1]

Finally, the patient's $PaCO_2$ is often allowed to increase (**permissive hypercapnia**) as a trade-off to protect the lungs from high airway pressures. In most cases, an increased ventilatory rate adequately offsets the decreased tidal volume used in the management of ARDS. The $PaCO_2$, however, should not be permitted to increase to the point of severe acidosis (e.g., a pH below 7.2).[2]

To summarize, the therapeutic goal of mechanical ventilation of the ARDS patient is to maintain (1) a low tidal volume, between 6 to 8 mL/kg; (2) a high respiratory rate, but not greater than 35 breaths/min; (3) an alveolar plateau pressure between 25 and 30 cm H_2O; (4) an oxygenation level between PaO_2 55 and 80 mm Hg or an SpO_2 between 88% and 95%, and (5) the pH between 7.30 and 7.45.

Other Treatment Methods

- *Inhaled nitric oxide (iNO):* iNO may be used as a bridge to other interventions in cases of profound hypoxemia. Prolonged use is not recommended.
- *Extracorporeal membrane oxygenation (ECMO):* In severe cases, and where skilled ECMO services are available, ECMO use may be considered. The most appropriate time to apply it in life support is not clear, and its use involves considerable patient risk.
- *Prone ventilation:* Prone ventilation is ventilation that is delivered with the patient lying in the prone position. Prone ventilation may be used for the treatment ARDS mostly as a strategy to improve oxygenation when the more traditional modes of ventilation have failed.

---

[1]To review the complete recommendations of ARDSnet mechanical ventilation protocol, criteria for another mechanical ventilation, oxygenation goals, plateau pressure goals, pH goals, and mechanical ventilation weaning protocol, go to http://www.ardsnet.org.

[2]Permissive hypercapnia defined: Mechanical ventilation was traditionally applied with the goal of normalizing arterial blood gas values, particularly the arterial carbon dioxide tension ($PaCO_2$). However, this is no longer the primary objective of mechanical ventilation. Today, the emphasis is on maintaining adequate gas exchange while—and, importantly—minimizing the risks for ventilator-associated injuries (VALIs) (see discussion on VALI in Chapter 11, Respiratory Insufficiency, Respiratory and Failure, and Ventilator Management). Common strategies used to reduce the complications of mechanical ventilation include (1) low tidal volume ventilation to protect the lung from VALI in patients with acute lung injury (e.g., ARDS) and (2) reduction of the tidal volume, respiratory rate, or both to minimize intrinsic positive end-expiratory pressure (i.e., auto-PEEP) in patients with obstructive lung disease (e.g., COPD). Although these mechanical ventilation strategies may result in an increased $PaCO_2$ level (hypercapnia), they do help protect the lung from barotauma (i.e., shear stress damage to lung tissues caused by excessive gas pressures). The lenient acceptance of the hypercapnia is called *permissive hypercapnia*. In most cases, the patient's $PaCO_2$ is adequately maintained by an increased ventilatory rate that offsets the decreased tidal volume. The $PaCO_2$, however, should not be permitted to increase to the point of severe acidosis. The most current consensus suggests it is safe to allow pH to fall to at least 7.20 (http://www.ARDSsnet.org).

ARDSNET* MECHANICAL VENTILATION PROTOCOL SUMMARY

Criteria for Mechanical Ventilation

Acute Onset of:

- PaO_2/FIO_2 <300
- Bilateral infiltrates consistent with pulmonary edema
- No Clinical evidence of left atrial hypertension

Ventilation Setup and Adjustments

- Calculate predicted body weight (PBW)
  - Males = 50 + 2.3 [height (inches) − 60]
  - Females = 45.5 + 2.3 [height (inches) − 60]
- Select any ventilator mode
- Set ventilator settings to achieve initial V_T = 8 mL/kg PBW
- Reduce V_T by 1 mL/kg at intervals <2 hours until V_T = 6 mL/kg PBW
- Set initial RR to approximate patient baseline minute ventilation (not >35 bpm)
- Adjust V_T and RR to achieve pH and plateau pressure goals as shown below:
  - Plateau Pressure (Pplat) Goals: <30 cm H_2O
    - Check Pplat (0.5 second inspiratory pause) at least q4h and each change in PEEP or V_T
    - If Pplat >30 cm H_2O: decrease V_T by 1 mL/kg steps (minimum = 4 mL/kg)
    - If Pplat <25 cm H_2O & VT <6 mL/kg: increase V_T by 1 mL/kg until Pplat >25 cm H_2O or V_T = 6 mL/kg
    - If Pplat <30 and breath stacking of asynchrony occurs: May increase V_T in 1 mL/kg increments to 7 or 8 mL/kg if Pplat remains <30 cm H_2O

Oxygenation Goal: PaO_2 55–80 mm Hg or SpO_2 88%–95%

Use a minimum PEEP of 5 cm H_2O. Consider use of incremental FIO_2/PEEP combinations such as shown below (not required) to achieve goal.

Lower PEEP With Higher FIO_2

FIO_2	0.3	0.4	0.4	0.5	0.5	0.6	0.7	0.7
PEEP	5	5	8	8	10	10	10	12

Higher PEEP With Lower FIO_2

FIO_2	0.3	0.3	0.3	0.3	0.3	0.3	0.4	0.4
PEEP	5	8	10	12	14	14	16	16

pH Goal: 7.30–7.45

- **Acidosis Management (pH <7.30):**
  - **If pH 7.15–7.30:** Increase RR until pH >7.30 or $PaCO_2$ <25 mm Hg (maximum set RR = 35)
  - **If pH <7.15:** Increase RR to 35
    - If pH remains <7.15, V_T may be increased in 1 mL/kg steps until pH >7.15 (Pplat target of 30 cm H_2O may be exceeded.)
    - May give $NaHCO_3$
- Alkalosis management (pH >7.45):
  - Decrease RR if possible

I:E Ratio Goal

- Recommend that duration of inspiration be < duration than expiration.

RR = respiratory rate, Pplat = plateau pressure (airway pressure), V_T = tidal volume, PEEP = positive end expiratory pressure.

*To review the complete recommendations of ARDSnet mechanical ventilation protocol, criteria for mechanical ventilation, oxygenation goals, plateau pressure goals, pH goals, and mechanical ventilation weaning protocol, go to: http://www.ardsnet.org

PROTOCOL 28.1

CASE STUDY Acute Respiratory Distress Syndrome

Admitting History and Physical Examination

This comatose 47-year-old woman was admitted to the emergency department (ED) of a small community hospital. Her husband found her lying in bed with an empty bottle of "sleeping pills" and a "goodbye note" on the bedside table. She had a long history of depression.

In the ED she was found to be in a moderately deep coma, responding to deep painful stimulation but otherwise nonresponsive. She was of average size and, according to her husband, had previously been in good physical health. She did not smoke or drink and was taking no other medication. Her blood pressure and pulse were within normal limits, but her respirations were shallow and noisy. The ED physician attempted to lavage her stomach. During the introduction of the nasogastric tube, the patient vomited and aspirated liquid gastric contents. At this time it was decided to transfer her by ambulance to a tertiary care medical center about 30 miles away. The pH of the gastric contents was not determined.

On arrival at the medical center, the patient was comatose but responsive to mild painful stimulation. Her weight was 50 kg, and her rectal temperature was 101.5°F (38.6°C). Her blood pressure was 100/60 mm Hg, heart rate 114 beats/min, and respirations 10 breaths/min and shallow. On auscultation, there were fine crackles over the left lung, and coarse crackles over the right side. A chest radiograph showed bilateral moderate fluffy infiltrates, mostly on the right side. Blood gases on a nonrebreather oxygen mask were pH 7.29, $PaCO_2$ 56 mm Hg, HCO_3^- 26 mEq/L, PaO_2 52 mm Hg, and SaO_2 80%.

At the time the respiratory therapist recorded the following SOAP note.

Respiratory Assessment and Plan

S N/A

O Patient is comatose. BP 100/60; HR 114; RR 28; T 101.5°F (38.6°C). Auscultation: Fine crackles over the left lung, and coarse crackles over the right side. CXR: Bilateral infiltrates, worse on right side. Arterial blood gas values (ABGs) on nonrebreather oxygen mask were pH 7.29, $PaCO_2$ 56, HCO_3^- 26, PaO_2 52, and SaO_2 80%.

A • Sedative drug overdose with coma (history)
• Aspiration pneumonitis without previous history of pulmonary disease (aspiration observed)
• Possible early stages of ARDS (history and x-ray)
• Acute ventilatory failure with moderate hypoxemia (ABGs)

P Contact physician stat regarding acute ventilatory failure. Manually ventilate and oxygenate patient until the physician's orders are completed. Repeat ABGs 1 hour after intubation and PRN.

Over the next 30 minutes, the patient was transferred to the intensive care unit, intubated, and mechanically ventilated for possible early stages of mild ARDS. The initial ventilator settings were V_T 400 mL (8 mL × 50 kg), rate 15 breaths/min, FIO_2 0.50, and 10 cm H_2O of PEEP. The Pplat was 26 cm H_2O. An arterial line was placed in her left radial artery, and an intravenous infusion was started with lactated Ringer solution.

Over the next 15 hours, the patient's oxygenation status continued to deteriorate, in spite of a progressive increase in the delivered FIO_2, PEEP, and pressure-controlled mechanical ventilation. When the arterial oxygen tension did not improve appreciably on an FIO_2 of 1.0 and a PEEP of 20 cm H_2O, a Swan-Ganz catheter was placed in the pulmonary artery. In view of the PEEP, the pressure readings were difficult to interpret. A mean pulmonary artery pressure of 27 mm Hg, however, did suggest increased pulmonary vascular resistance.

A chest radiograph revealed ARDS with bilateral diffuse infiltrates and atelectasis. The heart was not enlarged. At this time, the physician charted "severe ARDS" in the patient's progress notes. The respiratory therapist decreased the tidal volume on the ventilator to 300 mL (6 mL × 50 kg) and increased the rate to 20 breaths/min. The FIO_2 remained at 1.0, and the PEEP was increased to 22 cm H_2O. Twenty minutes later the patient's ABGs were pH 7.31, $PaCO_2$ 49 mm Hg, HCO_3^- 24 mEq/L, PaO_2 38 mm Hg, and SaO_2 65%. Her PaO_2/FIO_2 ratio was 38 (38 ÷ 1.0 = 38). She had coarse crackles and bronchial breath sounds throughout all lung fields. Moderate to large amounts of purulent sputum were frequently suctioned from the endotracheal tube. Her blood pressure was 90/60, and her heart rate was 130 beats/min. Her temperature was 100.2°F (37.9°C).

At this time, the respiratory therapist charted the following SOAP note.

Respiratory Assessment and Plan

S N/A (patient comatose)

O Patient remains comatose. BP 90/60, HR 130, T 100.2°F (37.9°C). Bilateral coarse crackles and bronchial breath sounds. ABGs on decreased V_T of 300 mL, rate 20, FIO_2 1.0, and +22 PEEP: pH 7.31, $PaCO_2$ 49, HCO_3^- 24, PaO_2 38, and SaO_2 65%. PaO_2/FIO_2 ratio: 38. CXR: ARDS with bilateral diffuse infiltrates and atelectasis, worse on the right side. Purulent sputum. PA pressure (mean) 27 mm Hg.

A • Severe ARDS (symptoms associated with ARDS: bilateral infiltrates on CXR, PaO_2/FIO_2 ratio is 38 on ventilator settings that include PEEP >20 cm H_2O).
• Persistent coma (physical examination)
• Aspiration pneumonitis—progressing to ARDS with bilateral infiltrates and atelectasis (CXR, bronchial breath sounds)
• Increasing airway secretions with infection (fever, coarse crackles, and purulent sputum)
• Acute ventilatory failure on present ventilator settings (but acceptable hypercapnia in this case)
• Severe hypoxemia (ABGs, extremely low PaO_2/FIO_2 ratio: 38)

P Call physician to discuss worsening PaO_2 and to confirm an acceptable hypercapnia level and PEEP upper limit. Airway Clearance Therapy Protocol (suction PRN). Adjust Mechanical Ventilation Protocol (titrate tidal volume and rate to raise $PaCO_2$ to permissive hypercapnia range). Repeat Gram stain and culture sputum. Closely monitor and reevaluate.

After 3 hours it was apparent that current management would not be successful; the physician decided to alert the extracorporeal membrane oxygenation (ECMO) team and place the patient on extracorporeal membrane oxygenation. This was done, and the patient was maintained on ECMO for 13 hours, when she developed ventricular tachycardia followed by ventricular fibrillation. Attempts to reestablish normal cardiac function were not successful, and the patient was pronounced dead 45 minutes later.

Discussion

This was possibly a preventable death. *Gastric lavage should never be performed on an unconscious patient unless the airway is first protected with a cuffed endotracheal tube.* This is one of the very few categoric imperatives in pulmonary medicine. The following three causative factors known to produce ARDS may have been operative in this patient: (1) drug overdose, (2) aspiration of gastric contents, and (3) breathing an excessive FIO_2 for a long period. As time progressed, the patient's lungs

became stiffer and physiologically nonfunctional as a result of the anatomic alterations associated with ARDS. The PaO_2/FIO_2 ratio helped detect this and raises the point that an initial (or very early) ABG at a known FIO_2 should be established in patients who are acutely ill.

As documented in the first assessment, her crackles, refractory hypoxemia, and radiograph findings all reflected the pathophysiologic changes seen in patients with atelectasis (see Fig. 10.7) and/or increased alveolar-capillary membrane thickening (see Fig. 10.9). Aggressive lung expansion therapy (see Protocol 10.3), in the form of PEEP, was used with mechanical ventilation from the start. Unfortunately, severe ARDS was confirmed 15 hours later—that is, when the respiratory symptoms associated with ARDS were present in less than 1 week, bilateral infiltrates were seen on the chest radiograph, and the PaO_2/FIO_2 ratio was only 38 on ventilator settings that include PEEP greater than 20 cm H_2O (see Box 28.3, The Berlin Definition of Acute Respiratory Distress Syndrome). The respiratory therapist's immediate reduction in the tidal volume of the patient to 300 mL, increase in respiratory rate to 20 breaths/min, and permissive hypercapnia were all clearly indicated and appropriate.

Unfortunately, these therapeutic techniques and use of ECMO to manage the condition were not enough in the final analysis.

SELF-ASSESSMENT QUESTIONS

1. In response to injury, the lungs of a patient with ARDS undergo which of the following changes?
   1. Atelectasis
   2. Decreased alveolar-capillary membrane permeability
   3. Interstitial and intraalveolar edema
   4. Hemorrhagic alveolar consolidation
      a. 1 and 3 only
      b. 2 and 4 only
      c. 1, 2, and 4 only
      d. 1, 3, and 4 only

2. Which of the following is/are recommended ventilation strategies for most patients with ARDS?
   1. High tidal volumes
   2. Low respiratory rates
   3. High respiratory rates
   4. Low tidal volumes
      a. 1 only
      b. 3 and 4 only
      c. 1 and 3 only
      d. 2 and 4 only

3. Common chest assessment findings in ARDS include the following:
   1. Diminished breath sounds
   2. Dull percussion note
   3. Bronchial breath sounds
   4. Crackles
      a. 1 only
      b. 3 only
      c. 2 and 3 only
      d. 2, 3, and 4 only

4. During the early stages of ARDS, the patient commonly demonstrates which one of the following arterial blood gas values?
   a. Decreased pH
   b. Decreased $PaCO_2$
   c. Increased HCO_3^-
   d. Normal PaO_2

5. Which of the following oxygenation indices is/are associated with ARDS?
   a. Increased $\dot{V}O_2$
   b. Decreased DO_2
   c. Increased $S\bar{v}O_2$
   d. Decreased $\dot{Q}_s/\dot{Q}_T$

Chapter Objectives

After reading this chapter, you will be able to:

- List the anatomic alterations of the lungs associated with Guillain-Barré syndrome.
- Describe the etiology and epidemiology of Guillain-Barré syndrome.
- List the cardiopulmonary clinical manifestations associated with Guillain-Barré syndrome.
- Describe the general management of Guillain-Barré syndrome.
- Describe the clinical strategies and rationales of the SOAPs presented in the case study.
- Define key terms and complete self-assessment questions at the end of the chapter and on Evolve.

Key Terms

Acute Inflammatory Demyelinating Polyradiculopathy (AIDP)
Acute Motor and Sensory Axonal Neuropathy (AMSAN)
Acute Motor Axonal Neuropathy (AMAN)
Albuminocytologic Dissociation (Spinal Fluid)
Areflexia
Ascending Paralysis
Autonomic Dysfunction
Campylobacter jejuni Infection
Cytomegalovirus (CMV) Infection
Demyelination
Dysautonomia
Electromyography (EMG)

Guillain-Barré Syndrome (GBS)
Hydrotherapy (Whirlpool Therapy)
Hyporeflexia
Intravenous Immune Globulin (IVIG)
Landry's Paralysis
Maximum Inspiratory Pressure (MIP)
Miller Fisher Syndrome
Nerve Conduction Studies (NCS)
Nonsteroidal Antiinflammatory Drugs (NSAIDs)
Paresthesia or Dysesthesias
Plasma Exchange
Plasmapheresis
Stryker Frame

Chapter Outline

Anatomic Alterations of the Lungs Associated With Guillain-Barré Syndrome
Etiology and Epidemiology
Clinical Presentation
  Diagnosis
Overview of Cardiopulmonary Clinical Manifestations Associated With Guillain-Barré Syndrome
General Management of Guillain-Barré Syndrome
  Respiratory Care Treatment Protocols
  Physical Therapy and Rehabilitation
Case Study: Guillain-Barré Syndrome
Self-Assessment Questions

Anatomic Alterations of the Lungs Associated With Guillain-Barré Syndrome[1]

Guillain-Barré syndrome (GBS) is an autoimmune disease that causes an acute peripheral nervous system disorder (called *polyneuropathy*) that results in a flaccid paralysis of the skeletal muscles and loss of muscle reflexes. Box 29.1 lists other names in the literature for GBS. In severe cases, paralysis of the

diaphragm and ventilatory failure can develop. Clinically, this is a medical emergency. In these cases, mechanical ventilation is required. If the patient is not properly managed (e.g., via the Airway Clearance Therapy Protocol, Protocol 10.2, Ventilator Initiation and Management Protocol, Protocol 11.1, and Ventilator Weaning Protocol, Protocol 11.2), mucus accumulation with airway obstruction, alveolar consolidation, and atelectasis may develop.

The major pathologic or structural changes of the lungs associated with poorly managed GBS are as follows:

- Mucus accumulation
- Airway obstruction

---

[1]The Guillain-Barré syndrome is named after the French physicians Georges Guillain and Jean Alexandre Barré, who described it in 1916.

TABLE 29.1 Subtypes of Guillain-Barré Syndrome*

Acute inflammatory demyelinating polyneuropathy (AIDP)	AIDP is the most common form of GBS in North America and Europe, representing about 75% to 80% of cases. AIDP falls into the classic category that affects motor, sensory, and autonomic nerves in a symmetric fashion.
Acute motor axonal neuropathy (AMAN)	AMAN is similar to AIDP, but without sensory symptoms, affects the motor axons of the nerves.
Acute motor and sensory axonal neuropathy (AMSAN)	AMSAN is a severe variant of GBS that is more prevalent in Asia, Central America, and South America. AMSAN causes severe, rapid destruction to nerves throughout the body.
Miller Fisher syndrome (MFS)	MFS is characterized by double vision, loss of balance, and loss of deep tendon reflexes

*All share the characteristic of being "rapid onset."
From GBS/CIDP Foundation: Everything you need to know. Retrieved from https://www.gbs-cidp.org/gbs/all-about-gbs/.

- Alveolar consolidation
- Atelectasis

Etiology and Epidemiology

GBS occurs worldwide with an overall incidence of 1 to 2 per 100,000 people. The incidence of GBS is slightly more frequent in males than in females. The incidence is greater in people over 50 years of age. GBS is 50% to 60% more common in whites than blacks. There is no obvious seasonal clustering of cases. As shown in Table 29.1, there are several different subtypes of GBS.

Although the precise cause of GBS is not fully understood, it is known that all forms of GBS are autoimmune diseases that develop from an immune response to foreign antigens

(e.g., an infectious agent) that attack the nerve tissues. For example, **acute inflammatory demyelinating polyradiculopathy (AIDP)** is thought to be caused by an immunologic attack that results in peripheral nerve demyelination and inflammation. Lymphocytes and macrophages appear to attack and strip off the myelin sheath of the peripheral nerves and leave swelling and fragmentation of the neural axon. It is believed that the myelin sheath covering the peripheral nerves (or the myelin-producing Schwann cell) is the actual target of the immune attack. Microscopically, the nerves show **demyelination**, inflammation, lymphocytes, macrophages, and edema. As the anatomic alterations of the peripheral nerves intensify, the ability of the neurons to transmit impulses to the muscles decreases, and eventually paralysis ensues (Fig. 29.1).

In about two-thirds of the cases, the onset of GBS occurs 1 to 4 weeks after a febrile episode caused by a mild respiratory or gastrointestinal viral or bacterial infection. Although the precise infectious cause of GBS is not fully understood, it is known that many patients with GBS have had a *Campylobacter jejuni* or **cytomegalovirus (CMV) infection** before developing GBS.

Other precipitating factors include infectious mononucleosis, parainfluenza 2, vaccinia, variola, measles, mumps, hepatitis A and B viruses, *Mycoplasma pneumoniae*, *Salmonella typhi*, and *Chlamydia psittaci*. Although the significance of the association is controversial, during the nationwide immunization campaign in the United States in 1976, more than 40 million adults were vaccinated with swine influenza vaccine and more than 500 new cases of GBS were reported among the vaccinated individuals, with 25 deaths. Today, about 2% to 3% of patients with GBS die.

Clinical Presentation

The general clinical history of patients with GBS is (1) symmetric muscle weakness in the distal extremities accompanied by **paresthesia** (tingling, burning, shocklike sensations) or **dysesthesias** (unpleasant, abnormal sense of touch), (2) pain (throbbing, aching, especially in the lower back, buttocks, and leg), and (3) numbness. The muscle paralysis then spreads upward (**ascending paralysis**) to the arms, trunk, and face. The muscle weakness and paralysis may develop within a single day or over several days. The muscle paralysis generally peaks in about 2 weeks. Deep tendon reflexes are commonly absent. More than half of patients experience severe pain, and about two-thirds have autonomic symptoms.

The patient often drools and has difficulty chewing, swallowing, and speaking. The management of oral secretions may be a problem. Oculomotor weakness occurs in about 15% of cases. In 10% to 30% of cases, respiratory muscle paralysis develops, followed by acute ventilatory failure (hypercapnic respiratory failure). Although GBS is typically an ascending paralysis—that is, moving from the lower portions of the legs and body upward—in about 10% of cases, muscle paralysis affects the facial and arm muscles first and then moves downward.

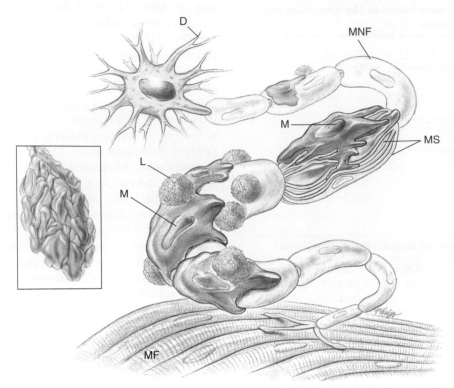

FIGURE 29.1 Guillain-Barré syndrome. Lymphocytes and macrophages attacking and stripping away the myelin sheath of a peripheral nerve. *D,* Dendrite; *L,* lymphocyte; *M,* macrophage; *MF,* muscle fiber; *MNF,* myelinated nerve fiber; *MS,* myelin sheath (cross-sectional view; note the macrophage attacking the myelin sheath). Inset, Atelectasis, a common secondary anatomic alteration of the lungs.

Although the weakness is commonly symmetric, a single arm or leg may be involved before paralysis spreads. The paralysis also may affect all four limbs simultaneously. Progression of the paralysis may stop at any point. After the paralysis reaches its maximum, it usually remains unchanged for a few days or weeks. Improvement generally begins spontaneously and continues for weeks or, in rare cases, months. Between 10% and 20% of patients have permanent residual neurologic deficits. About 90% of patients make a full recovery, but the recovery time may be as long as 3 years.

Diagnosis

If diagnosed early, patients with GBS have an excellent prognosis. The diagnosis is typically based on (1) the patient's clinical history (e.g., sudden ascending paralysis), (2) cerebrospinal fluid (CSF) findings (obtained through a lumbar spinal puncture), and (3) thorough neurophysiology studies by way of an **electromyography (EMG)** or a **nerve conduction studies (NCS)**. Neurophysiology studies are usually not required for the diagnosis.

- *Spinal fluid:* In 80% to 90% of cases, the typical CSF finding is an elevated protein level (100 to 1000 mg/dL) with a normal white blood cell count. This is called **albuminocytologic dissociation of the spinal fluid.**

- *Neurophysiology:* Directly assessing the patient's nerve conduction of electrical impulses can exclude other causes of acute muscle weakness and distinguish the different types of Guillain-Barré syndromes. Needle EMG results typically show evidence of an acute polyneuropathy with demyelinating characteristics in acute inflammatory demyelinating polyneuropathy (AIDP). Other EMG findings may include features that are predominantly axonal in acute motor axonal neuropathy (AMAN), or acute sensorimotor axonal neuropathy (AMSAN). Box 29.2 provides the diagnostic criteria for GBS developed by the National Institute of Neurological Disorders and Stroke (NINDS). These criteria are based on expert consensus and are widely used today in clinical practice.[2]

Also shown in Box 29.2, note that glycolipid antibodies may be associated with some GBS subtypes. For example, antibodies against GQ1b (a ganglioside component of nerve) are found in 85% to 90% of patients with **Miller Fisher syndrome**. Antibodies to GM1, GD1a, GalNac-GD1a, and GD1b are mostly associated with axonal subtypes of GBS.

---

[2]These diagnostic criteria have been used for years in research studies and are applicable to about 80% or 90% of patients with GBS in North America and Europe, particularly those with the AIDP form of GBS.

OVERVIEW of the Cardiopulmonary Clinical Manifestations Associated With Guillain-Barré Syndrome

The following clinical manifestations result from the pathologic mechanisms caused (or activated) by atelectasis (see Fig. 10.7), alveolar consolidation (see Fig. 10.8), and excessive bronchial secretions (see Fig. 10.11)—the major anatomic alterations of the lungs associated with GBS, which may occur when the patient is not properly managed via the Airway Clearance Therapy Protocol, Protocol 10.2, and Ventilator Initiation and Management Protocol, Protocol 11.1, and Ventilator Weaning Protocol, Protocol 11.2 (see Fig. 29.1).[1]

CLINICAL DATA OBTAINED AT THE PATIENT'S BEDSIDE

The Physical Examination

Respiratory Rate
- Varies with the degree of respiratory muscle paralysis
- Apnea (in severe cases)
- Anxiety

Cyanosis

Chest Assessment Findings
- Diminished breath sounds
- Crackles

CLINICAL DATA OBTAINED FROM LABORATORY TESTS AND SPECIAL PROCEDURES

Pulmonary Function Test Findings[2]
(Restrictive Lung Pathology)

FORCED EXPIRATORY VOLUME AND FLOW RATE FINDINGS

FVC	FEV_T	FEV_1/FVC ratio	$FEF_{25\%-75\%}$
↓	N or ↓	N or ↑	N or ↓

$FEF_{50\%}$	$FEF_{200-1200}$	PEFR	MVV
N or ↓	N or ↓	N or ↓	N or ↓

LUNG VOLUME AND CAPACITY FINDINGS

V_T	IRV	ERV	RV
↓	↓	↓	↓

VC	IC	FRC	TLC	RV/TLC ratio
↓	↓	↓	↓	N

MAXIMUM INSPIRATORY PRESSURE (MIP) ↓

Arterial Blood Gases
Moderate to Severe Guillain-Barré Syndrome

Acute Ventilatory Failure With Hypoxemia[3] (Acute Respiratory Acidosis)

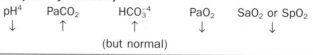

pH^4	$PaCO_2$	HCO_3^{-4}	PaO_2	SaO_2 or SpO_2
↓	↑	↑ (but normal)	↓	↓

Oxygenation Indices[5]

$\dot{Q}_S/\dot{Q}_T$	DO_2^6	$\dot{V}O_2$	$C(a-\bar{v})O_2$	O_2ER	$S\bar{v}O_2$
↑	↓	N	N	↑	↓

RADIOLOGIC FINDINGS

Chest Radiograph
- Normal, or
- Increased opacity (when atelectasis or consolidation are present)

If the ventilatory failure associated with GBS is properly managed (e.g., via the Airway Clearance Therapy Protocol, Protocol 10.2, Ventilator Initiation and Management Protocol, Protocol 11.1, and Ventilator Weaning Protocol, Protocol 11.2), the chest radiograph should appear normal. However, if the patient is not properly managed, mucous accumulation, alveolar consolidation, and atelectasis may develop. In these cases, the chest radiograph will show an increased density of the lung segments affected.

AUTONOMIC NERVOUS SYSTEM DYSFUNCTIONS

Dysautonomia (autonomic dysfunction) occurs in about 70% of cases. Symptoms include:
- Cardiac arrhythmias
  - Tachycardia (the most common)
  - Bradycardia, ventricular tachycardia, atrial flutter, atrial fibrillation, and asystole
- Urinary retention
- Hypertension alternating with hypotension
- Orthostatic hypotension
- Obstruction of the intestines (ileus)
- Loss of sweating

---

[1]It should be noted that the clinical manifestations associated with Guillain-Barré may occur over hours or days, depending on how quickly the paralysis progresses.

[2]Progressive worsening of these values is key to anticipating the onset of ventilatory failure.

[3]See Fig. 5.3 and Table 5.5 and related discussion for the acute pH, $PaCO_2$, and HCO_3^- changes associated with acute ventilatory failure.

[4]When tissue hypoxia is severe enough to produce lactic acid, the pH and HCO_3^- values will be lower than expected for a particular $PaCO_2$ level.

[5]$C(a-\bar{v})O_2$, Arterial-venous oxygen difference; DO_2, total oxygen delivery; O_2ER, oxygen extraction ratio; $\dot{Q}_S/\dot{Q}_T$, pulmonary shunt fraction; $S\bar{v}O_2$, mixed venous oxygen saturation; $\dot{V}O_2$, oxygen consumption.

[6]The DO_2 may be normal in patients who have compensated to the decreased oxygenation status with (1) an increased cardiac output, (2) an increased hemoglobin level, or (3) a combination of both. When the DO_2 is normal, the O_2ER is usually normal.

General Management of Guillain-Barré Syndrome[3]

GBS is a potential medical emergency, and patients must be monitored closely after the diagnosis has been made. About 30% of cases develop acute ventilatory failure and require mechanical ventilation. The primary treatment should be directed at stabilization of vital signs and supportive care for the patient. Close respiratory monitoring with frequent measurements of the patient's forced vital capacity (FVC), **maximum inspiratory pressure (MIP)**, maximum expiratory pressure (MEP), blood pressure, oxygenation saturation, and, when indicated, arterial blood gases (ABGs) should be performed. Mechanical ventilation should be initiated when the clinical data demonstrate impending or acute ventilatory failure.

Good clinical indicators of impending acute ventilatory failure include the following:

- FVC <20 mL/kg
- MIP <−30 cm H_2O: In other words, the patient is unable to generate a maximum inspiratory pressure of −30 cm H_2O or more. For example, an MIP of only −15 cm H_2O would

confirm severe muscle weakness and, importantly, that acute ventilatory failure is likely.

- MEP <40 cm H_2O
- $PaCO_2$ >45 mm Hg
- pH <7.35

The primary treatment modalities for GBS are (1) **plasmapheresis** (also called **plasma exchange**) and (2) **intravenous immune globulin (IVIG)**. These two treatments have been shown to be equally effective. Plasmapheresis, or plasma exchange (PE), has been shown to be effective in decreasing the morbidity and shortening the clinical course of GBS. Plasmapheresis entails the removal of damaged antibodies from the patient's blood plasma, followed by the transfusion of blood. It is believed that plasmapheresis removes the antibodies from the plasma that contribute to the immune system attack on the peripheral nerves. This procedure has been shown to reduce circulating antibody titers during the early stages of the disorder. High-dose IVIG has been demonstrated to be at least as effective, and possibly more, than plasmapheresis. IVIG is a blood product that contains the pooled immunoglobulins (IgG) from thousands of donors. The effects of IVIG last between 2 weeks and 3 months. IVIG products are used to treat multiple conditions, including GBS. Glucocorticoids are not recommended.

As in any patient who is paralyzed or immobilized for prolonged periods, the risk for thromboembolism increases. Because of this danger, the patient commonly receives anticoagulants, elastic stockings, and passive range-of-motion exercises (every 3 to 4 hours) for all extremities. To prevent skin breakdown, the patient should be turned frequently. **Nonsteroidal antiinflammatory agents (NSAIDs)** are helpful for pain control. A rotary bed or **Stryker frame** may be required. Blood pressure disturbances and cardiac arrhythmias require immediate attention. For example, episodes of bradycardia are commonly treated with atropine.

Respiratory Care Treatment Protocols

Oxygen Therapy Protocol

Oxygen therapy is used to treat hypoxemia, decrease the work of breathing, and decrease myocardial work. Because of the hypoxemia that may develop in GBS, supplemental oxygen may be required. However, because of the alveolar consolidation and atelectasis associated with GBS, capillary shunting may be present. Hypoxemia caused by capillary shunting is refractory to oxygen therapy (see Oxygen Therapy Protocol, Protocol 10.1).

Airway Clearance Therapy Protocol

Because of the excessive mucous accumulation, airway obstruction, alveolar consolidation, and atelectasis associated with GBS, a number of airway clearance modalities may be used to enhance the mobilization of bronchial secretions (see Airway Clearance Therapy Protocol, Protocol 10.2).

Lung Expansion Therapy Protocol

Lung expansion measures are commonly administered to offset the alveolar consolidation and atelectasis associated with GBS (see Lung Expansion Therapy Protocol, Protocol 10.3).

---

[3]About 80% of GBS cases have a complete recovery within a few months. Even with treatment, about 5% to 10% of cases have a prolonged course with very prolonged and incomplete recovery. About 2% to 3% die despite intensive care. In addition, relapse occurs in up to 10% of patients.

Mechanical Ventilation Protocol

Mechanical ventilation may be necessary to provide and support alveolar gas exchange and eventually return the patient to spontaneous breathing. Because acute ventilatory failure is seen in patients with severe GBS, continuous mechanical ventilation is often required. Continuous mechanical ventilation is justified because the acute ventilatory failure is thought to be reversible. Noninvasive positive-pressure ventilation (NIPPV) may be helpful if carefully monitored (see Ventilator Initiation and Management Protocol, Protocol 11.1, and Ventilator Weaning Protocol, Protocol 11.2).

Physical Therapy and Rehabilitation

Physical therapy usually begins long before the patient recovers from the effects of GBS, often while the patient is still being mechanically ventilated. In long-term cases, for example, the arms and legs of the patient will be manually moved on a regular basis to keep the muscles flexible. After recovery, the patient frequently requires physical therapy to regain full strength and normal mobility. **Hydrotherapy (whirlpool therapy)** is commonly used to relieve pain and facilitate limb movement. Full recovery may occur in as little as a few weeks or as long as 3 years.

CASE STUDY Guillain-Barré Syndrome

Admitting History and Physical Examination

A 48-year-old career US Navy physician visited the base hospital clinic because of the acute onset of severe muscle weakness. He had joined the Navy immediately after medical school. Throughout his time in the service, he had the opportunity to pursue his passion—competitive water-ski jumping. For many years he was the first-place winner at most tournaments, including the nationals held yearly. For almost 25 years, he progressed through the age divisions, always remaining the top seed, always capturing the highest title.

The man was in outstanding physical condition. He was an avid runner and weightlifter, and during the off-season he often traveled to a warm climate to practice his water-ski jumping. He had never smoked and had never been hospitalized. He had an occasional "cold." About 2 years previously, he had begun to focus all his attention on his 19-year-old son, who was quickly following in his father's footsteps, having just captured the Men's Division I championship in collegiate ice hockey.

The man stated that he had felt good until 3 weeks before his admission, at which time he experienced a flulike syndrome for 3 days. About 10 days after returning to work, he noticed a tingling and burning sensation in his feet during his morning patient rounds. By dinner time that same day, the tingling and burning had radiated from his feet to about the level of his knees. Thinking that he was just tired from being on his feet all day, he went to bed early that evening. The next morning, however, his legs were completely numb, although he could still move them. Alarmed, he asked his son to drive him to the clinic. After examining him, his doctor (a personal friend) admitted him for a diagnostic workup and observation.

Over the next 3 days, the laboratory results showed that the patient's CSF had an elevated protein concentration with a normal cell count. The electrodiagnostic studies showed a progressive ascending paralysis of the man's legs and arms. He began to have difficulty eating and swallowing his food. The respiratory therapist, who was monitoring his forced vital capacity (FVC), maximum inspiratory pressure (MIP), pulse oximetry, and arterial blood gas values (ABGs), reported a progressive deterioration in all the values. A provisional diagnosis of Guillain-Barré syndrome was recorded in the patient's chart.

When the man's ABGs showed pH 7.29, $PaCO_2$ 53 mm Hg, HCO_3^- 23 mEq/L, PaO_2 86 mm Hg, and SaO_2 96% (on a 2 L/min oxygen nasal cannula), the respiratory therapist called the attending physician and reported his assessment of acute ventilatory failure. The doctor transferred the patient to the intensive care unit (ICU), intubated him, and placed him on a mechanical ventilator. The initial ventilator settings were synchronized intermittent mandatory ventilation (SIMV) mode, 12 breaths/min, tidal volume 750 mL, and FIO_2 0.50, without added PEEP.

About 15 minutes after the patient was committed to the ventilator, he appeared comfortable. No spontaneous breaths were noted between the 12 set breaths/min. His vital signs were blood pressure 126/82 mm Hg and heart rate 68 beats/min. He was afebrile. A portable chest radiograph confirmed that the endotracheal (ET) tube was in a good position and the lungs were adequately aerated. Normal vesicular breath sounds were auscultated over both lung fields. His ABGs were pH 7.51, $PaCO_2$ 29 mm Hg, HCO_3^- 22 mEq/L, PaO_2 204 mm Hg, and SaO_2 98%. On the basis of these clinical data, the following SOAP was documented.

Respiratory Assessment and Plan

S N/A (intubated on ventilator)

O Vital signs: BP 126/82, HR 68, RR 12 (SIMV); afebrile; no spontaneous breaths; CXR: normal; normal breath sounds; ABGs (on FIO_2 0.50) pH 7.51, $PaCO_2$ 29, HCO_3^- 22, PaO_2 204, SaO_2 98%

A • Acute alveolar hyperventilation with excessive oxygenation on ventilator (ABGs)

  • FIO$_2$ too high (ABGs)

P Adjust mechanical ventilator settings (decrease tidal volume to 650 mL and FIO$_2$ to 0.40) according to Mechanical Ventilation Protocol and Oxygen Therapy Protocol. Monitor closely and reevaluate.

Three Days After Admission

The patient's cardiopulmonary status had been unremarkable. No improvement was seen in his muscular paralysis. No changes had been made in his ventilator settings over the previous 48 hours. His skin color appeared good. Palpation and percussion of the chest were unremarkable. On auscultation, however, coarse crackles could be heard over both lung fields.

Moderate amounts of thick, whitish, clear secretions were being suctioned from the patient's endotracheal tube regularly. His vital signs were blood pressure 124/83 mm Hg, heart rate 74 beats/min, and rectal temperature 37.7°C (99.8°F). A recent portable chest radiograph revealed no significant pathologic process. His ABGs on an FIO$_2$ of 0.40, a respiratory rate of 12 breaths/min, and tidal volume of 650 were pH 7.44, PaCO$_2$ 35 mm Hg, HCO$_3^-$ 24 mEq/L, PaO$_2$ 98 mm Hg, and SaO$_2$ 97%. On the basis of these clinical data, the following SOAP was documented.

Respiratory Assessment and Plan

S N/A (intubated on ventilator)

O Skin color good; coarse crackles over both lung fields; moderate amount of whitish, clear secretions being suctioned regularly; vital signs BP 124/83, HR 74, T 37.7°C (99.8°F); CXR: unremarkable; ABGs (FIO$_2$ 0.4) pH 7.44, PaCO$_2$ 35, HCO$_3^-$ 24, PaO$_2$ 98, SaO$_2$ 97%.

A • Normal acid-base and oxygenation status on present ventilator settings (ABGs)

  • Excessive sputum accumulation; possible progression to mucous plugging and atelectasis (coarse crackles, whitish and clear secretions)

P Begin Airway Clearance Therapy Protocol (PRN tracheal suctioning and obtain sputum stain and culture). Begin Lung Expansion Therapy Protocol (+10 cm H$_2$O positive end-expiratory pressure [PEEP] to offset any early development of atelectasis). Monitor and reevaluate (4 × per shift). Continue Mechanical Ventilation Protocol and Oxygen Therapy Protocol.

Five Days After Admission

The patient remained alert and comfortable, except for the presence of the ET tube. His muscular paralysis remained unchanged. His skin color appeared good, and no abnormalities were noted during palpation and percussion of the chest. Although coarse crackles could still be heard over both lung fields, they were not as intense as they had been 48 hours earlier. A small amount of clear secretions was suctioned from the patient's ET tube. His vital signs were blood pressure 118/79 mm Hg, heart rate 68 beats/min, and temperature normal. Results of a recent portable chest radiograph appeared normal. His ABGs on an FIO$_2$ of 0.40, a respiratory rate of 12 breaths/min, a tidal volume of 650, and PEEP of +10 cm

H$_2$O were pH 7.42, PaCO$_2$ 37 mm Hg, HCO$_3^-$ 24 mEq/L, PaO$_2$ 97 mm Hg, and SaO$_2$ 97%. The sputum culture was unremarkable. On the basis of these clinical data, the following SOAP note was recorded.

Respiratory Assessment and Plan

S N/A (intubated on ventilator)

O Skin color good; coarse crackles over both lung fields improving; small amount of clear secretions suctioned; vital signs BP 118/79, HR 68, T normal; no spontaneous respirations; CXR: normal; ABGs (FIO$_2$ 0.4) pH 7.42, PaCO$_2$ 37, HCO$_3^-$ 24, PaO$_2$ 97, SaO$_2$ 97%.

A • Normal acid-base and oxygenation status on present ventilator settings (ABGs)

  • Respiratory insufficiency (no spontaneous respirations)

  • Secretion control improving (coarse crackles, clear secretions)

P Continue Mechanical Ventilation Protocol. Continue Airway Clearance Therapy Protocol. Continue Lung Expansion Therapy Protocol. Monitor and reevaluate (SpO$_2$, maximum inspiratory pressure, and forced vital capacity 2 × per shift).

Discussion

Guillain-Barré syndrome is a neuromuscular paralysis that ensues after infection with a neurotropic virus. This patient had a classic history of ascending paralysis and paresthesia and the diagnostic finding of elevated protein concentration in the spinal fluid. In this setting, serial measurements of the patient's forced vital capacity (FVC), maximum inspiratory pressure (MIP), blood pressure, oxygen saturation, and arterial blood gases (ABGs) must be measured and charted.

Once respiratory failure develops, intubation and respiratory support on a ventilator became necessary. As discussed in this chapter, good clinical indicators of acute ventilatory failure include FVC less than 20 mL/kg, MIP below −30 cm H$_2$O, pH less than 7.35, and PaCO$_2$ greater than 45 mm Hg. As noted by the respiratory therapist, a progressive deterioration was observed in all of these clinical indicators over a 3-day period.

As shown during the first assessment, when acute ventilatory failure developed, the patient was transferred to the ICU, intubated, and placed on a mechanical ventilator. Shortly after the patient was placed on the ventilator, his ABG values showed hyperoxia and acute alveolar hyperventilation, both of which were caused by the ventilator settings. The appropriate response was to immediately adjust the ventilator settings by reducing the tidal volume or frequency (or both) and the FIO$_2$. At the time of the assessment, the patient exhibited no evidence of airway obstruction or secretions. Therefore the Airway Clearance Therapy Protocol (Protocol 10.2) was not indicated. Indeed, all that needed to be done at that time was to ensure adequate ventilation and oxygenation on the ventilator.

However, 3 days later, at the time of the second assessment, coarse crackles were heard over all lung fields. There was no indication of fluid overload. Clearly the time had come to initiate the Airway Clearance Therapy Protocol (Protocol 10.2). Because of the risk for atelectasis, the Lung Expansion

Therapy Protocol (Protocol 10.3), in the form of PEEP on the ventilator, was indicated. In such a case, the sputum should be cultured to see whether any infectious organisms were present.

At the time of the final assessment (2 days later), the clinical indicators for airway secretions had decreased—the crackles could no longer be heard over the lung fields, and the small amount of sputum suctioned appeared clear. At that point down-regulation of the Airway Clearance Therapy Protocol (Protocol 10.2) was indicated.

Serial SpO$_2$, FVC, or MIP measurements would continue to be made until the patient was ready to be extubated and thereafter for at least several days. Indeed, extubation occurred about 3 weeks after the initiation of mechanical ventilation. The patient recovered without incident and returned to his active lifestyle within a year.

SELF-ASSESSMENT QUESTIONS

1. In Guillain-Barré syndrome, which of the following pathologic changes develop in the peripheral nerves?
   1. Inflammation
   2. Increased ability to transmit nerve impulses
   3. Demyelination
   4. Edema
      a. 2 and 3 only
      b. 3 and 4 only
      c. 2, 3, and 4 only
      d. 1, 3, and 4 only

2. Which of the following is(are) associated with Guillain-Barré syndrome?
   1. Alveolar consolidation
   2. Mucus accumulation
   3. Alveolar hyperinflation
   4. Atelectasis
      a. 1 and 2 only
      b. 3 and 4 only
      c. 1, 2, and 4 only
      d. 2, 3, and 4 only

3. Guillain-Barré syndrome is more common in:
   1. People older than 50 years of age
   2. Blacks
   3. Males than in females
   4. Early childhood
      a. 1 only
      b. 4 only
      c. 1 and 3 only
      d. 3 and 4 only

4. Which of the following are possible precursors to Guillain-Barré syndrome?
   1. Mumps
   2. Swine influenza vaccine
   3. Infectious mononucleosis
   4. Measles
      a. 2 and 4 only
      b. 3 and 4 only
      c. 2, 3, and 4 only
      d. 1, 2, 3, and 4

5. Full recovery from Guillain-Barré syndrome is expected in approximately what percentage of cases?
   a. 30%
   b. 40%
   c. 50%
   d. 90%

6. Which of the following are indicators for intubation and mechanical ventilation in patients with Guillain-Barré syndrome?
   1. pH >7.40
   2. PaCO$_2$ >45
   3. FVC <20 mL/kg
   4. MIP <−30 cm H$_2$O
      a. 1 and 2 only
      b. 3 and 4 only
      c. 2, 3, and 4 only
      d. 1, 2, and 3 only

Chapter Objectives

After reading this chapter, you will be able to:

- List the anatomic alterations of the lungs associated with myasthenia gravis.
- Describe the etiology and epidemiology of myasthenia gravis.
- Discuss the screening for and diagnosis of myasthenia gravis.
- List the cardiopulmonary clinical manifestations associated with myasthenia gravis.
- Describe the general management of myasthenia gravis.
- Describe the clinical strategies and rationales of the SOAPs presented in the case study.
- Define key terms and complete self-assessment questions at the end of the chapter and on Evolve.

Key Terms

Acetylcholine (ACh)
Acetylcholinesterase inhibitors
Anticholinesterase Inhibitors
Binding AChR Antibodies Test
Chronic Immunotherapies
CMAP Amplitude
Decremental Response
Diplopia
Edrophonium (Tensilon) Test
Electromyography
Generalized Myasthenia Gravis
Ice Pack Test
Immunoglobulin G (IgG) Antibodies
Inadvertent Right Mainstem Bronchial Intubation
Intravenous Immune Globulin (IVIG)
Muscle-specific receptor tyrosine kinase (MuSK)
Myasthenic Crisis
Mycophenolate Mofetil

Neuromuscular Junction
Ocular Myasthenia Gravis
Ophthalmoparesis
Ophthalmoplegia
Plasmapheresis
Ptosis
Pyridostigmine (Mestinon)
Rapid Immunotherapies
Repetitive Nerve Stimulation (RNS)
Seronegative Myasthenia Gravis
Seropositive Myasthenia Gravis
Single-Fiber Electromyography (SFEMG)
Symptomatic Treatment
Thymectomy
Thymoma

Chapter Outline

Anatomic Alterations of the Lungs Associated With Myasthenia Gravis

Myasthenia gravis is the most common chronic disorder of the **neuromuscular junction**. The disorder interferes with the chemical transmission of **acetylcholine (ACh)** between the axonal terminal and the receptor sites of voluntary muscles (Fig. 30.1). The hallmark clinical feature of myasthenia gravis is fluctuating skeletal muscle weakness, often with true muscle fatigue. The fatigue and weakness usually improve after rest.

There are two clinical types of myasthenia gravis: *ocular* and *generalized.* In **ocular myasthenia gravis**, the muscle weakness is limited to the eyelids and extraocular muscles. In **generalized myasthenia gravis**, the muscle weakness involves a variable combination of (1) muscles of the mouth and throat responsible for speech and swallowing (called *bulbar muscles*), (2) limbs, and (3) respiratory muscles. Neck extensor and flexor muscles are commonly affected, producing a "dropped head syndrome." The facial muscles are often involved, causing the patient to appear expressionless. Generalized myasthenia gravis may, or may not,

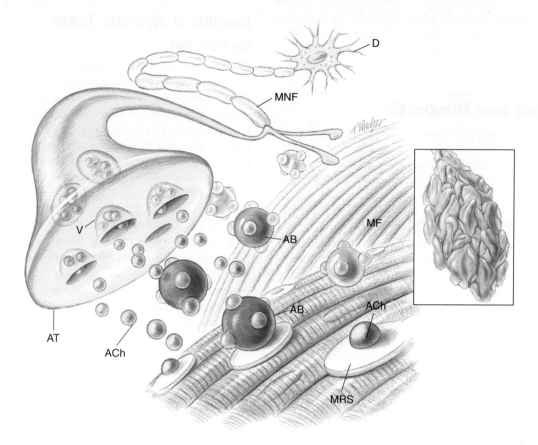

FIGURE 30.1 Myasthenia gravis, a disorder of the neuromuscular junction that interferes with the chemical transmission of acetylcholine. *AB,* Antibody; *ACh,* acetylcholine; *AT,* axonal terminal; *D,* dendrite; *MF,* muscle fiber; *MNF,* myelinated nerve fiber; *MRS,* muscle receptor site; *V,* vesicle. Note that the antibodies have a physical structure similar to that of ACh, which permits them to connect to (and block ACh from) the muscle receptor sites. Inset, Atelectasis, a common secondary anatomic alteration of the lungs.

involve the ocular muscles. Because the disorder affects only the myoneural (motor) junction, sensory function is not lost.

The abnormal weakness may be confined to an isolated group of muscles (e.g., the drooping of one or both eyelids), or it may manifest as a generalized weakness that in severe cases includes the diaphragm. When the diaphragm is involved, ventilatory failure can develop, producing **myasthenic crisis**. In these cases, mechanical ventilation is required. If the patient is not properly managed (e.g., via the Airway Clearance Therapy Protocol, Protocol 10.2, Ventilator Initiation and Management Protocol, Protocol 11.1, and Ventilator Weaning Protocol, Protocol 11.2), mucus accumulation with airway obstruction, alveolar consolidation, and atelectasis may develop.

The major pathologic or structural changes of the lungs associated with a poorly managed myasthenic crisis are as follows:

• Mucus accumulation
• Airway obstruction
• Alveolar consolidation
• Atelectasis

Etiology and Epidemiology

The cause of myasthenia gravis appears to be related to ACh receptor (AChR) antibodies (**immunoglobulin G [IgG]**

antibodies) that block the nerve impulse transmissions at the neuromuscular junction. Patients who have detectable antibodies to the AChR, or to **muscle-specific receptor tyrosine kinase (MuSK)**, are said to have **seropositive myasthenia gravis**, whereas those lacking both AChR and MuSK antibodies on standard assays are said to have **seronegative myasthenia gravis**. About 50% of patients with only ocular myasthenia gravis are seropositive. About 90% of cases of generalized myasthenia gravis are seropositive.

It is believed that the IgG antibodies disrupt the chemical transmission of ACh at the neuromuscular junction by (1) blocking the ACh from the receptor sites of the muscular cell, (2) accelerating the breakdown of ACh, and (3) destroying the receptor sites (see Fig. 30.1). Receptor-binding antibodies are present in 85% to 90% of persons with myasthenia gravis. Although the specific events that activate the formation of the antibodies remain unclear, the thymus gland is often abnormal; it is generally presumed that the antibodies arise within the thymus or in related tissue.

According to the Myasthenia Gravis Foundation of America, there are between 36,000–60,000 cases of myasthenia gravis in the United States (20 per 100,000 population). The disease usually has a peak age of onset in females of 15 to 35 years, compared with 40 to 70 years in males. The clinical manifestations associated with myasthenia gravis are often provoked by emotional upset, physical stress, exposure to extreme temperature changes, febrile illness, and pregnancy. Death caused by myasthenia gravis is possible, especially during the first few years after onset.

Screening and Diagnosis

Screening methods and tests used to diagnose myasthenia gravis include (1) clinical presentation and history, (2) bedside tests, (3) immunologic studies, (4) electrodiagnostic studies, and (5) evaluation of conditions associated with myasthenia gravis.

Clinical Presentation and History

The hallmark of myasthenia gravis is chronic muscle fatigue. The muscles become progressively weaker during periods of activity and improve after periods of rest. Signs and symptoms include facial muscle weakness; **ptosis** (drooping of one or both eyelids); **diplopia** (double vision); **ophthalmoplegia** (paralysis or weakness of one or more of the muscles that control eye movement); difficulty in breathing, speaking, chewing, and swallowing; unstable gait; and weakness in arms, hands, fingers, legs, and neck brought on by repetitive motions. The muscles that control the eyes, eyelids, face, and throat are especially susceptible and are usually affected first. The respiratory muscles of the diaphragm and chest wall can become weak and impair the patient's ventilation. Impairment in deep breathing and coughing predisposes the patient to retain bronchial secretions, atelectasis, and pneumonia.

The signs and symptoms of myasthenia gravis during the early stages are often elusive. The onset can be subtle, intermittent, or sudden and rapid. The patient may (1) demonstrate normal health for weeks or months at a time, (2) show signs of weakness only late in the day or evening, or (3) develop a sudden and transient generalized weakness that includes the diaphragm. Because of this last characteristic, ventilatory failure is always a sinister possibility. In most cases, the first noticeable symptom is weakness of the eye muscles (droopy eyelids) and a change in the patient's facial expressions. As the disorder becomes more generalized, weakness develops in the arms and legs. The muscle weakness is usually more pronounced in the proximal parts of the extremities. The patient has difficulty in climbing stairs, lifting objects, maintaining balance, and walking. In severe cases, the weakness of the upper limbs may be such that the hand cannot be lifted to the mouth. Muscle atrophy or pain is rare. Tendon reflexes almost always remain intact.

Bedside Diagnostic Tests

Ice Pack Test

The **ice pack test** is a very simple, safe, and reliable procedure for diagnosing myasthenia gravis in patients who have ptosis (droopy eye). In addition, the ice pack test does not require special medications or expensive equipment and is free of adverse effects. The test consists of the application of an ice pack to the patient's symptomatic eye for 3 to 5 minutes (Fig. 30.2). The test is considered positive for myasthenia gravis when there is improvement of the ptosis (an increase of at least 2 mm in the palpebral fissure from before to after the test).

A major disadvantage of the ice pack test is that it is useful only when ptosis is present. Even though the symptoms associated with diplopia (double vision) also may improve with the ice pack test, the reliability of the ice pack test in patients with diplopia without ptosis is usually questionable because the patient's personal impression of the diplopia is subjective. Therefore caution should be exercised in patients with isolated diplopia without ptosis. The ice pack test may be especially useful in patients in whom the edrophonium test is contraindicated by either cardiac status or age.

Edrophonium (Tensilon) Test

The **edrophonium (Tensilon) test** is used in patients with obvious ptosis or **ophthalmoparesis**. Edrophonium, a short-acting drug, blocks cholinesterase from breaking down ACh after it has been released from the terminal axon. This action increases the myoneural concentration of ACh, which in turn offsets the influx of antibodies at the neuromuscular junction. When muscular weakness is caused by myasthenia gravis, a dramatic transitory improvement in muscle function (lasting about 10 minutes) is seen after the administration of edrophonium. A disadvantage of the edrophonium test is that it can be complicated by cholinergic side effects that include cardiac arrhythmias and cardiopulmonary arrest. Cardiac monitoring, or avoiding this test altogether, is suggested in the elderly or those with a history of arrhythmia or heart disease. Although the sensitivity of the Tensilon test for the diagnosis of myasthenia gravis is in the 80% to 90% range, it is associated with many false-negative and false-positive results.

Immunologic Studies

Serologic tests to detect the presence of circulating acetylcholine receptor antibodies (AChR-Abs) is the first step in the laboratory confirmation of myasthenia. There are three AChR-Ab

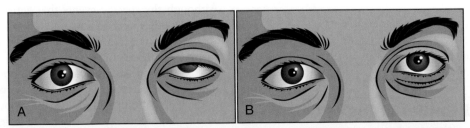

FIGURE 30.2 Ice pack test. (A) Myasthenia gravis in a patient who has ptosis (droopy left eye). (B) Same patient after 5-minute application of an ice pack. Note that the patient's left eye lid is no longer droopy.

assays: binding, blocking, and modulating. The **binding AChR antibodies test** is highly specific for myasthenia gravis (80% to 90%). Most experts use the term *AChR-Abs* as synonymous with the binding antibodies. In some patients, assays for blocking and modulating antibodies also may be helpful. Blocking AChR-Abs are found in about 50% of patients with generalized myasthenia gravis. Assays for modulating AChR-Abs increase the diagnostic sensitivity by about 5% when combined with the binding studies. When AChR-Abs are negative, an assay for the antibodies to MuSK proteins should be performed.

Electrodiagnostic Studies

The **repetitive nerve stimulation (RNS)** and **single-fiber electromyography (SFEMG)** tests are important diagnostic supplements to the immunologic studies. The RNS study is the most frequently used electrodiagnostic test for myasthenia gravis. The RNS study is performed by electrically stimulating the motor nerve of selected muscles 6 to 10 times at low rates (2 or 3 Hz). In the normal muscle, there is no change in the compound muscle action potential (CMAP) amplitude. In patients with myasthenia gravis, there may be a progressive decline in the **CMAP amplitude** within the first four to five stimuli—called a **decremental response**. The RNS is considered positive when the decrement is greater than 10%.

The SFEMG is the most sensitive diagnostic test for myasthenia gravis, although it is technically more difficult. A specialized needle electrode allows simultaneous recording of the action potential of two muscle fibers innervated by the same motor axon. The variability in time between the two action potentials is called *jitter*. In patients with myasthenia gravis, the jitter is increased. The SFEMG is positive in more than 95% of patients with generalized myasthenia gravis. The sensitivity of the SFEMG ranges between 85% and 95% in ocular myasthenia gravis.

Evaluation of Conditions Associated With Myasthenia Gravis

Thymic Tumors and Other Malignancies

Thymic abnormalities are often seen in patients with myasthenia gravis. Computed tomography (CT) or magnetic resonance imaging (MRI) scans may be used to identify an abnormal thymus gland or the presence of a **thymoma** (a usually benign tumor of the thymus gland that may be associated with myasthenia gravis). A **thymectomy** has been shown to reduce symptoms of myasthenia gravis. In fact, a thymectomy may be recommended even when there is no tumor. The removal of the thymus seems to improve the condition in many patients.

Differential Diagnosis

Studies to rule out other disease in the differential diagnosis of myasthenia gravis are indicated in some patients. For example, in cases with ocular or bulbar symptoms, an MRI of the brain is indicated. CT scanning or ultrasound of the orbits is helpful in the differential diagnosis of ocular myasthenia and thyroid ophthalmopathy. A lumbar puncture may be helpful in ruling out lymphomatous or carcinomatous

meningitis in some cases. Blood tests should include thyroid function tests. In patients who have symptoms associated with a rheumatologic disorder, assays for antinuclear antibodies and rheumatoid factor should be performed.

Pulmonary Function Testing

Pulmonary function testing may be performed to help evaluate the patient's ventilatory status and the possibility of ventilatory failure—that is, a myasthenic crisis. Serial testing is advised.

Table 30.1 provides a widely accepted clinical classification system of myasthenia gravis, which was developed by the Myasthenia Gravis Foundation of America.

TABLE 30.1 Clinical Classifications of Myasthenia Gravis

Class I	Any ocular muscle weakness; may have weakness of eye closure; all other muscle strength is normal
Class II	Mild weakness affecting other ocular muscles; may also have ocular muscle weakness of any severity
Class IIa	Predominantly affecting limb, axial muscles, or both; may also have lesser involvement of oropharyngeal muscles
Class IIb	Predominantly affecting oropharyngeal, respiratory muscles, or both; may also have lesser or equal involvement of limb, axial muscles, or both
Class III	Moderate weakness affecting other ocular muscles; may also have ocular muscle weakness of any severity
Class IIIa	Predominantly affecting limb, axial muscles, or both; may also have lesser involvement of oropharyngeal muscles
Class IIIb	Predominantly affecting oropharyngeal, respiratory muscles, or both; may also have lesser or equal involvement of limb, axial muscles, or both
Class IV	Severe weakness affecting other ocular muscles; may also have ocular muscle weakness of any severity
Class IVa	Predominantly affecting limb, axial muscles, or both; may also have lesser involvement of oropharyngeal muscles
Class IVb	Predominantly affecting oropharyngeal, respiratory muscles, or both; may also have lesser or equal involvement of limb, axial muscles, or both; use of a feeding tube without intubation
Class V	Defined by the need for intubation, with or without mechanical ventilation, except when used during routine postoperative management

From Jaretzki A, Barohn RJ, Ernstoff RM, et al. Myasthenia gravis: recommendations for clinical research standards. Task Force of the Medical Scientific Advisory Board of the Myasthenia Gravis Foundation of America. *Neurology*. 2000; 55(1):16-23.

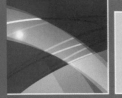

OVERVIEW of the Cardiopulmonary Clinical Manifestations Associated With Myasthenia Gravis

The following clinical manifestations result from the pathologic mechanisms caused (or activated) by atelectasis (see Fig. 10.7), alveolar consolidation (see Fig. 10.8), and excessive bronchial secretions (see Fig. 10.11)—the major anatomic alterations of the lungs associated with myasthenia gravis, which may occur when the patient is not properly managed via the Airway Clearance Therapy Protocol, Protocol 10.2, Ventilator Initiation and Management Protocol, Protocol 11.1, and Ventilator Weaning Protocol, Protocol 11.2 (see Fig. 30.1).[1]

CLINICAL DATA OBTAINED AT THE PATIENT'S BEDSIDE

The Physical Examination

Respiratory Rate

- Varies with the degree of respiratory muscle paralysis
- Apnea (in severe cases)

Cyanosis (in Severe Cases)

Chest Assessment Findings

- Diminished breath sounds
- Crackles

CLINICAL DATA OBTAINED FROM LABORATORY TESTS AND SPECIAL PROCEDURES

Pulmonary Function Test Findings[2]
(Restrictive Lung Pathology)

FORCED EXPIRATORY VOLUME AND FLOW RATE FINDINGS

FVC	FEV_T	FEV_1/FVC ratio	$FEF_{25\%-75\%}$
↓	N or ↓	N or ↑	N or ↓

$FEF_{50\%}$	$FEF_{200-1200}$	PEFR	MVV
N or ↓	N or ↓	N or ↓	N or ↓

LUNG VOLUME AND CAPACITY FINDINGS

V_T	IRV	ERV	RV
↓	↓	↓	↓

VC	IC	FRC	TLC	RV/TLC ratio
↓	↓	↓	↓	N

MAXIMUM INSPIRATORY PRESSURE (MIP) ↓

Arterial Blood Gases
Moderate to Severe Myasthenia Gravis

Acute Ventilatory Failure With Hypoxemia[3]
(Acute Respiratory Acidosis)

pH[4]	$PaCO_2$	HCO_3^- [4]	PaO_2	SaO_2 or SpO_2
↓	↑	↑ (but normal)	↓	↓

Oxygenation Indices[5]

$\dot{Q}_S/\dot{Q}_T$	DO_2[6]	$\dot{V}O_2$	$C(a-\bar{v})O_2$	O_2ER	$S\bar{v}O_2$
↑	↓	N	N	↑	↓

RADIOLOGIC FINDINGS

Chest Radiograph

- Normal, or
- Increased opacity (when atelectasis or consolidation are present)

If the ventilatory failure associated with myasthenia gravis is properly managed (e.g., via the Airway Clearance Therapy Protocol, Protocol 10.2, Ventilator Initiation and Management Protocol, Protocol 11.1, and Ventilator Weaning Protocol, Protocol 11.2), the chest radiograph should appear normal. However, if the patient is not properly managed, mucus accumulation, alveolar consolidation, and atelectasis may develop—as part of the **myasthenic crisis**. In these cases, the chest radiograph will show an increased density of the lung segments affected.

---

[1]It should be noted that the clinical manifestations associated with myasthenia gravis may occur over hours or days, depending on how quickly the paralysis progresses.

[2]Progressive worsening of these values is key to anticipating the onset of ventilatory failure.

---

[3]See Fig. 5.3 and Table 5.5 and related discussion for the acute pH, $PaCO_2$, and HCO_3^- changes associated with acute ventilatory failure.

[4]When tissue hypoxia is severe enough to produce lactic acid, the pH and HCO_3^- values will be lower than expected for a particular $PaCO_2$ level.

[5]$C(a-\bar{v})O_2$, Arterial-venous oxygen difference; DO_2, total oxygen delivery; O_2ER, oxygen extraction ratio; $\dot{Q}_S/\dot{Q}_T$, pulmonary shunt fraction; $S\bar{v}O_2$, mixed venous oxygen saturation; $\dot{V}O_2$, oxygen consumption.

[6]The DO_2 may be normal in patients who have compensated to the decreased oxygenation status with (1) an increased cardiac output, (2) an increased hemoglobin level, or (3) a combination of both. When the DO_2 is normal, the O_2ER is usually normal.

General Management of Myasthenia Gravis

In the past, many patients with myasthenia gravis died within the first few years of diagnosis of the disease. Today, a number of therapeutic measures provide most patients with marked relief of symptoms and allow them to live a normal life. Close respiratory monitoring with frequent measurements of the patient's forced vital capacity (FVC), maximum inspiratory pressure (MIP), maximum expiratory pressure (MEP), blood pressure, oxygen saturation, and, when indicated, arterial blood gases (ABGs) should be performed. Mechanical ventilation should be initiated when the clinical data demonstrate impending or acute ventilatory failure.

Good clinical indicators of impending acute ventilatory failure include the following:

- FVC less than 20 mL/kg
- MIP below −30 cm H_2O—In other words, the patient is unable to generate a maximum inspiratory pressure of −30 cm H_2O or more. For example, an MIP of only −15 cm H_2O would confirm severe muscle weakness and, importantly, that acute ventilatory failure is likely.
- MEP less than 40 cm H_2O
- $PaCO_2$ greater than 45 mm Hg
- pH less than 7.35

The four basic therapy modalities used to treat myasthenia gravis are (1) **symptomatic treatment (acetylcholinesterase inhibitors)**, (2) **chronic immunotherapies** (e.g., glucocorticoids and other immunosuppressive drugs), (3) **rapid immunotherapies** (plasma exchange and intravenous immune globulins [IVIG]), and (4) **thymectomy**.

Symptomatic Treatment: Acetylcholinesterase Inhibitors

Acetylcholinesterase inhibitors are recommended as the first line of treatment for symptomatic myasthenia gravis. **Pyridostigmine (Mestinon)** is usually the first choice. Pyridostigmine inhibits the function of acetylcholinesterase. This action increases the concentration of ACh to compete with the circulating anti-ACh antibodies, which interfere with the ability of ACh to stimulate the muscle receptors. Although the **anticholinesterase inhibitors** are effective in mild cases of myasthenia gravis, they are not completely effective in severe cases.

Chronic Immunotherapies

Most patients with myasthenia gravis need some form of immunotherapy in addition to an acetylcholinesterase inhibitor (see previous section). It is recommended that immunotherapy be administered to patients who remain significantly symptomatic while on an acetylcholinesterase inhibitor or who become symptomatic after a temporary response to an acetylcholinesterase inhibitor. Common immunotherapy agents include glucocorticoids, azathioprine, **mycophenolate mofetil**, and cyclosporine. Immunotherapy agents are usually used for more severe cases. The patient's strength often improves strikingly with steroids. Patients receiving long-term steroid therapy, however, may develop serious complications such as diabetes, cataracts, steroid myopathy, gastrointestinal bleeding, infections, aseptic necrosis of the bone, osteoporosis, and psychoses.

Rapid Immunotherapies

Rapid immunotherapies are also immunomodulating, but are unique because of their quick onset, transient benefit, and use in select situations. These therapies are used most often for the following situations:

- Myasthenic crisis
- Preoperatively before thymectomy or other surgery
- As a bridge to slower acting immunotherapies
- To help maintain remission in hard-to-control patients.

Rapid immunotherapy modalities include plasmapheresis and IVIG therapy.

Plasmapheresis (plasma exchange) directly removes the AChR antibodies from the patient's blood. The beneficial effects of plasmapheresis basically correlate to the decrease in the AChR antibodies. Immunotherapy (e.g., glucocorticoids) is typically administered concurrently to offset an AChR antibody level rebound. Plasmapheresis is a well-established treatment selection for seriously ill patients in a myasthenic crisis. Plasmapheresis can be a life-saving intervention in the treatment of myasthenia gravis. However, it is time-consuming and is associated with many side effects, such as low blood pressure, infection, and blood clots.

Intravenous immune globulin (IVIG) entails the administration of pooled immunoglobulins (IgG) from multiple donors. Although the precise mechanism of IVIG therapy is uncertain, the benefits are typically seen in less than a week and can last for 3 to 6 weeks. Similar to plasmapheresis, IVIG therapy is used to quickly reverse an exacerbation of myasthenia gravis. IVIG therapy also provides an alternative to plasmapheresis or immunosuppressive agents in certain patients with refractory myasthenia gravis, or as a preoperative treatment before a thymectomy, or as a "bridge" to slower acting immunotherapy agents. Transfusion reactions to rapid administrations of IVIG are not uncommon.

Thymectomy

Although controversial, a thymectomy may be recommended for some patients with generalized myasthenia gravis who are younger than 60 years of age and without thymoma. The thymus is the source of the anti-ACh receptor antibodies. Although a thymectomy may improve muscle strength in some patients, the full benefits of this procedure usually take several years to accumulate.

Respiratory Care Treatment Protocols
Oxygen Therapy Protocol

Oxygen therapy is used to treat hypoxemia, decrease the work of breathing, and decrease myocardial work. Because of the hypoxemia that may develop in myasthenia gravis, supplemental oxygen may be required. However, because of the alveolar consolidation and atelectasis associated with myasthenia gravis, capillary shunting may be present. Hypoxemia caused by capillary shunting is refractory to oxygen therapy (see Oxygen Therapy Protocol, Protocol 10.1).

Airway Clearance Therapy Protocol

Because of the excessive mucous production and accumulation associated with myasthenia gravis, a number of airway clearance therapies may be used to enhance the mobilization of bronchial secretions (see Airway Clearance Therapy Protocol, Protocol 10.2).

Lung Expansion Therapy Protocol

Lung expansion measures are commonly administered to prevent or offset the alveolar consolidation and atelectasis associated with myasthenia gravis (see Lung Expansion Therapy Protocol, Protocol 10.3).

Mechanical Ventilation Protocol

Mechanical ventilation may be needed to provide and support alveolar gas exchange and eventually return the patient to spontaneous breathing. Because acute ventilatory failure is often seen in patients with severe myasthenia gravis, continuous mechanical ventilation may be required. Continuous mechanical ventilation is justified when the acute ventilatory failure is thought to be reversible. Noninvasive positive-pressure ventilation (NIPPV) may be helpful if carefully monitored (see Ventilator Initiation and Management Protocol, Protocol 11.1, and Ventilator Weaning Protocol, Protocol 11.2).

CASE STUDY Myasthenia Gravis

Admitting History

A 35-year-old Spanish-American woman was a schoolteacher with a 3-year-old son and an unemployed husband who was still "finding his real place in life." The woman was a high achiever. She had recently received her doctoral degree in education, but she continued to work in the classroom with the grade-school children she loved so much. She was named Teacher of the Year in the large city where she lived. Her colleagues at school considered her a nonstop worker. She had never smoked.

At home, she was always on the move. She had just finished remodeling her kitchen and two bathrooms. She also did her own backyard landscaping on the weekends, a job she particularly enjoyed. She read and played with her son whenever they had time together. Although she enjoyed cooking (a skill she learned from her mother), she did not like to shop for groceries. Fortunately, this was a chore that her husband enjoyed.

Three weeks before the current admission, the woman noticed that her eyes "felt tired." She began to experience slight double vision. Thinking that she was working too hard, she slowed down a bit and went to bed earlier for about a week. However, she progressively felt weaker. Her legs quickly became tired, and she began having trouble chewing her food. Concerned, the woman finally went to see her doctor. After reviewing the woman's recent history and performing a careful physical examination, the physician admitted her to the hospital for further evaluation and treatment.

Over the next 48 hours, the woman's physical status declined progressively. At the patient's bedside, an ice pack test was positive for myasthenia gravis when her ptosis improved by 5 mm. She also indicated that her diplopia was better for about 10 minutes after the test. After the administration of edrophonium, her muscle strength increased significantly for about 10 minutes. **Electromyography** disclosed extensive

muscle involvement and a high degree of fatigability in all the affected muscles. A diagnosis of myasthenia gravis was recorded in the patient's chart.

The woman began to choke and aspirate food during meals, and a nasogastric feeding tube was inserted. Her speech became increasingly more slurred. Both her upper eyelids drooped, and she was unable to hold her head off her pillow on request. The respiratory therapists who monitored her forced vital capacity, maximum inspiratory pressure, pulse oximetry, and arterial blood gas values (ABGs) reported a progressive worsening in all parameters.

When the woman's ABGs were pH 7.32, $PaCO_2$ 51 mm Hg, HCO_3^- 23 mEq/L, PaO_2 59 mm Hg, and SaO_2 88% (on room air), the respiratory therapist called the physician and reported an assessment of acute ventilatory failure. The doctor had the patient transferred to the intensive care unit, intubated (no. 7 endotracheal tube with a tube length charted at 23 cm at the lip), and placed on a mechanical ventilator. The initial ventilator settings were synchronized intermittent mechanical ventilation (SIMV) mode, frequency 10 breaths/min, tidal volume 600 mL, FIO_2 0.50, and positive end-expiratory pressure (PEEP) of +5 cm H_2O.

On these ventilator settings, her ABG values were pH 7.28, $PaCO_2$ 64 mm Hg, HCO_3^- 29 mEq/L, PaO_2 52 mm Hg, and SaO_2 81%. About 45 minutes after the patient was placed on the ventilator, she appeared agitated. No spontaneous ventilations were seen. Her vital signs were blood pressure 132/86 mm Hg, heart rate 90 beats/min, and rectal temperature 38°C (100.5°F). A portable chest radiograph had been taken, but the image was still being processed. Normal vesicular breath sounds were auscultated over the right lung, and diminished-to-absent breath sounds were auscultated over the left lung. On the basis of these clinical data, the following SOAP was recorded.

Respiratory Assessment and Plan

S N/A (patient intubated)

O No spontaneous ventilations; vital signs: BP 132/86, HR 90, RR 10 (controlled), T 38°C (100.5°F); normal breath sounds over right lung; diminished-to-absent breath sounds over left lung; ABGs (on FIO_2 0.50) pH 7.28, $PaCO_2$ 64, HCO_3^- 29, PaO_2 52, and SaO_2 81%.

A • Myasthenic crisis
  • Endotracheal tube possibly placed in right mainstem bronchi (diminished-to-absent breath sounds over left lung, ABGs)
  • Acute ventilatory failure with moderate hypoxemia—on present ventilatory settings (ABGs)
  • Worsening condition likely caused by misplacement of endotracheal tube

P Notify physician stat. Check CXR. Pull endotracheal tube back until breath sounds can be auscultated over both lungs. Confirm initial placement of the endotracheal tube when radiograph is available. Mechanical Ventilation Protocol (increase tidal volume to 750 mL and increase FIO_2 to 1.0). Monitor and reevaluate immediately.

Forty-Five Minutes Later

After the patient's endotracheal tube was pulled back 3 cm to 20 cm at the lip, normal vesicular breath sounds could be auscultated over both lungs. The first chest radiograph examination confirmed that the endotracheal tube had indeed been inserted too far into the patient's right main-stem bronchus. A follow-up chest radiograph examination confirmed that the endotracheal tube was now appropriately positioned about 2 cm above the carina. Her vital signs were blood pressure 123/75 mm Hg, heart rate 74 beats/min, and temperature normal. On the new ventilatory settings per the last SOAP (see earlier), the ABGs were pH 7.53, $PaCO_2$ 27 mm Hg, HCO_3^- 22 mEq/L, PaO_2 376 mm Hg, and SaO_2 98%. On the basis of these clinical data, the following SOAP was written.

Respiratory Assessment and Plan

S N/A (patient intubated on ventilator)

O Vital signs: BP 123/75, HR 74, T normal; normal bronchovesicular breath sounds over both lung fields; CXR: No. 7 endotracheal tube in good position (20 cm at lip); lungs adequately ventilated; ABGs pH 7.53, $PaCO_2$ 27, HCO_3^- 22, PaO_2 376, and SaO_2 98%.

A Acute ventilator-induced alveolar hyperventilation (respiratory alkalosis), with overly corrected hypoxemia (ABGs)

P Adjust present settings per Mechanical Ventilation Protocol (decrease tidal volume to 650 mL). Down-regulate Oxygen Therapy Per Protocol (decrease FIO_2 to 0.30). Monitor and reevaluate (e.g., SpO_2, maximum inspiratory pressure [MIP], and forced vital capacity (FVC) 2 × per shift).

Three Days Later

No changes in the patient's ventilator settings were made since the SOAP shown above. No remarkable information was noted during the past 72 hours. However, on this day the woman appeared pale and her vital signs were blood pressure 146/88 mm Hg, heart rate 92 beats/min, and temperature 37.9°C (100.2°F). Large amounts of thick, yellowish sputum were being suctioned from her endotracheal tube about every 30 minutes. No improvement was seen in her muscular paralysis.

Coarse crackles were auscultated over both lung fields. A sputum sample was obtained and sent to the laboratory to be cultured. A portable chest radiograph revealed a new infiltrate in the right lower lobe consistent with pneumonia or atelectasis. The ABGs (on FIO_2 0.30, tidal volume 650 mL, respiratory rate of 10, and PEEP of +5) were pH 7.28, $PaCO_2$ 36 mm Hg, HCO_3^- 16 mEq/L, PaO_2 41 mm Hg, and SaO_2 69%. On the basis of these clinical data, the following SOAP was recorded.

Respiratory Assessment and Plan

S N/A

O No improvement seen in muscular paralysis; skin: pale; vital signs: BP 146/88, HR 92, T 37.9°C (100.2°F); large amounts of thick, yellowish sputum; coarse crackles over both lung fields. CXR: Pneumonia and atelectasis in right lower lobe. ABGs pH 7.28, $PaCO_2$ 36, HCO_3^- 16, PaO_2 41, and SaO_2 69%.

A • Excessive bronchial secretions (coarse crackles, sputum)
  • Infection likely (yellow sputum, fever, CXR: pneumonia)
  • Metabolic acidosis with moderate to severe hypoxemia (ABGs)
  • Acidosis likely caused by lactic acid (ABGs)

P Up-regulate Airway Clearance Therapy Protocol (med. neb. with 0.5 mL albuterol in 2 mL normal saline, q4h; therapist to suction patient frequently; sputum culture check in 24 and 48 hours). Up-regulate Lung Expansion Therapy Protocol (+10 cm H_2O PEEP). Up-regulate Oxygen Therapy Protocol (increase FIO_2 to 0.60). Monitor closely and reevaluate (check ABGs in 30 minutes).

Discussion

As with the patient with Guillain-Barré syndrome, this case of myasthenia gravis provides another chance to discuss ventilatory failure secondary to neuromuscular disease. The presentation of this patient with double vision (diplopia), difficulty in swallowing (dysphagia), and progressive muscle weakness is classic for this condition. The positive edrophonium test noted in the history was necessary for a final diagnosis. Also important to note is that aspiration of gastric contents is not uncommon in such cases.

In the first assessment the therapist correctly recognized that this case was more than simple respiratory failure. The reader sees that the patient was intubated and that breath sounds no longer were present in the entire left lung (**inadvertent right mainstem bronchial intubation**). The therapist appropriately responded quickly and pulled the endotracheal tube back until breath sounds could be auscultated over both lung fields. The inappropriate positioning of the tube was confirmed 45 minutes later in the patient's chest radiograph. The patient's respiratory status could have been seriously compromised if the therapist had waited a full 45 minutes before pulling the tube above the carina. This event further demonstrates the importance of good bedside assessment skills.

In addition, because lactic acidosis was probably present at this time, oxygenating the patient was of primary importance. In fact, increasing the FIO_2 to 1.0 would have been appropriate in this case.

The second assessment reflected that the patient was improving and was now hyperventilated and hyperoxygenated on the current ventilator settings. The therapist adjusted the ventilator settings accordingly and began the process of longitudinal evaluation of forced vital capacity and maximum inspiratory pressure so that the Mechanical Ventilation Protocol was appropriate for this condition.

The final assessment suggested that the patient had taken another turn for the worse. The sputum was now purulent, coarse crackles were heard over both lung fields, and a right lower lobe pneumonia or atelectasis had developed. The patient had an uncompensated metabolic acidemia that required evaluation. The fact that the patient's PaO_2 was only 41 provided a significant clinical indicator that the cause of the metabolic acidosis was probably lactic acid generated from a low tissue oxygen level. It was clearly appropriate for the respiratory therapist to focus on the patient's oxygenation status. This was done by up-regulating the Oxygen Therapy Protocol (Protocol 10.1) (increasing the FIO_2 to 0.60) and starting the Lung Expansion Therapy Protocol (Protocol 10.3) (the addition of 10 cm H_2O PEEP to ventilator settings).

The therapist should have anticipated this development, obtained appropriate cultures, and, if not done before, prophylactically started the Airway Clearance Therapy Protocol (Protocol 10.2) and Aerosolized Medication Therapy Protocol (Protocol 10.4)—with frequent suctioning, percussion, postural drainage, and possibly mucolytics. Finally, for a better understanding of lactic acidosis, the reader may wish to review other possible causes of metabolic acidemia at this time (e.g., diabetic ketoacidosis, renal failure) (see Chapter 5, Blood Gas Assessment).

Unfortunately the patient's pulmonary condition progressively deteriorated, and she died 3 weeks later.

SELF-ASSESSMENT QUESTIONS

1. The onset of the signs and symptoms of myasthenia gravis is(are):
   1. Slow and insidious
   2. Sudden and rapid
   3. Intermittent
   4. Often elusive
      a. 1 only
      b. 2 only
      c. 2 and 4 only
      d. 1, 2, 3, and 4

2. Myasthenia gravis:
   1. Is more common in young men
   2. Has a peak age of onset in females of 15 to 35 years
   3. Is often provoked by emotional upset and physical stress
   4. Is associated with receptor-binding antibodies
      a. 1 only
      b. 2 and 4 only
      c. 2, 3, and 4 only
      d. 1, 2, 3, and 4

3. Which of the following is associated with myasthenia gravis?
   1. Bronchospasm
   2. Mucus accumulation
   3. Alveolar hyperinflation
   4. Atelectasis
      a. 1 and 2 only
      b. 2 and 4 only
      c. 1, 2, and 4 only
      d. 2, 3, and 4 only

4. When monitoring the patient with myasthenia gravis, *all* of the following are indicators of acute ventilatory failure *except*:
   a. pH: 7.31
   b. $PaCO_2$: 55 mm Hg
   c. FVC: 25 mL/kg
   d. MIP: −15 cm H_2O

5. Which of the following antibodies is believed to block the nerve impulse transmissions at the neuromuscular junction in myasthenia gravis?
   a. IgG
   b. IgE
   c. IgA
   d. IgM

Cardiopulmonary Assessment and Care of Patients with Neuromuscular Disease

Chapter Objectives

After reading this chapter, you will be able to:

- Describe the etiology and epidemiology of various neuromuscular diseases, including spinal cord injury, amyotrophic lateral sclerosis, stroke, muscular dystrophy, and head injury.
- List the cardiopulmonary manifestations associated with neuromuscular diseases.
- Describe the general management of neuromuscular diseases.
- Describe strategies for the respiratory care of patients with neuromuscular disease.
- Describe the clinical strategies and rationales of the SOAPs presented in the case studies.
- Define key terms and complete self-assessment questions at the end of the chapter and on Evolve.

Key Terms

Amyotrophic Lateral Sclerosis (ALS)
Ataxic (Biot)
Bi-level Positive Airway Pressure (BPAP)
Breath Stacking
Bulbar Dysfunction
Cerebral Perfusion Pressure (CPP)
Cheyne-Stokes Respiration
Diaphragm Pacing
Duchenne Muscular Dystrophy (DMD)
Dysarthria
Dysphagia
Emery-Dreifuss Muscular Dystrophy
Facioscapulohumeral Dystrophy (FSHD)
Gower's Sign
Intracranial Pressure (ICP) Monitoring
Intubation Risk
Leak Speech
Limb-Girdle Muscular Dystrophy (LGMD)
Mouthpiece Ventilation (MPV)

Muscle Biopsy
Muscular Dystrophy
Myotonic Dystrophy
Neuromuscular Disease (NMD)
Obesity
Oropharyngeal Dysphagia
Paradoxical Abdominal Breathing
Pseudobulbar Palsy
Pseudohypertrophy of the Calf Muscles
Rapid Sequence Intubation (RSI)
Sialorrhea
Speaking Valve
Spinal Cord Injury (SCI)
Stroke
Talking Tracheostomy Tubes
Transient Ischemic Attacks (TIAs)
Tissue Plasminogen Activator (tPA)
Video-Assisted Thoracoscopic Surgery (VATS)
Volume-Assured Pressure Support (VAPS)

Chapter Outline

Chronic Neuromuscular Diseases
  Spinal Cord Injury
  Amyotrophic Lateral Sclerosis
  Muscular Dystrophies
  Stroke
  Head Injury
Overview of the Cardiopulmonary Manifestations Associated With Neuromuscular Diseases
General Management of Neuromuscular Disease
  Nutrition
Ventilatory Management of Patients With Neuromuscular Diseases
  Tracheostomy
  Ventilatory Support
Case Study: Amyotrophic Lateral Sclerosis
Self-Assessment Questions

Neuromuscular disease (NMD) is a generalized term used to describe disorders of the brain, spinal cord, peripheral nerves, neuromuscular junction, and muscles. These disorders are associated with a wide range of motor and sensory deficits; however, patients with NMD may develop significant cardiopulmonary issues. In fact, breathing disorders are the leading cause of death in patients with NMD. Thus it is important for the respiratory therapist to be familiar with these conditions and their effect on the respiratory system. Table 31.1 includes a list of acute and chronic NMDs that affect the respiratory system. This chapter will focus specifically on spinal cord injury, amyotrophic lateral sclerosis, muscular dystrophies,

TABLE 31.1 Acute and Chronic Neuromuscular Diseases That Affect the Respiratory System

Cerebral Cortex	Brainstem/Basal Ganglia	Spinal Cord	Motor Nerves/ Anterior Horn Cell	Neuromuscular Junction	Myopathies
Stroke (acute)	Stroke (acute)	Trauma (acute)	Motor neuron disease	Myasthenia gravis	Muscular dystrophies
Malignancy	Malignancy	Infarction	Postpolio syndrome	Lambert-Eaton myasthenic syndrome	Polymyositis
Seizures	Central alveolar hypoventilation	Hemorrhage	Amyotrophic lateral sclerosis	Drugs Antibiotics Anticholinesterase inhibitors Corticosteroids Lithium	Dermatomyositis
Cerebral degeneration	Multiple system atrophy	Disk compression	Vasculitis		
	Parkinson disease	Malignancy	Spinal muscular atrophy		
	Dyskinesias	Demyelinating disease	Metabolic disorders		

stroke, and head injuries. Other neuromuscular disorders will be covered in other chapters.

Chronic Neuromuscular Diseases

Spinal Cord Injury

Etiology and Epidemiology

Spinal cord injury (SCI) is a relatively common and devastating event associated with significant morbidity and mortality (Fig. 31.1). According to the National Spinal Cord Injury Statistical Center (NSCSC) in 2018, the annual incidence of spinal cord injury (SCI) was about 17,700 new cases each year. New SCI cases do not include those who die at the location of the indecent that caused the SCI. The number of people with SCI living in the United States is currently estimated to be approximately 288,000 persons. The average age at injury has increased from 29 years during the 1970s to 43 years currently. About 78% of new SCI cases are male. Vehicle crashes are currently the leading cause of SCI injuries, closely followed by falls. Acts of violence (primarily gunshot wounds) and sports/recreation activities are also relatively common causes. Table 31.2 lists causes of nontraumatic SCI.

Clinical Presentation

Patients with disorders of the spinal cord will present with a variety of clinical signs and symptoms that vary depending on the level of injury. Damage to the lumbosacral spinal cord results in lower extremity weakness/paralysis, spasticity, and dysfunction of the bowel and bladder. Cervical nerves C3 through C5 innervate the diaphragm via the phrenic nerve. Thus injuries at or above this level will result in significant respiratory compromise and even death without immediate intervention. Thoracic cord injuries will have lower extremity symptoms as well; however, despite sparing the phrenic nerve,

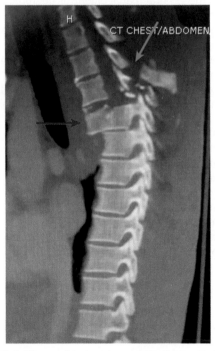

FIGURE 31.1 A 53-year-old man who sustained a severe T4 vertebral injury after a motor vehicle collision. Note the anterior displacement of the thoracic spine (red arrow) and the fracture of the spinous process (green arrow).

injuries at this level can affect breathing by impairing function of respiratory muscles. Impairment of these muscles will also contribute to poor coughing, which can increase the risk for developing pulmonary infections. These muscles are displayed in Fig. 31.2.

Additionally, the rib cage stiffens in the months after an SCI. This results in decreased thoracic compliance and atelectasis, with an increased compliance of the abdomen. Patients with cervical or thoracic injuries may develop a rapid shallow breathing pattern and a **paradoxical abdominal**

TABLE 31.2 Nontraumatic Causes of Spinal Cord Injury

Congenital	Spinal dysraphism
	Arnold-Chiari malformations
	Skeletal malformations
	Syringomyelia
Genetic	Hereditary spastic paraplegias
	Spinal muscular atrophies
	Adrenoleukodystrophy
	Amyotrophic lateral sclerosis
	Friedreich ataxia
Acquired	Malignancy
	Paraneoplastic syndromes
	Infections
	Degenerative vertebral disease
	Vascular disorders
	Spinal cord infarction
	Vascular malformations
	Spinal epidural hematoma
	Autoimmune disorders
	Transverse myelitis
	Sarcoidosis
	Toxic-metabolic disorders
	Radiation myelopathy
	Copper deficiency
	Decompression sickness myelopathy
	Subacute combined degeneration
	Hepatic myelopathy
	Vitamin C deficiency

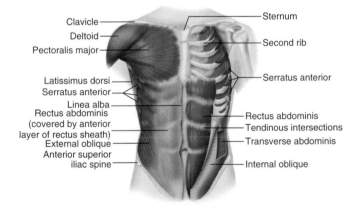

FIGURE 31.2 The muscles of respiration. (From Patton, K. T., Thibodeau, G. A., & Douglas, M. M. (2012). *Essentials of anatomy and physiology.* St. Louis, MO: Elsevier.)

breathing pattern in which the chest wall moves inward during inspiration because of isolated diaphragmatic breathing. Autonomic dysfunction is also common in patients with SCI and can manifest as hypotension, hypertensive crises, and tachycardia.

The American Spinal Injury Association (ASIA) Impairment Scale classifies the extent of SCIs into the following categories:

A = Complete: No sensory or motor function is preserved in sacral segments S4-S5.

B = Incomplete: Sensory, but not motor, function is preserved below the neurologic level and extends through sacral segments S4-S5.

C = Incomplete: Motor function is preserved below the neurologic level, and most key muscles below the neurologic level have a muscle grade less than 3.

D = Incomplete: Motor function is preserved below the neurologic level, and most key muscles below the neurologic level have a muscle grade that is 3 or greater.

E = Normal: Sensory and motor functions are normal.

Diagnosis

SCIs may not always be readily recognizable. Evaluation for possible SCI should be performed in patients who experience traumatic injuries, including head injuries, pelvic fractures, penetrating injuries involving the spine, and falls from heights. X-rays are a quick, portable, and inexpensive way to evaluate the bony structures of the spine. However, they are insensitive for diagnosing most disorders of the spinal column. Computed tomography (CT) scanning of the spine can be used to identify vertebral fractures (see Fig. 31.1), epidural hematomas and fluid collections, and other injuries involving the spinal cord. It can be done quickly, which makes it an appropriate initial evaluation in patients with suspected spinal injury. Magnetic resonance imaging (MRI) is much more sensitive and better evaluates the spinal cord, nerve roots, ligaments, and disk spaces compared with CT. Electromyography and nerve conduction studies are generally unnecessary to make the diagnosis.

Management

The treatment of SCIs involves a multidisciplinary approach. Prompt assessment is important to prevent additional injury and initiate the appropriate treatment in a timely fashion. Comorbid injuries, such as abdominal or thoracic trauma, should be sought and managed accordingly. Maintaining proper cervical alignment using skull traction or other forms of mechanical stabilization will help prevent secondary injury and improve prospects for recovery. Specific injuries may be best treated with prompt surgical intervention by a neurosurgeon or orthopedic surgeon who is trained in the management of SCIs.

Autonomic dysfunction may require intravenous fluid resuscitation and possibly vasoactive medications to maintain adequate tissue perfusion. Anticoagulation should be initiated to prevent venous thromboembolism. Those with neurogenic bowel and bladder will require assistance with defecation and urination. Flaccid rectal tone may necessitate the use of digital rectal stimulation, suppositories, or enemas to treat constipation. Repeated bladder catheterization or insertion of a chronic indwelling suprapubic catheter may be considered.

Patients with injuries below the level of C5 generally do not require ventilatory support; however, significant injuries at the C5 level and above will have diaphragmatic impairment (and impairment of other respiratory muscles) necessitating additional respiratory support. Intubation and mechanical ventilation should be instituted in patients with evidence of impending respiratory failure, including tachypnea, rising $PaCO_2$ levels, and hypoxemia. Manual or mechanically assisted coughing, respiratory physiotherapy, and breathing exercises can help clear bronchial secretions and prevent pulmonary infection. An abdominal binder can be used to decrease work of breathing by reducing the paradoxical breathing pattern.

The **intubation risk** for patients with cervical SCIs is significant. Extension of the neck can lead to worsening cervical injury. Additionally, patients with traumatic cervical SCIs may have facial trauma that will make orotracheal intubation difficult. It is not uncommon for these patients to require emergent tracheostomy placement for further long-term airway management.

Diaphragm pacing is a potential treatment option for selected patients with SCI who are dependent on mechanical ventilation. It can be an effective modality to eliminate the need for or reduce dependence on mechanical ventilation. A thoracic surgeon may perform a laparoscopy to place electrodes within the muscle of the diaphragm or use **video-assisted thorascopic surgery (VATS)** to place leads directly on the phrenic nerve. These electrodes are connected to an external transmitting box that can be used to control the frequency, amplitude, and duration of pacing. Once the device is placed, the patient will undergo a conditioning period of weeks to months during which the pacemaker settings are adjusted based on minute ventilation, gas exchange, and patient comfort. The optimal timing for evaluation is unknown; however, it is generally accepted that patients with a cervical SCI should not be evaluated until at least 3 months after their injury because there may be partial or complete recovery of phrenic nerve function. Diaphragm pacing is challenging when the phrenic nerve or the diaphragm is not functional, and phrenic nerve transplantation has poor success rates at this time. Much of the experience with diaphragm pacing comes from observational studies and published case series.

Amyotrophic Lateral Sclerosis

Etiology and Epidemiology

Amyotrophic lateral sclerosis (ALS) is a progressive neurologic disorder characterized by degeneration of upper and lower motor neurons. The disease is also known as *Lou Gehrig disease*, named after the famous baseball player who was diagnosed with this condition in the 1930s.

The exact cause is unknown; however, research has suggested that the pathogenesis of ALS centers around genetic mutations in genes involved in protein homeostasis, RNA homeostasis and trafficking, and cytoskeletal dynamics. Both familial and sporadic cases have been reported and have similar pathologic features. The National ALS Registry estimates that the overall prevalence of ALS in the United States is 4.7 to 5.0 per 100,000 people. In Europe and the United States, there are approximately 1 or 2 new cases of ALS per year per 100,000 people. The majority of new cases are sporadic in origin, with only about 10% being familial. The average survival time from diagnosis to death is 3 to 5 years. The leading cause of death in ALS is respiratory failure.

Clinical Presentation

ALS affects both upper and lower motor neurons. The disorder typically begins with limb findings (arm or leg weakness, gait instability, etc.); however, up to one-third of patients present with bulbar findings such as **dysphagia**, **dysarthria** (difficulty with speech), and difficulty chewing. Table 31.3 lists common neurologic findings in patients with ALS. **Pseudobulbar palsy**, characterized by emotional lability, facial spasticity, and inappropriate laughing or crying, suggests involvement of the

TABLE 31.3 Neurologic Signs and Symptoms in Amyotrophic Lateral Sclerosis

	Upper Motor Neuron	Lower Motor Neuron
Limb findings	Limb spasticity	Fasciculations
	Limb weakness	Gait disorder
	Spastic gait	Muscle atrophy
	Incoordination of movements	Foot drop
	Spontaneous clonus	Poor rise from chair
	Spontaneous flexor spasms	Cramps
	Increased reflexes	
	"Preserved" reflexes in weak/atrophic muscles	
	Hoffman sign	
	Upgoing toe	
	Distal spread of arm reflexes	
	Triple flexion	
Bulbar findings	Spastic dysarthria	Tongue wasting
	Brisk gag and jaw reflex	Tongue weakness
	Facial asymmetry	Tongue fasciculations
	Increased facial reflexes	Nasal speech
	Slow tongue movement	Hoarse speech
	Dysphagia	Weak cough
	Laryngospasm	Difficulty maintaining jaw closure
	Pseudobulbar affect	Incomplete eye closure
	Mood incongruent	Poor lip closure and seal
	Inappropriate laughing, crying, and/or yawning	Difficulty chewing
	Sialorrhea (drooling)	
	Difficulty managing secretions	

frontopontine motor neurons. The disease typically involves the diaphragm and can cause dyspnea, impaired cough, and respiratory failure. Cognitive symptoms also may be present. It is important to note that there are several variants of ALS that have different presentations, including isolated bulbar ALS, brachial amyotrophic diplegia ("man-in-the-barrel syndrome"), and leg amyotrophic diplegia. Patients can present with purely upper motor neuron (UMN) or lower motor neuron (LMN) signs and symptoms. ALS-plus syndrome encompasses the same UMN and LMN findings as ALS accompanied by other disorders, including frontotemporal dementia, autonomic insufficiency, Parkinsonism, and/or sensory loss.

Diagnosis

The diagnosis of ALS is typically made on clinical grounds. There are no laboratory or other diagnostic markers that are pathognomonic for ALS. Multiple diagnostic criteria exist. However, the most widely accepted and validated criteria are the revised El Escorial World Federation of Neurology criteria. The diagnosis of ALS requires the evidence of LMN degeneration, the presence of UMN degeneration, and progressive spread of symptoms or signs within a region or to other regions as determined by history of physical examination. LMN and UMN degeneration may be identified by clinical examination, electrophysiologic testing, or neuropathologic examination. Furthermore, electrophysiologic or pathologic evidence of other disease processes that can explain the LMN and/or UMN degeneration and neuroimaging evidence of another disease process that could explain the clinical and electrophysiologic findings must be absent. In the absence of pathologic confirmation, the certainty of the diagnosis may be classified as clinically definite, clinically probable, and clinically possible ALS. This diagnostic approach has been validated pathologically and has been shown to have acceptable interobserver agreement. It is important to note that as many as 21% of patients die from ALS without ever meeting the revised El Escorial criteria. Some patients, particularly those in the intensive care unit, may not be able to undergo electromyography and nerve conduction studies or may not have access to a neurologist to perform the necessary evaluation. For a respiratory therapist, **sialorrhea** (drooling) and tongue fasciculations are two important clinical cues that should prompt one to consider a diagnosis of ALS.

Electromyography will demonstrate signs of acute and chronic denervation. Nerve conduction studies are often normal, but compound motor action potential amplitudes may be reduced in more severe disease. Repetitive nerve stimulation, which assesses the integrity of the neuromuscular junction, may be normal or abnormal in ALS, but it remains a useful test to help exclude diseases that primarily target the neuromuscular junction such as myasthenia gravis or Lambert-Eaton myasthenic syndrome (see Chapter 30). MRI of the brain and spinal cord is helpful to exclude other disorders that may manifest with UMN findings.

Muscle biopsy is not a routine test performed in the diagnosis of ALS, but it may be performed to exclude other diagnoses that cause myopathy. Small, angular fibers are indicative of neurogenic atrophy. There also may be findings consistent with reinnervation. These findings are not specific for ALS.

Management

There is currently no cure for ALS. Riluzole is a medication that has been shown to slow ALS disease progression. Its exact mechanism of action in ALS is unknown; however, experimental data suggest that riluzole has effects on neural activity. Riluzole is thought to inhibit glutamate-induced excitotoxicity by inhibiting neurotransmitter release, antagonizing N-methyl-D-aspartate (NMDA) receptors, and inhibiting the action of sodium channels. The American Academy of Neurology recommends riluzole for patients with definite or probable ALS who have had symptoms less than 5 years, have a vital capacity greater than 60% of predicted, and do not have a tracheostomy. Potential side effects include asthenia, dizziness, elevated liver enzymes, gastrointestinal upset, weakness, worsening muscular weakness. Edaravone (Radicava) is a new intravenous medication approved by the US Food and Drug Administration for treatment of ALS. Its mechanism of action is unknown. It has been shown to slow the decline in physical function; however, edaravone has not been shown to improve respiratory parameters in patients with ALS.

Symptom management involves close monitoring of respiratory function to determine the appropriate timing to initiate supportive ventilation. Airway clearance therapy to assist cough and improve clearance of secretions will help reduce the incidence of pneumonia. Management of comorbid conditions, including insomnia, depression, pain, and sialorrhea, is also important. Patients should have discussions regarding their goals of care and advance directives early in the course of the disease. Referral to hospice care is advised in the terminal phase of disease.

Muscular Dystrophies

Etiology, Epidemiology, and Clinical Presentation

Muscular dystrophy is a term that is composed of several genetic disorders characterized by pathologic changes within muscles affecting the limbs, face, and sometimes respiratory and cardiac muscles as well. They are distinguished from other neuromuscular disorders in that they are primary myopathies, are progressive, manifest degeneration of muscle fibers pathologically, and have a genetic origin. Muscular dystrophies may manifest at different times throughout life with different degrees of severity. These disorders can be transmitted as autosomal dominant, autosomal recessive, or X-linked traits. Sporadic cases can occur as well. Table 31.4 lists different forms of muscular dystrophy and their typical age of onset, clinical manifestations, and life expectancies. Advances in medical therapy, particularly in the management of respiratory and cardiac complications, have resulted in significant increases in life expectancy for many of these patients.

Duchenne muscular dystrophy (DMD) is the most common inherited neuromuscular disorder. Guillaume Benjamin Amand Duchenne de Boulogne, a French neurologist, was the first to describe the disease when he reported a series of 13 boys with progressive muscular weakness in the 1860s.

TABLE 31.4 Muscular Dystrophies

Disease	Inheritance Pattern	Onset of Symptoms	Pattern of Skeletal Muscle Involvement	Extraskeletal Manifestations	Life Expectancy
Duchenne muscular dystrophy	XLR	1–3 yr	Proximal muscle weakness and lower limbs affected first, followed by upper limbs and distal muscles	Cardiomyopathy, intellectual impairment, seizures, autism-like behavior, respiratory failure	40–50 yr
Becker muscular dystrophy	XLR	Childhood to early 20s	Proximal muscles	Dilated cardiomyopathy, respiratory failure	30–50 yr
Myotonic dystrophy	AD	Childhood to adulthood (depending on size of trinucelotide repeat)	Type 1: Facial, neck, forearm, hand, foot dorsiflexor Type 2: Neck flexor, elbow extensor, finger flexor, hip flexor	Cardiac arrhythmias, hypersomnia, excessive daytime sleepiness, primary hypogonadism, dysphagia, gallbladder disease, cognitive dysfunction, cataracts, abnormal liver function, hypogammaglobulinemia, premature balding	Mildly reduced (type 1) Normal (type 2)
Emery-Dreifuss muscular dystrophy	XLR AD/AR forms are rare	5–15 yr	Humeroperoneal distribution	Dilated cardiomyopathy, arrhythmia, stroke	Variable
Limb-girdle muscular dystrophies	AD, AR	Childhood to adulthood	Scapulohumeral, pelvifemoral, or both	Cardiomyopathy, arrhythmias	Variable
Facioscapulohumeral muscular dystrophy	AD	Late childhood to middle adulthood	Facial, shoulder girdle (scapular winging), foot extensors, pelvic girdle	Arrhythmia, cognitive impairment, hearing loss, epilepsy, retinal vasculopathy, pain	Normal
Oculopharyngeal Muscular Dystrophy	AD; AR form is less common	Third decade of life	Extraocular, pharyngeal	Dysphagia, ptosis	Normal

AD, Autosomal dominant; AR, autosomal recessive; XLR, X-linked recessive.

DMD is inherited as an X-linked recessive trait, which means it is much more likely to occur in males than in females. However, 30% of cases arise from de novo mutations. The incidence is estimated to be 1 in 3600 live male births in the United States. Some women are asymptomatic carriers of the mutation. DMD is caused by mutations in the dystrophin gene at the Xp21.1 locus. Dystrophin is a cytoplasmic protein that plays a vital role in attaching the cytoskeleton of a muscle fiber to its surrounding extracellular matrix. Abnormal dystrophin is associated with other forms of muscular dystrophy, including Becker myotonic dystrophy, which manifests in adulthood.

Infants born with DMD are generally asymptomatic but may have hypotonia. Poor head control in infancy may be an early sign of disease. **Pseudohypertrophy of the calf muscles** occurs because of fatty infiltration of the muscle. This is typically accompanied by muscle wasting of the thighs. Children with DMD, and those with other forms of muscular dystrophy, exhibit the **Gower sign** at approximately 3 years of age (use of hands and arms to "walk up" their own body from a squatting position). This is indicative of proximal muscle weakness, particularly of the hips and thighs.

As muscle weakness progresses, patients will have difficulty ambulating and performing activities of daily living (ADLs). Respiratory muscle weakness will result in dyspnea, weak coughing, a nasal voice quality, and an increased risk for aspiration. Contractures of the ankles, knees, hips, and elbows may occur. From 50% to 80% of patients develop cardiomyopathy. Intellectual impairment with an intelligence quotient (IQ) below 70 is present in as many as 30% of patients. Epilepsy and autism-like behavior also have been described.

Myotonic dystrophy is the second most common form of muscular dystrophy. The estimated prevalence is 1 in 8000 worldwide. The incidence ranges from 1 in 100,000 to 1 in 300,000 in developed nations. Types 1 and 2 myotonic dystrophy are each caused by genetic mutations resulting from expansions of repeating nucleotides on specific chromosomes. Type 2 tends to be milder than type 1.

Myotonic dystrophy manifests at any age. Patients may have facial wasting, hypotonia, an arched palate (secondary to weakness of the temporal and pterygoid muscles), and progressive weakness that begins in the distal muscles. Weakness begins as mild in the first few years but progresses slowly throughout childhood and into adulthood. Wasting occurs in the dorsal forearms, anterior lower legs, neck, and tongue muscles. Patients do have difficulty with ambulation and exhibit the Gower sign. Speech is commonly impaired as well.

Myotonia, a very slow relaxation of muscles after contraction, can be elicited by asking patients to make a tight fist and quickly open their hand. It can also be elicited through percussion of the thenar eminence of the hand. Myalgias are not present in myotonic dystrophy. Extraskeletal manifestations include complete heart block, ventricular arrhythmias, thyroid dysfunction, low immunoglobulin levels, cataracts, diabetes mellitus, and intellectual impairment. Type 2 myotonic dystrophy shares many of the same features, but it is typically milder and not associated with a shortened life span.

Emery-Dreifuss muscular dystrophy, also known as *scapuloperoneal* or *scapulohumeral muscular dystrophy*, is transmitted in X-linked, autosomal recessive, and autosomal dominant fashions. The overall prevalence of disease is unknown. Symptoms typically begin between the ages of 5 and 15 years and progress relatively slowly in most cases. Patients typically exhibit muscle weakness and wasting in a scapulohumeroperoneal distribution. They develop contractures at the elbows and ankles early in the course of the disease. Muscular pseudohypertrophy does not occur. In fact, patients may exhibit atrophy of the peroneal muscles. Facial weakness may also be present. Intellectual function is normal. Dilated cardiomyopathy is severe and is often associated with significant arrhythmias, including sudden ventricular fibrillation. Implantable cardiac defibrillators may be required to prevent sudden cardiac death.

Limb-girdle muscular dystrophy (LGMD) is a heterogeneous group of disorders characterized by a proximal distribution of weakness. There are many forms of the disease that can be inherited in autosomal recessive or autosomal dominant fashion. Multiple genetic mutations can occur on different chromosomes and lead to the various disease states. The estimated prevalence is about 1 in 20,000 individuals. Patients generally present with progressive weakness and muscle atrophy of the shoulder girdle, pelvic girdle, or both. Onset of symptoms can begin in childhood or adulthood. Adult-onset cases typically manifest with progressive proximal muscle weakness leading to difficulty with mobility. Facial weakness can be mild, but extraocular muscles are spared. Most types have spared distal muscle strength initially; however, distal muscles eventually develop weakness. Calf pseudohypertrophy and ankle contractures develop in some forms of LGMD. Cardiopulmonary involvement and dysphagia are also common.

Facioscapulohumeral dystrophy (FSHD) is an autosomal dominant form of muscular dystrophy. It is the third most common form of muscular dystrophy, with an estimated prevalence of 4 to 12 cases per 100,000 population. Symptoms begin in infancy to middle age, with most becoming symptomatic by the age of 20 years. As the name implies, muscle weakness predominantly affects the muscles of the face, scapula, and upper arms. Facial manifestations include inability to close the eyes tightly, inability to smile or whistle, and characteristic facial expressions. Weakness also involves the abdominal muscles. The distribution of muscle weakness tends to be asymmetric. Dysphagia and respiratory failure are rare. In some instances, patients with respiratory involvement may require noninvasive ventilation (NIV), usually nocturnally. Other manifestations include chronic pain, visual disturbances, retinal vasculopathy, progressive hearing loss, cardiac arrhythmias, and cognitive impairment.

Diagnosis

The diagnosis of muscular dystrophy combines physical examination, laboratory testing, and muscle biopsy findings. Clinical findings of muscular weakness, fatigue, muscle wasting, or dysphagia should prompt evaluation for a myopathic disorder. A thorough family history should be obtained when muscular dystrophy is suspected. In circumstances in which the clinical presentation and inheritance pattern are consistent with a diagnosis, additional testing may not be necessary. Creatine kinase and aldolase are proteins that, if elevated, may suggest muscle damage.

Many, but not all, muscular dystrophies are associated with elevations in creatine kinase and aldolase. In Duchenne and Becker muscular dystrophies, genetic testing of the dystrophin gene can be diagnostic and obviate the need for muscle biopsy. Molecular genetic testing is available for other forms of muscular dystrophy as well. A muscle biopsy is indicated when the clinical scenario suggests a myopathic process and the likelihood of obtaining a diagnosis through less invasive means is unlikely. The muscle on which the biopsy is to be performed should be one affected by the disorder. It is important to note that severely affected muscles may only show end-stage morphology that will not be sufficient to provide a diagnosis. Myopathic changes seen on biopsy often show generalized features of muscle damage with superimposed changes consistent with a specific disorder. Table 31.4 also includes histopathologic findings associated with several forms of muscular dystrophy.

Management

There is no cure for any form of muscular dystrophy. Management of muscular dystrophies requires a multidisciplinary approach. A 2016 Cochrane Database meta-analysis evaluated the effect of corticosteroids in Duchenne muscular dystrophy. Corticosteroids were associated with improved muscle strength and function compared with placebo in the short term (6 months to 2 years). Areas of improvement included time to rise from the floor, timed walk, four-stair climbing time, ability to lift weight, leg function grade, quality of life, and forced vital capacity. Deflazacort was shown to stabilize muscle strength versus placebo. Very few studies compared prednisone with deflazacort, and at this time no conclusions can be drawn regarding which steroid is more effective. Corticosteroids are associated with significant side effects, including weight gain, behavioral abnormalities, excessive hair growth, diminished bone density, poor wound healing, and impaired glucose control.

Physical and occupational therapy can improve strength, functional status, and quality of life. Range-of-motion exercises are important to help prevent and treat limb contractures. Patients with severe contractures may require surgical intervention. Gene therapy, using viral or nonviral vectors, is a promising modality for treatment of muscular dystrophies that is still under investigation.

Monitoring for pulmonary complications is important because many forms of muscular dystrophy are associated with respiratory muscle weakness, impaired coughing, and ventilatory failure. NIV improves outcomes and quality of life in patients with respiratory failure. Airway clearance therapy is important to prevent atelectasis and subsequent pulmonary infection. Congestive heart failure should be managed according to established guidelines with administration of beta-blockers, angiotensin converting enzyme (ACE) inhibitors, and appropriate management of salt and fluid intake.

Patients with significant risk for fatal arrhythmias (primarily ventricular arrhythmias) may benefit from antiarrhythmic medications. Automated implantable cardioverter-defibrillators are necessary for primary and secondary prevention of ventricular arrhythmias and to prevent sudden cardiac death. Ventricular assist devices (VADs) should be considered for patients with end-stage cardiomyopathy. However, heart transplantation may be challenging for those with muscular dystrophy because of the risk for respiratory failure and potential need for tracheostomy.

Stroke

Etiology and Epidemiology

Stroke, also known as *acute brain attack* or *cerebrovascular accident*, is a condition characterized by decreased perfusion to the brain resulting in cellular damage or cellular death. The two main categories of stroke are hemorrhagic and ischemic. Of acute strokes, 80% result from thrombosis or embolism and the other 20% are the result of hemorrhagic conditions (i.e., subarachnoid hemorrhage or intracerebral hemorrhage). According to the Centers for Disease Control and Prevention (CDC), approximately 800,000 Americans have a stroke each year, and about 140,000 of these individuals will die from this condition. *This disorder is currently the fifth leading cause of death in the United States. Furthermore, stroke is a leading cause of long-term disability and results in billions of dollars of health care spending each year.* Risk factors for stroke development include hypertension, diabetes mellitus, tobacco use, elevated cholesterol, peripheral arterial disease, and atrial fibrillation.

Clinical Manifestations

The clinical manifestations of a stroke are related to the location of the insult and the degree of ischemia. The onset of symptoms is classically acute. Patients may report a history of **transient ischemic attacks** (TIAs) with temporary neurologic symptoms in the weeks to months preceding an acute stroke.

Patients who experience a stroke typically experience changes in vital signs with elevation in blood pressure, decreased respiratory rate (because of increased intracranial pressure [ICP] causing decreased respiratory drive), and fever. Weakness of muscles of the face or extremities is common and may be accompanied by sensory, visual, or cognitive impairment. Infarcts involving the middle cerebral artery (MCA) will affect the parietal lobe, resulting in contralateral sensory/motor impairment, contralateral lower face weakness, ataxia, speech impairment, and visual deficits.

Strokes of the anterior circulation will cause sensory and motor impairment of the lower extremities, akinetic mutism, and incontinence. Posterior cerebral artery (PCA) strokes may result in contralateral hemiplegia (paralysis), chorea, hemiballismus, visual field deficits, memory deficits, and visual hallucinations. Strokes impairing the midbrain generally cause cranial nerve deficits (e.g., double vision, taste disturbances, hearing loss, dizziness, and difficulty swallowing). Patients may have strokes involving multiple brain areas, resulting in variable signs and symptoms.

Stroke is associated with several respiratory complications. Acute central nervous system injury can result in acute pulmonary edema with associated tachycardia, tachypnea, and hypoxemia. Pneumonia frequently occurs in patients who have had a stroke. Aspiration of food particles or oral secretions represents the most common cause of pneumonia in these patients. This may occur because of stroke-related **oropharyngeal dysphagia** and a decreased level of consciousness resulting in impaired cough reflex and ability to protect the airway. The development of pneumonia after a stroke is associated with increased mortality and worse long-term outcomes. The respiratory therapist must recognize the importance of oral secretion management in the prevention of pulmonary complications.

Abnormal breathing patterns (see Chapter 2, The Physical Examination) are common after an acute infarct. Many of these breathing patterns are not prognostic, nor do they result from infarcts in specific locations within the brain or spinal cord. *Obstructive and central sleep apnea are both consequences of and risk factors for developing a stroke.* **Cheyne-Stokes respiration** describes a cyclical pattern of breathing in which the respiratory rate and tidal volume gradually increases then decreases in a crescendo-decrescendo pattern with apneic periods between each cycle. This pattern of breathing is seen in patients with congestive heart failure, hypoxia, hypocapnia, and diffuse cerebral injury. **Ataxic (Biot)** respiration describes chaotic, irregular periods of rapid, deep respirations followed by irregular periods of apnea that last 10 to 30 seconds. Apneustic breathing is characterized by prominent end-inspiratory pauses interrupted by occasional short expirations. This pattern of breathing localizes to the lower half of the pons but also may occur in meningitis, hypoxia, and hypoglycemia. Kussmaul respirations may occur in patients with metabolic acidosis. Agonal respirations occur frequently in patients with bilateral medullary injury or those with terminal brain injury.

Diagnosis

The initial evaluation of patients suspected of having a stroke should be conducted in an emergent fashion. The sooner a diagnosis can be made, the sooner interventions can be undertaken to improve cerebral ischemia and prevent further neurologic deficits. A thorough neurologic examination can identify clinical findings that may help localize the area of ischemia. CT or MRI studies of the brain are necessary to determine if the stroke is hemorrhagic or ischemic. These imaging modalities also will give information regarding the degree of ischemia and can offer clues to the underlying cause (e.g., identifying cerebrovascular aneurysms or atherosclerosis). Oxygen saturation should be monitored, and supplemental oxygen should be provided to prevent hypoxia. Patients with ischemic stroke require higher blood pressures to prevent worsening of ischemia. In selected patients **intracranial pressure (ICP) monitoring** may be required.

Management

Patients with ischemic strokes may require **tissue plasminogen activator (tPA)** to lyse clots and reestablish cerebral perfusion. tPa should be administered within 4.5 hours of the onset of stroke symptoms provided there are no contraindications. Specialized stroke centers may have trained interventionalists who can remove thrombi from within cerebral vessels. Antiplatelet therapy with aspirin and clopidogrel reduces mortality and helps prevent subsequent ischemic strokes. Hyperthermia requires treatment with acetaminophen or external cooling to normalize core body temperatures.

Those with a Glasgow Coma Scale score of 8 or less or worsening mental status with concern for airway protection will require emergent airway control. Patients with increased ICP are at high risk for complications during intubation, including hypotension, an exaggerated sympathetic response to airway manipulation, or further increases in ICP. Preoxygenation is important to prevent hypoxia, which can worsen ICP and cerebral ischemia. Intubation should be performed by an experienced provider to prevent multiple attempts at intubation and delays in securing a stable airway. Pretreatment with an opioid can diminish the rise in ICP caused by **rapid sequence intubation (RSI)**. Topical anesthetics and sedating medications should be used in patients with a decreased level of consciousness because they may still cough and increase their ICP with laryngoscopy. Supplemental oxygen should be used to prevent hypoxemia. When using mechanical ventilation it is important to be mindful that high levels of positive end-expiratory pressure (PEEP) may reduce mean arterial pressure (MAP) and ultimately decrease **cerebral perfusion pressure (CPP)**. CCP is defined as the MAP minus the ICP.

Prevention of respiratory complications is an important component of poststroke care. Bronchial hygiene with incentive spirometry, positive expiratory pressure (PEP) devices, and other airway clearance techniques can prevent atelectasis and pneumonia. Ambulation, when possible, will also improve airway hygiene. Atropine drops given sublingually and botulinum toxin (Botox) injections into salivary glands can reduce oral secretions and decrease the risk for aspiration pneumonia. NIV is used to treat patients with sleep apnea and hypoventilation syndromes. The respiratory therapist should be aware of the abnormal breathing patterns that occur after a cerebral injury, especially Cheyne-Stokes respirations, so the appropriate ventilatory support can be provided.

Head Injury

Respiratory therapists are frequently involved in the care of patients with head injuries. According to the CDC, traumatic brain injury (TBI) contributes to approximately 30% of all injury deaths in the United States. In 2013, about 2.8 million TBI-related emergency department visits, hospitalizations, and deaths occurred in the United States; falls account for the majority of those injuries. Brain injury can result in multiple respiratory complications. Patients with TBI typically exhibit a depressed level of consciousness, which significantly raises the risk for aspiration. These patients can develop apnea through multiple mechanisms, including functional airway obstruction in the setting of loss of consciousness. Aspiration events and apnea can result in hypoxemia and hypercapnia, which can further compromise cerebral oxygen delivery.

Management

The initial step in the management of patients with TBI is an assessment of the patient's ability to *protect the airway*. A focused but thorough assessment should be performed to identify additional injuries that might have an effect on airway management, particularly maxillofacial or spinal cord trauma. There is a high incidence of peri-intubation hypoxemia and cardiac arrest (defined as occurring within 60 minutes after initiation of airway management), hypocapnia, and hemodynamic instability in patients with head injuries; therefore intubation should be performed by experienced providers. Maneuvers such as a jaw thrust, use of temporary bag-mask ventilation (BMV), or a supraglottic airway may be lifesaving in emergent situations before placing an endotracheal tube. RSI is the most common technique for airway management in these patients. It is not uncommon for patients to develop peri-intubation hypotension related to induction agents and use of positive pressure ventilation, particularly in a trauma setting in which patients may have acute blood loss.

Attempts should be made to adequately resuscitate patients with packed red cell transfusions or administration of intravenous crystalloid to prevent peri-intubation hemodynamic instability. An awake intubation with a topical anesthetic should be considered for selected patients with an anticipated difficult airway or concern for potentially significant hemodynamic compromise related to RSI. Early tracheostomy should be considered for patients with severe brain injuries who are felt to require prolonged ventilatory support.

Prevention of increases in ICP are important. *Head of bed elevation* to at least 30 degrees minimizes venous outflow resistance and promotes cerebrospinal fluid displacement into the spinal compartment, reducing ICP in the process. Hypoxemia should be promptly corrected to ensure adequate cerebral oxygenation. **Carbon dioxide tension** *plays an important role in cerebral blood flow. Hypercapnia has been shown to cause vasodilation of cerebral blood vessels, which increases cerebral blood flow and ICP. For patients with increased ICP, careful hyperventilation can be used in emergency situations to decrease cerebral blood flow. However, it is important to note that hypocapnia has the opposite effect, and the resultant vasoconstriction can cause cerebral ischemia. Under most circumstances eucapnia is the goal.*

A limited volume of exogenous tissue, cerebrospinal fluid, blood, or edema fluid can be added to the intracranial contents without significantly raising the ICP. Death or severe worsening may follow increases in ICP with a shift in intracranial contents if CPP is elevated or vital brain stem centers are displaced. CPP is the force that drives circulation across and through the brain's capillary system. An ICP pressure port is illustrated

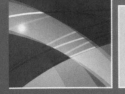

Neuromuscular diseases (NMDs) are associated with multiple cardiopulmonary manifestations. Respiratory impairment results from weakness of the muscles of respiration, from either loss of normal innervations or direct muscle dysfunction. Atelectasis (see Fig. 10.7) develops from lack of deep breathing, weak coughing, and/or poor chest wall compliance. These factors contribute to the development of alveolar consolidation (see Fig. 10.8) and excessive bronchial secretions (see Fig. 10.11). These patients are also at an increased risk for developing pulmonary infections because of the inability to expectorate secretions effectively. The Airway Clearance Therapy Protocol (for the newborn), Protocol 33.2; Lung Expansion Therapy Protocol (for the newborn), Protocol 33.3; Airway Clearance Protocol (for the pediatric patient), Protocol 34.2; Ventilator Initiation and Management Protocol, Protocol 11.1; and Ventilator Weaning Protocol, Protocol 11.2, are important in preventing these complications.

As respiratory muscle weakness progresses in NMDs, acute ventilatory failure may develop. Patients with severe neuromuscular disorders are at risk for acute ventilatory failure in a variety of settings, including invasive procedures (as a result of receiving sedation or general anesthesia) and critical illness.

CLINICAL DATA OBTAINED AT THE PATIENT'S BEDSIDE

The Physical Examination

Respiratory Rate
- Varies with the degree and etiology of respiratory muscle weakness
- Increased in moderate to severe cases (rapid shallow breathing pattern)

Paradoxical Abdominal Respirations
- Caused by decreased chest wall compliance and increased abdominal compliance
- During inspiration the chest wall moves inward instead of outward
- Seen in more severe cases of NMD

Diminished Breath Sounds at the Lung Bases

Egophony
- Can indicate atelectasis or consolidation. Have the patient repeat the "ee" sound while performing auscultation with stethoscope. If the sound changes to an "ay" sound, then egophony is present.

Crackles

Babinski Sign
- Reflex great toe extension and fanning of other toes with lateral plantar stimulation
- Sign of upper motor neuron (UMN) disease, such as stroke (not specific to ALS)
- Present in approximately 50% of patients with ALS

CLINICAL DATA OBTAINED FROM LABORATORY TESTS AND SPECIAL PROCEDURES

Pulmonary Function Test Findings[1]
(Restrictive Lung Pathology)

FVC[2]	FEV_T	FEV_1/FVC ratio	$FEF_{25\%-75\%}$
↓	N or ↓	N or ↑ (>0.70)	N or ↓

$FEF_{50\%}$	$FEF_{200-1200}$	PEFR	MVV
N or ↓	N or ↓	N or ↓	N or ↓

LUNG VOLUME AND CAPACITY FINDINGS

V_T	IRV	ERV	RV
↓	↓	↓	↓

VC	IC	FRC	TLC	RV/TLC ratio
↓	↓	↓	↓	N

MAXIMUM INSPIRATORY PRESSURE (MIP) ↓

Arterial Blood Gases
Moderate to Severe Neuromuscular Diseases

Acute Ventilatory Failure With Hypoxemia[3]
(Acute Respiratory Acidosis)

pH[4]	$PaCO_2$	HCO_3^-[4]	PaO_2	SaO_2 or SpO_2
↓	↑	↑	↓	↓
		(but normal)		

---

[1]Progressive worsening of these values is key to anticipating the onset of ventilatory failure.

[2]Patients with neuromuscular disease may exhibit a decline in FVC when in a supine position.

[3]See Fig. 5.2 and Table 5.4 and related discussion for the acute pH, $PaCO_2$, and HCO_3^- changes associated with acute ventilatory failure.

[4]When tissue hypoxia is severe enough to produce lactic acid, the pH and HCO_3^- values will be lower than expected for a particular $PaCO_2$ level.

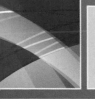
Severe Neuromuscular Diseases

Chronic Ventilatory Failure With Hypoxemia[5] (Compensated Respiratory Acidosis)

pH	$PaCO_2$	HCO_3^-	PaO_2	SaO_2 or SpO_2
N	↑	↑	↓	↓
		(significantly)		

ACUTE VENTILATORY CHANGES SUPERIMPOSED ON CHRONIC VENTILATORY FAILURE[6]

Because acute ventilatory changes may be seen in patients with chronic neuromuscular disease, the respiratory therapist must be familiar with—and alert for—the following two dangerous arterial blood gas findings:

- Acute alveolar hyperventilation superimposed on chronic ventilatory failure that should further alert the respiratory therapist to document the following important ABG assessment: *Possible impending acute ventilatory failure*
- *Acute ventilatory failure (acute hypoventilation) superimposed on chronic ventilatory failure*

---

[5]See Table 5.6 and related discussion for the acute pH, $PaCO_2$, and HCO_3^- changes associated with chronic ventilatory failure.

[6]See Table 5.7, Table 5.8, and Table 5.9 and related discussion for the pH, $PaCO_2$, and HCO_3 changes associated with acute ventilatory changes superimposed on chronic ventilatory failure.

---

in Fig. 31.3. The catheter is inserted into the brain through a burr hole drilled into the skull. *Acceptable ICP is 5 to 10 mm Hg.* ICP greater than 20 mm Hg suggests that a volume of cerebral fluid is under significant pressure and should be treated. High amounts of PEEP may impair cerebral perfusion by decreasing venous return and cardiac output. Moderate levels of PEEP are typically well tolerated by patients who need them (e.g., patients with acute respiratory distress syndrome provided that the MAP is maintained).

Elevated ICPs are prevented by head of the bed elevation, sedation with benzodiazepine agents or propofol, avoidance of stimulation such as encouraged coughing or suctioning, and/or intravenous mannitol or hypertonic saline. The aim is to keep the $PaCO_2$ at 35 to 40 mm Hg.

Airway clearance therapy is important to prevent atelectasis and respiratory infection. Bronchodilators and chest physiotherapy are acceptable initial measures to improve airway clearance. Devices such as a cough assist, the MetaNeb System,[1] or high-frequency chest wall oscillators (vest therapy) may be contraindicated in patients with a concern for increased ICP or unstable head/neck injuries. These devices can be introduced after resolution of increased ICP and clinical stabilization.

Early mobilization and physical therapy should be implemented whenever feasible as another means to improve bronchial hygiene. Patients with a tracheostomy should receive standard tracheostomy care.

General Management of Neuromuscular Disease

Nutrition

Nutrition is a vital, and often underestimated, aspect in the care of patients with NMD. Weight loss and malnutrition are poor prognostic factors in several NMDs, especially muscular dystrophies and ALS. Muscle wasting is associated with an increased energy expenditure and creates an overall catabolic state that promotes disability and further functional decline. Furthermore, dysphagia contributes a great deal to the inability of these patients to adequately consume enough calories to meet their resting energy needs. Protein calorie malnutrition increases the risk for infection and is associated with worsening morbidity and mortality. It is also associated with worsening respiratory function. Respiratory therapists, in conjunction with speech pathologists and dietitians, are important in monitoring for nutritional issues and swallowing complications in NMDs.

Patents should undergo regular assessment of their swallowing and have their weight monitored closely, especially early in

---

[1]The MetaNeb System consists of the following three modes: (1) continuous positive expiratory pressure (CPEP), (2) continuous **high-frequency chest wall oscillation**, and (3) aerosol mode.

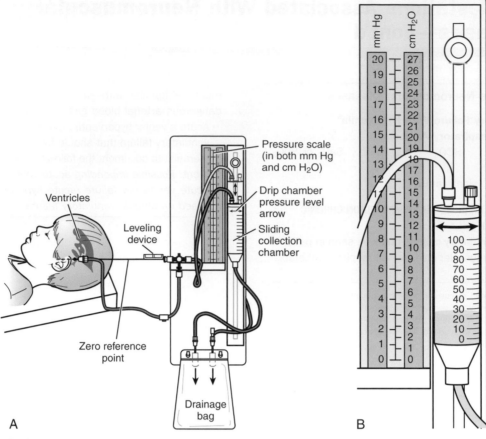

FIGURE 31.3 Intraventricular intracranial pressure (ICP) monitoring system with an external ventricular drainage system for controlled drainage of cerebrospinal fluid. A, The system consists of an intraventricular catheter joined by tubing to a drainage system with adjustable height and a drainage bag. The system also typically has a stopcock, an injection sampling port, and a clamp. The zero reference point for the system is typically between the outer canthus of the eye and the external auditory canal (see leveling device placed at that level). B, The drip chamber pressure level (horizontal arrow) is placed at a prescribed height (in cm) above this zero reference point. The drainage stopcock can allow continuous drainage or be turned to allow only intermittent drainage when the patient's ICP exceeds a prescribed threshold. If the system is functioning and the stopcock is turned to drainage, CSF will drain from the patient's ventricle into the collection chamber and ultimately into the drainage bag once the patient's ICP is sufficiently high. If the drip chamber is placed 27.2 cm (rounded to 27 cm) above the child's ventricles, drainage should occur if the patient's ICP equals 27.2 cm H_2O or 20 mm Hg (1.36 cm H_2O pressure = 1 mm Hg pressure; 27.2 cm H_2O pressure = 20 mm Hg pressure). (Redrawn and modified from Owen, A. [2009]. *Clinical guideline: external ventricular drainage.* [Revised, September, 2009]. London, UK: Great Ormond Street Hospital for Sick Children, Institute of Children's Health and University College of London. In Hazinski, M. F. [2013]. *Nursing care of the critically ill child* [3rd ed.]. St. Louis, MO: Elsevier.)

their disease. Calorie counting provides an objective measure of caloric intake. Patients experiencing fatigue with meals may benefit from a lung volume recruitment maneuver to reduce the work of breathing associated with swallowing. In addition, nutritional supplements, usually in liquid form, may provide additional calories in a method that is less fatiguing.

Gastrostomy tube placement may be required to supplement nutritional needs and provide enteral access for medication administration. Studies have not consistently proven a survival benefit in many forms of NMD; however, gastrostomy insertion has been shown to reduce anxiety among patients with poor oral intake and their caregivers. The optimal timing of gastrostomy tube placement is uncertain. In ALS some sources recommend that a 5% decrease in premorbid weight should prompt consideration of a percutaneous endoscopic gastrostomy (PEG) tube and initiation of enteral feedings. The American Academy of Neurology recommends PEG placement before the forced vital capacity drops below 50% of predicted to prevent respiratory complications during the procedure. Ultimately the decision to insert a feeding tube should be based on multiple factors (e.g., patient preference, weight trends, objective measurements of caloric intake, age, and underlying disease process).

Although much of the attention regarding nutritional assessments in NMD focuses on weight loss, it is important to note that too much weight gain can be just as harmful. **Obesity** increases risk for development of cardiovascular disease such as stroke or heart attack. Increased abdominal girth can cause worsening restrictive thoracic disease and impair respiratory function, especially in patients with respiratory muscle weakness. Obesity also further impairs mobility and increases the risk for developing diabetes mellitus and hyperlipidemia, both of which are risk factors for cardiovascular disease. Patients with muscular dystrophy who are on corticosteroids are at an even higher risk for developing obesity and obesity-related complications. This highlights the importance of a balanced diet that is high in protein to promote growth of lean muscle mass.

Ventilatory Management of Patients With Neuromuscular Disease

Mechanical ventilation is an important part of the care for patients with NMD who have respiratory insufficiency. Traditionally, tracheostomy placement and invasive mechanical ventilation was the mainstay of chronic ventilatory management in this population; however, in recent years it has been demonstrated that NIV can be an acceptable strategy for long-term ventilatory support. An understanding of not only the indications for ventilatory support but also the various modalities available is important for the respiratory therapist caring for these patients. Protocol 11.1 outlines a general approach to the initiation of ventilatory support of patients.

Mechanical ventilatory support is indicated for patients with signs and symptoms that are concerning for hypoventilation. It has been shown to prolong survival in ALS and DMD, and it improves quality of life in most forms of NMD. Subjective symptoms that may suggest chronic hypoventilation include dyspnea on exertion, orthopnea, morning headaches, fatigue, daytime somnolence, impaired cognition, and frequent nighttime awakenings. Paradoxical breathing, tachycardia, diaphoresis, and accessory muscle use are signs of respiratory insufficiency and should warrant further evaluation. An arterial blood gas (ABG) determination may show evidence of hypercapnia (PaCO$_2$ greater than 45 mm Hg) with or without metabolic compensation. Patients may have hypoxemia as well.

Spirometry is a useful tool to both identify patients with respiratory insufficiency and monitor disease progression over time. FVC and MIP are typically decreased. *Additionally, patients may have normal spirometry while upright but may exhibit a sharp decline when testing is performed in the supine position.* Recurrent episodes of acute respiratory failure requiring intubation is an indication for initiation of chronic NIV even in the absence of ABG or spirometry data. The Centers for Medicare & Medicaid Services (CMS) produced the Respiratory Assist Device (RAD) Qualifying Guidelines for the use of NIV for multiple disorders (Box 31.1).

Tracheostomy

The choice between a tracheostomy with invasive ventilation and prolonged NIV involves a multitude of clinical factors and patient and caregiver preference. Smaller designs have improved ventilator portability and made chronic mechanical ventilation a much more feasible option. Tracheostomies should be considered when patients have difficulty clearing secretions, impaired mental status (obtunded or uncooperative), uncontrolled seizure disorders, inability to tolerate NIV, NIV failure, or failure to wean from invasive mechanical ventilation. Tracheostomies have the added benefit of immediate airway

---

> **BOX 31.1 Respiratory Assist Device Qualifying Guidelines for Noninvasive Ventilation Use**
>
> 1. Diagnosis of a neuromuscular disease
> 2. At least one of the following:
>   - ABG values (done while awake) with a PaCO$_2$ ≥45 mm Hg
>   - Sleeping oxygen saturation ≤88% for ≥5 minutes with a minimum of 2 hours recording time
>   - Forced vital capacity <50% of predicted or a MIP <60 cm H$_2$O (for patients with neuromuscular disease)

---

access to invasive mechanical ventilation in the event of acute respiratory decompensation.

Tracheostomies can be performed using local anesthetic and NIV support in patients with hypercapnia. Long-term use of a tracheostomy tube can result in tracheal stenosis, necrosis, hemorrhage, stomal infections, and even tracheoesophageal fistula formation. Tracheostomy tube use requires humidification and daily respiratory care management, which can be cumbersome for home caregivers. Swallowing and speech mechanics may be impaired, although devices and ventilatory techniques can allow for verbal communication while on a ventilator in selected individuals. Tracheostomy use is also associated with an increase in bacterial airway colonization and an increased risk for ventilator-associated pneumonia. The optimal timing for tracheostomy placement varies from patient to patient, and is basically unknown.

Speech in Patients With a Tracheostomy

When counseling patients regarding tracheostomy placement it is important to bear in mind that there are options to restore verbal communication. Under normal circumstances, a subglottic pressure of at least 2 cm H$_2$O and air flow through the upper airway of about 50 to 300 mL/s is required. As shown in Fig. 31.4, **talking tracheostomy tubes** are now available (e.g., the Passy Muir type of **speaking valve**). However, the voice quality is poor. One-way speaking valves placed on the proximal end of the tracheostomy tube allows for much improved speech quality by allowing exhaled air to escape through the vocal cords. It should be noted that their use requires the cuff to be completely deflated, thus increasing a risk for aspiration and impairment in gas exchange while speaking.

Some patients with speaking valves can speak during inspiration and expiration. Patients can also achieve the ability to speak with **leak speech**. With a deflated tracheostomy cuff, approximately 15% of the delivered tidal volume will leak around the tube and out through the vocal cords. Using PEEP and a prolonged inspiratory time will increase the tracheal pressure and therefore improve the ability to speak, and as much as 60% to 80% of the respiratory cycle can be used for speech. Both volume and pressure modes can be used effectively to provide speech to mechanically ventilated individuals. In volume modes, increasing the tidal volume can help compensate for the air leak. Selecting patients who are appropriate for speech communication while being ventilated specialist requires

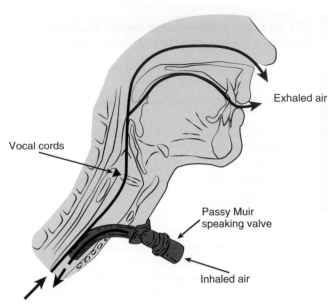

Vocal cords

Exhaled air

Passy Muir
speaking valve

Inhaled air

FIGURE 31.4 Mechanism of action of the Passy Muir type of speaking valve. The valve is a unidirectional valve that occludes air outflow through the tracheotomy cannula during expiration, thereby forcing air through vocal cords. (From Fernández-Carmona, A., Peñas-Maldonado, L., Yuste-Osorio E, et al. [2012]. Exploration and approach to artificial airway dysphagia. *Medicina Intensiva* 36(6), 423-433.)

collaboration between speech-language pathology specialist and respiratory therapists. Those with increased secretions, significant hypoxemia, and significant ventilatory needs may not be appropriate candidates.

Ventilatory Support

NIV can be used as a primary method of ventilatory support in patients with ventilatory failure. Case series have described patients successfully using NIV for ventilatory support 24 hours per day. Reports have also described its use in weaning patients from tracheostomy-assisted ventilation. NIV is most commonly used with a face mask, nasal mask, or nasal pillows.

Ventilatory support is generally initiated nocturnally, with additional use during the day for patients with ongoing respiratory weakness. Several sources recommend volume-cycled ventilation to allow for breath stacking maneuvers; however, patients can be adequately and comfortably ventilated with pressure-cycled ventilation, in particular **bi-level positive airway pressure (BPAP)**. A pressure-controlled style of BPAP is most helpful in NMD by ensuring a complete inspiratory time with each breath.

PEEP can be set to a minimum value (i.e., 2 cm H_2O) unless the patient has concomitant obstructive sleep apnea or other pulmonary pathologic process. When using bilevel ventilation the inspiratory time should be prolonged, generally at least 1 s, to provide an adequate inspiratory volume. It is important to note that spontaneous (S) or spontaneous timed (ST) modes of ventilation can result in premature inspiration-expiration cycling in patients with NMD. This occurs because in these modes patients dictate their own inspiratory time for all spontaneous breaths. In this situation assisted modes of ventilation allow the provider to set a specific inspiratory time for all breaths received by the patient.

Volume-assured pressure support (VAPS) devices are frequently used for NIV in patients with acute and chronic hypoventilation syndromes. This nonconventional ventilatory strategy attempts to combine volume- and pressure-controlled ventilation by adjusting the pressure support within a prespecified range to target a specific tidal volume. It can be used in S, ST, and PC modes. Clinical trials have found VAPS to be as efficacious, and in some cases more beneficial, for the management of patients with different forms of hypoventilation, including NMD, restrictive thoracic disorders, obesity hypoventilation, and COPD.

The devices automatically adjust the inspiratory pressure within the preset range to achieve a desired tidal volume or minute ventilation, as opposed to conventional bilevel ventilation, which uses one set inspiratory pressure during the entire delivered breath. This ultimately ensures more consistent tidal volumes in the setting of a varying patient respiratory effort and chest wall compliance. It also tends to be more comfortable.

Respiratory therapists should be aware that specific details of modes of NIV will vary across device manufacturers. Therapists will need to become familiar with exact devices that may be available to them. In general, when using S or ST modes, the inspiratory time will not be adjustable or may only become applicable if the patient becomes apneic. In PC mode, an inspiratory time will be fixed and will apply to all breaths, whether spontaneous or delivered by the device. Several VAPS devices are available.

These devices differ primarily in the algorithm used to automatically adjust settings. Specifics of these modes vary depending on the manufacturer. In general, devices are designed to target either exhaled tidal volume or alveolar ventilation. These goals are reached by augmenting pressure support and adjusting the backup respiratory rate. Newer devices may also auto-adjust the expiratory positive pressure airway pressure (EPAP) to eliminate obstructive events.

In those with NMD, when using VAPS technology it is important to adjust trigger, cycle, and inspiratory time to ensure patient comfort and ease of ventilation. In NMD, patients will need these settings to be adjusted at the bedside. Automatic ventilator operation algorithms are frequently incapable of meeting the needs of these patients. The trigger should be highly sensitive and the inspiratory time prolonged to optimize patient-ventilatory synchrony.

Mouthpiece ventilation (MPV), also known as *sip and puff ventilation* or *sip ventilation*, is a less commonly used ventilatory strategy in NMD. In mouthpiece ventilation, a mouthpiece connected to ventilator can be inserted into the mouth, allowing the patient to take a ventilator-assisted breath intermittently. This is most commonly used for daytime support and can be coupled with nighttime NIV via an alternative interface. MPV reduces the risk for infection compared with that with tracheostomy.

Compared with NIV, using traditional interfaces MPV results in less skin breakdown, facilitates speech, facilitates coughing, facilitates swallowing, has a better appearance, and may have less of a psychological effect on patients. MPV requires active patient participation and may not be appropriate for patients with significant bulbar disease, because of inability to make a seal with the mouthpiece. The ventilator is typically set to assist control (AC) mode and volume control (VC) with a set tidal volume of 10 to 15 mL/kg of ideal body weight. Volume-controlled modes are preferred because it allows for **breath stacking**, though pressure control (PC) may be preferred when gastric inflation is severe. The respiratory rate and PEEP should be set to zero. Triggering the breath should be made as easy as possible (i.e., flow triggering set at 1 L/min). The apnea alarm should be set to its highest threshold or turned off to prevent unnecessary alarms. The low-pressure alarm should be set to the minimum setting. Box 31.2 provides sample ventilator settings for MPV.

Noninvasive ventilatory support can be started in the sleep laboratory, the inpatient setting (usually an intensive care unit), or at home. Overnight pulse oximetry and ABGs can be used to objectively titrate ventilator settings. The goal of therapy should be to not only normalize objective values but also to improve symptoms and optimize patient comfort.

BOX 31.2 Sample Mouthpiece Ventilator Settings

AC/VC or AC/PC

Flow pattern: Square waveform (can use ramp if more comfortable for patient)

Tidal volume: 10 to 15 mL/kg IBW or 1.5 × FVC

Inspiratory time: 1.2 to 1.5 seconds (can increase up to 2.0 seconds based on patient comfort)

Respiratory rate: 0 bpm

PEEP: 0 cm H_2O

Low inspiratory pressure: 1 to 2 cm H_2O (disable alarm when possible, otherwise minimize to lowest setting)

High inspiratory pressure: Up to 70 cm H_2O (disable alarm when possible, otherwise maximize to highest setting)

Apnea alarm: Disabled (or set to longest time possible)

Trigger: 1 L/min flow

AC/PC, Assist control/pressure control; *AC/VC*, assist control/volume control; *FVC*, forced vital capacity; *IBW*, ideal body weight; *PEEP*, positive end-expiratory pressure.

CASE STUDY Amyotrophic Lateral Sclerosis

Admitting History

A 53-year-old female physician with known ALS presented to the emergency department (ED) with progressive dyspnea and generalized fatigue. Over the course of 6 months, the patient noted worsening dyspnea on exertion, which had limited her ability to work. These symptoms had forced her to significantly decrease her workload. At this time, she only saw patients 2 half days per week in her primary care clinic. Being unable to work full time had been both an emotional and a financial strain on her and her family. She reported frequent coughing with meals. Her friends had commented that her voice appeared softer and her cough sounded weaker but more congested. Three months earlier the patient had been hospitalized for right lower lobe pneumonia. No evaluation of her swallowing was performed at that time, and she recovered fully with antibiotic therapy. At discharge her arterial blood gas (ABG) values were all normal.

The patient confirmed multiple falls at home. The patient added that while walking she occasionally stumbled and "tripped over her own feet." These falls were not associated with palpitations, lightheadedness, dizziness, or syncopal symptoms. Additionally, she had noted some "muscle twitching" of her tongue. Her medical history was significant for hypertension and hyperlipidemia. Her medications included an antihypertensive and a lipid-lowering agent. She had never smoked and denied the use of alcoholic beverages. She had no family history of respiratory or other neurologic conditions.

Physical Examination

In the ED the patient was calm and alert. She appeared to be in moderately acute respiratory distress. Her vital signs were blood pressure 138/86 mm Hg, pulse 96 beats/min, respiratory rate 28 to 32 breaths/min and shallow, and temperature 37.0°C. On room air, her SpO_2 was noted to be 87%. At this time, the respiratory therapist started her on supplemental oxygen via a 2 L/min nasal cannula. Neurologic examination notes showed decreased motor strength in the arms and legs, increased bilateral patellar tendon reflexes, and fasciculation of the tongue. There was notable muscle wasting of the extremities. The patient's voice was strained with decreased intelligibility of speech. On auscultation, there were fine and coarse crackles throughout her lung bases. Her cough was weak and congested. No sputum was observed. The cardiac examination was unremarkable. Blood was drawn for laboratory testing, and a chest x-ray film was obtained. The chest x-ray film showed atelectasis at the bases without signs of infection or pneumothorax. There was no consolidation or signs of interstitial edema. At this time the patient was admitted to the hospital for treatment and observation.

Two days later, the head nurse sent out a stat call to the physician and respiratory therapist. On observation, the patient was obtunded and nonresponsive to aggressive painful stimuli. Her vital signs were blood pressure 164/96 mm Hg, pulse 121 beats/min, and respiratory rate 16 breaths/min and shallow. The nurse stated that the night shift had reported that the patient was now coughing up moderate amounts of yellow sputum. On a 2 L/min nasal cannula, an ABG sample was drawn and showed pH 7.04, $PaCO_2$ 106 mm Hg, HCO_3^- 25, PaO_2 58 mm Hg, and SaO_2 68%, which was immediately assessed by the respiratory therapist as acute ventilatory failure with moderately severe hypoxemia.

The patient was emergently intubated because of the acute hypercapnic respiratory failure and inability to protect her airway. The initial ventilator settings were volume-controlled intermittent mandatory ventilation (IMV), respiratory rate 12 breaths/min, tidal volume 500 mL, PEEP 5 cm H_2O, an FIO_2 0.4, and a decelerating flow at 60 L/min. A chest x-ray film confirmed that the end of the endotracheal tube was 2.0 cm above the carina and the presence of bilateral atelectasis. The patient appeared to be comfortable without evidence of ventilator-patient dyssynchrony. Some spontaneous breathing was noted—about 4 to 6 breaths/min. A repeat ABG sample 20 minutes after intubation and mechanical ventilation showed pH 7.37, $PaCO_2$ 43 mm Hg, HCO_3^- 24, PaO_2 109 mm Hg, and SaO_2 96%. Her vital signs were blood pressure 134/77 mm Hg, pulse 90 beats/min, respiratory rate 12 breaths/min (mechanical ventilation and 4 to 6 spontaneous). Moderate amounts of yellow and green sputum were being suctioned. On auscultation fine and coarse bilateral crackles could be heard in the lung bases.

Respiratory Assessment and Plan

S N/A (intubated and sedated)

O Vital signs: BP 134/77, HR 90, RR IMV 12 (4 to 6 spontaneous breaths). ABGs: pH 7.37, $PaCO_2$ 43, HCO_3^- 24, PaO_2 109, and SaO_2 96%. CXR: Bilateral atelectasis. AUS: Bilateral crackles could be heard in the lung bases. Moderate amounts of yellow and green sputum.

A • Acute ventilatory failure secondary to ALS
  • Acid-base and oxygenation status within normal range on present ventilator settings (ABG)
  • Atelectasis (x-ray, bilateral crackles in lung bases)
  • Excessive bronchial secretions with evidence of infection (yellow and green sputum suctioned)

P Mechanical Ventilation Protocol: Continue on ventilator settings as now adjusted. Airway Clearance Protocol (e.g., suctioning, PEP devices, increased PEEP). Perform daily a spontaneous breathing trial to assess for readiness for extubation. Monitor SpO_2 closely.

Four Days After Admission

The patient remained on the mechanical ventilator. She had been receiving aggressive airway clearance therapy and had minimal secretions. She had clear lung sounds bilaterally and no peripheral edema. Her x-ray film showed resolution of basilar atelectasis. On this morning a spontaneous breathing trial was performed. Ventilator settings were pressure support of 5 cm H_2O, FIO_2 of 21%, and PEEP of 5 cm H_2O. After 2 hours on these settings, her average exhaled tidal volume was approximately 400 mL with a respiratory rate of 21, giving a rapid shallow breathing index (RSBI) of 52. On physical examination she was following commands.

At this time, the patient was successfully extubated and liberated from the mechanical ventilator without difficulty. She initially received supplemental oxygen at

2.0 L/min via nasal cannula with a goal saturation of 88% to 92%.

Unfortunately, after about 2 hours it was noted that her respiratory rate increased to 35 breaths/min. She complained that it was difficult to catch her breath even at rest. On auscultation, her lungs were clear and without wheezes or crackles. Even though the patient was oriented to person, time, and place, she appeared very anxious. Her vital signs were blood pressure 144/88 mm Hg, respiratory rate 35 breaths/min and shallow, and heart rate 102 beats/min. On a 2 L/min nasal cannula, an ABG sample showed a pH of 7.16, $PaCO_2$ of 83 mm Hg, HCO_3^- 28, PaO_2 62 mm Hg, and SpO_2 80%.

The respiratory therapist paged the attending physician stat and informed her of the patient's recurrent acute ventilatory failure with moderate hypoxemia and the need for ventilatory support. The patient was reintubated, and a chest x-ray was ordered. At this time, the following SOAP was documented.

Respiratory Assessment and Plan

S Patient states it is difficult to catch her breath

O Appears drowsy but follow commands appropriately. Vital signs BP 144/88, RR 35 & shallow, HR 102 beats/min. ABGs on 2 L/min nasal cannula pH 7.16, $PaCO_2$ 83, HCO_3^- 28, PaO_2 62, and SpO_2 80%. CXR: No report at this time.

A • Acute ventilatory failure with moderate hypoxemia secondary to neuromuscular weakness

P Mechanical Ventilation Protocol: Initiate noninvasive ventilation. Start with pressure control (PC) ventilation, IPAP 20, EPAP 5, inspiratory time 1.2 s, respiratory rate 15. Monitor the exhaled tidal volume achieved with these settings, and adjust the inspiratory pressure, driving pressure (IPAP – EPAP), and inspiratory time to achieve the goal minute ventilation with resolution of tachypnea. Continue Airway Clearance Therapy Protocol (e.g., suctioning, PEP devices, increased PEEP).

Over the next 3 days the patient was again liberated from the ventilator. Her strength returned, and she was discharged from the hospital with additional patient and family education for ventilatory support for her symptomatic hypoventilation—nocturnal noninvasive ventilation (NIV).

Discussion

ALS is a progressive neuromuscular disorder associated with upper and lower motor neuron findings. The patient in this clinical case had signs and symptoms compatible with ALS, although she had not had a formal evaluation before her presentation. Before her first mechanical ventilation, her ABGs were consistent with acute ventilatory failure with moderately severe hypoxemia.

Although it very possible that patients with severe neuromuscular disorders can develop chronic ventilatory failure (also called *compensated respiratory acidosis*) during the advanced severe stages, this was not the case in this patient at this time. Nevertheless—and precisely like the patient with chronic obstructive pulmonary disease (COPD)—it is important for the respiratory therapist to be on the alert for acute ventilatory changes superimposed on chronic ventilatory failure when confronted with patients with severe NMD (see Acute Ventilatory Changes Superimposed on Chronic Ventilatory Failure, Chapter 5, page 78). Similar to the patient with severe COPD, patients with chronic respiratory muscle weakness caused by NMD are also at high risk for developing acute hypercapnia (i.e., on top of chronic ventilatory failure) when exposed to excessive supplemental oxygen. Be careful not to overoxygenate these patients.

Our patient met several criteria for the initiation of ventilatory support, including respiratory distress, altered mental status, and acute ventilatory failure with moderately severe hypoxemia. Clearly on day 2 mechanical ventilation was justified with a pH of 7.04, $PaCO_2$ 106 mm Hg, HCO_3^- 25, PaO_2 58 mm Hg, and SaO_2 68%. Note how quickly her blood gases returned to normal once she was placed on ventilatory support. On day 5, the objective data strongly supported that she be discontinued from the ventilation—for example, average exhaled tidal volume of 400 mL, respiratory rate of 21, a RSBI of 52, following commands, and clear lung sounds bilaterally. Unfortunately, in this case, additional ventilatory support was needed after the patient was liberated from the mechanical ventilator on day 5, because of the postextubation acute ventilatory failure.

After another 3 days of mechanical support and routine airway clearance therapies, the patient was successfully liberated from the ventilator. On discharge, the attending physician documented the following in the patient's progress notes:

After recovery from her acute illness episode, the patient will likely require additional ventilatory support at home for her symptomatic hypoventilation. The following is recommended: Nocturnal non-invasive ventilation (NIV) because symptoms of hypoventilation (such as dyspnea, shallow breathing, somnolence, and fatigue) and acute changes in arterial blood gas measurements can improve with nocturnal NIV. I will discuss this recommendation with the patient and family. This will be followed by arrangements to have the NIV equipment placed in the patient's home. Patient and family education for the nocturnal NIV will be prescribed—both before discharge and in the patient's home.

Nocturnal NIV improves overall survival and quality of life. ALS is a progressive disease, and as respiratory muscle weakness evolves, the patient may need more than just nocturnal respiratory support. In some clinical practices, patients are instructed to use their noninvasive ventilation after meals or other physically exhausting activities. In end-stage ALS, patients may require ventilatory support 24 hours a day, which can be accomplished both invasively (with a tracheostomy) and noninvasively (generally with nasal pillows or sip ventilation).

Our patient had evidence of **bulbar dysfunction** (i.e., strained voice and slurred speech) on clinical examination. Furthermore, atelectasis of the bases was present, which was the result of inability to take full, deep breaths. Adding airway clearance techniques as part of the patient and family education program would be helpful and allow for better aeration of the lower lobes of the lungs—thus reducing the risk for pulmonary infection.

SELF-ASSESSMENT QUESTIONS

1. Which of the following is an indication for ventilatory support in a patient with neuromuscular disease?
   a. Awake $PaCO_2$ ≥45 mm Hg
   b. MIP <60 cm H_2O
   c. Sleeping oxygen saturation ≤88% for ≥5 minutes with a minimum of 2 hours recording time
   d. FVC <50% predicted
   e. All of the above

2. Spinal cord injuries involving the upper thoracic area affect breathing in which of the following ways?
   a. Impairment in diaphragm function
   b. Altering respiratory drive
   c. Impairment of the intercostal muscles, abdominal muscles, and scalenes.
   d. Increased airway resistance
   e. All of the above

3. What is the most common cause of death in patients with ALS?
   a. Respiratory failure
   b. Cardiovascular disease
   c. Traumatic injury
   d. Cerebrovascular disease (e.g., stroke)

4. Which of the following is not a finding typically seen in muscular dystrophy?
   a. Calf pseudohypertrophy
   b. Gower sign
   c. Tongue fasciculations
   d. Limb contractures

5. You are caring for a patient with ALS who was recently started on noninvasive ventilation to treat chronic hypoventilation. You choose Pressure Control, Average Volume-Assured Pressure Support (AVAPS) as your initial ventilatory mode. The settings are RR 10, targeted tidal volume 500 mL, IPAP min 10 cm H_2O, IPAP max 15 cm H_2O, EPAP 5 cm H_2O, inspiratory time 0.8 s, rise time 3. The patient states the settings are comfortable, but she is not taking as large of a breath as she would want. You check the ventilator and note that the patient is only achieving exhaled tidal volumes of 300 mL with those settings. The maximum pressure of each breath is at 15 cm H_2O. Which of the following adjustments will increase the patient's exhaled tidal volume?
   a. Increase IPAP max to 25 cm H_2O
   b. Increase set tidal volume to 800 mL
   c. Increase the inspiratory time to 1.2 s
   d. Decrease the respiratory rate to 8 breaths/min
   e. b and d
   f. a and c

32 | Sleep Apnea

Chapter Objectives

After reading this chapter, you will be able to:

- List the major classifications of sleep disorders.
- Define the commonly used terms and phrases associated with sleep-related disorders.
- Describe the derived measurements used to calculate the frequency of respiratory disturbances during sleep.
- Differentiate between obstructive sleep apnea, central sleep apnea, and mixed sleep apnea.
- Describe the anatomic alterations of the lungs associated with sleep apnea.
- Explain the signs and symptoms associated with obstructive sleep apnea.
- List the common risk factors associated with obstructive sleep apnea.
- Differentiate between hyperventilation-related central sleep apnea and hypoventilation-related sleep apnea.
- Differentiate between the advantages and disadvantages of polysomnography and in-home portable monitoring in the diagnosis of sleep apnea.
- Explain the diagnostic criteria for obstructive and central sleep apnea.
- Differentiate among the criteria for mild, moderate, and severe obstructive sleep apnea.
- List the cardiopulmonary clinical manifestations associated with sleep apnea.
- Describe the management of obstructive sleep apnea.
- Describe the management of central sleep apnea.
- Describe the clinical strategies and rationales of the SOAPs presented in the case study.
- Define key terms and complete self-assessment questions at the end of the chapter and on Evolve.

Key Terms

Adaptive Servoventilation (ASV)
Alpha Wave
Apnea-Hypopnea Index (AHI)
Atrial Fibrillation
Autotitrating Positive Airway Pressure (APAP)
Basal Metabolic Index (BMI)
Beta Waves
Bi-level Positive Airway Pressure (BPAP)
Brady-Tachy Syndrome
Cardiopulmonary Complications of Sleep Apnea
Central Sleep Apnea (CSA)
Cheyne-Stokes Breathing Pattern
COHb-corrected Oximetry O_2 Saturation

Confusional Arousals
Continuous Positive Airway Pressure (CPAP)
CPAP Compliance/Adherence
CPAP Titration Polysomnogram
Delta Waves
Drug-Induced Sleep Endoscopy (DISE)
Electroencephalogram (EEG)
Electromyogram (EMG)
Electrooculogram (EOG)
Epoch
Epworth Sleepiness Scale
Fatigue Severity Scale (FSS)
Fricative Breathing
Home Sleep Test (HST)
Hyperventilation-Related CSA
Hypopneas
Hypoventilation-Related CSA
Implantable Upper Airway Stimulator
K Complexes
Laser-Assisted Uvulopalatoplasty
Mallampati Classification
Mixed Apnea
Nocturnal Low-Flow Oxygen Therapy
Non–Rapid Eye Movement (Non-REM) Sleep
Obstructive Apneas
Obstructive Sleep Apnea (OSA)
Overlap Syndrome
Oxygen Desaturation Index
Pickwickian Syndrome
Polysomnogram (PSG)
Polysomnography
Positive End-Expiratory Pressure (PEEP)
Primary Central Sleep Apnea
Pulmonary Hypertension
Radiofrequency Ablation
Rapid Eye Movement (REM) Sleep
Respiratory Disturbance Index (RDI)
Respiratory Effort Index (REI)
Respiratory Effort–Related Arousals (RERAs)
Sawtooth Wave Pattern
Secondary Central Sleep Apnea
Sleep Apnea Screening Programs
Sleep-Related Hypoventilation and Hypoxemia Syndromes (SRHHSs)
Sleep Spindles
Sleep Stages
Sleep Stage Latency

Sleep-related breathing disorders are characterized by abnormal breathing patterns during sleep and include (1) **obstructive sleep apnea** (OSA) syndrome (Fig. 32.1), (2) central sleep apnea syndrome, (3) mixed sleep apnea, and (4) **sleep-related hypoventilation** and **hypoxemia syndromes**. According to the American Academy of Sleep Medicine (AASM),[1] sleep disorders can be classified into eight major groups (Box 32.1). Of particular interest to the respiratory therapist is the category of *sleep-related breathing disorders* and, importantly, the ability to pursue additional education, training, and, finally, certification through the National Board for Respiratory Care,[2] or the Board of Registered Polysomnographic Technologists (RPSGT)[3] as a *sleep disorder specialist (SDS)* (Fig. 32.2). Table 32.1 provides commonly used terms and phrases associated with sleep-related breathing disorders.

Table 32.2 shows derived measurements used to determine the frequency of respiratory disturbances during sleep. Based on the type and frequency of the respiratory events, the following syndromes of sleep-related breathing disorders can be established.

Obstructive Sleep Apnea

Obstructive sleep apnea (OSA) is a common sleep disorder that often requires lifelong care. Cardinal features include **obstructive apneas, hypopneas,** and **respiratory effort–related arousals (RERAs)**, which are caused by recurring collapse of

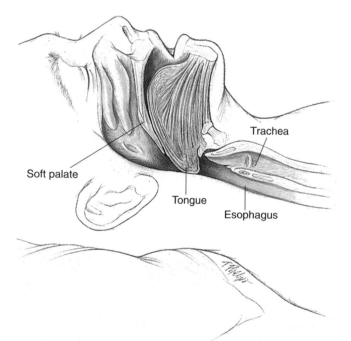

FIGURE 32.1 Obstructive sleep apnea. When the genioglossus muscle fails to oppose the forces that tend to collapse the airway passage during inspiration, the tongue moves into the oropharyngeal area and obstructs the airway.

Soft palate

Trachea

Tongue

Esophagus

BOX 32.1 Sleep Disorder Categories

- Sleep-related breathing disorders
- Insomnia
- Hypersomnias of central origin
- Circadian rhythm sleep disorders
- Parasomnias
- Sleep-related movement disorders
- Isolated symptoms and normal variants
- Other sleep disorders

Modified from American Academy of Sleep Medicine. (2014). *International classification of sleep disorders: Diagnostic and coding manual* (3rd ed.). Darien, IL: American Academy of Sleep Medicine.

---

[1]American Academy of Sleep Medicine (AASM) (http://www.aasmnet.org).

[2]National Board for Respiratory Care, Inc. (http://www.nbrc.org).
[3]Board of Registered Polysomnographic Technologists (http://www.brpt.org/).

TABLE 32.1 Common Terms and Phrases Associated With Sleep-Related Breathing Disorders (Sleep Events)

Term and/or Phrase	Definition
Apnea	The cessation, or near cessation, of air flow. Apnea exists when air flow is less than 10% of pre-event baseline for at least 10 seconds in adults. Apneas can be associated with arousals from sleep, increased arterial carbon dioxide, and decreased oxygen levels.
Obstructive apnea	Air flow is absent or nearly absent, but ventilatory effort persists. It is caused by complete, or near complete, upper airway obstruction.
Central apnea	The absence of both air flow and ventilatory efforts (i.e., diaphragmatic contraction as measured by electromyography and esophageal manometry).
Mixed apnea	A period during which there is no ventilatory effort (i.e., central apnea pattern) followed by a period during which there are obstructed respiratory efforts (obstructive apnea pattern).
Hypopnea	Is present when the following three criteria are present: Air flow decreased ≥30% from pre-event baseline The decreased air flow lasts ≥10 seconds The decreased air flow is accompanied by ≥3% SpO_2 desaturation from preevent baseline or an arousal*
Obstructive hypopnea	Is present when any of the following occur: Snoring during the event Increased inspiratory flattening of the nasal pressure waveform or air flow compared with baseline An associated thoracoabdominal paradox during the event but not during preevent breathing
Central hypopnea	The hypopnea is called *central* when none of the three criteria for obstructive hypopnea (snoring, increased inspiratory flattening of nasal pressure waveform, or thoracoabdominal paradox) is present during the event.
Arousals	Arousals range from full awakenings to 3-second transient electroencephalography shifts to a lighter stage of sleep (alpha, theta, and/or frequencies above 16 Hz (but not **sleep spindles**) with at least 10 seconds of stable sleep preceding the change.
Respiratory effort–related arousals (RERAs)	Said to be present when: 1. There are a series of ventilatory patterns that have a duration of 10 seconds or longer. 2. The ventilatory pattern is characterized by increasing ventilatory effort or flattening of the nasal pressure waveform, followed by an arousal from sleep *and* 3. The ventilatory patterns do not meet the criteria for an apnea or hypopnea. 4. RERAs are often associated with a terminal snort or an abrupt change in ventilatory measures.
Hypoventilation	An increase in the arterial carbon dioxide ($PaCO_2$) to a value greater than 55 mm Hg for at least 10 minutes or a 10 mm Hg or greater rise in the $PaCO_2$ during sleep (compared with awake supine level) above the patient's normal $PaCO_2$ level, exceeding 50 mm Hg for at least 10 minutes.
Cheyne-Stokes breathing	At least three consecutive central apneas and/or central hypopneas, followed by crescendo-decrescendo breathing, with a cycle length (i.e., time from the beginning of a central apnea or hypopnea to the beginning of the next apnea or hypopnea) of at least 40 seconds. In addition, there must be at least five apneas or hypopneas per hour associated with the crescendo-decrescendo breathing pattern.

*Previous definitions endorsed by the American Academy of Sleep Medicine (AASM) and still used by the Centers for Medicare and Medicaid Services use a 4% cutoff for SpO_2 desaturation.

the upper airway during sleep (see Fig. 32.1). During periods of airway obstruction, patients commonly appear quiet and still, as though they are holding their breath, followed by increasingly desperate efforts to inhale. Often the apneic episode ends only after an intense struggle. A snorting sound called *fricative breathing* may be heard at the end of the apneic periods. In severe cases, the patient may suddenly awaken, sit upright in bed, and gasp for air. Patients with OSA usually demonstrate perfectly normal and regular breathing patterns when awake.

In fact, a large number of patients with OSA demonstrate what is commonly called the **Pickwickian syndrome** (named after a character in Charles Dickens' *The Posthumous Papers of the Pickwick Club*, published in 1837). Dickens' description

of Joe, "the fat boy" who snored and had excessive daytime sleepiness, included many of the classic features of what is now recognized as sleep apnea syndrome with hypercapnia, or the obesity hypoventilation syndrome. It should be noted, however, that many patients with sleep apnea are not obese, and therefore clinical suspicion should not be limited to this group. Box 32.2 provides common signs and symptoms associated with OSA. Table 32.3 provides the more common risk factors associated with OSA.

Central Sleep Apnea

Central sleep apnea (CSA) is a disorder characterized by the repetitive stopping or reduction of both air flow and ventilatory

TABLE 32.2 Derived Measurements Used to Calculate the Frequency of Respiratory Disturbances During Sleep

Measures	Definition
Apnea index (AI)	The total number of apneas per hour of sleep.
Apnea hypopnea index (AHI)	The total number of apneas and hypopneas calculated per hour of total sleep. The AHI also may be calculated per hour of **non–rapid eye movement (REM) sleep**, per hour of **rapid eye movement (REM) sleep**, or per hour of sleep in a certain position. The AHI may provide information regarding the sleep stage dependency, or sleep position dependency, of the sleep-related breathing disorder.
Respiratory disturbance index (RDI)*	The total number of events (e.g., apneas, hypopneas, and RERAs) per hour of sleep. The RDI is usually greater than the AHI. This is because the RDI includes the frequency of RERAs; the AHI does not.
Oxygen desaturation (SpO₂)	The drop in hemoglobin oxygenation caused by periods of apnea and hypopnea. Serial measurements are normally used to quantify the severity of the desaturation and should be included on the polysomnogram report.
Oxygen desaturation index (ODI)	The total time that the oxygen saturation falls by more than 3 percentage points per hour of sleep or of total recording time.
Arousal index (ArI)	The total number of arousals per hour of sleep.
Total sleep time (TST)	The total duration of light sleep (stages N1 and N2), deep sleep (stage N3), and REM sleep.
Total recording time (TRT)	The total duration of recording time only.
Sleep efficiency (SE)	The TST divided by the total recording time (i.e., time in bed).
Sleep stage percentage (SSP)	The duration of a particular stage divided by the TST.
Sleep stage latency	The duration from the onset of sleep to the initiation of any stage of sleep.

*The American Academy of Sleep Medicine Prefers respiratory effort index (REI).

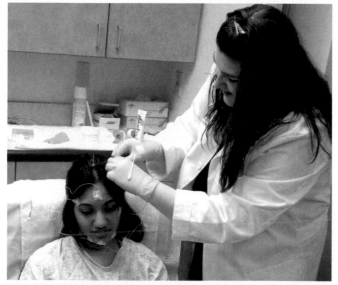

FIGURE 32.2 A sleep disorder specialist (SDS) setting up scalp electrodes on a patient to be studied. While the patient sleeps, the SDS (1) monitors brain waves, eye movements, muscle activity, multiple breathing patterns, and blood oxygen levels using specialized recording equipment; (2) interprets the recordings as they happen and responds appropriately to any emergencies; (3) instructs the patient in recording and maintaining a sleep diary of wake/sleep cycles; and (4) provides support services related to the treatment of sleep-related problems, including helping the patient use various treatment devices for breathing problems during sleep. (Courtesy George G. Burton, MD, Sleep Disorders Center, Kettering Medical Center, Dayton, Ohio.)

BOX 32.2 Signs and Symptoms Associated With Obstructive Sleep Apnea

- Loud snoring
- Observed episodes of breathing cessation during sleep
- Abrupt awakenings accompanied by shortness of breath
- Difficulty staying asleep (insomnia)
- Moodiness or irritability
- Lack of concentration
- Memory impairment
- Awakening with a dry mouth or sore throat
- Morning headache
- Nausea
- Excessive daytime sleepiness (hypersomnia)
- Intellectual and personality changes
- Depression
- Nocturnal enuresis
- Sexual impotence
- Night sweats

effort during sleep. CSA can be classified as **primary central sleep apnea** (idiopathic or unknown cause) or **secondary central sleep apnea**. Examples of conditions associated with secondary CSA include Cheyne-Stokes breathing (congestive heart failure), medical conditions (e.g., encephalitis, brain stem neoplasm, brain stem infarction, spinal surgery, hypothyroidism, drug or substance abuse), and high-altitude periodic breathing. CSA is further categorized as either **hyperventilation-related CSA** or **hypoventilation-related CSA**.

Hyperventilation-related CSA is the most common. It includes primary CSA and CSA associated with

TABLE 32.3 Risk Factors Associated With Obstructive Sleep Apnea

Excess weight	More than 50% of patients diagnosed with obstructive sleep apnea (OSA) are overweight. Fat deposits around the upper airway may obstruct breathing.
Neck size	OSA is often seen in patients with a large neck size. A neck circumference larger than 17 inches in males and 16 inches in females increases the risk for OSA.
Hypertension	OSA is commonly seen in patients with high blood pressure.
Anatomic narrowing of upper airway	Common causes of anatomic narrowing of the upper airway include excessive pharyngeal tissue, **tonsillar hypertrophy** or adenoids, deviated nasal septum, laryngeal stenosis, vocal cord dysfunction, and a Mallampati classification score of 3 or 4 (see Fig. 32.4).
Chronic nasal congestion	OSA occurs twice as often in patients with chronic nasal congestion from any cause.
Diabetes	Patients with diabetes are three times more likely to have OSA than persons who do not have diabetes.
Male sex	Men are twice as likely to have OSA as women.
Age older than 65 years	OSA is two to three times greater in people older than 65 years.
Age under 35 years, and black, Hispanic, or Pacific Islander heritage	Among individuals under the age of 35, the incidence of OSA is greater in blacks, Hispanics, and Pacific Islanders.
Menopause	The risk for OSA is greater after menopause.
Family history of sleep apnea	Individuals who have one or more family members with OSA are also at greater risk for developing it.
Alcohol, sedatives, or tranquilizers	Depressive agents relax the muscles of the upper airway.
Smoking	Smokers are almost three times more likely to develop OSA.

Cheyne-Stokes breathing pattern (see Table 2.4), medical conditions such as congestive heart failure, or high-altitude periodic breathing. Patients with hyperventilation-related CSA develop alternating cycles of apnea—or hypopneas—with hyperpnea (i.e., increased rate and depth of breathing) during sleep. As a result, this condition produces a sequence of abnormal respiratory events, including periods of ventilatory overshoot, hypocapnia, central apnea, hypercapnia, and recurrent hyperpnea. Carbon dioxide sensing is fundamental to this process as opposed to hyopventilatory CSA. This group does not have an elevated baseline carbon dioxide.

Hypoventilation-related CSA is usually a secondary problem related to an underlying condition, such as a central nervous system disease, central nervous system–suppressing drugs or substances (e.g., alcohol, acute use of opiates, barbiturates, benzodiazepines, and various tranquilizers), neuromuscular disease (e.g., Guillain-Barré syndrome or myasthenia gravis), or severe disorders of pulmonary mechanics (e.g., chronic obstructive pulmonary disease [COPD]). During sleep, the patient no longer has the wakefulness stimulus to breathe and, as a result, alveolar hypoventilation and central apnea occur. The patient's breathing is restored during arousal from sleep, but again decreases when sleep resumes, resulting in cyclic periods of normal ventilation, hypoventilation, and apnea. The choice of therapy is based on whether the patient's central apneas are hyperventilation- or hypoventilation-related (see Management of Sleep Apnea, page 470).

Mixed Apnea

Mixed apnea is a combination of OSA and CSA. These episodes are *events* and not a condition. It usually *begins* as central apnea followed by the onset of ventilatory effort without air flow (obstructive apnea). Clinically, patients with predominantly mixed apnea are classified (and treated) as having OSA. Fig. 32.3 illustrates the patterns of air flow, respiratory effort (reflected in this illustration through the esophageal pressure tracing), and arterial oxygen saturation in central, obstructive, and mixed apneas. Respiratory effort is classically measured from "effort detections" around the thorax and/or abdomen. *It is essential that the respiratory therapist recognize the differences among these three entities.*

Sleep-Related Hypoventilation and Hypoxemia Syndromes

Sleep-related hypoventilation and hypoxemia syndromes (SRHHSs) include a broad range of sleep disorders. Some are quite common, such as obesity hypoventilation syndrome (also known as *Pickwickian syndrome*) or coexisting with COPD, the **overlap syndrome**. Others are rather rare, such as congenital central hypoventilation syndrome and neuromuscular and chest wall disorders. However, all share the characteristic of abnormal gas exchange that worsens or may be present only during sleep or sedation. Such abnormalities are usually caused by hypoventilation and result in hypercapnia and hypoxemia. Pulmonary disorders, such as chronic bronchitis or emphysema, are not considered "stand-alone" sleep-related breathing disorders. However, they are known to cause hypoventilation—and hypercapnia and hypoxemia—during sleep. In these cases, the diagnosis of sleep-related hypoventilation or hypoxemia should be considered. Unfortunately, the diagnosis of the overlap syndrome is often missed in critically ill, hospitalized patients.

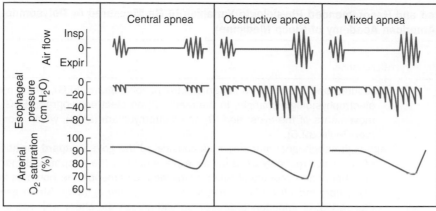

FIGURE 32.3 Patterns of air flow, respiratory efforts (reflected through the esophageal pressure), and arterial oxygen saturation produced by central, obstructive, and mixed apneas.

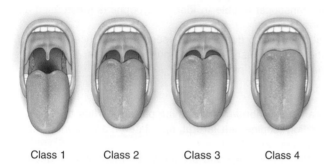

| Class 1 | Class 2 | Class 3 | Class 4 |

FIGURE 32.4 Mallampati classification. Class 1: Soft palate, fauces, uvula, pillars are easily seen. Class 2: Soft palate, fauces, portion of uvula are seen. Class 3: Soft palate, only the base of uvula are seen. Class 4: Only the hard palate is seen.

Diagnosis of Obstructive Sleep Apnea

The diagnosis of OSA begins with a comprehensive sleep evaluation, which includes a history from the patient and/or the patient's bed partner, especially noting the presence of snoring, sleep fragmentation, periods of apnea during sleep, nonrefreshing sleep, and persistent daytime sleepiness. The **Epworth Sleepiness Scale** is routinely used as a validated measure of daytime sleepiness. Sleepiness must be differentiated from fatigue, which can be semiquantitated with the use of the **Fatigue Severity Scale (FSS)** or the **Visual Analogue Fatigue Scale (VAFS)**. This is followed by a careful examination of the upper airway and perhaps by pulmonary function studies (especially by analysis of the flow-volume loop) to determine whether upper airway obstruction is present. Abnormalities in the posterior pharynx include a large uvula, enlarged tonsils, a long soft palate, redundant lateral pharyngeal walls, macroglossia (enlarged tongue), and the presence of an overbite of the upper teeth with a posterior placement of the mandible. The **Mallampati classification** score is frequently used in physician notes to describe abnormalities of the soft palate and uvula (Fig. 32.4).

The patient's blood may be evaluated for the presence of polycythemia, reduced thyroid function, and bicarbonate retention. Arterial blood gas (ABG) values may be obtained to determine resting, wakeful oxygenation, and acid-base status.

When possible, a carboxyhemoglobin level should be obtained. It should be noted that the pulse oximeter used routinely in polysomnography assumes that the patient has normal hemoglobin, PaO_2, and SpO_2 relationships. If carboxyhemoglobin is present, it should be subtracted from the pulse oximeter reading. For example, if the pulse oximeter gives an SpO_2 of 90% and the patient has 7% carboxyhemoglobin, the true **COHb-corrected oximetry oxygen saturation** would be 83% (90% − 7% = 83%). A chest x-ray film, electrocardiogram (ECG), and echocardiogram are helpful in evaluating the presence of **pulmonary hypertension**, the state of right and left ventricular compensation, cardiac arrhythmias, and the presence of any other cardiopulmonary disease.

Finally, in patients suspected of having sleep apnea, the diagnosis and type of sleep apnea are confirmed by either polysomnography or in-home portable monitoring

These diagnostic methods are discussed in more detail below.

Polysomnography

Polysomnography (PSG) is a specialized sleep test that monitors and records a number of physiologic parameters that occur during sleep. The test result is called a **polysomnogram** (which is also abbreviated PSG). The PSG may be administered as either a full-night, attended, in-laboratory polysomnograph or a split-night, attended, in-laboratory polysomnograph. The *full-night, attended, in-laboratory PSG* is considered the gold-standard diagnostic test for OSA. It is performed on selected patients overnight in a sleep laboratory with a technologist (i.e., SDS) in attendance.

In a *split-night, attended, in-laboratory PSG*, the diagnosis of OSA is established during the first portion of the study, followed by a form of positive airway pressure (CPAP, BPAP, VPAP) treatment called a *CPAP (or BPAP or VPAP) titration polysomnogram*. The positive airway pressure is applied to prevent upper airway obstruction or central apneas during sleep for the remaining time. This test is both diagnostic and therapeutic. Because of the perceived cost-effectiveness, there is a growing trend to perform split-night studies if the patient's total sleep time allows.

Table 32.4 provides the physiologic variables that are *required*, and recommended, by the AASM during a PSG. Table 32.5 illustrates the stages of sleep recorded during a

TABLE 32.4 Required and Recommended Physiologic Variables to Be Measured by Polysomnography (According to the American Academy of Sleep Medicine)

Required Physiologic Variable	Description
Sleep stages	Measured and recorded via (1) an electroencephalogram (EEG), which measures the electrophysiologic changes in the brain; (2) an electrooculogram (EOG), which records the movements of the eyes; and (3) an electromyogram (EMG), which monitors muscle activity (see Table 32.5).
Respiratory efforts	Although esophageal manometry is considered the gold standard for assessing respiratory effort, it not routinely used because placement of the esophageal manometer is invasive. The American Academy of Sleep Medicine recommends the noninvasive method of *respiratory inductive plethysmography* and *electromyography*. Strain gauges, piezo electrodes, or impedance devices spread across the chest wall and abdomen are also acceptable options.
Air flow	Measured via nasal prongs connected to a pressure transducer that detects inspiratory flow. Because the pressure transducer is unable to sense air flow through the mouth, a thermistor is added to detect air flow at the mouth by sensing alterations in heat exchange. Thus the nasal pressure transducer is able to identify hypopneas (decreased air flow), and the thermistor can diagnose apneas.
Snoring	Measured via a microphone placed at the neck to detect the presence or absence of snoring.
Pulse oximetry (SpO₂)	Measures the oxyhemoglobin saturation continuously during the polysomnogram.
Electrocardiogram	Detects arrhythmias during sleep. Lead II alone is preferred.

Recommended Physiologic Variable

Body position	In some patients, the body position can cause abnormal breathing patterns. Thus the monitoring of the patient's body position (supine, left lateral, right lateral, and prone) with a position sensor and/or video monitor may be helpful.
Limb movements	An electromyogram of the anterior tibialis of both legs and arms may be monitored to detect leg movements. Used to diagnose periodic limb movement of sleep (PLMS)

TABLE 32.5 Stages of Sleep and Electroencephalogram Waveforms

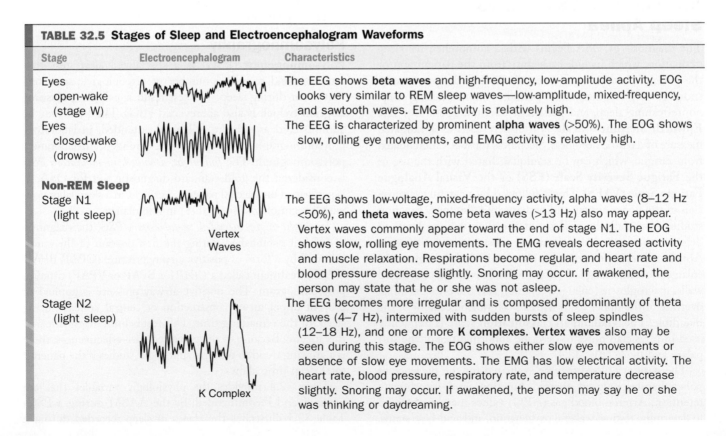

Stage	Electroencephalogram	Characteristics
Eyes open-wake (stage W)		The EEG shows **beta waves** and high-frequency, low-amplitude activity. EOG looks very similar to REM sleep waves—low-amplitude, mixed-frequency, and sawtooth waves. EMG activity is relatively high.
Eyes closed-wake (drowsy)		The EEG is characterized by prominent **alpha waves** (>50%). The EOG shows slow, rolling eye movements, and EMG activity is relatively high.
Non-REM Sleep		
Stage N1 (light sleep)	Vertex Waves	The EEG shows low-voltage, mixed-frequency activity, alpha waves (8–12 Hz <50%), and **theta waves**. Some beta waves (>13 Hz) also may appear. Vertex waves commonly appear toward the end of stage N1. The EOG shows slow, rolling eye movements. The EMG reveals decreased activity and muscle relaxation. Respirations become regular, and heart rate and blood pressure decrease slightly. Snoring may occur. If awakened, the person may state that he or she was not asleep.
Stage N2 (light sleep)	K Complex	The EEG becomes more irregular and is composed predominantly of theta waves (4–7 Hz), intermixed with sudden bursts of sleep spindles (12–18 Hz), and one or more **K complexes**. **Vertex waves** also may be seen during this stage. The EOG shows either slow eye movements or absence of slow eye movements. The EMG has low electrical activity. The heart rate, blood pressure, respiratory rate, and temperature decrease slightly. Snoring may occur. If awakened, the person may say he or she was thinking or daydreaming.

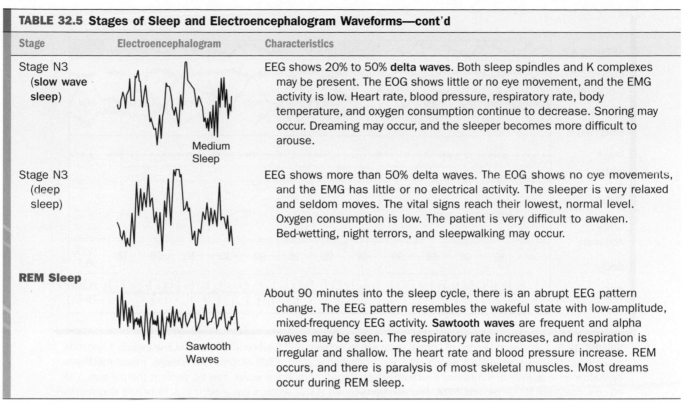

TABLE 32.5 Stages of Sleep and Electroencephalogram Waveforms—cont'd

Stage	Electroencephalogram	Characteristics
Stage N3 (slow wave sleep)	*Medium Sleep*	EEG shows 20% to 50% **delta waves**. Both sleep spindles and K complexes may be present. The EOG shows little or no eye movement, and the EMG activity is low. Heart rate, blood pressure, respiratory rate, body temperature, and oxygen consumption continue to decrease. Snoring may occur. Dreaming may occur, and the sleeper becomes more difficult to arouse.
Stage N3 (deep sleep)		EEG shows more than 50% delta waves. The EOG shows no eye movements, and the EMG has little or no electrical activity. The sleeper is very relaxed and seldom moves. The vital signs reach their lowest, normal level. Oxygen consumption is low. The patient is very difficult to awaken. Bed-wetting, night terrors, and sleepwalking may occur.
REM Sleep	*Sawtooth Waves*	About 90 minutes into the sleep cycle, there is an abrupt EEG pattern change. The EEG pattern resembles the wakeful state with low-amplitude, mixed-frequency EEG activity. **Sawtooth waves** are frequent and alpha waves may be seen. The respiratory rate increases, and respiration is irregular and shallow. The heart rate and blood pressure increase. REM occurs, and there is paralysis of most skeletal muscles. Most dreams occur during REM sleep.

EEG, Electroencephalogram; *EMG,* electromyelogram; *EOG,* electrooculogram; *REM,* rapid eye movement.

BOX 32.3 Diagnostic Criteria for Obstructive Sleep Apnea

During a polysomnogram, obstructive sleep apnea is confirmed when either of the following two conditions exists:
- Fifteen or more apneas, hypopneas, or respiratory effort–related arousals (RERAs) per hour of sleep (i.e., the apnea-hypopnea index [AHI] or respiratory disturbance index [RDI] greater than 15 events per hour) in an asymptomatic patient. More than 75% of the apneas and hypopneas must be obstructive.
- Five or more apneas, hypopneas, or RERAs per hour of sleep (i.e., the AHI or RDI is more than five events per hour) in patients with symptoms (e.g., sleepiness, fatigue, and inattention) or signs of disturbed sleep (e.g., snoring, restless sleep, and respiratory pauses). More than 75% of the apneas and hypopneas must be obstructive.

PSG. Each sleep stage is associated with characteristic **electroencephalogram (EEG), electrooculogram (EOG), electromyogram (EMG)**, behavioral, and breathing patterns. Fig. 32.5 provides a representative period of a sleep study PSG (called an **epoch**) of REM sleep. Box 32.3 shows the diagnostic criteria for OSA. Box 32.4 provides the criteria for mild, moderate, and severe OSA.

Diagnosis of Central Sleep Apnea

CSA is diagnosed when the majority of the respiratory events are central apnea or hypopneas. On the PSG, there is an absence of nasal or oral air flow *and* thoracoabdominal

movements. Patients diagnosed with CSA are evaluated carefully for the presence of cardiac disease and lesions involving the cerebral cortex and the brain stem. Atrial fibrillation is also associated with CSA. The treatment for CSA depends on its specific cause.

In-Home, Unattended, Portable Monitoring

The AASM endorses *in-home, unattended, portable monitoring*— commonly called a **home sleep test (HST)**—as a reasonable cost-effective alternative for patients who have a high likelihood of either moderate or severe OSA. According to their guidelines, an HST for the diagnosis of OSA should be performed only in conjunction with a comprehensive clinical sleep evaluation supervised by a practitioner with board certification in sleep medicine or eligible for the sleep medicine certification examination. Box 32.5 reviews the advantages and disadvantages of in-home, unattended, portable monitoring.

Over the past several years, the effectiveness of the in-laboratory PSG versus the HST has stimulated much debate. Some have argued that many of the advantages of HST—such as that it can be performed in the comfort of the patient's home, it can diagnose moderate or severe OSA, and it is more cost-effective—justify its use. Others counter that the quality of the HST often can be compromised, resulting in erroneous, misleading, or completely missed diagnostic information.

For example, in some cases the HST monitors consist of electrodes that are actually placed on the patient in the sleep laboratory by a polysomnographic technician, and then the patient is sent home; in other cases, the electrodes are shipped to the patient's home, with instructions on how to attach them to the body, a process that often can be problematic. In

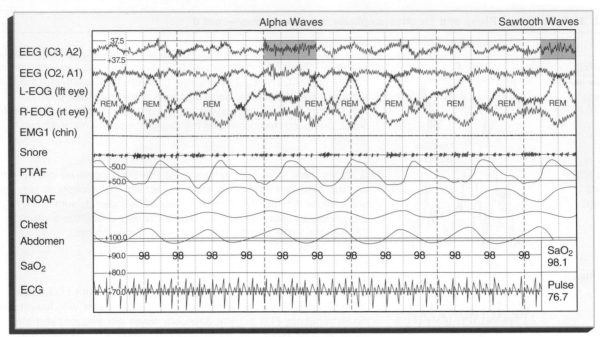

FIGURE 32.5 A 30-second epoch of normal rapid eye movement (REM) sleep (each vertical line equals 1 second), resembling the eyes open-wake epoch. The electroencephalogram (EEG) records low-voltage, mixed electroencephalographic activity and frequent sawtooth waves (brown bar). Alpha waves may be present (purple bar). The electrooculogram (EOG) records REM. The electromyogram (EMG) records low electrical activity and documents a temporary paralysis of most of the skeletal muscles (e.g., arms, legs). The breathing rate increases and decreases irregularly. During REM sleep, the heart rate becomes variable, with episodes of increased and decreased rates. Snoring may or may not be present. REM sleep is not as restorative as non-REM sleep. REM is also known as *paradoxical sleep*. Most dreams occur during REM sleep. *ECG,* Electrocardiograph; *PTAF,* pneumotachograph air flow; *TNOAF,* thermistor nasal/oral air flow; *SaO2,* Oximetry.

BOX 32.4 Diagnostic Criteria for Mild, Moderate, and Severe Obstructive Sleep Apnea

- *Mild obstructive sleep apnea (OSA)* is defined as an AHI between 5 and 15 respiratory events per hour of sleep. These patients are often asymptomatic or report occasional wake time sleepiness during quiet, nonstimulating periods. Such daytime sleepiness usually does not impair daily life activities.

- *Moderate OSA* is defined as an AHI between 15 and 30 respiratory events per hour of sleep. The patient is usually aware of daytime sleepiness and frequently feels the need to take a nap throughout the day. These patients are able to perform their daily activities but usually at a reduced level. Job malperformance is noted. These patients have an increased probability of having motor vehicle violations and accidents. Systemic hypertension may exist.

- *Severe OSA** is defined as an AHI of more than 30 respiratory events per hour of sleep and/or an SpO_2 below 90% for more than 20% of the total sleep time. These patients have significant daytime sleepiness that interferes with their daily activities. They often fall asleep during the day—commonly in the sitting position—and are at a high risk for accidental injury related to sleepiness. In addition, because of the chronic hypoxemia associated with severe OSA, the patient's condition is often further compromised by cardiopulmonary failure, pulmonary hypertension, cardiac arrhythmias, nocturnal angina, polycythemia, and/or cor pulmonale.

*It is not uncommon for patients to have 100 to 150 episodes of apnea and hypopnea per hour of sleep during a polysomnographic sleep study. Transient nocturnal SpO_2 desaturations to levels less than 30% are occasionally seen in the polysomnograms of individuals with severe sleep apnea. Fortunately, these episodes are self-limited when the patient wakens at the end of the apnea. Apneas may last for longer than 120 seconds.

---

addition, the standard HST records only nasal air flow, pulse rate, chest or abdominal effort, and oximetry. Snoring noise is not routinely recorded by most systems. Because of these limitations, there are many significant sleep disorders that can be easily missed. Box 32.6 lists sleep disorders not readily diagnosed with HST devices.

Another significant limitation of HST devices is that an EEG is not recorded—thus sleep staging and scoring are not possible. The HST surrogate for *total sleep time (TST)* is the *total recording time (TRT)*. Thus in the HST the SDS must calculate a **respiratory disturbance index (RDI)**[4] instead of an **apnea-hypopnea index (AHI)**, as follows:

---

[4]The AASM prefers the term **respiratory effort index (REI)** in place of RDI.

BOX 32.5 In-Home Portable Monitoring

Advantages

- It can be done in the patient's home and/or in areas without ready access to sleep centers
- Convenience
- Patient acceptance
- Easily can be performed over multiple nights
- Decreased cost

Disadvantages

- Absence of a trained technologist to correct and clarify recording artifacts and to make ongoing equipment adjustments

- Inability to intervene in medically unstable patients
- Possible data loss or distortion
- The potential for interpretation errors resulting from limited data
- Inability to perform subsequent multiple sleep latency testing according to standard protocol
- Varied sensor technology
- No published standards for scoring or interpretation

Physiologic Measurement Limitations of the Portable Monitor Compared With Polysomnogram (PSG)

PSG (type I) (in-laboratory studies) has:

- Electroencephalogram, measures arousals and true sleep
- Electrooculogram
- Electromyogram (chin and limbs)
- Electrocardiogram—rate, rhythm, and morphology
- Respiratory effort at thorax and abdomen
- Air flow from nasal cannula thermistor or CO_2 detector
- Pulse oximetry
- Addition channels for continuous positive airway pressure/bilevel positive airway pressure levels, CO_2, etc.

Portable monitoring (home sleep test) (type III) has:

- Respiratory movement
- Air flow (and snoring)
- Electrocardiogram (rate only)
- Pulse oximetry

BOX 32.6 Sleep Disorders That Cannot Be Diagnosed With Home (Portable) Sleep Testing Devices

- Type of sleep apnea (obstructive versus central conditions, versus mixed events)
- Insomnia (approximately 30% to 35% of patients with insomnia may need polysomnogram)
- Nocturnal seizure disorders
- Narcolepsy/hypersomnia
- Periodic limb movement disorder
- Nocturnal cardiac arrhythmias (home sleep test only measures heart rate)
- Rapid eye movement (REM) and position-dependent sleep apnea syndrome
- REM behavior disorder
- Other parasomnias, such as sleep walking, sleep talking, and **confusional arousals**

For the in-laboratory sleep study, the calculation is:

$$AHI = \frac{Number\ of\ apneas\ and\ hypopneas}{TST\ (hours)}$$

Example: If there are 100 apneas and hypopneas in a measured total sleep time of 8.0 hours, the AHI would be

12.5 per hour ($100 \div 8.0 = 12.5$), whereas in the HST, the calculation is:

$$RDI = \frac{Number\ of\ apneas\ and\ hypopneas}{TST\ (hours)}$$

A true measure of sleep time is not available with the HST. The patient may sleep for a very short time but be recorded for a long time. As a result, the patient's RDI can often be falsely low. Thus the HST can lead to miscalculations in estimating the severity of the patient's sleep-disordered breathing problems. It should not be used in patients with comorbidities such as cardiopulmonary disease, seizure disorders, etc.[5]

---

[5]The HST device was originally proposed for use in remote, medically underserved areas and as a screening device for hospitalized, critically ill patients, such as those with COPD and congestive heart failure. Much of the insurance industry however, has seized on HST as the new gold standard for sleep diagnostic testing, which has paradoxically reduced access to sleep medicine services in many locations because, in short, the insurance industry has made "prior authorization" for PSGs extremely time-consuming and tedious. Despite all of this, HST has indeed become the "preferred" diagnostic sleep study—at least by the insurance industry—in patients with a high probability of moderate or severe OSA.

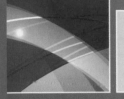

OVERVIEW of the Cardiopulmonary Clinical Manifestations Associated With Sleep Apnea

CLINICAL DATA OBTAINED AT THE PATIENT'S BEDSIDE

The Physical Examination (see also Box 32.2 and Table 32.3)

Apnea or Hypopnea

Cyanosis

CLINICAL DATA OBTAINED FROM LABORATORY TESTS AND SPECIAL PROCEDURES

Pulmonary Function Test Findings

The following findings are expected in patients who are obese or who have congestive heart failure—that is, restrictive pathophysiology.

LUNG VOLUME AND CAPACITY FINDINGS

V_T	IRV	ERV[1]	RV
N or ↓	↓	↓	↓

VC	IC	FRC	TLC	RV/TLC ratio
↓	↓	↓	↓	N

Obviously, pulmonary function cannot easily be studied during sleep. However, patients with OSA may demonstrate a sawtooth pattern on maximal inspiratory and expiratory flow-volume loops (Fig. 32.6). Also characteristic of OSA is a ratio of expiratory-to-inspiratory flow rates at 50% of the vital capacity ($FEF_{50\%}/FIF_{50\%}$) that exceeds 1.0 in the absence of obstructive pulmonary disease.

In addition, because the muscle tone of the intercostal muscles is low during periods of rapid eye movement (REM)-related apneas, the large swings in intrapleural pressure generated by the diaphragm often cause a magnified paradoxical motion of the rib cage—that is, during inspiration the tissues between the ribs move inward, and during expiration they bulge outward. This paradoxical motion of the rib cage may cause the vital capacity (VC), expiratory reserve volume (ERV), functional residual capacity (FRC), and total lung capacity (TLC) to decrease further—that is, toward restrictive pulmonary function pathophysiology as described earlier. Along with obesity-related atelectasis, this further contributes to the nocturnal hypoxemia seen in patients with sleep apnea syndrome.

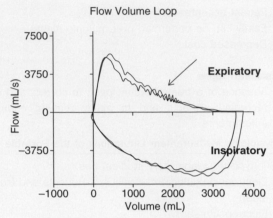

Flow Volume Loop

FIGURE 32.6 Sawtooth pattern. The expiratory limb of the flow volume loop shows fluttering in the midflow portion. This vibratory motion (fluttering) of the soft palate is known as the *sawtooth* pattern (see red arrow). The sawtooth pattern may be seen during obstructive sleep apnea (OSA). The arrow highlights the airway fluttering during exhalation. Note similar but less pronounced inspiratory fluttering. Contemporary pulmonary function testing equipment tends to "smooth" the expiratory fluttering that is characteristic of the phenomenon. The absence of sawtoothing does not exclude sleep apnea and neither does its presence rule it in; if present, sawtoothing should prompt a clinician to consider OSA and consider further testing. (From Charles Atwood, MD, VA Pittsburgh Healthcare System and University of Pittsburgh Medical Center, Pittsburg, PA. https://www.thoracic.org/professionals/clinical-resources/sleep/sleep-fragments/fluttering-on-a-flow-volume-loop.php.)

Arterial Blood Gases

SEVERE OBSTRUCTIVE SLEEP APNEA

Chronic Ventilatory Failure With Hypoxemia[2] (Compensated Respiratory Acidosis)

pH	$PaCO_2$	HCO_3^-	PaO_2	SaO_2 or SpO_2
N	↑	↑	↓	↓
		(significantly)		

Acute Ventilatory Changes Superimposed on Chronic Ventilatory Failure[3]

Because acute ventilatory changes are frequently seen in patients with chronic ventilatory failure, the respiratory therapist must be familiar with—and alert for—the following dangerous ABG findings:

- Acute alveolar hyperventilation superimposed on chronic ventilatory failure, which should further alert the respiratory therapist to record the following important ABG assessment: possible *impending acute ventilatory failure*
- Acute ventilatory failure (acute hypoventilation) superimposed on chronic ventilatory failure

---

[1]A decreased ERV is the hallmark of centripetal obesity.

[2]See Table 5.6 and related discussion for the pH, $PaCO_2$, and changes associated with chronic ventilatory failure.

[3]See Table 5.7, Table 5.8, and Table 5.9 and related discussion for the pH, $PaCO_2$, and changes associated with acute ventilatory changes superimposed on chronic ventilatory failure.

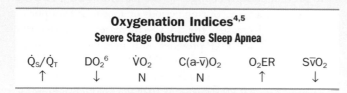

Oxygenation Indices[4,5]
Severe Stage Obstructive Sleep Apnea

$\dot{Q}_S/\dot{Q}_T$	DO_2[6]	$\dot{V}O_2$	$C(a-\bar{v})O_2$	O_2ER	$S\bar{v}O_2$
↑	↓	N	N	↑	↓

Hemodynamic Indices[7]
Severe Obstructive Sleep Apnea (With Cor Pulmonale)

CVP	RAP	$\overline{PA}$	PCWP	CO	SV
↑	↑	↑	N or ↓	N or ↑	N or ↓

SVI	CI	RVSWI	LVSWI	PVR	SVR
↓	↓	↑	↑	↑	↑

Brady-Tachy Syndrome

The presence of upper airway obstruction during apneic episodes often is accompanied by bradycardia and temporary reduction in cardiac output. This is unusual because hypoxemia usually causes tachycardia. In sleep apnea, oxygen transport ($\dot{Q}_T \times CaO_2 \times 10$) falls and results in electrocardiographic **brady-tachy syndrome** episodes and swings in heart rate and blood pressure secondary to surges of adrenaline in an attempt to compensate for tissue hypoxia.

The carotid body peripheral chemoreceptors are probably responsible for this response—that is, when ventilation is kept constant or is absent (e.g., during an apneic episode), hypoxic stimulation of the carotid body peripheral chemoreceptors slows the cardiac rate. Therefore it follows that when the lungs are unable to expand (e.g., during periods of obstructive apnea), the depressive effect of the carotid bodies on the heart rate predominates. The increased heart rate noted when ventilation resumes is activated by the excitation of the pulmonary stretch receptors.

Although changes in cardiac output during periods of apnea have been difficult to study, several studies have reported a reduction in cardiac output (about 30%) during periods of apnea, followed by an increase (10% to 15% above controls)

---

[4]$C(a-\bar{v})O_2$, Arterial-venous oxygen difference; DO_2, total oxygen delivery; O_2ER, oxygen extraction ratio; $\dot{Q}_S/\dot{Q}_T$, pulmonary shunt fraction; $S\bar{v}O_2$, mixed venous oxygen saturation; $\dot{V}O_2$, oxygen consumption.

[5]The abnormal oxygenation indices may develop as a result of hypoventilation and/or atelectasis.

[6]The DO_2 may be normal in patients who have compensated to the decreased oxygenation status with (1) an increased cardiac output, (2) an increased hemoglobin level, or (3) a combination of both. When the DO_2 is normal, the O_2ER is usually normal.

[7]CO, Cardiac output; CI, cardiac index; CVP, central venous pressure; $LVSWI$, left ventricular stroke work index; $\overline{PA}$, mean pulmonary artery pressure; $PCWP$, pulmonary capillary wedge pressure; PVR, pulmonary vascular resistance; RAP, right atrial pressure; $RVSWI$, right ventricular stroke work index; SV, stroke volume; SVI, stroke volume index; SVR, systemic vascular resistance.

after termination of apnea. *Both pulmonary and systemic arterial blood pressures increase in response to the nocturnal oxygen desaturation that develops during periods of sleep apnea.* The magnitude of the *pulmonary hypertension* is related to the severity of the alveolar hypoxia and hypercapnic acidosis. Repetition of these transient episodes of pulmonary hypertension many times a night every night for years may contribute to the development of the right ventricular hypertrophy, cor pulmonale, and eventual cardiac decompensation seen in such patients.

Episodic systemic vasoconstriction secondary to sympathetic adrenergic neural activity is thought to be responsible for the *elevation in systemic blood pressure* that is commonly seen during apneas. In normal individuals, blood pressures drop during sleep, a phenomenon known as blood pressure dipping. This often fails to occur in patients with sleep apnea, who are termed blood pressure nondippers. Sleep apnea is now recognized as one of the most frequent and correctable causes of systemic hypertension.

RADIOLOGIC FINDINGS
Chest Radiograph
- Often normal
- Right- or left-sided heart failure

Because of the pulmonary hypertension and polycythemia associated with persistent periods of apnea, right- and/or left-sided heart failure may develop. This condition may be identified as an enlargement of the heart on a chest radiograph or an echocardiogram and may help in diagnosis.

CARDIAC ARRHYTHMIAS
- Brady-tachy syndrome
- Sinus arrhythmia
- Sinus bradycardia
- Sinus pauses
- Atrioventricular block (second-degree)
- Premature ventricular contractions
- Supraventricular tachycardia
- Ventricular tachycardia
- **Atrial fibrillation**
- Sick sinus syndrome

In severe cases of sleep apnea, sudden arrhythmia-related death is always possible. Periods of apnea commonly are associated with sinus arrhythmia, sinus bradycardia, and sinus pauses (longer than 2 seconds). The extent of sinus bradycardia is directly related to the severity of the oxygen desaturation. Obstructive apneas usually are associated with the greatest degrees of cardiac slowing. To a lesser extent, atrioventricular heart block (second-degree), premature ventricular contractions, and ventricular tachycardia are also seen. Apnea-related ventricular tachycardia is viewed as a life-threatening event. Atrial fibrillation is extremely common in central sleep apnea.

General Management of Obstructive Sleep Apnea

Once the diagnosis of OSA is confirmed and its severity determined, the patient should be educated about the risk factors, natural history, and long-term consequences of OSA. Importantly, the patient should be warned about the potential danger and consequences of driving or operating other equipment or tools while sleepy. The types of therapy for OSA include the following.

Behavior Modification

Behavior modification is indicated for all patients who have OSA and modifiable risk factors. Helpful behavior modification areas include weight loss (if overweight or obese), exercise, changing sleep position (e.g., OSA often worsens in the supine position), abstaining from alcohol, and avoidance of certain medications when possible (e.g., medications that inhibit the central nervous system, such as benzodiazepines, benzodiazepine receptor agonists, and barbiturates).

Positive Airway Pressure

Positive airway pressure therapy is considered the first-line therapy for OSA. As discussed earlier, the cause of many cases of OSA is related to an anatomic malconfiguration of the pharynx and the decreased muscle tone that normally develops in the pharynx during REM sleep. When the patient with OSA inhales, the pharyngeal muscles (and surrounding tissues) are sucked inward as a result of the negative airway pressure generated by the contracting diaphragm. Positive airway pressure is useful in preventing the collapse of the hypotonic and obstructed airway and is the standard treatment for most cases of OSA. Positive airway pressure can be delivered as **continuous positive airway pressure (CPAP), bilevel positive airway pressure (BPAP), autotitrating positive airway pressure (APAP),** or **positive end-expiratory pressure (PEEP)**:

CPAP: The most common and arguably the most effective treatment for OSA. A CPAP device provides positive airway pressure at a level that remains constant throughout the ventilatory cycle in a spontaneously breathing patient (Fig. 32.7). Fig. 32.8 provides a useful protocol algorithm to help improve CPAP adherence in patients with sleep apnea/hypopnea syndrome.[6]

BPAP[7]: With a backup respiratory rate, is often very beneficial in patients with OSA who have frequent apneas and hypopneas during sleep. The backup respiratory rate works to prevent sudden changes in the patient's PaO_2, $PaCO_2$, and pH values (i.e., during periods of apneas or hypopneas, the PaO_2 decreases, the PCO_2 increases, and the pH decreases). The BPAP provides both an adjustable inspiratory positive airway pressure (IPAP) setting and an adjustable expiratory positive pressure airway pressure (EPAP) setting. The EPAP portion of BPAP actually functions as a PEEP. BPAP is particularly effective in obese OSA patients who demonstrate CO_2 retention.

APAP (also called autoPAP): Increases or decreases the level of positive airway pressure in response to a change in air flow, a change in circuit pressure, or a vibratory snore. Although APAP has not proved to be more effective than CPAP, patients may prefer it more. The use of APAP is indicated while a formal polysomnographic diagnosis of the precise type of sleep apnea is being made and thus is of use in hospitalized, not yet fully diagnosed, patients with sleep apnea or in the context of a "home sleep testing model."

PEEP: Defined as positive pressure at the end of expiration during either spontaneous breathing or mechanical ventilation. In

---

[6]It is estimated that between 30% and 80% of patients with sleep apnea are nonadherent to CPAP therapy, when nonadherence is defined as a mean of 4 hours or less of use per night. The mean duration of use is only 3 hours per night—on those nights when it is used—among patients who are nonadherent. The AASM recommends 5 hours per night, every night, for optimal **CPAP compliance/adherence**. Even one night without CPAP can diminish the benefits of therapy, which includes the number of apneas and hypopneas and daytime mood and concentration. In short, the patient's use of the CPAP device is both therapeutically critical and potentially problematic. Today, many CPAP devices have downloadable compliance features that provide periodic updates of patient compliance. Objective documentation of the patient's CPAP compliance is increasingly being required by third-party insurance agencies if payment for the CPAP device is to be made. New, evidence-based definitions of compliance and adherence are being evaluated.

[7]BPAP should not be confused with BiPAP, which is the brand name of a single manufacturer and is just one of many devices that can be used for BPAP.

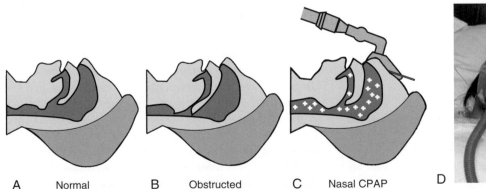

| A   Normal | B   Obstructed | C   Nasal CPAP | D |

FIGURE 32.7 (A) Normal airway. (B) Obstructed nasal airway during sleep. (C) Nasal continuous positive airway pressure (CPAP) generates a positive pressure and holds the airway open during sleep. (D) CPAP set-up in a patient in the sleep center. (Courtesy George G. Burton, MD, Sleep Disorders Center, Kettering Medical Center, Dayton, Ohio.)

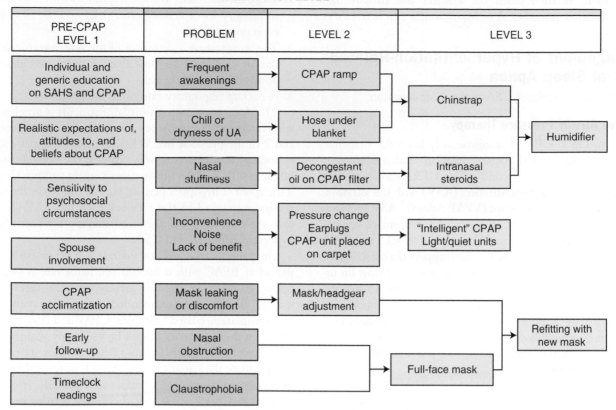

FIGURE 32.8 Protocol algorithm to help improve continuous positive airway pressure adherence. (Modified from Engleman, H. M., Wild, M. R. [2003]. Improving CPAP use by patients with the sleep apnoea/hypopnoea syndrome [SAHS]. *Sleep Medicine Review, 7,* 81.)

most cases, however, the term implies that the patient is also receiving mandatory breaths from a ventilator. When PEEP is used for treating OSA, it can be achieved via a disposable nasal device that permits unimpeded inspiration but provides increased resistance on expiration.

Oral Appliances

Most oral appliances fall under one of the following two categories: a mandibular-repositioning device or a tongue-retaining device. The mandibular-repositioning devices are the most popular. They are designed to reposition the mandible forward and down slightly. The tongue-retaining devices hold the tongue in a more anterior position. Either design works to position the soft tissues of the oropharynx away from the posterior pharyngeal wall. Recent literature has been increasingly favorable toward the use of such appliances in carefully selected, carefully fitted patients.

Surgery

Surgery is most effective in nonobese patients who have OSA because of a severe, surgically correctable, upper airway–obstructing lesion. For example, *tonsillectomy* is a reasonable approach in a patient with OSA caused by tonsillar hypertrophy, particularly in children but occasionally in adults. In patients without a strictly defined anatomic lesion, **uvulopalatopharyngoplasty (UPPP)** is one of the most common surgical procedures used to treat snoring and sleep apnea. The posterior third of the soft palate and the uvula are removed. The pillars of the palatoglossal arch and the palatopharyngeal arch are

tied together, and the tonsils are removed if present. As much excess lateral posterior wall tissue is removed as possible. The success rate of this type of surgery is 30% to 50%. **Laser-assisted uvulopalatoplasty** and **radiofrequency ablation** are less invasive alternatives to UPPP. Other possible surgical procedures for OSA include septoplasty, rhinoplasty, nasal turbinate reduction, nasal polypectomy, palatal advancement pharyngoplasty, adenoidectomy, palatal implants, tongue reduction (partial glossectomy, lingual tonsillectomy), genioglossus advancement, and maxillomandibular advancement.

Implantable Upper Airway Stimulator

Recently, studies have shown the effectiveness of an **implantable upper airway stimulator** device that stimulates the hypoglossal nerve (XII), which in turn activates the genioglossal muscle (the tongue) to contract and increase the patency of the upper airway. In selected patients who are refractory to CPAP therapy, and in whom complete concentric collapse of the retrolalatal airway can be demonstrated during **drug-induced sleep endoscopy (DISE)**, this technique shows promise.

General Management of Central Sleep Apnea

For all patients diagnosed with CSA, the initial treatment is directed at the conditions that may be causing the sleep apnea (e.g., congestive heart failure, encephalitis, or brain stem neoplasm). If the CSA continues after such therapy, management is then based on whether the patient has hyperventilation-related CSA or hypoventilation-related CSA.

Management of Hyperventilation-Related Central Sleep Apnea

Hyperventilation-related CSA is the most common.

Positive Airway Pressure Therapy

Similar to OSA, CPAP has customarily been the first-line therapy for patients with hyperventilation-related CSA.

Patients who do not respond well to CPAP should receive a trial of **adaptive servoventilation (ASV)** with the **variable positive airway pressure adapt (VPAP Adapt)**.[8] ASV provides ventilator support to treat all forms of CSA, mixed apnea, and periodic breathing (Cheyne-Stokes respiration). The VPAP Adapt responds by increasing pressure support during a central event when the patient's minute ventilation falls below his or her target ventilation (which is 90% of the patient's minute ventilation). To determine the degree of pressure support, the ASV algorithm continuously calculates target ventilation. The algorithm uses the following three factors to achieve synchronization between the needed pressure support and the patient's breathing pattern:

[8]From ResMed Corporation; http://www.resmed.com.

1. The patient's recent average respiratory rate, including the inspiratory-to-expiratory ratio (I:E) and the time of any expiratory pause
2. The instantaneous direction of air flow, magnitude, and rate of change of air flow that are measured at specific points during each breath
3. A backup respiratory rate of 15 breaths/min

The ASV ensures that ventilator support is synchronized with the patient's ventilatory efforts by means of numbers 1 and 2 in the previous list. When the patient experiences an episode of central apnea or hypopnea, the pressure support initially works to reflect the patient's recent pattern. However, if the apnea or hypopnea persists, the ASV increases the backup respiratory rate (3 in the previous list). Fig. 32.9 illustrates this. ASV is often the preferred therapy for patients with hyperventilation-related CSA.

For patients who do not tolerate CPAP or ASV, a trial period of BPAP with a backup ventilator rate is suggested before abandoning positive airway pressure therapy. The use of BPAP is recommended only for patients with hyperventilation-related CSA after CPAP and ASV has failed. BPAP in these patients should be used only with a backup respiratory rate. This is because BPAP, with a set rate, may overventilate the patient during periods of normal breathing or hyperpnea, causing discomfort and arousals. It can even cause more CSA events. ASV should not be used in patients with heart failure who have an ejection fraction below 45%.

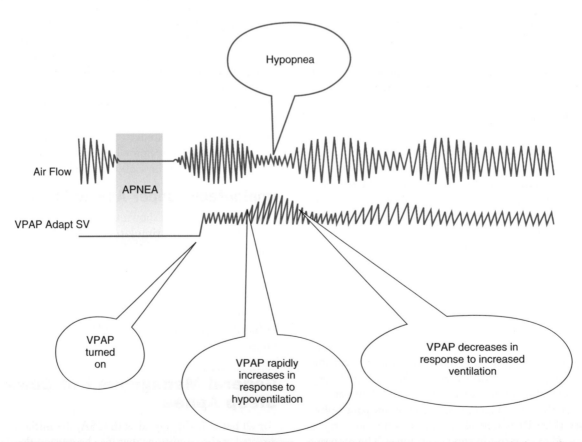

FIGURE 32.9 The variable positive airway pressure (VPAP) adaptive servoventilator responds to apnea by increasing pressure support. Note the progressive dampening of the Cheyne-Stokes cycles with the continued administration of VPAP.

Management of Hypoventilation-Related Central Sleep Apnea

BPAP, with a backup respiratory rate, is the first-line therapy for patients with hypoventilation-related CSA. Most patients with ventilatory failure tolerate BPAP well.

To automate PAP therapy for hypoventilation, VAPS can be used. The VAPS devices will optimize pressure support until a targeted exhaled tidal volume and/or alveolar ventilation is achieved. Because VAPS algorithms augment ventilation for hypoventilation, the devices are appropriate for disorders such as neuromuscular disease or scoliosis. The devices are not appropriate for Cheyne-Stokes respiration.

Other Treatments for Sleep Apnea

Oxygen Therapy

Because of the hypoxemia-related **cardiopulmonary complications of sleep apnea** (arrhythmias and pulmonary hypertension), **nocturnal low-flow oxygen therapy** is sometimes used alone to offset or minimize the oxygen desaturation (see Oxygen Therapy Protocol, Protocol 10.1). The reasoning behind the effectiveness of nasal oxygen therapy is that the airway is continually "flooded" with oxygen, which will be inspired during the nonapneic episodes—in effect, "preoxygenating" the patient in anticipation of the apnea events. Usually, no improvement in sleep fragmentation or hypersomnolence occurs with the use of supplemental oxygen.

All of the positive airway pressure devices listed in the foregoing section generally use room air as the airway-distending gas. Supplemental oxygen can be "bled" into any of them, if device-related manipulations of inspiratory and expiratory pressure and backup rate fail to adequately oxygenate the patient.

Recent literature has called the whole concept of oxygen supplementation into question. At the present time, Medicare will not supply oxygen to patients with OSA unless it can be shown that positive airway pressure therapy alone is insufficient.

Pharmacologic Therapy

In any patient who does not tolerate or benefit from positive airway pressure or supplemental oxygen during sleep, a respiratory stimulant such as acetazolamide or theophylline may be tried in patients with CSA, though the results are extremely variable. The use of other pharmacologic agents in OSA is, at present, experimental.

CASE STUDY Obstructive Sleep Apnea

Admitting History

A 55-year-old man with a history of moderate to severe chronic obstructive pulmonary disease (COPD) had been in the US Marine Corps for more than 25 years when he retired with honors at 46 years of age with the rank of sergeant. He had completed tours in Vietnam, Grenada, and Beirut. His last assignment had been in Iraq and Kuwait during Operation Desert Storm. During his military career he had received several medals, including a Purple Heart for a leg wound he incurred in Vietnam when he pulled a fellow Marine to safety. During his last 3 years in the service, he had been assigned to a desk job, working with new recruits as they progressed through boot camp.

Although retirement was not mandatory, he felt that "it was time." He had gained a great deal of weight over the years, and his ability to meet the physical challenge of being a Marine had become progressively more difficult. In addition, when he was doing paperwork at his office, he had become aware that he was "catnapping" while on the job. He knew that if he had observed a fellow Marine doing the same, he would have been quick to issue a severe reprimand. In view of these developments, he regretfully retired from the service.

For a few years after he retired, he continued to work for the Marines as a volunteer at a local recruitment office. At first he had enjoyed this job a great deal. He often found that his military experiences enhanced his ability to talk in a meaningful way to new recruits. Over the past few years, however, working had become progressively more difficult for him and his attendance had become increasingly sporadic. He was often tardy. He told the other recruitment volunteers that he was always tired and was experiencing severe morning headaches. His co-workers frequently found him irritable and quick to anger.

The man was having trouble at home, too. Several months before the admission under discussion, his wife had begun sleeping in a room vacated by their daughter. His wife said that she no longer could sleep with her husband because of his loud snoring and constant thrashing in bed. At about this time, he became clinically depressed and sexually impotent. Despite much discussion with and encouragement from his wife, he did not seek medical advice until a few hours before the admission under discussion, when he became extremely short of breath.

Physical Examination

On observation in the emergency department (ED), the man appeared to be in severe respiratory distress. He was 5 feet 11 inches tall. He was obese, weighing more than 160 kg (355 lb), and perspiring profusely. His **basal metabolic index (BMI)** (weight [kg]/height [m^2]) was 50. His skin appeared cyanotic, and his neck veins were distended. He had +4 edema of his feet and legs, extending to midcalf. His blood pressure was 164/100 mm Hg, heart rate was 78 beats/min, respiratory rate was 22 breaths/min, and temperature was normal. Although the man was in obvious discomfort, he stated that he was breathing "OK." His wife quickly piped up, "There's that damn Marine coming out again!"

The patient had diminished breath sounds, which were believed to result primarily from his obesity. Palpation of the chest was unremarkable, and percussion was unreliable because of the obesity. A chest radiograph showed cardiomegaly; the lungs appeared unremarkable. To treat the presumed cor pulmonale, the treating physician immediately started the patient on diuretics. His awake ABG values on room air were pH 7.54, $PaCO_2$ 58 mm Hg, HCO_3^- 48 mEq/L, PaO_2 52 mm Hg, and SaO_2 91%.

Because of the patient's history and present clinical manifestations, the ED physician diagnosed OSA and requested a full-night, attended, in-laboratory polysomnographic split study. The physician asked the respiratory therapist to document her assessment.

The following SOAP was charted.

Respiratory Assessment and Plan

S "I'm breathing OK."

O Weight: 160 kg (355 lb); skin: flushed and cyanotic; distended neck veins and edema of feet and legs (4+) to midcalf; vital signs BP 164/100, HR 78, RR 22, T normal; oropharyngeal examination typical for obstructive sleep apnea; diminished breath sounds, likely because of obesity; chest radiograph: cor pulmonale; lungs appear normal; ABGs (on room air) pH 7.54, $PaCO_2$ 58, HCO_3^- 48, PaO_2 52, and SaO_2 91%.

A • Obstructive sleep apnea likely (history, cor pulmonale, ABGs, physical appearance)
  • Acute alveolar hyperventilation superimposed on chronic ventilatory failure with moderate hypoxemia (ABGs and history)
  • Impending ventilatory failure

P Place patient on alarming oximeter, set to alarm at 85%. Initiate Oxygen Therapy Protocol (Venturi oxygen mask at FIO_2 0.24). Monitor and reevaluate (vital signs, ECG, ABGs, and SpO_2 q4h closely); patient is a CO_2 retainer.

Over the Next 72 Hours

A clinical diagnosis of severe OSA was quickly established with a split-night PSG study the next night. Along with the patient's classic history of OSA, the polysomnogram documented more than 325 periods of obstructive apnea or hypopnea during the study night. His apnea-hypopnea index (AHI) was 64. The **CPAP titration polysomnogram** indicated that 12 cm H_2O CPAP was required to effectively treat the apneic syndrome. In addition to the patient's short muscular neck and extreme obesity, an oropharyngeal examination revealed a small mouth and large tongue for his body size. The free margin of the soft palate hung low in the oropharynx, nearly obliterating the view behind it (Mallampati class 3). The uvula was widened (4+) and elongated, and the tonsillar pillars were widened (3+). Air entry through the nares was reduced bilaterally. The patient's hematocrit was 51% and hemoglobin 17 g/dL.

Results of a complete pulmonary function test showed severe restrictive pulmonary disorder. In addition, a sawtooth pattern was seen in the maximal inspiratory and expiratory flow-volume loops. A chest x-ray film obtained on the patient's second day of hospitalization showed reduced heart size and clear lungs. A brisk diuresis was in process. The patient stated that he was breathing much better.

On inspection the patient no longer appeared short of breath. Although he still appeared flushed, he did not look as cyanotic as he had on admission. His neck veins were no longer distended, and the peripheral edema of his legs and feet had improved. His breath sounds were clear but diminished. His ABGs on an FIO_2 of 0.24 were pH 7.36, $PaCO_2$ 82 mm Hg, HCO_3^- 45 mEq/L, PaO_2 66 mm Hg, and SaO_2 92%. The physician again called for a respiratory care evaluation. On the basis of these clinical data, the following SOAP was recorded.

Respiratory Assessment and Plan

S "I'm breathing much better."

O Recent diagnosis: OSA: More than 325 periods of obstructive apnea or hypopnea documented during baseline sleep study (AHI: 64); short muscular neck; narrow upper airway; obesity; Hct 51%; Hb 17 g/dL; pulmonary function tests: severe restrictive disorder; sawtooth pattern on maximal inspiratory and expiratory flow-volume loops; no longer appearing short of breath; cyanotic appearance improved; clear but diminished breath sounds; ABGs (on room air) pH 7.36, $PaCO_2$ 82, HCO_3^- 45, PaO_2 66, SaO_2 92%.

A • Severe OSA confirmed (history, polysomnographic study, ABGs)
  • Chronic ventilatory failure with mild hypoxemia
  • Cor pulmonale improved

P Continue Oxygen Therapy Protocol (via Venturi oxygen at FIO_2 0.24 during the daytime). Start Continuous Positive Airway Pressure (12 cm H_2O via mask) at bedtime. Ensure that patient sleeps in the head-up position and refrains from sleeping on his back. Start process to have CPAP device set up at patient's home. Monitor and reevaluate.

Discussion

Although the diagnosis of OSA is made most frequently in the outpatient setting, it often may be diagnosed in the course of an acute hospitalization. A recent study showed that 78% of more than 1000 patients admitted with acute decompensated heart failure (left ventricular ejection fraction less than 45%) had either OSA or CSA, *and they had never been diagnosed with sleep-disordered breathing.* CSA was an independent predictor of cardiac readmission at 1, 3, and 6 months. In the case under discussion, although the patient was first seen in the ED, it soon became clear that he was ill enough to be admitted and his workup proceeded from there.

In the first assessment the therapist needed to perform and record a more careful examination of the patient's nasopharynx and oropharynx and his chest. The typical upper airway anatomy of OSA was visible and should have been described in more detail—that is, tongue size? Overbite? Tonsillar enlargement? Uvular enlargement? Mallampati classification score? While the patient's polysomnogram and CPAP titration study were in progress, the therapist appropriately ensured the patient's oxygenation (FIO_2 0.24 Venturi oxygen mask) and attempted to prevent alveolar hypoventilation. In as classic a case as this, a **split-night polysomnogram** (half standard PSG, half CPAP titration) was certainly in order.

The patient's neck vein distention, polycythemia, cardiomegaly, and peripheral edema all suggested cor pulmonale. This condition would improve once the patient's overall hypoventilation and oxygenation were treated. Many physicians would go ahead and give the patient a bicarbonate-losing diuretic, watching for metabolic acidosis while this was being done. The therapist (in the first assessment) correctly analyzed the situation as being potentially hazardous and noted impending ventilatory failure, which was a real possibility.

After the second assessment the diagnosis was made. Pulmonary function tests showed upper airway obstruction and a restrictive disorder. Based on the pH value of 7.36, the patient's $PaCO_2$ appeared to be at its normal baseline level. It is not uncommon for patients with severe OSA to have chronic ventilatory failure (compensated respiratory acidosis). The therapist elected to have the patient refrain from sleeping on his back and to sleep in the head-up position instead. In addition, the physician would likely ask for a nutrition consultation at that time because the patient needed to begin a drastic weight-loss program.

At the end of the assessment and treatment period, the patient's condition still was not markedly improved, and he awaited the long-term benefits of CPAP therapy and weight loss. Indeed, the CPAP therapy was eventually helpful. The patient had a 9-kg (20-lb) diuresis during the first week of combined CPAP and diuretic use, and good oxygenation was achieved with 10 cm H_2O CPAP pressure.

A diagnosis of OSA often can complicate other primary respiratory disorders, such as COPD (overlap syndrome), pneumonia, atelectasis, or chest wall deformity. In these settings, care is more complicated and, if anything, should be even more data-driven, with careful examination of all subjective and objective findings.

Patients with OSA have a significant risk for cardiovascular and central nervous system morbidity and mortality (myocardial infarctions, arrhythmias, hypertension, and cerebrovascular accidents). Psychiatric effects such as depression, sleep-related job malperformance, and daytime motor vehicle accidents also are seen. Current evidence suggests that such patients need not experience these effects if the sleep disorder–related breathing problems are diagnosed early and treated effectively. Most good respiratory care departments now have **sleep apnea screening programs** in place for all hospitalized patients. Compliance with CPAP therapy is important but difficult to achieve. Close clinical monitoring is important if good therapeutic outcomes are to be achieved consistently.

SELF-ASSESSMENT QUESTIONS

1. What is(are) another name(s) for non–rapid eye movement (non-REM) sleep?
   1. Slow-wave sleep
   2. Active sleep
   3. Dreaming sleep
   4. Quiet sleep
      a. 1 only
      b. 3 only
      c. 4 only
      d. 1 and 4 only

2. During non-REM sleep, ventilation becomes slow and regular during which stage?
   a. Eyes open wake
   b. Stage N1
   c. Stage N2
   d. Stage N3

3. Moderate sleep apnea is said to be present when the apnea-hypopnea index (AHI) is:
   a. 3 to 5 episodes/hour
   b. 3 to 10 episodes/hour
   c. 15 to 30 episodes/hour
   d. 30 to 60 episodes/hour

4. During periods of apnea, the patient commonly demonstrates which of the following at the termination of apnea events?
   1. Systemic hypotension
   2. Decreased cardiac output
   3. Increased heart rate
   4. Transient pulmonary hypertension
      a. 1 and 3 only
      b. 2 and 4 only
      c. 3 and 4 only
      d. 1, 2, and 3 only

5. Periods of severe sleep apnea are commonly associated with which of the following?
   1. Ventricular tachycardia
   2. Sinus bradycardia
   3. Premature ventricular contraction
   4. Sinus arrhythmia
      a. 2 and 3 only
      b. 3 and 4 only
      c. 2, 3, and 4 only
      d. 1, 2, 3, and 4

6. **During REM sleep, there is paralysis of the:**
   1. Arm muscles
   2. Upper airway muscles
   3. Leg muscles
   4. Intercostal muscles
   5. Diaphragm
      a. 4 only
      b. 5 only
      c. 4 and 5 only
      d. 1, 2, 3, and 4 only

7. **Normally, REM sleep constitutes about what percentage of the total sleep time?**
   a. 5% to 10%
   b. 10% to 20%
   c. 20% to 25%
   d. 25% to 30%

8. **Which of the following therapy modalities is(are) therapeutic for obstructive sleep apnea?**
   1. Phrenic pacemaker
   2. CPAP
   3. Theophylline
   4. Negative-pressure ventilation
      a. 1 only
      b. 2 only
      c. 3 and 4 only
      d. 1 and 4 only

9. **Which of the following has customarily been the first-line therapy for patients with hyperventilation-related CSA.**
   a. Negative-pressure ventilation
   b. VPAP
   c. CPAP
   d. Tracheostomy

10. **How long do normal periods of apnea during REM sleep last?**
    a. 0 to 5 seconds
    b. 5 to 10 seconds
    c. 10 to 15 seconds
    d. 15 to 20 seconds

11. **While a formal polysomnographic diagnosis of the precise type and severity of sleep apnea is being made (i.e., obstructive, central, or mixed sleep apnea), which of the following respiratory care modalities would be most safely used?**
    a. VPAP
    b. Low-flow nasal oxygen therapy
    c. CPAP
    d. APAP

CHAPTER

33

Newborn Assessment and Management[1]

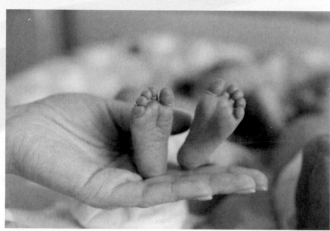

(© Shutterstock.com.)

Chapter Objectives

After reading this chapter, you will be able to:
- Describe fetal lung development.
- Describe the flow routing and major components of the fetal circulation in utero.
- Discuss the flow routing and major anatomic changes of the fetal circulation at birth.
- Discuss delivery room management of the newborn and include:
  - Risk factors
  - Apgar score
  - Neonatal resuscitation program
  - Birth transition goals
  - Primary apnea versus secondary apnea
  - Early resuscitation techniques
- Describe the assessment of the newborn, and include signs of respiratory distress.
- Discuss other special newborn conditions and topics and include:
  - Persistent pulmonary hypertension of the newborn (PPHN)
  - Oxygen toxicity
- Describe the respiratory protocols commonly used to treat the newborn patient.
- Define key terms and complete self-assessment questions at the end of the chapter and on Evolve.

Key Terms

Acute Alveolar Hyperventilation (Acute Respiratory Alkalosis) With Hypoxemia
Acute Ventilatory Failure (Acute Respiratory Acidosis) with Hypoxemia
Alveolar Hypoxia
Alveolar Phase
Apgar Score
Apnea
Apnea of Infancy
Apnea of Prematurity
Arterial Blood Gas (ABG)
Ballard Score
Bubble Nasal CPAP (B-NCPAP)
Canalicular Phase
Capillary Blood Gases (CBGs)
Capnometry
"Chest Wiggle"
Chronic Lung Disease of Infancy (CLDI)
Ductus Arteriosus
Ductus Venosus
Echocardiography
Embryonic Phase
Endothelin-1
End-Tidal Carbon Dioxide (ETCO$_2$)
Epoprostonol Sodium (Flolan)
Expiratory Grunting
Extracorporeal Membrane Oxygenation (ECMO)
Foramen Ovale
Fossa Ovalis
High-Frequency Jet Ventilation (HFJV)
High-Frequency Oscillatory Ventilation (HFOV)
High-Frequency Ventilation (HFV)
Inhaled Nitric Oxide (iNO)
Intercostal Retractions
Lateral Umbilical Ligaments
Ligamentum Arteriosus
Ligamentum Venosum
Maladaptation Abnormalities
Maldevelopment Abnormalities
Meconium Aspiration Syndrome (MAS)
Meconium Staining
Nasal Flaring
Neonatal Resuscitation Program
Non-invasive Positive Pressure Ventilation (NIPPV)
Oxygenation Index (OI)

[1]The authors would like to thank the Respiratory Care Department at Dayton Children's Hospital, Dayton, Ohio for providing their newborn and pediatric protocols.

Chapter Outline

To be fully safe and competent in the management of the newborn with respiratory disorders—both in the delivery room and during the neonatal period (i.e., the first month of life)—the respiratory therapist must have a strong knowledge and understanding of (1) fetal lung development, (2) fetal circulation, (3) normal circulatory changes at birth, (4) delivery room management of the newborn and the risk factors associated with perinatal complications, (5) early resuscitation techniques (6) respiratory assessment of the newborn and common clinical manifestations associated with cardiopulmonary disorders, (7) persistent pulmonary hypertension of the newborn, and (8) Newborn Protocols for application of respiratory care.

Fetal Development and Transition at Birth

Fetal lung development determines whether extrauterine life is possible at a given gestational age. Lung development occurs in the following five phases in utero: embryonic, pseudoglandular, canalicular, terminal saccular, and alveolar phase, which extends into childhood (Fig. 33.1).

The **embryonic phase** begins at approximately the 26th day after conception and continues to the 6th week of gestation. Initially, a ventral respiratory diverticulum (lung bud) appears as an outpouching of the primitive foregut (Fig. 33.2). This lung bud will continue to grow and divide into two bronchial

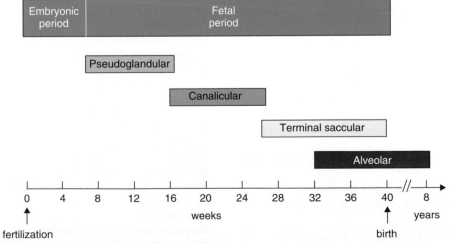

FIGURE 33.1 Major phases of respiratory development. (From Kacmarek, R. M., Stoller, J. K., & Heuer, A. J. [2017]. *Egan's fundamentals of respiratory care* [11th ed.]. St. Louis: Elsevier.)

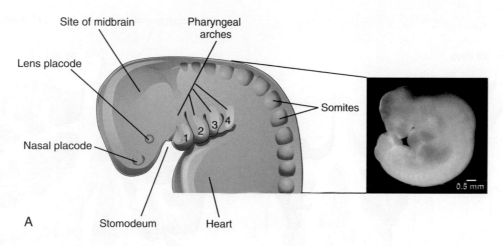

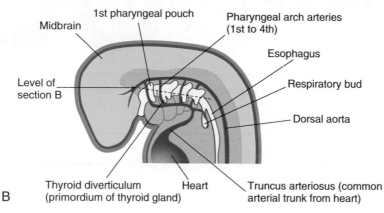

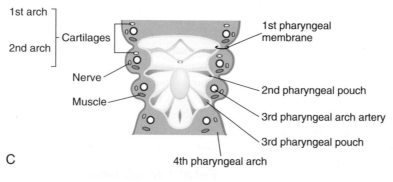

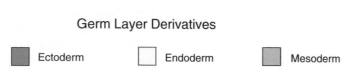

Germ Layer Derivatives

■ Ectoderm □ Endoderm ■ Mesoderm

FIGURE 33.2 Schematic drawing showing the lung bud that emerges as an outpouching of the primitive foregut, eventually forming the lung. The three primary germ layers from which all tissues and organs arise are illustrated. (From Moore, K. L., Persaud, T. V. N., & Torchia, M. G. [2016]. *The developing human: Clinically oriented embryology* [10th ed.]. Philadelphia: Elsevier.)

buds and the trachea. By the end of the embryonic phase, the major bronchi are present, which consist of 10 branches in the right lung and 9 branches in the left lung (Fig. 33.3). By the end of this phase, the pulmonary arteries and veins, segmental bronchioles, subsegmental bronchioles, and diaphragm are all in their early stage of development.

The **pseudoglandular phase** is between the 52nd day after conception and the 16th week. Repeated branching of the

bronchi and bronchioles occur during this period, forming the conducting airways, and the lungs resemble exocrine glands, thus the basis for the name pseudoglandular. By the end of this phase, the terminal bronchioles and associated pulmonary vessels, connective tissue cells, and capillaries appear (Fig. 33.4A). In addition, the submucosal glands, cilia, and goblet cells in the epithelial lining are present and developing. Furthermore, portions of the pulmonary lymphatic

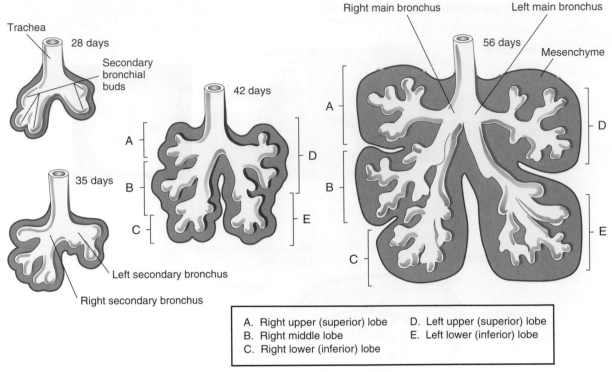

Trachea
28 days
Secondary bronchial buds
35 days
Left secondary bronchus
Right secondary bronchus

42 days
A
B
C
D
E

Right main bronchus
Left main bronchus
56 days
Mesenchyme
A
B
C
D
E

A. Right upper (superior) lobe
B. Right middle lobe
C. Right lower (inferior) lobe
D. Left upper (superior) lobe
E. Left lower (inferior) lobe

FIGURE 33.3 Various stages in the growth of the bronchi as the lungs enter the pseudoglandular period of development. (From Moore, K. L., Persaud, T. V. N., & Torchia, M. G. [2016]. *The developing human: Clinically oriented embryology* [10th ed.]. Philadelphia: Elsevier.)

network, smooth muscle fibers, elastic tissue, and cartilage can be seen through the conducting airways during this stage. By the end of this period, the diaphragm and heart formation are complete and the fetal circulation system is starting to form.

The **canalicular phase** begins at approximately the 17th week and continues to the 26th week of gestation. During this period, terminal bronchioles, respiratory bronchioles, and terminal saccules appear and proliferate, forming the basic structure of the gas-exchange unit, the acinus (see Fig. 33.4B). Pulmonary capillaries begin to form their network around the alveoli. In addition, the alveoli differentiate into type I and type II cells and pulmonary surfactant begins to appear. A fetus born prematurely at the end of this stage (between 24 to 26 weeks' gestation) may survive with intensive neonatal care support.

The **terminal saccular phase** is the period between the 26th and 36th weeks of gestation. During this stage, the terminal bronchioles, respiratory bronchioles, and terminal saccules continue to expand and form cylindrical terminal saccules (see Fig. 33.4 C). The terminal saccules then further subdivide to form subsaccules, which subsequently change into alveoli. The walls of the alveoli become thinner as the alveolar capillaries continue to proliferate. Elastin fiber is present around the acinus, and the alveolar cells continue to differentiate into type I and type II cells. The type II cells progressively increase the production of pulmonary **surfactant**. By the end of this stage, the lungs should be able to provide adequate gas exchange.

The **alveolar phase**—the final phase—begins at about 36 weeks' gestation and extends through childhood (about 8 to 10 years of age). At birth, approximately 50 million alveoli are present. At this time, the alveolar-capillary membranes are ready to adequately exchange oxygen and carbon dioxide (see Fig. 33.4D). By the age of 10 years, the number of alveoli-capillary units increases to about 300 million. This remarkable increase in the number of alveoli with aging helps explain why young children who experience various lung traumas during the neonatal and pediatric periods often "outgrow" their lung problems.

Table 33.1 provides an overview of each lung development stage and the clinical significance associated with any problems that may occur during each of these periods.

Fetal Circulation

Fetal circulation differs from circulation after birth for the following main reason: fetal blood must exchange oxygen and carbon dioxide and obtain nutrients from the maternal blood instead of from fetal lungs and digestive organs. Structures outside the fetus that accomplish these functions are the two umbilical arteries, the umbilical vein, and the placenta (Fig. 33.5). In addition, the following structures located within the body of the fetus play an important part in the fetal circulation: the ductus venosus, foramen ovale, and ductus arteriosus (Fig. 33.6). A brief description of each of these six structures required for life-sustaining fetal circulation follows.

- The two fetal **umbilical arteries** are branches of the internal iliac (hypogastric) arteries. They return deoxygenated blood from the fetus to the placenta. Normally, the PO_2 in the umbilical arteries is about 20 torr, and the PCO_2 is about 55 torr. The umbilical arteries wrap around the umbilical vein (see Fig. 33.5).

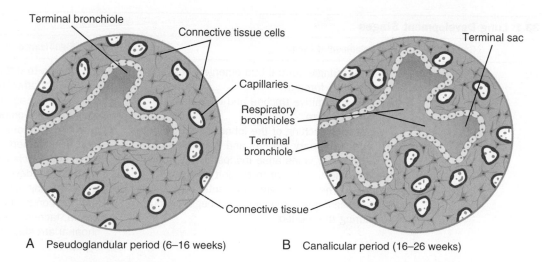

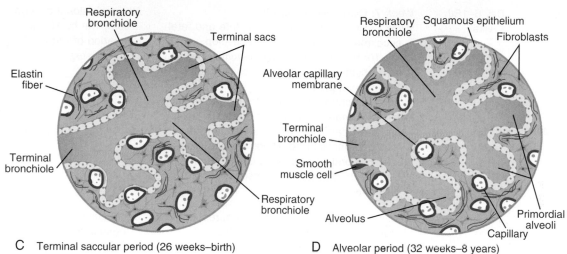

A Pseudoglandular period (6–16 weeks)

B Canalicular period (16–26 weeks)

C Terminal saccular period (26 weeks–birth)

D Alveolar period (32 weeks–8 years)

FIGURE 33.4 Histologic changes that illustrate various periods of airway development. (A and B) There is considerable distance between the air within the airways and blood within the capillaries. The air-blood distance is considerably thinner and more supportive of effective air breathing (C and D). (From Moore, K. L., Persaud, T. V. N., & Torchia, M. G. [2016]. *The developing human: Clinically oriented embryology* [10th ed.]. Philadelphia: Elsevier.)

- The **placenta** is attached to the (maternal) uterine wall. Throughout fetal life, the placenta transfers maternal oxygen and nutrients to the fetus and moves waste products from the fetal circulation. No mixing of maternal and fetal blood occurs (see Fig. 33.5).

- The **umbilical vein** returns oxygenated blood and nutrients from the placenta to the fetus (see Fig. 33.6). Normally, the PO$_2$ in the umbilical vein is about 30 to 35 torr, and the PCO$_2$ is close to maternal—low 30s torr during the last trimester of pregnancy. The umbilical vein enters the navel of the fetus and ascends anteriorly to the liver. The two umbilical arteries and the umbilical vein together constitute the **umbilical cord**.

- About half of the blood enters the liver, and the rest flows through the **ductus venosus** and enters the fetal **inferior vena cava** (see Fig. 33.6). This results in oxygenated blood (from the placenta) mixing with deoxygenated blood from the lower parts of the fetal body. The newly mixed blood then travels up the inferior vena cava and enters the right atrium of the heart, where it again mixes with deoxygenated blood from the **superior vena cava**.

- Once in the *right atrium*, a portion of the blood moves directly into the *left atrium* through the **foramen ovale**. While in the left atrium, the fetal blood mingles with a small amout of deoxygenated blood from the pulmonary veins (see Fig. 33.6).

- The remaining blood in the right atrium moves into the right ventricle, where it is then pumped into the pulmonary artery. Once in the pulmonary artery, a small amount of blood (about 15%) in the pulmonary artery flows through the fetal lungs and returns to the left atrium via the pulmonary veins. Most of the blood in the pulmonary artery moves through the **ductus arteriosus** and empties directly into the descending aorta (see Fig. 33.6). At this point, the PO$_2$ is about 20 torr as it moves downstream toward the common iliac arteries, which branch into the external and internal iliacs. The blood in the internal iliac branch moves into the umbilical arteries and back to the placenta.

Normal Circulatory Changes at Birth

Shortly after birth and after the normal extrauterine cardiopulmonary, renal, digestive, and liver functions are established, the

TABLE 33.1 Lung Development Stages

Stage	Gestational Age	Developmental Events	Clinical Significance
Embryonic stage	Day 26–6th wks	*Day 26:* Single ventral bud emerges from the primitive foregut. *Week 4:* Primitive trachea and mainstem bronchi form. *Week 5:* Branching of the lobar bronchi begins, and pulmonary arteries and veins emerge. Pulmonary veins arise independently from the lung and return to the left atrium. *Week 6:* The diaphragm, segmental and subsegmental bronchioles all begin to form during this period.	Airways begin to differentiate. Branching abnormalities (airway and esophageal) can occur this early in development. Agents or conditions that disrupt fetal development (e.g., drugs, infections, or chemicals) may disrupt fetal development and result in congenital anomalies, such as congenital diaphragmatic hernia, tacheoesophageal fistula, choanal atresia, and pulmonary hypoplasia.
Pseudoglandular stage	Day 6–16th wks	*Week 7:* Diaphragm complete. *Week 8:* Heart formation is complete and fetal circulation network begins to develop. *Week 10:* Progressive airway branching begins as bronchi and terminal bronchioles form. Submucous glands, cilia and goblet cells, and pulmonary lymphatic structures develop. *Week 14:* Smooth muscle fibers, elastic tissue and early cartilage can be seen along the tracheobronchial tree. Major arteries form. *Week 16:* Conducting airways complete and terminal bronchioles and associated pulmonary vessels appear.	All subdivisional airways are complete by 16 wks. Herniation of the diaphragm occurs in this stage.
Canalicular stage	17–26th wks	*Weeks 17–20:* Terminal bronchioles, respiratory bronchioles, and terminal saccules proliferate, and acini begin to appear. *Week 22:* Pulmonary capillaries begin to form a network around the acini. *Weeks 24–26:* There is rapid proliferation of the pulmonary capillary bed, an increase in the respiratory epithelium as alveolar ducts and saccules form. Alveolar cells differentiate into type I and type II cells, and immature surfactant begins to appear in lung fluid.	Conducting airways continue luminal development. The gas exchange structures (respiratory bronchioles and alveolar ducts) begin. By 22 wks, surface-active phospholipid can be detected. By 24 wks, the membrane between the alveoli and the capillaries allow sufficient gas exchange to support life.
Saccular stage	26–40th wks	*Weeks 26–28:* The terminal bronchioles, respiratory bronchioles, and terminal saccules continue to expand and form cylindrical terminal saccules. The terminal saccules then further subdivide to form subsaccules, which, subsequently, change into alveoli. *Weeks 34–40:* The principal surfactant compound (phosphatidylcholine) is present and increases dramatically.	Extrauterine life possible with support. Delivery after 36 wks is preferred because there is a marked increase in surface area for gas exchange.
Alveolar stage	32 wks to 8–10 yrs	Alveoli continue to increase in number, shape, and size, maximizing surface area for gas exchange.	Infants who sustain lung injury as a neonate can outgrow their disability.

six structures that serve fetal circulation are no longer needed (Fig. 33.7). These structural changes are briefly described below:

- As soon as the umbilical cord is cut, the mother sheds the umbilical arteries, umbilical vein, and placenta as the *afterbirth*.

The sections of these vessels that remain in the infant's body eventually become fibrous cords and remain throughout life. The two *umbilical arteries* atrophy and become the **lateral umbilical ligaments**. The *umbilical vein* becomes the **round ligament** (**ligamentum teres**) of the liver.

- The *ductus venosus* becomes the **ligamentum venosum**, which is a fibrous cord in the liver.
- The flap on the *foramen ovale* functionally closes (as a result of increased left atrial blood pressure) soon after the newborn takes the first breath and full circulation through the lungs becomes established. The closed foramen ovale becomes a depression—the **fossa ovalis**—in the interatrial septum.
- The *ductus arteriosus* contracts as soon as respirations are established and the PO_2 increases. The newborn's PO_2 must increase to greater than 45 to 50 torr for the ductus arteriosus to close. Under normal conditions, the ductus arteriosus atrophies and becomes the **ligamentum arteriosum**. If this PO_2 is not reached, the ductus arteriosus will remain open. This condition results in persistent pulmonary hypertension of the newborn (PPHN), previously known as *persistent fetal circulation*.
- Finally, it should be noted that when the neonate's PO_2 increases sufficiently to close the ductus arteriosus, but then decreases within the first 24 to 48 hours after birth (e.g., because of meconium aspiration, respiratory distress syndrome, or a congenital heart defect), the ductus arteriosus will again reopen, and PPHN may again ensue. (See discussion of PPHN at the end of this chapter.)

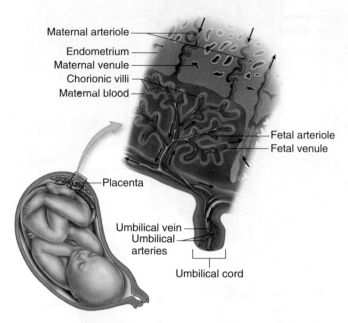

FIGURE 33.5 Placental circulation. The placenta is an organ that permits exchange of blood gases (O_2 and CO_2), nutrients, and waste between fetal blood and maternal blood. Note that fetal and maternal blood are separated by the chorionic villi. Other special features of fetal circulation are shown in Figs. 33.6 and 33.7. (From Patton, K. T., & Thibodeau, G. A. [2016]. *Anatomy & physiology* [9th ed.]. St. Louis: Elsevier.)

Delivery Room Management of the Newborn

The respiratory therapist is a valuable member of a high-risk delivery team. The respiratory therapist must be prepared for complications that could interfere with a normal delivery and outcome. Advance knowledge of the maternal risk factors and intrapartum risks allows the therapist to anticipate interventions. Box 33.1 provides common risk factors associated with neonatal complications at birth. The most common assessment tool used at birth in the delivery room is the **Apgar score** (Fig. 33.8). The Apgar score is a rating system for rapid identification of newborn infants requiring immediate intervention or transfer to a neonatal intensive care unit (NICU).

BOX 33.1 Risk Factors Associated With Neonatal Complications at Birth

Maternal Factors
- Diabetes
- Hypertension
- Preeclampsia
- Chronic hypertension
- Cardiac, renal, pulmonary, neurologic, or thyroid disease
- Bleeding in second or third trimester
- Infection
- Previous neonatal/fetal death
- Substance abuse
- Unknown gestational age
- Post-term gestation
- Multiple gestation
- Adrenergic agonist use
- Premature rupture of membranes
- No prenatal care
- Age older than 35 years
- Previous fetal malformations
- Diminished fetal activity
- Fetal hydrops
- Confirmed fetal congenital malformations

Intrapartum Factors
- C-section
- Forceps or vacuum-assisted delivery
- Breech presentation
- Preterm labor
- Precipitous labor
- Prolonged labor longer than 24 hours
- Prolonged rupture of membranes (longer than 18 hours)
- General anesthesia
- Narcotics within 4 hours of delivery
- Placental abruption
- Prolapsed cord
- Placenta previa
- Intrapartum bleeding
- Meconium-stained amniotic fluid
- Fetal heart rate changes
- Macrosomia (baby with excessive weight)
- Chorioamnionitis (intra-amniotic infection)

Modified from American Academy of Pediatrics Neonatal Resuscitation Program (http://www.aap.org).

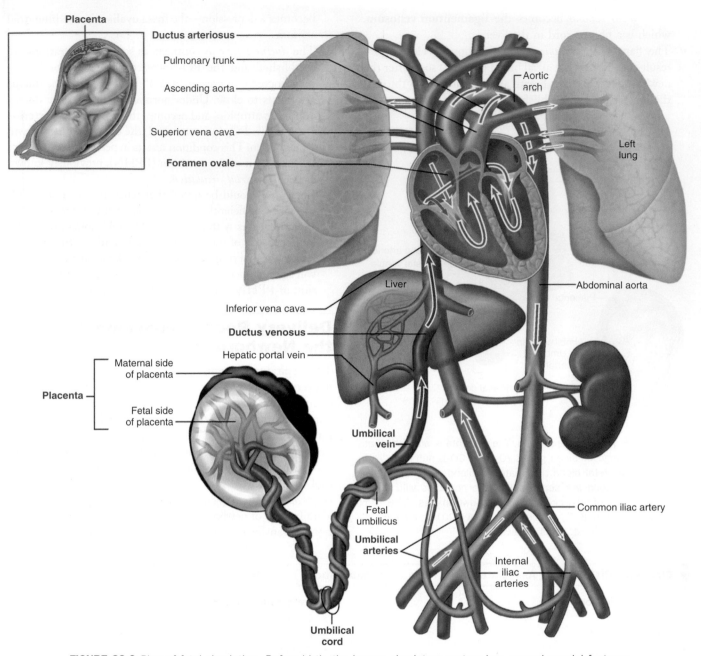

Placenta

Ductus arteriosus

Pulmonary trunk

Ascending aorta

Superior vena cava

Foramen ovale

Aortic arch

Left lung

Liver

Abdominal aorta

Inferior vena cava

Ductus venosus

Hepatic portal vein

Maternal side of placenta

Placenta

Fetal side of placenta

Umbilical vein

Common iliac artery

Fetal umbilicus

Umbilical arteries

Internal iliac arteries

Umbilical cord

FIGURE 33.6 Plan of fetal circulation. Before birth, the human circulatory system has several special features that adapt the body to life in the womb. These features (in red) include two umbilical arteries, one umbilical vein (carrying oxygenated blood), ductus venosus, foramen ovale, ductus arteriosus, and umbilical cord. The placenta, another essential feature of the fetal circulatory plan, is shown in Fig. 33.5. (From Patton, K. T., & Thibodeau, G. A. [2016]. *Anatomy & physiology* [9th ed.]. St. Louis: Elsevier.)

The American Academy of Pediatrics (**Neonatal Resuscitation Program [NRP]**) recommends asking these four questions of the obstetrics team when called to attend a delivery:

- *What is the expected gestational age?*
  - Lung development, surfactant production, and adequacy of the alveolar-capillary membrane improve with increased gestational age.
- *Is the amniotic fluid clear?*
  - Meconium-stained fluid or evidence of infection may require special interventions.
- *How many babies are expected?*
  - Multiple births add risk and require adequate supplies, equipment, and personnel.

- *Are there additional risk factors?*
  - Maternal, known fetal conditions, or delivery-specific concerns.

Team work and effective communication are extremely important to the successful management of the high-risk newborn. Communication has been shown to be the root cause of poor outcomes in preventable infant deaths. Supplies and equipment should be stocked, and the location known by the team. Box 33.2 provides the delivery room equipment and supply list recommended by the Neonatal Resuscitation Program.

Roles and clinical responsibilities should be assigned in advance, and the method of access to additional in-house

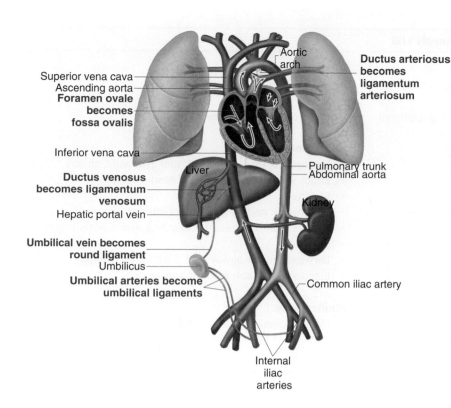

Superior vena cava
Ascending aorta
Foramen ovale becomes fossa ovalis

Inferior vena cava

Ductus venosus becomes ligamentum venosum

Hepatic portal vein

Umbilical vein becomes round ligament

Umbilicus

Umbilical arteries become umbilical ligaments

Aortic arch

Ductus arteriosus becomes ligamentum arteriosum

Liver

Pulmonary trunk
Abdominal aorta

Kidney

Common iliac artery

Internal iliac arteries

FIGURE 33.7 Changes in circulation after birth (shown in red). Within the first year after birth, certain changes in the circulatory plan occur to adapt the body to life outside the womb. The placenta and portions of the umbilical vessels outside the infant's body are removed or fall off at, or shortly after, the time of birth. The internal portion of the umbilical vein constricts and becomes fibrous, eventually forming the round ligament of the liver. Likewise, the internal umbilical arteries become umbilical ligaments, the ductus venosus becomes the ligamentum venosum, and the ductus arteriosus becomes the ligamentum arteriosum. The fetal foramen ovale closes, forming a thin region of the atrial wall called the *fossa ovalis*. (From Patton, K. T., & Thibodeau, G. A. [2016]. *Anatomy & physiology* [9th ed.]. St. Louis: Elsevier.)

	0	1	2	1 minute	5 minutes	10 minutes
Heart rate	Absent	Slow, irregular	More than 100 beats per minute			
Respiratory effort	Apnea	Irregular, slow, shallow, gasping	Strong cry			
Muscle tone	Flaccid/limp	Some flexion of extremities	Well flexed			
Reflex irritability	None/no response to stimulus	Grimace (withdraws)	Crying			
Skin color	Pale, blue (shock)	Blue hands and feet, body pink	Pink all over			

FIGURE 33.8 Apgar score interpretation (add the points in the 1-minute and 5-minute columns): 0 to 3 = distress; 4 to 6 = moderate distress; 7 to 10 = mild to no distress.

The Apgar evaluation is performed 1 minute after birth and again 5 and 10 minutes later. It is based on a rating of five factors that reflect the infant's ability to adjust to extrauterine life. The infant's heart rate, respiratory effort, muscle tone, reflex irritability, and color are scored from a low value of 0 to a normal value of 2. Each of the five assessments are scored individually and then combined for a total score. A total score of 0 to 3 represents severe depression, a total score of 4 to 6 indicates moderate concern, and a total score of 7 to 10 represents normal adaptation to extrauterine life. The totals are recorded at 1, 5, and 10 minutes. For example, an Apgar score of 7/9/10 is a score of 7 at 1 minute, 9 at 5 minutes, and 10 at 10 minutes.

The 5- and 10-minute scores are normally higher than the 1-minute score. A low 1-minute score requires immediate intervention, including oxygen administration and oral and nasal suctioning. A baby with a low score that remains low after 5 minutes requires expert care, which may include transfer to the NICU, continuous positive airway pressure, umbilical catheterization, and mechanical ventilation.

In the newborn who is lethargic, apneic, pale, cyanotic, and bradycardic at birth, and in whom resuscitation efforts are being done correctly and effectively, assessments typically follow this order: First, the heart rate returns to normal. This is followed by spontaneous respiratory movements and improved color. The last important response to be noted is improved tone and reflex irritability.

BOX 33.2 Delivery Room Equipment and Supply List

Warming Supplies
- Preheated radiant warmer with temperature probe
- Warm towels, infant hat
- Infant bag or wrap for less than 32 weeks' gestational age
- Thermal mattress

Airway Clearance Supplies
- Bulb syringe
- 10 to 12 French suction catheter with wall suction
- Meconium aspirator

Ventilation Supplies
- Flowmeter
- Blender set to 21% for infants older than 35 weeks and 21% to 30% for infants younger than 35 weeks
- Newborn- and premie-sized positive pressure masks
- Positive pressure device (bag or T-piece device)
- 8 French nasogastric tube and syringe

Oxygen Supplies
- Nasal cannula
- Mask
- Pulse oximeter and newborn probe

Intubation Supplies
- Laryngoscopes sizes 00, 0, and 1 straight blades
- Endotracheal tubes (2.5–3.5 mm)
- Stylette
- Colormetric carbon dioxide detector
- Tape or fixation device for securing endotracheal tube
- Scissors
- Laryngeal mask airway size 1 with 5-mL syringe
- Electrocardiograph monitor and leads

Medications
- Normal saline and 1:10,000 epinephrine

Modified from American Academy of Pediatrics Neonatal Resuscitation Program (http://www.aap.org).

support (i.e., anesthesia) must be verified in advance. Closed loop communication between the team members and the provider leading the team keeps everyone in situational awareness. For example, the leader is encouraged to think out loud—for example, "What is the heart rate?" Or, during all assessments, the practitioner may call out: "The heart rate is increasing." Or "The heart rate is not increasing." Or, during therapeutic interventions the respiratory therapist may say out loud: "I am suctioning the mouth" as this task is being performed. This allows the leader to monitor the ongoing performance and anticipate the need for additional team members earlier in the course of care.

Birth Transition Goals

As the newborn transitions from uterine to extrauterine life, the lungs will transition from fluid filled to fluid absorbing. Clamping the umbilical cord after birth will increase the systemic blood pressure and vascular resistance. The infant's inhalation distends the alveoli and stretches the pulmonary vasculature, which in turn drops the pulmonary vascular resistance. As a general rule, the infant's SpO_2 during the first minute after birth should be greater than 60%. In the normal infant, the SpO_2 progressively increases over time. As a general rule, the normal preductal oxygenation saturation during the first 10 minutes after birth should be as follows:
- 1 minute >60%
- 5 minutes >80%
- 10 minutes >85%

Good oxygenation will improve and support a strong cardiovascular system.

Some abnormal conditions can disrupt the normal cardiopulmonary transition at birth—for example, if the infant is not breathing, the infant's blood pressure is low because of hypovolemia, or the infant's pulmonary vasculature remains constricted (PPHN). When this happens, the infant typically demonstrates a decreased respiratory drive or tachypnea, poor muscle tone, low systemic blood pressure, low SpO_2, and bradycardia.

Primary Apnea Verses Secondary Apnea

When the infant presents at birth with **apnea**, it is important to discern **primary apnea** from **secondary apnea**. *Primary apnea* results from labor and delivery perinatal stress. It is an early sign of oxygen deprivation. It commonly manifests as periods of rapid breathing, followed by apnea. During the apnea periods, bradycardia develops while the infant's blood pressure typically is maintained. In primary apnea, the infant responds to tactile stimulation such as vigorous drying and rubbing of the infant's trunk and extremities, slapping the infant's feet, or suctioning. Secondary apnea occurs when oxygen deprivation continues. It commonly manifests as several gasps, followed by apnea. *Bradycardia occurs and the blood pressure falls and can quickly progress to asystole.* Tactile simulation does not help, and assisted ventilation is required. Types of apnea are discussed later in this chapter.

Resuscitation Techniques

A newborn who presents with a good, vigorous cry will unlikely need intervention and can stay at its mother's side after delivery. However, if a newborn is less than 37 weeks' gestation or presents with poor muscle tone or poor respiratory effort or

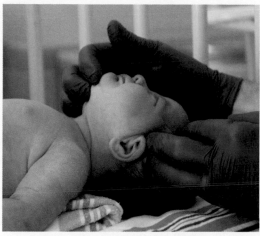

FIGURE 33.9 Sniffing position for resuscitation. (Courtesy Dayton Children's Hospital, Dayton, Ohio.)

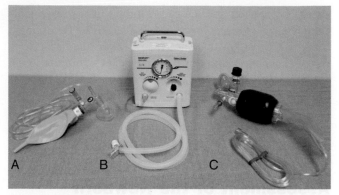

FIGURE 33.10 Lung inflation support (CPAP) devices. (A) a flow inflating bag (anesthesia type bag) with a gas source and manometer, (B) an infant T-piece resuscitator device with a manometer, and (C) a self-inflating bag, with a gas source, and attached positive end-expiratory pressure (PEEP) valve and manometer. (Courtesy Dayton Children's Hospital, Dayton, Ohio.)

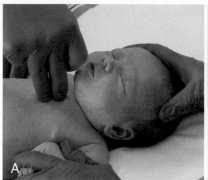
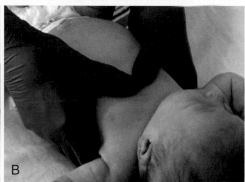

FIGURE 33.11 (A) Cardiopulmonary resuscitation (CPR) two finger technique. (B) CPR thumb technique. (Courtesy Dayton Children's Hospital, Dayton, Ohio.)

apnea, the infant should be whisked to the radiant warmer for assessment and possible intervention. This includes the following:

- Warming the infant under the radiant warming lights
- Positioning the head in a sniffing position (Fig. 33.9)
- Clearing the mouth and then nares with suction[2]
- Drying the infant to reduce evaporative heat loss
- Stimulating the infant by rubbing the back and trunk

All of these should take about 30 seconds. At this point, respirations can be assessed. If the infant is not breathing, resuscitation with positive pressure ventilation (PPV) is required. In addition, the infant's heart rate should be auscultated and electrocardiograph leads applied. If heart rate is below 100, even if the infant has breathing effort, PPV should continue.

Pulse oximetry should be used to assess hypoxemia, because color is not a reliable indicator of oxygenation in the newborn. The probe should be placed on the right hand or wrist to obtain a preductal reading. The FIO_2 should be adjusted to meet the preductal SpO_2 goals. In the spontaneously breathing infant who cannot reach the SpO_2 goals with 100% oxygen, lung inflation support (continuous positive airway pressure [CPAP]) can be applied with (1) a flow-inflating bag (anesthesia type bag) with a gas source and manometer, (2) an infant T-piece resuscitator device with a manometer, or (3) a self-inflating

bag, with a gas source, and attached positive end-expiratory pressure (PEEP) valve and manometer (Fig. 33.10).

For the newborn who is not breathing, or has bradycardia, continue positive pressure ventilation should be used at a rate of 40 to 60/min, with a positive inspiratory pressure (PIP) of 20 to 25 cm H_2O[3] and a PEEP of 5 cm H_2O to start.

Successful mask ventilation supports a return of heart rate greater than 100 BPM. Laryngeal mask airways (LMAs) can be used as an airway adjunct to improve ventilation. However, endotracheal intubation is necessary if the HR does not improve or if direct suctioning of the trachea is needed. For example, intubation may be required in neonates with significant meconium aspiration syndrome (MAS), in babies with congenital diaphragmatic hernia (CDH) with life-threatening gastric distention, or in infants requiring surfactant administration.

Cardiac compressions are required when the newborn's heart rate drops below 60 beats/min after 30 seconds of effective PPV. Compressions are applied to the lower third of the sternum, just below an imaginary line connecting the infant's nipples and above the tip of the xiphoid. The compressor can use two fingers or the thumb technique. The thumb technique is preferred, with the compressor using both thumbs to compress the sternum while the hands encircle the thorax, fingers supporting the baby's spine (Fig. 33.11). Compressions

---

[2]See Chapter 35, Meconium Aspiration Syndrome, for details of meconium aspiration management.

[3]An H_2O of 30 to 40 cm of pressure may be needed for the first initial breaths.

should be applied at a rate of 90/min, giving three rapid compressions plus one breath every 2 seconds—for example, "One-two-three-breathe, one-two-three-breathe." The depth of compression is one third of the infant's anteroposterior chest diameter. Complete pressure release must occur with each compression to allow for cardiac refill, without fingers or thumbs leaving the chest. Compressions are continued until the spontaneous heart rate returns to greater than 60 beats/min.

Assessment of the Newborn

Signs of Respiratory Distress

Respiratory disorders are the leading cause of admission to the NICU. As shown in Table 33.2, the *early* signs of respiratory distress in the newborn include apnea, tachypnea, intercostal and substernal retractions, expiratory grunting, **nasal flaring**, stridor, cyanosis, decreased breath sounds, fine and course crackles, asymmetry of the chest, and acute alveolar hyperventilation with hypoxemia. The *late,* ominous manifestations include lethargy, a decreased respiratory rate, gasping respirations, apnea, bradycardia, decreased systemic blood pressure, and acute ventilatory failure with severe hypoxemia.

Many of the pathophysiologic mechanisms and clinical manifestations presented by the newborn with a respiratory disorder are identical to those seen in the older child or adult.

The common signs of respiratory distress are discussed in more detail in the following section.

Vital Signs

Table 33.3 provides the normal values for vital signs in the neonatal patient. Common abnormalities associated with Table 33.3 include the following:

- Increased respiratory rate (tachypnea).
- All newborns have an irregular breathing pattern. For example, the newborn infant often has a breathing rate between 70 and 80 breaths/min for 10 to 20 seconds, then slows to a rate of 20 to 30 breaths/min for a short period, and then breathes at a faster rate again. The normal average breathing rate for the newborn over several minutes is between 30 and 60 breaths/min.
- *Apnea* is defined as an unexplained cessation of breathing for 20 seconds or longer, or a short respiratory pause associated with bradycardia, cyanosis, pallor, and marked hypotonia. Infants are believed to be susceptible to episodes of apnea because of the immature functioning of the chemoreceptors function, inadequate function of the airway receptors, and immaturity of the central nervous system that regulates oxygenation and carbon dioxide levels. Box 33.3 lists factors that trigger apneic episodes. Types of apnea include the following:
  - **Apnea of prematurity** is the cessation of breathing for longer than 20 seconds or any apnea duration associated

TABLE 33.2 Signs of Respiratory Distress in the Neonatal Patient

	Apnea	Tachypnea	Retractions	Grunting	Nasal Flaring	Stridor	Cyanosis	Breath Sounds	Other Findings
Respiratory distress syndrome		++	++	++	++		+	Decreased, crackles	Premature infants, infants of diabetic mothers
Pneumothorax		++	+	+	+		+	Decreased, asymmetric	Asymmetry of the chest, PMI shifted
Pneumonia	+	++	++	++	++		+	Crackles and rhonchi	
Upper airway obstruction	+	±	±	++	+	++	±		Gasping or labored breathing
Diaphragmatic hernia		++		+	++		++	Bowel sounds in chest	Scaphoid abdomen, often associated with pneumothorax
Meconium aspiration	+	++	++	+	+		+	Decreased	Hyperexpansion of chest, atelectasis, pneumothorax
Transient tachypnea		++	+	+	+			Fine crackles	Resolves in <24 h
Apnea of prematurity	+++		±				±	Normal	Bradycardia

From Walsh, B. K. (2014). *Neonatal and pediatric respiratory care* (4th ed.). St. Louis: Elsevier.
PMI, Point of maximal cardiac impulse; + = mild; ++ = moderate; +++ = severe; ± = varible.

TABLE 33.3 Normal Values for Vital Signs in the Neonatal Patient

Weight (g)	Systolic/Diastolic Blood Pressure (mm Hg)	Systemic Mean Blood Pressure (mm Hg)	Respiratory Rate (Breaths/Min) Older Than 12 Hours	Heart Rate (Beats/Min)
>600	45/20	25	30–60	120–170
>1000	48/25	35		
>2000	50/30	40		
>3000	50/35	45		
>4000	65/50	50		
Older than 12 hours	75/50	60		

with cyanosis or bradycardia in an infant younger than 37 weeks' gestation. Apnea of prematurity is due to the immaturity of the brainstem's respiratory centers, which results in a reduced response to C02 and a paradoxical response to hypoxia—i.e., the hypoxia causes more episodes of apnea and the hypoxia, in turn, worsens. About 75% of premature babies weighing less than 1250 g experience severe apnea. More than 25% of infants weighing more than 1500 g manifest severe apnea. In general, the more premature the infant, the greater is the number of apneic episodes that may occur.

- **Apnea of infancy** refers to apnea occurring in infants who are 37 weeks' gestation or older.
- **Periodic breathing** is a normal variation of breathing seen in premature and full-term infants. It occurs when the infant's breathing pauses for no more than 10 seconds at a time, followed by a burst of rapid, shallow breaths for 20 seconds or less. Then the breathing returns to normal without any stimulation or intervention. Although the precise cause of periodic breathing is not known, it is suggested that inactivity of the peripheral chemoreceptors may play a role.
- Primary and secondary apnea (see discussion under Delivery Room Management of the Newborn).
- **Brief Resolved Unexplained Event (BRUE)**: An event occurring in an infant under 1 year when the observer reports a sudden, brief and now resolved episode of one or more of the following: (1) cyanosis or pallor; (2) absent, decreased or irregular breathing; (3) marked change in tone, either hyper- or hypotonia; and (4) altered level of responsiveness. A BRUE is diagnosed only when there is no explanation for a qualifying event after completing a history and physical exam.
- **Sudden infant death syndrome (SIDS)** is defined as the sudden, unexplained death of a child younger than 1 year of age. The diagnosis requires that the cause of death remains unknown even after a thorough autopsy and detailed death scene investigation. SIDS usually occurs during sleep.

Cyanosis

Infants in respiratory distress commonly have cyanosis. Normal infant ABG values are: SpO_2 of 91%–96% and a PaO_2 of 60–80 mm Hg. Cyanosis may appear when mild, moderate, and severe hypoxemia is present. Table 33.4 provides normal oxygenation and hypoxemia values in the newborn.

TABLE 33.4 Normal Oxygenation and Hypoxemia Parameters in the Newborn

Oxygenation Status	SpO_2 (%)	PaO_2
Normal	91–96	60–80
Mild hypoxemia	88–90	55–60
Moderate hypoxemia	85–89%	50–59
Severe hypoxemia	<85%	<49

Modified from American Academy of Pediatrics Neonatal Resuscitation Program (http://www.aap.org).

Intercostal and Substernal Retractions

The *thorax* of the newborn infant is very flexible—that is, the compliance of the infant's thorax is high. This flexibility is a result of the large amount of cartilage (compared with bone in the adult) found in the skeletal structure of newborns. Although the thoracic compliance of the newborn is high, there are several common newborn respiratory disorders—such as, surfactant deficiency with prematurity, respiratory distress syndrome, and neonatal pneumonia—that result in low lung compliance. The low lung compliance, in turn, requires the infant to generate a greater negative intrapleural pressure to offset this decreased lung compliance during inspiration. As illustrated in Fig. 33.12, greater negative intrapleural pressures cause the following:

- **Intercostal retractions**
- **Substernal retraction**
- **Seesaw chest and abdominal motion**
  - The substernal area retracts, and the abdominal area protrudes outward. On expiration, the chest moves outward and the abdominal moves downward. This is referred to as a *seesaw* motion.

Nasal Flaring

- Nasal flaring is frequently observed in infants in respiratory distress (see Fig. 33.12). This clinical manifestation is probably a facial reflex to facilitate the movement of gas into the tracheobronchial tree. The dilator naris, which originates from the maxilla and inserts into the ala of the nose, is the muscle responsible for this movement. When activated, the dilator naris pulls the alae laterally and widens the nasal aperture, providing a larger orifice and, thereby, reducing airway resistance for gas to enter during inspiration.

BOX 33.3 Factors That Trigger Apnea in the Infant

Control of Ventilation
- Rapid eye movement sleep
- Decreased hypoxic and hypercapnic response
- Congenital central hypoventilation syndrome (Ondine curse, idiopathic alveolar hypoventilation)

Reflex Stimulation
- Suctioning of the nasopharynx and trachea
- Laryngeal stimulation
- Bowel movements (vagal response)
- Hiccups

Environmental Conditions
- Ambient temperature changes

Neurologic Disorders
- Seizures
- Intracranial hemorrhage
- Meningitis
- Drug-induced

Drug-Induced Respiratory Depression
- Sedatives
- Analgesics
- **Prostaglandins**

Primary Respiratory Disorders
- Respiratory distress syndrome
- Pneumonia
- Transient tachypnea of the newborn
- Meconium aspiration syndrome
- Bronchopulmonary dysplasia
- Diaphragmatic hernia

Primary Cardiac Disorders
- Patent ductus arteriosus
- Congestive heart failure
- Right-to-left intracardiac shunting

Systemic Disease Processes
- Hypothermia
- Hypoglycemia
- Hyponatremia
- Hypocalcemia
- Sepsis (group B *Streptococcus*)

Body Position
- Head flexion

Anatomic Abnormalities
- Micrognathia
- Choanal atresia
- Macroglossia

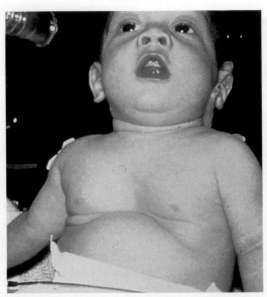

FIGURE 33.12 Five-month-old child with nasal flaring and substernal retractions. (Courtesy Dayton Children's Hospital, Dayton, Ohio.)

Expiratory Grunting

An audible **expiratory grunt** is frequently heard in infants with respiratory problems. Depending on the listener's auditory perception, the expiratory grunt may sound like an expiratory cry. It often is first detected on auscultation. The expiratory grunt is a natural physiologic mechanism that generates (high) positive pressures in the alveoli, which, at least in part, counteracts the alveolar collapse (atelectasis) and hypoventilation associated with the disorder (e.g., respiratory distress syndrome, discussed in detail in Chapter 35, Meconium Aspiration Syndrome). In short, as the gas pressure in the alveoli increases, the infant's PaO_2 increases. During exhalation the infant's epiglottis covers the glottis, which causes the intrapulmonary air pressure to increase. When the epiglottis abruptly opens, gas rushes past the infant's vocal cords and produces an expiratory grunt or cry.

Blood Gas Monitoring in Newborns

Common abnormal arterial blood gases in the newborn are:
- **Acute alveolar hyperventilation (acute respiratory alkalosis) with hypoxemia**
- **Acute ventilatory failure (acute respiratory acidosis) with hypoxemia**

A newborn in critical condition is likely to have an umbilical arterial catheter in place for arterial blood gas sampling. In older critically ill infants and children, an arterial line may be placed for frequent blood gas sampling.

For intermittent sampling, because of the difficulty of obtaining **arterial blood gas (ABG)** samples from newborn and pediatric patients, **capillary blood gas (CBG)** samples may be used to determine the pH, $PaCO_2$, and HCO_3^- (i.e., the acid-base and ventilation status only). *Capillary PO_2 values are unreliable and should not be used for clinical analysis.* The standard way to evaluate the oxygenation status in these young patients is pulse oximetry (SpO_2).

Proper Capillary Blood Gas Technique

Proper capillary sampling technique is needed to obtain a reliable, well-perfused sample. The lateral heel is the site of choice for newborns. The puncture site is warmed for 3 to 5 minutes using an activated heel warmer or warmed washcloth wrap. The site is then cleaned with a povidone-iodine preparation and wiped dry with a 2 × 2 gauze. A puncture is made with a lancet device that is appropriate for infants (a maximum puncture depth of 0.85 to 1.0 mm for newborns). The first drop of blood is wiped away with the gauze. The capillary tube is placed in the center of the drop of blood, keeping the capillary tube horizontal to avoid air entering the sample. If air enters, the tube should be tilted to release the air before proceeding. The capillary tube is filled to capacity. The foot may require some gentle "milking" to increase blood flow; however, there should be no squeezing at the puncture site. Samples must be analyzed immediately to avoid clotting.

Reliable Pulse Oximetry Sampling

To obtain a reliable pulse oximetry (SpO_2) measurement the oximeter probe is typically placed on the newborn's wrist, the medial surface of the palm, or the foot. Adequate cardiac output and skin blood perfusion are essential for accurate SpO_2 measurements. *In addition, the pulse rate shown on the oximeter should correlate with the patient's actual pulse for accurate SpO_2 measurements.*

For the newborn in respiratory distress, pulse oximetry is often used to monitor both the **preductal SpO_2** and the **postductal SpO_2**. To measure the preductal SpO_2, the oximeter probe is placed on the right hand or wrist; to measure the postductal SpO_2, the probe is placed on either foot (Fig. 33.13). *A large difference between the two readings (greater than 10%) indicates a right-to-left shunt.* See Table 33.5 for an overview of the SpO_2 and PaO_2 relationship in the newborn.

To summarize, the respiratory therapist must be careful in assessing the results of CBG measurements. The CBG provides a relatively accurate reading of the patient's pH, $PaCO_2$, and HCO_3^- status (the acid-base and ventilation status) but not the PO_2 or oxygenation status. Pulse oximetry (SpO_2) is used to monitor and evaluate the patient's oxygenation status.

Other noninvasive techniques that may be used to monitor blood gases include transcutaneous monitoring and capnometry.

Transcutaneous gas monitoring requires the application of miniaturized oxygen and carbon dioxide electrodes to the infant's chest, abdomen, or back. The electrode sensor is warmed to increase the capillary blood flow beneath, allowing for the measurement of the partial pressure of oxygen ($PtcO_2$) and carbon dioxide ($PtcCO_2$) through the skin's surface. It is most commonly used for monitoring when used with high-frequency ventilation.

Capnometry uses infrared radiation to measure **end-tidal carbon dioxide ($etCO_2$)** in the exhaled gas. Mainstream devices direct an infrared beam through the exhaled gas; sidestream devices use a vacuum pump to pull exhaled gas into the measuring chamber. An airway adapter is placed on the endotracheal tube in the intubated patient for capnometry. A special cannula is used for the spontaneously breathing patient; this requires a sidestream sampling device. Continuous $etCO_2$ monitoring is not always used in intubated newborns because of the dead space created by mainstream adapters and the dilution of exhaled gas with sidestream sampling.

Additional Assessment Scoring Tools

To supplement the bedside physical examination data and various laboratory assessment tools (e.g., pulse oximetry, capillary blood gas), the **Silverman Scoring System** and the **Ballard Score** are commonly used. The Silverman Scoring System measures the following five aspects of breathing during inspiration: chest and abdominal expansion, intercostal retractions, substernal (xiphoid) retractions, nasal flaring, and expiratory grunting. Fig. 33.14 provides a modified example of the Silverman Scoring System. The Ballard Score is used to assess the infant's gestational age base on external physical and neurologic findings (Fig. 33.15).

Special Newborn Conditions and Topics

Persistent Pulmonary Hypertension of the Newborn

Persistent pulmonary hypertension of the newborn (PPHN) is described as a condition in which there is an abnormally high **pulmonary vascular resistance (PVR)** after birth. As a result, the elevated PVR causes an increased right atrial pressure, which causes the foramen ovale to remain open. Because of these pathophysiologic changes, deoxygenated systemic venous blood, returning to the right heart, moves through the following fetal heart structures in this order: the *foramen ovale, left atrium, ductus arteriosus,* and into the *aorta.* Thus, as just outlined, the secondary pathophysiologic consequences of PPHN are as follows:
1. The venous blood (deoxygenated blood) moves from the right atrium through the foramen ovale to the left atrium—a *right-to-left shunt*—and mixes with the oxygenated blood returning to the left atrium from the lungs (venous admixture).

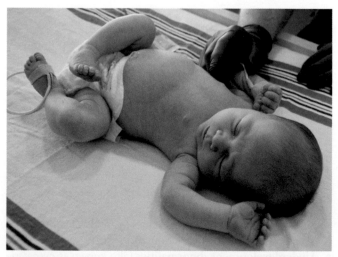

FIGURE 33.13 Pulse oximetry. To measure the preductal SpO_2, the oximeter probe is placed on the right hand or wrist; to measure the postductal SpO_2, the probe is placed on either foot. (Courtesy Dayton Children's Hospital, Dayton, Ohio.)

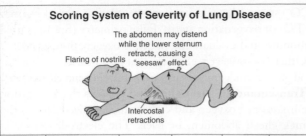

Scoring System of Severity of Lung Disease

Flaring of nostrils

The abdomen may distend while the lower sternum retracts, causing a "seesaw" effect

Intercostal retractions

Score	Anterior Chest and Abdomen Movement	Posterior Intercostal Retractions	Substernal Retraction	Nasal Flaring	Expiratory Grunting
Grade 0	Chest and abdomen both rise during inspiration	None	None	None	None
Grade 1	Chest outward movement lags behind abdomen outward movement during inspiration	Mild	Mild	Mild	Heard During Auscultation Only
Grade 3	Chest moves inward, and the abdomen moves outward during inspiration (sea-saw)	Severe	Severe	Severe	Heard Without Auscultation

FIGURE 33.14 Modified Silverman scoring system for evaluating the severity of lung disease in premature infants. It scores five aspects of breathing: (1) anterior chest movement compared to abdominal movement during inhalation; (2) retraction of the posterior intercostal muscles; (3) substernal (xiphoid) retraction during inspiration; (4) flaring of the nares with inhalation; and (5) grunting on exhalation. The score reflects the sum of these five factors graded individually as 0, 1, or 2. Adequate ventilation is indicated by the lowest score 0 and the most severe respiratory distress is indicated by the highest score of 15.

2. A large portion of the blood in the right atrium via the pulmonary arteries takes the path of least resistance and moves through the ductus arteriosus and empties into the aorta (another venous admixture).
3. The newly mixed blood in the aorta—with a decreased PaO_2 and oxygen content—moves through the systemic circulation.

Etiology and Epidemiology

PPHN occurs primarily in term or late preterm infants (≥34 weeks' gestation). The prevalence of PPHN is estimated at 1.9 per 1000 births in the United States. Box 33.4 lists factors commonly associated with PPHN.

Conditions that disrupt the normal decline in the **pulmonary/systemic vascular resistance ratio (PVR/SVR ratio)**, which in turn prolong the transitional circulation of the newborn and result in PPHN, can generally be classified as one of three abnormalities: *maladaptation, underdevelopment,* and *maldevelopment.*

- **Maladaptation abnormalities** (also known as *acute pulmonary vasoconstriction conditions*) are the most commonly encountered clinical scenarios of PPHN. Although the lungs are fully developed, the pulmonary system can be affected by a variety of perinatal conditions that cause acute pulmonary arterial vasoconstriction. As a result of the acute

BOX 33.4 Factors Associated With Persistent Pulmonary Hypertension of the Newborn

Maternal Factors
- Diabetes
- Cesarean section
- Hypoxia

Cardiovascular Factors
- Systemic hypotension
- Congenital heart disease
- Shock

Fetal Factors
- Intrauterine stress
- Hypoxia
- Decreased pH
- Placental vascular abnormalities

Hematologic Factors
- Increased hematocrit
- Septicemia
- Maternal-fetal blood loss
- Placental abruption
- Placenta previa
- Acute blood loss

Respiratory Factors
- Meconium aspiration syndrome
- Respiratory distress syndrome
- Pneumonia

Other Factors
- Central nervous system disorders
- Hypoglycemia
- Hypocalcemia
- Neuromuscular disorders

American Academy of Pediatrics. (2016). *Textbook of neonatal resuscitation* (7th ed.). Itaska, IL.

pulmonary vasoconstriction, the normal postnatal decrease in PVR is delayed and PPHN ensues. Acute pulmonary vasoconstriction is also commonly caused by:
- **Alveolar hypoxia** secondary to parenchymal lung disease (such as meconium aspiration syndrome)
  - Respiratory distress syndrome
  - Pneumonia
  - Bacterial infections, especially those caused by group B *Streptococcus*
  - Hypoventilation and alveolar hypoxia may also be caused by neurologic conditions or use of maternal depressants
  - Hypothermia and hypoglycemia can also lead to acute pulmonary vasoconstriction and PPHN
- **Underdevelopment abnormalities** (also known as *hypoplasia of the pulmonary vascular bed conditions*) involve situations that reduce the cross-sectional area of the pulmonary vascular bed, resulting in a fixed elevation of the PVR.

Neuromuscular maturity

	−1	0	1	2	3	4	5
Posture							
Square window (wrist)	>90°	90°	60°	45°	30°	0°	
Arm recoil		180°	140°–180°	110°–140°	90°–110°	<90°	
Popliteal angle	180°	160°	140°	120°	100°	90°	<90°
Scarf sign							
Heel to ear							

Physical maturity

Skin	Sticky Friable Transparent	Gelatinous red, translucent	Smooth pink, visible veins	Superficial peeling &/or rash, few veins	Cracking pale areas, rare veins	Parchment, deep cracking, no vessels	Leathery, cracked, wrinkled
Lanugo	None	Sparse	Abundant	Thinning	Bald areas	Mostly bald	
Plantar surface	Heel-toe 40-50 mm: −1 <40 mm: −2	>50 mm no crease	Faint red marks	Anterior transverse crease only	Creases anterior 2/3	Creases over entire sole	
Breast	Imperceptible	Barely perceptible	Flat areola, no bud	Stippled areola, 1-2 mm bud	Raised areola, 3-4 mm bud	Full areola, 5-10 mm bud	
Eye/ear	Lids fused loosely: −1 tightly: −2	Lids open; pinna flat, stays folded	Sl. curved pinna; soft, slow recoil	Well-curved pinna; soft but ready recoil	Formed & firm; Instant recoil	Thick cartilage; ear stiff	
Genitals (male)	Scrotum flat, smooth	Scrotum empty, faint rugae	Testes in upper canal, rare rugae	Testes descending, few rugae	Testes down, good rugae	Testes pendulous, deep rugae	
Genitals (female)	Clitoris prominent, labia flat	Prominent clitoris, small labia minora	Prominent clitoris, enlarging minora	Majora & minora equally prominent	Majora large, minora small	Majora cover clitoris & minora	

Maturity rating

score	weeks
−10	20
−5	22
0	24
5	26
10	28
15	30
20	32
25	34
30	36
35	38
40	40
45	42
50	44

FIGURE 33.15 The Ballard score assesses neuromuscular maturity looking at 6 different aspects of muscle tone, grading each aspect on a scale from −1 to 5, with 5 being most mature. Six aspects of physical maturity is also rated −1 to 5 each. The lower the overall score, the less mature the baby. The lowest score of −10 score would indicate 20 weeks gestation whereas the highest score of 50 would indicate 44 weeks gestation (From Walsh, B. K. [2015]. *Neonatal and pediatric respiratory care* [4th ed.]. St. Louis: Elsevier.)

Causes of underdevelopment abnormalities and subsequent PPHN include congenital diaphragmatic hernia, cystic adenomatoid malformation of the lung, oligohydramnios with accompanying obstructive uropathy, and intrauterine growth restriction.

- **Maldevelopment abnormalities** (also known as *idiopathic pulmonary hypertension conditions*) include thickening of the muscle layer of the pulmonary arterioles and the extension of this muscle layer into small vessels that usually have thin walls and no smooth muscle cells. In addition, the extracellular tissue that surrounds the pulmonary vessels may be thicker than normal. In newborns with PPHN caused by a maldevelopment abnormality, there is favorable remodeling of the pulmonary vascular bed that usually occurs during the first 7 to 14 days after birth, with an accompanying fall in PVR.

Causes of maldevelopment abnormalities are unclear, but vascular mediators are thought to play a role. For example, infants with PPHN are thought to have a higher plasma concentration of the vasoconstrictor **endothelin-1** and a lower concentration of cyclic guanosine monophosphate, a vasodilator. In addition, a genetic predisposition may influence the availability of the precursors for nitric oxide (NO), a vasodilator, which further impedes cardiopulmonary vascular adaptation at birth. Conditions associated with vascular maldevelopment and PPHN include postterm delivery, **meconium staining**, and meconium aspiration. In these disorders, the pulmonary vasculature usually responds poorly to therapies that normally decrease PVR, such as increased arterial oxygen tension and effective alveolar ventilation.

In addition, conditions that cause an excessive perfusion of the fetal lung are believed to predispose the pulmonary vasculature to maldevelopment. Such fetal conditions include premature closure of the ductus arteriosus (e.g., caused by maternal use of nonsteroidal antiinflammatory drugs such as ibuprofen), premature closure of the foramen ovale (e.g., caused by high placental vascular resistance), and total anomalous pulmonary venous drainage.

Diagnosis

The diagnosis of PPHN always should be suspected in any infant with nonresponsive or ongoing hypoxemia and cyanosis that are out of proportion to the degree of pulmonary disease, oxygen requirement, and mean airway pressure (MAP) support. The diagnosis of PPHN is confirmed by **echocardiography**. When PPHN is present, echocardiography demonstrates evidence of pulmonary hypertension (e.g., flattended or leftwardly displaced ventricular septum). Doppler studies show *right-to-left* shunting through the patent ductus arteriosus and/or foramen ovale.

Clinical Manifestations

The newborn with PPHN generally presents with cyanosis and tachypnea. PPHN should be strongly considered in any neonate with severe cyanosis. PPHN also should be suspected when certain prenatal risk factors (such as heart abnormalities and meconium-stained amniotic fluid) or when specific respiratory disorders (such as **meconium aspiration syndrome**, pneumonia, respiratory distress, diaphragmatic hernia, and pulmonary hypoplasia) are present.

The pulse oximeter often demonstrates a significant difference between the preductal and postductal oxygen saturation.[4] A difference of more than 10% between the preductal and postductal oxygen saturation indicates right-to-left shunting. The chest radiograph is usually normal when no other pulmonary condition is present.

PPHN is confirmed by echocardiography. The echocardiogram typically demonstrates normal cardiac structure and evidence of pulmonary hypertension. The differential diagnosis of PPHN includes cyanotic congenital heart disease, other pulmonary disorders, and sepsis.

Management

The **oxygenation index (OI)** is often used to assess the severity of hypoxemia in PPHN and other critical conditions to help determine the need for more aggressive therapies, such as **high-frequency ventilation (HFV)**, inhaled nitric oxide (iNO) administration, or extracorporeal membrane oxygenation (ECMO) support. The OI is calculated as follows:

$$OI = [(\text{mean airway pressure} \times FIO_2) \div PaO_2] \times 100.$$

In most cases of PPHN, the OI criteria are used while the infant is already receiving an FIO_2 of 1.0 and is being mechanically ventilated. Thus the OI can be easily calculated from

TABLE 33.5 Oxygenation Index Range

Clinical Severity of Hypoxemia	Range
Mild	5–15
Moderate	16–25
Severe	26–40
Very severe	>40

the MAP shown on the ventilator and the PaO_2. For example, if a newborn infant with PPHN is receiving ventilatory support with a MAP of 15 cm H_2O, an FIO_2 of 1.0, and a PaO_2 of 60, the OI would be calculated as follows:

$$OI = \frac{15 \times 1.0}{60} \times 100$$
$$= 25$$

NOTE: Because of the awkwardness of the mathematic notation associated with the result of the OI calculation—that is, cm H_2O/mm Hg—the units are typically not included as part of the OI answer (in this case, 25). *It should also be noted here that the OI discussed above is different from the oxygen desaturation index (ODI) discussed in Chapter 32, Sleep Apnea.*

Table 33.5 provides the OI ranges for mild, moderate, severe, and very severe hypoxemia. Infants with a severe OI (25 to 40) should receive care in a center where high-frequency ventilation, iNO, and ECMO are readily available in addition to general supportive care. In the infant with an OI less than 25 and echocardiography that shows PPHN, a trial period of iNO may be administered to determine its effectiveness in reversing the PPHN and reducing the required MAP support. In general, management strategies include the following:

- *Oxygen* is a pulmonary vasodilator and should be administered in a concentration of 100% in an effort to reverse pulmonary vasoconstriction. However, because high concentrations of oxygen may eventually cause lung injury (**pulmonary oxygen toxicity**), the FIO_2 should be adjusted downward as soon as possible.[5] Efforts should be made to maintain the PaO_2 in the range of 70 to 90 mm Hg (SaO_2 95% or greater). If adequate oxygenation cannot be achieved, more aggressive and invasive measures are required—for example, HFV support, iNO, or ECMO.

- *Ventilatory support* is used to prevent or reverse hypercarbia and acidosis, which both increase PVR. In newborns requiring high peak inspiratory pressures (e.g., greater than 30 cm H_2O) or high MAP (e.g., greater than 15 cm H_2O), the use of HFV should be considered to reduce barotrauma and associated air leak syndrome. HFV in newborns may be accomplished with **high-frequency oscillatory ventilation (HFOV)** or **high-frequency jet ventilation (HFJV)**. During ventilatory support, attempts to achieve and maintain the $PaCO_2$ at 40 to 45 mm Hg and the pH between 7.35 and 7.45 are recommended. However, **permissive hypercapnia** may be used to prevent lung damage in patients with significant disease. The ultimate strategy of ventilator support is based on the presence or absence of

---

[4]See discussion of preductal and postductal oxygenation saturation under Arterial Blood Gases in Newborns and Infants, page 494.

[5]See more on this topic in Chapter 37, Respiratory Distress Syndrome.

pulmonary parenchymal disease and the infant's response to treatment. Sedation and analgesia with opioids are often required to achieve and maintain adequate mechanical ventilation in infants with PPHN.

- **Inhaled nitric oxide (iNO)** provides a rapid relaxation of the smooth muscles of the pulmonary vascular system and reduces PVR. The administration of iNO is recommended in infants with an OI of 25 or greater or documented pulmonary hypertension as noted on the echocardiogram. It is a gas easily administered through the ventilator's inspiratory limb with an injector that ensures an accurate "parts per million" (ppm) dose per breath. The initial recommended concentration of iNO is 20 ppm. In infants who respond to iNO, oxygenation is usually improved within a few minutes. Once the patient is stabilized, iNO should be gradually weaned to prevent rebound pulmonary vasoconstriction. Most tertiary nurseries have iNO weaning protocols that allow the respiratory therapist to daily evaluate continued need for iNO. This promotes timely weaning because iNO is very costly. Although iNO is the most common pulmonary vasodilator administered in the NICU, other drugs also can be nebulized, such as **epoprostenol sodium (Flolan)**, to effectively treat PPHN. Long-term treatment may include oral sildenafil for infants with **chronic lung disease of infancy (CLDI)**.

- **Extracorporeal membrane oxygenation (ECMO)** is needed in approximately 40% of infants with severe PPHN who remain hypoxemic despite full ventilatory support and the administration of iNO. One criterion for the institution of ECMO is an elevated OI (consistently 40 or greater) in a patient resistant to iNO. However, when the baby is receiving HFV, the MAPs are typically higher than those seen with conventional ventilation. In these cases, the criterion to start ECMO is usually an OI of 60 or greater. Common pulmonary disorders associated with the need for ECMO are meconium aspiration and congenital diaphragmatic hernia. The goal of ECMO is to maintain adequate tissue oxygenation and avoid irreversible lung injury from mechanical ventilation while the infant's PVR decreases and the PPHN resolves. Infants with severe PPHN requiring ECMO therapy are at increased risk for developmental delay, motor disability, and hearing deficits. ECMO also may be used as a bridge therapy until lung transplantation is possible, in selected cases.

- *Circulatory support* is often required to reduce right-to-left shunting and augment tissue oxygenation. As discussed earlier, right-to-left shunting increases in PPHN because of the increased PVR. When the SVR is low or the cardiac output is poor, the right-to-left shunting will be even greater. Because the pulmonary mean arterial BP in infants with PPHN is at, or near, normal the systemic mean arterial BP, the systemic MAP goal is at the infant's upper limits of normal: MAP between 45 and 60 mm Hg. This is accomplished by (1) ensuring adequate vascular volume via intravenous fluids and transfusion of packed red blood cells and (2) providing vasopressor support, such as dopamine (most common), dobutamine, epinephrine, or norepinephrine.

Oxygen Toxicity

Hyperoxia should be avoided in newborns to prevent the resulting oxidative stress that can cause significant toxicity. The damage is caused by cytotoxic oxygen metabolites or free oxygen radicals. Adult lungs have intact antioxidant enzymes that can detoxify these radicals. However, premature infants lack these enzymes and can develop O_2 radical-induced chronic lung disease.

Hyperoxia (high PaO_2 levels) also contributes to another newborn complication, **retinopathy of prematurity**. Retinal vessels develop at 40 to 42 weeks' gestation. Premature infants with very low birth weight are at risk for developing retinal scarring, retraction, or detachment because oxygen promotes disorganized new vascularization and fibrovascular changes in the retina. The Vermont Oxford Network recently reported a 36% incidence of retinopathy of prematurity in such infants (500 to 1500 g). The American Academy of Pediatrics **Neonatal Resuscitation Program** (NRP) does not recommend the use of 100% oxygen in initial resuscitation, citing a series of human randomized and quasi-randomized studies over the past 20 years that have demonstrated that resuscitation with 21% oxygen is as effective as resuscitation with 100% oxygen. A meta-analysis of these studies showed a statistically significant decrease in mortality among babies resuscitated with 21% oxygen.

Newborn Treatment Protocols

Fig. 33.16 provides a nice overview of the objective data, assessment, and treatment plans commonly associated with newborn respiratory disorders.

Examples of Oxygen Therapy, Airway Clearance, Lung Expansion Therapy, Mechanical Ventilation and Ventilator Weaning, and Surfactant Administration Protocols that are commonly used to treat newborn are provided in the following pages.[6]

---

[6]The authors would like to thank the Respiratory Care Department at Dayton Children's Hospital, Dayton, Ohio, for providing their newborn and pediatric treatment protocols.

HISTORY	OBJECTIVE DATA — Clinical manifestations that commonly develop in response to respiratory disease				ASSESSMENT	PLAN
	Inspection	Auscultation	ABGs/ Pulse Oximetry	Chest Radiograph	COMMON CAUSES OF CLINICAL INDICATORS	
Prematurity, maternal diabetes, C-section, multiple births, sibling with RDS	• Retractions • Nasal flaring • Paradoxical (see-saw) respirations • Cyanosis or pallor	• Expiratory grunting • Poor air entry • May have crackles	↓PO_2/SpO_2 while on ↑FIO_2 (Note: premature infants need PO_2 in 60-80 range) Avoid SpO_2 >95%	Reticulogranular, ground-glass appearance with air bronchograms	RESPIRATORY DISTRESS SYNDROME (RDS) • Surfactant deficiency • Atelectasis	• Oxygen therapy • Hyperinflation therapy (CPAP/PEEP) • Mechanical ventilation • Surfactant administration
Prematurity, history of RDS, mechanical ventilation	• Decreased chest movement	• Diminished or distant breath sounds	Further ↓PO_2/SpO_2 while on ↑FIO_2	Small cystic areas with possibly flattened diaphragms	PULMONARY INTERSTITIAL EMPHYSEMA (PIE) • Air trapping	• Oxygen therapy • Decrease ventilator pressures • Permissive hypercapnia • Possibly high frequency ventilation and/or selective mainstem intubation • Monitor for barotrauma
Low birth weight, RDS, prolonged mechanical oxygen, slow growth	• Cyanosis if off O_2 • Barrel chest	• Wheezes • Crackles	↑PCO_2 with normal pH, ↓PO_2/SpO_2	Cystic pattern	BRONCHOPULMONARY DYSPLASIA (BPD) • Airtrapping • Wheezing	• Oxygen therapy • Steroids • Airway clearance • Permissive hypercapnia • Fluid management • Increased calorie and caffeine intake
Usually full term, possibly C-section, perinatal complications	• Tachypnea • Retractions	• Crackles	↓PCO_2, ↓PO_2/SpO_2	Perihilar streaking with enlarged cardiac silhouette	TRANSIENT TACHYPNEA OF THE NEWBORN • Airway fluid	• Oxygen therapy • CPAP
Stress and/or asphyxia in utero, meconium noted in amniotic fluid, usually full term to post-term	• Dyspnea • Meconium-stained umbilical cord or fingernails	• Crackles	↓PCO_2 (May increase as patient fatigues), ↓PO_2/SpO_2	Hyperaeration	MECONIUM ASPIRATION SYNDROME (MAS) • Airway secretions • Air trapping	• Suction oropharynx, and endotrachea before delivery • Oxygen therapy • Airway clearance • Possible hyperventilation (to further ↓PCO_2 and ↑pH) if hypertension likely • May need to consider ECMO, HFV, iNO • Monitor for barotrauma
Possible underlying problem with meconium aspiration, congenital heart disease, or perinatal asphyxia. Minimal ↑ PO_2 with 100% O_2 challenge	• Persistent cyanosis disproportionate to degree of pulmonary disease on CXR • Tachypnea	• Corresponds to underlying cardiopulmonary disorder	Fluctuations in PO_2 /SpO_2	Normal to mild pulmonary parenchymal disease	PERSISTENT PULMONARY HYPERTENSION OF THE NEWBORN (PPHN) • Pulmonary vasoconstriction • Reopening of fetal circulation pathways	• Oxygen therapy • Mechanical ventilation • Treat underlying cause • May need to consider ECMO, HFV, iNO
May have normal pregnancy and delivery (full term), may have dusky, cyanotic episodes. Minimal ↑ PO_2 with 100% O_2 challenge.	• May be normal in appearance if Left → Right shunt present • Cyanotic if Right → Left shunt present	• Heart murmur may be present	PO_2 may vary widely depending on heart lesion: low with Right → Left shunt; more normal with Left → Right	May have irregular heart shape (e.g., boot or egg) depending on lesion	CONGENITAL HEART DISEASE • Pulmonary shunting	• Evaluation to identify problem • Echocardiogram • Surgery; pre- and post-op supportive care • Cardiac MRI
Problems with breathing; difficulty with eating and breathing (e.g., dusky with feeding), noisy breathing	• Varies with lesion • Respiratory distress, drooling, gastric distension	• Varies with lesion	Usually ↓PCO_2 and ↓PO_2, extent of which varies with lesion	Normal to highly irregular, depending on lesion	CONGENITAL ANOMALIES of the respiratory system • Airway obstruction	• Evaluation to identify problem • Radiographic procedures/operative procedures to diagnose and treat • Pre- and post-op supportive care

FIGURE 33.16 Common neonatal clinical manifestations (objective data), assessments, and treatment plans. See similar information for the pediatric patient in Figure 34.7. (Used with permission of author, Terry Des Jardins.)

Oxygen Therapy Protocol

For the Newborn
PROTOCOL 33.1

Order for Oxygen Therapy Protocol

Evaluate for Indications

- Room air SpO_2 desired range or less
- Room air PaO_2 desired range or less
- Acute situation in which hypoxemia is likely, as in significant respiratory distress
- Trauma with shock, hemorrhage
- Short-term postsedation
  WARNING: Avoid high SpO_2 in LBW and VLBW infants who are prone to retinopathy of prematurity (ROP).

SpO_2 Goals

- VLBW newborn <1000 g: High risk for ROP; maintain at 85% to 95%. Avoid high SpO_2.
- LBW newborn >1000 g: Moderate risk for ROP. Maintain at 85% to 95%.
- Term infant: 88% to 98%.
- PPHN: 95% or greater.
- CHD: To be determined by managing physician based on patient history.
- BPD: 88% to 98%; may need to keep toward the higher range to prevent BPD "fits" with transient hypoxia.

Choose Device

Bag and Mask Blow-by or Assist

- Commonly used on a short-term basis for the newborn who is unstable and has the potential to deteriorate requiring either continuous positive airway pressure (CPAP) or assisted ventilation.
- Delivery gas may be blended 21% to 100% oxygen.
- Anesthesia-type bags will deliver 100% of the source gas.
- The use of a pressure limited device is recommended for extended ventilator support in the delivery room.

Nasal Cannula

- Most common device used for the delivery of low to moderate concentrations of oxygen to newborns. Commercially available adhesive disks allow for the cannula to be gently taped to the newborn's cheeks to prevent dislodging.
- An air-oxygen blender is commonly used with the nasal cannula. The blender is set to an FIO_2 to achieve the desired SpO_2 at a flow rate of 0.5 to 1.0 L/min. Decrease FIO_2 to wean to room air. Home-going oxygen will require the newborn to be placed directly on oxygen. Oxygen flow rates may be adjusted in increments of 0.1 L/min for home use with a special infant regulator.

High-Flow Nasal Cannula

- High-flow oxygen system applied via nasal cannula at 100% relative humidity at body temperature.

- An air-oxygen blender is used to adjust FIO_2.
- High flow rates provide expiratory resistance and **intermittent** positive pressure (insufflation therapy) to reduce work of breathing and fatigue (flows 4–8 lpm)
- Pharyngeal pressure varies with breathing cycle and leak through mouth. Proper fitting cannula allows for leakage at the nares.
- Unlikely to reverse atelectasis or increase functional residual capacity, but can be helpful in reducing work of breathing and preventing fatigue-related respiratory failure.

Oxygen Hood

- Used for short-term oxygen delivery in newborns.
- Accurate FIO_2 when total flow rate exceeds infant's inspiratory flow rate, up to 100% oxygen.
- Hood limits access to face; FIO_2 fluctuates when hood is opened.
- May be used postoperatively for infants with upper airway surgery, such as choanal atresia repair.

Isolette

- Rarely used in newborn care for oxygen delivery
- Difficult to maintain FIO_2 with opening of side ports to access patient.

Assess Effectiveness of Oxygen Therapy

An oxygenation assessment should always include a respiratory assessment along with SpO_2. The frequency of assessments depends on the patient's acuity and stability: from continuous monitoring in critical care, to intermittent 2 hourly for patient who has the potential to deteriorate or is labile, 4 hourly for acute respiratory admission, 4 to 6 hourly for the stable acute patient, 6 hourly when weaning, and 8 hourly for chronic patient until stable.

Adjustment

Oxygen flow rate or FIO_2 should be adjusted to meet the SpO_2 goals.

Documentation and Communication

Document all respiratory assessments with SpO_2 in the medical record along with it any adjustments in oxygen administration. Any time oxygen is initiated, increased significantly, and/or the FIO_2 exceeds 0.40, and/or the patient's SpO_2 does not reach the desired goal, the medical team should be notified to discuss additional treatment and/or diagnostics (chest x-ray, laboratory tests, etc.) to identify and treat the underlying condition.

BPD, Bronchopulmonary dysplasia; *CF*, cystic fibrosis; *CHD*, congenital heart disease; *LBW*, low birth weight (less than 2500 g); *PPHN*, persistent pulmonary hypertension of the newborn; *VLBW*, very low birth weight (less than 1500 g).

Airway Clearance Protocol
For the Newborn
PROTOCOL 33.2

Evaluate for Indications
- Difficulty with secretion clearance
- Evidence of retained bronchial secretions
- Chest x-ray (CXR) demonstrates atelectasis secondary to mucus plugging

Suctioning
- Endotracheal suctioning is applicable in newborns with an endotracheal tube or tracheostomy tube (as needed).
- Hypopharyngeal suction is applicable in newborns with airway secretions.
- Noninvasive suction (bulb [BBG, etc.]) is often used as an adjunct to gently remove secretions from the mouth or the stoma area in chronic tracheostomy patients (as needed).

Lung Expansion Therapy Protocol
For the Newborn
PROTOCOL 33.3

Newborn Applications/indications
Goals
- To reduce work of breathing in respiratory distress syndrome (RDS) or transient tachypnea of the newborn (TTN).
- To improve functional residual capacity in restrictive lung disease.
- To prevent or treat microatelectasis.
- To stent airways (tracheomalacia or bronchomalacia) until airway matures or is surgically corrected.

Common Newborn Treatment Modalities
High-Flow Nasal Cannula
- High-flow oxygen is applied via nasal cannula at 100% humidity at body temperature.
- An air-oxygen blender is used to adjust FIO_2.
- High flow rates provide expiratory resistance and **intermittent** positive pressure (insufflation therapy) to reduce work of breathing and fatigue (flows 4–8 lpm)
- Assists the infant in maintaining functional residual capacity.
- Good postextubation adjunct.

Bubble Nasal CPAP (B-NCPAP)
- Medical gas at desired FIO_2 is bubbled through water creating a vibratory, high-frequency oscillatory CPAP; expiratory limb is immersed in water at the level of pressure desired (e.g., 4 cm H_2O).
- Applied via nasal prongs.
- Effective in the management of newborns with mild to moderate respiratory distress after delivery.

Nasal CPAP via Ventilator (V-NCPAP)
- CPAP applied through nasal prongs via a conventional ventilator.

Medications to Facilitate Airway Clearance
- In the newborn with meconium aspiration syndrome, surfactant is indicated to help mobilize debris.

Bronchoscopy
- Assist with diagnostic and therapeutic bronchoscopy in nonresolving atelectasis.

Assess Clinical Improvement Techniques After Each Treatment
Clinical Improvement Includes
- Breath sounds clear after suctioning.
- FIO_2 decreases, SpO_2 increases.
- Subjective improvement.
- Objective improvement: Infant tolerates feeds.
  - Chest x-ray images improve.
  - On ventilator, airway resistance and lung compliance improve.

- Pressures of 6 to 9 cm H_2O are effective.
- Specific FIO_2 is controlled and weaned to desired SpO_2.

CPAP by Bag and Mask or T-piece Resuscitator
- Often used in the delivery room or when an infant is unstable and may require assisted ventilation.
- Only for short-term use.
- Monitor CPAP pressure with a manometer.

Endotracheal CPAP
- CPAP through endotracheal tube via a conventional ventilator.
- Pressures of 5 to 6 cm H_2O are often effective.
- Often combined with pressure support to overcome airway resistance of the endotracheal tube during spontaneous breathing.
- Specific FIO_2 is controlled and weaned to desired SpO_2.
- May be used postoperatively to prevent atelectasis or as an interim step between synchronized intermittent mechanical ventilation and extubation.

Frequency
- These are all continuous therapies and should be accompanied by continuous pulse oximetry and as-needed suctioning of the airway to remove secretions and elicit cough.

Assessment
FIO_2, flow rate, and CPAP levels should be documented with a patient physical assessment every 2 to 8 hours. Weaning the flow rate of a high-flow nasal cannula (HFNC) or CPAP pressure may begin once the patient's FIO_2 is below 0.30 and chest x-ray (CXR) findings are improved. Use of CPAP for the treatment of airway malacia is often long term and may require continued home use. In premature infants with respiratory distress syndrome, these therapies are applied in conjunction with surfactant administration.

Modes

- **Noninvasive positive pressure ventilation (NIPPV)** is preferred over invasive ventilation when it is effective in assisting ventilation in the spontaneously breathing infant. Special nasal interfaces/cannulas are available to support non-invasive bilevel ventilation with certain ventilators in newborn care.
  - A volume-targeted mode for newborn ventilation is ideal to maintain consistent ventilation in the face of changing compliance. The actual mode chosen may be pressure controlled or pressure regulated because airway leaks may prevent the use of a volume-controlled mode. In the pressure-control mode, the therapist must ensure that pressure is adjusted to reach the desired weight-based tidal volume as well as to avoid overdistention and ventilator-associated lung injury.
- Pressure support is generally used when available to counter the airway resistance associated with small endotracheal tubes used with spontaneous breathing.
- High-frequency ventilation (HFV) should be considered when positive inspiratory pressure (PIP) rises above 30 cm H_2O pressure or when air leak is possible.
- Sedation and sometimes paralysis may be necessary in infants requiring significant control of mean airway pressure (MAP).

Settings

- *Delivered tidal volume (V_T):* 4 to 6 mL/kg, as set in a volume mode or as the targeted exhaled volume in pressure modes. Newer ventilators can be set to correct for compressible tubing volume to improve the accuracy of exhaled volume.
- *Inspiratory time (IT)*:* 0.25 to 0.5 seconds, with higher inspiratory times used with obstructive conditions such as meconium aspiration syndrome and lower with restrictive disease such as respiratory distress syndrome.
- *Respiratory rate (RR)*:* Usually set to 20 to 40 breaths/min, higher with restrictive disease, slower with obstructive disease. Higher rates may be necessary in cases in which higher MAP is needed and raising PIP or PEEP is not desirable.
- *FIO_2:* Adjust to reach desired SpO_2 after setting appropriate ventilator parameters.
- *Peak inspiratory pressure (PIP):* Adjust initially to achieve an "easy breath" with good bilateral aeration and chest rise; when exhaled volume is measured, adjust to reach target of 4 to 6 mL/kg. Usually 18 to 25 cm H_2O pressure is adequate to begin; higher PIP may be necessary for

---

*Consider **respiratory time constant**: This is the infant's airway resistance (R_{aw}) × lung compliance (V/P). Newborns with RDS have low R_{aw} and low compliance, requiring shorter inspiratory times and faster rates. Patients with high airway resistance and higher compliance, such as in meconium aspiration syndrome, may need a longer inspiratory time and slower rates to ventilate.

NIPPV or with poor compliance as with significant pulmonary hypoplasia.

- *Positive end-expiratory pressure (PEEP):* Generally started at 4 to 5 cm H_2O for most newborn conditions. *NOTE:* This parameter has the most impact on MAP. Infants with very low birth weight may require less (3 to 4 cm H_2O), especially after surfactant administration.

Monitoring

- Newborns with respiratory distress at birth will often have an **umbilical artery catheter** (UAC) placed for central monitoring of arterial blood gases (ABGs). This line will remain in use until the patient improves, or generally up to 7 days.
- Infants who require ventilation, without the availability of a UAC, should be monitored with **capillary blood gases** and pulse oximetry, or a peripheral arterial line if critically unstable.
- Transcutaneous electrodes may be placed on the infant's chest or abdomen to monitor $PtcCO_2$ continuously.
- Newer ventilators for infants will give continuous feedback: exhaled volume with ventilator breaths, exhaled volume with spontaneous breaths, wave forms to demonstrate inspiratory effort, loops to show overdistention with prolonged inspiratory time, MAP trends, etc. This feedback should be used by the respiratory therapist to adjust ventilator settings.

Adjustments and Weaning in Infants Who Demonstrate Clinical Improvement

- Because surfactant quickly improves the infant's lung compliance, frequent monitoring and adjustments should be made to reduce PIP and, possibly, IT to reach the 4 to 6 mL/kg tidal volume goal as soon possible after surfactant delivery. Weaning of the FIO_2 is usually needed to prevent overoxygenation.
- Chest x-ray (CXR) is helpful in determining the adequacy of ventilation. PIP and/or PEEP may need to be increased to achieve an adequate FRC or reduced to prevent overdistention. The diaphragm generally should be at the level of T8.
- Controlled or synchronized intermittent mandatory ventilation rate should be reduced incrementally to allow infants to assume more of their own minute ventilation. Pressure support prevents fatigue with spontaneous breaths.
- The FIO_2 should be adjusted downward toward room air as soon as possible, following the SpO_2 goals for the newborn's gestational age and weight.
- Active weaning should occur with each assessment and blood gas check, with active communication with the medical management team.
- Assessing Extubation Readiness in the Weaning Newborn:
  - An extubation readiness tool (ERT) can be used each shift to determine an infant's readiness for a short spontaneous breathing trial (SBT). The goal of the ERT and SBT efforts is to reduce the number of unnecessary intubated days, reduce unplanned extubations and reduce ventilator associated events.

Protocol 33.4 cont'd on page 500

- The ERT takes into consideration the infant's spontaneous ventilation effort, moderate ventilator settings, oxygen requirement, clinical stability, required sedation, and needs, such as continue mechanical ventilation based on medical necessity or upcoming surgical procedures, etc. The infant either passes of fails this assessment; failing any one criteria = a failed ERT. If the infant passes all criteria, an SBT will be conducted.
- The SBT is performed on a moderate level of CPAP for a very short interval, i.e, 5–10 minutes. The infant's ability to maintain a targeted tidal volume and oxygenation (SPO_2) at the current FiO_2 while demonstrating cardiovascular stability (HR, RR, BP, etc.) without respiratory distress during the SBT indicates a successful test. Nursing is always involved in the SBT timing and assessment.
- The infant's readiness (Pass or Fail) ERT and the (Pass or Fail) outcome of their daily SBT when indicated and completed, is shared daily with the medical management team at rounds and documented in the EHR.

Adjustments for Patients With Worsening Clinical Condition (Higher MAP, PIP, PEEP Required)

- Inline suction should be placed in the ventilator circuit to avoid drops in MAP during suctioning.

- As the required PIP approaches 30 cm H_2O pressure to achieve adequate tidal volume or FRC on CXR, HFV should be considered in restrictive lung diseases.
- The oxygenation index (OI) should be assessed using ABG PaO_2 and MAP and reported to the medical team.
- If HFOV is initiated, settings should begin with MAP set at 3 above the conventional setting, rate at 9 to 12 Hz (540 to 720 oscillations/min), IT at 33%, and amplitude set to produce the classic "**chest wiggle**" down to the umbilicus. The **chest wiggle factor** is defined as a visual bilateral vibration from the nipple line to the umbilicus seen during HFOV; it signals that the chest wall is actively vibrating and suggests effective ventilation on the current power setting or Amplitude/Delta P (change of pressure).
- Permissive hypercapnia may be required to protect the lungs.
- Sedation and paralysis may be necessary to manage the infant's ventilation and MAP.
- Persistent pulmonary hypertension of the newborn (PPHN) should be assessed by echocardiogram; a trial of iNO may determine effectiveness in reversing shunt-related hypoxemia.
- If underlying condition requires surgical repair, immediate surgery may be necessary.
- Extracorporeal membrane oxygenation (ECMO) may be necessary for infants whose OIs are 40 or higher.

Surfactant Administration Protocol
PROTOCOL 33.5

- Transport standing order for surfactant administration with specific drug and dosage.
- Order in electronic medical record for surfactant administration with specific drug and dosage.

Verify Indications

- Newborn exhibiting respiratory distress at birth
- Premature infants under 30 weeks' gestation
- Surfactant deficiency with presence of reticulogranular ground-glass appearance on chest x-ray (CXR) film
- Meconium aspiration
- No contraindication is present, such as significant air leak (tension pneumothorax requiring immediate treatment) or known nonviable condition.

Procedure

1. Intubate infant with appropriate-sized endotracheal tube (ET):

<1000 g and <28 weeks' gestation	2.5 mm
1000–2000 g and 28–34 weeks' gestation	3.0 mm
>2000 g and >34 weeks' gestation	3.5 mm

If a large leak around the tube is present, the infant should be reintubated with the next larger size tube.

2. Assess ET position to ensure it is not in the esophagus or in the right or left mainstem bronchus.
   - Good symmetric chest movement with each positive pressure breath
   - Equal breath sounds bilaterally
   - CXR shows tip of ET tube at T1 to T2
3. Place infant on mechanical ventilator and continuously monitor with pulse oximetry. Manual ventilation with pressure monitoring also may be used if a ventilator is not available.
4. Suction patient before surfactant administration.
5. Inspect the surfactant vial for discoloration; normal surfactant is off-white. Gently swirl the vial if drug has settled during storage. Do not shake. The drug should be at room temperature for 20 minutes or warmed by hand for at least 8 minutes.
6. Dosing is specific to the type of surfactant used. For example, initial Curosurf (poractant alfa) dose is 2.5 mL/kg per dose. Curosurf comes in 3-mL vials, so more than one vial is needed when the infant is over 1200 g. Slowly draw up the surfactant using an 18- to 19-gauge needle and a 5 mL-syringe.
7. Verify the infant's weight and the ordered dose with the infant's nurse before administration.
8. Bolus dosing procedure (routine)
   - Attach the feeding tube to the surfactant syringe.
   - Connect the multiaccess catheter adapter to the ET; reattach the ventilator wye to continue ventilation.
   - Position the infant supine with the head midline.

Protocol 33.5 cont'd

- Insert the feeding tube through the multiaccess port to the length required to just reach the end of the ET.
- Quickly inject half of the dose. Remove the feeding tube.
- Roll the infant laterally for 1 to 2 minutes.
- Reposition the infant supine with the head and ET midline. Insert the feeding tube to the appropriate length.
- Quickly inject the second half of the dose and remove the feeding tube.
- Roll the patient to the other side for 1 to 2 minutes.
- Replace the multiaccess adapter with the original ET 15 mm-adapter and attach to ventilator wye to continue ventilation.

9. *Drip dosing procedure:* This option may be considered when the infant is unstable and bolus delivery could add to instability. This is an older technique, using a 15-mm ET adapter with a Luer-Lok side port for the surfactant syringe attachment. The surfactant is instilled slowly with each mechanical inspiration, two half doses over 5 to 10 minutes each, with right and left side positioning after each half dose. If at any time the infant's SpO_2 drops significantly, dosing is paused and the PIP is increased (4 to 5 cm H_2O) and the FIO_2 is increased for several minutes until recovery.

10. After dosing:
- Reevaluate the ET position to ensure it was not dislodged during dosing.

- Because surfactant will quickly improve the infant's lung compliance, chest expansion, color, exhaled tidal volume, and SpO_2 must be monitored closely for 30 minutes after dosing. Frequently wean PIP and FIO_2 to avoid hyperventilation and hyperoxia. Tidal volume goal is 4 to 6 mL/kg. Obtain blood gas at 30 minutes.
- Infants should not be suctioned for at least 1 hour after surfactant administration unless clinically necessary.

11. *Documentation:* Document the indication for the surfactant administration, the method of administration, and the patient's tolerance and response. Relay any concerns to the medical team.

12. *Concerns:*
- If the infant continues to have a supplemental oxygen requirement (i.e., over 30% to 40%) or increasingly significant ventilator support, a second dose of surfactant may be ordered based on the drug's specific recommended frequency. (Some surfactant preparations may recommend a repeat dose at 6 or 12 hours.) A second dose requires an additional order and dosage—for example, Curosurf is dosed at half the initial dose at 1.25 mL/kg if given a second time
- Watch for signs of pulmonary hemorrhage. This is a possible complication with surfactant administration, because the rapid improvement of lung compliance can result in pulmonary hyperperfusion. This occurs in the first few days of life.

SELF-ASSESSMENT QUESTIONS

1. Which of the following trigger(s) apneic episodes?
   1. Hypoglycemia
   2. Nasotracheal suctioning
   3. Head flexion
   4. MAS
      a. 4 only
      b. 2 and 3 only
      c. 2, 3, and 4 only
      d. 1, 2, 3, and 4

2. A newborn baby with PPHN is receiving ventilator support with a mean airway pressure of 10 cm H_2O, an FIO_2 of 1.00, a pH of 7.31, a $PaCO_2$ of 49, HCO_3^- 24, and a PaO_2 of 50. Based on this information, what is the patient's oxygenation index?
   a. 10
   b. 15
   c. 20
   d. 25

3. When resuscitation of the newborn is being done correctly, which of the following begins to improve first?
   a. Tone
   b. Heart rate
   c. Reflex irritability
   d. Respiratory movements

4. Which of the following is(are) associated with PPHN?
   1. Hypoglycemia
   2. Decreased pH
   3. Hypercalcemia
   4. Systemic hypotension
      a. 1 only
      b. 3 only
      c. 2 and 4 only
      d. 1, 2, and 4 only

5. The Apgar evaluation is performed 1 minute after birth, 5 minutes after birth, and again:
   a. 7 minutes after birth
   b. 10 minutes after birth
   c. 15 minutes after birth
   d. 20 minutes after birth

Pediatric Assessment and Management[1]

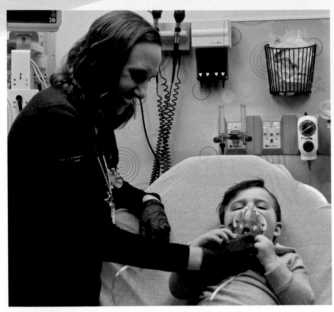

(Courtesy Dayton Children's Hospital, Dayton, Ohio.)

Chapter Objectives

After reading this chapter, you will be able to:

- Discuss the special challenges to assessing and managing infants and children requiring respiratory care.
- Describe popular communication tools used for pediatric patient care concerns.
- List the common infant and pediatric cardiopulmonary disorders.
- Discuss the assessment of the pediatric patient with respiratory disease.
- Describe the special considerations for pediatric assessment and care, including:
  - Infant and pediatric airways
  - Compliant chest wall
  - Inability to increase lung volume resulting in tachypnea
  - Special assessment tools used to direct care
  - Pediatric emergencies
  - Sizing of pediatric respiratory equipment
- Describe the respiratory protocols commonly used to treat the pediatric patient.
- Define key terms and complete self-assessment questions at the end of the chapter and on Evolve.

Key Terms

Arterial Blood Gases (ABGs)
Asthma
Bacterial Tracheitis

Bronchiolitis
Broselow Tape and Broselow Cart
Capillary Blood Gas (CBG)
Cough Assist Device
Croup
Cystic Fibrosis (CF)
Endotracheal Suctioning
Epiglottitis
Expiratory Grunting
Flutter Valve
Foreign Body Aspiration
Glasgow Coma Score (GCS)
Head Bobbing
Huff Cough
Hypopharyngeal Suctioning
Intercostal Retractions
Large Volume Medication Nebulizer
Modified Glasgow Coma Score
Nasal Flaring
Oscillatory Positive Expiratory Pressure
Pari LC Nebulizer
Pediatric Advanced Life Support (PALS)
Pediatric Early Warning Score (PEWS)
Percussive Vest Therapy
Pertussis
Pneumonia
Respiratory Syncytial Virus Infection
Situation, Background, Assessment and Recommendation Technique (SBAR)
Vibrating Mesh Nebulizer

Chapter Outline

Special Challenges in Pediatric Care
    Parents as the Patient Representative
    Family Involvement to Gain Patient Cooperation
    Popular Communication Tools Used for Pediatric Patient Care Concerns
Common Infant and Pediatric Cardiopulmonary Disorders
Assessment of the Infant and Pediatric Patient
    Age-Specific Vital Signs
    Signs of Respiratory Distress
    Level of Consciousness
    Arterial Blood Gases in Children
    Proper Capillary Blood Gas Technique for the Infant and Pediatric Patient
    Special Considerations for Pediatric Assessment and Care
Pediatric Treatment Protocols
Self-Assessment Questions

[1]The authors would like to thank the Respiratory Care Department at Dayton Children's Hospital, Dayton, Ohio for providing their newborn and pediatric protocols.

Special Challenges in Pediatric Care

Parents as the Patient Representative

As discussed in Chapter 1, subjective patient data is typically based on the patient interview to determine his chief complaint and reason for seeking care. However, with infants (1 to 12 months) and pediatric patients (1 to 14 years), the "patient" interview is often not possible. Subjective assessments and complaints are often provided by the parents, guardian or caregiver.

The respiratory therapist should always take the parent's concerns seriously, particularly when assessing a child with chronic disease. Fortunately, parents are usually very reliable and can identify when and how their child is "not acting like himself/herself." In the absence of a primary caregiver with a nonverbal infant or child, the subjective assessment given in hand-off may be minimal (e.g., from the emergency medical services [EMS] squad in the emergency department [ED]). Respiratory therapists will need to use his or her expert objective assessment skills to determine the concerns at hand and recommendations for appropriate respiratory care.

Family Involvement to Gain Patient Cooperation

Involving the family or caregiver is key to effectively managing the child's respiratory care. The respiratory therapist should always acknowledge both the child and the family and introduce him- or herself; this shows the respect needed to begin a professional relationship. It is important to explain what you are going to do before you begin, to get the parent's buy-in and assistance—particularly needed with smaller, frightened children. Asking them how their child best tolerates his or her therapy can be helpful in gaining the child's cooperation. The respiratory therapist may need to reinforce appropriate standards of delivery with the family to ensure effective care. Certain breathing maneuvers may need to be adapted to the child's level of development. Blowing bubbles, for example, is a good way to get a toddler to deep breathe.

Always anticipate resistance or lack of cooperation with therapy that may be fear-provoking or uncomfortable to a child. Such therapy may require a second pair of hands. For example, having a parent or another health care professional securing an infant's head position for suctioning is much safer and more effective than allowing the infant to flail and shake his or her head while inserting a suction catheter. However, even toddlers will cooperate when they know the aerosol or metered dose inhaler (MDI) you are administering makes them feel better. Remember, kids are kids. Teens can be as obstinate as they are at home and try to manipulate their care. In addition, kids with chronic disease will probably prefer the therapist who talks to them about fun things over one who speaks to them only about their illness.

Popular Communication Tools Used for Pediatric Patient Care Concerns

Any assessment concerns, lack of patient cooperation, recommendations for alternative care or unexpected outcomes, such as deterioration in a child's condition, should be effectively communicated to the multidisciplinary health care team to establish an effective plan of care.

A popular multidisciplinary communication tool used in the clinical setting is the *Situation, Background, Assessment,* and *Recommendation* approach—the **SBAR** technique (Table 34.1). The benefit of the SBAR format is that it quickly and succinctly communicates the assessments, concerns, and recommendations to appropriate members of the health care team, particularly the physicians and providers who are responsible for and have the authority for directing care. Box 34.1 provides an example of the SBAR communication method. This techniques can be used in conjunction with the SOAP format described in chapter 12.

In summary, caring for infants and children requires strong clinical assessment skills because patients are often nonverbal. Parents and guardians are generally reliable informants on their child's condition and behavior. Respiratory therapists should engage the family when assessing their patients and planning strategies for effective care delivery. Reports of physical assessments, patient cooperation and tolerance of care, effectiveness of ordered therapy, and the need to advance care are succinctly communicated to the medical management team using the SBAR format.

TABLE 34.1 SBAR Communicator Technique

S	Situation Briefly describe the situation. Give a succinct overview.
B	Background Briefly state pertinent history. What got us to this point?
A	Assessment Summarize the facts. What do you think is going on?
R	Recommendation What are you asking for? What needs to happen next?

BOX 34.1 SBAR Communication Method Example*

S: Situation: (Concern)
- Amy Dixon, a 2-year-old female patient in room 342 with chronic muscle weakness, is now requiring 4 L/min per nasal cannula to achieve an SPO_2 of 92%.

B: Background: (Recent History)
- She was comfortable overnight and earlier today on 1.5 L/min with SPO_2 values between 92% and 95%.

A: Assessment: (Current)
- She is more tachypneic this afternoon, and breath sounds in her left lower lung are diminished; her temperature is 38.5°C.

R: Recommendation/request:
- I think a chest x-ray may be helpful to assess the extent of her atelectasis and what lung expansion therapy would be best for her; e.g., continuous positive airway pressure, or noninvasive ventilation.

*See Table 34.1 for SBAR template.

Common Infant and Pediatric Cardiopulmonary Disorders

Pediatric respiratory disorders fall into a relatively short list of common conditions: **asthma** (Chapter 14); **Respiratory Syncytial Virus Infection** (Chapter 39); **pneumonia** (Chapter 18); **cystic fibrosis** (Chapter 15); **croup, epiglottitis,** and **bacterial tracheitis** (Chapter 43); and **foreign body aspiration**.[2] In addition, and as discussed in Box 34.2, **pertussis** is very prevalent in the infant and pediatric population. The respiratory therapist is also involved in the care of infants and children with chronic conditions, which may result in respiratory compromise or respiratory emergencies. These conditions include neuromuscular weakness or breathing control disorders, sleep disorders, congenital abnormities, and children who experienced birth trauma. These patients may require significant respiratory care including ventilatory assistance. Additionally, children may present with acute respiratory emergencies that require the respiratory therapist to provide stabilization. Box 34.3 provides an overview of pediatric conditions that often require respiratory care.

Assessment of the Infant and Pediatric Patient

Age-Specific Vital Signs

The respiratory therapist must know the age-specific normal values for respiratory rate (RR), heart rate (HR), and blood pressure (millimeters of mercury [mm Hg]) when managing pediatric patients. Table 34.2 provides an overview of **Pediatric Advanced Life Support (PALS)** normals for respiratory and heart rate values and defined levels of hypotension in children. Some hospitals use the **Pediatric Early Warning Score (PEWS)** as an early indicator of those hospitalized children at risk for deterioration. The PEWS system objectively uses the patient's vital signs, level of consciousness, oxygen saturation, glucose level, white blood cell (WBC) count, and urine output (Table 34.3). A higher PEWS score indicates concern and triggers an escalation of this concern to the medical management team for a new assessment and intervention plan.

Signs of Respiratory Distress

Similar to the newborn neonate (see Chapter 33, Newborn Assessment and Management), infants and young children exhibit many of the exact same signs of respiratory distress. Box 34.4 provides an overview of the early and late signs of respiratory distress common to the newborn infant and pediatric patient. Some signs of respiratory distress, however, are unique to the older infant, child, and adult. For example, **head bobbing** is a sign of severe respiratory distress and fatigue seen only in the older infant, child, and adult.[3] Head bobbing occurs during periods of respiratory distress when the sternocleidomastoids—the neck muscles that flex and rotate the head—attempt

---

[2]Children younger than 3 years of age are especially at risk for choking because they explore the environment by putting objects in their mouth. Among children, the most common causes of choking include food, coins, toys, and balloons.

[3]Head bobbing is not seen in the newborn because they do not have developed neck muscles.

BOX 34.2 Pertussis

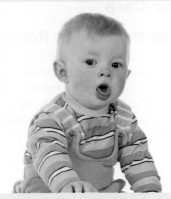

(© Shutterstock.com.)

Pertussis, also known as whooping cough, is a very contagious respiratory illness caused by the bacterium *Bordetella pertussis,* which spreads from person to person by coughing or sneezing or sharing the same breathing space. According to the Centers for Disease Control and Prevention (CDC), although pertussis is found in all age groups, infants younger than 1 year are at the greatest risk for serious disease and death. Symptoms of pertussis usually appear within 5 to 10 days after exposure. The bacteria attach to the cilia of the airways that line the upper respiratory tract. The bacteria release toxins that damage the cilia and cause the airways to swell. Infected people are most contagious up to about 2 weeks after the cough begins.

Early symptoms can last for 1 to 2 weeks and include the following:

- Runny nose
- Low-grade fever
- Mild, occasional cough
- Apnea (in babies)

Pertussis in its early phase appears like the common cold. Pertussis is often missed until more severe symptoms develop. After 1 to 2 weeks, and as the disease progress, the traditional symptoms of pertussis appear. The later stage symptoms of pertussis include the following:

- Paroxysms (fits) of many rapid coughs followed by a high-pitched "whoop" sound
- Vomiting during or after a coughing spell.
- Extreme exhaustion after coughing fits

Coughing fits caused by pertussis infection can last up to 10 weeks or more. In China, pertussis is known as the "100-day cough."

The most effective way to prevent pertussis is through vaccination with diphtheria-tetanus-pertussis (DTaP) for babies and children and with tetanus-diphtheria-pertussis (Tdap) for preteens, teens, and adults. Vaccination of pregnant women with Tdap is especially important to help protect babies.

BOX 34.3 Pediatric Conditions Often Requiring Respiratory Care

- Congenital malformations, including congenital heart disease and spina bifida
- Genetic or Chromosomal Defect: Cystic fibrosis, trisomy 21 (Down syndrome)
- Conditions acquired because of prematurity: Bronchopulmonary dysplasia (BPD), chronic lung disease of infancy (CLDI)
- Conditions acquired at birth: Anoxic brain injury, cerebral palsy
- Neuromuscular weakness: Muscular dystrophy, spinal muscular atrophy
- Neurologic disorders: Seizures, anoxic brain injury after arrest, brain tumors
- Airway disorders: Tracheal stenosis, airway malacias
- Chronic ventilator assistance and tracheostomy
- Sleep-related airway obstruction or hypoventilation
- Viral illnesses: Croup, bronchiolitis
- Allergic reactions: Asthma, anaphylaxis
- Bacterial infections: Pneumonia, bacterial tracheitis, epiglottitis
- Foreign body aspiration
- Ingestions: Hydrocarbon, poisons, opioids
- Burns, smoke inhalation, carbon monoxide poisoning
- Near-drowning
- Trauma: Closed head injury, multiple trauma, child abuse
- Shock: Septic, hypovolemic, cardiogenic, obstructive (tamponade)
- Cardiac arrhythmias/arrest: Bradycardia, supraventricular tachycardia (SVT), asystole, pulseless electrical activity (PEA)

to counteract decreased lung compliance, increased airway resistance, or a combination of both by contracting during inspiration, causing the head to move downward and the clavicles and rib cage to move upward. Because the child's neck extensor muscles are not strong enough to stabilize the head, the head bobs forward during each inspiration. Head bobbing with a decreased level of consciousness is an ominous sign of respiratory fatigue and failure.

TABLE 34.2 Normal Respiratory Rate and Heart Rate Values and Defined Levels of Hypotension in Children

Normal Respiratory Rates by Age

Age	Breaths/Min
Infant <1 yr	30–53
Toddler 1–3 yrs	24–40
School age 6–12 yrs	18–25
Adolescent 13–18 yrs	12–20

Normal Heart Rates by Age

Age	Awake	Asleep
Newborn to 3 mos	100–205	90–160
Toddler 1–3 yrs	98–140	80–120
School age 6–12 yrs	75–118	58–90
Adolescent 13–18 yrs	60–100	58–90

Hypotension in Children

Age	Systolic Blood Pressure (mm Hg)
Term neonates (0–28 days)	<60
Infants (1–12 mo)	<70
Children 1–10 y	<70 + (age in years × 2)
Children >10 y	<90

Modified from Pediatric Advanced Life Support (PALS).

TABLE 34.3 Pediatric Early Warning Score

	2	1	Normal 0	1	2	Score
Respiratory rate per minute	<8	8–9	10–20	21–27	>28	
Heart rate per minute	<50	51–59	60–100	101–119	>120	
Systolic blood pressure	<90	91–99	100–150	151–179	>180	
Temperature (°F)	<96.8	96.9–97.4	97.5–100.3	100.4–101	>101	
Level of consciousness (LOC)	Agitation Confusion Acute change in LOC		Baseline status		Unresponsive to voice or pain	
Oxygen saturation	<90	91–95	96–100			
Glucose level (mg/dL)	<60 symptomatic	60–73 or <60 nonsymptomatic	74–140	140–180	>180 for two consecutive readings	
White blood cell count		<4000	4.5–11.0	>12,000		
Hourly urine for 2 hours	<30 mL/h	<45 mL/h	0.5–1 mL/kg/h Note normal minimum output			

Note: 0 represents normal baseline. Numbers to the right or left represents early warning signs.

Level of Consciousness

The common cause of respiratory failure in children is fatigue caused by the increased WOB; therefore a diminished level of consciousness (LOC) is a key indicator of impending acute ventilatory failure. Infants and pediatric patients who are alert and anxious are of concern, but they are of less concern than those who are somnolent and difficult to arouse while still struggling to breathe. As a general rule, the LOC ranges from being alert, to being actively anxious, to slipping into unconsciousness and lethargy. The lethargic state is quickly followed by alveolar hypoventilation, an increased $PaCO_2$, and a decreased pH and oxygenation level—in short, acute ventilatory failure with severe hypoxemia.

The therapeutic goal in managing respiratory distress is to intervene early in the course of care to reduce WOB and prevent such progression to fatigue. As shown in Table 34.4A, the **Glasgow Coma Score** (GCS) is an important tool to assess the patient's LOC. It is used to assess neurologic status of infants and children, evaluating eye opening, best verbal response, and best motor response. In addition, a **Modified Glasgow Coma Score** can be used for infants and children who are nonverbal (see Table 34.4B). Any child who presents with decreased consciousness—that is, acute head injury, metabolic disorders, or postingestion—should have a GCS assessment to determine the ability to effectively manage the airway. *A GCS of 8 or less represents a loss of airway control and requires endotracheal intubation to protect the airway.*

BOX 34.4 Early and Late Signs of Respiratory Distress Common to Newborn, Infant, and Pediatric Patients*

Early signs
- Increased respiratory rate (tachypnea)
- Cyanosis
- Intercostal and substernal retractions
- Nasal flaring
- Expiratory grunting
- Acute alveolar hyperventilation (acute respiratory alkalosis) with hypoxemia

Late signs
- Lethargy
- Decreased respiratory rate
- Gasping respirations, apnea
- Head bobbing[†]
- Bradycardia
- Decreased blood pressure
- Acute ventilatory failure with severe hypoxemia.

*See Chapter 33, The Newborn Disorders, for a further discussion on these early signs of respiratory distress common to both the newborn neonate and the infant and pediatric patient.

[†]Head bobbing is not seen in newborns, because their neck muscles to head bob are not yet developed.

Arterial Blood Gases in Children

Arterial lines are often used for sampling of **arterial blood gases (ABGs)** in the intensive care unit (ICU) for pediatric patients in critical condition with hemodynamic instability

---

TABLE 34.4 Glasgow Coma Score

A. Glasgow Coma Score			B. Modified Children's Coma Score		
Behavior	**Response**	**Score**	**Behavior**	**Response**	**Score**
Eye opening	Spontaneously	4	Eye opening	Spontaneously	4
	To speech	3		To speech	3
	To pain	2		To pain	2
	No response	1		No response	1
Best verbal response	Orientated to time, place, and person	5	Verbal	Coos, babbles	5
				Irritable	4
	Confused	4		Cries to pain	3
	Inappropriate words	3		Moans to pain	2
	Incomprehensible sounds	2		None	1
	No response	1			
Best motor response	Obeys commands	6	Motor	Normal spontaneous movements	6
	Moves to localized pain	5		Withdraws to touch	5
	Flexion withdrawal from pain	4		Withdraws to pain	4
	Abnormal flexion (decorticate)	3		Abnormal flexion	3
	Abnormal extension (decerebrate)	2		Abnormal extension	2
				Flaccid	1
	No response	1			
Total Score	Best response	15	Total Score	Best response	15
	Comatose client	8 or less		Comatose client	8 or less
	Totally unresponsive	3		Totally unresponsive	3

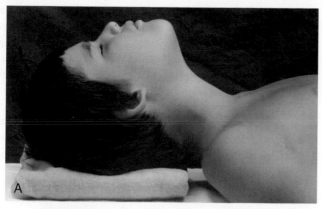
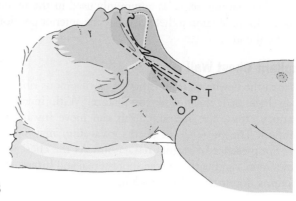

FIGURE 34.1 Correct positioning for ventilation and tracheal intubation. When patient is lying flat on the bed or operating table, the extension of the patient's head as shown in (A) results in the alignment of the oral (O), pharyngeal (P), and tracheal (T) axes as shown in (B). (From Coté, C. J., Lerman, J., & Anderson, B. [2019]. *A practice of anesthesia for infants and children* [6th ed.]. St. Louis: Elsevier.)

or significant ventilator settings. Routine arterial punctures are typically not ordered in general pediatric care because of the difficulty in obtaining an ABG[4] sample from an active, uncooperative child. Like the neonate, capillary blood gases (CBGs) are usually obtained to assess the pH, $PaCO_2$, and HCO_3^- values (the acid-base and ventilation status), and pulse oximetry (SpO_2) is used to monitor and assess the patient's oxygenation status.

Proper Capillary Blood Gas Technique for the Infant and Pediatric Patient

A properly obtained **capillary blood gas (CBG)** sample, from a well-perfused heel, finger, or toe of an infant or child, can safely and accurately reflect the patient's arterial pH, $PaCO_2$, and HCO_3^- level. Remember, the PO_2 reading of a CBG sample varies significantly from the arterial value and should not be used for clinical analysis. Typically, the PO_2 value in a CBG sample is much lower than the actual arterial PO_2 level (see Chapter 33, Newborn Assessment and Management, for the proper CBG sampling technique of the newborn). Although the sampling site of the newborn is limited to the heel, the fingers can be used in the pediatric population, with the puncture on either side of the fingertip. Toes are also an option but can be very wiggly in the conscious child.

Oxygenation is determined by pulse oximetry. To obtain a reliable SpO_2 value, the oximeter probe is typically placed on the child's finger or toe. Adequate cardiac output and skin blood perfusion are essential for accurate SpO_2 measurements. In addition, the pulse rate shown on the oximeter should correlate with the patient's actual pulse for accurate SpO_2

measurements. Common CBG and SpO_2 findings associated with early childhood respiratory disorders are acute alveolar hyperventilation (acute respiratory alkalosis) with hypoxemia and acute ventilatory failure (acute respiratory acidosis) with hypoxemia.

To summarize, the respiratory therapist must be careful in assessing the results of CBG measurements. The CBG provides a relatively accurate reading of the patient's pH, $PaCO_2$, and HCO_3^- status (the acid-base and ventilation status), but not the PO_2 or oxygenation status. Pulse oximetry\(SpO_2) is used to monitor and evaluate the patient's oxygenation status. See Chapter 33, Newborn Assessment and Management, for discussion of other noninvasive techniques that may be used to monitor blood gases.

Special Considerations for Pediatric Assessment and Care

Infant and Pediatric Airway

The infant and young child both have narrowed airways, which predisposes them to significant upper or lower airway obstruction from viral illnesses such as croup or bronchiolitis. Infants with congenital or acquired airway stenosis or malacia will likely become less symptomatic as their airways grow in diameter. Because infants are very sensitive to vagal stimulation—which, for example, can cause bradycardia and a drop in blood pressure—the respiratory therapist should avoid any contact with the infant's vocal cords when suctioning. In infants and toddlers, the trachea is very anterior and is not easily visualized with a laryngoscope during endotracheal intubation.

To offset this problem, it is best to place the infant's head in a sniffing position without hyperextension of the neck. The head should be flexed forward at the level of the shoulders, with the external ear canal slightly anterior to the shoulder. In the older child, a folded towel under the child's occiput will allow just the right elevation of the head to align the axes of the mouth, pharynx, and trachea (Fig. 34.1). A Miller

---

[4]An ABG "stick" is generally reserved for the newborn or pediatric patient who is critically unstable or who has an unstable circulatory system. A poor circulatory system makes the peripheral CBG and SpO_2 measurements less likely to be accurate. In these infants, an in-line arterial catheter is typically inserted to minimize needlesticks and to allow for easy and rapid ABG monitoring.

straight blade laryngoscope is commonly used in the infant population for intubation to help visualize the anterior position of the vocal cords.

Compliant Chest Wall

Similar to the newborn, infants have a cartilaginous rib cage and an increased chest wall compliance. With increased respiratory effort, the sternum itself can move inward on inspiration. The presence of pectus excavatum may falsely mimic the presence of sternal retractions. As the chest wall becomes more rigid with age, the suprasternal and **intercostal retractions** dominate as in the adult.

Inability to Increase Lung Volume Results in Tachypnea

Without the rigidity of the chest wall, the "bucket handle effect" limits the volume and depth of each breath. Thus the infant is able to only increase his/her respiratory rate to generate a greater minute ventilation. An increased tidal volume causes an increased negative intrapleural pressure, which in turn causes the infant's compliant chest to limit lung expansion. The WOB is often assessed by noting the number of words a child can speak or babble before having to take a breath.

Special Scoring Tools Used to Direct Care

Respiratory assessment of children with respiratory disease often involves a severity scoring system that takes into consideration all of the previously mentioned vital signs, WOB assessments, level of consciousness (LOC), oxygenation status, etc. For example, scoring systems are used in a number of respiratory disorders to determine the type and frequency of therapy indicated per protocol—for example, the stepwise asthma management protocol (see Fig. 14.7), respiratory syncytial virus (Bronchiolitis Scoring System) (see Table 39.1 and Table 39.2), and croup (See Table 43.2, Laryngotracheobronchitis Scoring System).

Pediatric Emergencies

Pediatric respiratory emergencies will require the respiratory therapist to use the PALS approach to assessment and stabilization. These conditions include near-drowning, hydrocarbon aspiration, smoke inhalation, burns, closed head injury, seizure disorders, septic shock, diabetic ketoacidosis, cardiac arrhythmias, multiple trauma, child abuse, and cardiac arrest. These emergencies often require critical interventions such as supplemental oxygen, airway management, ventilation, and cardiopulmonary resuscitation in extreme cases. Box 34.5 provides common mechanisms of acute ventilatory failure in the pediatric patient and common respiratory interventions. Table 34.5 provides an overview of the recommended PALS guidelines from the American Heart Association Guidelines for CPR and Emergency Cardiovascular Care.

Sizing of Pediatric Respiratory Equipment

The practice of pediatric respiratory care requires the additional knowledge of the appropriate sizes of various respiratory devices (e.g., airways, endotracheal tubes, suction catheters) used with different ages. Table 34.6 provides the approximate sizes of commonly used items in pediatric respiratory care. Because children with chronic conditions do not always follow normal growth curves, it is often best to assess both a child's weight and age. It is always best to bring a couple of sizes to the bedside when trying fit a device to the child's size. In pediatric respiratory emergencies, the **Broselow tape** and **Broselow cart** commonly uses a color-coded grouping of appropriately sized equipment based on the child's length and weight. (Fig. 34.2).

BOX 34.5 Mechanisms of Ventilatory Failure in the Pediatrics Patient and Common Interventions

Upper Airway Obstruction (Loss of Airway, Asphyxia)

- Anaphylaxis: Reverse anaphylaxis with epinephrine, provide airway if needed
- Croup: Decadron, vaponephrine aerosol if severe, heliox inhalation
- Bacterial tracheitis: Antibiotics and intubate if needed
- Airway trauma, foreign body, airway burns, neurologic loss of airway control: Intubate, cricothyrotomy, or tracheostomy to secure airway

Lower Airway Obstruction (Fatigue, Hypoxemia)

- Asthma: Reduce work of breathing (WOB) with bronchodilators and steroids
- Bronchiolitis: Reduce WOB with airway clearance and oxygen therapy
- Cystic fibrosis: Reduce WOB with bronchodilators, antibiotics, oxygen therapy, ventilator support if needed

Parenchymal Disease (Hypoxemia)

- Infectious pneumonia, acute respiratory distress syndrome, chemical pneumonitis, aspiration pneumonitis, pulmonary edema
- Provide oxygen therapy and close monitoring, antibiotics if indicated, positive pressure support as needed to reverse hypoxemia.

Disordered Control of Breathing (Ineffective Breathing, Hypoventilation)

- Head injury, spinal injury: Assess adequacy of ventilation; intubate to control airway, and initiate mechanical ventilation if needed
- Poisoning: Maintain airway and ventilation until reversal or effect wears off
- Opioid ingestion: Narcan, airway and ventilatory support until reversal
- Neuromuscular weakness: Assess pulmonary function and sleep hypoventilation. Provide ventilatory assistance as needed, using noninvasive options as long as possible

TABLE 34.5 Overview of Pediatric Cardiopulmonary Resuscitation: PALS Guidelines

	Infant	Child	Adolescents and Adults
Age	1 month to 1 year	1 year to puberty	>8 y
Airway position	Sniffing position, towel under shoulder, external ear canal anterior to the shoulder	Towel under occiput, head elevated so that external ear canal is anterior to the shoulder	Head tilt, chin lift
Breathing	8–10 per minute 1 second per breath	8–10 per minute 1 second per breath	8–10 per minute 1 second per breath
Pulse check	Brachial artery	Carotid or femoral artery	Carotid artery
Compression rate	At least 100–120 per minute	At least 100–120 per minute	At least 100–120 per minute
Compression depth	At least ⅓ anteroposterior (AP) diameter, about 1½ inch	At least ⅓ AP diameter, about 2 inches	At least 2 inches
Compression to ventilation ratio	30:2 with one rescuer, 15:2 with two rescuers	30:2 with one rescuer, 15:2 with two rescuers	30:2 with one or two rescuers

Modified from Pediatric Advanced Life Support (PALS). For the most recent American Heart Association Guidelines for CPR and Emergency Cardiovascular Care, www.heart.org/cpr.

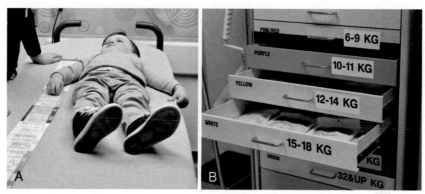

FIGURE 34.2 (A) Color-coded Broselow tape. (B) Color-coded Broselow cart.

Pediatric Treatment Protocols

Fig. 34.3 provides a nice overview of the objective data, assessment, and treatment plans commonly associated with pediatric respiratory disorders.

Examples of Oxygen Therapy, Airway Clearance Therapy, Lung Expansion Therapy, Aerosolized Medication, and Mechanical Ventilation and Ventilator Weaning Protocols that are commonly used to treat the pediatric patient are provided in following pages.[5]

---

[5]The authors would like to thank the Respiratory Care Department at Dayton Children's Hospital, Dayton, Ohio, for providing their newborn and pediatric treatment protocols.

TABLE 34.6 Sizes of Equipment Used in Pediatric Respiratory Care

Device	Premature Newborn	Newborn <1 mo, <5 kg	Infant 1–12 mo, 6–9 kg	Toddler 1–3 y 10–14 kg	Pre-Schooler 4–5 y 15–23 kg	School Age 6–12 y 24–44 kg	Adolescent 13–18 y >45 kg	Comments
Oral Guedel airway	00	0	1	2	2	3–4	5–6	Guedel is best for the child's proportionally large tongue.
Nasopharyngeal airway	2.5 ETT	3.0 ETT	3.5 ETT	3.5–4.5 ETT	18 Fr	20–22 Fr	24 Fr	Measure length from nares to tragus of the ear. Size used will vary with size of nares. Use ETT in infants and toddlers inserted to the appropriate depth.
ETT size (mm)	2.5	3.0	3.5	3.5–4.5	5.0–5.5	5.5–6.5	6.5–7.5	Age/4 + 4 = Uncuffed size Age/4 + 3.5 = Cuffed size. Use Broselow tape to guide. Cuffs are typically required for 5.5 or larger, but can be used in smaller sizes with suspected poor lung compliance.
ETT depth in cm	6–8	8–9	9–11	11–13.5	15–16.5	16.5–19	19–22	3 × ETT size
Laryngoscope blade	0–00 Miller	0–1 Miller	1 Miller	1–2 Miller	2 Miller	2 Mac or Miller	3 Mac or Miller	Miller blades are used for infants.
Laryngeal mask airway (LMA)		1.0 <5 kg	1.5 5–10 kg	2.0 10–20 kg	2.5 20–30 kg	3.0–4.0 30–70 kg	4.0–5.0 50–100 kg	LMA sizes are based on kilogram weight.
King airway		0 <5 kg	1 5–12 kg	2 12–25 kg	2 12–25 kg	2.5 25–35 kg	4–5–6	Adolescent is based on height: 4: 4–5 ft 5: 5–6 ft 6: >6 ft
Tracheostomy tubes	2.5 N	3.0 N	3.5 N	3.5 P	4.0	4.0–6.0	6.0–7.0	Appropriate sizes vary significantly with the child's size and condition. Length varies as well or may be custom.

Equipment								Notes
Suction catheters (French)	6	6–8	8	8	10	10–12	14	In smaller ETTs, you may not be able to follow the 50% of ETT rule.
Bag-valve-mask, self-inflating / Flow-inflating bag	Infant 500 mL	Infant 500 mL	Infant 500 mL	Infant 500 mL	Pediatric 1000 mL	Pediatric to adult 1000–2000 mL	Adult 2000 mL	Make sure to use adequate flow and adjust pop-off to control pressure
Positive pressure mask	Premie	Newborn	Infant	Small child	Child	Small adult	Adult	Large enough to cover nose and mouth and easily sealed. Use sizing charts for CPAP/BPAP masks.
Ventilator circuit	Infant	Infant	Infant	Pediatric	Pediatric	Pediatric to adult	Adult	Infant <10 kg. Pediatric <40 kg. Some manufacturers establish circuit size based on tidal volume.
Noninvasive ventilation interface	Cannula	Cannula	Cannula or Infant Gel	Infant Gel	Small child mask	Child mask	Small adult to adult prongs or mask	Use any sizing tools available.
Oxygen mask	Infant	Infant	Infant	Toddler: Pediatric	Pediatric	Pediatric	Adult	Flows will vary with age to achieve a moderate FIO$_2$.
Nasal cannula	Premie	Infant	Infant	Pediatric	Pediatric	Pediatric to adult	Adult	Depends on application; high-flow nasal cannula should be sized to 50% of nares diameter.
Metered dose inhaler with spacer	N/A	Mask	Mask	Mask	Mask	Mouthpiece	Mouthpiece	Developmental age will determine ability to use.

Modified from Pediatric Advanced Life Support (PALS). For the most recent American Heart Association Guidelines for CPR and Emergency Cardiovascular Care, go to http://www.heart.org/cpr.

PEDIATRIC RESPIRATORY CARE POCKET CARD

HISTORY	OBJECTIVE DATA Clinical manifestations that commonly develop in response to respiratory disease				ASSESSMENT	PLAN
	Inspection	Auscultation	ABGs/ Pulse Oximetry	Chest Radiograph	COMMON CAUSES OF CLINICAL INDICATORS	
Infant or young child (usually newborn–3 y.o.), upper respiratory infection, barking cough	• Tachypnea • Retractions • Nasal flaring • May have cyanosis	• Barking cough • Stridor	↓PCO_2 and ↓PO_2/SpO_2	Subglottic edema on neck radiograph–*steeple* sign	LARYNGOTRACHEO-BRONCHITIS (CROUP) (*typically parainfluenza viruses, occasionally bacterial in origin*) • Laryngeal edema	• Oxygen therapy • Cool mist • Racemic epinephrine • Steroids
Toddler or school age child (usually 2 y.o. or >), acute onset of fever and respiratory distress, non-immunized fever patient	• Stridor • Dyspnea • Drooling • May have cyanosis	• Stridor	↓PCO_2 and ↓PO_2/SpO_2	Epiglottis appears as large, round, soft tissue density on neck radiograph–*thumb* sign	EPIGLOTTITIS (*H. influenzae Type B; vaccine available*) • Edema	• Emergency attention • Oxygen therapy • Intubation in OR or tracheostomy in OR • Antibiotics
Upper respiratory infection, apnea (newborn–2 y.o. or older child with chronic cardiopulmonary condition)	• Tachypnea, retractions, nasal flaring, nasal secretions • Cyanosis if severe	• Wheezes	↓PO_2/SpO_2	May vary from normal to streaky infiltrates or hyperaeration	BRONCHIOLITIS (*typically RSV organism*) • Airway secretions • Bronchospasm possible • Airway inflammation/edema	• Supportive • Oxygen therapy • Suction • Trial of bronchodilator therapy if significant respiratory distress. • Mechanical ventilation; HFNC, CPAP
Upper respiratory infection, late onset of fever, may c/o earache	• Tachypnea, retractions, nasal flaring, nasal secretions • Cyanosis if severe	• Crackles • Wheezes • Bronchial sounds	↓PO_2/SpO_2	Infiltrates and/or consolidation	PNEUMONIA • Consolidation • Airway secretions	• Supportive as above if viral • Antibiotics if bacterial with supportive care also provided
Wheezing, family history of asthma/allergies, frequent respiratory infections, or chronic unexplained cough	• Accessory muscle use • Decreased chest excursion • Pursed-lip breathing	• Wheezes, • Prolonged expiration • Crackles	↓PCO_2 (increasing PCO_2 is an ominous sign), ↓PO_2/SpO_2	May be normal or show hyperaeration	ASTHMA (*most common chronic disease in childhood; see Expert Guidelines ref. below*) • Inflammation • Reversible airway obstruction/bronchospasm	(*See Expert Guidelines ref. below*) • Plan varies with severity • Inhaled β_2 agonists, steroids, anticholinergics, mast cell stabilizers, leukotriene modifiers, PEF or FEV_1 assessments, oxygen therapy, possible mechanical ventilation • Discharge teaching of med use, peakflow self-monitoring, and school management plan
Meconium ileus at birth, excessive thick respiratory secretions, frequent respiratory infections, failure to thrive	• Accessory muscle use • Barrel chest • Clubbed fingertips	• Wheezes • Crackles	May have ↓PO_2/SpO_2	Hyperaeration, peribronchial thickening, bronchiectasis, increased AP diameter	CYSTIC FIBROSIS (*one of the most common hereditary disorders*) • Excessive secretions • Air trapping	• Bronchial hygiene therapy (postural drainage and percussion, PEP mask therapy, mucolytics) • Bronchodilators • Antibiotics if indicated • Oxygen therapy • Nutritional support • May need to consider lung transplant
Previously healthy, acute onset of choking, coughing. Occasionally chronic unexplained cough	• Drooling • Stridor • May have cyanosis	• Asymmetrical breath sounds • Wheezes	May be normal, May have ↓PO_2/SpO_2	Asymmetrical expansion of chest with forced expiratory film	FOREIGN BODY OBSTRUCTION • Airway obstruction	Rigid bronchoscopy with anesthesia, followed by bronchial hygiene therapy and bronchodilator therapy
Presence of underlying disorder such as shock, sepsis, near drowning, aspiration	• Dyspnea • Tachypnea progressing to cyanosis • Irritability	• Crackles • Bronchial sounds	↓PCO_2 (PCO_2 increases as disease progresses), ↓PO_2/SpO_2, which continues to worsen despite treatment	Normal early in course, progressively shows fluffy infiltrates and patchy, nodular densities	ADULT RESPIRATORY DISTRESS SYNDROME (ARDS) • Increased alveolar-capillary membrane • Atelectasis • Consolidation	• Oxygen therapy • Hyperinflation therapy (CPAP) • Mechanical ventilation • May need to consider HFV, ECMO • Monitor for barotrauma

FIGURE 34.3 Common pediatric clinical manifestations (objective data), assessments, and treatment plans. See similar information for the neonatal patient in Figure 33.16. (Used with permission of author, Terry Des Jardins.)

Oxygen Therapy Protocol
For the Pediatric Patient
PROTOCOL 34.1

Order for Oxygen Therapy Protocol
Evaluate for Indications
- Room air SpO_2 at desired range or less
- Room air PaO_2 at desired range or less
- Acute situation in which hypoxemia is likely, as in significant respiratory distress
- Trauma with shock, hemorrhage
- Short-term postsedation
- Carbon monoxide poisoning

SpO_2 Goals: Generally Specific to Unit Policy or Respiratory Care Protocol
- Coronary heart disease: To be determined by managing physician based on patient history
- BPD/CLDI: 93% to 97%; may need to keep toward the higher range to prevent BPD "fits" with transient hypoxia.
- Bronchiolitis: 91% to 94% or higher.
- Asthma 92% to 94% or higher.
- Pneumonia 92% to 94% or higher.
- Chronic cystic fibrosis: 88% to 92% or higher.
- Carbon monoxide poisoning: Ignore SpO_2 and deliver 100% oxygen until measured carboxyhemoglobin level drops to desired normal range (<5%).

Choose Device
Bag and Mask Blow-by or Assist
- Commonly used on a short-term basis for the infant or child who is unstable and has the potential to deteriorate requiring high-flow nasal cannula (HFNC), continuous positive airway pressure (CPAP), or assisted ventilation.
- Delivery gas may be 100% oxygen or blended.
- Anesthesia-type bags will deliver 100% of the source gas.
- Flow must be adequate to achieve effectiveness 5 to 10 L/min.

Nasal Cannula
- Most common device used for the delivery of low to moderate concentrations of oxygen to children. Commercially available adhesive disks allow for the cannula to be gently taped to the infant's/toddler's cheeks to prevent removal.
- Bronchiolitis infants (generally younger than 6 months of age) requiring oxygen by cannula should be set up on incrementally lower flowrates (i.e., 0.25 to 0.5 L/min, etc.) with oxygen flow titrated to desired SpO_2. Flows greater than 1.5 L/min reflect significant FIO_2 in this age group— that is, 1500 mL/min or 25 mL/s, may provide the majority of the inspired flow and fill physiologic dead space, providing an FIO_2 of 0.60 or greater. Flowrates in excess of 1.5 L/min may reflect the need for increased flowrate to support positive pharyngeal pressure to reduce work of breathing (WOB); such flowrates contribute to drying of secretions and dehydration. A high-flow nasal cannula (HFNC) may be a better delivery device at these flows.

- Older pediatric patients can be managed with nasal cannula oxygen; higher flowrates, 4 to 6 L/min, may suggest a need to evaluate the patient's actual FIO_2 with a Venturi mask challenge. Using the Venturi mask, adjust the FIO_2 and flowrate to get the desired SpO_2. Report this to the managing medical team to quantify the child's degree of hypoxemia.

High-Flow Nasal Cannula
- High-flow oxygen system is applied by nasal cannula at 100% relative humidity at body temperature.
- An air-oxygen blender is commonly used to adjust FIO_2.
- High flow rates provide expiratory resistance and **intermittent** positive pressure (insufflation therapy) to reduce work of breathing and fatigue (flows 4–8 lpm in infants, 15–40 lpm in older children)
- High flowrates flush the hypopharynx and can aid carbon dioxide elimination.
- Pharyngeal pressure varies with breathing cycle and leak through the mouth, but can be positive with sufficient flowrates.
- Unlikely to reverse atelectasis or increase functional residual capacity (FRC) but can be helpful in reducing WOB and preventing fatigue-related respiratory failure.

Simple Mask
Used primarily for short-term, moderate oxygen use, possibly during a procedure or sedation. It may be used in the emergency department (ED) or in an emergency until a specific oxygen requirement is determined and a more comfortable device (nasal cannula, HFNC, cool aerosol face mask, etc.) is set up. Flow must be adequate to flush carbon dioxide from the added dead space of the mask (i.e., 3 to 5 L/min for the pediatric and 6 to 10 L/min for the adult mask).

Venturi Mask
The Venturi mask is used for pediatric and adult-sized patients for short-term, high-flow oxygen delivery; precise FIO_2 delivery is helpful in quantifying the child's degree of ventilation-perfusion mismatch for the clinical team. Dry gas limits its long-term use.

Nonrebreather Mask
Used for quick pediatric application of high-flow oxygen or specialty gas delivery in the ED or intensive care unit (ICU). Flow should be set high enough to meet patient's inspiratory demand. Often used in trauma and carbon monoxide poisoning. It can be used to deliver heliox. Dry gas prevents long-term use.

Cool Aerosol Face Mask or Face Tent
- Allows for delivery of continuous bland aerosol with accurate FIO_2 when total flowrate exceeds patient's inspiratory demand.
- Appropriate for cooperative pediatric patients.
- Face tent offers aerosol and FIO_2 control without direct contact to oronasal region and is desirable with some trauma or surgical cases.

Protocol 34.1 cont'd on page 514

Protocol 34.1 cont'd
Oxygen Hood

- Used for short-term oxygen delivery in younger infants who are unable to roll over.
- Accurate FIO_2 when total flowrate exceeds infant's inspiratory flowrate, up to 100% oxygen.
- Hood limits access to face; FIO_2 fluctuates when hood is opened.
- May be used postoperatively for infants with upper airway surgery—for example, in choanal atresia repair.

Mist Tent

- Rarely used in pediatric care for oxygen delivery since the introduction of adhesive disks that allow cannulas to be secured to an infant or child's cheeks.
- Difficult to maintain FIO_2 when opening tent to access patient.

Assess Effectiveness of Oxygen Therapy

An oxygenation assessment should always include a respiratory assessment along with SpO_2; the frequency of assessments depends on the patient's acuity and stability: from continuous monitoring in critical care, intermittent Q2H for the patient who has the potential to deteriorate or is labile, Q4H for acute respiratory admission, Q4H to Q6H for the stable acute patient, Q6H when weaning, and Q8H for the chronic patient until stable. Continuous SpO_2 monitoring of general care patients often leads to nuisance alarms and has been shown to lengthen hospitalization stays.

Adjustment

Oxygen flowrate or FIO_2 should be adjusted to meet the SpO_2 goals or until a specific clinical goal is reached (e.g., carboxyhemoglobin level less than 5%). Generally, as the FIO_2 requirement drops, masks are transitioned to the nasal cannula for its ease of use during feeding, ambulation, etc.

Documentation and Communication

Document all respiratory assessments with SpO_2 in the medical record along with any adjustments in oxygen administration. Any time oxygen is initiated, the need for it has increased significantly, and/or the FIO_2 exceeds 0.40 or the patient's SpO_2 does not reach the desired goal, the medical team should be notified to discuss additional treatment and/or diagnostic examinations (chest x-ray, laboratory tests, etc.) to identify and treat the underlying condition.

Airway Clearance Protocol
For the Pediatric Patient
PROTOCOL 34.2

Order for Airway Clearance Protocol

Evaluate for Indications

- Difficulty with secretion clearance
- Muscle weakness impairing normal airway clearance
- Sedation impairing normal cough and airway clearance
- Evidence of retained bronchial secretions
- Chest x-ray (CXR) demonstrates atelectasis secondary to mucous plugging
- Cystic fibrosis (CF), primary ciliary dyskinesia
- Accumulation of purulent secretions in bronchopneumonia
- Residual secretions and debris after foreign body removal

Choose Applicable Techniques Based on Patient Age, Cooperation, Ability to Cough, and Disease Process

Suctioning

- **Endotracheal suctioning** is applicable to infants and children with an endotracheal tube or tracheostomy tube (PRN).
- **Hypopharyngeal suction** is applicable to infants or children with airway secretions who are unable to cough on demand because of age, muscle weakness, or mental capacity (PRN).
- Noninvasive suction (use of olive-tipped suction catheter [i.e., BBG] or Yankauer catheter) is often used as an adjunct to gently remove secretions from the nares of small infants, the mouths of children with limited ability to cough, or the stoma area of chronic tracheostomy patients (PRN).

Cough Assist

- Applicable to a child with muscle weakness or lack of motor control to produce an effective cough (spinal muscular atrophy or muscular dystrophy). A **cough assist device** will deliver a pressurized breath and then apply negative pressure to bring lower airway secretions into the upper airway for removal by oral suction. Frequency based on Neuromuscular Disorder Score.
- Inspiratory/expiratory pressures of 30 to 40 cm H_2O are needed for effective therapy.
- Contraindicated in patients with an effective cough.

Cough and Deep Breathing

- Indicated in all children who are able to cooperate and cough on demand with every encounter.
- Diaphragmatic breathing with pursed lip breathing is often used to relax an asthmatic child or a child with CF.
- **Huff cough** is used for effective coughing with CF patient's therapies.
- Adjuncts may be used to encourage deep breathing and mobilization of secretions (e.g., incentive spirometry, blowing bubbles, blowing pinwheels, laughing). Choose technique that matches the child's age and ability to perform.

Flutter Valve, Positive Expiratory Pressure, and Oscillatory Positive Expiratory Pressure

- These techniques are used in cooperative children to encourage deep breathing and mobilization of secretions. Frequency depends on patient presentation. Any secretion-related atelectasis with hypoxemia requiring supplemental

Protocol 34.2 cont'd on page 515

oxygen should increase treatment to Q4H or more frequently. Routine care at BID to QID.

- Effective in patients with secretion-related atelectasis, bronchopneumonia, and/or chronic obstructive pulmonary disease.
- These therapies can be used for home therapy as well.
- These techniques encourage active participation in patients who may be passive with other therapies.

Chest Physical Therapy, Postural Drainage, and Percussion

Indications

- Secretion-related atelectasis, bronchitis, CF, and other childhood conditions in which lower airway secretions are retained. Q4H for acute presentation, and BID to QID for chronic condition.
- May be used for localized removal of secretions or debris after foreign body removal.
- Choice of chest physiotherapy or postural drainage because the method of bronchial hygiene depends on history of effectiveness, patient preference, ability to actively cough with each position, and risk versus benefit of positioning (i.e., risk for extubation while on ventilator).
- Medicated aerosol therapy may be helpful before or after this procedure.
- Postural drainage is routinely used for airway clearance in patients with neuromuscular disease and cystic fibrosis.

Contraindications

- Manual or mechanical percussion technique with positioning is currently contraindicated in newborns and young infants with highly compliant chest walls.
- A meta-analysis of chest physical therapy in bronchiolitis and asthma showed that it is not effective.
- Gastrophangeal reflux and the risk for intraventricular hemorrhage in newborns and young infants make positioning in a head-down position contraindicated.
- Generally not performed when active hemoptysis is present.

Percussive Vest Therapy

- Alternative to chest physical therapy and postural drainage in secretion-related atelectasis (Q4H to QID). BID for chronic care.
- Size of vest may limit use in younger patients.
- Alternative "wrap" vest may allow for easy application in ventilated patients.
- Common method for airway clearance in chronic patients while hospitalized and at home.
- Patient may be able to take aerosol treatment during vest therapy.
- Vest does not require gravity-dependent positioning.

Intrapulmonary Percussive Ventilation or MetaNeb

- These intrapulmonary percussive or high-frequency oscillatory ventilation techniques are generally used with older cooperative pediatric patients. The patient uses a mouthpiece to inspire from a self-activated manifold. These devices deliver aerosolized medication while pulsating to mobilize secretions and stimulate cough (Q4H in acute care, BID to QID in chronic care).
- For younger or less cooperative patients, use a positive pressure mask.
- Patient preference and history of effectiveness determine use.
- Both devices also can be placed in line with a ventilator to mobilize secretions.
- Contraindications: This device delivers a pressure that could be dangerous in patients with a pneumothorax or at risk for air leak.
- Endotracheal application in smaller infants could contribute to unplanned extubation.

Medications to Facilitate Airway Clearance

- Bronchodilators are used to improve aeration in patients with reactive airways disease and to promote an effective cough (Q4H or BID to QID as an adjunct to airway clearance).
- Hypertonic saline (3%) is an option for the treatment of copious secretions in bronchiolitis after several days of admission (TID).
- Hypertonic saline 3% to 7% has been recommended for the mobilization of secretions in CF and primary ciliary dyskinesia (BID to QID).
- DNAse Pulmozyme (dornase alfa) is a mucolytic that breaks down the DNA of white blood cells to thin secretions in CF (QD or BID).

Bronchoscopy

- Assist with bronchoscopy in nonresolving atelectasis.

Assess Clinical Improvement Techniques After Each Treatment

Clinical Improvement Includes

- Breath sounds clear after treatment
- FIO_2 decreases, SpO_2 increases
- Subjective improvement
- Objective improvement: Patient up and playing
- CXR improves
- On ventilator, airway resistance and lung compliance improve.

Weaning of Therapy

- Reduce frequency of therapy to daytime hours (QID, TID, BID) or at least Q6H at night.
- The Neuromuscular Disease Score is used in spinal muscular atrophy to determine frequency of airway clearance.
- Discontinue treatment in acute conditions if improvement is sustained over 24 hours treatment.
- Decrease treatment frequency to home regimen in chronic pulmonary conditions.
- Consider lung expansion therapy if bronchial hygiene therapy is too painful for patient cooperation.

Lung Expansion Therapy Protocol
For the Pediatric Patient
PROTOCOL 34.3

Goals
- To encourage cough and deep breathing
- To prevent postoperative atelectasis
- To reverse lung consolidation
- To treat obstructive sleep apnea (continuous positive airway pressure [CPAP])

Is the patient cooperative and able to breathe without assistance? Yes or No?

If yes, consider the following common pediatric treatment modalities.

Incentive Spirometry
- Primarily a technique for deep breathing and coughing.
- Can be a lung expansion technique in an older, cooperative child to prevent and treat atelectasis.
- Alternative deep-breathing therapies to substitute for younger children include blowing bubbles, blowing a pinwheel, laughing, etc. Emphasize the deep breathing before blowing.
- Encourage active coughing and expectoration.
- Frequency is usually (Q2H to Q4H) and supervised in the beginning and then tapered as the patient and family are able to assume care and the patient is not requiring oxygen.
- Reevaluate effectiveness Q24H.

Positive Expiratory Pressure or Oscillatory Positive Expiratory Pressure Therapy
- Indicated when there is evidence of lung consolidation with mild oxygen requirement.
- Positive expiratory pressure supports lower airway integrity and improves ventilation distribution.
- Effective in mobilizing secretions, particularly in cystic fibrosis.
- Encourages active coughing and expectoration.
- Frequency of Q2H to Q4H and supervised in the beginning; wean to QID once oxygen is no longer required to maintain SpO_2.

Is the patient cooperative and able to deep breathe without assistance? Yes or No?

If no, consider these common treatment modalities.

Intermittent Positive Pressure Breathing Therapy
CAUTION: *Active application of positive pressure is contraindicated when there is evidence of untreated air leak, such as pneumomediastinum, pneumothorax, subcutaneous air, etc.*
- Intermittent application of positive airway pressure on inspiration; patient triggers breath with inspiratory effort for a 15-minute treatment.
- Pressure is adjusted to achieve good breath sounds and may be volume targeted to achieve one-third of predicted inspiratory capacity.

- May be applied by mask in patients unable to cooperate or by mouthpiece for cooperative patients.
- Generally used when there is chest x-ray (CXR) evidence of volume-related atelectasis.
- Patient may be positioned to elevate involved segment for better aeration.
- Frequency may be Q2 to Q4H at first, then tapered to Q4H to Q6H until CXR improves or oxygen requirement subsides.

Continuous Positive Airway Pressure Therapy
- Generally applied noninvasively via nasal mask, oronasal mask, or full-face mask.
- Provides continuous positive airway pressure to build functional residual capacity and reverse atelectasis in the spontaneously breathing patient.
- Requires continuous pulse oximetry for acute use.
- CPAP pressure is adjusted to patient comfort, degree of atelectasis, and oxygen requirement, generally 5 to 10 cm H_2O pressure.
- May be applied during sleep for children with obstructive sleep apnea at the CPAP pressure prescribed after a CPAP titration sleep study.
- Pressures above 15 cm H_2O should be avoided because it can interfere with venous return.

Reevaluate the Patient's Progress Toward Specific Goals with Every Intervention
Improvement is suggested by the following:
- Decreased respiratory rate
- Normal pulse rate
- Absence of fever
- Improved aeration over affected segment/lung field per breath sounds
- Resolution of atelectasis on CXR
- Improved muscle strength and effective cough
- Patient ambulation
- No supplemental oxygen required for SpO_2 goal

If goals are reached and patient's condition is improving: Reduce frequency and wean to most appropriate therapy for level of cooperation and participation. Consider family-directed care.

If patient does not improve: Advance care to intermittent positive pressure breathing or noninvasive CPAP or bilevel positive airway pressure (BPAP). Consult with medical team for possible invasive support via mechanical ventilation with PEEP.

Document all assessments and communicate with medical team frequently if the patient does not progress as expected.

Recommend arterial blood gas examination when ineffective ventilation is a suspected cause of hypoxemia.

NOTE: *In premature infants with respiratory distress syndrome, these therapies are applied in conjunction with surfactant administration.*

Aerosolized Medication Protocol

For the Pediatric Patient
PROTOCOL 34.4

Indications

- To reverse bronchospasm and reduce work of breathing
- To determine response to bronchodilators or the presence of reversible airways disease (trial)
- To maximize ventilation before bronchial hygiene
- To reduce airway edema in croup
- To liquefy and mobilize secretions
- To reduce airway inflammation and reactivity
- To provide topical antibiotics for treatment or prophylaxis

Methods of Delivery

Medicated Aerosol by Hand-Held Nebulizer

- These aerosolized medications are commonly delivered by nebulizer: Tobi (tobramycin solution for inhalation), DNase, hypertonic saline, racemic epinephrine, Duo-Neb (albuterol/ipratropium).
- The nebulizer used may be specific to the drug, because the U.S. Food and Drug Administration (FDA) approval of the drug includes the nebulizer used in the clinical trial (e.g., Budesonide Respules, Tobi, and DNase are to be nebulized in the Pari LC nebulizer*).
- A mouthpiece is preferred over a mask for improved medication delivery; a mask may be used in a young, uncooperative child.
- Breath-activated nebulizers have been shown to improve drug delivery.

*The **Pari LC nebulizer** is an effective jet nebulizer that is breath-enhanced and produces consistent respirable particle size.

Metered Dose Inhaler With Valved Holding Chamber or Spacer

- Use of metered dose inhaler (MDI) with valved holding chamber (VHC) in the hospital allows the patient to practice proper technique for home use with each treatment.
- Infants can be treated effectively with MDI-VHC with mask.
- If policy is to provide asthma patients with individual MDI during hospital stay, this will ensure that the patient has an understanding of the MDI and VHC at discharge for continued care.

Dry Powder Inhalers

- Several parasympatholytics, inhaled corticosteroids, and combination long-acting bronchodilators/inhaled corticosteroids come in a dry powder with a unique inhaler, which requires a coordinated breathing effort and a high peak inspiratory flowrate. These may not be suitable for young children under 6 years of age.

Continuous Albuterol Aerosol

- Children in status asthmaticus are often advanced to a continuous albuterol aerosol, which can run for hours until symptoms subside.
- Dosing can vary from 5 to 20 mg/h, using a syringe pump and a **vibrating mesh nebulizer** or a large-volume medication nebulizer.
- Continuous electrocardiographic monitoring is required, and often this care is provided in an intensive care unit or emergency department (see the Procedure for Continuous Albuterol Aerosol Administration in this protocol).

Disease-Specific Drugs in Hospitalization

Disease	Type of Medication	Drug	Method	Frequency
Asthma/reactive airways disease	Rescue bronchodilator	Albuterol	Aerosol or MDI-VHC	Q20 minutes in emergency department, Q2H to Q6H inpatient, continuous in status. Up to 20 mg/h (see the Procedure for Continuous Albuterol Aerosol Administration in this protocol) (some institutions use higher concentrations)
	Controller	Inhaled corticosteroids	MDI DPI aerosol	QD or BID
Bronchiolitis caused by viral illness	Bronchodilator	Albuterol	Aerosol	Rescue trial only for high bronchiolitis score, although not recommended for routine care

Protocol 34.4 cont'd on page 518

Disease	Type of Medication	Drug	Method	Frequency
	Bronchodilator with alpha effect that causes vasoconstriction and reduces edema	Racemic epinephrine	Aerosol	Rescue trial only for high bronchiolitis score, although not recommended for routine care
Croup	Bronchodilator with alpha effect that causes vasoconstriction and reduces edema	Racemic epinephrine	Aerosol	PRN for croup score in moderate range
Cystic fibrosis	Bronchodilator	Albuterol	Aerosol	QID and PRN
	Mucolytic	Hypertonic saline	Aerosol or intrapulmonary percussive delivery	QID
	Mucolytic	DNase	Aerosol	QD or BID
	Antibiotic	Variety of antibiotics specific to the patient's sensitivity: for example, Tobi, colistin, Cayston (aztreonam), amphotericin	Aerosol	QD or BID
HIV positive/ immunosuppressed patient	Antibiotic prophylaxis	Pentamidine	Aerosol via filtered circuit and HEPA[†] system	Q30 days

[†]High-efficiency particulate absorption (HEPA) refers to a filter used to protect the caregiver (e.g., HEPA hood) during treatment or clearing the room (room HEPA filter) after a treatment.

DPI, Dry powder inhaler; *MDI,* metered dose inhaler; *VHC,* valved holding chamber.

Assessment and Weaning

- Patients who are receiving aerosolized medications for acute relief are assessed at every encounter. Frequency of therapy is actively weaned using disease-specific scoring systems, such as asthma, bronchiolitis, or croup protocol.
- Any time patient does not progress as expected or needs to increase the frequency of aerosols to gain relief, the medical team must be notified to discuss need for additional treatment or diagnostic examinations.
- Chronic patients are weaned to their home regimen.

Education

During assessments or treatments, particularly in the case of families with infants or children with chronic respiratory disease, the respiratory therapist should reinforce proper breathing technique, medication delivery, trigger avoidance, airway clearance, and when to seek medical help.

Procedure for Continuous Albuterol Aerosol Administration

Method 1

Using a **large-volume medication nebulizer,** such as a HEART nebulizer: see Table below

Drug Dose (mg/h)	IV Pump Rate (mL/h)	Albuterol (mL)	Saline (mL)	Total Volume (mL)	Duration (h)
5	12	4	44	48	4
10	12	8	40	48	4
15	12	12	36	48	4
20	12	16	32	48	4

Protocol 34.4 cont'd on page 519

- Place 100 mL of normal saline into the HEART nebulizer.
- Add 16 mL of 0.5% albuterol (5 mg/mL × 16 mL = 80 mg of albuterol).
- Set flowmeter for the source gas at 10 L/min. At this flowrate, the nebulizer will nebulize over 4 hours, delivering approximately 20 mg of albuterol/h.

Method 2

Using a medication syringe pump with a small volume vibrating mesh nebulizer, such as the Aerogen:

- Determine desired albuterol dosing per hour.
- Using the following chart, mix specific albuterol volume with the normal saline volume and draw the mixture in a 60-mL syringe.
- Attach the intravenous tubing to the syringe and the nebulizer.
- Prime the intravenous tubing, pushing the syringe until the solution reaches the nebulizer.
- Place the syringe in the pump and set the pump to 12 mL/h.

Mechanical Ventilation and Ventilator Weaning
For the Pediatric Patient
PROTOCOL 34.5

Modes

- Modes will vary as significantly as in adult care because of the wide range of conditions requiring ventilation—for example, trauma, chronic and acute obstructive respiratory disease, neuromuscular weakness, respiratory depression, restrictive or parenchymal pulmonary disease, congenital disorders, infectious disease, acute respiratory distress syndrome (ARDS), etc. Follow Oxygen Therapy Protocol, Protocol 11.1 (see Chapter 11), for choice of ventilator mode.
- A ventilator with newborn, pediatric, and adult modes and capabilities is best suited to the pediatric intensive care unit. These ventilators must have the sensitivity to (1) detect the inspiratory effort of a small infant to an adult-sized teen, (2) deliver an accurate tidal volume across the newborn to adult spectrum, and (3) have a range of flowrates to meet both the minimal inspiratory demands of a newborn and the largest, air-hungry teen (e.g., Servo-i, Avea, PB 840, Drager V500, Hamilton G5).
- The choice of ventilator mode and method of triggering will depend on airway leaks, patient breathing effort, use of sedation or paralysis, and underlying disease state.
- Nasal intermittent positive pressure ventilation is preferred to invasive ventilation when it can assist the spontaneously breathing patient. Many critical care ventilators have noninvasive modes that are applicable through a variety of mask interfaces. Gaining a child's cooperation to wear a mask takes time and supervision to ensure continued use.
- Most pediatric intensive care units have both conventional and high-frequency options for providing ventilation to those children with severe hypoxemia requiring higher mean arterial pressures (MAPs).
- Generally, infant ventilator circuits accommodate tidal volumes up to 120 mL; pediatric/adult circuits are used for tidal volumes above 80 to 100 mL.
- Acute ventilator patients are typically monitored continuously with pulse oximetry and capnography.

Settings

Delivered tidal volume (V_T)[†]: 6 to 10 mL/kg. Generally, 6 to 8 mL is the common starting point, unless the patient has obstructive lung disease, in which case higher volume may be preferred because of increased physiologic dead space. Lower volumes are preferred when resulting PIP exceeds 35 cm H_2O pressure.

Inspiratory time (IT): 0.5 to 1.2 seconds with the shorter IT for infants and longer IT for older patients or children with obstructive disease.

Respiratory rate (RR): Age appropriate to produce a normal ventilation pattern, usually 12 to 30 breaths/min, with 30 for infants and as low as 12 for teens. Higher rates may be used when there is a need to increase MAP in patients who cannot tolerate increased PEEP or PIP.

Peak inspiratory pressure (PIP): In pressure cycled modes, adjust PIP to a pressure that produces an easy breath, bilateral aeration, and normal chest rise; when exhaled volume measurement is available, adjust PIP to achieve desired V_T of 6 to 10 mL/kg.

Positive end-expiratory pressure (PEEP): Generally, this should be set with the patient's lung condition in mind: 4 to 5 cm H_2O is a common starting point for nearly all patients. In restrictive disease, the PEEP may need to be significantly increased, watching the patient's pressure-volume hysteresis curve and volume delivery to achieve optimal PEEP. In obstructive disease, the PEEP is typically set to 4 to 5 cm H_2O to provide airway stenting; IT and rate need to be adjusted to avoid auto-PEEP (air trapping), which can occur with insufficient expiratory time.

Pressure support: Commonly used to overcome endotracheal resistance with spontaneous breathing. Level is set to provide an easy, unlabored breath with spontaneous efforts.

[†]*NOTE:* Newer ventilators can be set to correct for compressible tubing volume—that is, the volume that expands the ventilator tubing that is not delivered to the patients. In older machines, compressible volume should be calculated, particularly in the younger patient. It is calculated as (PIP-PEEP) in centimeters of water pressure × tubing factor (i.e., 1 to 3 mL/cm H_2O pressure depending on the size of circuit used); subtract this volume from the displayed exhaled volume to determine the actual delivered tidal volume.

Protocol 34.5 cont'd on page 520

Adjustment and Weaning of Patients With Clinical Improvement

- The child's clinical condition will affect the speed of weaning. Those receiving ventilation for respiratory depression (i.e., postseizure, postoperative, postnarcotic overdose) will typically wean quickly as soon as the respiratory depression reverses.
- Those who have chronic pulmonary disease with an acute exacerbation or a condition such as acute respiratory distress syndrome (ARDS), an immunosuppressive disorder, a neuromuscular weakness, or congenital heart disease may require a longer weaning period, requiring a variety of modes to reach weaning goals.
- Follow adult Ventilator Weaning Protocol, Protocol 11.2.
- Assessing Extubation Readiness in the Weaning Infant or Child:
  - An extubation readiness tool (ERT) can be used each shift to determine a patient's readiness for a spontaneous breathing trial (SBT). The goal of the ERT and SBT efforts is to reduce the number of unnecessary intubated days, reducing unplanned extubations and ventilator associated events.
  - The ERT takes into consideration the patient's spontaneous ventilation effort, moderate ventilator settings, moderate oxygen requirement, clinical stability, required sedation, and needs, such as continued mechanical ventilation based on medical necessity or upcoming surgical procedures, etc. The infant either passes of fails this ERT assessment; failing any one criteria causes the patient to fail.
  - The spontaneous breathing trial is on a moderate level of CPAP with pressure support, i.e., 8cm H_2O/5 cm H_2O for one hour. The patient's ability to maintain his oxygenation (SPO_2) at the current FiO2 while demonstrating cardiovascular stability (HR, RR, BP, etc.) without increased respiratory distress during the SBT indicates a successful test. Nursing is always involved in the SBT timing and assessment.

- The patient's extubation readiness (assessment per ERT) and the (pass or fail) outcome of their daily SBT when indicated and completed, is shared daily at with the medical management team at rounds and documented in the EHR.

Adjustment and Weaning of Patients With Worsening Condition

- For patients who worsen because of ARDS or consolidation, lung recruitment strategies are needed. This typically involves higher PEEP to increase functional residual capacity (FRC) and a raised MAP.
- Airway pressure-release ventilation (APRV) and high-frequency ventilation (HFV) are ventilator strategies that may be considered when the PIP exceeds 35 cm H_2O pressure (plateau pressure above 30 cm H_2O) or when oxygenation index exceeds 24 (see Oxygen Therapy Protocol, Protocol 34.1).
- Sedation and paralysis may be required in patients requiring a significantly high MAP.
- If high-frequency oscillatory ventilation (HFOV) is initiated, settings should begin with MAP at 5 above the conventional setting, rate at 5 to 6 Hz (300 to 360 oscillations/min), inspiratory time at 33%, and amplitude set to produce the classic "chest wiggle" down to the midthigh region. Lower frequency hertz will increase bulk movement and help with carbon dioxide elimination. Children over 35 kg need an oscillator with increased flow capacity and power.
- Permissive hypercapnia becomes a physiologic goal when ventilation parameters increase and become more likely to induce ventilator-associated lung injury.
- Volumetric carbon dioxide monitoring may be helpful in adjusting ventilator settings in patients who may be difficult to manage with increased physiologic dead space.
- Neurally adjusted ventilatory assistance (NAVA) may be helpful in weaning patients who are weak or who have problems with asynchrony with spontaneous breathing efforts.

SELF-ASSESSMENT QUESTIONS

1. According to the Glasgow Coma Scale, a patient is considered comatose with a score of:
   a. 15 or less
   b. 10 or less
   c. 8 or less
   d. Below 3

2. The normal respiratory rate of a toddler is:
   a. 12 to 16 breaths/min
   b. 18 to 30 breaths/min
   c. 22 to 34 breaths/min
   d. 24 to 40 breaths/min

3. The cause of whooping cough is:
   a. *Bordetella pertussis*
   b. Parainfluenza type I
   c. *Haemophilus influenzae* type B
   d. *Staphylococcus aureus*

4. Which of the following muscle causes head bobbing in the child with respiratory distress?
   a. Internal oblique
   b. Sternocleidomastoids
   c. Pectoralis major
   d. Trapezius

5. Which of the following is most indicated for a child who is having (1) difficulty with secretion clearance, (2) muscle weakness impairing normal airway clearance, and (3) evidence of retained bronchial secretions?
   a. Oxygen therapy protocol
   b. Airway clearance protocol
   c. Lung expansion therapy protocol
   d. Aerosolized medication protocol

35 Meconium Aspiration Syndrome

Chapter Objectives

After reading this chapter, you will be able to:

- List the anatomic alterations of the lungs associated with meconium aspiration.
- Describe the causes of meconium aspiration.
- List the cardiopulmonary clinical manifestations associated with meconium aspiration syndrome.
- Describe the general management of meconium aspiration.
- Describe the clinical strategies and rationales of the SOAPs presented in the case study.
- Define key terms and complete self-assessment questions at the end of the chapter and on Evolve.

Key Terms

"Ball-Valve" Effect
Capillary Blood Gas (CBG) Samples
Chemical Pneumonitis
Colorimetric CO_2 Detector
Extracorporeal Membrane Oxygenation (ECMO)
High-Frequency Oscillatory Ventilation (HFOV)

Inhaled Nitric Oxide (iNO)
High-Frequency Jet Ventilation (HFJV)
Meconium
Meconium Aspiration Syndrome (MAS)
Meconium Stained Amniotic Fluid
Neonatal Resuscitation Program (NRP) Guidelines
Persistent Pulmonary Hypertension of the Newborn (PPHN)
Pneumomediastinum
Pneumothorax
Umbilical Arterial Catheter
Upper Airway Obstruction (UAO)

Chapter Outline

Anatomic Alterations of the Lungs
Etiology and Epidemiology
Overview of the Cardiopulmonary Clinical Manifestations
    Associated With Meconium Aspiration Syndrome
General Management of Meconium Aspiration Syndrome
Case Study: Meconium Aspiration Syndrome
Self-Assessment Questions

Anatomic Alterations of the Lungs

During normal intrauterine fetal development, the fetus periodically demonstrates normal rapid, shallow respiratory chest movements. This normal action moves pulmonary fetal fluid into and out of the oropharynx while the glottis remains closed. During periods of fetal hypoxemia, however, the fetus may demonstrate very deep, gasping inspiratory movements that may force the contents of the nasooropharynx to pass through the glottis into the airways. The aspiration of minimal amounts of clear amniotic fluid is not usually associated with serious anatomic or functional problems of the lungs. During fetal hypoxemia, however, the aspirate may contain **meconium** and amniotic fluid—hence the phrase **meconium aspiration syndrome (MAS)**.

MAS is a clinical entity seen primarily in full-term or post-term infants who have had some degree of fetal stress or hypoxemia either prenatally or during the birth process. Meconium is the material that collects in the intestine of the fetus and forms the first stools of the newborn. Meconium, an odorless, thick, sticky, blackish-green material, is a heterogeneous mixture of aspirated intestinal tract secretions, amniotic fluid, pulmonary fetal fluid, and intrauterine debris such as

epithelial cells, mucus, lanugo, blood, and vernix. When the fetus experiences in utero hypoxia, the intestinal response is vasoconstriction, increased gastrointestinal peristalsis, anal sphincter relaxation, and passage of meconium into the amniotic fluid. Aspiration of meconium leads to one or more of the following complications.

First, MAS causes **chemical pneumonitis**, which is characterized by an acute inflammatory reaction and edema of the bronchial mucosa and alveolar epithelium. This reaction commonly leads to excessive bronchial secretions and alveolar consolidation. Meconium also promotes the growth of bacteria, which in turn augments the development of alveolar pneumonitis, infection, and consolidation. Meconium aspiration can interfere with alveolar pulmonary surfactant production. When this occurs, respiratory distress syndrome may complicate MAS.

Second, the physical presence of the meconium may result in an **upper airway obstruction (UAO)** at birth because of the high viscosity of the meconium. In addition, if gasping inspirations are present after delivery, clumps of meconium can rapidly migrate past the glottis and penetrate the smaller airways (Fig. 35.1). However, it has been found that in most cases of MAS, meconium is already present in the distal airways at birth. Although MAS primarily causes a restrictive lung pathophysiology, when thick particulate meconium is aspirated into the small airways, the meconium can partially or totally obstruct the airways. Airways that are partially obstructed are affected by a **"ball-valve" effect**, in which air can enter but cannot readily leave the distal airways and alveoli. This condition, in turn, may lead to air trapping and alveolar hyperinflation. Excessive hyperinflation may lead to alveolar rupture and air leak syndromes (see Chapter 38, Pulmonary Air Leak Syndrome) such as **pneumomediastinum** or **pneumothorax**. Totally obstructed airways lead to alveolar shrinkage and atelectasis. This combination of areas of overexpanded alveoli adjacent to areas of atelectasis creates both an increased functional residual capacity (FRC) and a decrease in air flow during exhalation.

Third, because of the hypoxemia associated with MAS, infants with the condition often develop hypoxia-induced pulmonary arterial vasoconstriction and vasospasm, which cause pulmonary hypertension. This results in blood shunting from *right-to-left* through the ductus arteriosus and the foramen ovale; intrapulmonary shunts are also occasionally seen. Therefore the blood flow is diverted away from the lungs (pulmonary hypoperfusion), which worsens the hypoxemia. Clinically, this condition is referred to as **persistent pulmonary hypertension of the newborn (PPHN)**.

The major pathologic or structural changes associated with MAS are as follows:
- Physical presence of the meconium leading to:
  - Partially obstructed airways, air trapping, and alveolar hyperinflation
  - Pulmonary air leak syndromes (pneumomediastinum or pneumothorax)
  - Totally obstructed airways and absorption atelectasis
  - Edema of the bronchial mucosa and alveolar epithelium
  - Excessive bronchial secretions
  - Alveolar consolidation (or secondary infection)
  - Disrupted pulmonary surfactant production

Etiology and Epidemiology

Meconium-stained amniotic fluid (MSAF) complicates nearly 8% of deliveries. As shown in Fig. 35.2, the prevalence of severe MAS increases with gestational age. About 30% to 50% of infants with severe MAS will require mechanical ventilation or continuous positive airway pressure (CPAP). As discussed earlier, the fetal passage of meconium is caused by fetal hypoxemia and stress. Fetal hypoxemia causes a vagal response that relaxes anal sphincter tone and allows meconium to move into the amniotic fluid. MAS is rarely seen in infants born at less than 36 weeks' gestation because the release of meconium requires strong peristalsis and sphincter tone, which are not usually present in preterm infants. Thus postterm infants (infants born after 42 weeks' gestation) are especially at risk for MAS, because both strong peristalsis and sphincter tone are present in babies of this age.

Other infants who are at high risk for MAS are those who are small for gestational age, those who are delivered in the breech position, and those whose mothers are toxemic, hypertensive, or obese.

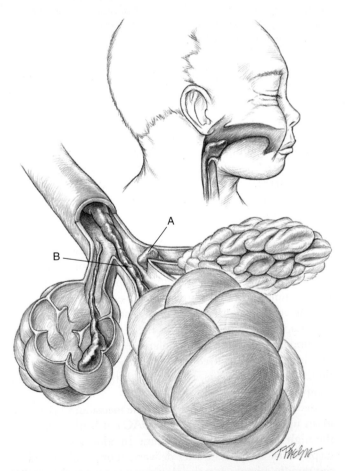

FIGURE 35.1 Meconium aspiration syndrome. (A) Total obstruction with meconium causing alveolar atelectasis. (B) Partial obstruction causing air trapping and alveolar hyperinflation.

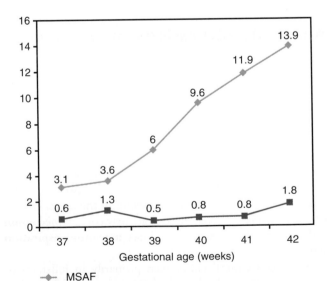

FIGURE 35.2 Percentage of meconium-stained amniotic fluid (MSAF) and meconium aspiration syndrome (MAS) in a retrospective review of 2000 to 2007 births in Burgundy, France. (From Fischer C, Rybakowski C, Ferdynus C, et al. A population-based study of meconium aspiration syndrome in neonates between 37 and 43 weeks of gestation. Int J Pediatric 2012;2012: 321545.)

The following clinical manifestations result from the pathologic mechanisms caused (or activated) by atelectasis (see Fig. 10.7), alveolar consolidation (see Fig. 10.8), excessive bronchial secretions and debris (see Fig. 10.11), and airway obstruction—the major anatomic alterations of the lungs associated with MAS (see Fig. 35.1).

CLINICAL DATA OBTAINED AT THE PATIENT'S BEDSIDE

The Physical Examination

Vital Signs

Increased Respiratory Rate (Tachypnea)

Normally, a newborn infant's respiratory rate is about 40 to 60 breaths/min. In MAS the respiratory rate generally is well over 60 breaths/min. Several pathophysiologic mechanisms operating simultaneously may lead to an increased ventilatory rate:

- Stimulation of the peripheral chemoreceptors (hypoxemia)
- Relationship of decreased lung compliance to increased ventilatory rate
- Stimulation of the central chemoreceptors
- Increased temperature

Increased Heart Rate (Pulse) and Blood Pressure

Apnea (see Box 33.3)

Clinical Manifestations Associated With More Negative Intrapleural Pressure During Inspiration

- Intercostal retractions
- Substernal retraction and abdominal distention (seesaw movement)
- Nasal flaring

Chest Assessment Findings

- Wheezes
- Crackles

Expiratory Grunting

Cyanosis

Common General Appearance

- **Meconium staining** (brownish-yellow color) on:
  - Skin
  - Nails
  - Umbilical cord
  - Wrinkles and creases in the skin

Barrel chest (when airways are partially obstructed)

CLINICAL DATA OBTAINED FROM LABORATORY TESTS AND SPECIAL PROCEDURES

Pulmonary Function Test Findings
(Extrapolated Data for Instructional Purposes)
(Primarily Restrictive Lung Pathophysiology)

The anatomic alterations of the lungs associated with MAS primarily cause a restrictive lung pathophysiology. For example, in moderate to severe cases the following lung volumes and capacities may be lower than normal.

RV	IRV	VC	FRC	TLC
↓	↓	↓	↓	↓

When thick particulate meconium is aspirated into the small airways, the meconium may cause partial obstruction, air trapping, and alveolar hyperinflation. In these cases, an obstructive lung pathophysiology may develop—for example, the following might be greater than normal.

RV	FRC
↑	↑

Arterial Blood Gases[1]

MILD TO MODERATE MECONIUM ASPIRATION SYNDROME
Acute Alveolar Hyperventilation With Hypoxemia[2]
(Acute Respiratory Alkalosis)

pH	PaCO$_2$	HCO$_3^-$	PaO$_2$	SaO$_2$ or SpO$_2$
↑	↓	↓ (but normal)	↓	↓

SEVERE MECONIUM ASPIRATION SYNDROME
Acute Ventilatory Failure With Hypoxemia[3]
(Acute Respiratory Acidosis)

pH[4]	PaCO$_2$	HCO$_3^-$[4]	PaO$_2$	SaO$_2$ or SpO$_2$
↓	↑	↑ (but normal)	↓	↓

[1]*NOTE:* A critically ill newborn is likely to have an **umbilical arterial catheter** in place for arterial blood gas (ABG) sampling. In older critically ill infants and children, an arterial line may be placed for frequent ABG sampling. For intermittent sampling, because of the difficulty of obtaining ABG samples from newborn and pediatric patients, **capillary blood gas (CBG) samples** may be used to determine the pH, PaCO$_2$, and HCO$_3^-$ (i.e., the acid-base and ventilation status only). Capillary PO$_2$ values are unreliable and should not be used for clinical analysis. The standard way to evaluate the oxygenation status in these infants is pulse oximetry (SpO$_2$) (see Chapter 33, Newborn Assessment and Management).
[2]See Fig. 5.2 and Table 5.4 and related discussions for the acute pH, PaCO$_2$, and HCO$_3^-$ changes associated with acute alveolar hyperventilation.
[3]See Table 5.5 and related discussion for the acute pH, PaCO$_2$, and HCO$_3^-$ changes associated with acute ventilatory failure.
[4]When tissue hypoxia is severe enough to produce lactic acid, the pH and HCO$_3^-$ values will be lower than expected for a particular PaCO$_2$ level.

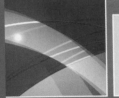
Oxygenation Indices[5]

$\dot{Q}_S/\dot{Q}_T$	DO_2[6]	$\dot{V}O_2$	$C(a\text{-}\bar{v})O_2$	O_2ER	$S\bar{v}O_2$
↑	↓	N	N	↑	↓

RADIOLOGIC FINDINGS
Chest Radiograph

When alveolar atelectasis and consolidation are present, the chest radiograph shows irregular densities throughout the lungs. Although the chest radiograph is clearly different from that seen in respiratory distress syndrome, it is difficult to differentiate the radiograph appearance of MAS from that of pneumonia (Fig. 35.3).

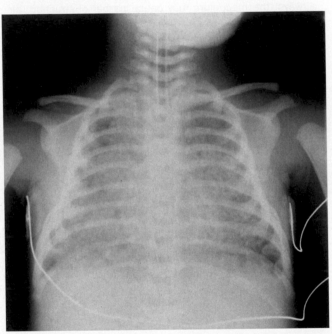

FIGURE 35.3 Chest radiograph of an infant with meconium aspiration syndrome. Patchy areas of increased density are observed in both lungs. (From Taussig, L. M., & Landau, L. I. [2008]. *Pediatric respiratory medicine* [2nd ed.]. St. Louis, MO: Elsevier.)

The chest radiograph may show local or generalized problem areas. When significant partial airway obstruction, air trapping, and alveolar hyperinflation are present, the chest radiograph appears hyperlucent and the diaphragm may be depressed. The respiratory therapist should be alert for the sudden development of a pneumothorax or pneumomediastinum in infants with MAS (Fig. 35.4).

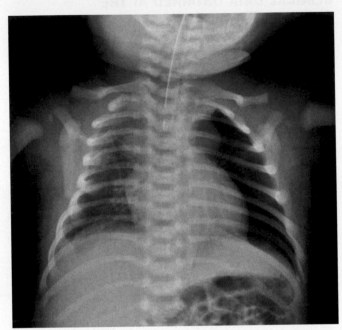

FIGURE 35.4 Meconium aspiration with left-sided pneumothorax. (Courtesy Dayton Children's Hospital, Dayton, Ohio.)

---

[5]$C(a\text{-}\bar{v})O_2$, Arterial-venous oxygen difference; DO_2, total oxygen delivery; O_2ER, oxygen extraction ratio; $\dot{Q}_S/\dot{Q}_T$, pulmonary shunt fraction; $S\bar{v}O_2$, mixed venous oxygen saturation; $\dot{V}O_2$, oxygen consumption.

[6]Because the newborn normally has a higher hemoglobin level at birth (16.8 to 18.9 g/dL), the DO_2 may actually be better than indicated by PaO_2 or SpO_2 alone (see Chapter 6, Assessment of Oxygenation).

General Management of Meconium Aspiration Syndrome

The **Neonatal Resuscitation Program (NRP) Guidelines** recommend using gentle oral suctioning for babies with meconium-stained fluids who are having difficulty clearing their airway and who are not breathing or crying. Elective intubation for the clearance of meconium-stained fluid is no longer recommended. During a resuscitation, if adequate chest rise is not able to be obtained, intubation and suctioning through the endotracheal tube may be required.

After the infant has been stabilized and transported to the neonatal intensive care unit, suctioning of the airways should be performed as needed (see Airway Clearance Protocol, Protocol 33.2). Although postural drainage and percussion may seem an appropriate therapy for the removal of thick meconium in the airway, the marginal effectiveness of this technique on a newborn's compliant chest wall is not worth the risk for overstimulation in these very ill infants.

Appropriate oxygen therapy should be administered per protocol (see Oxygen Therapy Protocol, Protocol 33.1); in severe cases, CPAP (see Lung Expansion Therapy Protocol, Protocol 33.3) or mechanical ventilation (see Ventilator Initiation and Management Protocol, Protocol 33.4) may be necessary. As already mentioned, however, mechanical ventilation should be avoided or applied cautiously to prevent the possibility of dislodging unseen particulate meconium and pushing it further down the infant's airways. In addition, a high incidence of pneumothorax is associated with MAS. If mechanical ventilation is necessary, an inspiration-to-expiration ratio that permits a long exhalation time (to allow expired gas enough time to flow past partially obstructed airways) should be used.

Finally, the infant should be monitored closely for possible superimposed infection. Antibiotics may be indicated, and steroids may be required to offset the inflammatory response in chemical pneumonitis. Because meconium aspiration disrupts normal surfactant production, exogenous pulmonary surfactant is often administered to infants with MAS (see Surfactant Administration Protocol, Protocol 33.5). Exogenous surfactant is also helpful because its low surface tension helps wash out meconium particles while replacing surfactant stores. Current evidence shows that the use of surfactant with MAS within 2 hours of delivery reduces the need for **extracorporeal membrane oxygenation (ECMO)** and decreases infant mortality.

In the event that the infant develops persistent pulmonary hypertension of the newborn, **inhaled nitric oxide (iNO)** is administered via mechanical ventilation. iNO is an inhaled gas and a potent pulmonary vasodilator. It is effective in dilating the pulmonary capillaries, which, in turn, decreases the pulmonary vascular resistance adjacent to effectively ventilated alveoli. This effect can greatly improve oxygenation by improving the ventilation-perfusion match in the ventilated regions of the damaged lung. iNO is administered in 1 to 20 parts/million (ppm) and titrated to the infant's oxygenation. When iNO fails to improve oxygenation in infants with MAS, ECMO may be required.

CASE STUDY Meconium Aspiration Syndrome

Admitting History and Physical Examination

A 38-week-gestation newborn male infant was delivered by emergency cesarean section because of sudden maternal vaginal hemorrhage. The mother, a primigravida, 19-year-old white woman, had no prenatal care. She was a heavy smoker and had an uncertain history of recreational psychopharmaceutical drug use during pregnancy. Rupture of membranes was believed to have occurred about 18 hours before delivery.

At delivery, the infant's umbilical cord was wrapped once around his neck. He was covered with meconium. He was limp and blue and did not show any spontaneous movement or respiratory effort when he was handed to the neonatologist, who was heading the resuscitation team, which also included a registered nurse and a registered respiratory therapist. With gentle suctioning, several clumps of meconium were suctioned from the infant's oral and pharyngeal areas.

Despite these efforts, the infant demonstrated no spontaneous respirations, and his heart rate was less than 60 beats/min. Because of this, manual ventilation could no longer be avoided. At this time, the respiratory therapist started positive pressure ventilation (PPV) with a bag-valve-mask resuscitation bag, at an FIO_2 of 0.21, PIP of 20 to 25 cm H_2O, and a respiratory rate of 40 breaths/min. After 30 seconds of PPV, the heart rate was less than 60, so the nurse began chest compressions at about 90 per minute, with a rhythm of three compressions to one breath. The FIO_2 was also increased to 1.0. Bilateral crackles were auscultated.

At 1 minute, the Apgar score was 1 for the heart rate. By the third minute, the heart rate was 80 beats/min. The infant was gasping occasionally and demonstrated improved color. Although compressions were stopped, bagging continued at 40 breaths/min. At 5 minutes, the Apgar score was 5 (heart rate 2, respirations 1, tone 1, reflex irritability 0, and color 1). At 10 minutes, the Apgar score was still 5. The neonatologist decided to intubate the baby with a 3.5-mm endotracheal tube (ET). The respiratory therapist confirmed the correct position of the ET by means of careful auscultation and the appearance of yellow on the **CO_2 Expiratory Gas Detector** (i.e., yellow confirms CO_2 and purple indicates no CO_2). The respiratory therapist then taped the tube at the 9.0-cm mark at the infant's lips. The baby was transferred to the neonatal intensive care unit and placed on a ventilator. Initial ventilator settings were respiratory rate (RR) 26, inspiratory time (T_I) 0.5 second, FIO_2 1.0, positive inspiratory pressure (PIP) +25, and positive end-expiratory pressure (PEEP) +5. The infant's SpO_2 was 94%. At that time the respiratory therapist documented the following in the infant's chart.

Respiratory Assessment and Plan

S N/A

O Apneic at birth, hypoactive, cyanotic, covered with meconium. Apgar score at 1 minute = 1, at 5 minutes = 5. Bilateral crackles. Meconium suctioned from oral and pharyngeal areas. SpO_2: 94%.

A • Possible MAS (meconium in airway)
- Airway secretions (meconium?) (crackles)
- Probable asphyxia episode; likely combined respiratory and metabolic acidosis (history, cyanosis)
- Adequate oxygenation and ventilation (SpO_2, auscultation, CO_2 detector)

P Mechanical Ventilation Protocol in combination with Oxygen Therapy and Lung Expansion Protocol (RR 26, FIO_2 100%, PIP +25, and PEEP 5). Airway Clearance Protocol (suction). Surfactant Protocol: Administer surfactant per physician order. Monitor closely, weaning PIP to maintain exhaled V_T of 6 mL/kg, oximetry, vital signs; watch for signs of acute air leak, pulmonary hemorrhage.

Over the next hour, an umbilical artery catheter (UAC) was inserted; it showed a pH of 7.19, $PaCO_2$ 37 mm Hg, HCO_3^- 14 mEq/L, PaO_2 87 mm Hg, and SpO_2 94%. Although the infant's skin was now completely pink, bilateral crackles were still present. The chest radiograph revealed hyperinflation in both the right and left lungs. There was whiteout of the right upper and middle lobes, most likely caused by atelectasis. Clumps of white patches of atelectasis (resembling small popcorn balls) were seen throughout the remainder of the lungs. The ET tip was at the clavicle level, and the UAC tip was appropriately positioned at T-8.

The following SOAP note was recorded.

Respiratory Assessment and Plan

S N/A

O Pink skin. Bilateral crackles. CXR: Atelectasis in the right upper and middle lobes. Air trapping right and left lower lobes. ABGs pH 7.19, $PaCO_2$ 37, HCO_3^- 14, PaO_2 87, and SpO_2 94% (on FIO_2 1.0).

A • Airway secretions (crackles)
- Atelectasis (CXR)
- Uncompensated metabolic acidosis (ABG)

P Continue Mechanical Ventilation Protocol in combination with Oxygen Therapy and Lung Expansion Therapy Protocols (RR 26, TI 0.5, FIO_2 1.0, wean PIP to +22 cm H_2O, and PEEP +5 cm H_2O). Continue Airway Clearance Protocol (suction PRN). Discuss with the neonatologist possible ways to correct the uncompensated metabolic acidosis. For example, in this sequence, bolus the infant with fluids, which may help correct the metabolic acidosis. If this does not suffice, sodium bicarbonate may be considered to support a pH of 7.25, or slightly higher. Monitor closely (vital signs, watch for signs of acute air leak, pulmonary hemorrhage).

Because the infant's mechanical ventilation was more than adequate (confirmed by a normal $PaCO_2$ of 37), the PIP was weaned to 22. The baby progressively improved over the next 4 days. On the fifth day, he was off the ventilator; on the seventh, he was discharged from the hospital. The mother was scheduled to see social services on a weekly basis.

Discussion

Inspection—the first step in the assessment process—was of the utmost importance in this case. The umbilical cord wrapped around the infant's neck, the presence of meconium, the blue skin, and the absence of spontaneous respirations were all important clinical indicators demonstrating the severity of the baby's condition. The fact that the baby was not manually ventilated, even though he had no spontaneous respirations, until after several clumps of meconium were suctioned from his oral and pharyngeal areas is paramount. Great care must be taken not to drive any meconium, blood, or amniotic fluid deeper down the tracheobronchial tree. The neonatal team must always be alert for the presence of a ball-valve meconium obstruction and the possibility of a pneumothorax. A ball-valve obstruction was verified in this case by the identification of alveolar hyperinflation on the chest radiograph. Fortunately, a pneumothorax did not develop. The early administration of surfactant to infants with MAS should be part of routine care.

As with adult subjects, several of the clinical manifestations in this case can be traced back through the "clinical scenarios" associated with atelectasis (see Fig. 10.7) and excessive bronchial secretions (see Fig. 10.11). For example, the increased lung density caused by the atelectasis was revealed on the chest radiograph, and the crackles were produced by the excessive airway secretions recorded in the second SOAP.

Although it was not used here, **high-frequency oscillatory ventilation (HFOV)** or **high-frequency jet ventilation (HFJV)** is often used in such cases. Either ventilator management approach appears to benefit the patient equally. Therapeutically, these techniques ventilate by air streams that flow down the center of the airways while gas leaving the lungs moves along the peripheral walls of the airways, thus moving meconium and secretions out of the lungs. However, both can have a negative effect in some cases in which there is significant airway obstruction, causing more gas trapping.

These babies are very sensitive to external stimuli. Great caution should be taken not to overstimulate them. They should be suctioned only as needed. Chest physical therapy is contraindicated. When suctioning is necessary, the respiratory therapist should not prolong the suctioning process. Often, these babies are given eye patches and earplugs to decrease external sensory stimulation. Occasionally, they will be paralyzed to minimize their reactions to stimuli and resistance to ventilation. Inhaled nitric oxide is used in severe cases, when persistent pulmonary hypertension of the newborn is verified. In extreme cases, if no improvement is seen with the previous treatments, including nitric oxide, extracorporeal membrane oxygenation may be considered.

1. When the fetus experiences in utero hypoxia, which of the following occur(s)?
   1. Vasoconstriction
   2. Inspiratory gasping
   3. Sphincter constriction
   4. Increased intestinal peristalsis
      a. 1 only
      b. 2 only
      c. 1, 2, and 4 only
      d. 2, 3, and 4 only
      e. 1, 2, 3, and 4

2. Aspiration of meconium may lead to which of the following?
   1. Ball-valve effect
   2. Atelectasis
   3. Total airway obstruction
   4. Alveolar hyperinflation
   5. Chemical pneumonitis
      a. 2 only
      b. 1, 2, and 4 only
      c. 2, 3, and 4 only
      d. 1, 2, 3, 4, and 5

3. Which of the following is associated with MAS when a ball-valve effect is present?
   a. Decreased RV
   b. Increased IRV
   c. Increased FRC
   d. All the lung volumes and capacities are decreased

4. Which of the following clinical manifestations are associated with meconium aspiration syndrome?
   1. Apnea
   2. Intercostal retractions
   3. Barrel chest
   4. Expiratory grunting
      a. 2 only
      b. 1, 2, and 4 only
      c. 2, 3, and 4 only
      d. 1, 2, 3, and 4

5. Which factors provide a higher risk for an infant to have Meconium Aspiration Syndrome?
   1. Post term infants.
   2. Infants born at less than 36 weeks.
   3. Mother is hypertensive.
   4. Baby is small for gestational age.
      a. 1 and 3 only.
      b. 2 and 4 only.
      c. 1, 3, and 4 only.
      d. 2, 3, and 4 only.

Transient Tachypnea of the Newborn

Chapter Objectives

After reading this chapter, you will be able to:

- List the anatomic alterations of the lungs associated with transient tachypnea of the newborn.
- Describe the causes of transient tachypnea of the newborn.
- List the cardiopulmonary clinical manifestations associated with transient tachypnea of the newborn.
- Describe the general management of transient tachypnea of the newborn.
- Describe the clinical strategies and rationales of the SOAP presented in the case study.
- Define key terms and complete self-assessment questions at the end of the chapter and on Evolve.

Key Terms

Apgar Score
Bubble CPAP
Capillary Blood Gas (CPG) Sampling
Dependent Cyanosis
Grunting

High Flow Nasal Cannula (HFNC)
Intercostal Retractions
Interstitial Edema
Macrosomia
Nasal flaring
Perihilar Streaking (Starbursts or Sunbursts)
Pulmonary Capillary Congestion
Rapid and Shallow Breathing Pattern (Hallmark Clinical Manifestation)
Substernal Retraction
Type II Respiratory Distress Syndrome
"Wet Lung" Syndrome

Chapter Outline

Anatomic Alterations of the Lungs
Etiology and Epidemiology
General Management of Transient Tachypnea of the Newborn
    Respiratory Care Treatment Protocols
Overview of the Cardiopulmonary Clinical Manifestations Associated With Transient Tachypnea of the Newborn
Case Study: Transient Tachypnea of the Newborn
Self-Assessment Questions

Anatomic Alterations of the Lungs

Transient tachypnea of the newborn (TTN) (also called **type II respiratory distress syndrome** and **"wet lung" syndrome**) was first described in the literature in 1966. Within the first 4 to 6 hours after birth, TTN produces clinical signs very similar to those associated with the early stages of respiratory distress syndrome (see Chapter 37, Respiratory Distress Syndrome). However, the anatomic alterations of the lungs associated with TTN are very different from the pulmonary pathology seen in respiratory distress syndrome. Although TTN can occur in premature infants, it is most commonly found in full-term infants between 37 and 42 weeks' gestation.

As shown in Fig. 36.1, the infant with TTN has a delay in pulmonary fluid absorption by the lymphatic system and pulmonary capillaries. As this condition worsens, the infant develops **pulmonary capillary congestion, interstitial edema**, fluid in the interlobular fissures, hyperexpansion, hypoxemia, and decreased lung compliance. In severe cases, the excessive fluid accumulation throughout the alveolar-capillary interstitial tissue may also compress the bronchial airways, leading to

air trapping and alveolar hyperinflation. Fortunately, these abnormal anatomic alterations of the lungs associated with TTN usually begin to resolve about 48 to 72 hours after birth.

The major pathologic or structural changes associated with TTN are as follows:

- Incomplete absorption of fetal lung fluid by pulmonary lymphatics
- Pulmonary capillary congestion
- Interstitial edema
- Air trapping and alveolar hyperinflation
- Compressed bronchial airways (from excessive alveolar-capillary interstitial fluid)

Etiology and Epidemiology

TTN affects 1% to 2% of all newborns. Classically, TNN is most often seen in full-term infants. Risk factors include elective cesarean section, delayed cord clamping, rapid delivery, excessive administration of fluids to the mother during labor, male gender, multiple gestations, and **macrosomia** (a newborn with excessive birth weight). The infant's history often includes

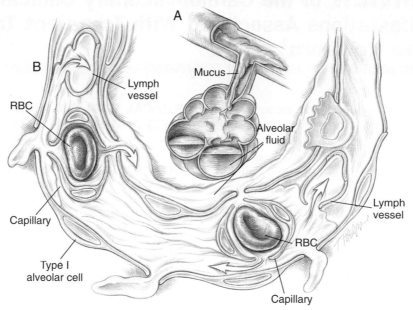

FIGURE 36.1 Transient tachypnea of the newborn. (A) Excessive alveolar fluid. (B) Cross-section of alveolus with interstitial edema and pulmonary capillary congestion.

maternal analgesia or anesthesia during labor and delivery or episodes of intrauterine hypoxia. TTN is also commonly associated with maternal bleeding, maternal diabetes, maternal asthma, and prolapsed cord. TTN is occasionally seen in very small infants.

TTN results from a delayed absorption of fetal lung fluid. It is thought that the lung epithelium is slow to transition from a fluid-secreting function to a fluid-absorbing function in the patient who presents with TTN. The process of reabsorption begins during labor. Normally a surge in fetal catecholamine secretion at birth stimulates the beta-adrenergic receptors, which improve lung fluid reabsorption. The typical baby with TTN usually has good **Apgar scores** at birth. During the next few hours, however, signs of respiratory distress develop. Early clinical manifestations include tachypnea, chest retractions, **nasal flaring**, **grunting**, and cyanosis. It is common to see respiratory rates greater than 60 breaths/min. *In fact, the rapid and shallow breathing pattern is often considered a hallmark clinical manifestation of TTN.* In addition, the infant may demonstrate a barrel chest and coarse crackles. Within 24 to 48 hours, the clinical manifestations of respiratory distress usually disappear.

Because there are several neonatal disorders that manifest early respiratory distress symptoms (e.g., respiratory distress syndrome, group B streptococcal pneumonia, and pulmonary hypertension of the newborn), TTN is often the differential diagnosis when all other disorders have been ruled out.

General Management of Transient Tachypnea of the Newborn

Because of the relatively short course of TTN, the treatment consists mostly of proper stabilization, close monitoring, and frequent and thorough evaluations to rule out other, more serious conditions that may develop. Oxygen therapy is provided to maintain adequate oxygenation, and suctioning (see Airway Clearance Protocol, Protocol 33.2) may be performed to keep the airways clear of bronchial secretions. Lung expansion therapy (CPAP) is often used as a preventive measure, but endotracheal intubation and mechanical ventilation usually are not required. Fluid restriction is usually ordered until the signs associated with TTN resolve. Oral feedings typically are started as soon as the infant is able to tolerate them (usually at a respiratory rate below 60). Nasogastric (NG) feeds may be started if the respiratory rate is elevated to provide nutrition and comfort. Use of diuretics is not indicated in the treatment of TTN and does not change the clinical course. In cases in which pneumonia is suspected, the use of antibiotics is indicated.

Respiratory Care Treatment Protocols

Oxygen Therapy Protocol

Oxygen therapy is used to treat hypoxemia, decrease the work of breathing, and decrease myocardial work. Because of the hypoxemia that often develops in TTN, supplemental oxygen may be required (see Oxygen Therapy Protocol, Protocol 33.1).

Airway Clearance Protocol

As a result of fluid accumulation, there may be some degree of airway narrowing, which may cause secretions to block the airways. Occasional suctioning may need to be performed if secretions cannot be cleared by the infant (see Airway Clearance Protocol, Protocol 33.2).

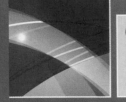

OVERVIEW of the Cardiopulmonary Clinical Manifestations Associated With Transient Tachypnea of the Newborn[1]

The following clinical manifestations result from the pathologic mechanisms caused (or activated) by increased alveolar-capillary membrane thickness (see Fig. 10.9), pulmonary vascular congestion, and airway obstruction—the major anatomic alterations of the lungs associated with transient tachypnea of the newborn (TTN) (see Fig. 36.1).

CLINICAL DATA OBTAINED AT THE PATIENT'S BEDSIDE

The Physical Examination

Vital Signs

Increased Respiratory Rate (Tachypnea)

Infants with TTN frequently breathe rapidly and shallowly. As mentioned earlier, this **rapid and shallow breathing pattern** often is considered a **hallmark clinical manifestation** of TTN. Normally, a newborn infant's respiratory rate is about 40 to 60 breaths/min. During the early stages of TTN, the respiratory rate is often 60 to 100 breaths/min. Several pathophysiologic mechanisms operating simultaneously may lead to an increased ventilatory rate:

- Stimulation of the peripheral chemoreceptors (hypoxemia)
- Relationship of decreased lung compliance to increased ventilatory rate
- Stimulation of the central chemoreceptors

Increased Heart Rate (Pulse) and Blood Pressure

Clinical Manifestations Associated With More Negative Intrapleural Pressure During Inspiration

- Intercostal retractions
- Substernal retraction and abdominal distention (seesaw movement)
- Nasal flaring
- **Expiratory Grunting**

Chest Assessment Findings

- Wheezes
- Crackles
- Expiratory grunting

Cyanosis

Barrel Chest (When Airways Are Partially Obstructed)

CLINICAL DATA OBTAINED FROM LABORATORY TESTS AND SPECIAL PROCEDURES

Pulmonary Function Test Findings
(Extrapolated Data for Instructional Purposes) (Primarily Restrictive Lung Pathophysiology)

The anatomic alterations of the lungs associated with TTN primarily cause a restrictive lung pathophysiology. For example, in moderate to severe cases, the following lung volumes and capacities may be lower than normal:

RV	IRV	VC	FRC	TLC
↓	↓	↓	↓	↓

When excessive pulmonary vascular fluid is present, air trapping and alveolar hyperinflation may develop. In these cases, an obstructive lung pathophysiology may develop—that is, the following might be greater than normal:

RV	FRC
↑	↑

Arterial Blood Gases[2]

MILD TO MODERATE TRANSIENT TACHYPNEA OF THE NEWBORN
Acute Alveolar Hyperventilation With Hypoxemia[3]
(Acute Respiratory Alkalosis)

pH	$PaCO_2$	HCO_3^-	PaO_2	SaO_2 or SpO_2
↑	↓	↓ (but normal)	↓	↓

SEVERE TRANSIENT TACHYPNEA OF THE NEWBORN
Acute Ventilatory Failure With Hypoxemia[4]
(Acute Respiratory Acidosis)

pH[5]	$PaCO_2$	HCO_3^-[5]	PaO_2	SaO_2 or SpO_2
↓	↑	↑ (but normal)	↓	↓

---

[2]*NOTE:* A critical ill newborn is likely to have an umbilical arterial catheter in place for arterial blood gas (ABG) sampling. In older critical infants and children, an arterial line may be placed for frequent ABG sampling. For intermittent sampling, because of the difficulty of obtaining ABG samples from newborn and pediatric patients, **capillary blood gas (CBG) sampling** may be used to determine the pH, $PaCO_2$, and HCO_3^- (i.e., the acid-base and ventilation status only). Capillary PO_2 values are unreliable and should not be used for clinical analysis. The standard way to evaluate the oxygenation status in these infants is pulse oximetry (SpO_2) (see Chapter 33, Newborn Assessment and Management).

[3]See Fig. 5.2 and Table 5.4 and related discussions for the acute pH, $PaCO_2$, and HCO_3^- changes associated with acute alveolar hyperventilation.

[4]See Table 5.5 and related discussion for the acute pH, $PaCO_2$, and HCO_3^- changes associated with acute ventilatory failure.

[5]When tissue hypoxia is severe enough to produce lactic acid, the pH and HCO_3^- values will be lower than expected for a particular $PaCO_2$ level.

---

[1]The clinical manifestations of TTN usually disappear in the first 24 to 48 hours. Severe TTN is rare.

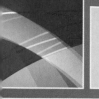
Oxygenation Indices[6]

$\dot{Q}_s/\dot{Q}_t$	DO_2[7]	$\dot{V}O_2$	$C(a\text{-}\bar{v})O_2$	O_2ER	$S\bar{v}O$
↑	↓	N	N	↑	↓

[6]$C(a\text{-}\bar{v})O_2$, Arterial-venous oxygen difference; DO_2, total oxygen delivery; O_2ER, oxygen extraction ratio; $\dot{Q}_s/\dot{Q}_t$, pulmonary shunt fraction; $S\bar{v}O_2$, mixed venous oxygen saturation; $\dot{V}O_2$, oxygen consumption.

[7]Because the newborn normally has a higher hemoglobin level at birth (16.8 to 18.9 g/dL), the DO_2 may actually be better than indicated by PaO_2 or SpO_2 alone (see Chapter 6, Assessment of Oxygenation).

RADIOLOGIC FINDINGS

Chest Radiograph

Initially, the chest radiograph appears normal. Over the next 4 to 6 hours, however, signs of pulmonary vascular congestion develop. These are revealed on the chest radiograph as prominent **perihilar streaking** (commonly called **starbursts or sunbursts**), air bronchograms, and fluid in the interlobular fissures. Air trapping and hyperinflation may occur and are manifested by peripheral hyperlucency, flattened diaphragms, and bulging intercostal spaces. Patches of infiltrates may be seen in some infants. Mild cardiomegaly and pleural effusions also may be seen (Fig. 36.2). Fig. 36.3 shows a radiograph of classic transient TTN with bilateral infiltration.

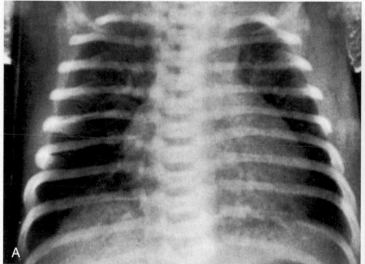
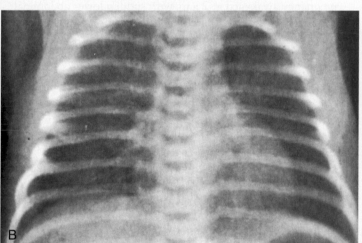

FIGURE 36.2 The large cardiovascular silhouette, air bronchogram, and streaky lung fields were seen at 2 hours of age (A) but had cleared by 24 hours of age (B), typical of transient tachypnea of the newborn or delayed clearance of lung liquid. (From Taeusch, W. H., Ballard, R. A., & Gleason, C. A. [2005]. *Avery's diseases of the newborn* [8th ed.]. Philadelphia: Saunders.)

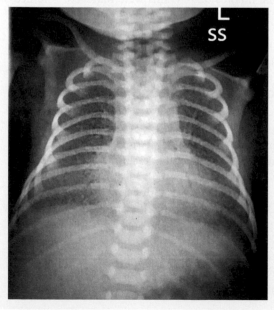

FIGURE 36.3 Classic radiograph of transient tachypnea of the newborn showing bilateral infiltration. (Courtesy Dayton Children's Hospital, Dayton, Ohio.)

Lung Expansion Therapy Protocol

Lung expansion measures, such as **bubble CPAP**, commonly are performed to offset the pulmonary capillary congestion and interstitial edema associated with TTN (see Lung Expansion Therapy Protocol, Protocol 33.3).

Mechanical Ventilation Protocol

Mechanical ventilation may occasionally be necessary to provide and support alveolar gas exchange and eventually return the patient to spontaneous breathing. Patients with TTN rarely require mechanical ventilation (see Ventilator Initiation and Management Protocol, Protocol 33.4).

CASE STUDY Transient Tachypnea of the Newborn

Admitting History and Physical Examination

A 27-year-old woman in the thirty-fifth week of her second pregnancy awakened at 2 a.m. with sudden lower abdominal pain and some vaginal bleeding. She had no contractions at the time. She woke her husband, who in turn called the obstetrician. The doctor instructed him to bring his wife to the hospital. On arrival at the hospital, she was immediately taken to the labor and delivery room. The nurse on duty placed an oxygen mask on the patient's face and started an intravenous line. The patient's vital signs were monitored closely. An ultrasound Doppler belt also was placed around the mother's lower abdominal area to monitor the baby's heart rate. Over the next 20 minutes, the mother continued to bleed, her blood pressure fell, and her heart rate increased. The baby's heart rate had increased from 155 beats/min to 170 beats/min.

The obstetrician called the operating room and asked the staff to prepare for an emergency cesarean section. The doctor also called for the neonatal resuscitation team (which consisted of a neonatologist, nurse, and respiratory therapist) and asked that they be on standby. The cesarean section was uneventful. The baby was a 3-kg girl. The neonatologist assessed the baby and gave a 1-minute Apgar score of 7 (2 heart rate, 2 respiratory rate, 1 tone, 1 reflex irritability, and 1 skin color) and a 5-minute Apgar score of 9 (2 heart rate, 2 respiratory rate, 2 tone, 2 reflex irritability, and 1 skin color). Within 30 minutes of delivery, the baby was tachypneic with a respiratory rate of 80 breaths/min. Auscultation revealed bilateral mild crackles and occasional coarse crackles. The baby was transferred to the neonatal intensive care unit (NICU).

In the NICU, the baby was placed in a warmed Isolette with continuous pulse oximetry; SpO_2 was noted to be 82% to 84%. An intravenous line and nasogastric tube were also placed. Warm, humidified oxygen was started via a **high-flow nasal cannula (HFNC)** [also called a *high-humidity nasal cannula*] at 4 L/min and an FIO_2 of 0.40. Ten minutes later the infant's vital signs were heart rate 155 beats/min, blood pressure 75/40 mm Hg (mean arterial pressure [MAP] 52), and respiratory rate 75 breaths/min. The infant's ventilatory pattern was described by the neonatologist as fast and shallow;

however, she did not appear to be working hard to breathe. She had no intercostal retractions or nasal flaring at this time. Capillary blood gas values were pH 7.33, $PaCO_2$ 31 mm Hg, and HCO_3^- 21 mEq/L. The baby's SpO_2 was 88%. The FIO_2 was increased to 0.60 to achieve an SpO_2 of 93%.

About 2 hours later, however, the baby started to show signs of worsening. Her vital signs were heart rate 170 beats/min, blood pressure 75/45 (55 MAP), and respiratory rate 100 breaths/min. She demonstrated abdominal respiratory efforts and nasal flaring. Her skin appeared pale and blue. Auscultation revealed moderate to severe bilateral crackles. On the same HFNC settings (4 L/min and an FIO_2 of 0.60), her SpO_2 had dropped to 84%. Capillary blood gas values revealed the following acid-base and ventilation status: pH 7.28, $PaCO_2$ 62 mm Hg, and HCO_3^- 23 mEq/L.

A chest radiograph showed areas of pulmonary vascular congestion throughout both lung fields, as well as prominent perihilar streaking (indicating fluid in the fissures). A starburst pattern was seen at the hilum of the lungs (indicating increased lymphatic fluid). The chest radiograph also showed air trapping and hyperinflation in the lower lobes (indicating fluid in the airways). The infant's diaphragms were flattened. The neonatologist charted a diagnosis of TTN in the baby's progress notes. The physician also stated that he did not want to mechanically ventilate the baby at this time. The respiratory therapist entered the following assessment in the baby's chart.

Respiratory Assessment and Plan

S N/A

O Vital signs: HR 170/min, BP 75/45 (55), and RR 100/min. Chest retractions, nasal flaring. Skin pale and blue. Moderate to severe bilateral crackles. CXR: Pulmonary vascular congestion and perihilar streaking in both lungs, generalized hyperinflation. CBG on HFNC at 4 L/min and FIO_2 0.60: pH 7.28, $PaCO_2$ 62 mm Hg, and HCO_3^- 23 mEq/L, SpO_2 84%.

A • TTN (neonatologist, CXR, history)
  • Pulmonary vascular congestion and perihilar streaking (CXR)
  • Air trapping (CXR)

- Excessive pulmonary fluid noted (bilateral crackles)
- Acute ventilatory failure (capillary blood gas) and moderate to severe hypoxemia

P Lung Expansion Therapy Protocol (nasal CPAP +5–6 cm H_2O). Increase Oxygen Therapy Protocol HFNC (FIO_2 0.60 via an increased CPAP +5–6 cm H_2O at set-up adjusting by Protocol to achieve desired SpO_2). Airway Clearance Protocol (suction PRN). Continue to monitor closely.

Over the next 48 hours, the baby's condition progressively improved. She no longer required oxygen therapy, and her breath sounds were normal. Her last room air capillary blood gas values showed a pH of 7.38, $PaCO_2$ 39 mm Hg, and HCO_3^- 24 mEq/L. Her SpO_2 was 94%. Her chest radiograph was normal. The baby was discharged the next day.

Discussion

This case reinforces the importance of observation and inspection in the assessment process. The respiratory therapist must continuously inspect and analyze infants with TTN. This baby, for example, born at 35 weeks, may have had respiratory distress syndrome (see Chapter 37), but the clinical symptoms ruled out the diagnosis. For example, babies with RDS have alveolar collapse and consolidation, whereas babies with TTN have airway trapping and alveolar hyperinflation. In addition, the respiratory pattern of babies with RDS is commonly described as hard, fast, and deep breathing; whereas infants with TTN usually breathe rapidly and shallowly. *This rapid and shallow breathing pattern often is considered a hallmark of TTN.* Certainly, the rapid shallow breathing seen in this baby was caused, in part, by the temporarily increased alveolar-capillary membrane thickness (see Fig. 10.9)—and decreased lung compliance—associated with TTN.

Although apnea may occur in these babies, it is not common. Therapeutically, most do quite well with just oxygen via an HFNC. Occasionally, nasal continuous positive airway pressure (CPAP) may be used. Caution, however, must be taken not to give the baby too high of an inspiratory pressure or prolonged exposure to CPAP. The lungs of these babies are usually already hyperinflated. Too high a CPAP pressure setting may expand the baby's lungs even more and may cause a tension pneumothorax. CPAP of +5 to 6 cm H_2O is usually safe. Mechanical ventilation rarely is needed for babies with TTN.

SELF-ASSESSMENT QUESTIONS

1. Which of the following is(are) associated with TTN?
1. Rapid and shallow breathing pattern
2. PPHN
3. Clinical signs similar to those of infant respiratory distress syndrome
4. Reduced DO_2
   a. 1 only
   b. 2 and 4 only
   c. 2, 3, and 4 only
   d. 1, 2, 3, and 4

2. The clinical manifestations associated with TTN usually disappear within:
a. 10 to 24 hours after birth
b. 24 to 48 hours after birth
c. 48 to 72 hours after birth
d. 2 weeks after birth

3. Which of the following is the hallmark clinical manifestation of TTN?
a. PPHN
b. Rapid and shallow breathing pattern
c. Substernal retraction and abdominal distention (seesaw movement)
d. Expiratory grunting

4. Radiologic findings associated with TTN include:
1. Flattened diaphragms
2. Starbursts
3. Air bronchograms
4. Deviated trachea
   a. 1 and 3 only
   b. 2 and 4 only
   c. 1, 2, and 3 only
   d. 1, 2, 3, and 4

5. Which of the following are the major anatomic alterations of the lungs associated with TTN?
1. Consolidation
2. Bronchospasm
3. Increased alveolar-capillary membrane thickness
4. Atelectasis
5. Excessive fluid
   a. 3 and 5 only
   b. 2 and 4 only
   c. 3, 4, and 5 only
   d. 1, 3, 4, and 5 only

6. Which maternal risk factors provide a higher risk for an infant to show signs of TTN?
1. Full term infants.
2. Elective cesarean section.
3. Multiple gestation.
4. Excessive administration of fluids to the mother during labor.
   a. 1 and 3 only.
   b. 2 and 4 only.
   c. 1, 2, and 3.
   d. 1, 2, 3, and 4.

Chapter Objectives

After reading this chapter, you will be able to:

- List the anatomic alterations of the lungs associated with respiratory distress syndrome.
- Describe the causes of respiratory distress syndrome.
- List the cardiopulmonary clinical manifestations associated with respiratory distress syndrome.
- Describe the general management of respiratory distress syndrome.
- Describe the clinical strategies and rationales of the SOAP presented in the case study.
- Define key terms and complete self-assessment questions at the end of the chapter and on Evolve.

Key Terms

Alveolar Type II Cells (Granular Pneumocytes)
Beractant (Survanta)
Bubble CPAP
Calfactant (Infasurf)
Exogenous Surfactant
Hyaline Membrane
Hyaline Membrane Disease

Infant Respiratory Distress Syndrome
INSURE Protocol
Lecithin-to-Sphingomyelin Ratio (L/S Ratio)
Neutral Thermal Environmental
Phosphatidylglycerol (PG)
Poractant Alfa (Curosurf)
Pulmonary Hyperperfusion
Pulmonary Hypoperfusion
Respiratory Distress Syndrome
Transient Pulmonary Hypertension
Volutrauma

Chapter Outline

Anatomic Alterations of the Lungs
Etiology and Epidemiology
Overview of the Cardiopulmonary Clinical Manifestations
    Associated With Respiratory Distress Syndrome
General Management of Respiratory Distress Syndrome
    Respiratory Care Treatment Protocols
Diagnosis
Case Study: Respiratory Distress Syndrome
Self-Assessment Questions

Respiratory distress syndrome (RDS) is the most common cause of respiratory failure in the preterm infant. Over the past several decades, a number of names have been used to identify infants with RDS (Box 37.1). A common thread running through most of the names is the term *respiratory distress*, which characterizes an immature lung disorder in a preterm infant caused by inadequate pulmonary surfactant. RDS is a major cause of morbidity and mortality in the premature infant born at fewer than 37 weeks' gestation. The introduction of exogenous surfactant therapy has greatly improved the clinical course of this disorder and reduced the morbidity and mortality rates.

Anatomic Alterations of the Lungs

On gross examination, the lungs of an infant with RDS are dark red and liver-like. Under the microscope the lungs appear solid because of countless areas of alveolar collapse. The pulmonary capillaries are congested, and the lymphatic vessels

---

> **BOX 37.1 Names Used to Identify Respiratory Distress Syndrome**
>
> - Infant respiratory distress syndrome
> - Idiopathic respiratory distress syndrome
> - Neonatal respiratory distress syndrome
> - **Respiratory distress syndrome**
> - Hyaline membrane disease

are distended. Extensive interstitial and intraalveolar edema and hemorrhage are evident.

In what appears to be an effort to offset alveolar collapse, the respiratory bronchioles, alveolar ducts, and some alveoli dilate. As the disease intensifies, the alveolar walls become lined with a dense, rippled **hyaline membrane** identical to the hyaline membrane that develops in adult acute respiratory distress syndrome (ARDS) (see Chapter 28, Acute Respiratory

Distress Syndrome). The membrane contains fibrin and cellular debris.

During the later stages of the disease, leukocytes are present and the hyaline membrane is often fragmented and partially ingested by macrophages. Type II cells begin to proliferate, and secretions begin to accumulate in the tracheobronchial tree. The anatomic alterations in RDS produce a restrictive type of lung disorder (Fig. 37.1).

As a consequence of the anatomic alterations associated with RDS, babies with this disorder often develop hypoxia-induced pulmonary arterial vasoconstriction and vasospasm, causing a state of **transient pulmonary hypertension**. This results in blood shunting from right to left through the ductus arteriosus and foramen ovale. Occasionally, intrapulmonary shunting may occur. As a consequence, the blood flow is diverted away from the lungs (**pulmonary hypoperfusion**), which worsens the hypoxemia. It should be noted that if this condition does not resolve within 24 hours or so, shunting will begin to flow from left to right through the patent ductus arteriosus. This condition can lead to excessive lung fluid, **pulmonary hyperperfusion**, and pulmonary edema.

The major pathologic or structural changes associated with RDS are as follows:

- Interstitial and alveolar edema and hemorrhage
- Alveolar consolidation
- Intraalveolar hyaline membrane
- Pulmonary surfactant deficiency or qualitative abnormality
- Atelectasis
- Hyperperfusion (leads to excessive lung fluid and pulmonary edema in cases lasting longer than 24 hours)
- Pulmonary arterial hypoxia-induced vasoconstriction and vasospasm

Etiology and Epidemiology

Although the exact cause of RDS is controversial, the most popular theory suggests that the early stages develop as a result of a pulmonary surfactant abnormality or deficiency and pulmonary hypoperfusion evoked by hypoxia, although the latter is probably a secondary response to the surfactant abnormality. The probable sequence of steps in the development of RDS is as follows:

1. Because of the pulmonary surfactant abnormality, alveolar compliance decreases, resulting in alveolar collapse.
2. The pulmonary atelectasis causes the infant's work of breathing to increase.
3. Alveolar ventilation decreases in response to the decreased lung compliance and infant fatigue, causing the alveolar oxygen tension (P_AO_2) to decrease.
4. The decreased P_AO_2 (alveolar hypoxia) stimulates a reflex pulmonary vasoconstriction.
5. Because of the pulmonary vasoconstriction, blood bypasses the infant's lungs through fetal pathways—the patent ductus arteriosus and the foramen ovale.
6. The lung hypoperfusion in turn causes lung ischemia and decreased lung metabolism.
7. Because of the decreased lung metabolism, the production of pulmonary surfactant is reduced even further, and a vicious circle develops (Fig. 37.2).

It is estimated that approximately 30,000 cases of RDS occur annually in the United States. RDS is the leading cause of death in preterm infants. About 50% of the neonates born at 26 to 28 weeks' gestation develop RDS. About 25% of the babies born at 30 to 31 weeks' gestation develop RDS. The condition occurs more often in male babies and is usually more severe than in female babies. The higher incidence and severity of RDS in male infants are explained by the increased circulating androgens in males, which in turn slow the maturation of the infant's lung. The delayed lung maturation results in immature **alveolar type II cells (granular pneumocytes)** and decreased pulmonary surfactant production.

RDS is also more commonly seen in infants of diabetic mothers (the high fetal insulin levels decrease lung surfactant and structural maturation), white preterm babies compared with black preterm infants, and infants delivered by cesarean section. RDS is also associated with low birth weight (1000 g

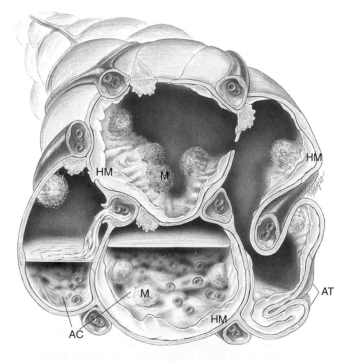

FIGURE 37.1 Respiratory distress syndrome. Cross-sectional view of alveoli in infant respiratory distress syndrome. *AC,* Alveolar consolidation; *AT,* atelectasis; *HM,* hyaline membrane; *M,* macrophage.

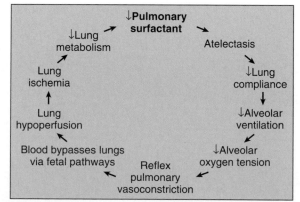

FIGURE 37.2 Early stages of respiratory distress syndrome.

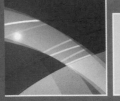

OVERVIEW of the Cardiopulmonary Clinical Manifestations Associated With Respiratory Distress Syndrome

The following clinical manifestations result from the pathologic mechanisms caused (or activated) by atelectasis (see Fig. 10.7), alveolar consolidation (see Fig. 10.8), and increased alveolar-capillary membrane thickness (see Fig. 10.9)—the major anatomic alterations of the lungs associated with respiratory distress syndrome (RDS) (see Fig. 37.1).

CLINICAL DATA OBTAINED AT THE PATIENT'S BEDSIDE

The Physical Examination

Vital Signs

Increased Respiratory Rate (Tachypnea)

Normally, a newborn infant's respiratory rate is about 30 to 60 breaths/min. During the early stages of RDS, the respiratory rate is generally well over 60 breaths/min. The respiratory pattern of a baby with RDS is commonly described as "hard, fast, and deep breathing." The following pathophysiologic mechanisms operating simultaneously may lead to an increased ventilatory rate:

- Stimulation of peripheral chemoreceptors (hypoxemia)
- Relationship of decreased lung compliance to increased ventilatory rate
- Stimulation of central chemoreceptors

Increased Heart Rate (Pulse) and Blood Pressure

Apnea (see Box 33.3)

Clinical Manifestations Associated With More Negative Intrapleural Pressures During Inspiration

- Intercostal retractions
- Substernal retraction and abdominal distention (seesaw movement)
- Nasal flaring

Chest Assessment Findings

- Bronchial (or harsh) breath sounds
- Fine crackles

Expiratory grunting

Cyanosis

CLINICAL DATA OBTAINED FROM LABORATORY TESTS AND SPECIAL PROCEDURES

Pulmonary Function Test Findings
(Extrapolated Data for Instructional Purposes)
(Primarily Restrictive Lung Pathophysiology)

The anatomic alterations of the lungs associated with RDS primarily cause a restrictive lung pathophysiology. For example, in moderate to severe cases, the following lung volumes and capacities may be lower than normal:

RV	IRV	VC	FRC	TLC
↓	↓	↓	↓	↓

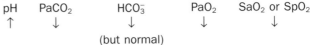

Arterial Blood Gases[1]

MILD TO MODERATE RESPIRATORY DISTRESS SYNDROME
Acute Alveolar Hyperventilation With Hypoxemia[2]
(Acute Respiratory Alkalosis)

pH	$PaCO_2$	HCO_3^-	PaO_2	SaO_2 or SpO_2
↑	↓	↓ (but normal)	↓	↓

SEVERE RESPIRATORY DISTRESS SYNDROME
Acute Ventilatory Failure With Hypoxemia[3]
(Acute Respiratory Acidosis)

pH[4]	$PaCO_2$	HCO_3^- [4]	PaO_2	SaO_2 or SpO_2
↓	↑	↑ (but normal)	↓	↓

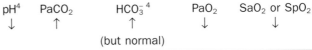

Oxygenation Indices[5]

$\dot{Q}_S/\dot{Q}_T$	DO_2[6]	$\dot{V}O_2$	$C(a-\bar{v})O_2$	O_2ER	$S\bar{v}O_2$
↑	↓	N	N	↑	↓

[1]NOTE: A critically ill newborn is likely to have an umbilical arterial catheter in place for arterial blood gas (ABG) sampling. In older critically ill infants and children, an arterial line may be placed for frequent ABG sampling. For intermittent sampling, because of the difficulty of obtaining ABG samples from newborn and pediatric patients, capillary blood gas (CBG) samples may be used to determine the pH, $PaCO_2$, and HCO_3^- (i.e., the acid-base and ventilation status only). Capillary PO_2 values are unreliable and should not be used for clinical analysis. The standard way to evaluate the oxygenation status in these infants is pulse oximetry (SpO_2) (see Chapter 33, Newborn Assessment and Management).

[2]See Fig. 5.2 and Table 5.4 and related discussion for the acute pH, $PaCO_2$, and HCO_3^- changes associated with acute alveolar hyperventilation.

[3]See Table 5.5 and related discussion for the acute pH, $PaCO_2$, and HCO_3^- changes associated with acute ventilatory failure.

[4]When tissue hypoxia is severe enough to produce lactic acid, the pH and HCO_3^- values will be lower than expected for a particular $PaCO_2$ level.

[5]$C(a-\bar{v})O_2$, Arterial-venous oxygen difference; DO_2, total oxygen delivery; O_2ER, oxygen extraction ratio; $\dot{Q}_S/\dot{Q}_T$, pulmonary shunt fraction; $S\bar{v}O_2$, mixed venous oxygen saturation; $\dot{V}O_2$, oxygen consumption.

[6]Because the newborn normally has a higher hemoglobin level at birth (16.8 to 18.9 g/dL), the DO_2 actually may be better than indicated by PaO_2 or SpO_2 alone (see Chapter 6, Assessment of Oxygenation).

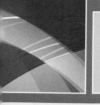

RADIOLOGIC FINDINGS
Chest Radiograph
· Increased opacity (ground-glass appearance)

On chest radiographs of infants with RDS, the air-filled tracheo-bronchial tree typically stands out against a dense opaque (or white) lung. This white density is often described as having a fine, ground-glass appearance throughout the lung fields. Because of the pathologic processes, the density of the lungs is increased. Increased lung density resists x-ray penetration and is revealed on the radiograph as increased opacity. Therefore the more severe the RDS, the whiter the radiographic image will be (Fig. 37.3).

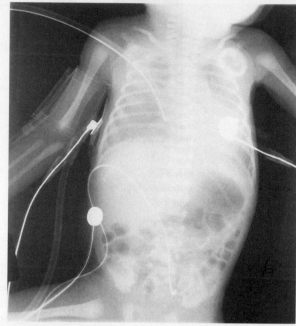

FIGURE 37.3 Whole body x-ray film of an infant with respiratory distress syndrome. Note the "whiteout," particularly of the left lower lobe and right upper lobe.

to 1500 grams), multiple births, prenatal asphyxia, prolonged labor, maternal bleeding, and second-born twins.

Diagnosis

There are two primary tests that can be performed *on amniotic fluid* to determine the lung maturity of the fetus: the lecithin-to-sphingomyelin ratio and the presence of phosphatidylglycerol.

The **lecithin-to-sphingomyelin ratio (L/S ratio)** is commonly used to test lung maturity. Lecithin, also called *dipalmitoyl phosphatidylcholine* (DPPC), is the most abundant phospholipid found in surfactant. When the concentration of lecithin is two times greater than sphingomyelin—an L/S ratio of 2:1—the infant's lung maturity is likely to be great enough that the lungs will produce adequate pulmonary surfactant at birth. Most infants with an L/S ratio less than 1:1 develop RDS. The L/S ratio is not reliable in pregnancies associated with diabetes and Rhesus (Rh) isoimmunization.

Phosphatidylglycerol (PG) is the second most abundant phospholipid found in surfactant. Because the PG level normally increases toward term, the presence of PG in the amniotic fluid indicates a low risk for RDS. When the amniotic fluid reveals an L/S ratio less than 2:1 and a lack of PG, the infant has a more than 80% risk for developing RDS. However, when the amniotic fluid shows an L/S ratio greater than 2:1 and when PG is present, the risk drops to almost zero.

General Management of Respiratory Distress Syndrome

During the early stages of RDS, continuous positive airway pressure (CPAP), **bubble CPAP**, or high-flow nasal cannula (HFNC) is the treatment of choice (**see Lung Expansion Therapy Protocol, Protocol 33.3**). Mechanical ventilation is usually avoided as long as possible. CPAP generally works well with these patients because it (1) increases the functional residual capacity, (2) decreases the work of breathing, and (3) works to increase the PaO_2 through alveolar recruitment while the infant is receiving a lower inspired concentration of oxygen. A PaO_2 of 40 to 70 mm Hg is normal for newborns. *No effort should be made to get an infant's PaO_2 within the normal adult range (80 to 100 mm Hg)*. This equates generally to a target SpO_2 of 85% to 95%. Special attention should be given to maintaining a **neutral thermal environment** for the infant with RDS because the infant's oxygenation can be further compromised if the body temperature is above or below normal.

Because of the decreased pulmonary surfactant associated with RDS, the administration of natural **exogenous surfactant** preparations, such as **beractant (Survanta)**, **calfactant (Infasurf)**, or **poractant alfa (Curosurf)** are now standard therapy for any infant with RDS who requires intubation. Surfactant is administered via an orotracheal tube with positive pressure ventilation (bagging or mechanical ventilation) to distribute the surfactant throughout the lungs. The term *exogenous*, used

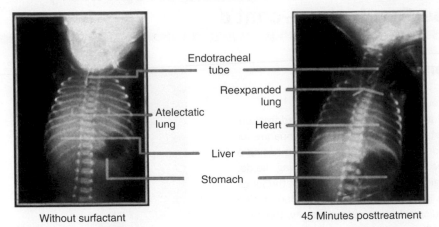

Surfactant function
Exogenous surfactant

Endotracheal
tube

Reexpanded
lung

Atelectatic
lung

Heart

Liver

Stomach

Without surfactant

45 Minutes posttreatment

FIGURE 37.4 Chest x-ray films of an infant with respiratory distress syndrome before and after exogenous surfactant treatments.

to describe these surfactant agents, indicates that these preparations are from outside the patient's body. Exogenous surfactant preparations originate from other humans, from animals, or from laboratory synthesis; natural surfactant preparations are preferred over synthetic preparations. These agents replace the missing pulmonary surfactant of the premature or immature lungs of the baby with RDS until the lungs are mature enough to produce adequate pulmonary surfactant themselves (see Surfactant Administration Protocol, Protocol 33.5).

Fig. 37.4 provides comparison chest radiographs of an infant without exogenous surfactant and the same infant 45 minutes after treatment. The use of exogenous surfactant at birth in premature infants has significantly reduced mortality and the incidence of pneumothorax and pulmonary interstitial emphysema previously associated with RDS. A surfactant administration protocol is often used to promote effective surfactant replacement therapy for prophylaxis and treatment (see Surfactant Administration Protocol, Protocol 33.5).

Respiratory Care Treatment Protocols

Oxygen Therapy Protocol

Oxygen therapy is used to treat hypoxemia, decrease the work of breathing, and decrease myocardial work. Because of the hypoxemia that often develops in RDS, supplemental oxygen is usually required (see Oxygen Therapy Protocol, Protocol 33.1).

Surfactant Administration Protocol

Surfactant replacement is essential to replace the missing pulmonary surfactant in the premature or immature lungs of infants with RDS. Studies have shown that routine intubation and prophylactic surfactant should be avoided to reduce the risks and complications of intubation and mechanical ventilation, unless the infant is less than 26 weeks gestation. These extremely premature infants have a much greater likelihood of failing CPAP before surfactant administration. The **INSURE protocol** (*IN*tubate-*SUR*factant-*E*xtubate) has been used with great success on many preterm infants. With this method, an infant is intubated, given surfactant, then extubated and placed on nasal or bubble CPAP for continued respiratory support. **Surfactant therapy occasionally may need to be repeated when there is a persistent or recurrent oxygen requirement of 30% or more 6 to 12 hours after the initial dose, depending on which type of surfactant is being used.** The protocol includes safeguards, such as confirming endotracheal tube position before surfactant administration, the method of administration, and dosing specifics for the type of surfactant used (see Surfactant Administration Protocol, Protocol 33.5).

Lung Expansion Therapy Protocol

Lung expansion therapies are commonly used to offset the pulmonary capillary congestion, interstitial edema, and atelectasis associated with RDS. CPAP or HFNC is commonly used (see Lung Expansion Therapy Protocol, Protocol, 33.3).

Mechanical Ventilation Protocol

Mechanical ventilation may be necessary to provide and support alveolar gas exchange and eventually return the patient to spontaneous breathing (see Mechanical Ventilation and Ventilator Weaning Protocol, Protocol 33.4).

CASE STUDY Respiratory Distress Syndrome

Admitting History and Physical Examination

A premature male infant was delivered after 28 weeks' gestation. The mother was a 19-year-old, unmarried primigravida patient who claimed to be in good health during the entire pregnancy until 6 hours before admission. At that time, she noticed the onset of painless vaginal bleeding. She called her obstetrician, who told her he would meet her in the emergency department of the medical center.

On examination she was found to be a healthy young woman, approximately 28 weeks pregnant, in early labor, and bleeding slightly from the vagina. Her vital signs were stable and within normal limits. A diagnosis of placental abruption, the premature separation of the placenta, was made. Because bleeding was minimal and both mother and fetus seemed to be doing well, it was decided to deliver the baby vaginally. She was monitored very closely, and labor progressed satisfactorily for about 8 hours, at which time she delivered the infant under epidural anesthesia without any obstetric complications. The baby weighed 1600 grams. The Apgar scores were 7 after 1 minute and 9 after 5 minutes. Physical examination findings were entirely normal for an infant of this size.

On admission to the newborn nursery 30 minutes after delivery, the infant was noted to have some moderate respiratory distress. His respiratory rate was 56 breaths/min with nasal flaring. A chest radiograph obtained at this time was read by the radiologist as having a "ground-glass appearance."

Within the next 30 minutes, the infant's respiratory distress became more marked with tachypnea, retractions, and grunting. The neonatologist was contacted. The respiratory therapist was called to the nursery to evaluate the infant for possible surfactant administration. On the therapist's arrival, the infant's respiratory rate was 64 breaths/min and heart rate 165 beats/min; auscultation of the infant's chest revealed bilateral fine crackles. The infant was grunting on $\frac{1}{2}$ L/min oxygen per nasal cannula, and nasal flaring was noted. A capillary blood gas sample showed pH 7.14, $PaCO_2$ 68 mm Hg, HCO_3^- 22 mEq/L. The infant's SpO_2 was 85%.

Respiratory Assessment and Plan

S N/A (newborn)

O Increased work of breathing with worsening hypoxemia. Retracting and using accessory muscles. Flaring of nostrils. Vital signs RR 64 with "grunting." HR 165. Bilateral fine crackles. CXR: Bilateral "ground-glass" haziness. CBGs on $\frac{1}{2}$ L/min oxygen: pH 7.14, $PaCO_2$ 68, HCO_3^- 22, SpO_2 85%.

A • **Respiratory respiratory distress syndrome** (history)
  • Alveolar hyaline membrane, atelectasis (CXR)
  • Acute ventilatory failure with severe hypoxemia (ABGs)

• Lactic acidosis likely (pH and HCO_3^- lower than expected for $PaCO_2$ of 68)

P Surfactant Administration Protocol: Apply CPAP by mask until intubation. Intubate, provide manual then mechanical ventilation; obtain chest radiograph to verify endotracheal tube placement. Draw up liquid surfactant using drug-specific mL per kg of infant's weight dose. Once endotracheal tube is in the correct position (T2-T3), administer surfactant per protocol in small doses to avoid "drowning" the airway while providing mechanical ventilation.

• Mechanical Ventilation Protocol: Ventilate using positive end-expiratory pressure (PEEP) per neonatal intensive care unit (NICU) ventilator protocol. Focus effort on weaning PIP to maintain 4 to 6 mL/kg tidal volume as the infant's lung compliance improves.

• Oxygen Therapy Protocol: Continuous pulse oximetry.

At this time, the baby was transferred to the NICU, intubated, and put on a ventilator. The initial ventilator settings were respiratory rate (RR) 40/min, inspiratory time (T_I) 0.35, FIO_2 0.40, positive inspiratory pressure (PIP) +25 cm H_2O, and PEEP +5 cm H_2O. Artificial surfactant was administered without complication. Fluid and electrolyte balance was maintained within normal levels. While maintaining the exhaled V_T at 4 to 6 mL per kilogram, the PIP was progressively decreased. At 7 days of age, the infant was weaned from mechanical ventilation and extubated to nasal CPAP. He was weaned off the nasal CPAP at 14 days of age. Chest x-ray examination on the 16th day was unremarkable. The baby was discharged after 10 weeks and has been healthy ever since.

Discussion

RDS is a fascinating disorder in which meticulous respiratory care of the infant is crucial. Most respiratory therapy students greatly look forward to and enjoy their NICU rotation. In these units the expertise of the respiratory therapist is crucial to the functioning of the unit because the majority of patients there have respiratory disorders. Indeed, many of the first reports of therapist-driven protocols came from this setting.

Many of the clinical manifestations seen in this case are associated with atelectasis (see Fig. 10.7) and increased alveolar-capillary membrane thickness (see Fig. 10.9). For example, the use of accessory muscles of inspiration was likely to be a compensatory mechanism activated to offset the increased stiffness of the lungs (decreased lung compliance) caused by the atelectasis and alveolar hyaline membrane. The atelectasis and alveolar hyaline membrane were objectively verified by the chest radiograph. In addition, the severity level of the anatomic alterations and clinical manifestations seen in this case was very high. This was objectively confirmed by the capillary blood gas analysis that identified the acute ventilatory failure with hypoxemia (SpO_2: 85%).

Thus the aggressive implementation of mechanical ventilation and use of artificial surfactant were certainly justified. Artificial surfactant has markedly improved the outlook for these infants. However, the respiratory therapist should be on the alert for sudden changes in lung compliance that often occur shortly after the administration of artificial surfactant. If the infant is on a pressure-cycled mode ventilator, it is especially important to avoid **volutrauma**.[1] As in adults with ARDS, in which the pathologic process is very similar, constant attention must be given to the possibility of nosocomial infection, fluid overload, and cardiovascular instability. In addition, lung protection strategies such as PEEP, permissive hypercapnia, and use of small ventilator tidal volumes are commonly used in RDS cases.

---

[1]*Volutrauma* is defined as damage to the lung caused by overdistention by a mechanical ventilator set for an excessively high tidal volume.

SELF-ASSESSMENT QUESTIONS

1. When transient pulmonary hypertension exists in respiratory distress syndrome, blood bypasses the infant's lungs through which of the following structures?
   1. Ductus venosus
   2. Umbilical vein
   3. Ductus arteriosus
   4. Foramen ovale
      a. 1 and 2 only
      b. 1 and 3 only
      c. 2 and 3 only
      d. 3 and 4 only

2. It is suggested that respiratory distress syndrome is a result of which of the following?
   1. Vernix membrane
   2. Prematurity
   3. Pulmonary surfactant deficiency
   4. Congenital alveolar dysplasia
      a. 1 and 3 only
      b. 2 and 3 only
      c. 1 and 4 only
      d. 2, 3, and 4 only

3. When an infant with respiratory distress syndrome creates more negative intrapleural pressure during inspiration, which of the following occurs?
   a. The soft tissue between the ribs bulges outward.
   b. The dependent blood vessels dilate and pool blood.
   c. The substernal area protrudes.
   d. The abdominal area retracts.

4. Infants with severe respiratory distress syndrome often have which of the following?
   1. Diminished breath sounds
   2. Bronchial breath sounds
   3. Hyperresonant percussion notes
   4. Fine crackles
      a. 1 and 4 only
      b. 3 and 4 only
      c. 2 and 3 only
      d. 2 and 4 only

5. Continuous positive airway pressure (CPAP) is often administered to infants with respiratory distress syndrome in an effort to do which of the following?
   1. Increase the infant's FRC
   2. Decrease the infant's work of breathing
   3. Increase the infant's PaO_2
   4. Decrease the FIO_2 necessary to oxygenate the infant
      a. 1 and 3 only
      b. 2 and 4 only
      c. 2, 3, and 4 only
      d. 1, 2, 3, and 4

Chapter Objectives

After reading this chapter, you will be able to:

- List the anatomic alterations of the lungs associated with pulmonary air leak syndromes.
- Describe the causes of pulmonary air leak syndromes.
- List the cardiopulmonary clinical manifestations associated with pulmonary air leak syndromes.
- Describe the general management of pulmonary air leak syndromes.
- Describe the clinical strategies and rationales of the SOAP presented in the case study.
- Define key terms and complete self-assessment questions at the end of the chapter and on Evolve.

Key Terms

Air Embolism
Blebs (Emphysema-Like)
Bronchopulmonary Dysplasia (Chronic Lung Disease of Infancy)
Cardiac Tamponade
Exogenous Surfactant
High-Frequency Ventilation (HFV)
Iatrogenic Pneumothorax
Intravascular Air Embolism
Needle Thoracentesis
Peak Inspiratory Pressure
Pericardiocentesis
Permissive Hypercapnia
Pneumomediastinum

Pneumopericardium
Pneumoperitoneum
Pneumothorax
Positive End-Expiratory Pressure (PEEP)
Positive Inspiratory Pressures (PIPs)
Pressure-Limited Resuscitation T-Piece Devices
Prolonged Inspiratory Time (T$_I$)
Pulmonary Air Leak Syndromes
Pulmonary Barotrauma
Pulmonary Interstitial Emphysema (PIE)
Pulmonary Volutrauma
Subcutaneous Emphysema
Syndrome of Inappropriate Antidiuretic Hormone (SIADH)
Tension Pneumothorax
Transillumination of the Chest
Vasovagal Reaction
Ventilator-Induced Lung Injury (VILI)

Chapter Outline

Anatomic Alterations of the Lungs
    Pulmonary Interstitial Emphysema
Etiology and Epidemiology
Overview of the Cardiopulmonary Clinical Manifestations
    Associated With Pulmonary Air Leak Syndromes
General Management of Pulmonary Air Leak Syndromes
    Respiratory Care Treatment Protocols
Case Study: Pulmonary Air Leak Syndromes
Self-Assessment Questions

Pulmonary air leak syndromes (also called **air block syndromes**) in the infant comprise a large spectrum of clinical entities, including **pulmonary interstitial emphysema (PIE)**, followed by (in severe cases), **pneumomediastinum, pneumothorax, pneumopericardium, pneumoperitoneum**, and, in rare cases, **intravascular air embolism**. Pulmonary air leak syndromes were common complications of mechanical ventilation in premature infants with respiratory distress syndrome before the introduction of **exogenous surfactant**. Infants who continue to be most at risk for pulmonary air leak are those born prematurely, or who develop respiratory distress syndrome or meconium aspiration syndrome, or any infant who requires resuscitation at birth.

It has long been known that mechanical ventilation can produce a variety of lung injuries referred to as **ventilator-induced lung injury (VILI), pulmonary volutrauma**, or **pulmonary barotrauma** (see discussion of ventilator hazards in Chapter 11, Respiratory Insufficiency, Respiratory Failure, and Ventilatory Management Protocols). *VILI* is defined as stress fractures of the pulmonary capillary endothelium, epithelium, and basement membrane, and, in severe cases, lung rupture. Lung ruptures can lead to leakage of fluid, protein, and blood into pulmonary tissue and air spaces or leakage of air into tissue spaces. This condition can be followed by an inflammatory response and possibly a reduced defense against infection. *Pulmonary volutrauma* is defined as damage to the lungs caused by overdistention secondary to the mechanical delivery of excessively high tidal volumes. *Pulmonary barotrauma* is defined as damage to the lungs caused by rapid or extreme pressures generated by mechanical ventilation.

Predisposing factors for VILI, pulmonary volutrauma, or pulmonary barotrauma include (1) mechanical ventilation with high peak inspiratory volumes and pressures, (2) mechanical ventilation with a high mean airway pressure, (3) structural immaturity of lung and chest wall, (4) surfactant insufficiency or inactivation, and (5) preexisting lung disease. Fortunately, newborn mechanical ventilator strategies today minimize lung injuries by keeping exhaled volumes low, accepting higher PCO_2 levels (**permissive hypercapnia**[1]) or switching to high-frequency ventilation when **positive inspiratory pressures (PIPs)** exceed safe limits. Pulmonary air leak syndrome, however, can still occur in certain clinical scenarios, especially when very high ventilator pressures are used or aggressive ventilation is applied during resuscitation. The respiratory therapist must alway be on alert for an **iatrogenic pneumothorax** when high ventilatory pressures are applied to the lungs of the newborn.

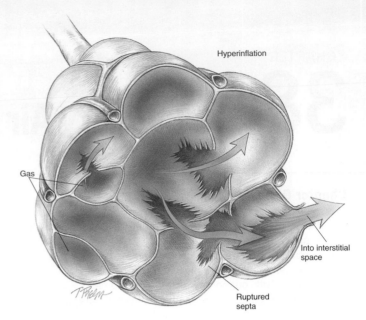

FIGURE 38.1 Pulmonary air leak syndromes.

Anatomic Alterations of the Lungs

Pulmonary Interstitial Emphysema

Virtually all pulmonary air leak syndromes begin with some degree of PIE. When high airway pressures are applied to an infant's lungs (e.g., during mechanical ventilation or excessive PEEP), the distal airways and alveoli often become overdistended—that is, they develop **blebs (emphysema-like)** areas and rupture (Fig. 38.1). In addition, gas trapping from an insufficient expiratory time or auto-PEEP can cause alveolar overdistention and rupture. Once the gas escapes, it is forced into the loose connective tissue sheaths that surround the airways and pulmonary capillaries and the interlobular septa containing pulmonary veins. In severe cases the gas continues to spread by dissecting along the peribronchial and perivascular spaces to the hilum of the lung, producing the classic radiographic appearance of PIE that shows bubbles of air in the interstitial cuffs (Figs. 38.2 and 38.3).

The overdistention associated with PIE forces the lungs into a full inflation position, which in turn decreases lung

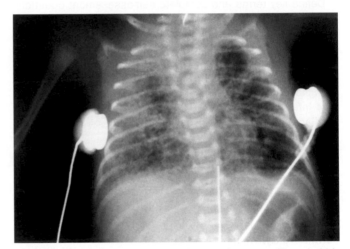

FIGURE 38.2 Pulmonary interstitial emphysema. Fine, bubbly appearance of the lungs in an infant with severe respiratory distress syndrome. (From Taussig, L. M., & Landau, L. I. [2008]. *Pediatric respiratory medicine* [2nd ed.]. St. Louis, MO: Elsevier.)

[1]Permissive hypercapnia defined: Mechanical ventilation was traditionally applied with the goal of normalizing arterial blood gas values, particularly the arterial carbon dioxide tension ($PaCO_2$). However, this is no longer the primary objective of mechanical ventilation. Today, the emphasis is on maintaining adequate gas exchange while—and, importantly—minimizing the risks of mechanical ventilation. Common strategies used to reduce the risk for mechanical ventilation include (1) low tidal volume ventilation to protect the lung from ventilator-associated lung injury in patients with acute lung injury (e.g., acute respiratory distress syndrome) and (2) reduction of the tidal volume, respiratory rate, or both to minimize intrinsic positive end-expiratory pressure (i.e., auto-PEEP) in patients with obstructive lung disease (e.g., chronic obstructive pulmonary disease). Although these mechanical ventilation strategies may result in an increased $PaCO_2$ level (hypercapnia), they do help protect the lung from barotrauma (i.e., physical damage to lung tissues caused by excessive gas pressures). The lenient acceptance of the hypercapnia is called *permissive hypercapnia*. In most cases, the patient's $PaCO_2$ is adequately maintained by an increased ventilatory rate that offsets the decreased tidal volume. The $PaCO_2$, however, should not be permitted to increase to the point of severe respiratory acidosis. The most current consensus suggests it is safe to allow the pH to fall as low as 7.20 (http://www.ARDSNet).

compliance (static lung compliance is reduced at *both* very low and very high lung volumes). Moreover, air trapped within the interstitial cuffs compresses the airways and increases airway resistance. In addition, the trapped air in the interstitial spaces impairs lymphatic function, resulting in fluid accumulation in the interstitial cuffs and alveoli, further decreasing lung compliance. Once the interstitial gas reaches the hilum of the lung, it either coalesces to form large hilar blebs or tracks beneath the visceral pleura to form large subpleural pockets of air. In either case, the accumulation of gas can be large enough to significantly compress the lung (i.e., atelectasis), or restrict mediastinal structures.

A **pneumomediastinum** may occur when the excessive air associated with a PIE continues to track and accumulate through the perivascular and peribronchial cuffs and causes the gas in the hilar area to rupture into the mediastinum. In

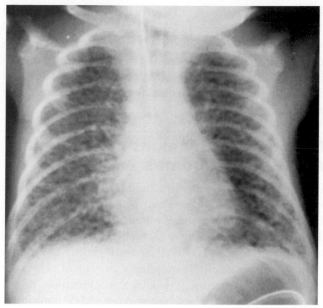

FIGURE 38.3 Pulmonary interstitial emphysema. The lung is grossly hyperinflated, with coarse radiolucencies extending from the pleura to the hilum. These radiolucencies represent bubbles of air in the perivascular and peribronchial interstitial cuffs. (From Gleason, C. A., & Juul, S. E. [2018]. *Avery's diseases of the newborn* [10th ed.]. Philadelphia: Elsevier.)

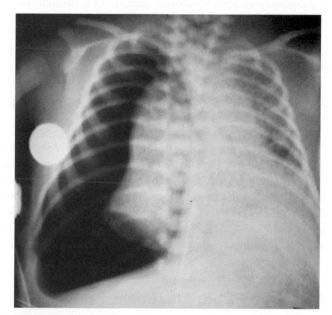

FIGURE 38.4 Tension pneumothorax. The lung on the involved (right) side is collapsed, and the mediastinum is shifted to the opposite side. Pleura can be seen bulging into the intercostal spaces. (From Gleason, C. A., & Juul, S. E. [2018]. *Avery's diseases of the newborn* [10th ed.]. Philadelphia: Elsevier.)

addition, the high gas pressures associated with a pneumomediastinum also may dissect into the pleural space and the fascial planes of the neck and skin, resulting in **subcutaneous emphysema,** presenting as crepitation and edema of the tissues.

A **pneumothorax** may occur because of the alveolar overdistention and subsequent rupture commonly associated with a PIE (Fig. 38.4). A **tension pneumothorax** is a life-threatening

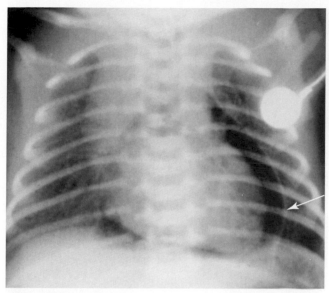

FIGURE 38.5 Pneumopericardium. A thin rim of pericardium (arrow) is visible and clearly separated from the heart by air within the pericardial sac. (From Gleason, C. A., & Juul, S. E. [2018]. *Avery's diseases of the newborn* [10th ed.]. Philadelphia: Elsevier.)

condition in which the air pressure in the thoracic cavity rises high enough to restrict systemic circulation, causing lung and circulatory collapse (see Chapter 23, Pneumothorax).

A **pneumopericardium** can develop from direct tracking of interstitial air along the great vessels into the pericardial sac (Fig. 38.5). Gas pressure in the pericardium restricts atrial and ventricular filling, resulting in a decreased stroke volume and, ultimately, a reduced cardiac output (**cardiac tamponade**) and systemic hypotension, which can be fatal if not treated.

A **pneumoperitoneum** may develop from the tracking of gas along the sheaths of the aorta and vena cava, which eventually may burst into the peritoneal cavity. Clinically, an infant with a pneumoperitoneum manifests the sudden onset of abdominal distention. The pneumoperitoneum may be large enough to block the descent of the diaphragm and may require drainage (Fig. 38.6). Finally, the excessive gas accumulation associated with a pneumoperitoneum may end up in the scrotum in male babies or the labia in females.

In very rare cases, an **intravascular air embolism** may occur. It is hypothesized that the air is actually pumped under high pressure through the pulmonary lymphatics into the systemic venous circulation. Intravascular air causes an abrupt cardiovascular collapse and is frequently diagnosed when air is observed in vessels on chest radiographs taken to establish the cause of cardiovascular collapse.

The major pathologic changes associated with pulmonary air leak syndromes are as follows:

- Collapsed alveoli adjacent to overdistended alveoli (e.g., blebs or emphysema-like area)
- Excessive bronchial secretions (late stages)
- Pneumothorax
- Pneumomediastinum
- Pneumoperitoneum
- Airway compression (caused by interstitial air accumulation)

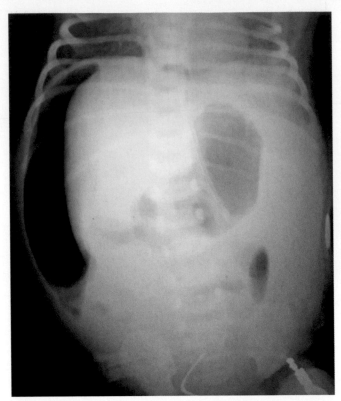

FIGURE 38.6 Pneumoperitoneum with right pneumothorax (decubitus view). (Courtesy Dayton Children's Hospital, Dayton, Ohio.)

BOX 38.1 Risk Factors for Neonatal Air Leak Syndrome

- Prematurity
- Very low birth weight
- Low Apgar score and need of resuscitation
- Positive pressure ventilation
- Use of high **peak inspiratory pressure**
- Use of high tidal volume
- Use of high inspiratory time
- Respiratory distress syndrome
- Meconium aspiration syndrome
- Amniotic fluid aspiration
- Pneumonia
- Pulmonary hypoplasia

Etiology and Epidemiology

Air leak syndrome occurs in 1% to 2% of all newborns; *the highest incidence is among infants with meconium aspiration syndrome*. In general, the incidence of air leak syndrome is inversely related to the birth weight of newborns, with infants with very low birth weights most at risk. Box 38.1 shows common risk factors for pulmonary air leak syndrome. Preterm infants who weigh less than 1000 grams at birth have an increased risk for the early occurrence of pulmonary air leak syndromes (often within the first 24 to 48 hours of life), especially because of the weak noncartilaginous structures of their distal airways. The most frequent cause of pulmonary air leak syndromes in preterm infants is the use of mechanical ventilation. Pulmonary air leak syndromes commonly result

from the use of high levels of **Positive End Expiratory Pressure (PEEP)**, high **Positive Inspiratory Pressures (PIPs)**, and **prolonged inspiratory time (T₁)**. The early use of surfactant and protective ventilator strategies, such as permissive hypercapnia, to minimize peak pressures has resulted in a significant decrease in the incidence of air leak syndromes in premature infants.

General Management of Pulmonary Air Leak Syndromes

Prevention is the best treatment for pulmonary air leak syndromes. These syndromes may be prevented by (1) using a manometer or **pressure-limited resuscitation T-piece device** for manual ventilation, (2) using the lowest mechanical ventilator pressures (PIP, PEEP) to reach patient-appropriate exhaled tidal volumes, (3) adopting a strategy of permissive hypercapnia, (4) securing radiologic confirmation of the appropriateness of PEEP and lung volumes, and (5) implementing high-frequency ventilation when required PIP exceeds 30 cm H_2O.

Selective intubation of the unaffected or less affected lung may allow the injured lung time to heal when PIE is present. **High-frequency ventilation (HFV)** has been successful in treating infants with pulmonary air leak syndromes. Survivors of pulmonary air leak syndromes may develop **bronchopulmonary dysplasia** (or **chronic lung disease of infancy**) (see Chapter 40, Chronic Lung Disease of Infancy) as a result of overly vigorous mechanical ventilation. Finally, the respiratory therapist always must be alert for signs and symptoms of subcutaneous emphysema, pneumothorax, pneumopericardium, pneumoperitoneum, pneumomediastinum, and intravascular air embolism.

Mechanical removal of free air from the intrathoracic cavity is necessary if the air accumulation is significant and prevents effective ventilation. Needle thoracentesis is a technique used to emergently relieve a significant or tension pneumothorax in these infants. Chest tube placement is the preferred method when a surgeon is present. A **pericardiocentesis** using a needle to tap and remove fluid or blood around the pericardium is performed when vascular collapse or cardiac tamponade is life-threatening.

Respiratory Care Treatment Protocols

Oxygen Therapy Protocol

Oxygen therapy is used to treat hypoxemia, decrease the work of breathing, and decrease myocardial work. Because of the hypoxemia that often develops in pulmonary air leak syndromes, supplemental oxygen is often required (see Newborn Oxygen Therapy Protocol, Protocol 33.1). Although 100% oxygen can be used in the acute treatment of an adult or older child with a pneumothorax to speed the reabsorption of inert nitrogen, it is not considered for this purpose in the management of newborns with pulmonary air leak.

Airway Clearance Protocol

If airway secretions and mucous accumulation are present with pulmonary air leak syndromes, suctioning may be used

OVERVIEW of the Cardiopulmonary Clinical Manifestations Associated With Pulmonary Air Leak Syndromes

The following clinical manifestations result from the pathologic mechanisms caused (or activated) by atelectasis (see Fig. 10.7) and decreased lung compliance—the major anatomic alteration of the lungs associated with pulmonary air leak syndromes (see Fig. 38.1).

CLINICAL DATA OBTAINED AT THE PATIENT'S BEDSIDE

The Physical Examination

Vital Signs

Increased Respiratory Rate (Tachypnea)

Normally, a newborn's respiratory rate is about 40 to 60 breaths/min. During the early stages of pulmonary air leak syndromes, the respiratory rate is generally well over 60 breaths/min. Several pathophysiologic mechanisms operating simultaneously may lead to an increased respiratory rate:

- Stimulation of peripheral chemoreceptors (hypoxemia)
- Relationship of decreased lung compliance to increased respiratory rate
- Stimulation of central chemoreceptors

Increased Heart Rate (Pulse) and Blood Pressure

Apnea (see Box 33.3)

Clinical Manifestations Associated With Increased Negative Intrapleural Pressures During Inspiration

- Intercostal retractions
- Substernal retraction and abdominal distention (seesaw movement)
- Flaring nostrils

Chest Assessment Findings

- Diminished breath sounds (decreased air exchange)
- Crackles

Expiratory Grunting

Cyanosis

Increased Transillumination

Transillumination of the chest is performed by placing a high-intensity fiberoptic light source against the infant's chest in a darkened room. When free air is present in the chest cavity (i.e., when a pneumothorax is present), an increased degree of transillumination is seen on the affected side.

CLINICAL DATA OBTAINED FROM LABORATORY TESTS AND SPECIAL PROCEDURES

Pulmonary Function Test Findings
(Extrapolated Data for Instructional Purposes)
(Primarily Restrictive Lung Pathophysiology)

The anatomic alterations of the lungs associated with pulmonary air leak syndromes primarily cause a restrictive lung pathophysiology. For example, in moderate to severe cases, the following lung volumes and capacities may be lower than normal:

RV	IRV	VC	FRC	TLC
↓	↓	↓	↓	↓

Arterial Blood Gases[1]

MILD TO MODERATE PULMONARY AIR LEAK SYNDROMES
Acute Alveolar Hyperventilation With Hypoxemia[2]
(Acute Respiratory Alkalosis)

pH	$PaCO_2$	HCO_3^-	PaO_2	SaO_2 or SpO_2
↑	↓	↓ (but normal)	↓	↓

SEVERE PULMONARY AIR LEAK SYNDROMES
Acute Ventilatory Failure With Hypoxemia[3]
(Acute Respiratory Acidosis)

pH[4]	$PaCO_2$	HCO_3^-[4]	PaO_2	SaO_2 or SpO_2
↓	↑	↑ (but normal)	↓	↓

---

[1]NOTE: A critically ill newborn is likely to have an umbilical arterial catheter in place for arterial blood gas (ABG) sampling. In older critically ill infants and children, an arterial line may be placed for frequent ABG sampling. For intermittent sampling, because of the difficulty of obtaining ABG samples, capillary blood gas (CBG) samples may be used to determine the pH, $PaCO_2$, and HCO_3^- (i.e., the acid-base and ventilation status only). Capillary PO_2 values are unreliable and should not be used for clinical analysis. The standard way to evaluate the oxygenation status in these young patients is pulse oximetry (SpO_2) (see Chapter 33, Newborn Assessment and Management).

[2]See Fig. 5.2 and Table 5.4 and related discussion for the acute pH, $PaCO_2$, and HCO_3^- changes associated with acute alveolar hyperventilation.

[3]See Table 5.5 and related discussion for the acute pH, $PaCO_2$, and HCO_3^- changes associated with acute ventilatory failure.

[4]When tissue hypoxia is severe enough to produce lactic acid, the pH and HCO_3^- values will be lower than expected for a particular $PaCO_2$ level.

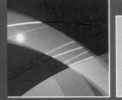
Oxygenation Indices[5]					
$\dot{Q}_S/\dot{Q}_T$	DO_2[6]	$\dot{V}O_2$	$C(a\text{-}\bar{v})O_2$	O_2ER	$S\bar{v}O_2$
↑	↓	N	N	↑	↓

RADIOLOGIC FINDINGS

Chest Radiograph

The chest radiograph may show focal or generalized problem areas. When significant partial airway obstruction, air trapping, and alveolar hyperinflation are present, the chest radiograph appears hyperlucent and the diaphragms may be depressed.

---

[5]$C(a\text{-}\bar{v})O_2$, Arterial-venous oxygen difference; DO_2, total oxygen delivery; O_2ER, oxygen extraction ratio; $\dot{Q}_S/\dot{Q}_T$, pulmonary shunt fraction; $S\bar{v}O_2$, mixed venous oxygen saturation; $\dot{V}O_2$, oxygen consumption.

[6]It should be noted that because the newborn normally has a higher hemoglobin (Hb) level at birth (16.8 g to 18.9 g/dL), the DO_2 may actually be better than the PaO_2 or SpO_2 alone (see Chapter 6, Assessment of Oxygenation).

The diagnosis of pulmonary interstitial emphysema (PIE) is commonly confirmed when the radiograph reveals lung hyperinflation and a fine, bubbly appearance (emphysema-like blebs) extending from the hilum to the pleura (see Fig. 38.2 and 38.3). PIE may affect both lungs or may be present in one lung or one lobe.

The respiratory therapist always should be alert for the sudden development of a pneumomediastinum or pneumothorax in infants with pulmonary air leak syndromes. When the excessive air associated with a PIE continues to track and accumulate through the perivascular and peribronchial cuffs, it may cause the gas in the hilar area to rupture into the mediastinum, resulting in a pneumomediastinum. A pneumothorax may occur because of the alveolar overdistention and subsequent rupture commonly associated with PIE (see Fig. 38.4).

Fig. 38.5 shows an infant with a pneumopericardium, which developed from the direct tracking of interstitial gas along the great vessels into the pericardial sac. Fig. 38.6 shows an infant with a pneumoperitoneum.

to enhance the mobilization of airway secretions (see Airway Clearance Protocol, Protocol 10.2).

Lung Expansion Therapy Protocol

Lung expansion measures commonly are administered cautiously to offset the pulmonary capillary congestion and interstitial edema and atelectasis associated with pulmonary air leak syndromes (see Lung Expansion Therapy Protocol, Protocol 33.3). Optimal PEEP strategies are needed to improve lung compliance and reduce the need for higher PIP.

Mechanical Ventilation Protocol

Mechanical ventilation may be necessary to provide and support alveolar gas exchange until the patient's condition improves. Prevention is the best treatment for pulmonary air leak syndromes. The respiratory therapist must watch the infant's tidal volume (V_T) and reduce the ventilating pressure (PIP) as the infant's lung compliance improves. The tidal volume is generally kept between 4 and 6 mL/kg to prevent volutrauma. Selective intubation and ventilation of the unaffected or less affected lung may allow the injured lung time to heal. High-frequency ventilation has been successful in treating infants with pulmonary air leak syndromes (see Newborn Mechanical Ventilation and Weaning Protocol 33.4).

Needle Thoracentesis

The **needle thoracentesis** technique is used to emergently relieve the life-threatening pressure caused by a significant pneumothorax or tension pneumothorax that is impeding effective ventilation. Once the presence of free air is determined by chest radiograph, transillumination, or absence of breath sounds in a rapidly deteriorating infant who is difficult to manually ventilate, a sheathed catheter or needle is inserted above the third intercostal space of the affected side at the midclavicular line or the midaxillary line (Fig. 38.7). The needle is advanced until it enters the pleural cavity, at which time a "pop" or release of air is heard. The needle is removed, and the catheter is taped in place and attached to a three-way stopcock for intermittent air removal by syringe. This emergency technique allows for pressure relief until a larger chest tube is placed.

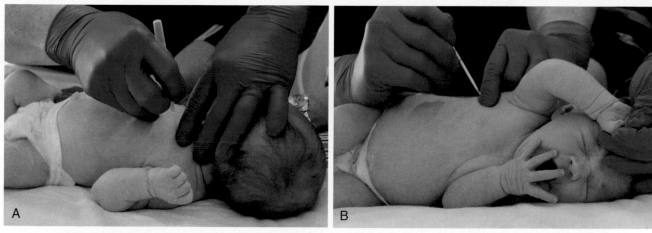

FIGURE 38.7 Needle thoracentesis is a technique used to emergently relieve a significant or tension pneumothorax in these infants. (A) Needle thoracentesis, midclavicle. (B) Needle thoracentesis, lateral. (Courtesy Dayton Children's Hospital, Dayton, Ohio.)

CASE STUDY Pulmonary Air Leak Syndromes

Admitting History and Physical Examination

A 32-week-gestation, preterm female infant was delivered by emergency cesarean section to a healthy 25-year-old mother. The infant weighed 2750 grams. The mother's admitting history showed her to be a primigravida with normal prenatal care with no history of illness during her pregnancy. The cesarean section was performed because of repeated and prolonged fetal heart rate decelerations that did not improve with maternal positioning or oxygen administration. At delivery, the infant was found to have the umbilical cord twice wrapped tightly around her neck. She was limp, appeared pale and cyanotic, and was apneic. She showed no response to tactile stimuli, and her heart rate was 65 beats/min. Her 1-minute Apgar score was 1 (color 0, pulse 1, grimace 0, reflex irritability 0, muscle tone 0, respiratory 0).

The neonatologist, nurse, and respiratory therapist immediately started chest compressions with manual ventilation with a bag-valve-mask and 30% oxygen. The 5-minute Apgar was 5 (color 1, pulse 2, grimace 0, reflex irritability 0, muscle tone 1, respiratory 1). Despite the fact that the baby's condition had started to improve, she suddenly took a turn for the worse. Her heart rate started to drop; she again appeared cyanotic, and her muscle tone decreased.

At this time, the respiratory therapist noted that the baby's breath sounds were absent over the right lung and severely decreased over the left upper and lower lobes. Her heart sounds were muffled and faint. Transillumination showed a large right pneumothorax. This was later confirmed by chest radiographic examination as a right tension pneumothorax. The neonatologist inserted a chest tube, and the baby was placed on a mechanical ventilator with the following settings: intermittent mandatory ventilation (IMV) rate of 30, FIO$_2$

1.0, positive inspiratory pressure (PIP) +25 cm H$_2$O, **positive end-expiratory pressure (PEEP)** +5 cm H$_2$O, and inspiratory time (T$_I$) 0.35 seconds.

Moments later, an umbilical artery catheter was inserted; it showed the following values: pH 7.19, PaCO$_2$ 77 mm Hg, HCO$_3^-$ 19 mEq/L, PaO$_2$ 31 mm Hg, and SaO$_2$ 47%. The ventilator rate was increased immediately to 40 breaths/min. ABG values 20 minutes later were as follows: pH 7.33, PaCO$_2$ 43 mm Hg, HCO$_3^-$ 22 mEq/L, PaO$_2$ 47 mm Hg, and SaO$_2$ 83%.

A second chest radiographic examination an hour later showed that the right lung had reexpanded, with scattered areas of segmental atelectasis throughout. At this time, the infant appeared pink and her vital signs were stable, with a heart rate of 155 beats/min and blood pressure of 68/35 mm Hg. Breath sounds revealed bilateral crackles. ABG values were pH 7.34, PaCO$_2$ 43 mm Hg, HCO$_3^-$ 22 mEq/L, PaO$_2$ 53 mm Hg, and SaO$_2$ 89%. The respiratory therapist recorded the following in the baby's chart:

Respiratory Assessment and Plan

S N/A

O Skin: Pink. HR 155 bpm, BP 68/35. Crackles throughout. ABGs pH 7.34, PaCO$_2$ 43, HCO$_3^-$ 22, PaO$_2$ 53, and SaO$_2$ 89%. CXR: Reexpanded right lung with scattered areas of segmental atelectasis throughout.

A • Preterm infant in respiratory distress at birth
 • Right tension pneumothorax, treated
 • Atelectasis—right lung (CXR)
 • Adequate ventilation and oxygenation on present ventilator settings (ABGs)
 • Excessive airway secretions (crackles and rhonchi)

P Continue Mechanical Ventilation Protocol. Attempt to reduce FIO_2 per Oxygen Therapy Protocol. Continue Lung Expansion Therapy Protocol (PEEP +5 cm H_2O). Start Airway Clearance Protocol (suction PRN). Monitor closely (vital signs, color, ABGs).

Discussion

A tension pneumothorax caused by a resuscitation effort is not uncommon during resuscitation of the newborn. This is especially true when staff is inexperienced or perform resuscitation too aggressively because of the anxiety and urgency of the situation. **Pressure limited resuscitation T-piece devices** used in most delivery rooms are good adjuncts for limiting manual ventilating pressures during neonatal resuscitation.

The respiratory therapist must be prepared to attend deliveries, to manage the infant's airway and provide ventilatory support when their presence is expected by the perinatal team. In fact, most departments expect staff to have one or more of the following credentials: Neonatal Resuscitation Program (NRP), Pediatric Advanced Life Support (PALS), or Registered Respiratory Therapist-Neonatal/Pediatric Specialist (RRT-NPS). With the simulation baby and other computerized training manikins available, many respiratory therapists are trained and ready to participate on such rapid response teams.

Since the advent of surfactant therapy, pneumothoraces in mechanically ventilated infants in neonatal intensive care units (NICUs) have decreased. Tension pneumothorax is a potentially life-threatening emergency, and the respiratory therapist who attends deliveries or is on a newborn transport team should always be alert for any signs or symptoms associated with this condition and know how to treat it.

In this case the clinical manifestations associated with a pneumothorax and/or atelectasis were quickly identified when the respiratory therapist noted the possibility of a pneumothorax by pointing out that the baby's breath sounds were absent over the right lung and severely decreased over the left upper and middle lobes. Transillumination further supported the presence of a pneumothorax. The chest radiograph confirmed a right lung pneumothorax. Caution should be used when evacuating air from a large pneumothorax because rapid reexpansion of a collapsed lung can cause a severe **vasovagal reaction**[2] and may result in transient pulmonary edema.

Finally, it is not uncommon for infants with pulmonary air leak syndromes to develop fluid in their lungs shortly after a pneumothorax has resolved (i.e., the chest tube is no longer sucking any air out of the baby's chest). When this occurs, these infants retain fluid evidenced by rapid weight gain, demonstrate crackles, and require a higher FIO_2 to maintain their desired PaO_2 levels. The reason for this is that babies who have iatrogenic tension pneumothoraces often develop a transient **syndrome of inappropriate antidiuretic hormone (SIADH)**. In other words, the pneumothorax causes the release of antidiuretic hormone, which inhibits urination. Some of the retained fluid accumulates in the baby's lungs. Often, a diuretic (such as furosemide), a little more airway pressure, an increased FIO_2, or an increased ventilator rate may need to be administered to offset this transient problem. The condition usually lasts only about 24 hours. The respiratory therapist should expect this condition and should not be overly concerned.

---

[2] A vasovagal reaction is defined as a reflex of the involuntary nervous system that causes the heart to slow down (bradycardia) and that, at the same time, affects the nerves to the blood vessels in the legs permitting those vessels to dilate (widen). As a result the heart puts out less blood, the blood pressure drops, and what blood is circulating tends to go into the legs rather than to the head. The brain is deprived of oxygen and the fainting episode occurs. The vasovagal reaction is also called a *vasovagal attack*.

SELF-ASSESSMENT QUESTIONS

1. The most frequent etiologic factor causing air leak syndromes in preterm infants is:
   a. Infants who weigh less than 1000 grams
   b. Mechanical ventilation
   c. Excessive bronchial secretions
   d. Increased expiratory grunting

2. During the advanced stages of pulmonary air leak syndromes, the infant demonstrates a(n):
   1. Increased $PaCO_2$
   2. Decreased HCO_3^-
   3. Increased pH
   4. Decreased PaO_2
      a. 1 and 4 only
      b. 2 and 3 only
      c. 1, 3, and 4 only
      d. 1, 2, 3, and 4

3. Infants with pulmonary air leak syndromes often have:
   1. Reduced urine output
   2. Increased transillumination
   3. Hypoxia-induced pulmonary arterial vasoconstriction
   4. Ventilator-induced lung injury
      a. 1 and 3 only
      b. 2 and 4 only
      c. 2, 3, and 4 only
      d. 1, 2, 3, and 4

4. Which of the following are associated with pulmonary air leak syndromes?
    1. Poor lung compliance
    2. Inadequate ventilation
    3. Hypoxemia
    4. Circulatory compromise
        a. 3 and 4 only
        b. 1, 3, and 4 only
        c. 2, 3, and 4 only
        d. 1, 2, 3, and 4

5. In pulmonary air leak syndromes, if the high interstitial lung pressure persists, the gas may:
    1. Continue to spread peripherally
    2. Remain localized and restrict the airway lumen
    3. Cause a pneumomediastinum or pneumopericardium
    4. Rupture the visceral pleura
        a. 1 and 3 only
        b. 2 and 4 only
        c. 2, 3, and 4 only
        d. 1, 2, 3, and 4

Respiratory Syncytial Virus Infection (Bronchiolitis)

Chapter Objectives

After reading this chapter, you will be able to:

- List the anatomic alterations of the lungs associated with respiratory syncytial virus infection.
- Describe how respiratory syncytial virus is contracted
- List the cardiopulmonary clinical manifestations associated with respiratory syncytial virus infection.
- Describe the general management of respiratory syncytial virus infection (Bronchiolitis).
- Describe the clinical strategies and rationales of the SOAPs presented in the case study.
- Define key terms and complete self-assessment questions at the end of the chapter and on Evolve.

Key Terms

"Ball-valve" Mechanism
Bronchiolitis
Enzyme Immunoassay (EIA)
Palivizumab (Synagis)

Pneumonitis
Polymerase Chain Reaction (PCR)
Respiratory Infectious Disease Panel (RIDP)
Syncytium

Chapter Outline

Anatomic Alterations of the Lungs
Etiology and Epidemiology
  Laboratory Testing for Respiratory Syncytial Virus
Overview of the Cardiopulmonary Clinical Manifestations Associated With Respiratory Syncytial Virus Infection
General Management of Respiratory Syncytial Virus Infection (Bronchiolitis)
  Monitoring
  Oxygen Therapy Protocol
  Respiratory Care Treatment Protocols
Case Study: Respiratory Syncytial Virus Infection (Bronchiolitis)
Self-Assessment Questions

Anatomic Alterations of the Lungs

The inhaled or aspirated respiratory syncytial virus (RSV) moves down the respiratory tract by means of cell-to-cell transfer, causing **bronchiolitis** and, in severe cases, atelectasis and pneumonia in the infant or child. The **syncytium** is defined as a "multinucleate mass of protoplasm produced by the merging of cells." At the level of the bronchioles the virus causes neighboring cells to fuse to form a syncytium, hence the name *respiratory syncytial virus*. The lower airways also may become infected when secretions from RSV-infected upper airways are aspirated.

RSV infection causes peribronchiolar mononuclear infiltration and necrosis of the epithelium of large and small airways. This condition leads to *edema of the small airways and increased production of mucus*. Airway clearance is impaired by loss of ciliated epithelial cells, and clearance of secretions becomes entirely cough dependent. As the condition worsens, the epithelium of the small airways becomes necrotic and desquamates into the airway lumen. The combination of sloughing necrotic tissue, airway edema, and accumulation of mucus leads to a decreased airway lumen and either a partially or a completely obstructed airway. Partial airway obstruction leads

to alveolar hyperinflation as a result of a **"ball-valve" mechanism** (Fig. 39.1).

Although RSV is primarily associated with obstructive lung pathophysiology, complete airway obstruction may lead to alveolar collapse or atelectasis. In these cases, pneumonic consolidation can result in **pneumonitis**. RSV is also referred to as *bronchiolitis* or *pneumonitis*, although bacterial superinfection is uncommon with RSV.

The following major pathologic or structural changes are associated with RSV infection:

- Inflammation and swelling of the peripheral airways
- Excessive airway secretions
- Sloughing of necrotic airway epithelium with loss of cilia
- Partial airway obstruction and alveolar hyperinflation
- Complete airway obstruction and atelectasis
- Consolidation

Etiology and Epidemiology

RSV is the most common viral respiratory pathogen seen in infancy and early childhood that leads to hospitalization. Although RSV infection can occur at any age, it is the small infant who presents with the most severe symptoms requiring

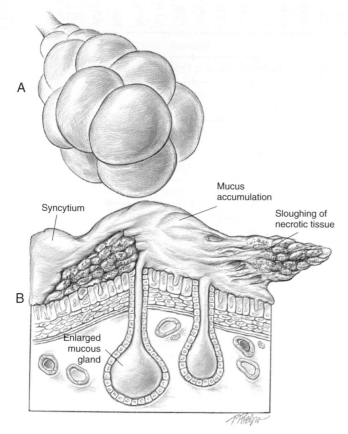

FIGURE 39.1 Bronchiolitis caused by respiratory syncytial virus. (A) Partial airway obstruction and alveolar hyperinflation. (B) Cross-section of inflamed airway.

Labels in figure: Syncytium, Mucus accumulation, Sloughing of necrotic tissue, Enlarged mucous gland, A, B

medical attention. Premature infants, infants younger than 6 months of age, and infants with congenital heart disease, cystic fibrosis, weakened immune systems, or neuromuscular disease have a greater risk for respiratory failure with RSV. Adults with compromised immune systems and those older than 65 years of age are also at risk.

RSV is commonly transmitted by young children who are infected with RSV and demonstrate the signs and symptoms of a mild upper respiratory tract infection or a "cold"—for example, coughing, sneezing, runny nose, decreased appetite, irritability, decreased activity, and respiratory distress. Ninety percent of children under 2 years of age have already contracted RSV, with 40% of those having lower respiratory tract involvement. RSV is easily transmitted when droplets containing the virus are coughed or sneezed into the air, although the primary mode of transmission is by contact. The lower respiratory tract is infected as the viral-laden nasopharyngeal secretions are aspirated.

Infection occurs when the particles touch the nose, mouth, or eyes of uninfected individuals in the immediate area. RSV also can spread from direct or indirect contact with nasal or oral secretions from an infected person. For example, RSV can be contracted by kissing the face or hands of a child infected with RSV who has a runny nose. Indirect contact may occur when touching the hard surface of a table, crib rail, or doorknob that has been touched by a person infected with RSV; RSV can remain infectious on countertops for more than 6 hours. Common areas of RSV transmission include

elementary schools and day care centers. Handwashing before and after contact is key; alcohol-based rubs are preferred to avoid skin breakdown for health care workers during the viral season. Frequent handwashing and wiping hard surfaces with a disinfectant may help stop the spread of RSV.

Infants and children infected with RSV usually develop symptoms within 4 to 6 days of infection (range 2 to 8 days). Hospital length of stay for bronchiolitis is difficult to predict because the infant's recovery depends on the disease severity, coinfections with other viruses, and when the family seeks medical treatment in the course of the disease. When care is sought later in the disease, the infant may present with more severe symptoms, such as dehydration and hypoxemia, but recovery may ensue quickly with supportive care. For those who seek medical attention early in the course of the disease, their mild symptoms may worsen over 3 to 5 days, resulting in repeated office or emergency department (ED) visits and readmission. Most patients will recover in 1 to 2 weeks, but about 25% will have symptoms after 21 days. Infected individuals are usually contagious for up to 8 days. Some patients with a weakened immune system may be contagious for as long as 4 weeks. Reinfections with RSV are common because there is no long-term immunity from having an RSV infection.

Most otherwise healthy children with RSV do not require hospitalization. However, according to the Centers for Disease Control and Prevention (CDC), 75,000 to 125,000 children under the age of 1 year are hospitalized each year in the United States because of RSV infection. Of this group, most are under 6 months old, with the highest age-specific rate of hospitalization at 30 to 60 days of age.

Although the outbreak of RSV cases varies by location each year, the number of RSV cases typically increases during the fall, winter, and early spring months. It is not fully known why RSV outbreaks occur in certain regions more than in others, but temperature, climate, and humidity appear to play a role. Fig. 39.2 shows the typical RSV season in the United States by region and in Florida according to the CDC.

Laboratory Testing for Respiratory Syncytial Virus

RSV infection should be suspected when the clinical manifestations correlate to the time of year, the presence of a local outbreak, age of the patient, history of the illness, and recent exposure. RSV can be diagnosed with commercially available antigen assay tests, typically ordered as an (RSV–**enzyme immunoassay [EIA]**). This test requires a nasopharyngeal aspirate or lavage sample, often obtained in the physician's office or ED. It is a rapid and usually reliable screen, but a negative RSV-EIA does not rule out RSV. A more definitive test is the **respiratory infectious disease panel (RIDP)** by **polymerase chain reaction (PCR)**. This test identifies RSV plus other respiratory viruses such as rhinovirus, influenza, parainfluenza, adenovirus, coronavirus, and human metapneumovirus, which also cause bronchiolitis. The EIA test is less sensitive in older children and adults, making the RIDP by PCR the more accurate test. The current AAP Clinic Practice Guidelines for RSV bronchiolitis discourages the routine use of laboratory studies (EIA and RIDP) during the RSV season, because treatment will not differ based on viral etiology. However, if hospitalization requires cohorting,

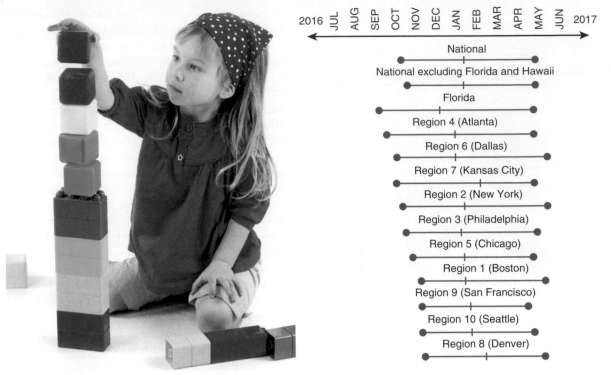

FIGURE 39.2 Respiratory syncytial virus season in the United States by region and in Florida, July 2016-June 2017. (Left, copyright Shutterstock.com. Right, data modified from Centers for Disease Control and prevention. Retrieved from https://www.cdc.gov/rsv/research/us-surveillance.html.)

viral etiology would be of interest to avoid additional viral exposures. It also may be of value if an infant receiving Synagis presents with bronchiolitis symptoms to see if the infant has contracted RSV despite therapy.

General Management of Respiratory Syncytial Virus Infection (Bronchiolitis)

The management of RSV bronchiolitis is largely supportive. Therapy includes carefully monitoring clinical status, providing adequate oxygenation, maintaining upper airway patency through frequent suctioning, delivering adequate hydration and nutrition, and providing parental education on home management. Table 39.1 shows an RSV bronchiolitis scoring system commonly used to objectively evaluate the patient's condition and, importantly, to up-regulate or down-regulate therapy according to the managing medical team. Table 39.2 provides a helpful overview of an RSV bronchiolitis management protocol based on the patient's bronchiolitis score (see Table 39.1).

Prophylaxis

Palivizumab (Synagis) is a monoclonal antibody (directed against the fusion protein of RSV) used as a preventive measure against RSV infection in high-risk infants. The American Academy of Pediatrics (AAP) 2014 guidelines recommend that premature infants (less than 29 weeks' gestation) and infants with hemodynamically significant heart disease or chronic lung disease of prematurity (who were less than 32 weeks' gestation and required greater than 21% oxygen

for at least 28 days of life) receive a monthly injection of palivizumab—an immunoglobulin prophylaxis—ideally for at least 5 months starting 2 months before the RSV season is likely to occur. Research has shown that the use of palivizumab has significantly reduced the number of hospitalizations and the duration of hospitalization in high-risk infants.

Monitoring

Close cardiopulmonary monitoring of the patient with RSV bronchiolitis is important in the detection of worsening clinical respiratory status, apnea, or bradycardia. CBGs to assess the patient's acid-base status and ventilation along with pulse oximetry (SpO_2) to evaluate oxygenation can be helpful in determining the severity of respiratory failure in patients who are in significant respiratory distress, require high FIO_2 levels, demonstrate apneic or bradycardic episodes, or are slow to improve with aggressive care.

Oxygen Therapy Protocol

Oxygen therapy is used to treat hypoxemia, decrease the work of breathing, and decrease myocardial work (see Oxygen Therapy Protocol, Protocol 34.1).

The oxygen therapy protocol for infants with RSV bronchiolitis includes the benefits provided by the high-humidity gas flow delivered with high-flow nasal cannula (HFNC) therapy. HFNC therapy provides a constant flow that washes out the infant's upper airway dead space, decreases inspiratory resistance, provides increased humidity to moisten secretions, and can provide positive pressure during the respiratory cycle, which can in turn decrease air trapping by stenting swollen airways. In general, the benefits of HFNC are as follows:

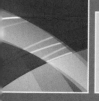

OVERVIEW of the Cardiopulmonary Clinical Manifestations Associated With Respiratory Syncytial Virus Infection

The following clinical manifestations result from the pathologic mechanisms caused (or activated) by atelectasis (see Fig. 10.7), alveolar consolidation (see Fig. 10.8), and excessive bronchial secretions (see Fig. 10.11)—the major anatomic alterations of the lungs associated with RSV infection (see Fig. 39.1).

CLINICAL DATA OBTAINED AT THE PATIENT'S BEDSIDE

The Physical Examination

Vital Signs

Increased Respiratory Rate (Tachypnea)

During the early stages of RSV infection, the respiratory rate is generally higher than normal (often 60 to 70 or more breaths/min). Several pathophysiologic mechanisms operating simultaneously may lead to an increased respiratory rate:

- Stimulation of peripheral chemoreceptors (hypoxemia)
- Relationship of decreased dynamic lung compliance to increased ventilatory rate
- Significantly increased dead space to tidal volume ratio
- Stimulation of central chemoreceptors
- Fever (increased temperature secondary to infection)

Increased Heart Rate (Pulse) and Blood Pressure

Apnea (see Box 33.3), generally in infants younger than 1 month of age or 48 weeks of gestational age for premature infants.

Clinical Manifestations Associated With Increased Negative Intrapleural Pressures During Inspiration

- Intercostal retractions
- Substernal retraction and abdominal distention (seesaw movement or paradoxical chest motion)
- Flaring nostrils

Chest Assessment Findings

- Wheezes secondary to airway narrowing with edema, secretions, and debris
- Crackles
- Upper airway noise from nasopharyngeal secretions that transmits throughout the chest during both inspiration and expiration.
- Increased resonance hyperresonance to percussion (in severe cases when airways are partially obstructed)

Bronchial Secretions (Copious)

Expiratory Grunting

Cyanosis

CLINICAL DATA OBTAINED FROM LABORATORY TESTS AND SPECIAL PROCEDURES

Pulmonary Function Test Findings
(Extrapolated Data for Instructional Purposes)
(Primarily an Obstructive Lung Pathophysiology)

The anatomic or structural changes of the lungs associated with RSV primarily cause an obstructive lung pathophysiologic process. For example, in moderate to severe cases, the following would be higher than normal.

RV	FRC	RV/TLC ratio
↑	↑	↑

NOTE: When alveolar consolidation and atelectasis are present, a primary *restrictive* lung pathophysiologic process may be present. In these cases, the following might be observed.

RV	IRV	VC	FRC	TLC
↓	↓	↓	↓	↓

Arterial Blood Gases[1]

MILD TO MODERATE RESPIRATORY SYNCYTIAL VIRUS INFECTION

Acute Alveolar Hyperventilation With Hypoxemia[2]
(Acute Respiratory Alkalosis)

pH	$PaCO_2$	HCO_3^-	PaO_2	SaO_2 or SpO_2
↑	↓	↓ (but normal)	↓	↓

SEVERE RESPIRATORY SYNCYTIAL VIRUS INFECTION

Acute Ventilatory Failure With Hypoxemia[3]
(Acute Respiratory Acidosis)

pH[4]	$PaCO_2$	HCO_3^-[4]	PaO_2	SaO_2 or SpO_2
↓	↑	↑ (but normal)	↓	↓

Oxygenation Indices[5]

$\dot{Q}_S/\dot{Q}_T$	DO_2	$\dot{V}O_2$	$C(a-\bar{v})O_2$	O_2ER	$S\bar{v}O_2$
↑	↓	N	N	↑	↓

NOTE: RSV bronchiolitis is such a dead space–producing disease that infants may have to increase their minute volume significantly to maintain normal PCO_2, leading to fatigue.

[1]NOTE: Because of the difficulty of obtaining arterial blood gas samples from newborn and pediatric patients, capillary blood gas (CBG) samples may be used to determine the pH, $PaCO_2$, and HCO_3^- (i.e., the acid-base and ventilation status only). Capillary PO_2 values are unreliable and should not be used for clinical analysis. The standard way to evaluate the oxygenation status of these young patients is pulse oximetry (SpO_2) (see Chapter 33, Newborn Assessment and Management).
[2]See Fig. 5.2 and Table 5.4 and related discussion for the acute pH, $PaCO_2$, and HCO_3^- changes associated with acute alveolar hyperventilation.
[3]See Table. 5.5 and related discussion for the acute pH, $PaCO_2$, and HCO_3^- changes associated with acute ventilatory failure.
[4]When tissue hypoxia is severe enough to produce lactic acid, the pH and HCO_3^- values will be lower than expected for a particular $PaCO_2$ level.
[5]$C(a-\bar{v})O_2$, Arterial-venous oxygen difference; DO_2, total oxygen delivery; O_2ER, oxygen extraction ratio; $\dot{Q}_S/\dot{Q}_T$, pulmonary shunt fraction; $S\bar{v}O_2$, mixed venous oxygen saturation; $\dot{V}O_2$, oxygen consumption.

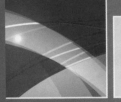

OVERVIEW of the Cardiopulmonary Clinical Manifestations Associated With Respiratory Syncytial Virus Infection—cont'd

RADIOLOGIC FINDINGS
Chest Radiograph

RSV infection appears as both bronchiolitis and bronchopneumonia in infants and young children. The chest radiograph commonly shows streaky peribronchial opacities associated with air trapping and hyperinflation. Lobar atelectasis also is frequently seen—particularly of the right upper lobe; alveolar and lobar pneumonic consolidation may occur (Fig. 39.3). Changes on chest radiographs may persist for up to 12 months after severe RSV infection. The American Association of Pediatrics (AAP) does not recommend routine radiographic studies in the infant who presents with mild to moderate disease.

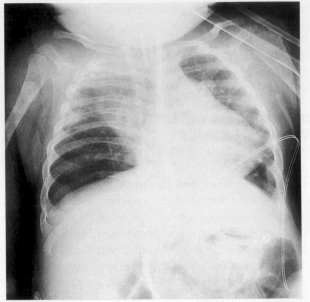

FIGURE 39.3 Chest x-ray film of a 6-month-old child with respiratory syncytial virus infection.

TABLE 39.1 Bronchiolitis Scoring System*

	0: Normal	1: Mild	2: Moderate	3: Severe
Respiratory rate	<40	40–50	50–60	>60
Color	Normal	Normal	Normal	Dusky, mottled
O₂ saturation on room air	>97%	94%–96%	90%–93%	<90%
Capillary refill	<2 sec	<2 sec	<2 sec Normal color on O₂ ≤1 L/min	≥3 sec Normal color on O₂ >1 L/min
Retractions/ work of breathing	None	Subcostal	Intercostal and subcostal when quiet	Supraclavicular and sternal paradoxical respiration
Air entry	Normal	Good entry	Fair air entry	Poor/grunting
wheezing	Breath sounds clear/good	End-expiratory wheeze ± crackles	Inspiration and expiration wheeze ± crackles	Inspiration and expiration wheeze ± crackles
Level of consciousness	Normal/alert	Mild irritability	Restless when disturbed, agitated	Lethargic, hard to arouse

Modified from Dayton Children's Hospital, Dayton, Ohio.
*Other factors used in evaluation of infants with suspected bronchiolitis:
- Signs of dehydration/difficulty feeding
- Parental ability to provide necessary care for child during acute infection
- Preexisting condition contributing to increased possibility of respiratory failure

- HFNC application is effective in reducing work of breathing.
- The benefits of HFNC are generally seen within 60 to 90 minutes of application.
- HFNC with a flow rate 2 L/kg per minute or higher in small infants generates a clinically relevant pharyngeal insufflation pressure.
- Clinically, 5 to 8 L/min O₂ is commonly used for these small infants (3 to 4 kg).

Respiratory Care Treatment Protocols
Airway Clearance Protocol

After oxygen therapy, secretion clearance by nasopharyngeal suctioning is the essential core therapy for RSV bronchiolitis. One-third of an infant's total airway resistance derives from the nose. A bulb or BBG (olive-tipped nasal aspirator) suctioning of the infant's nares can significantly improve air flow,

TABLE 39.2 General Overview: Management Protocol for Respiratory Syncytial Virus Based on Bronchiolitis Score

Score	Aerosolized Bronchodilators*	Other Therapy
Normal 0–4	Assess q6h	Bulb syringe suction for home
Mild 5–7	Assess q4h	Oxygen per protocol Suction PRN IV fluids if patient exhibits dehydration or failure to feed
Moderate 8–10	For scores ≥8, consult with medical staff about rescue aerosol × 1 (racemic epinephrine). Continue to assess the patient q2h.	Oxygen per protocol, including option for HFNC Capillary blood gas Suction IV fluids Consider CXR
Severe 11–15	Racemic epinephrine trial. Evaluate response. If severity persists, activate rapid response team for PICU transfer and therapy with HFNC.	Chest x-ray IV fluids Capillary blood gas If excessive PCO_2, acidosis, or hypoxia, transfer to ICU HFNC, CPAP NIV, mechanical ventilation

Modified from Dayton Children's Hospital, Dayton, Ohio.

*Aerosol bronchodilator trial: Patients will be suctioned if necessary, scored, given aerosol, and scored again. A positive response is defined as a decrease of the patient's postaerosol bronchiolitis score by 2 or more (decreased wheezing, work of breathing, respiratory rate, increased aeration). If the patient received an aerosol trial in the emergency department (ED), it is not necessary to repeat the trial when the patient is hospitalized.

NOTE: Racemic epinephrine (0.5 mL) is generally the recommended aerosol medication for trial in hospitalized patients, unless patient responded to albuterol in the ED.

CPAP, Continuous positive airway pressure; CXR, chest x-ray; HFNC, high-flow nasal cannula; ICU, intensive care unit; IV, intravenous; NIV, noninvasive ventilation; PICU, pediatric intensive care unit; PRN, as needed.

which is typically performed before feeding and as needed. Proper technique is key to effective nasopharyngeal suctioning. The infant must be held so that the head is stabilized while a lubricated suction catheter of appropriate size (generally 8 French) is inserted at the correct downward angle to enter the hypopharynx. This prevents harm to the infant's nasal mucosa while effectively clearing the nasal passages and stimulating a cough by "tickling" the hypopharynx. Nasotracheal or deep suctioning is not indicated in patients with RSV and could cause apnea or bradycardia with vagal stimulation.

In recent years, nebulized *hypertonic saline* (3%) has been suggested for bronchiolitic infants with documented copious secretions. The benefits of hypertonic saline include:

- Inducing an osmotic flow of water into the mucous layer
- Rehydrating the airway surface liquid and improving mucus clearance
- Breaking ionic bonds within the mucus gel, lowering viscosity and elasticity
- Stimulating ciliary beats
- Absorbing water from the mucosa and submucosa, reducing edema of the airway

According to the AAP Clinical Practice Guidelines, chest physiotherapy should not be performed on infants and children with a diagnosis of bronchiolitis. Infants with RSV bronchiolitis do not benefit from chest percussion and drainage. In fact, patient agitation associated with percussion therapy may exacerbate small airway obstruction (see Airway Clearance Protocol, Protocol 34.2).

Aerosolized Medication Protocol

Bronchodilators. Several studies and reviews have failed to demonstrate the benefit of bronchodilators in the treatment of RSV bronchiolitis. The 2014 AAP guidelines suggest that bronchodilators may be more harmful than beneficial. Infants who swallow aerosolized bronchodilators often demonstrate tachycardia and tremors while getting very little improvement in ventilation, resulting in further ventilation-perfusion mismatch and transient hypoxemia. Multiple aerosols contribute to the infant's hypoxemia. A review of the literature on the use of beta-agonists for children under 2 years of age showed no clear benefits from use. One recent study suggests a trial of racemic epinephrine could be used as needed only for rescue in the patient with severe respiratory distress, possibly before a trip to the intensive care unit, although a formal study is needed before a recommendation can be made. A trial typically entails a single aerosol of racemic epinephrine to determine improvement or lack of improvement. For the patient who does not demonstrate airway improvement, no further aerosolized bronchodilator therapy should be given. ED care may involve a single trial of albuterol, because the effect of racemic epinephrine is short-lived and not a drug for continued use at home if the infant responds positively (see Aerosolized Medication Protocol, Protocol 34.4).

Rehydration. The level of respiratory distress associated with RSV bronchiolitis often interferes with proper fluid intake and nutrition, especially when breathing rates exceed 70 breaths/min. In addition, infants have a hard time coordinating breathing, sucking, and swallowing. Fluid and nutrient depletion adds to the likelihood of fatigue. Infants with bronchiolitis should be given intravenous fluids or nasogastric feedings to maintain their strength. Fluid management and nutrition are very important to prevent respiratory failure. Nasogastric feeds satisfy the infant's hunger, which can reduce fussiness. Oxygen flow rates of greater than 1 to 1.5 L/min delivered via nasal cannula with bubble humidification to small infants also can contribute to a humidity deficit and dried secretions. Many children's hospitals have adopted protocols to begin HFNC therapy as the mode of oxygen delivery when the infant's oxygen requirements exceed 1 to 1.5 L/min. HFNC provides 100% relative humidity at body temperature at higher flowrates, preventing the humidity deficit caused by poorly humidified supplemental oxygen.

Corticosteroids

Steroid therapy given by inhalation or intravenous, intramuscular, or oral administration is not recommended for RSV bronchiolitis because of a lack of efficacy in numerous clinical trials. A small subset of infants with previous history of chronic respiratory disease or bronchopulmonary dysplasia may benefit from corticosteroids because of their underlying inflammatory disease.

Smoking Counseling

Tobacco smoke exposure increases the risk and severity of bronchiolitis. In fact, infants with bronchiolitis who are exposed to smoke are more than twice as likely of being hospitalized. Clinicians must inquire as to the smoking habits of those who live with and care for the infant with bronchiolitis. Material regarding the effects of second-hand must be provided for the family.

Asking the family to consider quitting smoking for the health of their infant is sometimes difficult to do, but nevertheless asking with respect while offering support can be effective.

CASE STUDY Respiratory Syncytial Virus Infection (Bronchiolitis)

Admitting History and Physical Examination

A 6-week-old male infant presented to the emergency department (ED) in respiratory distress. His mother noted that her son was unable to breast-feed because of his increasing congestion. His symptoms began 3 days earlier. She also reported that her nephew, whom they visited the previous weekend, was diagnosed with something called "RSV."

On examination, this 4.5-kg infant had a heart rate of 168 beats/min, respiratory rate of 72 breaths/min, and SpO_2 of 94% on room air. He exhibited moderate subcostal and intercostal retractions and nasal flaring, and white frothy secretions were visible in his nares. His breath sounds on auscultation showed good bilateral aeration with noisy, congested upper airway sounds transmitted throughout, making it difficult to assess lower airway sounds. The infant appeared a little dry; the mother noted that he had been nursing poorly and had not had a wet diaper for 6 hours. The ED physician requested a fluid bolus to improve the infant's hydration. The physician directed the nurse caring for the infant to suction his nasopharynx before inserting the intravenous line. The suctioning removed a moderate amount of tenacious white secretions. The physician explained to the mother that the infant would be observed for a few hours in the ED to see if the secretions reaccumulated and to assess his oxygen level during feeding and sleeping. During a nap in the ED, the infant's SpO_2 dropped into the high 80s. He was unable to breast-feed without difficulty because of secretions in his upper airway. A respiratory infectious disease panel (RIDP) was ordered to determine the cause of his viral bronchiolitis because both RSV and influenza A were present in the community.

The infant was then admitted for supportive care, fluids, and ¼ L/min oxygen by nasal cannula administration. Respiratory therapy was called to assess and make recommendations for care. On admission to the general pediatric floor, the patient had heart rate of 142 beats/min, respiratory rate 56 breaths/min, and SpO_2 of 90% on ¼ L/min oxygen per nasal cannula. Breath sounds revealed noisy upper airway sounds as a result of congestion, with bilateral wheezing and grunting on expiration. Moderate subcostal and intercostal retractions persisted with nasal flaring noted. The RIDP was positive for RSV only. The bronchiolitis score (see Table 39.1) was 8. The respiratory therapist wrote the following SOAP.

Respiratory Assessment and Plan

S N/A

O 6-week-old infant with viral bronchiolitis. RSV+ per RIDP. Vital signs: HR 142, RR 56, SpO_2 90% on ¼ L/min oxygen per nasal cannula. Moderate amount of tenacious white secretions. Persistent respiratory distress with subcostal and intercostal retractions, nasal flaring. Breath sounds: Bilateral wheezing with grunting noted on expiration. Irritable and fussy on examination.

A
- Wheezing—most likely because of mucosal edema
- Hypoxemia (SpO_2 90%)
- Excessive secretions (noisy upper airway sound resulting from congestion, tenacious white secretions)
- Possible atelectasis or $\dot{V}/\dot{Q}$ mismatch (history, positive for RSV, low SpO_2 during nap)
- Potential for fatigue with persistent increased work of breathing and irritability
- Bronchiolitis score = 8

P Airway Clearance Protocol: Effective suction to remove upper airway secretions
- Oxygen therapy protocol to achieve SpO2 of 91% to 94%
- Aerosolized Medication Protocol (Trial), if score remains 8 or above

- Consider request for chest radiograph if oxygen requirement continues to increase
- Recommend CPG to identify impending respiratory failure
- May need to implement HFNC or continuous positive airway pressure (CPAP) to stent airways to prevent respiratory fatigue/failure

After increasing the infant's oxygen to 1 L/min, the SpO_2 was 92%. His respiratory symptoms did seem to improve after nasopharyngeal suctioning. The respiratory therapist notified the medical team of the marginal improvement and told the mother that he would return in 2 hours to assess the infant again. One hour later, the infant's nurse called to report that the infant's SpO_2 had dropped to 84% after a brief feeding and he was now on 1.5 L/min by oxygen nasal cannula. An NPO order was initiated, and intravenous fluids were started.

One hour later, the infant demonstrated more significant respiratory distress, this time demonstrating subcostal and intercostal retractions with nasal flaring and head bobbing. The therapist arrived and suctioned a moderate amount of thick secretions from the infant's nasopharynx. The infant's heart rate was 176 beats/min and the respiratory rate was 72 breaths/min. Bilateral crackles and wheezing were heard on auscultation. The therapist called the physician and requested a CBG and chest radiograph. The CBG and pulse oximetry showed pH 7.33, $PaCO_2$ 57 mm Hg, HCO_3^- 29 mEq/L, and SpO_2 89% on 1.5 L/min oxygen per nasal cannula. The chest radiograph showed patchy atelectasis in the right upper and lower lobes and the left lower lobe. A bronchodilator trial with racemic epinephrine was given, with no apparent response.

At this time, the respiratory therapist documented the following SOAP.

Respiratory Assessment and Plan

S N/A

O Infant in severe distress. HR 176, RR 72, subcostal and intercostal retractions with nasal flaring, head bobbing. Breath sounds diminished in bases, crackles and wheezing present. CBG: pH 7.33, $PaCO_2$ 57, HCO_3^- 29. SpO_2: 89% on 1.5 L/min nasal cannula. The infant was less reactive to suctioning at this time.

A • Excessive secretions (crackles, suctioned thick secretions)
- Extensive atelectasis (CXR: Right upper and lower lobes and left lower lobe)
- Hypercarbia despite increased minute volume effort (CBG)
- Hypoxemia (SpO_2 89%)
- Impending respiratory failure (CBG and SpO_2)

P • Discontinue medicated aerosol trial; not effective in relieving symptoms
- Airway Clearance Therapy: Suctioned as needed
- Oxygen therapy: Need to advance to HFNC (5 to 8 L/min on FIO_2 0.40)
- Place CPAP/mechanical ventilation on standby, if HFNC unable to reverse impending respiratory failure.

With the approval of the attending physician, the therapist started the infant on HFNC at 6 L/min of 50% oxygen in his room with central monitoring (Fig. 39.4). Despite this level of support, the infant's respiratory rate did not improve,

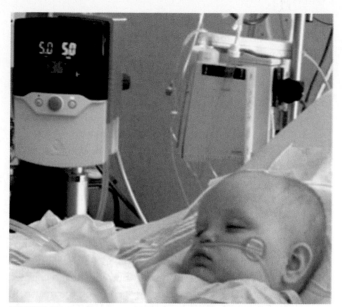

FIGURE 39.4 Infant on a high-flow nasal cannula (HFNC). (Courtesy Dayton Children's Hospital, Dayton, Ohio.)

continuing to track in the 60s. A repeat CBG after 60 minutes showed pH 7.31, $PaCO_2$ 60 mm Hg, and HCO_3^- 29 mEq/L. The SpO_2 was 91%. Because of the infant's general lack of improvement, he was transferred to the pediatric intensive care unit (PICU) and received noninvasive ventilation (NIV) with an inspiratory peak airway pressure (IPAP) of 24 and an expiratory positive airway pressure (EPAP) of 6 with an FIO_2 0.60 oxygen via nasal prongs. This noninvasive support was initiated to relieve the infant's work of breathing, increase his minute ventilation to effectively normalize his blood gases and reverse his lobar atelectasis. This also reduces physiologic dead space, improves alveolar ventilation, and effectively reduces hypercarbia during the acute phase of the illness.

Suctioning and fluids along with nasogastric feeds continued in the PICU for supportive care. After 3 days, NIV respiratory support was weaned to HFNC 6 L/min of 40% O_2, and eventually he was weaned off all supplemental oxygen.

Discussion

This case involves a 6-week-old infant who was exposed to the RSV virus by contact with another infant in the family. Family members could have easily transmitted RSV through hand contact. Strict attention to good hand hygiene is important for family members and medical personnel. Washing hands and using gloves, gowns, and masks are indicated when caring for an RSV-infected infant. The fact that multiple viruses were active in the community supported ordering the RIDP because several viruses can cause similar symptoms.

Most infants present with the inability to feed because of secretions. Nasopharyngeal suctioning with an intravenous fluid bolus to counter dehydration may be sufficient care in the ED, and the infant can be sent home after observation. The infant in this case was demonstrating hypoxemia, requiring oxygen therapy along with fluids. Signs of severe respiratory distress (grunting, nasal flaring with wheezing, and tachypnea) warranted a rescue bronchodilator trial (Aerosolized Medication Therapy Protocol). However, the effectiveness of bronchodilators in bronchiolitis has been shown to be only marginal in many of these infants. The trial of bronchodilators in this case did not show clinical improvement from preassessment to postassessment scores.

The implementation of airway clearance therapy (suctioning) was necessary to offset the excessive bronchial secretions (see Fig. 10.11) (see Airway Clearance Protocol, Protocol 34.2). Postural drainage and percussion are not recommended in these infants. The goal of suctioning is to reduce airway resistance, reduce the work of breathing, and prevent fatigue.

The Oxygen Therapy Protocol is usually required in the RSV bronchiolitis patient and is often the reason for hospitalization (see Oxygen Therapy Protocol, Protocol 34.1). The goal is to maintain the SpO_2 above 90%, ideally 91% to 94%. The use of HFNC, which delivers fully humidified and warmed gas mixtures, has had a dramatic positive effect on the treatment of many infants with RSV bronchiolitis. HFNC is generally considered in infants with RSV who require higher oxygen cannula flow rates (1.5 L/min or higher in infants). In addition, HFNC provides expiratory resistance and flow to the upper airway, thus washing out dead space and increasing pharyngeal insufflation pressure to help stent the airways. This can markedly decrease the work of breathing and improve air exchange in most infants. Patients with bronchiolitis who are on HFNC therapy should be managed where central monitoring is available. Infants with RSV bronchiolitis typically recover faster with early use of HFNC; the goal is to prevent fatigue and respiratory failure. Importantly, NIV by nasal prongs can be used to give support ventilation without the need for intubation (see Mechanical Ventilation and Ventilator Weaning Protocol, Protocol 34.5).

Intubation and mechanical ventilation may be necessary in the bronchiolitic infant who presents with persistent apnea or if fatigue with hypercapnia ensues despite HFNC or NIV intervention. Ventilation of the infant with RSV bronchiolitis often requires sedation and is generally required for several days.

Although palivizumab—an immune globulin prophylaxis—can be given once a month to high-risk infants to build their immunity against RSV and reduce the severity of symptoms, there is no vaccine available for all newborns. The cost of palivizumab limits its use to those born at 29 weeks' gestation or less. The development of a safe and effective vaccine to prevent RSV has been pursued for the past 50 years without great success. At present, there are vaccines for RSV under development and in clinical trials. Unfortunately, none of these potential vaccines will be effective in preventing RSV infection in infants under 6 months of age.

SELF-ASSESSMENT QUESTIONS

1. Which of the following are associated with RSV infection?
   1. Alveolar hyperinflation
   2. Atelectasis
   3. Excessive bronchial secretions
   4. Pneumonic consolidation
      a. 2 and 4 only
      b. 3 and 4 only
      c. 2, 3, and 4 only
      d. 1, 2, 3, and 4

2. Although the outbreak timing of RSV cases varies, the number of patients with RSV typically increases during:
   1. Summer
   2. Fall
   3. Winter
   4. Early spring
      a. 1 only
      b. 3 only
      c. 2, 3, and 4 only
      d. 1, 2, 3, and 4

3. How long is the typical patient with RSV usually contagious?
   a. 1 to 2 days
   b. 8 days
   c. 2 weeks
   d. 1 month

4. Although RSV infection can occur at any age, children younger than what age tend to be more severely affected?
   a. Less than 1 year old
   b. Less than 2 years old
   c. Less than 3 years old
   d. Less than 4 years old

5. Which of the following agents is(are) used to prevent RSV infection in high-risk babies?
   1. Virazole
   2. Synagis
   3. Streptomycin
   4. Ribavirin
      a. 1 only
      b. 2 only
      c. 3 only
      d. 1 and 4 only

Chapter Objectives

After reading this chapter, you will be able to:

- List the anatomic alterations of the lungs associated with chronic lung disease of infancy.
- Differentiate between the classic and "new" description of chronic lung disease of infancy.
- Describe the causes of chronic lung disease of infancy.
- List the cardiopulmonary clinical manifestations associated with chronic lung disease of infancy.
- Describe the general management of chronic lung disease of infancy.
- Describe the clinical strategies and rationales of the SOAP presented in the case study.
- Define key terms and complete self-assessment questions at the end of the chapter and on Evolve.

Key Terms

Alveolar Hypoplasia
Bronchopulmonary Dysplasia (BPD)
Canalicular Stage
Chronic Lung Disease of Infancy (CLDI)
Exogenous Surfactant
Gentle Ventilation
High-Frequency Oscillatory Ventilation (HFOV)
Hyaline Membrane Disease
Hyperplasia
Metaplasia
"New" Chronic Lung Disease of Infancy
Permissive Hypercapnia
Pulmonary Barotrauma
Pulmonary Volutrauma
Stage I CLDI
Stage II CLDI
Stage III CLDI
Stage IV CLDI
Ventilator-Induced Lung Injury (VILI)

Chapter Outline

Anatomic Alterations of the Lungs
    The "New" Chronic Lung Disease of Infancy
Etiology and Epidemiology
Overview of the Cardiopulmonary Clinical Manifestations
    Associated With Chronic Lung Disease of Infancy
General Management of Chronic Lung Disease of Infancy
    Respiratory Care Treatment Protocols
Case Study: Chronic Lung Disease of Infancy
Self-Assessment Questions

Anatomic Alterations of the Lungs

Chronic lung disease of infancy (CLDI), formerly known as **bronchopulmonary dysplasia (BPD),** was first described by Northway and colleagues in 1967 as a severe chronic lung injury in premature infants who survived **hyaline membrane disease** (i.e., respiratory distress syndrome [RDS] after being treated with high levels of mechanical ventilation and oxygen exposure for prolonged periods. At this time, Northway and colleagues described the following four pathologic stages of CLDI (again, previously called bronchopulmonary dysplasia during this period):

Stage I CLDI in the Northway classification was said to occur during the first 2 to 3 days of life. This stage is often indistinguishable from RDS. During this period, alveolar hyaline membranes, patches of atelectasis, and lymphatic dilation were seen. In addition, early signs of bronchial mucosal necrosis appeared (Fig. 40.1A). The chest radiographic findings revealed ground glass–like granular patterns and small lung volumes (Fig. 40.2A).

Stage II CLDI was said to occur 4 to 10 days after birth. Atelectasis was more extensive during this period. In addition, metaplasia of the normal lung tissue cells caused bronchial necrosis, cellular debris, partial airway obstruction, air trapping, and alveolar hyperinflation. The pathologic findings during stage II were commonly described as alternating areas of atelectasis and emphysema (see Fig. 40.1B). These changes appeared on the chest radiograph as patchy opaque areas of atelectasis next to areas of dark translucency (areas of hyperinflation) (see Fig. 40.2B).

Stage III CLDI was said to occur at 11 to 30 days of age. Pathologic findings included extensive bronchial and bronchiolar **metaplasia** and **hyperplasia** (an increased number of cells), interstitial fibrosis, and excessive bronchial

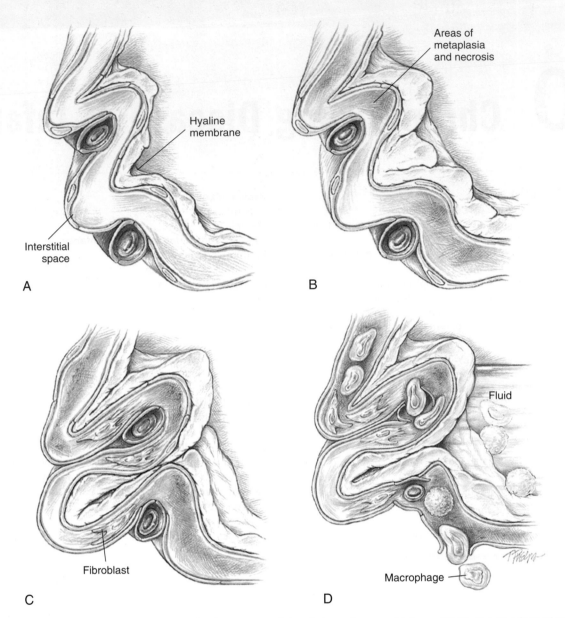

FIGURE 40.1 Alveolar changes during the four stages of chronic lung disease of infancy. (A) Stage I: The formation of hyaline membrane. (B) Stage II: The development areas of metaplasia and necrosis. (C) Stage III: Extensive metaplasia, hyperplasia, and interstitial fibrosis. (D) Stage IV: Progressive destruction of alveoli and airways.

airway secretions. In addition, the alveolar hyperinflation continued to form circular groups of emphysematous bullae that were surrounded by patches of atelectasis (see Fig. 40.1C). On the chest radiograph, the lungs began to show circular or cystic areas surrounded by patches of irregular density (see Fig. 40.2C).

Stage IV CLDI was said to occur after 30 days of life. During this stage, massive fibrosis of the lung and destruction of the bronchial airways, alveoli, and pulmonary capillaries occurred. Areas of emphysematous, or cystlike, regions continued to increase in size and number. Thin strands of atelectasis and normal alveoli were interspersed around emphysematous areas. In addition, pulmonary hypertension often developed, lymphatic and bronchial mucous gland deformation occurred, and excessive bronchial secretions continued (see Fig. 40.1D). The chest radiographs revealed

fibrosis and edema, with areas of consolidation adjacent to areas of overinflation (see Fig. 40.2D). Table 40.1 summarizes the original CLDI stages, with pathologic and radiologic correlates.

The major pathologic or structural changes of the lungs associated with earlier descriptions of CLDI were:

- Hyaline membrane formation
- Atelectasis
- Bronchial mucosal necrosis
- Excessive bronchial secretions
- Chronic alveolar fibrosis and bronchial smooth muscle hypertrophy
- Bronchial mucosal metaplasia and hyperplasia
- Alveolar hyperinflation
- Emphysematous areas surrounded by areas of atelectasis and normal alveoli

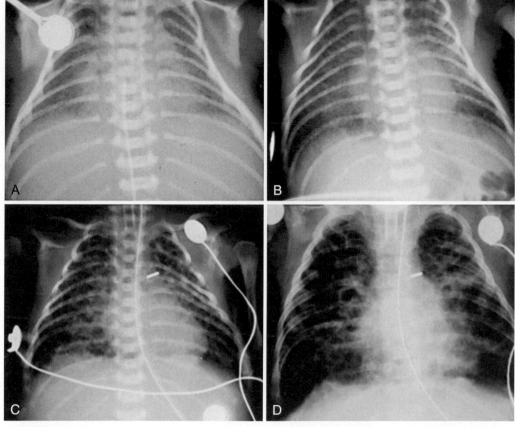

FIGURE 40.2 (A) Stage I: Occurs during the first 2 to 3 days of life. The chest radiographic findings show ground glass–like granular patterns and small lung volumes. (B) Stage II: Occurs 4 to 10 days after birth. The chest x-ray film shows patchy opaque areas with bronchograms (areas of atelectasis) next to areas of dark translucency (areas of hyperinflation). (C) Stage III: Occurs at 11 to 30 days of age. The chest radiograph shows circular or cystic areas surrounded by patches of irregular density. (D) Stage IV: Occurs after 30 days of life. The chest radiographs show fibrosis and edema with areas of consolidation adjacent to areas of overinflation. (From Taeusch, W. H., Ballard, R. A., & Gleason, C. A. [2005]. *Avery's diseases of the newborn* [8th ed.]. Philadelphia, PA: Saunders.)

TABLE 40.1 Chronic Lung Disease of Infancy Staging (Northway)

CLDI Stage	Period After Birth	Pathologic Findings
I	2–3 days	• Patches of atelectasis • Alveolar hyaline membranes • Lymphatic dilation • Mucosal necrosis • Chest radiograph—ground glass appearance
II	4–10 days	• More extensive atelectasis • Partial bronchial obstruction and air trapping (alveolar hyperinflation) • Commonly described as alternating lung areas of atelectasis and emphysema • Metaplasia and bronchial necrosis • Chest radiograph—patchy opaque (white) area adjacent to dark translucency areas of hyperinflation
III	11–30 days	• Extensive bronchial metaplasia and hyperplasia • Interstitial fibrosis • Excessive bronchial secretions • Emphysematous bullae surrounded by patches of atelectasis • Chest radiograph—cystic areas surrounded by patches of irregular density
IV	>30 days	• Massive fibrosis and destruction of bronchial airways, alveoli, and pulmonary capillaries • Cyst like areas increase in size and numbers • Thin strands of atelectasis and normal alveoli are interspersed around the cyst like areas • Pulmonary hypertension and lymphatic and bronchial mucous gland deformation • Chest radiograph—fibrosis, edema, and consolidation adjacent to emphysematous areas.

Data from Northway, W. H. Jr., Rosan, R. C., & Porter, D. Y. (1967). Pulmonary disease following respiratory therapy of hyaline-membrane disease: bronchopulmonary dysplasia. *The New England Journal of Medicine, 276,* 357-368.

The "New" Chronic Lung Disease of Infancy

Much has been learned about CLDI since it was first described in 1967. During the late 1960s, CLDI occurred predominantly in larger preterm infants born at 30 to 34 weeks' gestation, with a history of severe respiratory distress necessitating aggressive ventilatory support and high oxygen concentrations for prolonged periods.

Today, however, CLDI, as it was originally described in 1967, has virtually disappeared. Today, infants who develop CLDI typically have very low birth weights (less than 1500 grams) and are born at less than 28 weeks' gestation. They are now usually managed with several new and improved therapeutic techniques, including prenatal maternal steroids, postnatal **exogenous surfactant, gentle ventilation** techniques, controlled low oxygen concentrations, nasal continuous positive airway pressure (CPAP), fluid restriction, treatment of infection, vitamin A, enteral and parenteral nutritional support—diuretics, caffeine, postnatal corticosteroids, and pulmonary vasodilators.

Today, the pathologic findings of CLDI are described as more uniformly inflated alveoli with minimal airway injury or fibrosis. The major anatomic pathologic process is a decrease in alveolar *number*, called **alveolar hypoplasia**. In the very preterm infant with the **"new" chronic lung disease of infancy**, the lung is just completing the **canalicular stage** of development at the time of birth. Interruption of the canalicular stage is thought to significantly disrupt the progress of alveolar growth and likely contributes to the development of the new CLDI.

In response to awareness of the newly described CLDI, the National Institutes of Child Health and Human Development in 2001 sponsored a workshop on CLDI and a new definition of CLDI resulted. The new definition outlines specific diagnostic criteria, including the need for oxygen, positive pressure ventilation, and/or CPAP. It also includes the postnatal age to better assess the severity of CLDI. Table 40.2 provides an overview of the diagnostic criteria for the newly described CLDI.

Etiology and Epidemiology

CLDI is the most common form of chronic lung disease in children. It is estimated that about 10,000 to 15,000 infants are diagnosed with CLDI in the United States annually. Although exogenous surfactant reduced the incidence of CLDI in premature infants in randomized controlled trials in the 1980s, the number of infants under 28 weeks' gestation who survive today has increased. The current understanding is that multiple causative factors are associated with CLDI. Table 40.3 provides an overview of the primary causes of CLDI. Recent research has shown there is a high probability of genetics playing a role in the development of the condition.

TABLE 40-2 Diagnostic Criteria for the New Chronic Lung Disease of Infancy

	<32 Weeks Gestation	≥32 Weeks Gestation
Severity of **CLDI**	• 36 weeks' PMA, or • Discharge to home, whichever comes first	• >28 days but <56 days' postnatal age, or • Discharge to home, whichever comes first
	The newborn is treated with >21% oxygen for at least 28 days—**PLUS, ONE OF THE FOLLOWING**	
Mild **CLDI**	• Breathing room air at 36 weeks' PMA, or • Discharge to go home, whichever comes first	• Breathing room air by 56 days' postnatal age, or • Discharge to go home, whichever comes first
Moderate **CLDI**	• The infant requires <30% oxygen at 36 weeks' PMA, or • Discharge to go home, whichever comes first	• The infant requires <30% oxygen at 56 days' postnatal age, or • Discharge to go home, whichever comes first
Severe **CLDI**	• The infant requires ≥30% oxygen and/or PPV or NCPAP at 36 weeks' PMA, or • Discharge to go home, whichever comes first	• The infant requires ≥30% oxygen and/or PPV or NCPAP at 56 postnatal age, or • Discharge to go home whichever comes first

Modified from Jobe, A. H., & Bancalari, E. (2001). Bronchopulmonary dysplasia. *American Journal of Respiratory Critical Care Medicine, 163,* 1723-1729.
CLDI, Chronic lung disease of infancy; *NCPAP,* nasal continuous positive airway pressure; *PMA,* postmenstrual age; *PPV,* positive-pressure ventilation.

OVERVIEW of the Cardiopulmonary Clinical Manifestations Associated With Chronic Lung Disease of Infancy (CLDI)

The following clinical manifestations result from the pathologic mechanisms caused (or activated) by atelectasis (see Fig. 10.7), increased alveolar-capillary membrane thickness (see Fig. 10.9), and excessive bronchial secretions (see Fig. 10.11)—the major anatomic alterations of the lungs associated with CLDI (see Fig. 40.1).

CLINICAL DATA OBTAINED AT THE PATIENT'S BEDSIDE

The Physical Examination

Vital Signs

Increased Respiratory Rate (Tachypnea)

Normally, a newborn's respiratory rate is about 40 to 60 breaths/min. During the early stages of CLDI, the respiratory rate is generally well over 60 breaths/min. The following pathophysiologic mechanisms operating simultaneously may lead to an increased ventilatory rate:

- Increased stimulation of peripheral chemoreceptors (hypoxemia)
- Stimulation of central chemoreceptors
- Relationship of decreased lung compliance to increased ventilatory rate
- Temperature instability (secondary to infection)

Increased Heart Rate (Pulse) and Blood Pressure

Clinical Manifestations Associated With Increased Negative Intrapleural Pressures During Inspiration

- Intercostal retractions
- Substernal retraction and abdominal distention (seesaw movement)
- Nasal flaring

Chest Assessment Findings

- Diminished breath sounds
- Wheezes
- Crackles

Expiratory Grunting

Cyanosis

CLINICAL DATA OBTAINED FROM LABORATORY TESTS AND SPECIAL PROCEDURES

Pulmonary Function Test Findings:
(Extrapolated Data for Instructional Purposes)
(Primarily Restrictive Lung Pathophysiology)

The anatomic alterations of the lungs associated with CLDI primarily cause a restrictive lung pathophysiologic process. For example, in moderate to severe cases, the following lung volumes and capacities would be lower than normal.

RV	IRV	VC	FRC	TLC
↓	↓	↓	↓	↓

However, when the airways are partially obstructed, and/or bullae, and/or emphysematous changes are present (e.g., In stage IV CLDI), obstructive lung findings may be seen. In these cases, the following might be greater than normal.

RV	FRC	RV/TLC ratio
↑	↑	↑

Arterial Blood Gases[1]

MILD TO MODERATE CHRONIC LUNG DISEASE OF INFANCY
Acute Alveolar Hyperventilation With Hypoxemia[2]
(Acute Respiratory Alkalosis)

pH	$PaCO_2$	HCO_3^-	PaO_2	SaO_2 or SpO_2
↑	↓	↓ (but normal)	↓	↓

SEVERE CHRONIC LUNG DISEASE OF INFANCY
Chronic Ventilatory Failure With Hypoxemia[3]
(Compensated Respiratory Acidosis)

pH	$PaCO_2$	HCO_3^-	PaO_2	SaO_2 or SpO_2
N	↑	↑ (significantly)	↓	↓

ACUTE VENTILATORY CHANGES SUPERIMPOSED ON CHRONIC VENTILATORY FAILURE[4]

Because acute ventilatory changes are frequently seen in patients with chronic ventilatory failure, the respiratory therapist must be familiar with—and alert for—the following dangerous arterial blood gas finding:

- Acute alveolar hyperventilation superimposed on chronic ventilatory failure, which should further alert the respiratory therapist to record the following important ABG assessment: possible impending acute ventilatory failure
- Acute ventilatory failure (acute hypoventilation) superimposed on chronic ventilatory failure

[1]*NOTE:* Because of the difficulty of obtaining arterial blood gas samples from newborn and pediatric patients, capillary blood gas (CBG) samples may be used to determine the pH, $PaCO_2$, and HCO_3^- (i.e., the acid-base and ventilation status only). Capillary PO_2 values are unreliable and should not be used for clinical analysis. The standard way to evaluate the oxygenation status of these young patients is pulse oximetry (SpO_2) (see Chapter 33, Newborn Assessment and Management).

[2]See Fig. 5.2 and Table 5.4 and related discussion for the acute pH, $PaCO_2$, and HCO_3^- changes associated with acute alveolar hyperventilation.

[3]See Table 5.6 and related discussion for the acute pH, $PaCO_2$, and HCO_3^- changes associated with chronic ventilatory failure.

[4]See Tables 5.7, 5.8, and 5.9 and related discussion for the pH, $PaCO_2$, and HCO_3^- changes associated with acute ventilatory changes superimposed on chronic ventilatory failure.

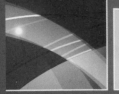

Oxygenation Indices[5]					
$\dot{Q}_S/\dot{Q}_T$	DO_2[6]	$\dot{V}O_2$	$C(a\text{-}\bar{v})O_2$	O_2ER	$S\bar{v}O_2$
↑	↓	N	N	↑	↓

RADIOLOGIC FINDINGS

Chest Radiograph

Using the classic description of the "new CLDI," Fig. 40.2 provides a radiographic overview of the four stages of CLDI. During stage I, the radiologic findings are analogous to those of severe respiratory distress syndrome (RDS) or neonatal pneumonia, showing a ground-glass granular pattern and small lung volume (see Fig. 40.2A). During stage II, patchy opaque areas with bronchograms (atelectasis) adjacent to areas of dark translucency (hyperinflation) appear. Identifying the precise cause of the haziness, whether pulmonary edema, alveolar consolidation, or atelectasis, is usually difficult (see Fig. 40.2B).

The radiologic findings during stage III are more specific to CLDI. Circular or cystlike areas of hyperlucency begin to appear and are surrounded by patches of irregular density areas caused by atelectasis. This condition generates a spongelike appearance of the lungs on the chest radiograph (see Fig. 40.2C). Stage IV shows an increase in the size and number of cystlike areas of hyperlucency (emphysematous bullae), surrounded by thin strands of radiodensity (atelectasis and interstitial fibrosis). The emphysematous bullae and interstitial fibrosis around the bullae create a honeycomb appearance on the chest radiograph. *Cor pulmonale may be seen during the advanced stages of CLDI* (see Fig. 40.2D).

[5]$C(a\text{-}\bar{v})O_2$, Arterial-venous oxygen difference; DO_2, total oxygen delivery; O_2ER, oxygen extraction ratio; $\dot{Q}_S/\dot{Q}_T$, pulmonary shunt fraction; $S\bar{v}O_2$, mixed venous oxygen saturation; $\dot{V}O_2$, oxygen consumption.

[6]Because the newborn normally has a higher hemoglobin level at birth (16.8 to 18.9 g/dL), the DO_2 may actually be greater than indicated by the PaO_2 or SpO_2 alone (see Chapter 5, Blood Gas Assessment).

TABLE 40.3 Causative Factors of Chronic Lung Disease of Infancy

Host susceptibility and genetic predisposition	The single most important causative factor associated with the development of chronic lung disease of infancy (CLDI) is prematurity. In addition, the restriction of intrauterine growth and a family history of respiratory distress syndrome and asthma put the infant at a higher risk for CLDI.
Oxygen toxicity	Even in the first cases of CLDI reported by Northway and colleagues in 1967, it was clear that exposure to high concentrations of oxygen was a factor in causing CLDI. Subsequent reports continue to show that prolonged exposure to high levels of supplemental oxygen puts infants at risk for CLDI.
Inflammation	A severe inflammatory response also plays a major role in the development of CLDI.
Neonatal infection	The development of postnatal bacterial sepsis or pneumonia puts the infant at risk for CLDI. Even airway microbial colonization without frank sepsis may increase the risk for CLDI.
Mechanical ventilation	The development of CLDI is strongly associated with mechanical ventilation. The major causative factors linked to mechanical ventilation are (1) high peak inspiratory pressures, (2) high mean airway pressures, and (3) overdistention of the lungs. Overinflation of the lungs causes stress fractures of the capillary endothelium, epithelium, and basement membranes. This mechanical injury in turn causes leakage of fluid into the alveolar spaces, with additional inflammation.
Pulmonary edema and patent ductus arteriosus	Abnormalities of lung fluid volume are associated with CLDI. Several reports have shown that patency of the ductus arteriosus has a high correlation with the incidence of CLDI.
Poor nutrition	All of the above causative factors are intensified by a poor nutritional status.

General Management of Chronic Lung Disease of Infancy

Several preventive methods are used today to avert or treat CLDI. Mothers in preterm labor are often given steroids to hasten the lung maturity of the infant in an attempt to avoid mechanical ventilation. The most significant treatment for the prevention of CLDI in the newborn is the administration of **exogenous surfactant**. This drug alone has significantly reduced the incidence of CLDI; original randomized controlled studies have shown a reduction in the incidence of CLDI from 55% to 26% with use of surfactant. Dosing the infant with surfactant soon after birth allows for effective ventilation at lower pressures with improved lung compliance (see Surfactant Administration Protocol, Protocol 33.5). Keeping the newborn's exhaled tidal volume at 4 to 6 mL/kg of body weight avoids volutrauma. This requires weaning the peak inspiratory pressure (PIP) as the infant's lung compliance improves.

Infants who may have coinfections or comorbidities that require higher ventilating pressures should be transitioned to **High-Frequency Oscillatory Ventilation (HFOV)** to avoid high PIPs while maintaining mean airway pressure (MAP) necessary for oxygenation. **Permissive hypercapnia**[1] (allowing the PCO_2 to rise above normal while keeping the pH around 7.2) is another method of avoiding lung injury (see Chapter 28, Acute Respiratory Distress Syndrome). Continuous pulse oximetry allows the respiratory therapist to adjust oxygen settings to the infant's desired SpO_2.

In general, the management of infants who are at high risk for development of CLDI or who have evolving CLDI is directed at (1) minimizing the administration of high concentrations of oxygen, (2) supporting airway clearance (3) minimizing the need for ventilatory support, (4) using low inspiratory pressures, (5) managing the MAPs, and (6) supporting and maintaining an adequate functional residual capacity with PEEP or CPAP. Additionally, vitamin A is important as a key regulator of normal lung growth that can increase functional alveoli and pulmonary vasculature. Caffeine has been shown to reduce the incidence of CLDI by acting as a respiratory stimulant and strengthening diaphragmatic function, both of which can improve the infant's weaning potential. Infants with severe CLDI also may have cor pulmonale (pulmonary hypertension), requiring treatment with pulmonary vasodilators, such as sildenafil, or inhaled nitric oxide for acute respiratory failure.

Respiratory Care Treatment Protocols

Oxygen Therapy Protocol

Oxygen therapy is used to treat hypoxemia, decrease the work of breathing, and decrease myocardial work. Because of the hypoxemia that often develops in CLDI, supplemental oxygen may be required (see Oxygen Therapy Protocol, Protocol 33.1). It should be noted that supplemental oxygen should be titrated to need to minimize complications of CLDI. In the past, some physicians preferred allowing lower than normal SaO_2 values in infants with low birth weight; however, a recent review demonstrated a higher risk for necrotizing enterocolitis and mortality when this practice was followed.

Airway Clearance Protocol

Because of the excessive airway secretions and accumulation associated with CLDI, suctioning of secretions will be necessary to reduce airway resistance (see Airway Clearance Protocol, Protocol 33.2).

Mechanical Ventilation Protocol

Mechanical ventilation may be necessary to provide and support alveolar gas exchange and eventually return the patient to spontaneous breathing (see Mechanical Ventilation and Ventilator Weaning Protocol, Protocol 33.4).[2]

Table 40.4 provides an overview of the therapeutic measures used to prevent or manage infants with CLDI.

---

[1]Permissive hypercapnia defined: Mechanical ventilation was traditionally applied with the goal of normalizing arterial blood gas values, particularly the arterial carbon dioxide tension ($PaCO_2$). However, this is no longer the primary objective of mechanical ventilation. Today, the emphasis is on maintaining adequate gas exchange while—and, importantly—minimizing the risks of mechanical ventilation. Common strategies used to reduce the risks of mechanical ventilation include (1) low tidal volume ventilation to protect the lung from ventilator-associated lung injury in patients with acute lung injury (e.g., ARDS) and (2) reduction of the tidal volume, respiratory rate, or both to minimize intrinsic positive end-expiratory pressure (i.e., auto-PEEP) in patients with obstructive lung disease (e.g., COPD). Although these mechanical ventilation strategies may result in an increased $PaCO_2$ level (hypercapnia), they do help protect the lung from barotrauma (i.e., physical damage to lung tissues caused by excessive gas pressures). The lenient acceptance of the hypercapnia is called permissive hypercapnia. In most cases, the patient's $PaCO_2$ is adequately maintained by an increased ventilatory rate that offsets the decreased tidal volume. The $PaCO_2$, however, should not be permitted to increase to the point of severe acidosis. The most current consensus suggests it is safe to allow pH to fall to as low as 7.20 (http://www.ARDSNet).

[2]It has long been known that mechanical ventilation can produce a variety of lung injuries referred to as **ventilator-induced lung injury (VILI)**, **pulmonary volutrauma**, or **pulmonary barotrauma**. *VILI* is defined as stress fractures of the pulmonary capillary endothelium, epithelium, and basement membrane and, in severe cases, lung rupture. Lung ruptures can lead to leakage of fluid, protein, and blood into tissue and air spaces or leakage of air into tissue spaces. This condition can be followed by an inflammatory response and possibly a reduced defense against infection. *Pulmonary volutrauma* is defined as damage to the lung caused by overdistention by a mechanical ventilator set for an excessively high tidal volume. *Pulmonary barotrauma* is defined as damage to the lungs caused by rapid or extreme pressures generated by mechanical ventilation. Predisposing factors for VILI, pulmonary volutrauma, or pulmonary barotrauma include (1) mechanical ventilation with high peak inspiratory volumes and pressures, (2) mechanical ventilation with a high mean airway pressure, (3) structural immaturity of lung and chest wall, (4) surfactant insufficiency or inactivation, and (5) preexisting lung disease. Fortunately, newborn mechanical ventilator strategies today minimize lung injuries by keeping exhaled volumes low, accepting higher PCO_2 levels, or switching to high-frequency ventilation when positive inspiratory pressures exceed safe limits. Pulmonary air leak syndrome (see Chapter 38, Pulmonary Air Leak Syndrome), however, can still occur in certain clinical scenarios, especially when very high ventilator pressures are used or in the delivery room with aggressive ventilation during resuscitation.

TABLE 40.4 Therapeutic Measures Used to Manage Infants With or Prevent Chronic Lung Disease of Infancy

Prenatal steroids	A single course of prenatal glucocorticoids administered to women who are at high risk for premature delivery results in a significant decrease in the mortality rate and in the morbidity associated with prematurity.
Gentle ventilation	Despite development of numerous sophisticated ventilators for the newborn, there is still no clear advantage to any one approach. The general approach is a ventilatory mode that prevents atelectasis, sustains or maintains functional residual capacity, uses a minimal tidal volume, and permits the infant to trigger his or her own ventilation as much as possible. Every effort should be made to minimize high peak inspiratory pressures, high mean airway pressures, and overdistention of the lungs. For example, high-frequency ventilation, low tidal volumes, and permissive hypercapnia are commonly used.
Low inspired oxygen concentrations	Every effort should be made to administer only the lowest concentration of oxygen that is necessary.
Nasal continuous positive airway pressure (CPAP)	Early application of nasal CPAP in high-risk respiratory distress syndrome and infants with chronic lung disease of infancy (CLDI) is highly recommended during postnatal care.
Fluid restriction	Because fluid overload is a causative factor associated with CLDI, fluid limitation may be helpful. However, care should be taken to avoid being overly aggressive when limiting fluids, because undernutrition is also associated with the development of CLDI.
Vitamin A	Vitamin A is an essential nutrient for maintaining the epithelial cells of the tracheobronchial tree.
Caffeine	Early initiation of caffeine in those at risk for CLDI has been shown to shorten the course of respiratory support and the incidence of CLDI.
Diuretics	In infants with severe CLDI, pulmonary edema is a major component. There is clear evidence that either daily or alternate-day therapy with furosemide improves lung mechanics and gas exchange in infants with established CLDI.
Bronchodilator therapy	Increased airway resistance is highly associated with CLDI. Short-term therapy with inhaled or parenteral beta$_2$-adrenergic agonists is occasionally administered to infants with CLDI.
Airway clearance therapy	Routine suctioning is beneficial.
Postnatal corticosteroids	The administration of postnatal corticosteroids to preterm infants has been shown to reduce lung inflammation and the incidence of CLDI. Postnatal corticosteroids are also believed to increase surfactant synthesis, enhance beta-adrenergic activity, increase antioxidant production, stabilize cell and lysosomal membranes, and inhibit prostaglandin and leukotriene synthesis. Side effects include increased incidence of hyperglycemia and infection.
Prenatal Surfactant	Per Surfactant Administration Protocol, Protocol 33.5

CASE STUDY Chronic Lung Disease of Infancy

Admitting History and Physical Examination

An 1100-gram baby boy was born at 28 weeks' gestation to a mother who received no prenatal care. The mother had used cocaine and marijuana and may have had a vaginal infection during her pregnancy. Because of the baby's clinical presentation, mechanical ventilation was started moments after birth. Exogenous surfactant was given to improve lung compliance and avoid a prolonged ventilator course.

The infant worsened over 24 hours. He was diagnosed with respiratory distress syndrome and group B streptococcal pneumonia. An intravenous line and umbilical artery catheter were placed. Antibiotics were started. He required higher concentrations of oxygen, positive inspiratory pressures (PIPs) greater than 30 cm H_2O, and higher levels of positive end-expiratory pressure (PEEP) to maintain oxygenation and adequate tidal volume.

He was placed on high-frequency oscillatory ventilation for 4 days and was eventually transitioned back to conventional ventilation. He was placed on high-flow nasal cannula oxygen at day 14. However, at day 20 he became tachypneic, with grunting and retractions, requiring an increase in FIO_2. A respiratory viral panel showed he was positive for influenza A, a virus contracted from his maternal grandmother who had been visiting the nursery. He developed pneumonia, requiring another intubation and ventilator support. At this time the clinical team was concerned that the infant has the potential to develop chronic lung disease of infancy (CLDI).

At 4 weeks, the baby was still on a pressure-cycled mechanical ventilator with the following settings: PIP +25 cm H_2O, respiratory rate (RR) 35 breaths/min, inspiratory time (T_I) 0.45, FIO_2 0.60, and PEEP +7 cm H_2O. His pulmonary mechanics showed increased airway resistance and decreased lung compliance. He demonstrated coarse bilateral crackles and some wheezes. Thick, clear mucus was suctioned. The chest radiograph showed patchy atelectasis and areas of pulmonary fibrosis. His arterial line ABGs on an FIO_2 of 0.60 were pH 7.31, $PaCO_2$ 55 mm Hg, HCO_3^- 27 mEq/L, PaO_2 50 mm Hg, and SaO_2 of 84%. The doctor wrote the following order in the baby's chart: "Respiratory therapy to assess patient and begin to wean from ventilator."

The respiratory therapist charted the following assessment.

Respiratory Assessment and Plan

S N/A

O Marginal pulmonary mechanics—decreased compliance and increased airway resistance. Coarse crackles and wheezes. CXR: Suggests CLDI with scattered areas of atelectasis and hyperinflation. ABGs on ventilator and FIO_2 0.60: pH 7.31, $PaCO_2$ 55, HCO_3^- 27, PaO_2 50, and SaO_2 84%.

A • Stiff lung with airway obstruction (pulmonary mechanics) suggests CLDI
 • Chronic ventilatory failure with moderate hypoxemia (ABGs)
 • Excessive bronchial secretions (crackles and suctioning results)
 • Possible bronchospasm (wheezes—maybe caused by bronchial secretions)
 • Appears ready for slow weaning trial

P Wean slowly per **Mechanical Ventilation and Ventilator Weaning Protocol** (decrease mandatory respiratory rate slowly; decrease need for pressure; transition to pressure support ventilation). Continue Oxygen Therapy Protocol (FIO_2 to meet SpO_2 goals). Continue suction PRN. Trial Bronchodilator Therapy Protocol (in-line neb with 0.25 mL of albuterol in 2.0 mL normal saline q4h) to assess effectiveness. Continue to monitor closely and assess frequently.

Over the next 10 weeks, the baby slowly improved. Five days before discharge, the mother was trained on respiratory and nursing procedures for home care. Over the next 4 years, the child's lungs continued to improve even though he had recurrent pneumonia and was seen monthly in the ED during the first 6 months. On one occasion, he was readmitted to the hospital for a week; he recovered and is now doing well. He is of normal weight and height for his age, runs and plays well with other children, and is about to enter preschool.

Discussion

Several comments should be made regarding this challenging pulmonary disorder of the newborn. First, infants with CLDI have limited pulmonary reserves. Their lungs are seriously damaged, scarred, and fibrotic. They have increased airway resistance and decreased lung compliance. Because their lung tissues are constantly being bombarded by inflammatory stimuli, their hearts and lungs have a limited ability to recover from stress. *These infants may be slow to recover from procedures such as tracheal or nasopharyngeal suctioning.* They are also prone to gastroesophageal reflux disease (GERD) and microaspiration. Therefore health care personnel should perform all therapeutic procedures as quickly and efficiently as possible.

Second, every attempt should be made to wean the baby off the ventilator because ventilator pressures, rates, and high oxygen concentrations are the main factors causing the pulmonary damage. The longer the baby is on the ventilator, the more the lungs are being damaged. Some neonatal intensive care units are now implementing criteria for extubation readiness testing to regularly assess infants for extubation, hoping to shorten their days on the ventilator.

Because chronic ventilatory failure with hypoxemia commonly occurs in infants with chronic CIDI, the respiratory therapist should not hurry to decrease the infant's $PaCO_2$ to the "normal" range of 35 to 45 mm Hg. Infants in the acute and chronic stages of CLDI often have a high $PaCO_2$ and normal pH (compensated). A $PaCO_2$ of 50 to 60 mm Hg may be tolerated well. Therefore the therapist must be prepared to accept chronically high $PaCO_2$ levels. As the baby's lungs deteriorate, moreover, the ability of blood to flow easily through the lungs progressively declines. As the condition worsens, the work of the right side of the heart increases. If the CLDI does not resolve, pulmonary hypertension and cor pulmonale may develop and require treatment.

CLDI is a disorder that requires a great deal of parental education and support at the time of the baby's discharge from the hospital. Therefore the importance of comprehensive home medical and respiratory care and regular assessment of their child's respiratory status must be stressed to the family. The respiratory therapist can be instrumental in working with the family both in the hospital and in the home to ensure the parents are prepared to support the infant's respiratory care needs. For example, the parents must understand the procedures of oral and nasal suctioning, and aerosolized medication administration at home. Feeding problems and GERD are very common in these infants. Infants with CLDI who have been discharged from the hospital commonly return to the hospital once or twice a year in acute respiratory distress. The majority of infants with severe CLDI will develop some degree of airway hyperresponsiveness or reactivity. Although CLDI infants have asthma-like symptoms as they age, they are less likely to demonstrate significant response to bronchodilators because of their fixed airway narrowing and bronchomalacias. Inhaled or chronic low-dose systemic steroid therapy may be necessary. Therefore the importance of comprehensive home medical and respiratory care and regular assessment of their child's respiratory status must be stressed to the family.

1. Which of the following is(are) associated with the cause of chronic lung disease of infancy?
   1. History of RDS
   2. Low positive pressure mechanical ventilation
   3. High concentrations of oxygen
   4. Infant's weight greater than 2000 grams
      a. 2 only
      b. 1 and 3 only
      c. 2, 3, and 4 only
      d. 1, 3, and 4 only

2. The anatomic alterations of the lungs associated with chronic lung disease of infancy are:
   1. Increased alveolar-capillary membrane thickness
   2. Atelectasis
   3. Excessive bronchial secretions
   4. Consolidation
      a. 2 and 4 only
      b. 3 and 4 only
      c. 1, 2, and 3 only
      d. 1, 2, 3, and 4

3. In what is referred to as the "new" chronic lung disease of infancy (new CLDI), the major anatomic pathologic process is a decrease in alveolar number, called:
   a. Patches of atelectasis
   b. State IV CLDI
   c. Alveolar hypoplasia
   d. Canalicular period of fetal development

4. Which of the following arterial blood gas values are associated with severe chronic lung disease of infancy?
   1. Decreased pH
   2. Increased $PaCO_2$
   3. Normal pH
   4. Decreased HCO_3^-
      a. 2 and 3 only
      b. 1 and 4 only
      c. 2, 3, and 4 only
      d. 1, 2, and 4 only

5. Which of the following clinical manifestations are associated with chronic lung disease of infancy?
   1. Crackles
   2. Intercostal retractions
   3. Hypoxemia
   4. Wheezes
      a. 1 and 4 only
      b. 2 and 3 only
      c. 1, 2, and 3 only
      d. 1, 2, 3, and 4

41 Congenital Diaphragmatic Hernia

Chapter Objectives

After reading this chapter, you will be able to:

- List the anatomic alterations of the lungs associated with congenital diaphragmatic hernia.
- Describe the causes of congenital diaphragmatic hernia.
- List the cardiopulmonary clinical manifestations associated with congenital diaphragmatic hernia.
- Describe the general management of congenital diaphragmatic hernia.
- Describe the clinical strategies and rationales of the SOAP presented in the case study.
- Define key terms and complete self-assessment questions at the end of the chapter and on Evolve.

Key Terms

Atelectasis
Bochdalek Foramen
Bochdalek Hernia
Congenital Diaphragmatic Eventration
Congenital Diaphragmatic Hernia (CDH)
Echocardiogram
Extracorporeal Membrane Oxygenation (ECMO)
Hemothorax
Inhaled Nitric Oxide (iNO) Therapy
Morgagni Hernia
Pneumothorax
Posterolateral Diaphragmatic Hernia
Prenatal Ultrasound
Pulmonary Hypertension
Pulmonary Hypoplasia
Scaphoid Abdomen
Total Absence of the Diaphragm

Chapter Outline

Anatomic Alterations of the Lungs
Etiology and Epidemiology
Overview of Cardiopulmonary Clinical Manifestations
  Associated With Congenital Diaphragmatic Hernia
General Management of a Congenital Diaphragmatic Hernia
Case Study: Diaphragmatic Hernia
Self-Assessment Questions

Anatomic Alterations of the Lungs

During normal fetal development, the diaphragm first appears anteriorly between the heart and liver and then progressively grows posteriorly. Between the eighth and tenth week of gestation, the diaphragm normally completely closes at the left **Bochdalek foramen**, which is located posteriorly and laterally on the left diaphragm. At about the tenth week of gestation (about the same time the Bochdalek foramen is closing), the intestines and stomach normally migrate from the yolk sac. If, however, the bowels reach this area before the Bochdalek foramen closes, a hernia results—a **congenital diaphragmatic hernia (CDH)** (also called **Bochdalek hernia** or **posterolateral diaphragmatic hernia**). Thus the Bochdalek hernia is an abnormal hole in the posterolateral corner of the left diaphragm that allows the intestines—and in some cases

the stomach—to move directly into the chest cavity and compress the developing lungs.[1]

As shown in Fig. 41.1, the effects of a diaphragmatic hernia are similar to the effects of a **pneumothorax** or

---

[1] About 90% of CDHs are Bochdalek hernias. Rare CDHs include **Morgagni hernia**, which compromises approximately 9% of CDHs, **total absence of the diaphragm**, and **congenital diaphragmatic eventration** of the diaphragm. Morgagni hernias are characterized by herniation through the foramina of Morgagni, which are located immediately adjacent to the xyphoid process of the sternum. Most Morgagni hernias occur on the right side of the body and depending on the amount of liver involvement, tend to have a higher mortality rate and require more **extracorporeal membrane oxygenation (ECMO)** support than left-sided CDH infants. A congenital diaphragmatic eventration is abnormal elevation of part or all of an otherwise intact diaphragm into the chest cavity. This rare form of CDH occurs when a region of the diaphragm is thinner (commonly caused by an incomplete muscularization of the diaphragm), which in turn allows the abdominal viscera to protrude upward.

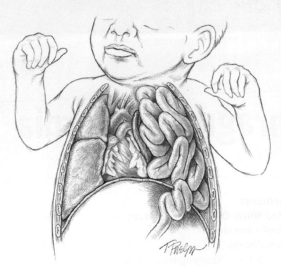

FIGURE 41.1 Diaphragmatic hernia.

hemothorax—that is, the lungs are compressed. As the condition becomes more severe, **atelectasis** and complete lung collapse may occur. When this happens, the heart and mediastinum are pushed to the right side of the chest. In addition, long-term lung compression in utero causes **pulmonary hypoplasia**, which is most severe on the affected (ipsilateral) side but also occurs on the unaffected (contralateral) side.

This pathologic process causes a marked reduction in the number of bronchial generations and alveoli per acinus. Concomitant increased muscularity of the small pulmonary arteries may contribute to the increased pulmonary vascular resistance and **pulmonary hypertension** commonly seen in these patients. Respiratory distress usually develops soon after birth. As the infant struggles to inhale, the increased negative intrathoracic pressure generated during each inspiration causes even more of the intestines to be sucked into the thorax.

Further compression of the lungs and heart occurs as the infant cries and swallows air, causing the intestine and stomach to distend further.

Finally, as a consequence of the hypoxemia associated with a diaphragmatic hernia, these babies often develop hypoxia-induced pulmonary arterial vasoconstriction and vasospasm, which also produce a state of pulmonary hypertension.

The major pathologic or structural changes associated with diaphragmatic hernia may include the following:

- Failure of the Bochdalek foramen of the diaphragm to close
- Migration of intestines and stomach into the thorax
- Atelectasis
- Complete lung collapse
- Mediastinal shift to the unaffected side of the thorax
- Reduction in the number of bronchial generations and alveoli per acinus
- Pulmonary hypoplasia
- Transient pulmonary hypertension

Etiology and Epidemiology

The overall incidence of CDH is 1 in 2500 to 3500 live births. The baby is usually mature, and two-thirds are male. About 90% of CDHs occur on the left side through the Bochdalek foramen. The mortality rate for infants with CDH, including spontaneous abortions, stillbirths, and prehospital deaths, is about 50% to 60%. The prognosis depends on (1) the size of the defect, (2) the degree of hypoplasia, (3) the condition of the lung on the unaffected side, and (4) the success of the surgical diaphragmatic closure. Most cases of CDH are now diagnosed by **prenatal ultrasound**, allowing the infant to be delivered at a hospital where surgical repair of the diaphragmatic hernia can occur very shortly after birth. A few pediatric centers are performing high-risk prenatal surgery (in-utero) to repair the diaphragm.

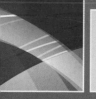
The following clinical manifestations result from the pathologic mechanisms caused (or activated) by atelectasis (see Fig. 10.7)—a common anatomic alteration of the lungs associated with diaphragmatic hernia (see Fig. 41.1).

CLINICAL DATA OBTAINED AT THE PATIENT'S BEDSIDE

The Physical Examination

Vital Signs

Increased Respiratory Rate (Tachypnea)

Normally, a newborn's respiratory rate is about 40 to 60 breaths/min. When a diaphragmatic hernia is present, the respiratory rate is generally well over 60 breaths/min. Several pathophysiologic mechanisms operating simultaneously may lead to an increased ventilatory rate:

- Stimulation of peripheral chemoreceptors (hypoxemia)
- Relationship of decreased lung compliance to increased ventilatory rate
- Stimulation of central chemoreceptors

Increased Heart Rate (Pulse) and Blood Pressure

Clinical Manifestations Associated With Greater Negative Intrapleural Pressures During Inspiration

- Intercostal retraction
- Substernal retraction
- Nasal flaring

Chest Assessment Findings

- Diminished or absent breath sounds over the affected side
- Bowel sounds over the affected side
- Apical heartbeat heard over the unaffected side (usually right)

Expiratory Grunting

Cyanosis

Barrel Chest Deformity

When the intestines are in the chest and distended with gas, the baby often demonstrates a barrel chest deformity.

Scaphoid Abdomen

Depending on the degree of intestinal displacement into the thorax, the infant's abdomen often appears flat or concave.

CLINICAL DATA OBTAINED FROM LABORATORY TESTS AND SPECIAL PROCEDURES

Pulmonary Function Test Findings
(Extrapolated Data for Instructional Purposes)
(Primarily Restrictive Lung Pathophysiology)

The anatomic alterations of the lungs associated with CDH primarily cause a restrictive lung pathophysiology. For example, in moderate to severe cases, the following lung volumes and capacities may be lower than normal.

RV	IRV	VC	FRC	TLC
↓	↓	↓	↓	↓

Arterial Blood Gases[1]

MILD TO MODERATE DIAPHRAGMATIC HERNIA

Acute Alveolar Hyperventilation With Hypoxemia[2]
(Acute Respiratory Alkalosis)

pH	$PaCO_2$	HCO_3^-	PaO_2	SaO_2 or SpO_2
↑	↓	↓	↓	↓
		(but normal)		

SEVERE DIAPHRAGMATIC HERNIA

Acute Ventilatory Failure With Hypoxemia[3]
(Acute Respiratory Acidosis)

pH[4]	$PaCO_2$	HCO_3^-[4]	PaO_2	SaO_2 or SpO_2
↓	↑	↑	↓	↑
		(but normal)		

Oxygenation Indices[5]

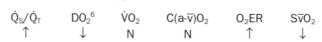

$\dot{Q}_S/\dot{Q}_T$	DO_2[6]	$\dot{V}O_2$	$C(a-\bar{v})O_2$	O_2ER	$S\bar{v}O_2$
↑	↓	N	N	↑	↓

---

[1]*NOTE:* A critically ill newborn is likely to have an umbilical arterial catheter in place for arterial blood gas (ABG) sampling. In older critically ill infants and children, an arterial line may be placed for frequent ABG sampling. For intermittent sampling, because of the difficulty of obtaining ABG samples from newborn and pediatric patients, capillary blood gas (CBG) samples may be used to determine the pH, $PaCO_2$, and HCO_3^- (i.e., the acid-base and ventilation status only). Capillary PO_2 values are unreliable and should not be used for clinical analysis. The standard way to evaluate the oxygenation status in these infants is pulse oximetry (SpO_2) (see Chapter 33, Newborn Assessment and Management).

[2]See Fig. 5.2 and Table 5.4 and related discussion for the acute pH, $PaCO_2$, and HCO_3^- changes associated with acute alveolar hyperventilation.

[3]See Table 5.5 and related discussion for the acute pH, $PaCO_2$, and HCO_3^- changes associated with acute ventilatory failure.

[4]When tissue hypoxia is severe enough to produce lactic acid, the pH and HCO_3^- values will be lower than expected for a particular $PaCO_2$ level.

[5]$C(a-\bar{v})O_2$, Arterial-venous oxygen difference; DO_2, total oxygen delivery; O_2ER, oxygen extraction ratio; $\dot{Q}_S/\dot{Q}_T$, pulmonary shunt fraction; $S\bar{v}O_2$, mixed venous oxygen saturation; $\dot{V}O_2$, oxygen consumption.

[6]Because the newborn normally has a higher hemoglobin level at birth (16.8 to 18.9 g/dL), the DO_2 may actually be greater than indicated by PaO_2 or SpO_2 alone (see Chapter 5, Blood Gas Assessment).

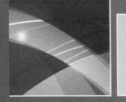

RADIOLOGIC FINDINGS

Chest Radiograph

Increased Opacity (Ground-Glass Appearance, Especially in Areas That Are Compressed)

A typical radiograph shows fluid- and air-filled loops of intestine in the chest and a shift of the heart and mediastinum to the unaffected side. Atelectasis and complete lung collapse may be present. The lungs may appear hypoplastic and may not expand to meet the chest wall. A nasogastric tube (in the patient's stomach, it is hoped!) may be seen on the chest radiograph. It is used to decompress the abdominal viscera. The presence of a diaphragmatic hernia on a chest radiograph usually confirms the need for surgery (Fig. 41.2).

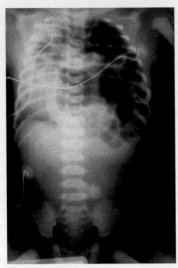

FIGURE 41.2 Chest radiograph of a left diaphragmatic hernia.

General Management of a Congenital Diaphragmatic Hernia

Severe diaphragmatic hernia used to be considered one of the most urgent neonatal surgical emergencies. Current practice is to make sure the patient has a stable cardiorespiratory status before undergoing surgical repair.

As soon as the diagnosis of a diaphragmatic hernia is made, a double-lumen oral gastric tube should be inserted with intermittent or low continuous suction. This reduces the amount of gas in the stomach and bowels and thereby reduces lung compression. Oxygen therapy should be started immediately (see Oxygen Therapy Protocol, Protocol 33.1). The infant also may be placed in the semi-Fowler position, which reduces intrathoracic pressure and facilitates the downward positioning of the abdominal viscera. Placing the infant on the affected side aids expansion of the good lung. *The infant must not be manually ventilated with a bag and mask because of the danger of air swallowing.*

The infant must, however, be intubated and ventilated. Mechanical ventilation should be applied with low peak airway pressures (less than 30 cm H_2O) and rapid respiratory rates. A typical set of ventilator parameters would be peak inspiratory pressure (PIP) +18 to +26 cm H_2O, respiratory rate 20 to 40, FIO_2 1.0, positive end-expiratory pressure (PEEP) +5 to +8 cm H_2O, and inspiratory time (T_I) 0.4. High-frequency oscillatory ventilation and high-frequency jet ventilation are other successful ventilation techniques to achieve adequate oxygenation and carbon dioxide elimination while keeping airway pressures lower (see Mechanical Ventilation and Ventilator Weaning Protocol, Protocol 33.4).

Because the infant's lungs are fragile and rupture easily, the incidence of pneumothorax is high. **Therefore the physician may need to insert one or more chest tubes during mechanical ventilation, if a pneumothorax occurs.** Paralysis with muscle relaxants and sedation are helpful at times. Paralysis eliminates air swallowing, which helps keep the gastrointestinal contents compressed. Suctioning may be necessary to maintain the infant's airways (see Airway Clearance Protocol, Protocol 33.2).

Occasionally, certain pharmacologic agents may be administered to offset the infant's pulmonary hypertension. Such drugs include tolazoline, prostacyclin, prostaglandin E1, sildenafil, and **inhaled nitric oxide (iNO)**, in combination with different inotropes, such as dopamine and dobutamine. The physiologic action of iNO is believed to be similar to that of the vasoactive substance, endothelium-derived relaxing factor. The use of iNO has significantly reduced the need for ECMO therapy.

The surgical procedure entails repositioning the abdominal contents into the abdomen and closing the diaphragmatic defect. In some infants the peritoneal cavity may be too small to contain the abdominal contents. In these cases, after the repair is completed, the surgeon will place a patch to close the surgical site. After surgery, the baby is placed back on the ventilator and weaned per ventilator protocol. Mechanical ventilation with PEEP and continuous positive airway pressure (CPAP) are commonly required to offset the atelectasis and hypoplasia associated with the disorder. Often, the lung on the affected side is hypoplastic, and days or weeks of therapy may be required for full expansion to occur (see Lung Expansion Therapy Protocol, Protocol 33.3).

Extracorpeal Membrane Oxygenation (ECMO) may be indicated to treat circulatory and respiratory complications after surgery for infants who do not respond favorably to conventional medical therapy. While on ECMO, the infant is put on ventilation with only 10 breaths/min to keep the lungs inflated.

Admitting History and Physical Examination

A full-term baby boy was delivered at 2:25 a.m. without complications to a mother who had received no prenatal care. After delivery, however, the baby made one cry and quickly became blue and limp, started to have bradycardia, and became apneic. The baby's 1-minute Apgar score was 3 (heart rate 1, respiration 0, tone 1, reflex irritability 1, color 0). The nurse handed the baby to a student intern, who immediately began manual ventilation. Both the respiratory therapist and the nurse noted that the baby's abdomen was scaphoid; the therapist stated that the baby might have a diaphragmatic hernia and that bagging should be stopped immediately. Moments later, the neonatologist entered the room, confirmed the **scaphoid abdomen**, noted that the lungs were very stiff in response to the bagging, and ordered a stat intubation with a 3.5-mm tube and a chest radiograph.

The infant was then transferred to the neonatal intensive care unit. The chest radiograph confirmed a left diaphragmatic hernia and hypoplastic left lung. At this time, a nasogastric tube was inserted and suction was begun. Initial ABGs were pH 7.19, $PaCO_2$ 63 mm Hg, HCO_3^- 23 mEq/L, PaO_2 37 mm Hg, and SaO_2 56%. The baby was sedated and placed on a pressure-limited mechanical ventilator. An intravenous line and umbilical artery catheter were then secured. The initial ventilator settings were respiratory rate 30 breaths/min, T_I 0.5, PEEP +5, PIP + 25, and FIO_2 1.0. No breath sounds could be heard over the infant's left chest.

The neonatologist diagnosed pulmonary hypertension of the newborn by **echocardiogram**. The respiratory therapist then adjusted the ventilator settings as follows: respiratory rate 35 breaths/min, T_I 0.4 second, PEEP +6, PIP +28 cm H_2O, and FIO_2 1.0. A second set of ABGs taken 15 minutes later showed pH 7.29, $PaCO_2$ 49 mm Hg, HCO_3^- 23 mEq/L, PaO_2 44 mm Hg, and SaO_2 74%.

The baby was started on iNO with little improvement in oxygenation. The team assumed this poor response was a result of the severe pulmonary hypoplasia. He was then placed on ECMO, with the ventilator set to minimal settings. Even though the ECMO was doing all the oxygenation, the baby's lungs were expanded by the ventilator 10 times a minute. Four days later, his pulmonary artery pressure was determined to be low enough for surgery. The diaphragmatic hernia was repaired, and the baby was returned to the unit. He was continued on a ventilator and ECMO.

The ventilator settings 3 days later were respiratory rate 10/min, T_I 0.6, PIP +20, PEEP +5, and FIO_2 0.45. His vital signs were heart rate 145 beats/min, **blood pressure 70/45 mm Hg and mean arterial pressure (MAP) of 53 mm Hg,** (In pediatrics, MAP is utilized routinely to evaluate blood pressure), respiratory rate 65 breaths/min (between ventilator breaths), and temperature 37°C (98.6°F). His skin was pink and normal. Good breath sounds were auscultated over the right lung, fine and coarse crackles could be heard over the left lung.

His ABGs at this time were pH 7.36, $PaCO_2$ 44 mm Hg, HCO_3^- 24 mEq/L, PaO_2 73 mm Hg, and SaO_2 94%. The baby's chest radiograph showed good lung expansion on the right side. Although the upper half of the left lung was well expanded, atelectasis and hypoplasia were still seen over the lower half of the left lung. A small amount of thin, clear secretions was suctioned from the baby's endotracheal tube three or four times an hour.

At that time the respiratory therapist wrote the following assessment in the infant's chart.

Respiratory Assessment and Plan

S N/A

O Vital signs: On ECMO HR 145, BP 70/45 (53), RR 65 (10 mechanical breaths), T 37°C (98.6°F). Skin: Pink and normal. Breath sounds: Right lung normal; left lung coarse crackles. ABGs pH 7.36, $PaCO_2$ 44, HCO_3^- 24, PaO_2 73, SaO_2 94%. CXR: Right lung normal; atelectasis and hypoplasia in left lower lung.

A • ECMO dependent on ventilator at minimal settings but improving (vital signs, skin color, ABGs)
   • Mild amount of large and small airway secretions (fine and coarse crackles)
   • Atelectasis and hypoplasia of the left lower lobe (CXR)
   • May be ready to wean from ECMO—check with physician

P **Mechanical Ventilation and Ventilator Weaning Protocol** (continue to wean per protocol—wean pressures first, then FIO_2). Lung Expansion Therapy Protocol (continue PEEP or CPAP per **Mechanical Ventilation and Ventilator Weaning Protocol**). Airway Clearance Protocol (continue suction PRN). Oxygen Therapy Protocol (keep SpO_2 at 97% as the FIO_2 is decreased. Do not decrease FIO_2 more than 0.10 per hour).

ECMO was discontinued. The baby continued to improve over the next 5 days. On day 6, he was off the ventilator and discharged from the hospital 2 weeks later. The baby continued to develop normally over the next 4 years; at the time of this writing, he was about to enter kindergarten.

Discussion

This case nicely illustrates the importance of good assessment skills. Most diaphragmatic hernias are identified before the baby is born by high-resolution ultrasound of the maternal abdomen, visualizing the fetus in utero during routine prenatal care. Unfortunately, this mother had no prenatal care, and as a result the baby's diaphragmatic hernia was a surprise. Fortunately, the respiratory therapist and nurse in this case quickly and correctly identified the possibility of the diaphragmatic hernia by noting the scaphoid abdomen. Had the student intern continued to bag the baby manually, more gas would have entered the stomach and intestines, compressing and compromising the infant's lungs even more. The atelectasis (see Fig. 10.7) caused by the enlarged intestines was objectively confirmed on the chest radiograph. The Lung Expansion Therapy Protocol was clearly justified to offset the atelectasis after the diaphragmatic hernia was repaired (see Lung Expansion Therapy Protocol, Protocol 33.3).

This case further illustrates that the first objective in the management of the infant born with a diaphragmatic hernia is correction of the pulmonary hypertension. Often, as in this case, treatment requires that the infant be given ECMO and other cardiorespiratory stabilization treatments for several days before surgery. After the pulmonary hypertension is controlled, the second objective is surgical repair of the hernia. Mechanical ventilation with PEEP is usually required after surgery to correct the atelectasis and hypoplasia associated with the disorder. Typically, weaning involves decreasing the FIO_2 while monitoring the baby's pulse oximetry. Ideally, the ventilator pressures are decreased first, followed by the ventilatory rates. Permissive hypercapnia is routinely used, with a target $PaCO_2$ of 55 mm Hg or less. An infant on a respiratory rate of 20 breaths/min, a peak inspiratory pressure of +20 cm H_2O or less, and a PEEP of +5 to 6 cm H_2O or less is usually ready for extubation. Infants who survive congenital diaphragmatic hernia require follow-up pulmonary care for the first years of life because they handle *pulmonary infections* poorly, owing to their smaller than normal lungs as a result of the prenatal lung hypoplasia.

SELF-ASSESSMENT QUESTIONS

1. The Bochdalek foramen closes at the:
   a. Fourth to sixth week of gestation
   b. Sixth to eighth week of gestation
   c. Eighth to tenth week of gestation
   d. Tenth to twelfth week of gestation

2. Which of the following are associated with a congenital diaphragmatic hernia?
   1. Females affected more than males
   2. Left side (90%)
   3. A scaphoid abdomen at birth
   4. Bowel sounds on the affected side of chest
      a. 1 and 3 only
      b. 2 and 4 only
      c. 2, 3, and 4 only
      d. 1, 2, 3, and 4

3. Which of the following arterial blood gas values is(are) associated with mild to moderate congenital diaphragmatic hernia?
   1. Increased pH
   2. Increased $PaCO_2$
   3. Increased PaO_2
   4. Increased HCO_3^-
      a. 1 only
      b. 1 and 4 only
      c. 2, 3, and 4 only
      d. 1, 2, and 4 only

4. Which of the following clinical manifestations is(are) associated with a congenital diaphragmatic hernia?
   1. Diminished or absent breath sounds
   2. Bowel sounds over the affected side
   3. Pulmonary hypertension
   4. Atelectasis
      a. 3 and 4 only
      b. 1 and 2 only
      c. 1, 2, and 3 only
      d. 1, 2, 3, and 4

5. Treatment of congenital diaphragmatic hernia may include:
   1. Inhaled nitric oxide
   2. ECMO
   3. Surgical repair
   4. High-frequency ventilation
      a. 1 and 4 only
      b. 2 and 3 only
      c. 1, 3, and 4 only
      d. 1, 2, 3 and 4

Chapter Objectives

After reading this chapter, you will be able to:

- List the anatomic alterations associated with common congenital heart diseases.
- Describe the etiology and epidemiology of common congenital heart diseases.
- Describe the testing of newborns to rule out "critical congenital heart defects" before hospital discharge.
- List the cardiopulmonary clinical manifestations associated with common congenital heart diseases.
- Describe the general management of the common congenital heart diseases.
- Describe the clinical strategies and rationales of the SOAPs presented in the case study.
- Define key terms and complete self-assessment questions at the end of the chapter and on Evolve.

Key Terms

Aortic Ejection Click
Atrial Septal Defect (ASD)
Balloon Atrial Septostomy (BAS)
Coeur-en-Sabot Appearance
Complex Transposition of the Great Arteries (Complex TGA)
Congenital Heart Diseases (CHDs)
Cyanotic Heart Defect
Critical Congenital Heart Defect (CCHD)
Dextrotransposition of the Great Arteries (d-TGA)
Differential Cyanosis
Doppler Color Flow Mapping
Foramen Ovale
Fossa Ovalis
"Hypercyanotic Spells"
Hypoplastic Left Heart Syndrome (HLHS)
Infundibular Stenosis
Ligamentum Arteriosum
Midsystolic Murmurs
Muscular Ventricular Septal Defect
Noncyanotic Heart Defect
Ostium Secundum ASD
Pansystolic Murmur
Patent Ductus Arteriosus (PDA)
Postductal
Preductal
Primum ASD
Prostaglandin E1
Pulmonary Flow to Systemic Flow ($\dot{Q}_P/\dot{Q}_T$) ratio
Pulse Oximetry Screening Test
Shunt Direction
Shunt Reversal
Simple Transposition of the Great Arteries (Simple TGA)

Stenosis of the Pulmonary Artery
Sub-atmospheric Oxygen Therapy
Subclavicular Thrill
Systolic Ejection
Systolic Thrill
Tetralogy of Fallot (TOF)
"Tet Spells"
Transposition of the Great Arteries (TGA)
Ultrasonography
Valvular Stenosis
Ventricular Septal Defect (VSD)

Chapter Outline

Patent Ductus Arteriosus (PDA)
  Anatomic Alterations of the Heart
  Etiology and Epidemiology
  Diagnosis
  Clinical Manifestations
  Treatment
Atrial Septal Defect (ASD)
  Anatomic Alterations of the Heart
  Etiology and Epidemiology
  Diagnosis
  Clinical Manifestations
  Treatment
Ventricular Septal Defect (VSD)
  Anatomic Alterations of the Heart
  Etiology and Epidemiology
  Diagnosis
  Clinical Manifestations
  Treatment
Tetralogy of Fallot (TOF)
  Anatomic Alterations of the Heart
  Etiology and Epidemiology
  Diagnosis
  Clinical Manifestations
  Treatment
Transposition of the Great Arteries (TGA)
  Anatomic Alterations of the Heart
  Etiology and Epidemiology
  Diagnosis
  Treatment
Hypoplastic Left Heart Syndrome (HLHS)
  Anatomic Alterations of the Heart
  Etiology and Epidemiology
  Diagnosis
  Treatment
Case Study: Transposition of the Great Arteries
Self-Assessment Questions

Congenital heart diseases (CHDs) (also known as *congenital heart defects*) are anatomic abnormalities of the heart that are present at birth. CHDs can involve the (1) interior walls of the heart, (2) valves inside the heart, and/or (3) arteries and veins that carry blood to and from the heart or body. According to the National Heart, Lung, and Blood Institute, CHDs are the most common type of birth defect, affecting 8 of every 1000 newborns. According to the Centers for Disease Control and Prevention (CDC), nearly 40,000 infants are born with a heart defect each year in the United States, and more than 1 million adults are living with CHD here.

There are several types of CHDs ranging from simple diseases with no symptoms to complex diseases with severe, life-threatening symptoms. Many of the simple diseases require no treatment or are relatively easy to repair. The complex diseases require medical care and surgical repair soon after birth. The ability to diagnose and treat CHDs has greatly improved over the past few decades. Today, nearly all children born with complex CHDs survive to adulthood and lead active, productive lives.

CHDs commonly encountered by the respiratory therapist include **patent ductus arteriosus (PDA), atrial septal defect (ASD), ventricular septal defect (VSD), tetralogy of Fallot (TOF), transposition of the great arteries (TGA),** and **hypoplastic left heart syndrome (HLHS)**. These CHDs can be further classified on the basis of **shunt direction** as either a **noncyanotic heart defect** (a left-to-right shunting heart defect), such as PDA, ASD, and VSD, or a **cyanotic heart defect** (a right-to-left shunting heart defect), such as TOF, TGA, and HLHS.

Approximately one-third of the infants with cardiac abnormalities are diagnosed after birth. Today, about two-thirds of fetal cardiac abnormalities (single ventricle lesions such as HLHS, TGA, and TOF) are diagnosed prenatally by obstetric screening with **ultrasonography**. Prenatal diagnosis allows for a scheduled delivery at a tertiary center where appropriate medical intervention can begin immediately after birth and cardiothoracic surgery physicians can be consulted.

Suspicion of CHD includes abnormal cardiac sounds (e.g., murmurs), presence of hypoxemia, and low systemic blood pressure or hypotension. Some infants present with hypoxemia and are nonresponsive to oxygen therapy. Any suspected cardiac abnormality requires a cardiologist to evaluate. Lesions are confirmed by visualization on echocardiogram, and, if necessary, cardiac computed tomography or magnetic resonance imaging. Cardiac catheterization in newborns is now limited to interventions such as a **balloon atrial septostomy (BAS)**.

Symptoms of CHD may not always be apparent in the first several days of life. Certain diseases may not be detected until the infant presents to the emergency department (ED) at 4 to 6 weeks in cardiogenic shock. In 2009 the American Heart Association and the American Academy of Pediatrics endorsed the use of pulse oximetry for early detection of **critical congenital heart defect (CCHD)**. In 2011 the US Secretary of Health and Human Services added newborn screening for CCHD to the Recommended Uniform Screening Panel. Presently, 46 states have adopted regulations requiring all infants cared for in nurseries to be screened for CHD before hospital discharge.

BOX 42.1 Critical Hypoxemic Congenital Heart Defects

Conditions that present with hypoxemia in the newborn period or that require treatment in the first few months:

Most Common
- Hypoplastic left heart syndrome
- Pulmonary atresia
- Tetralogy of Fallot
- Total anomalous pulmonary venous return
- Transposition of the great arteries
- Tricuspid atresia
- Truncus arteriosus

Least Common
- Coarctation of the aorta
- Double outlet right ventricle
- Ebstein anomaly
- Interrupted aortic arch
- Single ventricle

The **pulse oximetry screening test** is done by using two separate pulse oximeters with probes attached to the infant's right hand and right or left foot. The right hand is **preductal**, and the right or left foot is **postductal** (see Fig. 33.13)—that is, proximal or distal to the ductus arteriosis. If both SpO_2 readings are 95% or greater, the infant passes as normal. If the infant has an oxygen saturation of less than 90% on either extremity, the infant has a positive screen and is referred for cardiac evaluation. If the infant has an SpO_2 between 90% and 94% on either extremity or a 3% difference between the two readings, the test must be repeated three times 1 hour apart. If results remain abnormal, this is a positive screen and the infant is referred for cardiac evaluation.

The pulse oximetry test screening has been very successful in identifying both critical and serious cardiac defect, and—importantly—in preventing the poor outcomes that have been previously documented in EDs of babies with unidentified and untreated CHD. When combined with cardiac auscultation, the sensitivity of the pulse oximetry screening tests for CCHD is greater than 92%. Box 42.1 shows common CCHDs that present with hypoxemia in the newborn period or that require treatment in the first few months of life.

Patent Ductus Arteriosus (PDA)

Anatomic Alterations of the Heart

Patent ductus arteriosus is a congenital heart defect in which the ductus arteriosus, which is normally open during fetal life, fails to close shortly after birth. As a result, a portion of the oxygenated blood from the aorta (which has a higher blood pressure) flows through the open ductus back to the pulmonary artery (Fig. 42.1). The pathophysiologic effect of

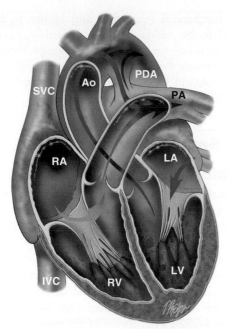

FIGURE 42.1 Patent ductus arteriosus (PDA) is a congenital heart defect in which the ductus arteriosus fails to close shortly after birth. The pathophysiologic effect of a PDA is a *left-to-right* shunt (noncyanotic disorder). When the infant has persistent hypertension of the newborn, a *right-to-left* shunt will develop (cyanotic disorder), resulting in a decreased PaO₂ and oxygen content. This figure illustrates both a left-to-right shunt and a right-to-left shunt. *Ao,* Aorta; *IVC,* inferior vena cava; *LA,* left atrium; *LV,* left ventricle; *PA,* pulmonary artery; *RA,* right atrium; *RV,* right ventricle; *SVC,* superior vena cava.

a PDA is a *left-to-right* shunt (noncyanotic disorder).[1] In other words, it allows blood from the systemic circulation to flow into the pulmonary circulation. Box 42.2 provides a brief review of the normal development and function of the ductus arteriosus.

A PDA results in excessive blood flow through the pulmonary circulation and hypoperfusion of the systemic circulation. Pulmonary engorgement results in decreased lung compliance—stiff lungs. Pulmonary blood flow can be up to three times greater than that of the systemic blood flow. The pathophysiologic consequences of the "ductal steal" depend on the size of the shunt and the response of the heart, lungs, and other organs affected by the shunt. In preterm infants, a clinically significant PDA is associated with an increased risk for pulmonary edema, pulmonary hemorrhage, bronchopulmonary dysplasia, and a decrease in pulmonary function requiring increased ventilator settings, such as increased positive end-expiratory pressure (PEEP) and mean airway pressure.

Etiology and Epidemiology

PDA is associated with prematurity, low birth weight, high altitude and low atmospheric oxygen tension, hypoxia, and a variety of chromosomal abnormalities. It is more common in premature than in full-term infants, occurring in about 8 of every 1000 premature babies, compared with 2 of every 1000 full-term babies. PDA is twice as common in girls than in boys. The prognosis is generally considered excellent in the newborn whose only problem is a PDA.

[1]When persistent pulmonary hypertension of the newborn is present, a right-to-left shunt will develop (cyanotic disorder), causing decreased PaO₂ and oxygen content (see Box 42.2, and Chapter 33, Newborn Assessment and Management, page 495).

Diagnosis

The diagnosis of PDA is usually based on its characteristic clinical findings—that is, a loud systolic/diastolic to-and-fro heart murmur at the upper left sternal border—and confirmed by echocardiography. The combination of two-dimensional echocardiographic imaging and Doppler color flow mapping is both sensitive and specific for the identification of PDA.

Clinical Manifestations

The patient with a PDA can present at any age. Typically, the newborn with a PDA is asymptomatic. The newborn with a moderate or large ductal PDA usually develops signs and symptoms during the first 2 to 3 days after birth, as the pulmonary vascular resistance decreases, which in turn increases the *left-to-right* shunting through the lungs. When PDA is complicated by *persistent pulmonary hypertension of the newborn*, the clinical manifestations include tachycardia, dyspnea, **differential cyanosis** (i.e., cyanosis of the lower extremities but not the upper body), low PaO_2 and SpO_2, increased $PaCO_2$, loud systolic/diastolic murmur at the upper left sternal border (the second heart sound [S_2] is often obscured by murmur), cardiomegaly, left **subclavicular thrill**, prominent left ventricular impulse, bounding pulse (related to the high left ventricular stroke volume, which may cause systolic hypertension), and widened pulse pressure. Suprasternal or carotid pulsations may be prominent. Complications of PDA in the newborn include pulmonary edema, congestive heart failure, intraventricular hemorrhage, necrotizing enterocolitis, and bronchopulmonary dysplasia as a result of prolonged ventilator and/or oxygen support. A PDA in a newborn with any of these resulting conditions will likely require an extended hospitalization.

PDA patients who are 3 to 6 weeks old commonly present with tachypnea, diaphoresis, inability to feed or difficulty with feeding, and weight loss or failure to gain weight. The patient with a moderate or large PDA may demonstrate a hoarse cry, cough, lower respiratory tract infection, atelectasis, or pneumonia. In the adult whose PDA has gone undiagnosed, the signs and symptoms include congestive heart failure, atrial arrhythmia, and differential cyanosis (i.e., cyanosis limited to the lower extremities).[2] The patient often reports decreased exercise tolerance.

Treatment

Medical treatment of the PDA is generally intravenous indomethacin; this drug can be given prophylactically to prevent a PDA or as treatment. Surgery (PDA ligation) may be needed to permanently close the ductus when medication is not effective and left-to-right shunting is prolonging the

need for mechanical ventilation and higher mean airway pressure. For the newborn, the standard respiratory care protocols are used—i.e., the Oxygen Therapy Protocol 33.1, Airway Clearance Protocol 33.2, Lung Expansion Therapy Protocol 33.4, and Mechanical Ventilation and Ventilatory Weaning 33.4 are all administered as needed.

Atrial Septal Defect (ASD)

Anatomic Alterations of the Heart

Atrial septal defect is a congenital heart defect in which there is a hole in the septal wall between the right and left atrium (Fig. 42.2). The two most common types of ASD are the ostium secundum ASD and the primum ASD.

The **ostium secundum ASD** is caused by arrested growth of the secundum septum or excessive absorption of the primum septum, resulting in an atrial septal wall defect. The secundum ASD presents as an isolated cardiac defect in the **fossa ovalis.** Box 42.3 provides a brief review of the normal development of the ostium secundum.

The **primum ASD** is caused by arrested growth of the apical portion of the atrial septum. It is associated with an anterior mitral valve cleft, which is often accompanied by mitral valve regurgitation. Box 42.4 provides a brief review of the normal development of the septum primum.

The degree of pathophysiology associated with an ASD depends on (1) the pulmonary and systemic vascular resistances, (2) the compliance of the left and right ventricles, and (3) the size of the ASD. At birth, the left atrial pressure becomes greater than right atrial pressure, resulting in a *left-to-right* shunt (noncyanotic disorder). Initially, the volume of blood

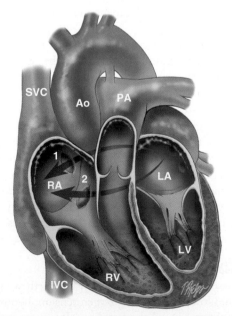

FIGURE 42.2 Atrial septal defect (ASD) is a congenital heart defect in which there is a hole in the septal wall between the right and left atrium. The two most common types of ASD are the ostium secundum ASD (1) and the primum ASD (2). *Ao,* Aorta; *IVC,* inferior vena cava; *LA,* left atrium; *LV,* left ventricle; *PA,* pulmonary artery; *RA,* right atrium; *RV,* right ventricle; *SVC,* superior vena cava.

---

[2]Differential cyanosis occurs when cyanosis is more evident in the lower extremities than the upper extremities and the head. Differential cyanosis is seen in patients with a patent ductus arteriosus (PDA). These patients commonly develop progressive pulmonary vascular disease, and pressure overload of the right ventricle occurs. When pulmonary pressure exceeds aortic pressure, a **shunt reversal** occurs—that is, a left-to-right shunt changes to a right-to-left shunt. The upper extremity remains pink because the brachiocephalic trunk, left common carotid trunk, and left subclavian trunk are given off proximal to the PDA.

shunted from left to right is small. This is because the right ventricle is still relatively thick and noncompliant. As the right ventricle remodels in response to the decreased pulmonary vascular resistance, its compliance increases, which in turn lowers the mean right atrial pressure. As a result, the left-to-right shunting increases in volume. In a large ASD, the **pulmonary flow to systemic flow ($\dot{Q}_P/\dot{Q}_T$) ratio** can be over 3:1. In other words, 75% of the blood returning to the left atrium from the lungs flows directly into the right atrium via the ASD and returns to the lungs and 25% of the blood in the left atrium flows into the left ventricle and out to the systemic system.

The increased pulmonary blood flow is usually well tolerated for years. Heart failure is unusual before age 30. Beyond this age, the prevalence of heart failure increases substantially. Other complications include atrial arrhythmias such as flutter and fibrillation.

Etiology and Epidemiology

ASDs are common and account for approximately 13% of all patients with CHD. According to the CDC, over 1900 infants in the United States are born each year with an ASD. Although the precise causes of ASDs are not known, abnormal genes in combination with certain maternal risk factors (e.g., environment, foods, and medicines) are believed to play a role.

Diagnosis

The diagnosis of ASD is usually based on its characteristic clinical manifestations and confirmed by echocardiography. The combination of two-dimensional echocardiographic imaging and **Doppler color flow mapping** is both sensitive and specific for the identification of ASD. Fig. 42.3 shows an echocardiograph of an ostium primum ASD in a 64-year-old man.

Clinical Manifestations

The patient with an ASD can present at any age. In a baby with a small ASD, there may not be any remarkable signs or symptoms. The clinical manifestations depend on the size of the defect and the degree of shunting between the atria. In some infants with a moderate to large ASD, the clinical manifestations include heart failure, tachypnea, respiratory distress, substernal and intercostal retractions, crackles, failure to thrive, recurrent respiratory infection, and hepatomegaly.

In the older patient, common signs and symptoms include exercise intolerance, dyspnea, fatigue, heart arrhythmias (e.g., atrial flutter and fibrillation), heart failure, and swollen feet and hands. In all ages, a moderate to large ASD may produce

---

BOX 42.3 Ostium Secundum

During fetal development, the ostium secundum (also called *foramen secundum* or the "second opening") is an atrial orifice that develops in the septum primum during normal development. At birth, this orifice is partially covered and sealed by the septum secundum. The oval orifice that remains in the atrial wall—the foramen ovale—is covered, but not sealed, on the left atrium side by a flexible flap that is part of the septum primum. The increased blood pressure that develops in the left atrium shortly after birth causes the flexible flap to functionally close. It will eventually form part of the fossa ovalis. Complete structural closure usually takes about 9 months or more.

BOX 42.4 Septum Primum

During fetal development, the cavity of the primitive atrium is subdivided into right and left chambers by a structure called the *septum primum,* which grows downward between the two atrial cavities. As the septum primum grows downward, the progressively smaller gap below it—before it fuses with the endocardial cushion—is called the *ostium primum* ("the first opening"). Eventually, the septum primum fuses with the endocardial cushion and closes the ostium primum off completely.

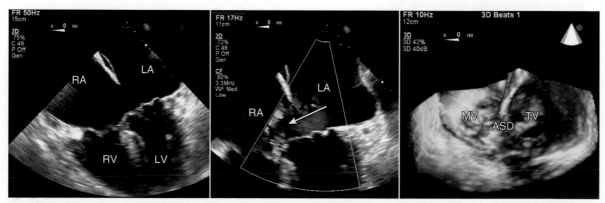

FIGURE 42.3 Echocardiograph of an ostium primum atrial septal defect (ASD) in a 64-year-old man. The transesophageal echocardiogram (TEE) four-chamber view (left) shows an ostium primum ASD with color Doppler (center) showing left-to-right flow across the large defect (see arrow). Three-dimensional imaging (right) shows the relationship between the ASD and the mitral valve (MV) and tricuspid valves (TV). *LA,* Left atrium; *LV,* left ventricle; *RA,* right atrium; *RV,* right ventricle. (From Otto, C. M. [2019]. *Textbook of clinical echocardiography* [6th ed.]. St. Louis, MO: Elsevier.)

a systolic murmur and a fixed split S$_2$, a QRS pattern suggestive of incomplete right bundle branch block, and a chest radiograph that shows cardiac enlargement and increased pulmonary vascularity. The heart murmur may be faint, and the diagnosis is easily overlooked, particularly in adults.

Treatment

Treatment is based on the seriousness of the signs and symptoms and the size of the ASD. Catheter-based procedures or surgery is required to repair the defect. Surgical risk and mortality are lowest when the ASD repair is performed under age 25 and before development of significant pulmonary hypertension.

For the newborn, the standard respiratory care protocols are used—that is, the Oxygen Therapy Protocol 33.1, Airway Clearance Protocol 33.2, Lung Expansion Therapy Protocol 33.3, and Mechanical Ventilation and Ventilatory Weaning 33.4 are all administered as needed.

Ventricular Septal Defect (VSD)

Anatomic Alterations of the Heart

A **ventricular septal defect** is a congenital heart defect in which there is an opening in the ventricular septum of the heart. There may be one or more openings in different locations of the ventricular septum. Common locations include the following:

- **Conoventricular ventricular septal defect:** Located where portions of the ventricular septum normally form below the pulmonary and aortic valves (see Fig. 42.4, 1)

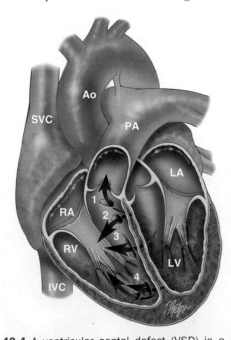

FIGURE 42.4 A ventricular septal defect (VSD) is a congenital heart defect in which there is an opening in the ventricular septum of the heart. Common VSDs are conoventricular ventricular septal defect (1), inlet ventricular septal defect (2), perimembranous ventricular septal defect (3), and muscular ventricular septal defect (4). *Ao,* Aorta; *IVC,* inferior vena cava; *LA,* left atrium; *LV,* left ventricle; *PA,* pulmonary artery; *RA,* right atrium; *RV,* right ventricle; *SVC,* superior vena cava.

- **Inlet ventricular septal defect:** Located near where blood enters the ventricles through the tricuspid and mitral valves. This congenital heart defect may be part of another heart defect called *atrioventricular septal defect (AVSD)* (see Fig. 42.4, 2).
- **Perimembranous ventricular septal defect:** Located in the upper portion of the ventricular septum (see Fig. 42.4, 3).
- **Muscular ventricular septal defect:** Located in the lower, muscular part of the ventricular septum. It is the most common type of VSD (see Fig. 42.4, 4).

The pathophysiology of a VSD depends on the size of the defect and the pulmonary vascular resistance. At birth, the following physiologic events normally occur: (1) an immediate fall in pulmonary vascular resistance, (2) the removal of the low-resistance placenta from circulation, and (3) the closure of the ductus arteriosus. In response to these normal physiologic changes, the left ventricle must contract against a higher systemic vascular resistance while, at the same time, the right ventricle contracts against a lower pulmonary vascular resistance. As a result of these vascular resistance changes, the pressure in the left ventricle quickly becomes greater (approximately 80 to 90 mm Hg) than the pressure in the right ventricle (approximately 20 mm Hg), which in turn causes blood flow from the left to the right ventricle during each contraction. In short, a *left-to-right* shunt develops (noncyanotic disorder) (see Fig. 42.4).

A VSD has the following two net effects: First, the influx of blood into the right ventricle from the left ventricle increases the right ventricular pressure and volume; in turn, this can lead to pulmonary hypertension, arrhythmias, and heart failure. Second, the circuitous route of blood through the lungs and back to the heart causes a volume overload and elevated pressure in the left ventricle as well.

Etiology and Epidemiology

VSD is the most common congenital heart disorder. It occurs in almost 50% of all patients with CHD. According to the CDC, the prevalence of VSD is about 42 in 10,000 babies each year. Although the precise causes of VSDs are not known, abnormal genes in combination with certain maternal risk factors (e.g., environment, foods, and medicines) are thought to play a role. VSDs are frequently associated with certain congenital conditions, such as Down syndrome.

Diagnosis

The diagnosis of VSD is usually based on its characteristic clinical findings and confirmed by echocardiography. The combination of two-dimensional echocardiographic imaging and **Doppler color flow mapping** is both sensitive and specific for the identification of VSD. Fig. 42.5 shows an echocardiograph of a large VSD in a 26-year-old woman.

Clinical Manifestations

The patient with a VSD can present at any age. The size of the VSD influences what signs and symptoms, if any, are present. Often, if the opening is small, it closes on its own and the baby will never show any signs of a VSD. When the VSD is moderate or large, the early clinical manifestations include tachycardia, tachypnea, increased work of breathing, poor weight gain, failure

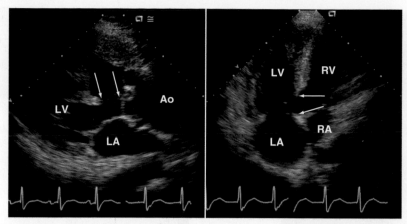

FIGURE 42.5 Echocardiograph of a large ventricular septal defect (VSD) in a 26-year-old woman. A large VSD (between arrows) is seen in a parasternal long-axis view (left) and an apical four-chamber view (right). Severe right ventricular hypertrophy is present. Doppler examination will show low-velocity bidirectional flow across the defect as a result of equalization of RV and LV pressures. *Ao,* Aorta; *LA,* left atrium; *LV,* left ventricle; *RA,* right atrium; *RV,* right ventricle. (From Otto, C. M. [2019]. *Textbook of clinical echocardiography* [6th ed.]. St. Louis, MO: Elsevier.)

to thrive, and diaphoresis. At 3 to 4 weeks of age, the baby usually manifests signs of heart failure, which include continued tachycardia and tachypnea, poor feeding (appears hungry, but tires easily and sweats with feeding), poor weight gain, hepatomegaly, pulmonary crackles, grunting, intercostal retractions, and pallor (from peripheral vasoconstriction).

Cardiac clinical manifestations include systolic murmurs at the mid-to-lower left sternal border, an increased S_2, diastolic murmurs at the apex (indicates a $\dot{Q}_P/\dot{Q}_T$ of 2:1 or greater), and diastolic murmurs at the mid-to-lower sternal border (indicating aortic or pulmonary regurgitation and left-to-right shunting). In addition, infants with a moderate to large VSD may develop a right ventricular heave as the pulmonary vascular pressure falls and the left-to-right shunt increases. In addition, the dilated pulmonary trunk and pulmonary valve closure may be palpable, the cardiac apex may be displaced outside the midclavicular line as the heart enlarges, and vigorous precordial activity and a dynamic left ventricular impulse may be present.

In patients with VSD and aortic regurgitation, the left ventricle is especially overloaded because of both the regurgitated volume from the aorta and the increased volume of blood returning to the left atrium from the pulmonary circulation. Clinical features include neck pulsations, bounding pulse, wide pulse pressure, early diastolic murmur, diaphoresis, and vigorous precordial movement (particularly in the left lateral recumbent position). The electrocardiographic findings may indicate increased volume and pressure loads on the left and right ventricles. The chest radiograph may show increased pulmonary vascular markings, and enlargement of the left atrium, left ventricle, and pulmonary artery. Magnetic resonance imaging may be helpful in showing how much blood is flowing to the lungs. Echocardiography is usually performed to confirm the diagnosis of a suspected VSD (see Fig. 42.5).

Treatment

Smaller congenital VSDs often close within the first year of life as the heart grows. Moderate or large VSDs, however, usually require surgical intervention to close the defect. Continuing care may involve medications to support the heart

(e.g., digitalis and diuretics) and close monitoring for early signs or symptoms of congestive heart failure. For the newborn, the standard respiratory care protocols are used—that is, the Oxygen Therapy Protocol 33.1, Airway Clearance Protocol 33.2, Lung Expansion Therapy Protocol 33.3, and Mechanical Ventilation and Ventilatory Weaning 33.4 are all administered as needed.

Tetralogy of Fallot (TOF)

Anatomic Alterations of the Heart

Tetralogy of Fallot is a congenital heart defect with the following four major anatomic alterations:

- **Stenosis of the pulmonary artery:** This defect is commonly described as a narrowing of the right ventricular outflow tract. The obstruction can occur at the pulmonary valve—called a **valvular stenosis** or just below the pulmonary valve—called an **infundibular stenosis**. The infundibular stenosis is primarily caused by hypertrophy of the myocardial wall. *NOTE: The degree of stenosis varies and is the primary determinant of symptoms and severity* (Fig. 42.6, 1).
- *Deviation of the aorta to the right* (also known as a *dextroposition of the aorta*): The aortic valve is situated directly over the VSD, and connected to both the right and left ventricles. The degree to which the aorta is attached to the right ventricle is referred to as its degree of "override." The degree of aortic override is quite variable; between 5% and 95% of the aortic valve may be connected to the right ventricle (see Fig. 42.6, 2).
- *Ventricular septal defect:* The defect is centered near the most superior portion of the ventricular septum and is usually a single, large hole (see Fig. 42.6, 3).
- *Right ventricular hypertrophy:* The right ventricle is more muscular than normal and causes a characteristic boot-shaped (**coeur-en-sabot appearance**) on the chest radiograph (Fig. 42.7). Because of the pulmonic stenosis and increased obstruction to the right outflow tract, the right ventricular wall increases in size. Right ventricular

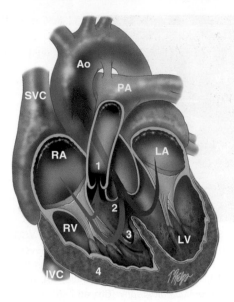

FIGURE 42.6 Tetralogy of Fallot (TOF) is a congenital heart defect that includes stenosis of the pulmonary artery (1), deviation of the aorta to the right (2), ventricular septal defect (3), and right ventricular hypertrophy (4). *Ao,* Aorta; *IVC,* inferior vena cava; *LA,* left atrium; *LV,* left ventricle; *PA,* pulmonary artery; *RA,* right atrium; *RV,* right ventricle; *SVC,* superior vena cava.

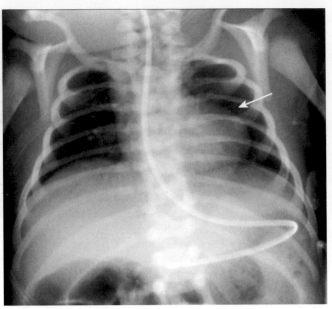

FIGURE 42.7 Tetralogy of Fallot (TOF). In TOF, the term *coeur-en-sabot* (French for "boot-shaped heart") is used to describe a radiologic silhouette of a heart that resembles that of a wooden shoe commonly seen in patients with TOF (see arrow). The "boot's toe" corresponds to an elevated cardiac apex, while the broad "foot" portion corresponds to an increased prominence of the left cardiac border caused by right cardiac hypertrophy. Coeur-en-sabot is the typical radiologic appearance of well-developed TOF—that is, infundibular pulmonary valve stenosis, ventricular septal defect, right ventricular hypertrophy, and dextroposition of the aorta. (Courtesy Dayton Children's Hospital, Dayton, Ohio).

hypertrophy is generally considered to be a secondary anomaly (see Fig. 42.6, 4).

The pathophysiologic effects and clinical symptoms of TOF largely depend on the degree of right ventricular outflow tract obstruction. The direction of blood flow across the VSD is determined by the path of least resistance, not the size of the VSD. For example, if the pulmonary vascular resistance is lower than the systemic vascular resistance, there will be a predominant left-to-right shunt; in this case, the patient will not likely be cyanotic (noncyanotic disorder). However, when there is a significant right ventricular outflow tract obstruction (i.e., a significant pulmonary stenosis), there will be a *right-to-left* shunt across the VSD and cyanosis will ensue (cyanotic disorder).

One of the unique physiologic features of TOF is that the right ventricular outflow tract obstruction often fluctuates in response to transient increases and decreases in the resistance caused by obstruction. The precise mechanism for this obstruction variation is unclear, although several mechanisms, such as increased infundibular contractility, peripheral vasodilation, hyperventilation, and stimulation of the right ventricular mechanoreceptors, have been proposed. During the most dramatic fluctuation events, there can be a near complete occlusion of the right ventricular outflow tract, resulting in very high resistance and significant right-to-left shunting with profound cyanosis. These episodes are referred to as **tet spells** or **hypercyanotic spells**. A typical tet spell is characterized by a sudden, marked increase in cyanosis, followed by syncope. Older children will often squat during a tet spell in an effort to increase systemic vascular resistance to help generate a temporary reversal of the right-to-left shunt.

Etiology and Epidemiology

The prevalence of TOF in the United States is about 4 per 10,000 live births, and it accounts for about 7% to 10% of

the CHDs. According to the CDC, about 1600 infants are born each year with TOF. *TOF is the most common congenital heart disorder to require intervention in the first year of life* and occurs equally in males and females. Although the precise causes of TOF are not known, abnormal genes in combination with certain maternal risk factors (e.g., environment, foods, and medicines) are believed to play a role.

Diagnosis

TOF is generally confirmed by echocardiography. Additional tests include electrocardiograms and chest radiography. However, findings from these studies are often suggestive but not conclusive for the diagnosis of TOF. Cardiac catheterization may be needed to further delineate the anatomic alterations and quantify the resulting hemodynamic pathology.

Clinical Manifestations

The clinical presentation of TOF depends on the degree of right ventricular outflow tract obstruction. Early signs and symptoms include episodes of pronounced cyanosis—that is, hypercyanotic or tet spells—especially during crying or feeding. Oxygen saturation during hypercyanotic spells is low, although in between spells it is often normal. Feeding is usually difficult, and the infant typically fails to thrive. Most infants are smaller than expected for their age.

On palpation, there may be a prominent right ventricular impulse and **systolic thrill** (i.e., a vibration felt by the examiner on palpation). Cardiac auscultation may reveal a single S_2

because the pulmonic component is rarely audible. An early systolic click (called an **aortic ejection click**) along the left sternal border may be heard, which is thought to be caused by flow into the dilated ascending aorta. Symptoms of heart failure may be present. Although the chest radiograph often appears normal, the classic "boot-shaped" heart (coeur-en-sabot) is the hallmark of the disorder (see Fig. 42.7).

A heart murmur is commonly heard primarily because of the right ventricular outflow tract obstruction, not the VSD. The murmur is described as a crescendo and decrescendo sound with a harsh systolic ejection quality. It is best heard along the left midsternal to upper sternal border. The murmur can have a more regurgitant quality that can be mistaken for a VSD. The murmur is effected by both the degree of obstruction and the amount of flow through the obstruction. Unlike an isolated pulmonary stenosis, in a TOF the amount of blood flow that can be pumped across the right ventricular outflow tract obstruction often varies—that is, the blood flow decreases as the obstruction increases and there is a right-to-left shunt. Thus, during periods of increased obstruction, the heart murmur will become softer. During severe hypercyanotic spells, the murmur may actually disappear as a result of the markedly diminished flow across the obstruction.

Treatment

The management of TOF entails initial medical care, surgical palliative care and intracardiac repair, and long-term postoperative care. The need for medical intervention depends on the degree of the right ventricular outflow tract obstruction. Severe cases may require intravenous prostaglandin therapy (alprostadil) to maintain ductal patency pending surgical repair. The stepwise management for patients who experience hypercyanotic (tet) spells includes knee-chest positioning to increase systemic vascular resistance, oxygen therapy, intravenous morphine and fluid bolus, and, if these measures fail, intravenous beta-blockers. Patients with symptoms of heart failure may require diuretic therapy (e.g., furosemide) and digoxin.

Intracardiac repair is typically performed by 3 months of age but can be performed earlier in the neonatal period. The surgery consists of a patch closure of the ventricular septal defect and enlargement of the right ventricular outflow tract. Chronic postoperative complications include pulmonary regurgitation with associated right ventricular enlargement, residual right ventricular outflow tract obstruction, right ventricular dysfunction, aortic root dilation and aortic valve insufficiency, and arrhythmias including atrial and ventricular tachycardia. Long-term follow-up care includes routine health care visits and cardiac testing (e.g., electrocardiogram, echocardiogram, Holter monitoring, exercise testing, and occasionally repeat cardiac magnetic resonance imaging or computed tomography).

The prognosis is poor for patients with uncorrected TOF. Surgical correction has shown excellent long-term survival. Patients who have surgery at a young age have a reported survival rate greater than 90% at 25 years after the surgical repair. Arrhythmias and heart failure are the most common causes of death after surgical repair.

For the newborn, the standard respiratory care protocols are used—that is, the Oxygen Therapy Protocol 33.1, Airway Clearance Protocol 33.2, Lung Expansion Therapy Protocol 33.3, and Mechanical Ventilation and Ventilatory Weaning 33.4 are all administered as needed.

Transposition of the Great Arteries (TGA)

Anatomic Alterations of the Heart

Transposition of the great arteries (also known as *transposition of the great vessels*) *is the most common cyanotic congenital heart lesion that presents in neonates.* TGA is a congenital heart defect in which the pulmonary artery and the aorta are switched in position or transposed. In short, the aorta arises from the right ventricle and the pulmonary artery arises from the left ventricle. The most common form of TGA is the **dextro-transposition of the great arteries (d-TGA)**, in which the origin of the aorta is anterior and to the right of the pulmonary artery (Fig. 42.8).

TGA results in a pulmonary and systemic circulation that functions in "parallel," rather than "series." In other words, the deoxygenated venous blood returning to the right atrium and right ventricle is pumped directly back into the systemic circulation via the aorta, which is connected to the right ventricle, completely bypassing the lungs. This heart defect produces a *right-to-left shunt*, a cyanotic disorder. The oxygenated blood returning to the left atrium and ventricle from the lungs is pumped directly back into the pulmonary circulation via the pulmonary artery, which is connected to the left ventricle, completely bypassing the systemic circulation.

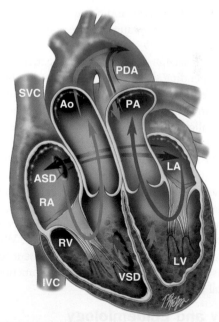

FIGURE 42.8 Transposition of the great arteries (TGAs) is a congenital heart defect in which the pulmonary artery and the aorta are switched in position, or transposed. TGA is commonly associated with an atrial septal defect, a ventricular septal defect, or a patent ductus arteriosus. *Ao,* Aorta; *ASD,* atrial septal defect; *IVC,* inferior vena cava; *LA,* left atrium; *LV,* left ventricle; *PA,* pulmonary artery; *PDA,* patent ductus arteriosus; *RA,* right atrium; *RV,* right ventricle; *SVC,* superior vena cava; *VSD,* ventricular septal defect.

The severity of the symptoms associated with a TGA depends on whether there are additional heart diseases that allow the two separate blood circulations to mingle and, as a result, provide an alternative pathway for oxygenated blood to enter the systemic circulation. Fortunately (relatively speaking), a TGA is usually accompanied by one or more additional heart diseases that provide a direct connection between these two circulations. The most common associated heart diseases are the following:

- *Atrial septal defect:* Is the most common. Depending on pressure differences between the right and left atrium at any given moment, blood may move in either direction through the ASD—that is, either a left-to-right or right-to-left shunt. When oxygenated blood from the left atrium moves into the right atrium (a left-to-right shunt) and mixes with the nonoxygenated blood, the newly mixed blood can move into the right ventricle and then on to the aorta and systemic circulation. However, when nonoxygenated blood moves from the right atrium into the left atrium (a right-to-left shunt) and mixes, some of this blood will move into the left ventricle and be pumped to the lungs via the pulmonary artery (see Fig. 42.8).

- *Ventricular septal defect:* Occurs in about 50% of TGA cases. Depending on pressure differences between the right and left ventricles at any given moment, blood may move in either direction through the VSD—that is, either a left-to-right or right-to-left shunt. When oxygenated blood from the left ventricle moves into the right ventricle (a left-to-right shunt) and mixes with the nonoxygenated blood, some of this blood will be pumped through the aorta and out to the body. However, when nonoxygenated blood moves from the right ventricle into the left ventricle (a right-to-left shunt) and mixes, some of this blood will be pumped to the lungs via the pulmonary artery (see Fig. 42.8).

- *Patent ductus arteriosus:* Is often seen in patients with TGA. Again, depending on the pressure differences between the ductus arteriosus and the aorta at any given moment, blood may flow in either direction. When additional heart diseases exist that allow oxygenated blood to enter the left ventricle, some of this blood may enter the systemic circulation when a right-to-left shunt is present (see Fig. 42.8).

Other heart diseases associated with TGA include a patent **foramen ovale**, left ventricular outflow tract obstruction, aortic arch obstruction, mitral and tricuspid valve abnormalities, and coronary artery anatomic variations. When no other heart diseases are present, it is called **simple TGA**. When other diseases are present, it is a **complex TGA**. The magnitude of these diseases may have an effect on cardiac function, mixing, and surgical approach.

Etiology and Epidemiology

The prevalence of TGA ranges from 2.3 to 4.7 per 10,000 live births in the United States. According to the CDC, approximately 1900 babies are born with TGA each year here. Although the precise cause of TGA is not known, it is associated with poor nutrition during pregnancy, rubella or other viral illness during pregnancy, alcoholism, maternal age over 40 years, and Down syndrome.

Diagnosis

The diagnosis of TGA is based on clinical suspicion of an underlying cyanotic CHD and is confirmed by echocardiography.

Clinical Manifestations

Infants with TGA commonly demonstrate cyanosis, tachypnea (respiratory rates greater than 60 breaths/min), poor feeding, and clubbing of fingers and toes. When there is a VSD, a **pansystolic murmur** (a murmur occupying the entire systolic interval, from S_1 to S_2) is usually present within a few days after birth, at the lower left sternal border. The intensity of the murmur depends on the turbulence of blood flow through the septal defect. In the patient with left ventricular outflow obstruction, there may be a systolic ejection murmur[3] along the upper left sternal border. The intensity of the murmur is a function of both the degree of obstruction and the amount of blood flow across the obstruction.

Treatment

The initial postnatal management of TGA is directed at stabilizing the patient's cardiac and pulmonary function and ensuring adequate systemic oxygenation. Therapy is focused on providing adequate mixing between the two circulatory systems. This can be accomplished by **prostaglandin E1** (alprostadil) therapy (to maintain patency of the ductus arteriosus), BAS,[4] and, ultimately, surgical repair. Surgical correction (e.g., arterial switch operation or atrial switch procedure) is ultimately necessary for survival in patients with TGA.

Complications of surgery include pulmonary artery stenosis, coronary artery insufficiency, neoaortic root dilation, neoaortic regurgitation, atrial arrhythmias, and progressive heart failure. Long-term follow-up care is required because of the potential complications. It entails a focused history; physical examinations; various tests such as echocardiography, electrocardiography, and angiography; and monitoring for atherosclerotic disease. Long-term survival is excellent, with more than 90% survival after 20 years. Although patients may have reduced exercise tolerance, their typical daily level of activity is usually not restricted.

For the newborn, the standard respiratory care protocols are used—that is, the Oxygen Therapy Protocol 33.1, Airway Clearance Protocol 33.2, Lung Expansion Therapy Protocol 33.3, and Mechanical Ventilation and Ventilatory Weaning 33.4 are all administered as needed.

---

[3]**Systolic ejection** or **midsystolic murmurs** are a result of turbulent forward flow across the right and left ventricular outflow tract, aortic or pulmonary valve, or through the aorta or pulmonary artery.

[4]Balloon atrial septostomy (BAS) (also known as the *Rashkind procedure*) is a life-saving technique used to enlarge a hole between the right atrium and the left atrium. It is often used to manage patients with transposition of the great arteries. The larger hole improves oxygenation of the blood. This is normally a palliative procedure used to prepare patients for, or sustain them until, corrective surgery.

Hypoplastic Left Heart Syndrome (HLHS)

Anatomic Alterations of the Heart

Hypoplastic left heart syndrome is a single ventricle defect that results from the left heart not forming correctly during pregnancy (Fig. 42.9). The associated defects include the following:

- An underdeveloped, small left ventricle
- A nonformed or very small mitral valve
- A nonformed or very small aortic valve
- An underdeveloped or very small ascending aorta/aortic arch
- Atrial septal defect (which is life-saving)

With these defects, the left side of the heart is not capable of pumping adequate oxygenated blood through the left ventricle and out the aorta. The degree of narrowing of the valves and structures can be critical. During the first few days of life, the PDA and the patent foramen ovale allow the right ventricle to pump oxygenated blood to the body via the pulmonary artery. Blood flow to the pulmonary vascular bed and the systemic circulation is determined by the balance of the systemic vascular resistance and the pulmonary vascular resistance. As the PDA and patent foramen ovale close, the condition becomes life-threatening. Survival is very tenuous, and surgical intervention is required.

Etiology and Epidemiology

The CDC estimates that about 960 babies are born with HLHS in the United States, with an incidence of 2.3 per 10,000 births. It accounts for 2% to 3% of CHD in newborns. As with all birth diseases, poor maternal nutrition, smoking, and alcohol use are risk factors.

Diagnosis

HLHS is most often diagnosed prenatally on obstetric screening. Echocardiograms are used to determine blood flow postnatally. Cardiac MRI is used to assess all involved structures before surgery.

Treatment

Surgical repair is the treatment for HLHS. Before surgery, prostaglandins are started immediately to keep the PDA open, and a balloon septostomy may be needed to ensure an open foramen ovale for blood flow across the atrial septum. **Sub-atmospheric oxygen** (17% to 19%) may be given to help balance the systemic and pulmonary circulation. Keeping the SPO_2 in the 70% to 80% range is critical to adequate systemic circulation. Three following separate surgeries are required:

- *Norwood procedure* (during the first 2 weeks of life) to create a "new" aorta that is connected to the right ventricle to allow the right ventricle to pump blood to the lungs and the rest of the body. Skin color will be bluish because of the venous admixture.
- *Bidirectional Glenn shunt procedure* (at 4 to 6 months of age) to create a direct connection between the pulmonary artery and the superior vena cava, decreasing the work of the right ventricle.
- *Fontan procedure* (18 months to 3 years of age) to connect the pulmonary artery and the inferior vena cava. This completely separates the deoxygenated blood from the oxygenated blood and color will improve.

Patients with HLHS typically have lifelong complications and are often candidates for heart transplant (see Newborn and Pediatric Respiratory Therapy Protocols, Chapters 33 and 34).

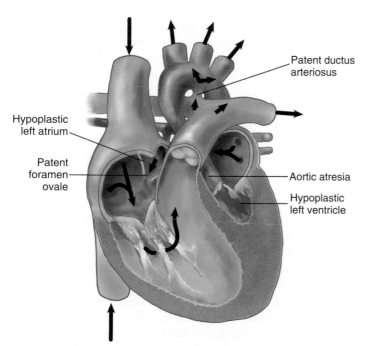

FIGURE 42.9 Hypoplastic left heart syndrome (HLHS). (In Hillegass, E. [2017]. *Essentials of cardiopulmonary physical therapy* [4th ed]. Philadelphia, PA: Elsevier. Redrawn from James, S. R., Nelson, K. W., & Ashwill, J. W. [2007]. *Nursing care of children: Principles and practice* [3rd ed.]. Philadelphia, PA: Saunders.)

Labels in figure: Patent ductus arteriosus; Hypoplastic left atrium; Patent foramen ovale; Aortic atresia; Hypoplastic left ventricle

CASE STUDY Transposition of the Great Arteries

Admitting History and Physical Examination

A 3.41-kg boy was delivered by vaginal delivery at 40 weeks to a 32-year-old mother. Although the mother had no prenatal care; her pregnancy was unremarkable. After being warmed and examined, the infant was taken to the regular nursery.

On arrival in the nursery, vital signs showed heart rate 150 beats/min, respiratory rate 50 breaths/min, blood pressure 70/35 mm Hg (mean arterial pressure [MAP] 52). The baby appeared to be comfortable, mildly tachypneic, and mildly cyanotic. Breath sounds were clear. No heart murmur was heard. A pulse oximeter was placed on the infant's right hand, and the SpO$_2$ was 70%.

The nurse called for the respiratory team leader to assess the infant; blow-by oxygen with a resuscitation bag was started. When the respiratory team leader arrived, he noted that the infant was breathing comfortably; there was no nasal flaring, no grunting, no stridor, and good aeration, with all lung fields clear. He checked the blow-by oxygen set-up to make sure that it was hooked up correctly to oxygen via the flowmeter in the nursery. It was set up correctly. The blow-by oxygen had raised the SpO$_2$ to 73%. The therapist also noted that, while placing his stethoscope on the infant's chest, the patient cried, and his color appeared cyanotic. At this time, the respiratory therapist charted the following SOAP note.

Respiratory Assessment and Plan

S N/A

O Term infant, HR 150, RR 50, BP 70/35, SpO$_2$ 73% and cyanotic on blow-by 100% oxygen. No apparent respiratory distress; no nasal flaring, grunting, or stridor. Mild tachypnea. Clear breath sounds in all fields. No heart murmur heard. Crying appears to make the infant more cyanotic.

A Newborn condition that appears to be refractory to oxygen. Stable at the moment. Good bilateral aeration and tachypnea. Need to rule out cardiac cause.

P The team leader told the infant's nurse that he was going to check the infant's preductal and postductal SpO$_2$. With one probe on the right hand and one on the right foot, both readings showed an SpO$_2$ of less than 75%. The neonatologist was contacted immediately.

The doctor requested a stat cardiology consult, chest radiograph, electrocardiogram, and echocardiogram. Luckily, a cardiologist was available to assess the infant. He ordered prostaglandin infusion until a more definitive diagnosis could be made. While the prostaglandins were being delivered from the pharmacy, the chest radiograph showed an "egg-shaped heart on a string," indicative of transposition of the great vessels. The cardiologist instructed the nursery charge nurse to arrange for transport of the infant to a tertiary pediatric center for cardiovascular surgery evaluation.

Discussion

When a respiratory therapist is faced with a cyanotic infant, he/she should first try to determine if the cause is respiratory, cardiac, or neurologic in origin. If an infant demonstrates respiratory distress with cyanosis, a respiratory cause always should be expected. Oxygen and possibly surfactant therapy with lung inflation/ventilation will be effective in treating this type of hypoxemia. If a cyanotic infant is born to a mother who is addicted to narcotics or overly sedated during delivery, the hypoxemia is likely the result of respiratory depression; the infant may present with apnea or ineffective respiratory effort. Manual ventilation or medications to reverse the narcotic effect can be used to improve oxygenation and ventilation until the infant recovers. The latter, however, may precipitate acute withdrawal symptoms in an infant born to an addicted mother.

An infant with CHD, who is cyanotic beyond the normal postdelivery period, generally presents with unlabored breathing and often tachypnea to compensate for a mild but growing metabolic acidosis. This infant will not respond to oxygen, because the blood is being shunted away from the pulmonary vascular bed. Pulse oximetry (preductal and postductal) demonstrated abnormal results reflective of CHD. Diseases of this magnitude warrant rapid evaluation by echocardiogram, medical treatment with prostaglandins, and possible balloon septostomy to maintain mixing between the arterial and venous circulation.

In the case presented, the infant was cyanotic and failed to respond to supplemental oxygen administration. In the absence of recognized pulmonary problems, these findings were all consistent with the presentation of severe CHD in the newborn. The chest radiograph was suggestive of transposition of the great vessels. The cardiologist initiated a prostaglandin infusion to prevent the ductus arteriosus from closing, which would markedly worsen the infant's oxygenation and metabolic acidosis. Transferring the infant to a center with a pediatric cardiologist will be key to improving outcome.

Today most severe CHD lesions are identified by prenatal ultrasound. Ideally these babies should be delivered at hospitals where pediatric cardiac services are available to diagnose and treat the newborn with CHD. *It is important to remember that the pregnant mother is still the best transport incubator ever devised!*

Note that technical accuracy in the delivery of oxygen is also important when treating infants with oxygen or using oxygen to help diagnose a shunt. This was why it was important for the respiratory team leader to make sure that the delivery gas was actually oxygen. It is possible in a nursery (where medical air is available) for staff to incorrectly connect their oxygen equipment to a medical air flowmeter. A mask attached to medical air would likely not improve the infant's SpO$_2$ and confuse the clinical team.

SELF-ASSESSMENT QUESTIONS

1. A critical congenital heart disease screening would be considered positive if:
   a. Either extremity has an SpO_2 less than 90%
   b. There is consistently a 3% difference between the SpO_2 readings in the two extremities
   c. The SpO_2 levels remain 90% to 94% on either extremity on repeated testing
   d. All of the above

2. In a ventricular septal defect (VSD), all the following are correct *except:*
   a. The defect may be a muscular VSD
   b. A right-to-left shunt develops
   c. The diagnosis is confirmed by echocardiography
   d. The patient with a VSD can present at any age

3. "Hypercyanotic" or "tet spells" are associated with which of the following disorders?
   a. Tetralogy of Fallot
   b. Ventricular septal defect
   c. Transposition of the great arteries
   d. Patent ductus arteriosus

4. During normal fetal development, the cavity of the primitive atrium is subdivided into right and left chambers by a structure called the:
   a. Septum secundum
   b. Ostium primum
   c. Ostium secundum
   d. Septum primum

5. In which of the following congenital disorders is a balloon atrial septostomy sometimes used as a palliative procedure until a corrective surgery can be performed?
   a. Transposition of the great arteries
   b. Ventricular septal defect
   c. Tetralogy of Fallot
   d. Atrial septal defect

Chapter Objectives

After reading this chapter, you will be able to:

- List the anatomic alterations of the lungs associated with inspiratory stridor (croup) syndrome.
- Describe the causes of inspiratory stridor (croup) syndrome.
- List the cardiopulmonary clinical manifestations associated with inspiratory stridor (croup) syndrome.
- Describe the general management of inspiratory stridor (croup) syndrome.
- Describe the clinical strategies and rationales of the SOAPs presented in the case studies.
- Define key terms and complete self-assessment questions at the end of the chapter and on Evolve.

Key Terms

Acute Epiglottitis
Anteroposterior Neck Radiograph
Bacterial Tracheitis
"Barking Seal" or Brassy Sounding Cough
Croup
Haemophilus Influenzae Type B
Heliox Therapy
Inspiratory Stridor
Laryngotracheobronchitis (LTB)
Lateral Neck Radiograph
Parainfluenza Viruses
Racemic Epinephrine
Spasmodic Croup
Steeple Point or Pencil Point (Lateral Neck Radiograph—LTB)
Subglottic Airway Obstruction
Subglottic Croup
Supraglottic Airway Obstruction
Supraglottic Croup
"Thumb Sign" (Lateral Neck Radiograph—Epiglottis)

Chapter Outline

Anatomic Alterations of the Upper Airway
  Laryngotracheobronchitis
  Bacterial Tracheitis
  Acute Epiglottitis
Etiology and Epidemiology
  Laryngotracheobronchitis
  Bacterial Tracheitis
  Acute Epiglottitis
Overview of the Cardiopulmonary Clinical Manifestations Associated With Laryngotracheobronchitis, Bacterial Tracheitis, and Epiglottitis
General Management of Laryngotracheobronchitis, Bacterial Tracheitis, and Epiglottitis
  Supplemental Oxygen
  Racemic Epinephrine
  Corticosteroids
  Antibiotic Therapy
  Heliox Therapy
  Endotracheal Intubation or Tracheostomy
Case Study 1: Laryngotracheobronchitis
Case Study 2: Acute Epiglottitis
Case Study 3: Bacterial Tracheitis
Self-Assessment Questions

The word **croup** is a general term used to describe the inspiratory barking or brassy sound associated with a partial upper airway obstruction. In other words, croup is actually a clinical sign (objective data) or a clinical manifestation—the **"barking seal" or brassy sound** associated with a partial upper airway obstruction. Technically, the inspiratory barking sound heard in a patient with a partial upper airway obstruction is more appropriately called an **inspiratory stridor**.

The anatomic alterations of the upper airway associated with croup—that is, the cause of the inspiratory stridor—can be subdivided into the following three types: laryngotracheobronchitis, bacterial tracheitis, and acute epiglottis. In addition, and as is discussed in further detail later, some sources refer to these three classifications as either **supraglottic croup** or **subglottic croup** based on where the inspiratory stridor sound originates. Laryngotracheobronchitis and bacterial tracheitis cause **subglottic airway obstruction**. Acute epiglottitis is a **supraglottic airway obstruction**.

Anatomic Alterations of the Upper Airway

Laryngotracheobronchitis

Most experts use the term *croup* and **laryngotracheobronchitis (LTB)** interchangeably. Because LTB primarily affects the lower laryngeal area, trachea, and occasionally the bronchi, the term *laryngotracheobronchitis* is used as a synonym for "classic" subglottic obstruction (Fig. 43.1B). Pathologically,

LTB is an inflammatory process that causes edema and swelling of the mucous membranes. Although the laryngeal mucosa and submucosa are vascular, the distribution of the lymphatic capillaries is uneven or absent in this region. Consequently, when edema develops in the upper airway, fluid spreads and accumulates quickly throughout the connective tissues, which in turn causes the mucosa to swell and the airway lumen to narrow. The inflammation also causes the mucous glands to increase their production of mucus and the cilia to lose their effectiveness as a mucociliary transport mechanism.

Because the subglottic area is the narrowest region of the larynx in an infant or small child, even a slight degree of edema can cause a significant reduction in the cross-sectional area of the airway. The edema in this area is further aggravated by the rigid cricoid cartilage, which surrounds the subglottic trachea and prevents external swelling as fluid engorges the laryngeal tissues. The edema and swelling in the subglottic region decrease the ability of the vocal cords to abduct (move apart) during inspiration. This further reduces the cross-sectional area of airway in this region. LTB is the most common cause of croup and croup-like symptoms.

Bacterial Tracheitis

Bacterial tracheitis is a life-threatening upper airway obstruction caused by an invasive bacterial infection of the soft tissues of the trachea. Although bacterial tracheitis is rare, it is more prevalent than acute epiglottitis. Bacterial tracheitis can affect children of any age and almost always in patients with preexisting upper respiratory tract viral infection (i.e., common cold, flu, or LTB). Bacterial tracheitis always should be considered

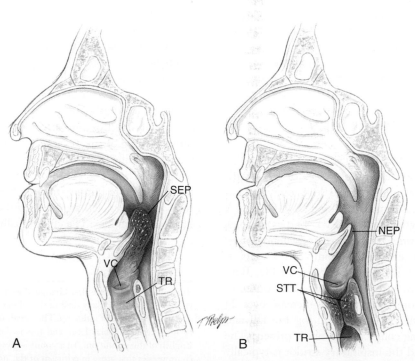

FIGURE 43.1 Laryngotracheobronchitis and acute epiglottitis. (A) Acute epiglottitis. (B) Laryngotracheobronchitis and/or bacterial tracheitis. *NEP,* Normal epiglottis; *SEP,* swollen epiglottis; *STT,* swollen tracheal tissue; *TR,* trachea; *VC,* vocal cords.

in any child with a presumed viral croup and who is not responding to conventional therapy.

The major site of bacterial tracheitis is at the subglottic level. It is characterized by inflammation and rapid edema with mucopurulent exudate and sloughing of the mucosa that adhere and obstruct the subglottic space. In some cases, there is involvement of the subglottic laryngeal structures—that is, extension into the upper bronchial tree or associated pneumonia. Other terms that have been used to describe bacterial tracheitis include *bacterial croup*, *membranous croup*, *pseudomembranous croup*, *acute laryngotracheobronchitis*, and *membranous laryngotracheobronchitis*.

Acute Epiglottitis

Acute epiglottitis is a life-threatening emergency. In contrast to LTB and bacterial tracheitis, epiglottitis is an inflammation of the supraglottic region, which includes the epiglottis, aryepiglottic folds, and false vocal cords (see Fig. 43.1A). Epiglottitis does not involve the pharynx, trachea, or other subglottic structures. As the edema in the epiglottis increases, the lateral borders curl and the tip of the epiglottis protrudes posteriorly and inferiorly. During inspiration, the swollen epiglottis is pulled (or sucked) over the laryngeal inlet. In severe cases, this may completely block the laryngeal opening. Clinically, the classic finding is a swollen, cherry-red epiglottis, severe respiratory distress, and drooling. Unlike LTB and bacterial tracheitis, which typically generate a loud and high-pitched brassy inspiratory stridor, acute epiglottitis commonly produces a lower pitch or a muffled or even absent sound.

To summarize, the major pathologic or structural changes associated with inspiratory stridor are as follows:

- *Laryngotracheobronchitis:* Airway obstruction caused by tissue swelling just *below* the vocal cords (subglottic)
- *Bacterial tracheitis:* Airway and obstruction caused by tissue swelling and mucopurulent membranous secretions below the vocal cords (subglottic)
- *Epiglottitis:* Airway obstruction caused by tissue swelling just *above* the vocal cords (supraglottic).

Etiology and Epidemiology

Laryngotracheobronchitis

The **parainfluenza viruses** cause most cases of LTB, with type 1 being the most common, type 3 less common, and type 2 infrequent. LTB also may be caused by influenza A and B, respiratory syncytial virus (RSV), herpes simplex virus, *Mycoplasma pneumoniae*, rhinovirus, and adenoviruses. LTB is primarily seen in children 6 months to 5 years of age, with peak prevalence in the second year of life. Boys are affected slightly more often than girls. The onset of LTB is slow (i.e., symptoms progressively increase over 24 to 48 hours), and it is most common during the fall and winter. A brassy or barking cough is commonly present. The child's voice is hoarse, and the inspiratory stridor is typically loud and high in pitch. The patient usually does not have a fever, drooling, swallowing difficulties, or a toxic appearance.

Although the diagnosis of LTB usually can be made on the basis of the patient's clinical history, a radiologic examination is helpful.

Bacterial Tracheitis

Bacterial tracheitis is most commonly caused by *Staphylococcus aureus* and frequently follows a recent viral upper respiratory tract infection such as a common cold, flu, or LTB. Other bacteria associated with bacterial tracheitis include *Haemophilus influenzae*, Beta-hemolytic *Streptococcus*, and *Streptoccus pyogenes*. *Moraxella catarrhalis* has been implicated with increased frequency and is associated with severe bacterial tracheitis. Although rare, some gram-negative organisms linked to bacterial tracheitis include the *Pseudomonas* and *Klebsiella* spp. High fever, toxic appearance, and elevated white blood cell count will indicate the presence of bacterial infection. Because of the link of bacterial tracheitis with viral epidemics, it is more commonly seen during the winter months. Males are more commonly affected. The **lateral neck radiograph** will rule out epiglottitis, showing only subglottic narrowing with an irregular mucosal surface. Direct visualization via laryngobronchoscopy of the airway is the most definitive method to diagnosis bacterial tracheitis.

Acute Epiglottitis[1]

Acute epiglottitis is a bacterial infection that historically was almost always caused by ***Haemophilus influenzae* type B**. It is transmitted via aerosol droplets. Since 1985, when vaccinations with *H. influenzae* type B vaccine became widespread, the number of reported cases of epiglottitis has decreased by more than 95%. *H. influenzae* type B, however, is still responsible for about 25% of the epiglottitis cases. Other bacteria now associated with epiglottitis include *H. parainfluenzae*, *Streptococcus pneumoniae*, and group A *S. pyogenes*. *Candida* and *Aspergillus* have been associated with epiglottitis in immunocompromised patients. Noninfectious causes of epiglottitis include aspiration of hot liquids and trauma from repeated intubation attempts.

Epiglottitis has no clear-cut geographic or seasonal incidence. Although acute epiglottitis may develop in all age groups (neonatal to adulthood), it most often occurs in children 2 to 6 years of age. Boys are affected more often than girls. The onset of epiglottitis is usually abrupt. Although the initial clinical manifestations are usually mild, they progress rapidly over 2 to 4 hours. A common scenario includes a sore throat or mild upper respiratory tract problems that quickly progresse to a high fever, lethargy, and difficulty in swallowing and handling secretions. The child usually appears frightened, pale,

---

[1]It is of interest to note that George Washington, the first president of the United States, most likely died in the winter of 1799 from acute epiglottitis during an epidemic of influenza. The details of the illness were fully recorded by his secretary, Tobias Lear, and this is the first published description in English of this condition. An account is given of the medical treatment and controversies that arose in criticism of the attendant doctors. (From Cohen, B. [2005]. The death of George Washington 1732–99: The history of cynanche. *Journal of Medical Biography, 13,* 225-231.)

TABLE 43.1 General History and Physical Findings of Laryngotracheobronchitis, Bacterial Tracheitis, and Acute Epiglottitis

	LTB	Bacterial Tracheitis	Epiglottitis
Age	6 mo–5 yrs (with the peak prevalence in the second year)	3 mo–13 yrs; more common 3–5 years	2–6 yrs
Incidence	Common	Rare	Very rare
Etiology	Parainfluenza type I	*Haemophilus influenzae* type B	*Staphylococcus aureus*
Onset	Usually slow or gradual (24–48 h)	Rapid	Abrupt (2–4 h)
Respiratory distress	Common	Common	Common
Fever	Absent	Common	Common
Voice	Hoarse	Very hoarse	Muffled
Drooling	Absent	Absent	Present
Preferred position	Supine	Supine	Tripod
Radiograph findings	Haziness in subglottic area, "pencil point" or "steeple point"	Irregular tracheal margins	Haziness in supraglottic area, "thumb sign"
Inspiratory stridor	High-pitched, brassy, loud sound	Present	Low-pitched and muffled, or absent
Cough	Present (barking or brassy cough)	Frequent	Absent
Swallowing difficulty	Absent	Absent	Present
White blood count	Normal (viral—parainfluenza viruses 1, 2, and 3; influenza A and B; respiratory syncytial virus)	Elevated; bandemia (immature white blood cells)	Elevated (bacterial—*Haemophilus influenzae* type B)
Endoscopic findings	Normal supraglottic area; edema of subglottic area	Erythema and edema supraglottic area (includes the epiglottis)	Normal supraglottic area; mucopurulent secretions, erythema of subglottic area

and septic. As the supraglottic area becomes swollen, breathing becomes noisy, the child will sit forward in a tripod position, the tongue is often thrust forward during inspiration, and the child may drool. Compared with LTB, the inspiratory stridor is usually softer and lower in pitch. A cough is usually absent with acute epiglottitis. The voice and cry are usually muffled rather than hoarse. Older children commonly complain of a sore throat during swallowing. Acute epiglottitis in adults is typically seen in patients with neck trauma (e.g., blunt force neck injury or aspiration of hot liquids), in those who have been intubated repeatedly, and in drug abuse (crack cocaine) cases.

The general history and physical findings of LTB, bacterial tracheitis, and epiglottitis are compared and contrasted in Table 43.1.[2]

[2]**Spasmodic coup:** For a complete discussion of croup-like syndromes, spasmodic croup must be included. Although it can be triggered by infection, it is thought to be an allergic form of croup that occurs in the absence of a viral illness. Spasmodic croup tends to come on suddenly and without fever, runny nose, or other evidence of cold-like symptoms. It usually affects children between 3 months and 3 years of age. It can be difficult to differentiate spasmodic croup from laryngotracheobronchitis. The characteristic seal-like barking cough is present and commonly occurs in the middle of the night and resolves by morning.

The following clinical manifestations result from the pathologic mechanisms caused (or activated) by an upper airway obstruction—the major anatomic alteration of the lungs associated with laryngotracheobronchitis (LTB), bacterial tracheitis, and epiglottitis (see Fig. 43.1).

CLINICAL DATA OBTAINED AT THE PATIENT'S BEDSIDE

The Physical Examination

Vital Signs

Increased Respiratory Rate (Tachypnea)

Several pathophysiologic mechanisms operating simultaneously may lead to an increased ventilatory rate:

- Increased stimulation of peripheral chemoreceptors
- Anxiety
- Increased temperature (secondary to infection)

Increased Heart Rate (Pulse) and Blood Pressure

Chest Assessment Findings

- Prolonged inspiratory phase
- Diminished breath sounds

Inspiratory Stridor

Under normal circumstances the slight narrowing of the upper (extrathoracic) airway that naturally occurs during inspiration is insignificant. Because the upper airway is relatively small in infants and children, however, even a slight degree of edema may become significant, particularly at the level of the cricoid cartilage. Thus when the cross section of the upper airway is reduced because of the edema, the child will generate stridor during inspiration, when the upper airway naturally becomes smaller. It also should be noted that if the edema becomes severe, the patient may generate both inspiratory and expiratory stridor.

Cyanosis

Intermittent coughing spells may produce intermittent cyanosis as secretions obstruct an already limited airway.

Use of Accessory Muscles During Inspiration

Substernal and Intercostal Retractions

CLINICAL DATA OBTAINED FROM LABORATORY TESTS AND SPECIAL PROCEDURES

Arterial Blood Gases[1]

Mild to Moderate Laryngotracheobronchitis, Bacterial Tracheitis or Epiglottitis

Acute Alveolar Hyperventilation With Hypoxemia[2]
(Acute Respiratory Alkalosis)

pH	$PaCO_2$	HCO_3^-	PaO_2	SaO_2 or SpO_2
↑	↓	↓	↓	↓
		(but normal)		

SEVERE LARYNGOTRACHEOBRONCHITIS, BACTERIAL TRACHEITIS, OR EPIGLOTTITIS

Acute Ventilatory Failure With Hypoxemia[3]
(Occurs in LTB with fatigue and epiglottitis with obstruction)
(Acute Respiratory Acidosis)

pH[4]	$PaCO_2$	HCO_3^-[4]	PaO_2	SaO_2 or SpO_2
↓	↑	↑	↓	↓
		(but normal)		

Oxygenation Indices[5]

$\dot{Q}_S/\dot{Q}_T$	DO_2[6]	$\dot{V}O_2$	$C(a-\bar{v})O_2$	O_2ER	$S\bar{v}O_2$
↑	↓	N	N	↑	↓

[1]*NOTE:* Because of the difficulty of obtaining arterial blood gas (ABG) samples from newborn and pediatric patients, capillary blood gas (CBG) samples are usually used to determine the pH, $PaCO_2$, and HCO_3^- (i.e., the acid-base and ventilation status only). Capillary PO_2 values are unreliable and should not be used for clinical analysis. The standard way to evaluate the oxygenation status in these young patients is pulse oximetry ($SpCO_2$) (see Chapter 33, Newborn Assessment and Management).

[2]See Fig. 5.2 and Table 5.4 and related discussion for the acute pH, $PaCO_2$, and HCO_3^- changes associated with acute alveolar hyperventilation.

[3]See Fig. 5.3 and related discussion for the acute pH, $PaCO_2$, and HCO_3^- changes associated with acute ventilatory failure.

[4]When tissue hypoxia is severe enough to produce lactic acid, the pH and HCO_3^- values will be lower than expected for a particular $PaCO_2$ level.

[5]$C(a-\bar{v})O_2$, Arterial-venous oxygen difference; DO_2, total oxygen delivery; O_2ER, oxygen extraction ratio; $\dot{Q}_S/\dot{Q}_T$, pulmonary shunt fraction; $S\bar{v}O_2$, mixed venous oxygen saturation; $\dot{V}O_2$, oxygen consumption.

[6]It should be noted that because the newborn normally has a higher hemoglobin (Hb) level at birth (16.8 to 18.9 g/dL), the DO_2 may actually be better than the PaO_2 or SpO_2 indicates (see Chapter 6, Assessment of Oxygenation).

LATERAL NECK RADIOGRAPH

- Haziness in the subglottic area (LTB and bacterial tracheitis)
- Haziness in the supraglottic area (epiglottitis)
- Classic "**thumb sign**" (epiglottitis)

ANTEROPOSTERIOR NECK RADIOGRAPH

- **Steeple point** or **pencil point** narrowing of the upper airway (LTB)

Although the diagnosis of epiglottitis or LTB generally can be made on the basis of the patient's clinical history, radiologic examinations are helpful, particularly with bacterial tracheitis. A **lateral neck radiograph** is usually done first to rule out the diagnosis of epiglottitis. Once this film is read as negative, an **Anteroposterior Neck Radiograph** is ordered to define the degree of subglottic edema. When the patient has acute epiglottitis, a white haziness is evident in the supraglottic area. In addition,

the epiglottitis often appears on a lateral neck radiograph as the classic **thumb sign**. The epiglottis is swollen and rounded, giving it an appearance of the distal portion of a thumb (Fig. 43.2). Fig. 43.3 shows an infant with new-onset leukemia and epiglottitis.

When the patient has LTB or bacterial tracheitis, a white haziness is demonstrated in the subglottic area; the AP neck will show the classic pencil point or steeple point narrowing at the level of the cricoid cartilage (Fig. 43.4). Bacterial tracheitis also may show irregularity in the tracheal margins. Fig. 43.5 shows subglottic narrowing in a child diagnosed with bacterial tracheitis. Also of importance is that a barky cough associated with partial airway obstruction can be caused by a foreign object in the airway, a not-so-infrequent cause in toddlers. Generally, the lateral and AP neck are helpful screens to suggest laryngoscopy in these cases.

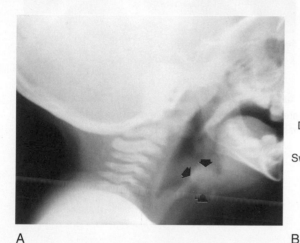

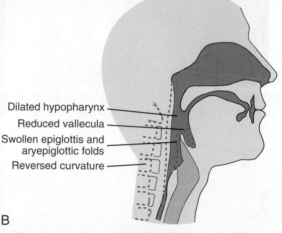

A   B

Dilated hypopharynx
Reduced vallecula
Swollen epiglottis and aryepiglottic folds
Reversed curvature

FIGURE 43.2 The classic "thumb sign" of an edematous epiglottis is evident in this lateral neck radiograph (see red arrows in [A]). The schematic illustrates the findings to look for in a lateral radiograph of a patient with suspected epiglottitis (B). Such radiographs are unnecessary in a child with the classic history, signs, and symptoms of epiglottitis; they can be of tremendous help, however, in diagnosing mild or questionable cases and explaining to parents the need for aggressive treatment. (From Ashcraft, C. K., & Steele, R. W. [1988]. Epiglottitis: A pediatric emergency. *Journal of Respiratory Disease, 9,* 48.)

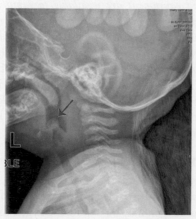

FIGURE 43.3 Young child with new-onset leukemia and epiglottitis (see red arrow). (Courtesy Dayton Children's Hospital, Dayton, Ohio.)

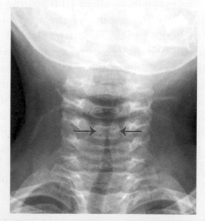

FIGURE 43.4 Classic "pencil point" or "steeple point" narrowing at the level of the cricoid cartilage (see red arrows). (Courtesy Dayton Children's Hospital, Dayton, Ohio.)

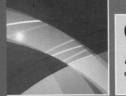

OVERVIEW of the Cardiopulmonary Clinical Manifestations Associated With **Laryngotracheobronchitis, Bacterial Tracheitis, and Epiglottitis—cont'd**

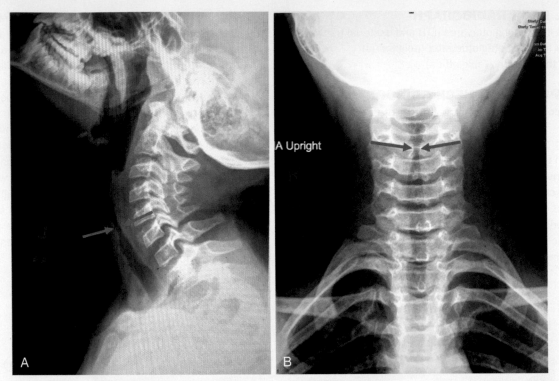

FIGURE 43.5 A. Lateral Neck Radiograph. B. Anterior-Posterial Radiograph. Red arrows shows sub-glottic narrowing. Young child diagnosed with bacterial tracheitis. (Courtesy Dayton Children's Hospital, Dayton, Ohio.)

General Management of Laryngotracheobronchitis, Bacterial Tracheitis, and Epiglottitis[3]

Treatment is based on the cause of the croup and croup-like syndromes. For example, excellent LTB scoring systems are available that allow the respiratory therapist to objectively assess and treat the patient. The typical LTB score table measures the patient's stridor, retractions, air movement, color, and level of consciousness (Table 43.2). In severe cases of bacterial tracheitis, the administration of intravenous antibiotics, the admission to the intensive care unit for intubation, and supportive ventilatory care are often required. The management of epiglottitis is very specific. Early recognition of epiglottitis may save a patient's life; it is a true airway emergency. Once the diagnosis is suspected or confirmed by the lateral neck radiograph, examination or inspection of the pharynx and larynx is to be done *only* in the operating room under general anesthesia with a fully trained team.

Under no circumstances should the mouth or throat be examined outside the operating room (even though depression of the tongue may reveal a bright red epiglottis and confirm the diagnosis) unless personnel and equipment are available to rapidly intubate or tracheostomize the patient. The patient usually maintains limited airway by sitting up and leaning forward with the chin protruding; having the patient lie down for examination will cause complete airway obstruction within minutes. The patient with a confirmed diagnosis of acute epiglottitis should be intubated immediately!

After the diagnosis of the croup and croup-like syndromes is established, the general management of LTB, bacterial tracheitis, and acute epiglottitis is as follows.

Supplemental Oxygen

Because hypoxemia and significant work of breathing is associated with LTB, bacterial tracheitis, and epiglottitis, supplemental oxygen may be required. Oxygen therapy should be started when the patient's SpO_2 is under 92% (see Pediatric Oxygen Therapy Protocol, Protocol 34.1).

---

[3]Although **cool aerosol mist** therapy was commonly used to treat patients with laryngotracheobronchitis in the past, it is rarely recommended today.

TABLE 43.2 Laryngotracheobronchitis Scoring System

Score	0	1	2	3
Stridor	None	Mild	Moderate at rest	Severe with insp/exp or none with markedly decreased air entry
Retractions	None	Mild	Moderate	Severe marked use of accessory muscles
Air entry	Normal	Mild decrease	Moderate decrease	Marked decrease
Color	Normal	Normal (0–score)	Normal (0–score)	Dusky or cyanotic
Level of consciousness	Normal	Restless when disturbed	Anxious, agitated, restless when undisturbed	Lethargic, depressed

Scoring Guidelines

Mild	0–2	See discussion under Racemic Epinephrine below.
Moderate	3–5	
Severe	6–11	
Impending ventilatory failure	>12	

Racemic Epinephrine

Aerosolized **racemic epinephrine** is administered to children with LTB based on the LTB Scoring System (see Table 43.2). Using the patient's LTB score, the administration of racemic epinephrine protocol is as follows:

- At ages 3 to 5: Consider racemic epinephrine
- At ages greater than 6: Administer racemic epinephrine 0.5 mL in 3 mL normal saline

This adrenergic agent is used for its vasoconstrictive effect on mucosal edema and is recognized as an effective and safe aerosol decongestant for in-hospital use.

Patients who present with LTB symptoms, but who have bacterial tracheitis, do not generally improve with racemic epinephrine. This is because their airway obstruction is complicated by purulent secretions. Poor response to racemic epinephrine should be immediately communicated to the medical team.

Corticosteroids

Corticosteroids, such as dexamethasone, have been shown to reduce the severity and duration of LTB and are generally given when the patient presents with moderate to severe symptoms (see Appendix V on the Evolve site).

Antibiotic Therapy

When bacterial tracheitis is suspected (or confirmed) a third-generation cephalosporin combined with a beta-lactamase–resistant penicillin (e.g., cloxacillin) is an appropriate first-line therapy.

If methicillin-resistant *S. aureus* is a concern, treatment should be extended to cover this organism (e.g., vancomycin). Because acute epiglottitis is usually caused by bacteria such as *H. influenzae* type B, appropriate antibiotic therapy is part of the treatment plan. Ceftriaxone (Rocephin) and ampicillin/sulbactam (Unasyn) are commonly prescribed to cover the most common organisms that cause acute epiglottitis.

Heliox Therapy

In severe cases of LBT, **heliox therapy** may be helpful. Heliox is a combination of helium and oxygen, generally 80% helium to 20% oxygen, which has a lower density than the density of room air. Breathing heliox lowers the airway resistance throughout the breathing cycle, reducing the child's work of breathing with airway obstruction and preventing fatigue. It must be delivered in a high-flow system, which provides all of the patient's inspiratory flow to be effective. Heliox via a high-flow nasal cannula is the best tolerated application in infants and small children. Heliox therapy can be used as a bridge therapy in patients with severe upper airway obstruction while awaiting the effects of corticosteroids. Because of the expense of Heliox, it is not typically first-line therapy in LTB management. It is reserved for those with higher croup scores.

Endotracheal Intubation or Tracheostomy

In the patient with suspected acute epiglottitis, **the examination or inspection of the pharyngeal and laryngeal areas is to be performed only in the operating room with a trained surgical team in attendance. This is because the epiglottis may obstruct completely in response to even the slightest touch or supine positioning during inspection**.

In the patient with suspected bacterial tracheitis, endotracheal intubation is also frequently required to stabilize the airway, especially in small children. Ideally, an anesthesiologist should be present. The endotracheal tube allows for direct suctioning of the purulent secretions that can continue to obstruct the airway. Management of endotracheal tubes placed in patients with airway obstruction requires extreme care to ensure that these "lifelines" do not become dislodged. The physician, nurse, and respiratory therapist should not leave the patient's intensive care unit bedside until the endotracheal tube is tightly secured at the proper depth of insertion. If the patient is anxious, restless, or uncooperative, proper restraints, sedation, and sometimes paralysis will be needed to prevent accidental extubation.

After intubation, the patient should be placed on continuous positive airway pressure (CPAP) or pressure support ventilation. Mechanical ventilation must be provided if paralysis is used to protect the airway in an uncooperative patient (see Mechanical Ventilation and Ventilator Weaning, Protocol 34.5).

CASE STUDY 1 Laryngotracheobronchitis

Admitting History and Physical Examination

An 18-month-old boy had a mild viral upper respiratory tract infection and some hoarseness. At 10 p.m. on the third day of his illness, he rapidly developed a brassy cough and high-pitched inspiratory stridor. He became moderately dyspneic. The child was restless and appeared frightened. The axillary temperature was 37°C. The mother claimed that the child was "blue" on two occasions during a coughing episode. She was going to take the child to the emergency department (ED), but the grandmother suggested that she try steam inhalation first. Accordingly, the child was taken to the bathroom, where the hot shower was turned on full force. The child was comforted by the grandmother and urged to breathe slowly and deeply. As the bathroom became filled with steam, the respiratory distress abated and within a few minutes the child was free of stridor, breathing essentially normally. The next day the same symptoms recurred, and the patient was taken to the ED.

Cough and inspiratory stridor were noted. Vital signs were blood pressure 90/60 mm Hg, pulse 160 beats/min, respiratory rate 32 breaths/min. The room air SpO_2 was 94%. The patient's inspiratory stridor (croup) score was 7. The anteroposterior neck radiograph showed narrowing of the subglottic airway. The respiratory therapist documented the following assessment and plan.

Respiratory Assessment and Plan

S Mother reports patient had cough and inspiratory stridor.
O Confirms above. Lungs clear except for stridor and tracheal breath sounds throughout. Vital signs BP 90/60, P 160/min, RR 32/min, T 37°C. Pallor noted. SpO_2 94% on room air. Inspiratory stridor (croup) score of 7. Soft tissue radiograph of neck suggests laryngotracheobronchitis.
A LTB, Lungs clear except for stridor and upper airway sounds throughout (history and inspiratory stridor).
P Notify the physician. Start Aerosolized Medication Protocol (med. neb. treatment with racemic epinephrine per protocol).

Discussion

Home remedies sometimes do work. Any parent who has had a child with LTB will find this scenario familiar. What may not be as widely recognized is that sometimes inhalation of warm or cool mist may improve this syndrome. When this approach failed, the parents were wise to bring their son to the ED for prompt vasoconstrictive therapy and oral steroids. This resulted in prompt improvement.

CASE STUDY 2 Acute Epiglottitis

Admitting History and Physical Examination

A 2-year-old girl whose parents had an objection to routine infant and childhood immunizations appeared quite well in the evening and was put to bed at the usual time. She woke up 2 hours later, and her parents were immediately aware that she was in serious respiratory distress. She was feverish, sitting up in bed, drooling, unable to speak or cry, and breathing noisily. The parents wrapped the child in warm blankets and drove her to the emergency department (ED) of the nearest hospital.

On inspection, the child demonstrated a puffy face, drooling, inspiratory stridor, and cyanotic nail beds. At this time, she was placed on a 4 L/min nasal cannula. The emergency physician looked at the girl and listened to her chest but did not examine her mouth. Respiratory rate was 36 breaths/min, blood pressure was 80/50 mm Hg, and pulse was 140 beats/min. The axillary temperature was 103.6°F (39.8°C). The physician ordered a lateral soft tissue radiograph of the neck, but while waiting for the radiograph, the child became increasingly dyspneic and more cyanotic. Her SpO_2 on 4 L/min nasal cannula was 88%. At this time, the following respiratory SOAP note was charted.

Respiratory Assessment and Plan

S Mother states that patient is in severe respiratory distress.

O RR 36/min, BP 80/50, P 140 regular. T 103.6°F (39.8°C). Child's face puffy, drooling. Inspiratory stridor (worsening). Nail beds cyanotic. On a 4 L/min nasal cannula: SpO$_2$ 88%. Soft tissue x-ray examination of neck pending.

A • Probable acute epiglottitis; no history of foreign body aspiration (general history)
   • Impending acute ventilatory failure (SpO$_2$ history, drooling, inspiratory stridor, and cyanosis)

P Stat page for anesthesiologist and ENT surgeon. Up-regulate the Oxygen Therapy Protocol (a nonrebreather with 100% oxygen [FIO$_2$ 1.0] if tolerated).

While the emergency page for the anesthesiologist and the ear, nose, and throat (ENT) surgeon went out, a nonrebreathing oxygen mask was immediately "lightly" held to the child's face by the respiratory therapist. As soon as the physicians arrived (after about 10 minutes), the child was taken to the operating room. The surgeon stood by to perform an emergency tracheostomy while the anesthesiologist attempted to intubate the child.

Fortunately, the anesthesiologist was successful in spite of an enlarged, cherry-red epiglottis partially obstructing the larynx. As soon as the endotracheal tube was in place, the child relaxed and soon went to sleep. She was admitted to the intensive care unit (ICU), sedated, and placed on +5 cm H$_2$O continuous positive airway pressure (CPAP). Intravenous ceftriaxone was administered. She was extubated the next day when she demonstrated a leak around her ET tube. She was discharged on the third hospital day. Blood cultures and a throat culture in the operating room were positive for *H. influenzae* (type B). She was discharged on a 7-day course of oral cefdinir (Omnicef).

Discussion

Acute epiglottitis is a life-threatening condition. The key point to remember is to refrain from examining the throat until a staff member qualified in pediatric intubation is nearby. Such manipulation is often unsuccessful, and unless qualified assistance is at hand, the child may asphyxiate. The treatment suitably selected here was placement of a nonrebreathing oxygen mask while the appropriate team was assembled. Typical of this disease is its abrupt onset, and once the airway is secured and antibiotics given, the symptoms and danger subside. Maintaining the intubated airway until a leak is heard is key to survival. In cases of acute epiglottitis, *H. influenzae* type B will grow from blood cultures, whereas airway or respiratory tract cultures will grow nontypeable *H. influenza*.

CASE STUDY 3 Bacterial Tracheitis

Admitting History and Physical Examination

A 7-month-old previously healthy white male presents to the emergency department (ED) in acute respiratory distress and inspiratory stridor. He was diagnosed with a common cold and flu 3 days previously by his primary care physician. There was no drooling. He had a 10-hour history of fever. Immunization were up to date. In the ED, he appeared pale and cyanotic and was febrile (39°C) and tachycardic (180 beats/min) and had a respiratory rate of 40 breaths/min. His blood pressure was 83/40 mm Hg. Oxygen saturation on room air was 88%. He was given racemic epinephrine and intramuscular dexamethasone before hospital admission.

Over the next 20 minutes, there was increased progression of stridor and his oxygen saturation dropped to 85%. The baby was placed on a 1 L/min of nasal cannula oxygen. A capillary blood gas pH was 7.35, PaCO$_2$ 42 mm Hg, and HCO$_3^-$ 24 mEq/L, and SpO$_2$ 90%. Complete blood count was remarkable for leukocytosis with significant bacteria. A lateral neck x-ray film showed an irregular subglottic trachea margin and narrowing. The attending physician documented the following in the baby's chart: Bacterial tracheitis is the likely cause of the croup-like symptoms.

The baby was then transferred to the pediatric intensive care unit (ICU) and placed on CPAP of +5 cm H$_2$0 and pressure support, and an FIO$_2$ 0.30 to maintain the baby's SaO$_2$ at 90%. Intravenous antibiotics were started and the baby was sedated to avoid accidental extubation. Purulent secretions were noted during tracheal suctioning. Frequent suctioning was required to maintain airway patency. The respiratory therapist recorded the following in the baby's chart.

Respiratory Assessment and Plan

S N/A (patient intubated)

O Inspiratory stridor. Appears cyanotic. Purulent secretions. HR 180 bpm, BP 83/40, RR 40. CBG on 1 L/min nasal cannula: pH 7.35, PaCO$_2$ 42, HCO$_3^-$ 24. SpO$_2$ 90%. Fever 39°C. Blood count: Leukocytosis with significant bacteria. Lateral neck x-ray: Irregular subglottic trachea margin and narrowing.

A
- Bacterial tracheitis (history, leukocytosis and bacteria findings, croup-like symptoms, lateral neck x-ray)
- Excessive airway secretions (purulent secretions observed)
- Good acid-base and oxygenation status (CBG on an FIO$_2$ 0.30)

P Lung Expansion Therapy Protocol: CPAP at 5 cm H$_2$0. Oxygen Therapy Protocol: FIO$_2$: 0.30. Airway Clearance Therapy Protocol: Suction PRN. Continue to monitor closely.

Over the next 28 hours the baby's condition improved. Secretions thinned and less suctioning was required. The FIO$_2$ was reduced to room air—with a room air SpO$_2$ of 94%. An air leak was detected with 20 cm H$_2$0 pressure by manual ventilation. At this time, the infant was extubated. He was observed for one more day before discharge.

Discussion

This case nicely illustrates several of the hallmark features of bacterial tracheitis. The baby's croup-like symptoms followed a common cold and flu. He had a fever, an elevated white blood count, and a bacterial infection. During intubation, purulent secretions were immediately observed during suctioning. The lateral neck x-ray film showed an irregular subglottic trachea margin and narrowing, which is a classic sign of bacterial tracheitis. The quick response to have the baby transferred to the pediatric ICU for elective intubation, routine airway maintenance, oxygen therapy, and intravenous antibiotics was very appropriate.

SELF-ASSESSMENT QUESTIONS

1. **The onset of LTB is usually:**
   a. 2 to 4 hours
   b. 5 to 10 hours
   c. 12 to 24 hours
   d. 24 to 48 hours

2. **Which of the following is(are) associated with epiglottitis?**
   1. Parainfluenza viruses
   2. *Haemophilus influenzae* type B
   3. RSV
   4. Influenza A and B
      a. 1 only
      b. 2 only
      c. 3 and 4 only
      d. 1, 3, and 4 only

3. **Which of the following is(are) a clinical manifestation(s) associated with LTB?**
   1. Haziness in supraglottic area on x-ray film
   2. High-pitched and loud inspiratory stridor
   3. Swallowing difficulty
   4. Drooling
      a. 2 only
      b. 3 only
      c. 1 and 3 only
      d. 1, 3, and 4 only

4. **The signs and symptoms associated with acute epiglottitis usually develop within:**
   a. 1 to 2 hours
   b. 2 to 4 hours
   c. 8 to 10 hours
   d. 12 to 24 hours

5. **Which of the following arterial blood gas values is(are) associated with mild to moderate LTB or epiglottitis?**
   1. Decreased pH
   2. Decreased PaCO$_2$
   3. Increased HCO$_3^-$
   4. Increased pH
      a. 1 only
      b. 4 only
      c. 2 and 4 only
      d. 1 and 3 only

6. **Bacterial tracheitis is most commonly caused by:**
   a. *Staphylococcus aureus*
   b. Parainfluenza type 1
   c. *Haemophilus influenzae* type b
   d. Influenza A

Chapter Objectives

After reading this chapter, you will be able to:
- List the anatomic alterations of the lungs associated with near drowning.
- Describe the causes of near drowning.
- List the cardiopulmonary clinical manifestations associated with near drowning.
- Describe the general management of near drowning.
- Describe the clinical strategies and rationales of the SOAPs presented in the case study.
- Define key terms and complete self-assessment questions at end of chapter and Evolve.

Key Terms

Dry Drowning
First Responder
Hypothermia
Laryngospasm
Near Drowning
Noncardiogenic Pulmonary Edema
Permissive Hypercapnia
Pulmonary Barotrauma
Pulmonary Volutrauma
Ventilator-Induced Lung Injury (VILI)
Warming Techniques
Wet Drowning

Chapter Outline

Anatomic Alterations of the Lungs
Etiology and Epidemiology
Overview of the Cardiopulmonary Clinical Manifestations
  Associated With Near Wet Drowning
General Management of Near Drowning/Wet Drowning
  The First Responder
  Management at the Hospital
Case Study: Near Wet Drowning
Self-Assessment Questions

Anatomic Alterations of the Lungs

Drowning is defined as suffocation and death as a result of submersion in liquid. Drowning may be classified further as **near drowning**, **dry drowning**, and **wet drowning**. *Near drowning* refers to the situation in which a victim survives a liquid submersion, at least temporarily. In *dry drowning* the glottis spasms and prevents water from passing into the lungs. The lungs of dry drowning victims are usually normal.

In *wet drowning* the glottis relaxes and allows water to flood the tracheobronchial tree and alveoli. When fluid initially is inhaled, the bronchi constrict in response to a parasympathetic-mediated reflex. As fluid enters the alveoli, the pathophysiologic processes responsible for **noncardiogenic pulmonary edema** begin—that is, fluid from the pulmonary capillaries moves into the perivascular spaces, peribronchial spaces, alveoli, bronchioles, and bronchi. As a consequence of this fluid movement, the alveolar walls and interstitial spaces swell, pulmonary surfactant concentration decreases, and the alveolar surface tension increases.

As this condition intensifies, the alveoli shrink and atelectasis develops. Excess fluid in the interstitial spaces causes the lymphatic vessels to dilate and the lymph flow to increase. In severe cases the fluid that accumulates in the tracheobronchial tree is churned into a frothy, white (sometimes blood-tinged) sputum as a result of air moving into and out of the lungs (generally by means of mechanical ventilation).

Finally, if the victim was submerged in unclean water (e.g., swamp, pond, sewage, or mud), a number of pathogens (e.g., *Pseudomonas*) and solid material may be aspirated. When this happens, pneumonia may occur, and in severe cases acute respiratory distress syndrome (ARDS) may develop. Although the theory has been controversial in the past, it is now believed that the major pathologic changes of the lungs are essentially the same in freshwater and seawater wet drownings; both result in a reduction in pulmonary surfactant, alveolar injury, atelectasis, and pulmonary edema (Fig. 44.1).

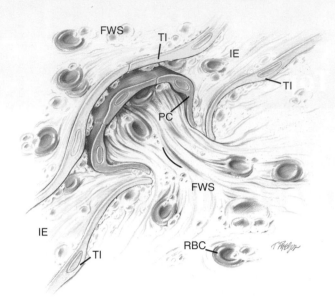

FIGURE 44.1 Near wet drowning. Cross-sectional, microscopic view of the alveolar-capillary unit. Illustration shows fluid moving from a pulmonary capillary to an alveolus. *FWS,* Frothy white secretions; *IE,* interstitial edema; *PC,* pulmonary capillary; *RBC,* red blood cell; *TI,* type I alveolar cell.

The major pulmonary pathologic and structural changes associated with wet drowning are as follows:

- **Laryngospasm**
- Interstitial edema, including engorgement of the perivascular and peribronchial spaces, alveolar walls, and interstitial spaces
- Decreased pulmonary surfactant with increased surface tension of alveolar fluid
- Frothy, white and pink secretions with stable bubbles throughout the tracheobronchial tree
- Alveolar shrinkage and atelectasis
- Alveolar consolidation
- Bronchospasm

Etiology and Epidemiology

According to the Centers for Disease Control and Prevention's most recent data, an average of 3536 fatal unintentional drownings (non–boating related) occur annually in the United States—about 10 deaths per day. About one in five people who die from drowning are children 14 and younger. For every child who dies from drowning, another five receive emergency department (ED) care for nonfatal submersion injuries. More than 50% of drowning victims treated in EDs

require hospitalization or transfer for further care (compared with a hospitalization rate of about 6% for all unintentional injuries). These nonfatal drowning injuries can cause severe brain damage that may result in long-term disabilities such as memory problems, learning disabilities, and permanent loss of basic functioning (e.g., permanent vegetative state). According to the World Health Organization (WHO), drowning is the third leading cause of death by unintentional injury worldwide. The WHO estimates that each year there are more than 360,000 drowning deaths worldwide.

Box 44.1 summarizes the general sequence of events that occurs in drowning or near drowning. Victims submerged in cold water generally demonstrate a much higher survival rate than victims submerged in warm water. Table 44.1 lists favorable prognostic factors in cold-water near drowning.

BOX 44.1 Drowning or Near Drowning Sequence

1. Panic and violent struggle to return to the surface
2. Period of calmness and apnea
3. Swallowing of large amounts of fluid, followed by vomiting
4. Gasping inspirations and aspiration
5. Seizures
6. Coma
7. Death

TABLE 44.1 Favorable Prognostic Factors in Cold-Water Near Drowning

Age	The younger, the better
Submersion time	The shorter, the better (60 minutes appears to be the upper limit in cold-water submersions)
Water temperature	The colder, the better (range, 27° to 70°F)
Water quality	The cleaner, the better
Other injuries	None serious
Amount of struggle	The less struggle, the better
Cardiopulmonary resuscitation (CPR) quality	Good CPR technique increases the survival rate
Suicidal intent	Lower survival rate among victims who attempted suicide than among victims of accidental submersion

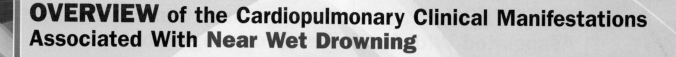

The following clinical manifestations result from the pathologic mechanisms caused (or activated) by atelectasis (see Fig. 10.7), alveolar consolidation (see Fig. 10.8), increased alveolar-capillary membrane thickness (see Fig. 10.9), bronchospasm (see Fig. 10.10), and excessive bronchial secretions (see Fig. 10.11)— the major anatomic alterations of the lungs associated with near wet drowning (see Fig. 44.1).

CLINICAL DATA OBTAINED AT THE PATIENT'S BEDSIDE

The Physical Examination

Apnea

Apnea is directly related to the length of time the victim is submerged and the temperature of the water. Cold water temperatures cause increased apnea. The longer the submersion, the more likely it is that the victim will not have spontaneous respiration. When spontaneous breathing is present, the respiratory rate is usually increased.

Vital Signs

Increased Respiratory Rate (Tachypnea)

Several pathophysiologic mechanisms operating simultaneously may lead to an increased ventilatory rate:

- Stimulation of peripheral chemoreceptors (hypoxemia)
- Relationship of decreased lung compliance to increased ventilatory rate
- Stimulation of J receptors
- Anxiety (conscious patient)

Increased Heart Rate (Pulse) and Blood Pressure

Cyanosis

Cough and Sputum Production (Frothy, White or Pink, Stable Bubbles)

Pallor (Extreme Paleness)—Particularly in Cold Water Episodes

Chest Assessment Findings

- Crackles

CLINICAL DATA OBTAINED FROM LABORATORY TESTS AND SPECIAL PROCEDURES

Pulmonary Function Test Findings
(Extrapolated Data for Instructional Purposes)
(Primary Restrictive Lung Pathophysiology)

FORCED EXPIRATORY VOLUME AND FLOW RATE FINDINGS

FVC	FEV_T	FEV_1/FVC ratio	$FEF_{25\%-75\%}$
↓	N or ↓	N or ↑	N or ↓

$FEF_{50\%}$	$FEF_{200-1200}$	PEFR	MVV
N or ↓	N or ↓	N or ↓	N or ↓

LUNG VOLUME AND CAPACITY FINDINGS

V_T	IRV	ERV	RV
N or ↓	↓	↓	↓

VC	IC	FRC	TLC	RV/TLC ratio
↓	↓	↓	↓	N

DECREASED DIFFUSION CAPACITY (DLCO)

Arterial Blood Gases

MODERATE AND ADVANCED STAGES OF WET DROWNING

Acute Ventilatory Failure With Hypoxemia[1]
(Acute Respiratory Acidosis)

pH[2]	$PaCO_2$	HCO_3^-[2]	PaO_2	SaO_2 or SpO_2
↓	↑	↑	↓	↓
		(but normal)		

Oxygenation Indices[3]

$\dot{Q}_S/\dot{Q}_T$	DO_2	$\dot{V}O_2$[4]	$C(a\text{-}\overline{v})O_2$[4]	O_2ER	$S\overline{v}O_2$
↑	↓	N	N	↑	↓

---

[1]See Table 5.5 and related discussion for the acute pH, $PaCO_2$, and HCO_3^- changes associated with acute ventilatory failure.
[2]When tissue hypoxia is severe enough to produce lactic acid (metabolic acidosis), the pH and HCO_3^- values will be lower than expected for a particular $PaCO_2$ level.
[3]$C(a\text{-}\overline{v})O_2$, Arterial-venous oxygen difference; DO_2, total oxygen delivery; O_2ER, oxygen extraction ratio; $\dot{Q}_S/\dot{Q}_T$, pulmonary shunt fraction; $S\overline{v}O_2$, mixed venous oxygen saturation; $\dot{V}O_2$, oxygen consumption.
[4]The $\dot{V}O_2$ and $C(a\text{-}\overline{v})O_2$ may be decreased in cold water drowning.

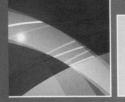
RADIOLOGIC FINDINGS
Chest Radiograph

· Fluffy infiltrates

The initial appearance of the radiograph may vary from being completely normal to showing varying degrees of pulmonary edema and atelectasis (Fig. 44.2). It should be emphasized, however, that an initially normal chest radiograph still may be associated with significant hypoxemia, hypercapnia, and acidosis. In any case, radiographic deterioration may occur in the first 48 to 72 hours.

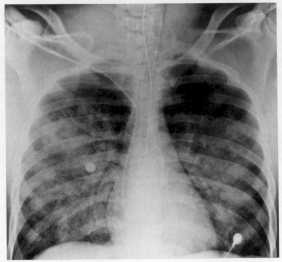

FIGURE 44.2 This radiograph of a young man, taken just after an episode of near drowning, shows a pulmonary edema pattern. Note the air bronchograms in both lungs reflecting atelectasis. (From Hansell, D. M., Lynch, D. A., McAdams, H. P., et al. [2010]. *Imaging of diseases of the chest* [5th ed.]. Philadelphia, PA: Elsevier.)

General Management of Near Drowning and Wet Drowning

The First Responder

For the **first responder**, the first objectives in treating a drowning victim are to remove the person from the water and, if the patient has no spontaneous ventilation and pulse, to call for help and immediately initiate cardiopulmonary resuscitation (CPR) with FIO_2 1.0. When the patient has been submerged for less than 60 minutes in cold water, fixed and dilated pupils do not necessarily indicate a poor prognosis. Because water is an excellent conductor of body heat (cold water can cool the body 25 times faster than air at the same temperature) and because evaporation further reduces an individual's body heat and produces **hypothermia**, the victim's wet clothing should immediately be removed and replaced with warm, dry coverings. High heat-loss areas of the body include the head and neck, axillae, and inguinal areas. The victim's vital signs, including rectal temperature, should be monitored closely during travel to the hospital. The victim's body temperature frequently falls during transport, and therefore measures to conserve the patient's body heat are extremely important. Victims with spontaneous ventilation should be monitored with pulse oximetry during transport, if at all possible.

Management at the Hospital

Treatment at the hospital is an extension of prehospital management. Virtually every near drowning victim suffers from hypoxemia, hypercapnia, and acidosis (acute ventilatory failure). Hypoxemia generally persists after aspiration of fluids in the airway (wet drowning) because of alveolar-capillary damage and continued intrapulmonary shunting. The degree of hypoxemia is directly related to the amount of alveolar-capillary damage. A chest radiograph should be obtained to help evaluate the magnitude of the alveolar-capillary injury. However, a normal initial chest radiograph does not rule out the possibility of alveolar-capillary deterioration during the first 24 hours.

Intubation and mechanical ventilation should be performed immediately for any victim with no spontaneous ventilations and for victims who are breathing spontaneously, but are unable to maintain a PaO_2 of 60 mm Hg with an FIO_2 of 0.50 or lower. Because of the nature of the alveolar-capillary injury seen in most wet drowning victims, mechanical ventilation with positive end-expiratory pressure (PEEP) or continuous positive airway pressure (CPAP) should be administered. It should be noted, however, that **pulmonary barotrauma, pulmonary volutrauma,**[1] and **ventilator-induced lung injury**

---

[1]It has long been known that mechanical ventilation can produce a variety of lung injuries referred to as *ventilator-induced lung injury (VILI)*, *pulmonary volutrauma*, and *pulmonary barotrauma*. VILI stress fractures of the pulmonary capillary endothelium, epithelium, basement membrane, and in severe cases lung rupture. Lung ruptures can lead to leakage of fluid, protein, and blood into tissue and air spaces or leakage of air into tissue spaces. This condition can be followed by an inflammatory response and possibly a reduced defense against infection. *Pulmonary volutrauma* is damage to the lung caused by overdistention by a mechanical ventilator set for an excessively high tidal volume. *Pulmonary barotrauma* is damage to the lungs caused by rapid or extreme pressures generated by mechanical ventilation. Predisposing factors for VILI, pulmonary volutrauma, and pulmonary barotrauma include (1) mechanical ventilation with high peak inspiratory volumes and pressures, (2) mechanical ventilation with a high mean airway pressure, (3) structural immaturity of lung and chest wall, (4) surfactant insufficiency or inactivation, and (5) preexisting lung disease (see Chapter 11).

(VILI) are common complications of ventilatory therapy in these patients. Low tidal volume ventilation and **permissive hypercapnia**[2] are ventilator management techniques to consider when appropriate. The patient also may benefit from inotropic agents and diuretics.

Finally, warming the victim should progress concomitantly with all the other treatment modalities. Nearly all near drowning victims are hypothermic to some degree. Depending on the severity of the hypothermia and on the available resources, a number of **warming techniques** may be employed. For example, the body temperature can be increased by the

intravenous administration of heated solutions; by heated lavage of the gastric, intrathoracic, pericardial, and peritoneal spaces; or by the administration of heated lavage to the bladder and rectum. Additional external heating techniques include warming of the patient's inspired air or gas mixtures, heating blankets, warm baths, and immersion in a heated Hubbard tank. In rare cases, extracorporeal circulation, with complete cardiopulmonary bypass and blood warming, has been successful. Resuscitation should not end even if the patient does not respond until a close approximation of normal body temperature is reached.

---

[2]Permissive hypercapnia: Mechanical ventilation was traditionally applied with the goal of normalizing arterial blood gas values, particularly the arterial carbon dioxide tension ($PaCO_2$). However, this is no longer the primary objective of mechanical ventilation. Today, the emphasis is on maintaining adequate gas exchange while—and, importantly—minimizing the risks of mechanical ventilation. Common strategies used to reduce the risk for mechanical ventilation include (1) low tidal volume ventilation to protect the lung from ventilator-associated lung injury in patients with acute lung injury (e.g., ARDS) and (2) reduction of the tidal volume, respiratory rate, or both to minimize intrinsic positive end-expiratory pressure (i.e.,

auto-PEEP) in patients with obstructive lung disease (e.g., COPD). Although these mechanical ventilation strategies may result in an increased $PaCO_2$ level (hypercapnia), they do help protect the lung from barotrauma (i.e., physical damage to lung tissues caused by excessive gas pressures). The lenient acceptance of the hypercapnia is called *permissive hypercapnia*. In most cases the patient's $PaCO_2$ is adequately maintained by an increased ventilatory rate that offsets the decreased tidal volume. The $PaCO_2$, however, should not be permitted to increase to the point of severe acidosis. The most current consensus suggests it is safe to allow pH to fall to at least 7.20 (http://www.ARDSNet) (see Chapter 11).

CASE STUDY Near Wet Drowning

Admitting History and Physical Examination

A 12-year-old boy had a prior history of a seizure disorder but had not taken his medication for almost a year. On the morning of admission, he participated in a regular swimming class in the junior high school pool. According to the coach on duty, there had been a "pool check" 30 seconds before the patient's partner reported that the patient seemed to stay under water "too long."

When taken from the water, he was unconscious and "blue." He was given mouth-to-mouth resuscitation, and by the time the emergency medical technician (EMT) squad arrived about 20 minutes later, he was comatose, but he was breathing at a rate of 10 breaths/min, although his lips and fingers were still cyanotic. He was placed on 5 L/min oxygen and taken to the nearest hospital.

On admission the patient's blood pressure was 100/60 and his pulse was 140 beats/min. Rectal temperature was 98°F (36.1°C). Auscultation of his chest revealed fine crackles bilaterally. Clear secretions were suctioned from his oral airway. A chest radiograph showed bilateral diffuse increase in density, which suggested pulmonary edema or possible hemorrhage. His SpO$_2$ was 72%. Plans were made to transfer him to a nearby tertiary care medical center. The respiratory therapist in the emergency department entered the following assessment moments before the patient transfer.

Respiratory Assessment and Plan

S N/A (patient comatose). History of near drowning.
O Comatose. Spontaneous breathing at 10/min, BP 100/60, P 140. Core temp 98°F (36.1°C) (normal). Crackles bilaterally. Nasotracheal suctioning yields clear fluid. Cyanotic. SpO$_2$ on 5 L/min O$_2$ per nasal cannula: 72%.
A • Near drowning. R/O seizure disorder (history)
　 • Increased airway secretions (suctioning of clear fluid)
　 • Poor oxygenation (cyanosis, SpO$_2$)
　 • Pulmonary edema (CXR)
P Stat ABG on FIO$_2$ 1.0, then titrate per Oxygen Therapy Protocol. Have equipment to intubate on standby. Bag-mask ventilate, and PRN. Provide continuous pulse oximetry. Will accompany on transfer.

After transfer to the tertiary care medical center, the patient was described as a well-developed, slightly obese adolescent in obvious respiratory distress. He was now alert, oriented, but extremely apprehensive. His vital signs were temperature (rectal) 100.8°F (38.2°C), blood pressure 112/70 mm Hg, pulse 140 beats/min, and respirations 60 breaths/min. The lips and fingertips were still cyanotic. The chest wall motion was paradoxical. There was marked substernal retraction. Breath sounds were diminished bilaterally, and loud crackles were heard over both lungs anteriorly.

Laboratory examination revealed a leukocytosis of 21,000/mm³ and 2+ albumin in the urine, but findings were otherwise within normal limits. There was no evidence of hemolysis. On bag-mask ventilation with an FIO_2 of 1.0, the arterial blood gas (ABG) values were pH 7.29, $PaCO_2$ 52 mm Hg, HCO_3^- 25 mEq/L, PaO_2 38 mm Hg, and SaO_2 67%. The patient's condition was rapidly deteriorating, and he developed even more severe crackles. He now had a spontaneous cough with frothy sputum production. The chest radiograph revealed pulmonary edema and nearly complete opacification of both lungs. The following was entered in the patient's chart.

Respiratory Assessment and Plan

S Anxious, dyspneic, crying. "I can't get my breath. Where am I? Am I going to die?"

O Afebrile. BP 112/70, P 140/min, RR 60/min. Cyanotic. Paradoxical chest/abdomen movements, sternal retraction. Crackles in both lungs anteriorly. Spontaneous cough with frothy sputum production, WBC 21,000/mm³. On FIO_2 1.0: pH 7.29, $PaCO_2$ 52, HCO_3^- 25, PaO_2 38, SaO_2 67%. CXR: "White-out."

A • Pulmonary edema secondary to near wet drowning (frothy sputum).
  • Acute ventilatory failure with severe hypoxemia (ABGs).

P Continue on FIO_2 1.0 and bag-mask ventilate. Page physician stat. Obtain intubation equipment and prepare to place patient on ventilator. Follow oximetry. Prepare to assist in placement of Swan-Ganz catheter.

The patient was intubated and paralyzed with succinylcholine. As soon as he was intubated, copious pink foam was aspirated from the endotracheal tube. He was alternately suctioned and ventilated with an Ambu bag. He was given 7 mg of morphine for sedation and was mechanically ventilated in continuous mechanical ventilation (CMV) mode at a rate of 10 breaths/min. On an FIO_2 of 1.0 and PEEP of 10 cm H_2O, his blood gases were pH 7.44, $PaCO_2$ 43 mm Hg, HCO_3^- 22 mEq/L, PaO_2 109 mm Hg, SaO_2 98%. At this time, the respiratory therapist started to slowly decrease the patient's FIO_2. Because he was still fighting the ventilator, he was paralyzed with pancuronium.

After several hours, the lungs were clear, the secretions were no longer present, and his blood gas values returned to normal on an FIO_2 of 0.50 and PEEP of 10 cm H_2O (pH 7.38, $PaCO_2$ 42 mm Hg, HCO_3^- 24 mEq/L, PaO_2 98 mm Hg, SaO_2 97%). His hemodynamic status was normal. The chest radiograph revealed considerable clearing of the earlier noted bilateral pulmonary infiltrates. A pulmonary artery catheter was not placed, because clinical improvement was clearly occurring. The respiratory therapist entered the following assessment and plan.

Respiratory Assessment and Plan

S N/A (patient sedated, paralyzed).

O Lungs clear. No secretions. On FIO_2 0.50 and +10 PEEP: pH 7.38, $PaCO_2$ 42, HCO_3^- 24, PaO_2 98, SaO_2 97%.

CXR: Considerable improvement in bilateral infiltrates. Swan-Ganz catheter not inserted because patient is improving.

A • Considerable improvement on CMV and PEEP (general improvement of clinical indicators)
  • Acceptable ventilation and oxygenation status on present ventilator settings (ABG)
  • Frothy airway secretions no longer present (clear lungs and no secretions)

P Contact physician to wean from muscle relaxant. Wean from mechanically ventilated breaths, FIO_2, and PEEP per Mechanical Ventilation Protocol. Change ventilator mode to synchronized intermittent mandatory ventilation (SIMV).

The patient was weaned from the ventilator over a period of 6 hours, after which he was extubated. The following morning, ABGs on an FIO_2 0.28 Venturi oxygen mask were pH 7.42, $PaCO_2$ 35 mm Hg, HCO_3^- 22 mEq/L, PaO_2 158 mm Hg, and SaO_2 98%. His chest radiograph was normal. An oxygen titration protocol was performed. He was discharged 2 days later.

Discussion

This case demonstrates initial worsening of the near wet drowning victim despite intensive respiratory care. The initial ABG values showed severe hypoxemia as a result of increased alveolar-capillary membrane thickness and alveolar flooding (see Fig. 44.1) and acute ventilatory failure and metabolic (probably lactic) acidosis. Bronchospasm never developed, and aggressive respiratory care prohibited the development of atelectasis and aspiration pneumonia.

When suctioning, supplemental oxygen, and bag ventilation were no longer successful, the patient was intubated and mechanical ventilation with PEEP was begun. Even on these modalities, the patient remained anxious and was ultimately paralyzed to allow better respiratory synchrony and diminish the chance of ventilatory-associated lung injury (barotrauma or volutrauma). Morphine was used for its sedative qualities and as a vascular afterload reducer. The fact that the patient was fighting the ventilator some time after succinylcholine had been administered reflects the fact that it is a very short-acting paralyzing agent. Pancuronium has a much longer half-life, and its use is standard in settings where longer effectiveness is required. Once the abnormal pathologic processes of the lungs associated with this case improved, the patient's cardiopulmonary status quickly returned to normal, and the respiratory therapist was able wean the patient from the ventilation in a relatively short time.

This case demonstrates the necessity for frequent reassessment of the patient and therapeutic adjustments to follow the findings so observed. Note that the therapist appropriately documented the reason that one of his suggestions (the Swan-Ganz catheter) was not placed. In the protocol-rich environment, such documentation is vital, if only for medical legal reasons.

SELF-ASSESSMENT QUESTIONS

1. In the United States, drowning is the:
   a. Leading cause of accidental death
   b. Second leading cause of accidental death
   c. Third leading cause of accidental death
   d. Fourth leading cause of accidental death

2. According to the Centers for Disease Control and Prevention, about how many people drown each year in the United States?
   a. 500
   b. 1000
   c. 1250
   d. >3000

3. Which of the following are the major anatomic alterations of the lungs associated with near drowning victims?
   1. Consolidation
   2. Bronchospasm
   3. Increased alveolar-capillary membrane thickness
   4. Atelectasis
   5. Excessive bronchial secretions
      a. 3 and 5 only
      b. 2 and 4 only
      c. 3, 4, and 5 only
      d. 1, 2, 3, 4, and 5

4. Which of the following clinical manifestations are associated with near drowning victims?
   1. Frothy, pink sputum
   2. Crackles
   3. Increased pH
   4. Increased $S\bar{v}O_2$
      a. 1 and 2 only
      b. 3 and 4 only
      c. 2, 3, and 4 only
      d. 1, 2, 3, and 4 only

5. Which of the following pulmonary function testing values are associated with near drowning victims?
   1. N or ↓ FEV_T
   2. ↓ FVC
   3. ↓ RV
   4. N or ↑ FEV_1/FVC ratio
      a. 1 and 2 only
      b. 3 and 4 only
      c. 2, 3, and 4 only
      d. 1, 2, 3, and 4

Smoke Inhalation, Thermal Lung Injuries, and Carbon Monoxide Intoxication

Chapter Objectives

After reading this chapter, you will be able to:

- List the anatomic alterations of the lungs associated with smoke inhalation and thermal injuries.
- Describe the causes of smoke inhalation, thermal injuries, and carbon monoxide intoxication.
- List the cardiopulmonary clinical manifestations associated with smoke inhalation, thermal injuries, and carbon monoxide intoxication.
- Describe the general management of smoke inhalation and thermal injuries.
- Describe the clinical strategies and rationales of the SOAPs presented in the case study.
- Define key terms and complete self-assessment questions at end of chapter and Evolve.

Key Terms

Acute Respiratory Distress Syndrome (ARDS)
Body Surface Burns
Bronchiolitis Obliterans Organizing Pneumonia (BOOP)
Bronchospasm
Carbon Monoxide Poisoning
Carbonaceous Sputum
Carboxyhemoglobin
Chest Wall Burns
COHB Half-Life
CO-Oximetry
Cyanide Blood Level
Cyanide Poisoning
Cryptogenic Organizing Pneumonia (COP)
Eschar
Facial Burns
First-Degree Burn
Hyperbaric Oxygenation (HBO) Therapy
Lactic Acidosis
Multiorgan Dysfunction Syndrome (MODS)
Noncardiogenic Pulmonary Edema
Parkland Formula (Fluid Resuscitation)
Pulmonary Embolism
Pyrolysis
Second-Degree Burn
Smoke Inhalation Injury
Steam Inhalation
Thermal Lung Injury
Third-Degree Burn

Chapter Outline

Anatomic Alterations of the Lungs
    Thermal Injury
    Smoke Inhalation Injury
Etiology and Epidemiology
Body Surface Burns
Overview of the Cardiopulmonary Clinical Manifestations Associated With Smoke Inhalation and Thermal Injuries
General Management of Smoke Inhalation and Thermal Injuries
    General Emergency Care
    Airway Management
    Bronchoscopy
    Hyperbaric Oxygen Therapy
    Treatment for Cyanide Poisoning
    Pharmacologic Treatment
    Respiratory Care Treatment Protocols
Case Study: Smoke Inhalation and Thermal Lung Injury
Self-Assessment Questions

Anatomic Alterations of the Lungs

The inhalation of smoke, hot gases, and **body surface burns**—in any combination—continue to be a major cause of morbidity and mortality among fire victims and firefighters. In general, fire-related pulmonary injuries can be divided into thermal and smoke (toxic gases) injuries.

Thermal Lung Injury

Thermal injury refers to injury caused by the inhalation of hot gases. Thermal injuries are usually confined to the upper airway—the nasal cavity, oral cavity, nasopharynx, oropharynx, and larynx. The distal airways and the alveoli are usually spared serious injury because of (1) the remarkable ability of the upper airways to cool hot gases, (2) reflex laryngospasm, and (3) glottic closure. The upper airway is an extremely efficient "heat sink." In fact, in 1945, Moritz and associates demonstrated that the inhalation of hot gases alone did not produce significant damage to the lung. Anesthetized dogs were forced to breathe air heated to 500°C through an insulated endotracheal tube. The air temperature dropped to 50°C by the time it reached the level of the carina. No histologic damage was noticed in the lower trachea or lungs.

Even though thermal injury may occur with or without surface burns, the presence of **facial burns** is a classic predictor of thermal injury. Thermal injury to the upper airway results in blistering, mucosal edema, vascular congestion, epithelial sloughing, and accumulation of thick secretions. Acute upper airway obstruction (UAO) occurs in about 20% to 30% of hospitalized patients with thermal injury and is usually most marked in the supraglottic structures (Fig. 45.1).

Inhalation of steam at 100°C or greater usually results in severe damage at all levels of the respiratory tract. This damage occurs because steam has about 500 times the heat energy content of dry gas at the same temperature. Thermal injury

to the distal airways results in mucosal edema, vascular congestion, epithelial sloughing, **cryptogenic organizing pneumonia (COP)**—also known as **bronchiolitis obliterans organizing pneumonia (BOOP)**—atelectasis, and pulmonary edema (see Chapter 27).

Therefore direct thermal injuries usually do not occur below the level of the larynx, except in the rare instance of **steam inhalation**. Damage to the distal airways is mostly caused by a variety of harmful products found in smoke.

Smoke Inhalation Injury

In **smoke inhalation injury** the pathologic changes in the distal airways and alveoli are mainly caused by the irritating and toxic gases, suspended soot particles, and vapors associated with incomplete combustion and smoke. Many of the substances found in smoke are extremely caustic to the tracheobronchial tree and poisonous to the body. The progression of injuries that develop from smoke inhalation and burns is described as the early stage, intermediate stage, and late stage.

Early Stage (0 to 24 Hours After Inhalation)

The injuries associated with smoke inhalation do not always appear right away, even when extensive body surface burns are evident. During the early stage (0 to 24 hours after smoke inhalation), however, the patient's pulmonary status often changes markedly. Initially, the tracheobronchial tree becomes more inflamed, resulting in **bronchospasm**. This process causes an overabundance of bronchial secretions to move into the airways, resulting in further airway obstruction. In addition, the toxic effects of smoke often slow the activity of the mucosal ciliary transport mechanism, causing further retention of mucus.

Smoke inhalation also may cause **acute respiratory distress syndrome (ARDS)**, (see Chapter 28), noncardiogenic high-permeability pulmonary edema, commonly referred to in smoke inhalation cases as *leaky alveoli*. **Noncardiogenic pulmonary edema** also may be caused by overhydration resulting from overzealous fluid resuscitation (see insert in Fig. 45.1). In severe cases, ARDS may occur early in the course of the pathology.

Intermediate Stage (2 to 5 Days After Inhalation)

Whereas upper airway thermal injuries usually begin to improve during the intermediate stage (2 to 5 days after smoke inhalation), the pathologic changes deep in the lungs continue to be a problem. For example, production of mucus continues to increase, whereas mucosal ciliary transport activity continues to decrease. The mucosa of the tracheobronchial tree frequently becomes necrotic and sloughs (usually at 3 to 4 days). The necrotic debris, excessive production of mucus, and retention of mucus lead to mucus plugging and atelectasis. In addition, the mucus accumulation often leads to bacterial colonization, bronchitis, and pneumonia. Organisms commonly cultured include gram-positive *Staphylococcus aureus* and gram-negative *Klebsiella, Enterobacter, Escherichia coli,* and *Pseudomonas*. If not already present, ARDS may develop at any time during this period.

When **chest wall burns** are present, the situation may be further aggravated by the patient's inability to breathe deeply and cough as a result of (1) pain, (2) the administration of

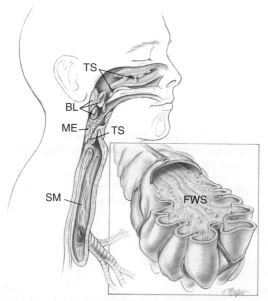

FIGURE 45.1 Smoke inhalation and thermal injuries. *BL,* Airway blister; *FWS,* frothy white secretions (pulmonary edema); *ME,* mucosal edema; *SM,* smoke (toxic gas); *TS,* thick secretions.

narcotics, (3) immobility, (4) increased airway resistance, and (5) decreased lung and chest wall compliance.

Late Stage (5 Days and Longer After Inhalation)

Infections resulting from burn wounds on the body surface are the major concern during the late stage (5 days and longer after smoke inhalation). These infections often lead to sepsis and **multiorgan dysfunction syndrome (MODS)**. Sepsis-induced MODS is the primary cause of death in seriously burned patients during this stage.

Pneumonia continues to be a major problem during this period. In addition, **pulmonary embolism** may develop within 2 weeks after serious body surface burns. Pulmonary embolism may develop from deep venous thrombosis secondary to a hypercoagulable state and prolonged immobility.

Finally, the long-term effects of smoke inhalation can result in restrictive and obstructive lung disorders. In general, a restrictive lung disorder develops from alveolar fibrosis and chronic atelectasis. An obstructive lung disorder is generally caused by increased and chronic bronchial secretions, bronchial stenosis, bronchial polyps, bronchiectasis, and bronchiolitis.

The major pathologic and structural changes of the respiratory system caused by thermal or smoke inhalation injuries are as follows:

Thermal injury (upper airway—nasal cavity, oral cavity, and pharynx):
- Blistering
- Mucosal edema
- Vascular congestion
- Epithelial sloughing
- Thick secretions
- Acute UAO

Smoke inhalation injury (tracheobronchial tree and alveoli):
- Inflammation of the tracheobronchial tree
- Bronchospasm
- Excessive bronchial secretions and mucous plugging
- Decreased mucosal ciliary transport
- Atelectasis
- Alveolar edema and frothy secretions (noncardiogenic pulmonary edema)
- ARDS (severe cases)
- COP (also called *bronchiolitis obliterans organizing pneumonia*)
- Alveolar fibrosis, bronchial stenosis, bronchial polyps, bronchiolitis, and bronchiectasis (severe cases)

Pneumonia (see Chapter 18, Pneumonia, Lung Abscess Formation, and Important Fungal Diseases) and pulmonary embolism (see Chapter 21, Pulmonary Vascular Disease: Pulmonary Embolism and Pulmonary Hypertension) often complicate smoke inhalation injury.

Etiology and Epidemiology

According to the National Fire Protection Association (NFPA),[1] more than 1.3 million fires were reported by fire departments in 2016, resulting in an estimated 3390 civilian deaths—the highest number of fatalities since 2008. The NFPA estimates that public fire departments in the United States responded to 1,342,000 fires during this period. In addition to the 3390 civilian deaths in 2016, there were an estimated 14,660 civilian fire injuries. NFPA estimates that the 1,342,000 fires in 2016 caused 10.6 billion dollars in property damage.

The prognosis of fire victims is usually determined by the (1) extent and duration of smoke exposure, (2) chemical composition of the smoke, (3) size and depth of body surface burns (Table 45.1), (4) temperature of gases inhaled, (5) age (the prognosis worsens in the very young or old), and (6) preexisting health status. When smoke inhalation injury is accompanied by a full-thickness or third-degree skin burn, the mortality rate almost doubles.

Smoke can result from either **pyrolysis** (smoldering in a low-oxygen environment) or combustion (burning, with visible flame, in an adequate-oxygen environment). Smoke is composed of a complex mixture of particulates, toxic gases, and vapors. The composition of smoke varies according to the chemical makeup of the material that is burning and the amount of oxygen being consumed by the fire. Table 45.2 lists some of the more common toxic substances produced by burning products that are frequently found in office, industrial, and residential buildings.

Although in some instances the toxic components of the smoke may be obvious, in most cases the precise identification of the inhaled toxins is not feasible. In general, the inhalation of smoke with toxic agents that have high water solubility (e.g., ammonia, sulfur dioxide, and hydrogen fluoride) affects the structures of the upper airway. In contrast, the inhalation of toxic agents that have low water solubility (e.g., hydrogen chloride, chlorine, phosgene, and oxides of nitrogen) affects the distal airways and alveoli. Many of the substances in smoke are caustic and can cause significant injury to the tracheobronchial tree (e.g., aldehydes [especially acrolein], hydrochloride, and oxides of sulfur).

Body Surface Burns

Because the amount and severity of body surface burns play a major role in the patient's risk for mortality and morbidity, an approximate estimate of the percentage of the body surface

TABLE 45.1 The Approximate Percentage of Body Surface Area (BSA) for Various Body Regions of Adults and Infants

Anatomic Region	BSA in Adults (%)	BSA in Infants (%)
Entire head and neck	9	18
Each arm	9	9
Anterior trunk	18	18
Posterior trunk	18	18
Genitalia	1	1
Each leg	18	13.5

NOTE: The "rule of nines" is used to estimate percentage of injury; each of the areas listed here represents about 9% or 18% of the body surface area. This rule does not apply to infants' legs.

[1]National Fire Protection Association: http://www.nfpa.org.

area burned is important. Table 45.1 lists the approximate percentage of surface area for various body regions of adults and infants. The severity and depth of burns are usually defined as follows:

- **First-degree burn** *(minimal depth in skin):* Superficial burn, damage limited to the outer layer of epidermis. This burn is characterized by reddened skin, tenderness, and pain. Blisters are not present. Healing time is about 6 to 10 days. The result of healing is normal skin.
- **Second-degree burn** *(superficial to deep thickness of skin):* Burns in which damage extends through the epidermis and into the dermis but is not of sufficient extent to interfere with regeneration of epidermis. If secondary infection results, the damage from a second-degree burn may be equivalent to that of a third-degree burn. Blisters are usually present. Healing time is 7 to 21 days. The result of healing ranges from normal to hairless and depigmented skin with a texture that is normal, pitted, flat, or shiny.
- **Third-degree burn** *(full thickness of skin including tissue beneath skin):* Burns in which both epidermis and dermis are destroyed, with damage extending into underlying tissues. Tissue may be charred or coagulated. Healing may occur after 21 days or may never occur without skin grafting if the burned area is large. The resultant damage heals with hypertrophic scars (keloids), chronic granulation, and contractures.

TABLE 45.2 Toxic Substances and Sources Commonly Associated With Fire and Smoke

Substance	Source
Aldehydes (acrolein, acetaldehyde, formaldehyde)	Wood, cotton, paper
Organic acids (acetic and formic acids)	
Carbon monoxide, hydrogen chloride, phosgene	Polyvinylchloride
Hydrogen cyanide, isocyanate	Polyurethanes
Hydrogen fluoride, hydrogen bromide	Fluorinated resins
Ammonia	Melamine resins
Oxides of nitrogen	Nitrocellulose film, fabrics
Benzene	Petroleum products
Carbon monoxide, carbon dioxide	Organic material
Sulfur dioxide	Sulfur-containing compounds
Hydrogen chloride	Fertilizer, textiles, rubber manufacturing
Chlorine	Swimming pool water
Ozone	Welding fumes
Hydrogen sulfide	Metal works, chemical manufacturing

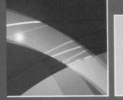

OVERVIEW of the Cardiopulmonary Clinical Manifestations Associated With Smoke Inhalation and Thermal Injuries

The following clinical manifestations result from the pathologic mechanisms caused (or activated) by atelectasis (see Fig. 10.7), alveolar consolidation (see Fig. 10.8), increased alveolar-capillary membrane thickness (see Fig. 10.9), bronchospasm (see Fig. 10.10), and excessive bronchial secretions (see Fig. 10.11)—the major anatomic alterations of the lungs associated with smoke inhalation and thermal injuries (see Fig. 45.1).

CLINICAL DATA OBTAINED AT THE PATIENT'S BEDSIDE

The Physical Examination

Vital Signs

Increased Respiratory Rate (Tachypnea)

Several pathophysiologic mechanisms operating simultaneously may lead to an increased ventilatory rate:

- Stimulation of peripheral chemoreceptors (hypoxemia)
- Relationship of decreased lung compliance to increased ventilatory rate
- Stimulation of J receptors
- Pain, anxiety
- Fever (with infection)

Increased Heart Rate (Pulse) and Blood Pressure

Assessment of Acute Upper Airway Obstruction (Thermal Injury)

- Obvious pharyngeal edema and swelling
- Inspiratory stridor
- Hoarseness
- Altered voice
- Painful swallowing

Because the inhalation of hot gases often results in severe upper airway edema, the respiratory therapist always should be alert for any clinical manifestations of acute upper airway obstruction, even when the patient shows no remarkable upper airway problems or upper body or facial burns at admission.

Cyanosis

Cough and Sputum Production

When the patient experiences upper airway thermal injuries, abnormally thick and sometimes excessive secretions usually result. During the early stage of recovery from smoke inhalation, the patient generally expectorates a small amount of black, sooty sputum (**carbonaceous sputum**). During the intermediate stage the patient may produce moderate to large amounts of frothy secretions. During the late stage, purulent mucus production is common.

Chest Assessment Findings

- Normal breath sounds (early stage)
- Wheezing
- Crackles

CLINICAL DATA OBTAINED FROM LABORATORY TESTS AND SPECIAL PROCEDURES

Pulmonary Function Test Findings
(Extrapolated Data for Instructional Purposes)
(Primarily Restrictive Lung Pathophysiology)

FORCED EXPIRATORY VOLUME AND FLOW RATE FINDINGS

FVC	FEV_T	FEV_1/FVC ratio	$FEF_{25\%-75\%}$
↓	N or ↓	N or ↑	N or ↓

$FEF_{50\%}$	$FEF_{200-1200}$	PEFR	MVV
N or ↓	N or ↓	N or ↓	N or ↓

LUNG VOLUME AND CAPACITY FINDINGS

V_T	IRV	ERV	RV^1
N or ↓	↓	↓	↓

VC	IC	FRC^1	TLC	RV/TLC ratio
↓	↓	↓	↓	N

DECREASED DIFFUSION CAPACITY (DLCO)

Arterial Blood Gases

EARLY STAGES OF SMOKE INHALATION

Acute Alveolar Hyperventilation With Hypoxemia[2]
(Acute Respiratory Alkalosis)

pH	$PaCO_2$	HCO_3^-	PaO_2	SaO_2 or SpO_2
↑	↓	↓ (but normal)	↓ or normal	↓ or normal

SEVERE SMOKE INHALATION AND BURNS WITH METABOLIC ACIDOSIS

COHb	pH^3	$PaCO_2^4$	HCO_3^{-3}	PaO_2	SaO_2 or SpO_2
↑	↓ (lactic acidemia)	↓	↓	↓ or normal (but tissue hypoxemia is present)	↓ or normal

COHb, Carboxyhemoglobin.

---

[1] ↑ When airways are partially obstructed.
[2] See Table 5.5 and related discussion for the acute pH, $PaCO_2$, and HCO_3^- changes associated with acute alveolar hyperventilation.
[3] When tissue hypoxia is severe enough to produce lactic acid, the pH and HCO_3^- values will be lower than expected for a particular $PaCO_2$ level.
[4] In severe burns with ARDS the $PaCO_2$ may be elevated and combined respiratory and metabolic acidosis may be present.

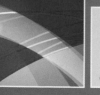

When carbon monoxide (CO) or cyanide poisoning is present, the pH may be decreased during the early stages of smoke inhalation. This decrease in pH occurs because patients with severe CO or cyanide poisoning commonly have **lactic acidosis** as a result of tissue hypoxia, even in the presence of a normal PaO_2. Therefore when CO or cyanide poisoning is present, the patient may demonstrate the following arterial blood gas values.

SEVERE SMOKE INHALATION AND BURNS WITH RESPIRATORY AND METABOLIC ACIDOSIS

Acute Ventilatory Failure (Acute Respiratory Acidosis) and Metabolic Acidosis

COHb	pH[5]	$PaCO_2$[6]	HCO_3^-[5]	PaO_2	SaO_2 or SpO_2
↑	↓	↑	↓	↓	↓
					or normal

COHb, Carboxyhemoglobin.

Oxygenation Indices
Smoke Inhalation and Burns

	Early and Intermediate Stages	Late Stage
DO_2	↓	↓
$\dot{V}O_2$	↑	↓
$C(a-\overline{v})O_2$	↑	↓
O_2ER	↑	↓
$S\overline{v}O_2$	↓	↓

When CO or cyanide poisoning is present, the oxygenation indices are unreliable because the PaO_2 is often normal in the presence of **carbon monoxide poisoning**, and when cyanide poisoning is present, the tissue cells are prevented from consuming oxygen. Both of these conditions cause falsely high pulse oximetry readings. For example, when CO is present, a normal DO_2 value may be calculated when, in reality, the patient's oxygen transport status is extremely low. When cyanide poisoning is present, the patient's $\dot{V}O_2$ may appear normal or increased, when in actuality the tissue cells are extremely hypoxic. Typically these problems are not present during the intermediate and late stages in the presence of appropriate treatment—that is, once the carbon dioxide and/or cyanide has been removed.

Hemodynamic Indices
Cardiogenic Pulmonary Edema[7]

Indices[8]	Early Stage	Intermediate Stage	Late Stage
CVP	↓	Normal	↓
RAP	↓	Normal	↓
$\overline{PA}$	↓	Normal	↓
PCWP	↓	Normal	↓
CO	↓	Normal	↓
SV	↓	Normal	↓
SVI	↓	Normal	↓
CI[8]	↓	Normal	↓
RVSWI	↓	Normal	↓
LVSWI	↓	Normal	↓
PVR	Normal	Normal	↑
SVR	↑	Normal	↑

In general, the hemodynamic profile in patients with body surface burns relates to the amount of intravascular volume loss (hypovolemia) that occurs as a result of third-space fluid shifts. For example, during the early stage, the decreased values shown for the CVP, RAP, $\overline{PA}$, CWP, CO, SV, SVI, CI, RVSWI, and LVSWI reflect the reduction in pulmonary intravascular and cardiac filling volumes. Hypovolemia causes a generalized peripheral vasoconstriction, which is reflected in an elevated SVR. When appropriate fluid resuscitation is administered, the patient's hemodynamic indices are usually normal during the intermediate stage.

CARBON MONOXIDE POISONING

When a patient has been exposed to smoke, *CO poisoning must be assumed.* Although CO has no direct injurious effect on the lungs, it can greatly reduce the patient's oxygen transport because CO has an affinity for hemoglobin that is about 210 times greater than that of oxygen. CO attached to hemoglobin is called **carboxyhemoglobin (COHb)**. Breathing CO at a partial pressure of less than 2 mm Hg can result in a COHb of 40% or greater. In other words, 40% or more of the hemoglobin oxygen transport system is then unavailable for oxygen transport.

In addition, high concentrations of COHb cause the oxyhemoglobin dissociation curve to move markedly to the left, which makes it more difficult for oxygen to leave the hemoglobin at

---

[5]When tissue hypoxia is severe enough to produce lactic acid, the pH and HCO_3^- values will be lower than expected for a particular $PaCO_2$ level.

[6]In severe burns with ARDS the $PaCO_2$ may be elevated and combined respiratory and metabolic acidosis may be present.

[7]When ARDS is present, noncardiogenic pulmonary edema findings may be present (see Chapter 28, Acute Respiratory Distress Syndrome).

[8]*CO,* Cardiac output; *CI,* cardiac index; *CVP,* central venous pressure; *LVSWI,* left ventricular stroke work index; *$\overline{PA}$,* mean pulmonary artery pressure; *PCWP,* pulmonary capillary wedge pressure; *PVR,* pulmonary vascular resistance; *RAP,* right atrial pressure; *RVSWI,* right ventricular stroke work index; *SV,* stroke volume; *SVI,* stroke volume index; *SVR,* systemic vascular resistance.

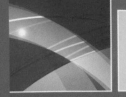
the tissue sites. In essence, the tissue cells are better oxygenated when 40% of the hemoglobin is absent (anemia) than when a COHb of 40% is present. Thus it should be stressed that SpO$_2$ and pulse oximeter–based oxygen content measurements are misleading and unreliable in the presence of COHb. ABG measurements (with **CO-oximetry**) provide important information regarding the presence of hypoxemia, widened alveolar-arterial oxygen gradient, acid-base status, and a correct measurement of both oxygen saturation (%) and COHb (%).

A COHb level in excess of 20% is usually considered CO poisoning, and a COHb level of 40% or greater is considered severe. A COHb level in excess of 50% may cause irreversible damage to the central nervous system. If available, hyperbaric oxygen (HBO) therapy is usually used at a COHb greater than 10%. Cigarette smokers may demonstrate COHb levels of 5% or greater to 7%; in cigar smokers levels can be as high as 15%.

Table 45.3 lists the clinical manifestations associated with CO poisoning.

CYANIDE POISONING

When smoke contains cyanide, oxygen transport may be further impaired. **Cyanide poisoning** should be suspected in comatose patients who have inhaled fumes from burning plastic (polyurethane) or other synthetic materials. Inhaled cyanide is easily transported in the blood to the tissue cells, where it bonds to the cytochrome oxidase enzymes of the mitochondria. This inhibits the metabolism of oxygen and causes the tissue cells to shift to an inefficient (anaerobic) form of metabolism. The end-product of anaerobic metabolism is lactic acid. Cyanide poisoning may result in lactic acidemia, which is caused by an inadequate *tissue* oxygen level, even though the PaO$_2$ and SpO$_2$ are normal or above normal. Clinically, cyanide concentrations

are easily measured with commercially available kits. A **cyanide blood level** in excess of 1 mg/L usually is fatal.

RADIOLOGIC FINDINGS
Chest Radiograph

- Usually normal (early stage)
- Pulmonary edema, ARDS (may be present during early stage)
- Patchy or segmental infiltrates (late stage)

During the early stage, the radiograph is generally normal. Signs of pulmonary edema and ARDS may be seen during the intermediate and late stages. The chest radiograph reveals dense, fluffy opacities and patchy or segmental infiltrates (Fig. 45.2).

TABLE 45.3 Blood Carboxyhemoglobin (COHb) Levels and Clinical Manifestations

COHb (%)	Clinical Manifestations
0–10	Usually no symptoms or mild fatigue
10–20	Mild headache, dilation of cutaneous blood vessels Cherry red skin—but not always
20–30	Throbbing headache, nausea, vomiting, impaired judgment
30–50	Throbbing headache, possible syncope, increased respiratory and pulse rates
50–60	Syncope, increased respiratory and pulse rates, coma, seizures, Cheyne-Stokes respiration
60–70	Coma, seizures, cardiovascular and respiratory depression, and possible death
70–80	Cardiopulmonary failure and death

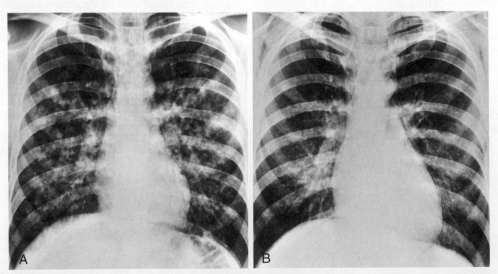

FIGURE 45.2 (A) Radiograph of a young man admitted after accidentally setting his kitchen on fire while intoxicated. (B) Prompt recovery after 72 hours. (From Hansell, D. M., Lynch, D. A., McAdams, H. P., et al. [2010]. *Imaging of diseases of the chest* [5th ed.]. Philadelphia, PA: Elsevier.)

General Management of Smoke Inhalation and Thermal Injuries

General Emergency Care

The principal goals in the initial care of patients with smoke inhalation injury and burns include the immediate assessment of the patient's airway, respiratory status, cardiovascular status, percentage of body burned, and depth of burns. An intravenous line should be started immediately to administer medications and fluids. Easily separated clothing should be removed, and any remaining clothing should be soaked thoroughly before removing. When present, burn wounds should be covered to prevent shock, fluid loss, heat loss, and pain. Infection control includes isolation, room pressurization, air filtration, and wound coverings.

Fluid resuscitation with lactated Ringer solution is usually initiated according to the **Parkland formula**—4 mL/kg of body weight for each percent of body surface area burned (see Table 45.1) over a 24-hour period. The patient's hemodynamic status will usually remain stable at this fluid replacement rate, with an average urine output target of 30 to 50 mL/h and a central venous pressure target of 2 to 6 mm Hg. Because this process may lead to overhydration and acute UAO and pulmonary edema, the patient's fluid and electrolyte status (weight, input and output, and laboratory values) must be monitored carefully.

Finally, knowledge of the exposure characteristics of the fire-related accident may be helpful in assessing the potential clinical complications. For example, did the accident involve a closed-space setting or entrapment? The amount and concentration of smoke are usually much greater under these conditions. What type of material was burning in the fire? Are the inhaled toxins known? Was CO or cyanide produced by the burning substances? Was the patient unconscious before entering the hospital? If the history warrants, tests for alcohol ingestion, poisoning, or drug overdose should be performed.

Airway Management

Early elective endotracheal intubation should be performed on the patient who has inhaled hot gases and demonstrates any signs of impending UAO (e.g., upper airway edema, blisters, inspiratory stridor, thick secretions). *This is a medical emergency.* Even though acute UAO is considered one of the most treatable complications of smoke inhalation, deaths still occur from UAO (hence the well-supported clinical guideline that states, "When in doubt, intubate.").

Securing an endotracheal tube often is difficult in the presence of facial burns (typically wet wounds). Adhesive tape may cause further trauma to the burn wounds. Ingenuity and creativity may be required. Securing the endotracheal tube without traumatizing the patient has been successful with use of umbilical tape and a variety of helmets, halo traction devices, and Velcro straps.

Because of the infections associated with body surface burns and smoke inhalation, a tracheostomy should be reserved for patients in whom an airway cannot be established otherwise or who will require prolonged mechanical ventilation.

Bronchoscopy

Therapeutic bronchoscopy often is used to clear the airways of mucus plugs and **eschar**.[2] In addition, early bronchoscopy often is performed for inspection and evaluation of the upper airways. Mucosal changes distal to the larynx serve as good predictors of subsequent respiratory problems.

Hyperbaric Oxygen Therapy

Hyperbaric oxygenation (HBO) therapy is useful in the rapid elimination of CO and the enhancement of skin graft viability. Its clinical utility, however, is still a matter of debate in the medical literature. Although a PaO_2 greater than 1500 mm Hg can be achieved with a hyperbaric chamber, it often is not possible or practical to institute this therapy. The chamber may not be immediately available. Can the patient be transported safely? Will the interruption of immediate therapy be detrimental?

Treatment for Cyanide Poisoning

The treatment for cyanide poisoning includes amyl nitrite inhalation and intravenous sodium thiosulfate.

Pharmacologic Treatment

Antibiotic Agents

Antibiotics are used to treat burn wounds and pulmonary infections (see Appendix III on the Evolve site).

Expectorants

Expectorants may be administered to facilitate expectoration (see Appendix V on the Evolve site).

Analgesic Agents

Analgesics generally are ordered when surface burns are present.

Prophylactic Anticoagulants

Heparin and other anticoagulants often are administered to patients with severe, long-term fire-related injuries to reduce the risk for pulmonary embolism. Immobile patients also are treated with this therapy.

Respiratory Care Treatment Protocols

Oxygen Therapy Protocol

Oxygen therapy is used to treat hypoxemia, decrease the work of breathing, and decrease myocardial work. Because of the hypoxemia and CO poisoning associated with smoke inhalation, a high concentration of oxygen should always be administered immediately. The **COHb half-life** when a patient is breathing room air at 1 atmosphere is approximately 5 hours. In other words, a 40% COHb decreases to about 20% in 5 hours and to about 10% in another 5 hours. Breathing 100% oxygen at 1 atmosphere reduces the COHb half-life to less than 1 hour. If available, HBO therapy is in order, especially in comatose

---

[2]An eschar is a slough or piece of dead tissue that is cast off from the surface of the skin or airway, particularly after a burn injury.

smoke inhalation victims with COHb levels greater than 10% (see Oxygen Therapy Protocol, Protocol 10.1).

Airway Clearance Therapy Protocol

Because of the excessive mucus production and accumulation in the intermediate and late stages of smoke inhalation injuries, a number of respiratory therapy modalities may be used to enhance the mobilization of bronchial secretions. However, even though chest physical therapy is an excellent treatment modality to mobilize secretions, patients with severe chest burns or recent skin grafts do not tolerate chest percussion and vibration. Intermittent percussive ventilation may be a reasonable alternative (see Airway Clearance Therapy Protocol, Protocol 10.2).

Lung Expansion Therapy Protocol

Lung expansion techniques are commonly used to offset the alveolar atelectasis and consolidation associated with smoke inhalation injuries. The administration of continuous positive airway pressure via an endotracheal tube or mask (when the patient has no facial or neck burns) may help minimize the development of pulmonary edema. Continuous positive airway pressure also supports the edematous airway and maintains or increases the patient's functional residual capacity (see Lung Expansion Therapy Protocol, Protocol 10.3).

Aerosolized Medication Protocol

Both sympathomimetic and parasympatholytic agents are used to produce vasoconstriction of the mucosa and to offset bronchial smooth muscle constriction. Inhaled gases must be humidified to aid in airway hydration and mobilization of secretions. Bland (saline) aerosols may be helpful. Mucolytics and antiinflammatory agents also may be administered as part of the Aerosolized Medication Protocol (see Aerosolized Medication Protocol, Protocol 10.4).

Mechanical Ventilation Protocol

Mechanical ventilation with positive end-expiratory pressure usually is required for patients who develop pulmonary edema, ARDS, and pneumonia. Mechanical ventilation should be implemented in the presence of acute or impending ventilatory failure (see Ventilator Initiation and Management Protocol, Protocol 11.1, and Ventilation Weaning Protocol, Protocol 11.2).

CASE STUDY   Smoke Inhalation and Thermal Injury

Admitting History and Physical Examination

A 21-year-old man, after smoking marijuana and falling asleep, suffered second- and third-degree burns on his face, chest, and abdomen after his bed caught fire. The extent of second- and third-degree burns was only 6% to 8% of his total body surface area. He had previously been in excellent health.

Shortly after admission, he developed respiratory distress and pulmonary edema. His blood pressure was 110/60 mm Hg, pulse 100 beats/min, and respiratory rate 30 breaths/min. His oral temperature was 98.8°F. Bilateral crackles and occasional wheezing were present. Spontaneous cough produced large amounts of thick, whitish-gray sputum. The chest radiograph revealed bilateral patchy infiltrates and consolidation. On 4 L/min oxygen, his arterial blood gas (ABG) values were pH 7.51, $PaCO_2$ 28 mm Hg, HCO_3^- 21 mEq/L, PaO_2 45 mm Hg, and SaO_2 86%. A COHb level was not obtained.

The patient was treated conservatively. He was placed on an oxygen mask, and the pulmonary edema progressively cleared over the next 48 hours. However, the respiratory distress and hypoxemia persisted, even on FIO_2 0.60 oxygen by Venturi mask. Three days after admission, his condition was worsening. The patient was agitated and complained of a productive cough, worsening shortness of breath, and substernal chest pain with deep breathing and coughing. Thick whitish-gray secretions were noted. Auscultation revealed bilateral crackles and expiratory wheezing. His vital signs were temperature 98.6°F (rectal), blood pressure 120/65 mm Hg, pulse 119 beats/min (regular sinus rhythm), respiratory rate 35 breaths/min. On an FIO_2 of 0.60, his ABG values were pH 7.54, $PaCO_2$ 25 mm Hg, HCO_3^- 20 mEq/L, PaO_2 38 mm Hg, and SaO_2 80%. His chest radiograph showed patchy infiltrates and some segmental consolidation. Fiberoptic bronchoscopy revealed extensive thermal damage and eschar in the trachea and large bronchi. A moderate amount of eschar and secretions was suctioned through the bronchoscope. At that time, the following respiratory assessment was documented.

Respiratory Assessment and Plan

S Complains of productive cough, substernal chest pain when coughing, and dyspnea.

O Afebrile. BP 120/65, P 119 and regular, RR 35. Bilateral crackles and expiratory wheezing. On FIO_2 0.60 O_2 by Venturi mask: pH 7.54, $PaCO_2$ 25, HCO_3^- 20, PaO_2 38, and SaO_2 80%. CXR: Bilateral patchy infiltrates and consolidation. No cardiomegaly. Bronchoscopy—blackish eschar in oropharynx; reddened and inflamed larynx, trachea, and large airways. Thick, whitish-gray secretions noted.

A • Smoke inhalation with thermal burns of the oropharynx, larynx, and large airways (history and bronchoscopy)
- Alveolar infiltrates and consolidation (CXR)
- Acute alveolar hyperventilation with severe hypoxemia (ABGs)
- Impending ventilatory failure (general history and clinical trend)
- Excessive and thick airway secretions (sputum, bronchoscopy and expectorate)

P Confer with attending physician to intubate and initiate mechanical ventilation care per Mechanical Ventilation Protocol. Oxygen Therapy Protocol: FIO_2 at 1.0 via nonrebreather mask. Aerosolized Medication Protocol and Airway Clearance Therapy Protocol: Albuterol premix 2 mL via med. nebulizer. q2h (alternate with racemic epinephrine 6 drops in 2 mL normal saline). Gentle PRN nasotracheal and oral suctioning after med. neb. treatments. Check I&O status and daily weights.

The patient was intubated and started on intravenously administered steroids. He was ventilated with an FIO_2 of 0.60, rate of 12, and positive end-expiratory pressure of +10 cm H_2O. Because of the upper body burns, chest physical therapy and postural drainage were prohibited. The bronchial secretions, however, were loosened and mobilized adequately with an in-line ultrasonic nebulizer and frequent endotracheal suctioning. In-line aerosolized steroids also were administered at this time.

The patient's vital signs and ABG values improved on this regimen. After 12 days of respiratory care, he was weaned to an FIO_2 of 0.40 and extubated. He continued to complain of exertional dyspnea with transfer activities but denied dyspnea at rest. Crackles were improved but still easily auscultated throughout all lung fields when the patient took deep breaths. Occasional expiratory wheezes also were heard.

Three days after extubation, on an FIO_2 of 0.35 via a Venturi oxygen mask, his pH was 7.45, $PaCO_2$ 36 mm Hg, HCO_3^- 24 mEq/L, PaO_2 63 mm Hg, and SaO_2 93%. On exercise, the SpO_2 fell to 85%. His peak expiratory flow rate (PEFR) was 40% of predicted. The infiltrates previously noted on chest radiograph were much improved. At that time, the respiratory therapist recorded the following assessment in the patient's chart.

Respiratory Assessment and Plan

S Complains of shortness of breath with any activity.
O Vital signs stable. Crackles heard over both lung bases. Some expiratory prolongation. ABGs (spontaneous breathing) (FIO_2 0.35 via Venturi mask): pH 7.45, $PaCO_2$ 36, HCO_3^- 24, PaO_2 63, and SaO_2 93%. SpO_2 falls to 85% with exercise. PEFR 40% of predicted. CXR: Improvement in patchy lung infiltrates.

A • Mild to moderate hypoxemia secondary to thermal injury to lung (ABGs and history)
- Moderate obstructive pulmonary disease (PEFR)

P Complete pulmonary function tests ordered. Up-regulate Oxygen Therapy Protocol (increase FIO_2 to 0.40 via Venturi mask). If patient is ambulatory, titrate oxygen therapy based on exercise SpO_2. If obstructive pulmonary disease is confirmed, restart Airway Clearance Therapy Protocol and Aerosolized Medication Protocol.

Pulmonary function studies showed severely reduced expiratory flows and a sharply decreased diffusion capacity. Chest radiographs taken at regular intervals thereafter began to show emphysematous changes. The diaphragms were flattened, and bilateral coarse reticular infiltrates were evident. Despite vigorous therapy over the next 6 weeks, the patient's cardiopulmonary status continued to worsen. He died on day 59, 2 months after his original thermal and inhalational injury. The postmortem diagnosis at autopsy was cryptogenic organizing pneumonia (COP)—also known as *bronchiolitis obliterans organizing pneumonia* (BOOP).

Discussion

At the time of the first assessment, the patient demonstrated most of the pathophysiologic correlates of smoke inhalation and thermal injuries to the lung. His dyspnea reflected the increased work of breathing associated with bronchospasm (see Fig. 10.10), increased alveolar-capillary membrane thickness (see Fig. 10.9), and excessive bronchial secretions (see Fig. 10.11). The bronchospasm was treated with the vigorous use of both bronchodilator (albuterol) and decongestant (epinephrine) aerosols. The excessive bronchial secretions were treated with ultrasonic bland aerosols and airway suctioning. No specific treatment was available for the changes that occurred in the alveolar-capillary membrane.

This interesting case is instructive for these reasons. Primarily, all patients with burns of the upper chest, neck, or face should have a careful oropharyngeal examination to determine whether burns have indeed occurred in the upper airway. The presence of soot or eschar in the oropharynx is diagnostic of this problem; respiratory distress almost certainly will ensue if such findings are present, although this does not happen immediately. A 24- to 72-hour lag may occur between the burn and clinical obstruction of the airway. Second, a dreaded complication of smoke and heat inhalation is COP, which developed in this patient and ultimately was fatal. Finally, failure to measure COHb on admission falls well below the standard of care.

This patient might have been considered a candidate for lung transplantation. This case study should remind the respiratory therapist that immediate intubation may be necessary over the diagnostic bronchoscope and that he or she should prepare accordingly.

1. About what percentage of hospitalized patients with thermal injury have an acute upper airway obstruction?
   a. 0% to 10%
   b. 10% to 20%
   c. 20% to 30%
   d. 30% to 40%

2. Except for the rare instance of steam inhalation, direct thermal injuries usually do not occur below the level of which of the following structures?
   a. Oral pharynx
   b. Larynx
   c. Carina
   d. Bronchi

3. When chest wall burns are present, the patient's pulmonary condition may be further aggravated by which of the following?
   1. Decreased lung and chest compliance
   2. Increased airway resistance
   3. Administration of narcotics
   4. Immobility
      a. 2 and 3 only
      b. 1 and 3 only
      c. 2 and 4 only
      d. 1, 2, 3, and 4

4. Which of the following is(are) the pulmonary-related pathologic change(s) associated with smoke inhalation?
   1. Pneumomediastinum
   2. Bronchospasm
   3. Pulmonary edema
   4. Pulmonary embolism
      a. 1 only
      b. 2 only
      c. 3 and 4 only
      d. 2, 3, and 4 only

5. Which of the following produce carbon monoxide when burned?
   1. Polyurethanes
   2. Wood, cotton, paper
   3. Organic material
   4. Polyvinylchloride
      a. 1 only
      b. 2 only
      c. 3 and 4 only
      d. 1, 2, and 3 only

6. Which of the following oxygenation indices is(are) associated with smoke inhalation and burns during the early and intermediate stages?
   1. Increased $\dot{V}O_2$
   2. Decreased $C(a-\bar{v})O_2$
   3. Increased DO_2
   4. Decreased $S\bar{v}O_2$
      a. 2 only
      b. 4 only
      c. 2 and 3 only
      d. 1 and 4 only

7. Which of the following hemodynamic indices is(are) associated with body surface burns during the early stage?
   1. Decreased CO
   2. Increased SVR
   3. Decreased $\overline{PA}$
   4. Increased PCWP
      a. 1 only
      b. 3 only
      c. 2 and 4 only
      d. 1, 2, and 3 only

8. If an adult's entire right arm, right leg, and anterior trunk have been burned, approximately what percentage of the patient's body surface area is burned?
   a. 15%
   b. 25%
   c. 35%
   d. 45%

9. Healing time for a second-degree burn is:
   a. 1 to 7 days
   b. 7 to 21 days
   c. 21 to 31 days
   d. 1 to 2 months

10. Breathing 100% oxygen at 1 atmosphere reduces the COHb half-life to less than:
    a. 1 hour
    b. 2 hours
    c. 3 hours
    d. 4 hours

Answers to Self-Assessment Questions

Chapter 1
1. A
2. B
3. B
4. D
5. C

Chapter 2
1. D
2. D
3. C
4. D
5. B
6. B

Chapter 3
1. C
2. B
3. D
4. B
5. D
6. C
7. D
8. D
9. D

Chapter 4
1. C
2. C
3. B
4. B
5. D
6. D
7. B
8. D
9. D
10. C

Chapter 5
1. C
2. D
3. B
4. A
5. B
6. B
7. B
8. D
9. C
10. D
11. D
12. D

13. C
14. D
15. D

Chapter 6
1. B
2. D
3. A
4. C
5. D
6. B
7. C
8. B
9. C
10. C
11. C
12. B
13. D
14. C
15. D

Chapter 7
1. D
2. D
3. B
4. D
5. C
6. B
7. B
8. C
9. C
10. B

Chapter 8
1. C
2. D
3. C
4. A
5. D
6. D
7. D
8. D
9. B
10. D

Chapter 9
1. C
2. B
3. C
4. C
5. A

6. B
7. A
8. C
9. D
10. D

Chapter 10
1. C
2. D
3. C
4. A
5. C
6. C
7. C
8. A
9. A
10. B

Chapter 11
1. C
2. D
3. C
4. A
5. C
6. C
7. C
8. A
9. A
10. B

Chapter 12
1. D
2. D
3. B
4. D
5. See text for answer.
6. See text for answer.
7. See text for answer.
8. See text for answer.
9. See text for answer.
10. See text for answer.

Chapter 13
1. B
2. D
3. C
4. B
5. D
6. D
7. B
8. B

9. D
10. C
11. D
12. C
13. D
14. D
15. B

Chapter 14
1. B
2. C
3. C
4. B
5. D
6. D
7. C
8. A
9. D
10. C

Chapter 15
1. D
2. C
3. C
4. D
5. D
6. D
7. B
8. D
9. B
10. D

Chapter 16
1. D
2. B
3. B
4. D
5. A
6. C
7. C
8. D
9. B
10. C
11. D

Chapter 17
1. B
2. B
3. D
4. D
5. C

Chapter 18
1. D
2. B
3. B
4. D
5. D
6. C
7. A
8. B
9. B
10. B
11. B
12. B
13. C
14. A
15. C

Chapter 19
1. D
2. D
3. D
4. D
5. C

Chapter 20
1. D
2. B
3. D
4. D
5. A
6. C

Chapter 21
1. C
2. D
3. C
4. B
5. A
6. D
7. D
8. B
9. C
10. A

Chapter 22
1. C
2. D
3. B
4. C
5. A

Chapter 23
1. D
2. C
3. D
4. D
5. A
6. D
7. D

8. B
9. B
10. D

Chapter 24
1. D
2. B
3. D
4. C
5. D

Chapter 25
1. A
2. C
3. C
4. A
5. D

Chapter 26
1. A
2. B
3. B
4. B
5. D

Chapter 27
1. B
2. C
3. A
4. D
5. C
6. C
7. D
8. C
9. B
10. D

Chapter 28
1. D
2. B
3. D
4. B
5. B

Chapter 29
1. D
2. C
3. C
4. D
5. D
6. C

Chapter 30
1. D
2. C
3. B
4. C
5. A

Chapter 31
1. E
2. C
3. A
4. C
5. F

Chapter 32
1. D
2. D
3. C
4. B
5. D
6. D
7. C
8. B
9. C
10. D
11. D

Chapter 33
1. D
2. C
3. B
4. D
5. B

Chapter 34
1. C
2. D
3. A
4. B
5. B

Chapter 35
1. C
2. D
3. C
4. D
5. C

Chapter 36
1. D
2. C
3. B
4. C
5. A
6. D

Chapter 37
1. D
2. B
3. B
4. D
5. D

Chapter 38
1. B
2. A

3. D
4. D
5. D

Chapter 39
1. D
2. C
3. B
4. A
5. B

Chapter 40
1. B
2. C
3. C
4. A
5. D

Chapter 41
1. C
2. C
3. A
4. D
5. D

Chapter 42
1. D
2. B
3. A
4. D
5. A

Chapter 43
1. D
2. B
3. A
4. B
5. C
6. B

Chapter 44
1. C
2. D
3. D
4. A
5. D

Chapter 45
1. C
2. B
3. D
4. D
5. C
6. D
7. D
8. D
9. B
10. A

Index

Page numbers followed by "*f*" indicate figures, "*t*" indicate tables, and "*b*" indicate boxes.